Abul K. Abbas, MBBS
Professor and Chair
Department of Pathology
University of California-San Francisco
San Francisco, California

Andrew H. Lichtman, MD, PhD
Associate Professor of Pathology
Harvard Medical School
Brigham and Women's Hospital
Boston, Massachusetts

Shiv Pillai, MBBS, PhD
Associate Professor of Medicine
Harvard Medical School
Massachusetts General Hospital Cancer Center
Boston, Massachusetts

Illustrations by David L. Baker, MA
Alexandra Baker, MS, CNT
DNA Illustrations, Inc.

CELLULAR AND MOLECULAR IMMUNOLOGY

6TH EDITION
Updated Edition

SAUNDERS

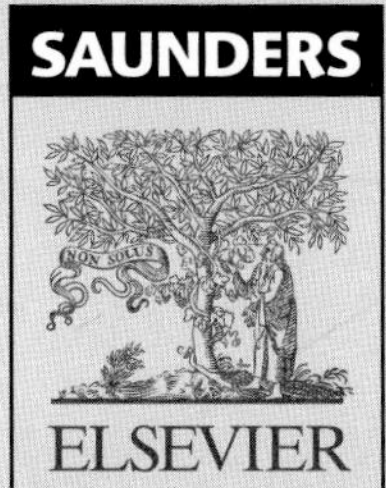

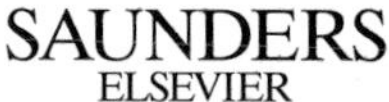

SAUNDERS
ELSEVIER

1600 John F. Kennedy Blvd.
Ste 1800
Philadelphia, PA 19103-2899

CELLULAR AND MOLECULAR IMMUNOLOGY, Updated 6/E ISBN: 978-1-4160-3123-9
International Edition ISBN: 978-0-8089-2411-1

Library of Congress Cataloging-in-Publication Data

Abbas, Abul K.
Cellular and molecular immunology / Abul K. Abbas, Andrew H. Lichtman, Shiv Pillai.—Updated 6th ed.
p. ; cm.
Includes bibliographical references and index.
ISBN 978-1-4160-3123-9
1. Cellular immunity. 2. Molecular immunology. I. Lichtman, Andrew H. II. Pillai, Shiv. III. Title.
[DNLM: 1. Immunity, Cellular. 2. Antibody Formation—immunology. 3. Antigens—immunology. 4. Immune System Diseases—immunology. 5. Lymphocytes—immunology. QW 568 A122c 2010]
QR185.5.A23 2010
616.07'97—dc22

2009008415

Executive Editor: William Schmitt
Managing Editor: Rebecca Gruliow
Publishing Services Manager: Joan Sinclair
Design Direction: Gene Harris

Printed in China

Last digit is the print number: 9 8 7 6 5 4 3 2 1

Cellular and Molecular Immunology

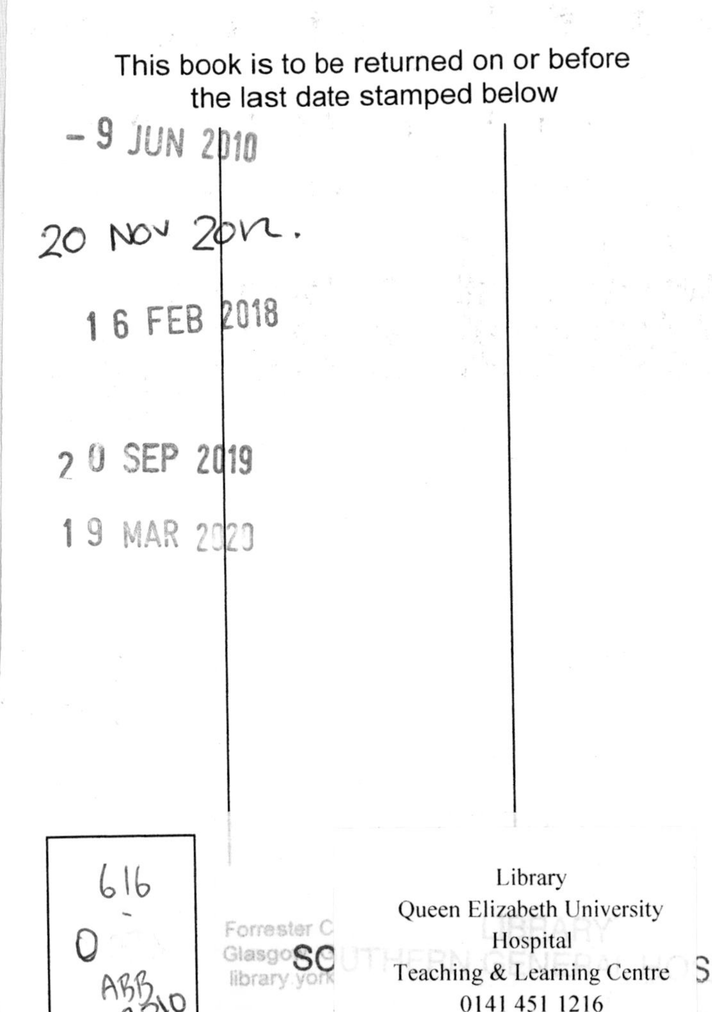

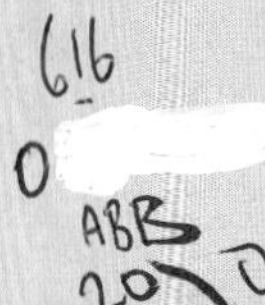

Preface

This sixth edition of *Cellular and Molecular Immunology* includes extensive revisions of the previous edition, which incorporate new discoveries in immunology and the constantly growing body of knowledge. It is remarkable and fascinating to us that new principles continue to emerge from analysis of the complex systems that underlie immune responses. Perhaps one of the most satisfying developments for students of human disease is that basic principles of immunology are now being used for rational development of new immunological therapies. Examples of areas in which our understanding has grown impressively since the last edition of this book include the recognition of microbial products by cytoplasmic and membrane sensors, the intricate organization of lymphoid tissues, the functional heterogeneity of subsets of dendritic cells and lymphocytes, and the roles of regulatory cells and inhibitory pathways in immune regulation. We have added new information while striving to emphasize important principles, and without increasing the length of the book. We have also changed many sections, when necessary, for increased clarity, accuracy, and completeness.

We have retained the design elements that have evolved through the previous editions to make the book easier to read. These include the use of bold italic text to highlight "take-home messages," presentation of experimental results in bulleted lists distinguishable from the main text, and the use of "In-depth" boxes (including several new ones) to present detailed information about experimental approaches, disease entities, and selected molecular or biological processes. We also constantly try to further improve the clarity of illustrations and tables.

Many individuals have made invaluable contributions to this edition. Drs. Michael Carroll, Jason Cyster, Moh Daha, and Richard Locklsey have been generous with advice and comments. Our illustrators, David and Alexandra Baker of DNA Illustrations, remain full partners in the book and provide invaluable suggestions for clarity and accuracy. Several members of the Elsevier Science staff have played critical roles. Our editor, Bill Schmitt, has been a source of support and encouragement. Our Developmental Editor, Rebecca Gruliow, shepherded the book through its preparation and production. Gene Harris was responsible for the design. Ellen Sklar took charge of the production and has been a constant source of good sense and efficiency. Our students were the original inspiration for the first edition of this book, and we remain continually grateful to them, because from them we learn how to think about the science of immunology, and how to communicate knowledge in the clearest and most meaningful way.

Abul K. Abbas

Andrew H. Lichtman

Shiv Pillai

Dedication

To
Ann, Jonathan, Rehana
Sheila, Eben, Ariella, Amos, Ezra
Honorine, Sohini

Contents

Section I

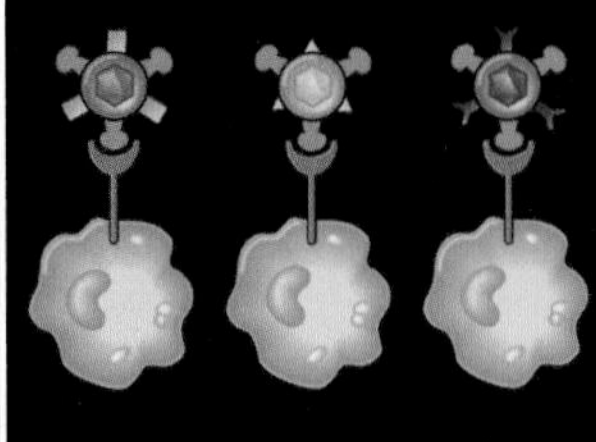

Introduction to the Immune System

The first three chapters of this book introduce the nomenclature of immunology and the components of innate and adaptive immune responses. In Chapter 1, we describe the types of immune responses and their general properties and present an overview of immune responses to microbes. In Chapter 2, we discuss the early innate immune response to infectious pathogens. Chapter 3 is devoted to a description of the cells and tissues of the adaptive immune system, with an emphasis on their anatomic organization and structure-function relationships. This section sets the stage for more thorough discussion of how the immune system recognizes and responds to antigens.

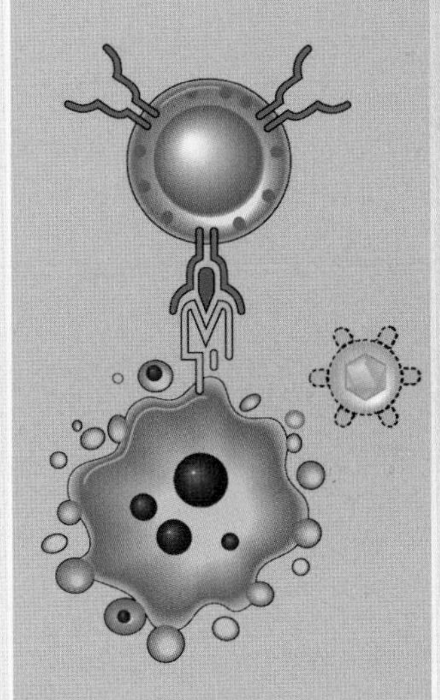

Chapter 1

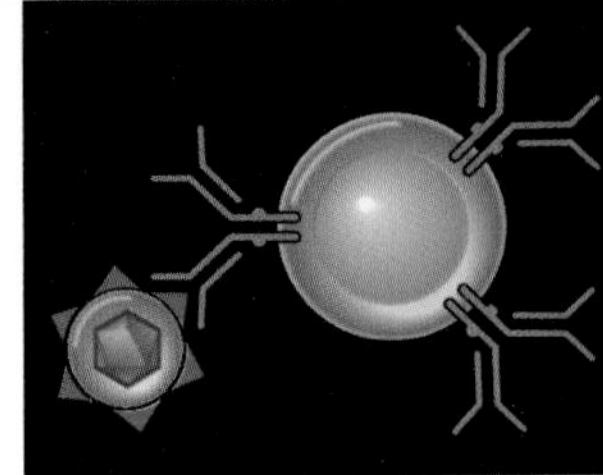

PROPERTIES AND OVERVIEW OF IMMUNE RESPONSES

The term *immunity* is derived from the Latin word *immunitas,* which referred to the protection from legal prosecution offered to Roman senators during their tenures in office. Historically, immunity meant protection from disease and, more specifically, infectious disease. The cells and molecules responsible for immunity constitute the **immune system,** and their collective and coordinated response to the introduction of foreign substances is called the **immune response.**

The physiologic function of the immune system is defense against infectious microbes. However, even noninfectious foreign substances can elicit immune responses. Furthermore, mechanisms that normally protect individuals from infection and eliminate foreign substances are also capable of causing tissue injury and disease in some situations. Therefore, a more inclusive definition of the immune response is a reaction to components of microbes as well as to macromolecules, such as proteins and polysaccharides, and small chemicals that are recognized as foreign, regardless of the physiologic or pathologic consequence of such a reaction. Immunology is the study of immune responses in this broader sense and of the cellular and molecular events that occur after an organism encounters microbes and other foreign macromolecules.

Historians often credit Thucydides, in Athens during the fifth century BC, as having first mentioned immunity to an infection that he called "plague" (but that was probably not the bubonic plague we recognize today). The concept of immunity may have existed long before, as suggested by the ancient Chinese custom of making children resistant to smallpox by having them inhale powders made from the skin lesions of patients recovering from the disease. Immunology, in its modern form, is an experimental science, in which explanations of immunologic phenomena are based on experimental observations and the conclusions drawn from them. The evolution of immunology as an experimental discipline has depended on our ability to manipulate the function of the immune system under controlled conditions. Historically, the first clear example of this manipulation, and one that remains among the most dramatic ever recorded, was Edward Jenner's successful vaccination against smallpox. Jenner, an English physician, noticed that milkmaids who had recovered from cowpox never contracted the more serious smallpox. On the basis of this observation, he injected the material from a cowpox pustule into the arm of an 8-year-old boy. When this boy was later intentionally inoculated with smallpox, the disease did not develop. Jenner's landmark treatise on **vaccination** (Latin *vaccinus,* of or from cows) was published in 1798. It led to the widespread acceptance of this method for inducing immunity to infectious diseases, and vaccination remains the most effective method for preventing infections (Table 1–1). An eloquent testament to the importance of immunology was the announcement by the World Health Organization in 1980 that smallpox was the first disease that had been eradicated worldwide by a program of vaccination.

Since the 1960s, there has been a remarkable transformation in our understanding of the immune system and its functions. Advances in cell culture techniques (including monoclonal antibody production), immunochemistry, recombinant DNA methodology, x-ray crystallography, and creation of genetically altered animals (especially transgenic and knockout mice) have changed immunology from a largely descriptive science into one in which diverse immune phenomena can be explained in structural and biochemical terms. In this chapter, we outline the general features of immune responses and introduce the concepts that form the cornerstones of modern immunology and that recur throughout this book.

Innate and Adaptive Immunity

Defense against microbes is mediated by the early reactions of innate immunity and the later responses of adaptive immunity (Fig. 1–1 and Table 1–2). **Innate immunity** (also called natural or native immunity) provides the early line of defense against microbes. It consists of cellular and biochemical defense mechanisms that are in place even before infection and are poised to respond rapidly to infections. These mechanisms react only to microbes (and to the products of injured cells), and they respond in essentially the same way to repeated infections. The principal components of innate immunity are (1) physical and chemical barriers, such as epithelia and antimicrobial substances produced at epithelial surfaces; (2) phagocytic cells (neutrophils, macrophages) and natural killer (NK) cells; (3) blood proteins, including members of the complement system and other mediators of inflammation; and (4) proteins called cytokines that regulate and coordinate many of the activities of the cells of innate immunity. The mechanisms of innate immunity are specific for structures that are common to groups of related microbes and may not distinguish fine differences between foreign substances.

In contrast to innate immunity, there are other immune responses that are stimulated by exposure to infectious agents and increase in magnitude and defensive capabilities with each successive exposure to a particular microbe. Because this form of immunity develops as a response to infection and adapts to the infection, it is called **adaptive immunity.** The defining characteristics of adaptive immunity are exquisite specificity for

Table 1–1. Effectiveness of Vaccines for Some Common Infectious Diseases

Disease	Maximum number of cases (year)	Number of cases in 2004	Percent change
Diphtheria	206,939 (1921)	0	-99.99
Measles	894,134 (1941)	37	-99.99
Mumps	152,209 (1968)	236	-99.90
Pertussis	265,269 (1934)	18,957	-96.84
Polio (paralytic)	21,269 (1952)	0	-100.0
Rubella	57,686 (1969)	12	-99.98
Tetanus	1,560 (1923)	26	-98.33
Haemophilus influenzae type B	~20,000 (1984)	16	-99.92
Hepatitis B	26,611 (1985)	6,632	-75.08

This table illustrates the striking decrease in the incidence of selected infectious diseases for which effective vaccines have been developed.

Adapted from Orenstein WA, AR Hinman, KJ Bart, and SC Hadler. Immunization. In Mandell GL, JE Bennett, and R Dolin (eds). Principles and Practices of Infectious Diseases, 4th ed. Churchill Livingstone, New York, 1995, and Morbidity and Mortality Weekly Report 53:1213–1221, 2005.

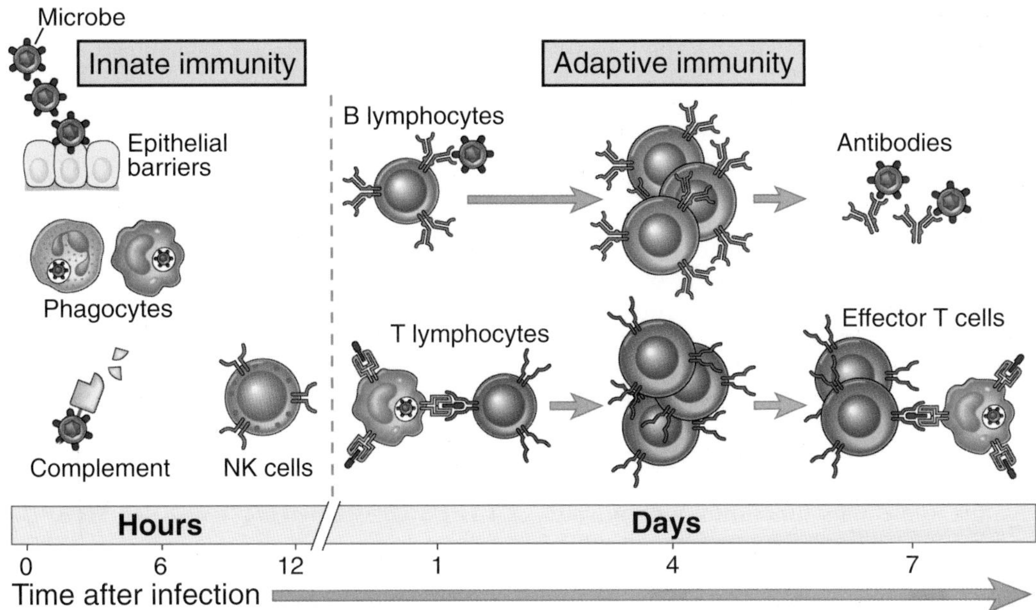

FIGURE 1–1 Innate and adaptive immunity. The mechanisms of innate immunity provide the initial defense against infections. Adaptive immune responses develop later and consist of activation of lymphocytes. The kinetics of the innate and adaptive immune responses are approximations and may vary in different infections.

Table 1–2. Features of Innate and Adaptive Immunity

	Innate	Adaptive
Characteristics		
Specificity	For structures shared by groups of related microbes	For antigens of microbes and for nonmicrobial antigens
Diversity	Limited; germline-encoded	Very large; receptors are produced by somatic recombination of gene segments
Memory	None	Yes
Nonreactivity to self	Yes	Yes
Components		
Cellular and chemical barriers	Skin, mucosal epithelia; antimicrobial chemicals	Lymphocytes in epithelia; antibodies secreted at epithelial surfaces
Blood proteins	Complement, others	Antibodies
Cells	Phagocytes (macrophages, neutrophils), natural killer cells	Lymphocytes

This table lists the major characteristics and components of innate and adaptive immune responses. Innate immunity is discussed in much more detail in Chapter 2.

distinct molecules and an ability to "remember" and respond more vigorously to repeated exposures to the same microbe. The adaptive immune system is able to recognize and react to a large number of microbial and nonmicrobial substances. In addition, it has an extraordinary capacity to distinguish between different, even closely related, microbes and molecules, and for this reason it is also called **specific immunity.** It is also sometimes called acquired immunity, to emphasize that potent protective responses are "acquired" by experience. The main components of adaptive immunity are cells called **lymphocytes** and their secreted products, such as antibodies. Foreign substances that induce specific immune responses or are the targets of such responses are called **antigens.**

Innate and adaptive immune responses are components of an integrated system of host defense in which numerous cells and molecules function cooperatively. The mechanisms of innate immunity provide an effective initial defense against infections. However, many pathogenic microbes have evolved to resist innate immunity, and their elimination requires the more powerful mechanisms of adaptive immunity. The innate immune response to microbes also stimulates adaptive immune responses and influences the nature of the adaptive responses. We will return to a more detailed discussion of the mechanisms and physiologic functions of innate immunity in Chapter 2.

Innate immunity is phylogenetically the oldest system of host defense, and the adaptive immune system evolved later (Box 1–1). In invertebrates, host defense against foreign invaders is mediated largely by the mechanisms of innate immunity, including phagocytes and circulating molecules that resemble the plasma proteins of innate immunity in vertebrates. Adaptive immunity, consisting of lymphocytes and antibodies, first appeared in jawed vertebrates and became increasingly specialized with further evolution.

Types of Adaptive Immune Responses

There are two types of adaptive immune responses, called humoral immunity and cell-mediated immunity, that are mediated by different components of the immune system and function to eliminate different types of microbes (Fig. 1–2). **Humoral immunity** is medi-

Box 1–1 ▪ IN DEPTH: EVOLUTION OF THE IMMUNE SYSTEM

Mechanisms for defending the host against microbes are present in some form in all multicellular organisms. These mechanisms constitute innate immunity. The more specialized defense mechanisms that constitute adaptive immunity are found in vertebrates only.

Various cells in invertebrates respond to microbes by surrounding these infectious agents and destroying them. These responding cells resemble phagocytes and have been called phagocytic amebocytes in acelomates, hemocytes in molluscs and arthropods, coelomocytes in annelids, and blood leukocytes in tunicates. Invertebrates do not contain antigen-specific lymphocytes and do not produce immunoglobulin (Ig) molecules or complement proteins. However, they contain a number of soluble molecules that bind to and lyse microbes. These molecules include lectin-like proteins, which bind to carbohydrates on microbial cell walls and agglutinate the microbes, and numerous lytic and antimicrobial factors such as lysozyme, which is also produced by neutrophils in higher organisms. Phagocytes in some invertebrates may be capable of secreting cytokines that resemble macrophage-derived cytokines in the vertebrates. Importantly, all multicellular organisms express cellular receptors resembling Toll-like receptors that sense microbes and initiate defense reactions against the microbes. Thus, host defense in invertebrates is mediated by the cells and molecules that resemble the effector mechanisms of innate immunity in higher organisms.

Many studies have shown that invertebrates are capable of rejecting foreign tissue transplants, or allografts. (In vertebrates, this process of graft rejection is dependent on adaptive immune responses.) If sponges (Porifera) from two different colonies are parabiosed by being mechanically held together, they become necrotic in 1 to 2 weeks, whereas sponges from the same colony fuse and continue to grow. Earthworms (annelids) and starfish (echinoderms) also reject tissue grafts from other species of the phyla. These rejection reactions are mediated mainly by phagocyte-like cells. They differ from graft rejection in vertebrates in that specific memory for the grafted tissue either is not generated or is difficult to demonstrate. Nevertheless, such results indicate that even invertebrates must express cell surface molecules that distinguish self from nonself, and such molecules may be the precursors of histocompatibility molecules in vertebrates. Recently, a family of polymorphic proteins belonging to the immunoglobulin superfamily has been isolated from marine chordates and shown to be responsible for rejection of organisms. These proteins may be precursors of mammalian histocompatibility molecules.

The hallmark of the vertebrate immune system is the expression of somatically rearranged antigen receptors. Such receptors appeared in jawed fish. Even some jawless fish express highly variable receptors that differ from one cell to another, but these are not generated by recombination of gene segments. It is believed that a transposon containing the gene(s) encoding the enzyme for recombination (RAG, or recombination activating genes, see Chapter 8) invaded a gene that encoded a

Continued on following page

protein resembling a variable (V) segment of an antibody molecule. This allowed V and related segments to be recombined to generate highly diverse and specific antigen receptors. Not only this feature, but most of the components of the adaptive immune system, including lymphocytes, antibodies and T cell receptors, MHC molecules, and specialized lymphoid tissues (but lacking germinal centers), all seem to have appeared quite suddenly and coordinately in jawed vertebrates (e.g., sharks) (see Table). A more primitive version of rearranged antigen receptors exists in jawless fish (lampreys). These receptors have been called "variable lymphocyte receptors," and are apparently generated by shuffling DNA segments in the absence of RAG genes and the more advanced somatic recombination machinery.

The immune system has also become increasingly specialized with evolution. For instance, fishes have only one type of antibody, called IgM; this number increases to two types in amphibians such as *Xenopus* and to seven or eight types in mammals. The presence of more types of antibodies increases the functional capabilities of the immune response.

	Innate immunity		Adaptive immunity	
	Phagocytes	NK cells	Antibodies	T and B lymphocytes
Invertebrates				
Protozoa	+	–	–	–
Sponges	+	–	–	–
Annelids	+	+	–	–
Arthropods	+	–	–	–
Vertebrates				
Elasmobranchs (sharks, skates, rays)	+	+	+ (IgM only)	+
Teleosts (common fish)	+	+	+ (IgM, others?)	+
Amphibians	+	+	+ (2 or 3 classes)	+
Reptiles	+	+	+ (3 classes)	+
Birds	+	+	+ (3 classes)	+
Mammals	+	+	+ (7 or 8 classes)	+

Key: +, present; –, absent

ated by molecules in the blood and mucosal secretions, called antibodies, that are produced by cells called B lymphocytes (also called B cells). Antibodies recognize microbial antigens, neutralize the infectivity of the microbes, and target microbes for elimination by various effector mechanisms. Humoral immunity is the principal defense mechanism against extracellular microbes and their toxins because secreted antibodies can bind to these microbes and toxins and assist in their elimination. Antibodies themselves are specialized, and different types of antibodies may activate different effector mechanisms. For example, some types of antibodies promote the ingestion of microbes by host cells (phagocytosis), and other antibodies bind to and trigger the release of inflammatory mediators from cells. **Cell-mediated immunity**, also called cellular immunity, is mediated by T lymphocytes (also called T cells). Intracellular microbes, such as viruses and some bacteria, survive and proliferate inside phagocytes and other host cells, where they are inaccessible to circulating antibodies. Defense against such infections is a function of cell-mediated immunity, which promotes the destruction of microbes residing in phagocytes or the killing of infected cells to eliminate reservoirs of infection.

Protective immunity against a microbe may be induced by the host's response to the microbe or by the transfer of antibodies or lymphocytes specific for the microbe (Fig. 1–3). The form of immunity that is induced by exposure to a foreign antigen is called **active immunity** because the immunized individual plays an active role in responding to the antigen. Individuals and lymphocytes that have not encountered a particular antigen are said to be naive, implying that they are immunologically inexperienced. Individuals who have responded to a microbial antigen and are protected from subsequent exposures to that microbe are said to be immune.

Immunity can also be conferred on an individual by transferring serum or lymphocytes from a specifically

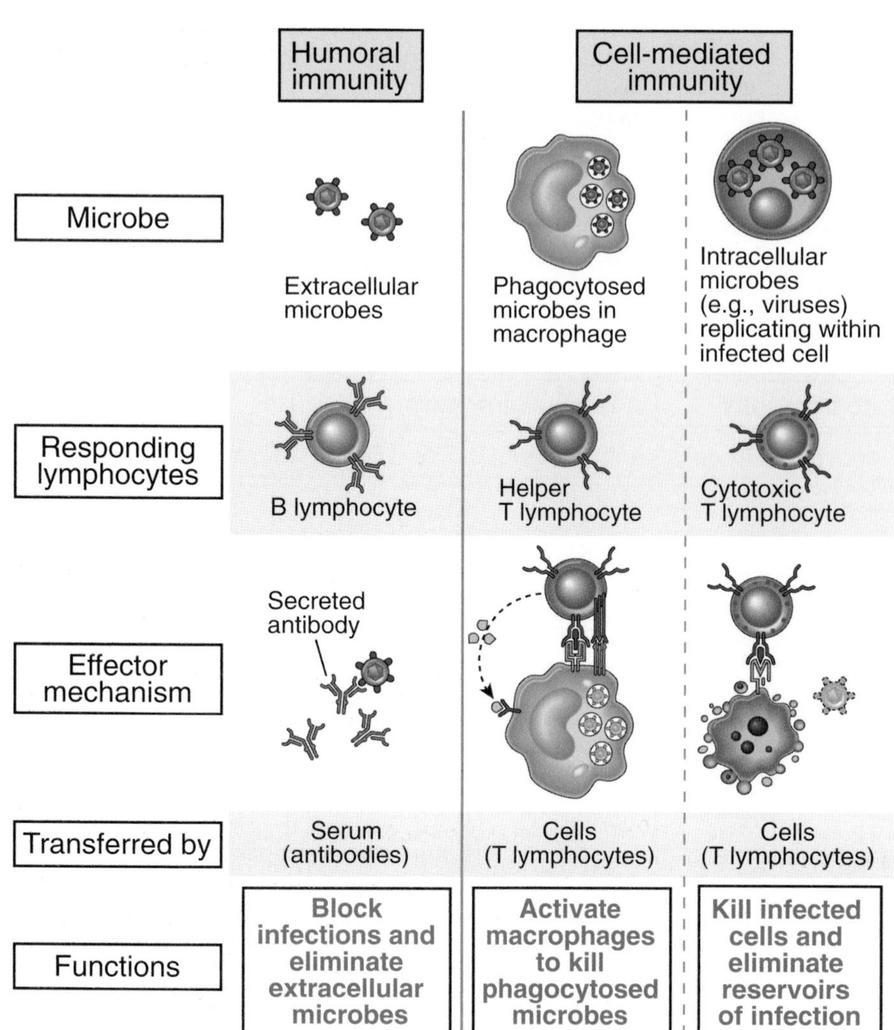

FIGURE 1–2 Types of adaptive immunity. In humoral immunity, B lymphocytes secrete antibodies that prevent infections by and eliminate extracellular microbes. In cell-mediated immunity, helper T lymphocytes activate macrophages to kill phagocytosed microbes or cytotoxic T lymphocytes (CTLs) directly destroy infected cells.

immunized individual, a process known as adoptive transfer in experimental situations. The recipient of such a transfer becomes immune to the particular antigen without ever having been exposed to or having responded to that antigen. Therefore, this form of immunity is called **passive immunity**. Passive immunization is a useful method for conferring resistance rapidly, without having to wait for an active immune response to develop. An example of passive immunity is the transfer of maternal antibodies to the fetus, which enables newborns to combat infections before they develop the ability to produce antibodies themselves. Passive immunization against bacterial toxins by the administration of antibodies from immunized animals is a lifesaving treatment for potentially lethal infections, such as tetanus and rabies. The technique of adoptive transfer has also made it possible to define the various cells and molecules that are responsible for mediating specific immunity. In fact, humoral immunity was originally defined as the type of immunity that could be transferred to unimmunized, or naive, individuals by antibody-containing cell-free portions of the blood (i.e., plasma or serum [once called humors]) obtained from previously immunized individuals. Similarly, cell-mediated immunity was defined as the form of immunity that can be transferred to naive animals with cells (T lymphocytes) from immunized animals but not with plasma or serum.

The first experimental demonstration of humoral immunity was provided by Emil von Behring and Shibasaburo Kitasato in 1890. They showed that if serum from animals that had recovered from diphtheria infection was transferred to naive animals, the recipients became specifically resistant to diphtheria infection. The active components of the serum were called antitoxins because they neutralized the pathologic effects of the diphtheria toxin. In the early 1900s, Karl Landsteiner and other investigators showed that not only toxins but also nonmicrobial substances could induce humoral immune responses. From such studies arose the more general term **antibodies** for the serum proteins that mediate humoral immunity. Substances that bound antibodies and generated the production of antibodies were then called **antigens**. (The properties of antibodies and antigens are described in Chapter 4.) In 1900, Paul Ehrlich provided a theoretical framework for the specificity of antigen-antibody reactions, the experimental proof for which came during the next 50

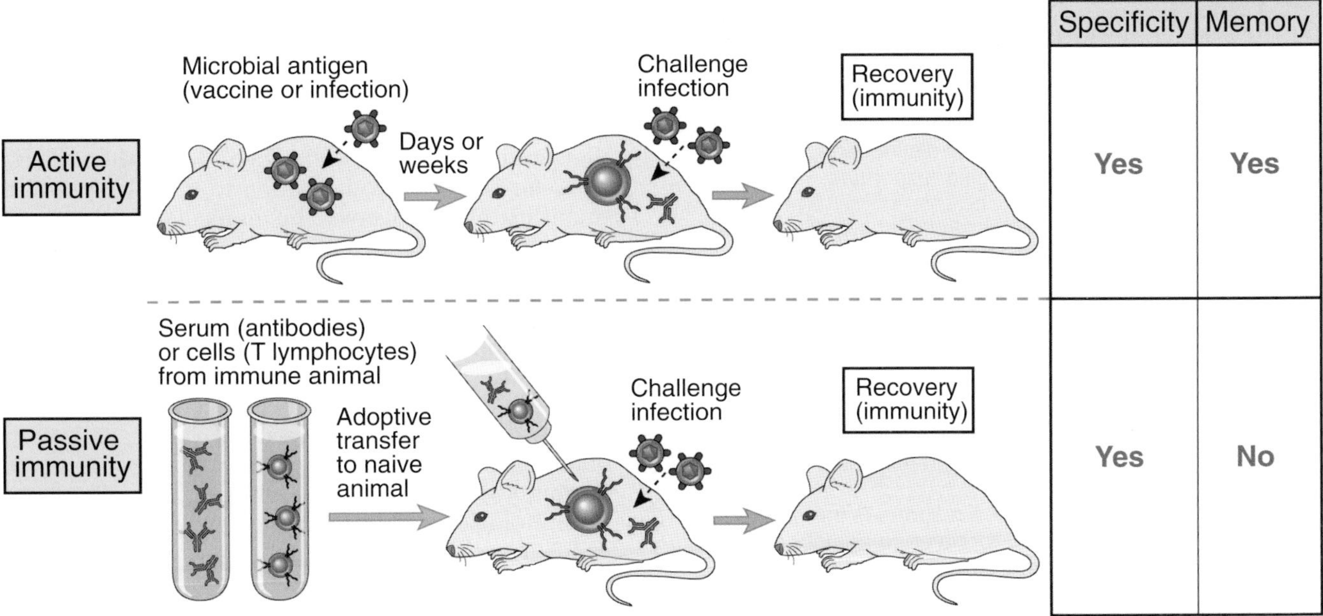

FIGURE 1–3 Active and passive immunity. Active immunity is conferred by a host response to a microbe or microbial antigen, whereas passive immunity is conferred by adoptive transfer of antibodies or T lymphocytes specific for the microbe. Both forms of immunity provide resistance to infection and are specific for microbial antigens, but only active immune responses generate immunologic memory.

years from the work of Landsteiner and others using simple chemicals as antigens. Ehrlich's theories of the physicochemical complementarity of antigens and antibodies are remarkable for their prescience. This early emphasis on antibodies led to the general acceptance of the humoral theory of immunity, according to which immunity is mediated by substances present in body fluids.

The cellular theory of immunity, which stated that host cells were the principal mediators of immunity, was championed initially by Elie Metchnikoff. His demonstration of phagocytes surrounding a thorn stuck into a translucent starfish larva, published in 1883, was perhaps the first experimental evidence that cells respond to foreign invaders. Sir Almroth Wright's observation in the early 1900s that factors in immune serum enhanced the phagocytosis of bacteria by coating the bacteria, a process known as opsonization, lent support to the belief that antibodies prepared microbes for ingestion by phagocytes. These early "cellularists" were unable to prove that specific immunity to microbes could be mediated by cells. The cellular theory of immunity became firmly established in the 1950s, when George Mackaness showed that resistance to an intracellular bacterium, *Listeria monocytogenes,* could be adoptively transferred with cells but not with serum. We now know that the specificity of cell-mediated immunity is due to lymphocytes, which often function in concert with other cells, such as phagocytes, to eliminate microbes.

In the clinical setting, immunity to a previously encountered microbe is measured indirectly, either by assaying for the presence of products of immune responses (such as serum antibodies specific for microbial antigens) or by administering substances purified from the microbe and measuring reactions to these substances. A reaction to a microbial antigen is detectable only in individuals who have previously encountered the antigen; these individuals are said to be "sensitized" to the antigen, and the reaction is an indication of "sensitivity." Although the reaction to the purified antigen has no protective function, it implies that the sensitized individual is capable of mounting a protective immune response to the microbe.

Cardinal Features of Adaptive Immune Responses

All humoral and cell-mediated immune responses to foreign antigens have a number of fundamental properties that reflect the properties of the lymphocytes that mediate these responses (Table 1–3).

- ***Specificity and diversity.*** Immune responses are specific for distinct antigens and, in fact, for different portions of a single complex protein, polysaccharide, or other macromolecule (Fig. 1–4). The parts of such antigens that are specifically recognized by individual lymphocytes are called **determinants** or **epitopes.** This fine specificity exists because individual lymphocytes express membrane receptors that are able to distinguish subtle differences in structure between distinct antigens. Clones of lymphocytes with different specificities are present in unimmunized individuals and are able to recognize and respond to foreign antigens. This concept is the basic tenet of the clonal selection hypothesis, which is discussed in more detail later in this chapter.

Table 1–3. Cardinal Features of Adaptive Immune Responses

Feature	Functional significance
Specificity	Ensures that distinct antigens elicit specific responses
Diversity	Enables immune system to respond to a large variety of antigens
Memory	Leads to enhanced responses to repeated exposures to the same antigens
Clonal expansion	Increases number of antigen-specific lymphocytes to keep pace with microbes
Specialization	Generates responses that are optimal for defense against different types of microbes
Contraction and homeostasis	Allows immune system to respond to newly encountered antigens
Nonreactivity to self	Prevents injury to the host during responses to foreign antigens

The features of adaptive immune responses are essential for the functions of the immune system.

The total number of antigenic specificities of the lymphocytes in an individual, called the **lymphocyte repertoire,** is extremely large. It is estimated that the immune system of an individual can discriminate 10^7 to 10^9 distinct antigenic determinants. This property of the lymphocyte repertoire is called **diversity.** It is the result of variability in the structures of the antigen-binding sites of lymphocyte receptors for antigens. In other words, there are many different clones of lymphocytes that differ in the structures of their antigen receptors and therefore in their specificity for antigens, contributing to a total repertoire that is extremely diverse. The molecular mechanisms that generate such diverse antigen receptors are discussed in Chapter 8.

- ***Memory.*** Exposure of the immune system to a foreign antigen enhances its ability to respond again to that antigen. Responses to second and subsequent exposures to the same antigen, called secondary immune responses, are usually more rapid, larger, and often qualitatively different from the first, or primary, immune response to that antigen (see Fig. 1–4). Immunologic memory occurs partly because each exposure to an antigen expands the clone of lymphocytes specific for that antigen. In addition, stimulation of naive lymphocytes by antigens generates long-lived memory cells (discussed in detail in Chapter 3). These memory cells have special characteristics that make them more efficient at responding to and eliminating the antigen than are naive lymphocytes that have not previously been exposed to the antigen. For instance, memory B lymphocytes produce antibodies that bind antigens with higher affinities than do antibodies produced in primary immune responses, and memory T cells react much more rapidly and vigorously to antigen challenge than do naive T cells.
- ***Clonal expansion.*** Lymphocytes undergo considerable proliferation following exposure to antigen. The

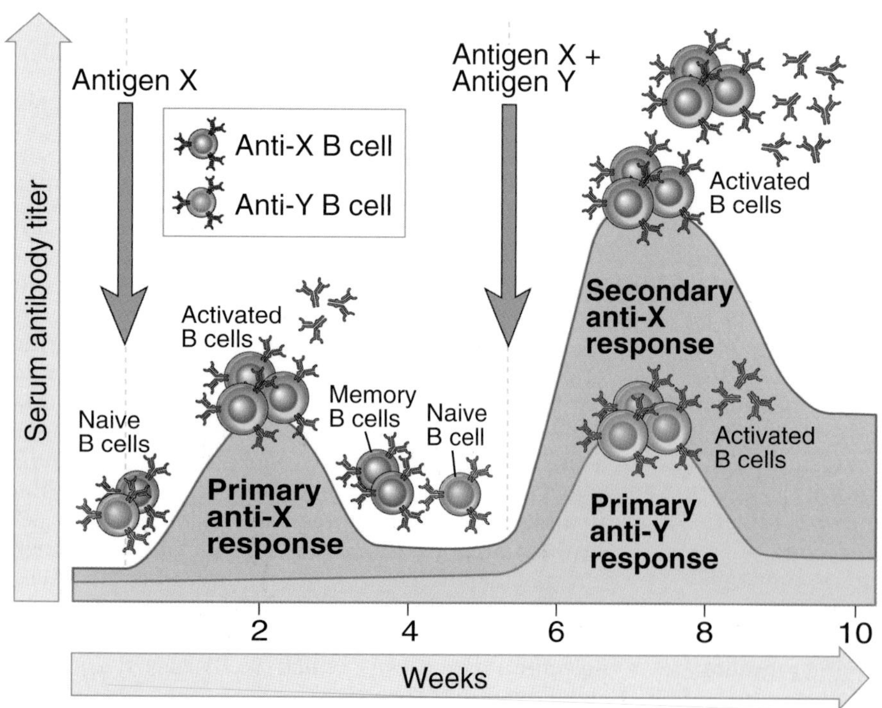

FIGURE 1–4 Specificity, memory, and contraction of adaptive immune responses. Antigens X and Y induce the production of different antibodies (specificity). The secondary response to antigen X is more rapid and larger than the primary response (memory). Antibody levels decline with time after each immunization (contraction, the process that maintains homeostasis). The same features are seen in cell-mediated immune responses.

term *clonal expansion* refers to an increase in the number of cells that express identical receptors for the antigen and thus belong to a clone. This increase in antigen-specific cells enables the adaptive immune response to keep pace with rapidly dividing infectious pathogens.

- ***Specialization.*** As we have already noted, the immune system responds in distinct and special ways to different microbes, maximizing the effectiveness of antimicrobial defense mechanisms. Thus, humoral immunity and cell-mediated immunity are elicited by different classes of microbes or by the same microbe at different stages of infection (extracellular and intracellular), and each type of immune response protects the host against that class of microbe. Even within humoral or cell-mediated immune responses, the nature of the antibodies or T lymphocytes that are generated may vary from one class of microbe to another. We will return to the mechanisms and functional significance of such specialization in later chapters.
- ***Contraction and homeostasis.*** All normal immune responses wane with time after antigen stimulation, thus returning the immune system to its resting basal state, a state that is called **homeostasis** (see Fig. 1–4). This contraction of immune responses occurs largely because responses that are triggered by antigens function to eliminate the antigens, thus eliminating the essential stimulus for lymphocyte survival and activation. Lymphocytes deprived of these stimuli die by apoptosis. The mechanisms of homeostasis are discussed in Chapter 11.
- ***Nonreactivity to self.*** One of the most remarkable properties of every normal individual's immune system is its ability to recognize, respond to, and eliminate many foreign (nonself) antigens while not reacting harmfully to that individual's own (self) antigenic substances. Immunological unresponsiveness is also called **tolerance.** Tolerance to self antigens, or self-tolerance, is maintained by several mechanisms. These include eliminating lymphocytes that express receptors specific for some self antigens and allowing lymphocytes to encounter other self antigens in settings that lead to functional inactivation or death of the self-reactive lymphocytes. The mechanisms of self-tolerance and discrimination between self and foreign antigens are discussed in Chapter 11. Abnormalities in the induction or maintenance of self-tolerance lead to immune responses against self antigens (autologous antigens), often resulting in disorders called **autoimmune diseases.** The development and pathologic consequences of autoimmunity are described in Chapter 18.

These features of adaptive immunity are necessary if the immune system is to perform its normal function of host defense (see Table 1–3). Specificity and memory enable the immune system to mount heightened responses to persistent or recurring stimulation with the same antigen and thus to combat infections that are prolonged or occur repeatedly. Diversity is essential if the immune system is to defend individuals against the many potential pathogens in the environment. Specialization enables the host to "custom design" responses to best combat particular types of microbes. Contraction of the response allows the system to return to a state of rest after it eliminates each foreign antigen and to be prepared to respond to other antigens. Self-tolerance is vital for preventing harmful reactions against one's own cells and tissues while maintaining a diverse repertoire of lymphocytes specific for foreign antigens.

Cellular Components of the Adaptive Immune System

The principal cells of the immune system are lymphocytes, antigen-presenting cells, and effector cells. Lymphocytes are the cells that specifically recognize and respond to foreign antigens and are therefore the mediators of humoral and cellular immunity. There are distinct subpopulations of lymphocytes that differ in how they recognize antigens and in their functions (Fig. 1–5). **B lymphocytes** are the only cells capable of producing antibodies. They recognize extracellular (including cell surface) antigens and differentiate into antibody-secreting plasma cells, thus functioning as the mediators of humoral immunity. **T lymphocytes,** the cells of cell-mediated immunity, recognize the antigens of intracellular microbes and function to destroy these microbes or the infected cells. T cells do not produce antibody molecules. Their antigen receptors are membrane molecules distinct from but structurally related to antibodies (see Chapter 7). T lymphocytes have a restricted specificity for antigens; they recognize only peptide antigens attached to host proteins that are encoded by genes in the major histocompatibility complex (MHC) and that are expressed on the surfaces of other cells. As a result, these T cells recognize and respond to cell surface–associated but not soluble antigens (see Chapter 6). T lymphocytes consist of functionally distinct populations, the best defined of which are **helper T cells** and **cytotoxic,** or **cytolytic, T lymphocytes** (CTLs). In response to antigenic stimulation, helper T cells secrete proteins called cytokines, whose functions are to stimulate the proliferation and differentiation of the T cells themselves, and activate other cells, including B cells, macrophages, and other leukocytes. CTLs kill cells that produce foreign antigens, such as cells infected by viruses and other intracellular microbes. Some T lymphocytes, which are called regulatory T cells, function mainly to inhibit immune responses. The generation and physiologic roles of these regulatory T cells are discussed in Chapter 11. A third class of lymphocytes, natural killer (NK) cells, is involved in innate immunity against viruses and other intracellular microbes. We will return to a more detailed discussion of the properties of lymphocytes in Chapter 3. Different classes of lymphocytes can be distinguished by the expression of surface proteins that are named "CD molecules" and numbered (Chapter 3).

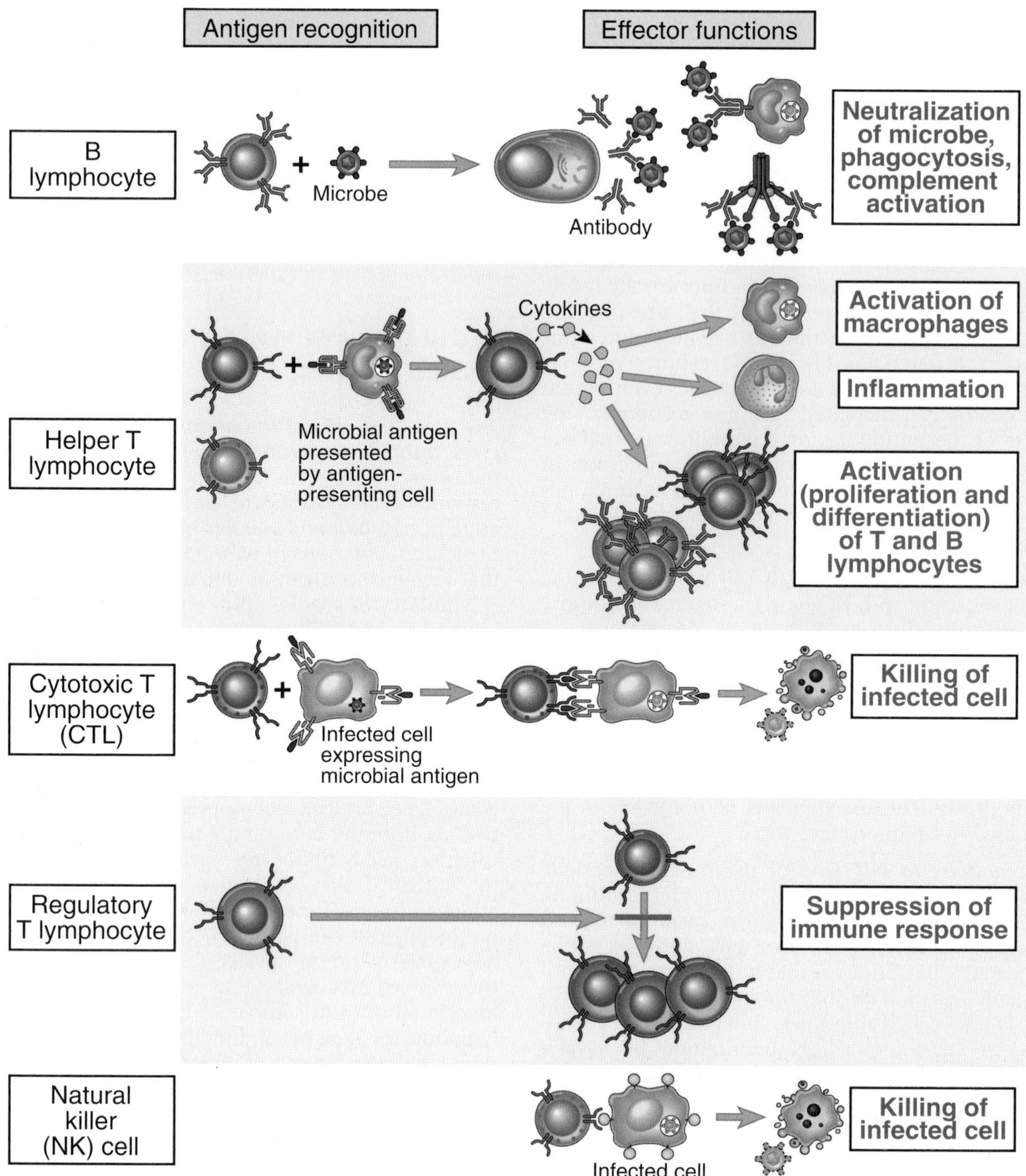

FIGURE 1–5 Classes of lymphocytes. B lymphocytes recognize soluble antigens and develop into antibody-secreting cells. Helper T lymphocytes recognize antigens on the surfaces of APCs and secrete cytokines, which stimulate different mechanisms of immunity and inflammation. CTLs recognize antigens on infected cells and kill these cells. Regulatory T cells suppress and prevent immune response, e.g. to self antigens. NK cells use receptors with more limited diversity than T or B cell antigen receptors to recognize and kill their targets, such as infected cells.

The initiation and development of adaptive immune responses require that antigens be captured and displayed to specific lymphocytes. The cells that serve this role are called **antigen-presenting cells** (APCs). The most specialized APCs are dendritic cells, which capture microbial antigens that enter from the external environment, transport these antigens to lymphoid organs, and present the antigens to naive T lymphocytes to initiate immune responses. Other cell types function as APCs at different stages of cell-mediated and humoral immune responses. We will describe the functions of APCs in Chapter 6.

The activation of lymphocytes by antigen leads to the generation of numerous mechanisms that function to eliminate the antigen. Antigen elimination often requires the participation of cells that are called **effector cells** because they mediate the final effect of the immune response, which is to get rid of the microbe.

Activated T lymphocytes, mononuclear phagocytes, and other leukocytes function as effector cells in different immune responses.

Lymphocytes and APCs are concentrated in anatomically discrete lymphoid organs, where they interact with one another to initiate immune responses. Lymphocytes are also present in the blood; from the blood, they can recirculate to lymphoid tissues and to peripheral sites of antigen exposure to eliminate the antigen (see Chapter 3).

Overview of Immune Responses to Microbes

Now that we have described the major components of the immune system and their properties, it is useful to summarize the principles of immune responses to different types of microbes. Such a summary will be a foundation for the topics that are discussed throughout the book.

The immune system has to combat many and diverse microbes. As we shall see shortly, some features of immune responses are common to all infectious pathogens, and others are unique to different classes of these microbes. How these adaptive immune reactions are initiated, orchestrated, and controlled are the fundamental questions of immunology. We start with a discussion of the innate immune response.

The Early Innate Immune Response to Microbes

The innate immune system blocks the entry of microbes and eliminates or limits the growth of many microbes that are able to colonize tissues. The main sites of interaction between individuals and their environment—the skin, and gastrointestinal and respiratory tracts—are lined by continuous epithelia, which serve as barriers to prevent the entry of microbes from the external environment. If microbes successfully breach the epithelial barriers, they encounter macrophages in the subepithelial tissue. Macrophages (and other phagocytic leukocytes) express on their surfaces receptors that bind and ingest microbes, and other receptors that recognize different microbial molecules and activate the cells.

Activated macrophages perform several functions that collectively serve to eliminate ingested microbes. These cells produce reactive oxygen species and lysosomal enzymes, which destroy microbes that have been ingested. Macrophages secrete cytokines that promote the recruitment of other leukocytes, such as neutrophils, from blood vessels to the site of infection. Cytokines are secreted proteins that are responsible for many of the cellular responses of innate and adaptive immunity, and thus function as the "messenger molecules" of the immune system. The local accumulation of leukocytes, and their activation to destroy the microbes, is part of the host response called inflammation. The innate immune response to some infectious pathogens, particularly viruses, consists of the production of anti-viral cytokines called interferons and activation of NK cells, which kill virus-infected cells.

Microbes that are able to withstand these defense reactions may enter the blood stream, where they are recognized by the circulating proteins of innate immunity. The most important plasma proteins of innate immunity are the members of the complement system. Complement proteins may be directly activated by microbial surfaces (the alternative pathway of activation), resulting in the generation of cleavage products that stimulate inflammation, coat the microbes for enhanced phagocytosis, and create holes in the microbial cell membranes, leading to their lysis. (As we shall see later, complement can also be activated by antibodies—called the classical pathway, for historical reasons—with the same functional consequences.)

The reactions of innate immunity are remarkably effective at controlling, and even eradicating, many infections. However, a hallmark of pathogenic microbes is that they have evolved to resist innate immunity and to successfully invade and replicate in the cells and tissues of the host. Defense against these pathogens requires the more powerful and specialized mechanisms of adaptive immunity.

The Adaptive Immune Response

The adaptive immune system uses three main strategies to combat most microbes.

- Secreted antibodies bind to extracellular microbes, block their ability to infect host cells, and promote their ingestion and subsequent destruction by phagocytes.
- Phagocytes ingest microbes and kill them, and helper T cells enhance the microbicidal abilities of the phagocytes.
- CTLs destroy cells infected by microbes that are inaccessible to antibodies.

The goal of the adaptive response is to activate one or more of these defense mechanisms against diverse microbes that may be in different anatomic locations, such as intestinal lumens, the circulation, or inside cells. A characteristic of the adaptive immune system is that it produces large numbers of lymphocytes during maturation and after antigen stimulation, and selects the most useful cells to combat microbes. Such selection maximizes the efficacy of the adaptive immune response. All adaptive immune responses develop in steps, each of which corresponds to particular reactions of lymphocytes (Fig. 1–6). We start this overview of adaptive immunity with the first step, which is the recognition of antigens.

The Capture and Display of Microbial Antigens

Because the number of naive lymphocytes specific for any antigen is very small (on the order of 1 in 10^5 or

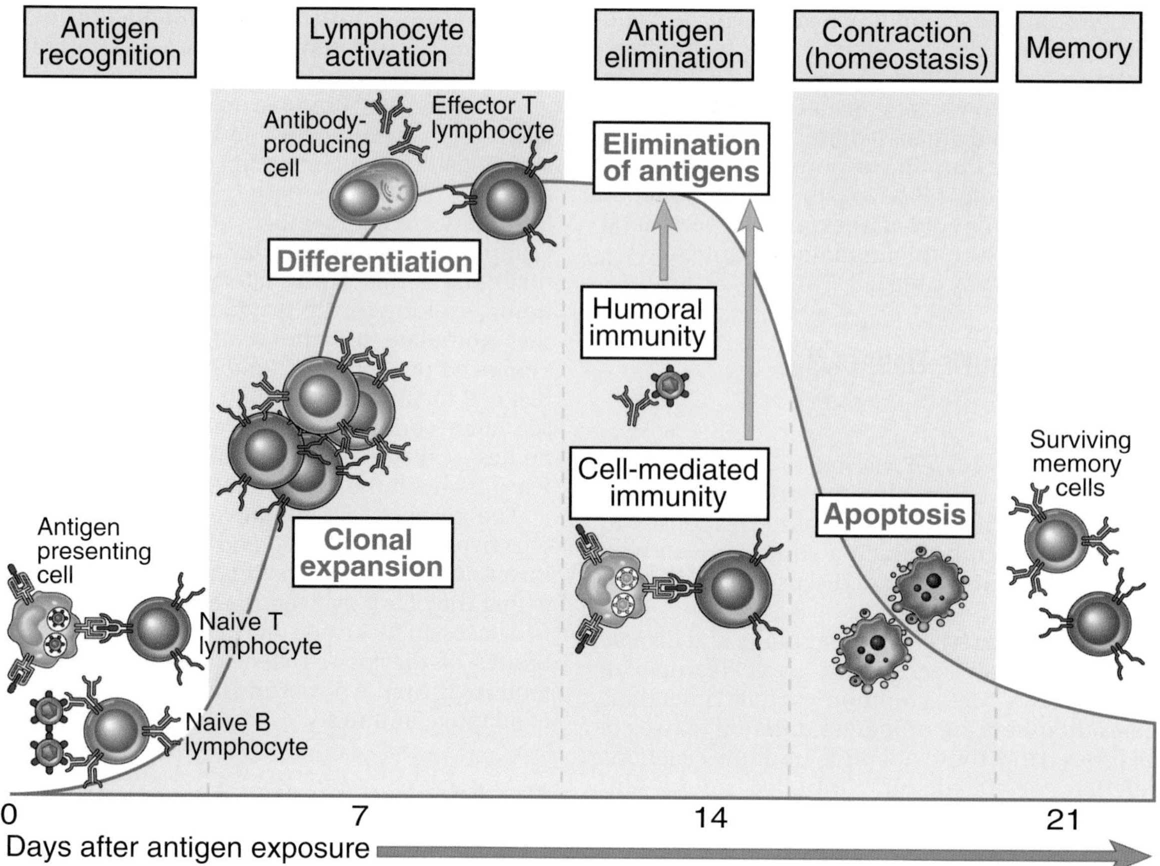

FIGURE 1–6 Phases of adaptive immune responses. Adaptive immune responses consist of distinct phases, the first three being the recognition of antigen, the activation of lymphocytes, and the elimination of antigen (the effector phase). The response contracts (declines) as antigen-stimulated lymphocytes die by apoptosis, restoring homeostasis, and the antigen-specific cells that survive are responsible for memory. The duration of each phase may vary in different immune responses. The y-axis represents an arbitrary measure of the magnitude of the response. These principles apply to humoral immunity (mediated by B lymphocytes) and cell-mediated immunity (mediated by T lymphocytes).

10^6 lymphocytes) and the quantity of the available antigen may also be small, special mechanisms are needed to capture microbes, concentrate them in the correct location, and deliver their antigens to specific lymphocytes.

Dendritic cells are the APCs that display microbial peptides to naive $CD4^+$ and $CD8^+$ T lymphocytes and initiate adaptive immune responses to protein antigens. Dendritic cells located in epithelia and connective tissues capture microbes, digest their proteins into peptides, and express on their surface these peptides bound to MHC molecules, which are specialized peptide display molecules. Dendritic cells carry their antigenic cargo to draining lymph nodes and take up residence in the same regions of the nodes through which naive T lymphocytes continuously recirculate. Thus, the chance of a lymphocyte with receptors for an antigen finding that antigen is greatly increased by concentrating the antigen in recognizable form in the correct anatomic location. Dendritic cells also display the peptides of microbes that enter other lymphoid tissues, such as the spleen.

Intact microbes or microbial antigens that enter lymph nodes and spleen are recognized in unprocessed (native) form by specific B lymphocytes. There are also specialized APCs that display antigens to B lymphocytes.

Antigen Recognition by Lymphocytes

Lymphocytes specific for a large number of antigens exist prior to exposure to the antigen, and when an antigen enters, it selects the specific cells and activates them (Fig. 1–7). This fundamental concept is called the **clonal selection hypothesis.** It was first suggested by Niels Jerne in 1955, and most clearly enunciated by Macfarlane Burnet in 1957, as a hypothesis to explain how the immune system could respond to a large number and variety of antigens. According to this hypothesis, antigen-specific clones of lymphocytes develop before and independent of exposure to antigen. The cells constituting each clone have identical antigen receptors, which are different from the receptors on the cells of all other clones. It is estimated that there are $>10^6$ different specificities in T and B lymphocytes, so that at least this many antigenic determinants can be recognized by the adaptive immune system. We will return to a more detailed discussion of clonal selection in Chapter 3.

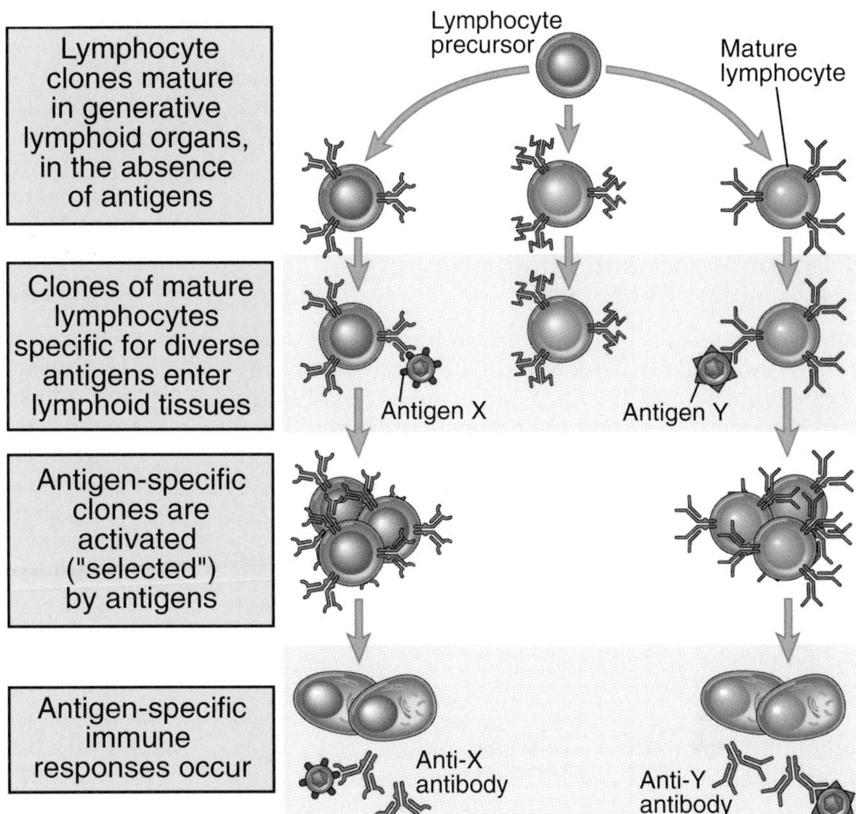

FIGURE 1–7 The clonal selection hypothesis. Each antigen (X or Y) selects a preexisting clone of specific lymphocytes and stimulates the proliferation and differentiation of that clone. The diagram shows only B lymphocytes giving rise to antibody-secreting effector cells, but the same principle applies to T lymphocytes.

The activation of naive T lymphocytes requires recognition of peptide-MHC complexes presented on dendritic cells. The nature of the antigen that activates T cells (i.e., peptides bound to MHC molecules) ensures that these lymphocytes can interact only with other cells (since MHC molecules are cell surface proteins) and not with free antigen. This, of course, is predictable, because all the functions of T lymphocytes are dependent on their physical interactions with other cells. In order to respond, the T cells need to recognize not only antigens but also other molecules, called costimulators, that are induced on the APCs by microbes. Antigen recognition provides specificity to the immune response, and the need for costimulation ensures that T cells respond to microbes (the inducers of costimulatory molecules) and not to harmless substances.

B lymphocytes use their antigen receptors (membrane-bound antibody molecules) to recognize antigens of many different chemical types.

Engagement of antigen receptors and other signals trigger lymphocyte proliferation and differentiation. The reactions and functions of T and B lymphocytes differ in important ways and are best considered separately.

Cell-Mediated Immunity: Activation of T Lymphocytes and Elimination of Intracellular Microbes

Activated $CD4^+$ helper T lymphocytes proliferate and differentiate into effector cells whose functions are mediated largely by secreted cytokines. One of the earliest responses of $CD4^+$ helper T cells is secretion of the cytokine interleukin-2 (IL-2). IL-2 is a growth factor that acts on the antigen-activated lymphocytes and stimulates their proliferation (clonal expansion). Some of the progeny differentiate into effector cells that can secrete different sets of cytokines, and thus perform different functions. These effector cells leave the lymphoid organs where they were generated and migrate to sites of infection and accompanying inflammation. When these differentiated effectors again encounter cell-associated microbes, they are activated to perform the functions that are responsible for elimination of the microbes. Some effector T cells of the $CD4^+$ helper cell lineage secrete the cytokine interferon-γ, which is a potent macrophage activator and induces production of microbicidal substances in macrophages. Thus, these helper T cells can recognize microbial antigens on macrophages that have phagocytosed the microbes and help the phagocytes to kill the infectious pathogens. Other $CD4^+$ effector T cells secrete cytokines that stimulate the production of a special class of antibody called immunoglobulin E (IgE) and activate leukocytes called eosinophils, which are able to kill parasites that may be too large to be phagocytosed. As we discuss below, $CD4^+$ helper T cells also stimulate B cell responses.

Activated $CD8^+$ lymphocytes proliferate and differentiate into CTLs that kill cells harboring microbes in the cytoplasm. These microbes may be viruses that infect many cell types, or bacteria that are ingested by macrophages but have learned to escape from phagocytic vesicles into the cytoplasm (where they are inaccessible to the killing machinery of phagocytes, which is largely confined to vesicles). By destroying the infected cells, CTLs eliminate the reservoirs of infection.

Humoral Immunity: Activation of B Lymphocytes and Elimination of Extracellular Microbes

Upon activation, B lymphocytes proliferate and differentiate into cells that secrete different classes of antibodies with distinct functions. Many polysaccharide and lipid antigens have multiple identical antigenic determinants that are able to engage many antigen receptor molecules on each B cell and initiate the process of B cell activation. The response of B cells to protein antigens requires activating signals ("help") from $CD4^+$ T cells (which is the historical reason for calling these T cells "helper" cells). B cells ingest protein antigens, degrade them, and display peptides bound to MHC molecules for recognition by helper T cells, which then activate the B cells.

Some of the progeny of the expanded B cell clones differentiate into antibody-secreting plasma cells. Each plasma cell secretes antibodies that have the same antigen binding site as the cell surface antibodies (B cell receptors) that first recognized the antigen. Polysaccharides and lipids stimulate secretion mainly of the antibody class called IgM. Protein antigens, by virtue of helper T cell actions, induce the production of antibodies of different classes (IgG, IgA, IgE). This production of functionally different antibodies, all with the same specificity, is called heavy chain class switching; it provides plasticity in the antibody response, enabling it to serve many functions. Helper T cells also stimulate the production of antibodies with increased affinity for the antigen. This process, called affinity maturation, improves the quality of the humoral immune response.

The humoral immune response combats microbes in many ways. Antibodies bind to microbes and prevent them from infecting cells, thus "neutralizing" the microbes. In this way, antibodies are able to prevent infections. In fact, antibodies are the only mechanisms of adaptive immunity that block an infection before it is established; this is why eliciting the production of potent antibodies is a key goal of vaccination. IgG antibodies coat microbes and target them for phagocytosis, since phagocytes (neutrophils and macrophages) express receptors for the tails of IgG. IgG and IgM activate the complement system, by the classical pathway, and complement products promote phagocytosis and destruction of microbes. Some antibodies serve special roles at particular anatomic sites. IgA is secreted from mucosal epithelia and neutralizes microbes in the lumens of the respiratory and gastrointestinal tracts (and other mucosal tissues). IgG is actively transported across the placenta, and protects the newborn until the immune system becomes mature. Most antibodies have half-lives of about 3 weeks. However, some antibody-secreting plasma cells migrate to the bone marrow and live for years, continuing to produce low levels of antibodies. The antibodies that are secreted by these long-lived plasma cells provide immediate protection if the microbe returns to infect the individual. More effective protection is provided by memory cells that are activated by the microbe.

Immunological Memory

An effective immune response eliminates the microbes that initiated the response. This is followed by a contraction phase, in which the expanded lymphocyte clones die and homeostasis is restored.

The initial activation of lymphocytes generates long-lived memory cells, which may survive for years after the infection. Memory cells are more effective in combating microbes than are naive lymphocytes because as mentioned earlier, memory cells represent an expanded pool of antigen-specific lymphocytes (more numerous than naive cells specific for the antigen), and memory cells respond faster and more effectively against the antigen than do naive cells. This is why generating memory responses is the second important goal of vaccination. We will discuss the properties of memory lymphocytes in more detail in Chapter 3.

In Sections II, III, and IV, we describe in detail the recognition, activation, regulation, and effector phases of adaptive immune responses. The principles introduced in this chapter recur throughout the book.

SUMMARY

- Protective immunity against microbes is mediated by the early reactions of innate immunity and the later responses of adaptive immunity. Innate immunity is stimulated by structures shared by groups of microbes. Adaptive immunity is specific for different microbial and nonmicrobial antigens and is increased by repeated exposures to antigen (immunologic memory).
- Humoral immunity is mediated by B lymphocytes and their secreted products, antibodies, and functions in defense against extracellular microbes. Cell-mediated immunity is mediated by T lymphocytes and their products, such as cytokines, and is important for defense against intracellular microbes.
- Immunity may be acquired by a response to antigen (active immunity) or conferred by transfer of antibodies or cells from an immunized individual (passive immunity).
- The immune system possesses several properties that are of fundamental importance for its normal

functions. These include specificity for different antigens, a diverse repertoire capable of recognizing a wide variety of antigens, memory of antigen exposure, the capacity for rapid expansion of clones of antigen-specific lymphocytes in response to the antigen, specialized responses to different microbes, maintenance of homeostasis, and the ability to discriminate between foreign antigens and self antigens.

- Lymphocytes are the only cells capable of specifically recognizing antigens and are thus the principal cells of adaptive immunity. The two major subpopulations of lymphocytes are B cells and T cells, and they differ in their antigen receptors and functions. Specialized antigen-presenting cells capture microbial antigens and display these antigens for recognition by lymphocytes. The elimination of antigens often requires the participation of various effector cells.

- The adaptive immune response is initiated by the recognition of foreign antigens by specific lymphocytes. Lymphocytes respond by proliferating and by differentiating into effector cells, whose function is to eliminate the antigen, and into memory cells, which show enhanced responses on subsequent encounters with the antigen. The activation of lymphocytes requires antigen and additional signals that may be provided by microbes or by innate immune responses to microbes.

- $CD4^+$ helper T lymphocytes help macrophages to eliminate ingested microbes and help B cells to produce antibodies. $CD8^+$ CTLs kill cells harboring intracellular pathogens, thus eliminating reservoirs of infection. Antibodies, the products of B lymphocytes, neutralize the infectivity of microbes and promote the elimination of microbes by phagocytes and by activation of the complement system.

Selected Readings

Burnet FM. A modification of Jerne's theory of antibody production using the concept of clonal selection. Australian Journal of Science 20:67–69, 1957.

Flajnik MF, and L du Pasquier. Evolution of innate and adaptive immunity: can we draw a line? Trends in Immunology 25:640–644, 2004.

Jerne NK. The natural-selection theory of antibody formation. Proceedings of the National Academy of Sciences U S A 41:849–857, 1955.

Litman GW, JP Cannon, and LJ Dishaw. Reconstructing immune phylogeny: new perspectives. Nature Reviews Immunology 5:866–879, 2005.

Silverstein AM. Paul Ehrlich's Receptor Immunology: The Magnificent Obsession. Academic Press, New York, 2001.

Silverstein AM. Cellular versus humoral immunology: a century-long dispute. Nature Immunology 4:425–428, 2003.

Van den Berg TK, JA Yoder, and GW Litman. On the origins of adaptive immunity: innate immune receptors join the tale. Trends in Immunology 25:11–16, 2004.

Chapter 2

INNATE IMMUNITY

Innate immunity is the first line of defense against infections. The mechanisms of innate immunity exist before encounter with microbes and are rapidly activated by microbes before the development of adaptive immune responses (see Chapter 1, Fig. 1–1). Innate immunity is also the phylogenetically oldest mechanism of defense against microbes and co-evolved along with microbes to protect all multicellular organisms, including plants and insects, from infections. Adaptive immunity mediated by T and B lymphocytes appeared in jawed vertebrates and is superimposed on innate immunity to improve host defense against microbes. In Chapter 1, we introduced the concept that the adaptive immune response enhances some of the antimicrobial mechanisms of innate immunity and provides both memory of antigen encounter and specialization of effector mechanisms. In this chapter, we describe the components, specificity, and functions of the innate immune system.

Innate immunity serves two important functions.

- ***Innate immunity is the initial response to microbes that prevents, controls, or eliminates infection of the host.*** The importance of innate immunity in host defense is illustrated by studies showing that inhibiting or eliminating any of several mechanisms of innate immunity markedly increases susceptibility to infections, even when the adaptive immune system is intact and functional. We will review examples of such studies later in this chapter and in Chapter 15 when we discuss immunity to different types of microbes. Many pathogenic microbes have evolved strategies to resist innate immunity, and these strategies are crucial for the virulence of the microbes. In infection by such microbes, innate immune defenses may keep the infection in check until the adaptive immune responses are activated. Adaptive immune responses, being more potent and specialized, are able to eliminate microbes that resist the defense mechanisms of innate immunity.

- ***Innate immunity to microbes stimulates adaptive immune responses and can influence the nature of the adaptive responses to make them optimally effective against different types of microbes.*** Thus, innate immunity not only serves defensive functions early after infection but also provides the "warning" that an infection is present against which a subsequent adaptive immune response has to be mounted. Moreover, different components of the innate immune response often react in distinct ways to different microbes (e.g., bacteria versus viruses) and thereby influence the type of adaptive immune response that develops. We will return to this concept at the end of the chapter.

Some components of innate immunity are functioning at all times, even before infection; these components include barriers to microbial entry provided by epithelial surfaces, such as the skin and lining of the gastrointestinal and respiratory tracts. Other components of innate immunity are normally inactive but poised to respond rapidly to the presence of microbes; these components include phagocytes and the complement system. We begin our discussion of innate immunity by describing, in general terms, how the innate immune system recognizes microbes and then proceed to the individual components of innate immunity and their functions in host defense.

FEATURES OF INNATE IMMUNE RECOGNITION

The specificity of the innate immune system for microbial products differs from the specificity of the adaptive immune system in several respects (Table 2–1).

- ***The components of innate immunity recognize structures that are characteristic of microbial pathogens and are not present on mammalian cells.*** The innate immune system recognizes only a limited number of microbial products, whereas the adaptive immune system is capable of recognizing a much wider array of foreign substances whether or not they are products of microbes. The microbial substances that stimulate innate immunity are called **pathogen-associated molecular patterns (PAMPs),** and the receptors that bind these conserved structures are called **pattern recognition receptors** (Table 2–2). Different classes of microbes (e.g., viruses, gram-negative bacteria, gram-positive bacteria, fungi) express different PAMPs. These structures include nucleic acids that are unique to microbes, such as double-stranded RNA found in replicating viruses or unmethylated CpG DNA sequences found in bacteria; features of proteins that are found in microbes, such as initiation by *N*-formylmethionine, which is typical of bacterial proteins; and complex lipids and carbohydrates that are synthesized by microbes but not by mammalian cells, such as lipopolysaccharides (LPS) in gram-negative bacteria, teichoic acids in gram-positive bacteria, and mannose-rich oligosac-

Table 2–1. Specificity of Innate and Adaptive Immunity

	Innate immunity	Adaptive immunity
Specificity	For structures shared by classes of microbes ("pathogen-associated molecular patterns") 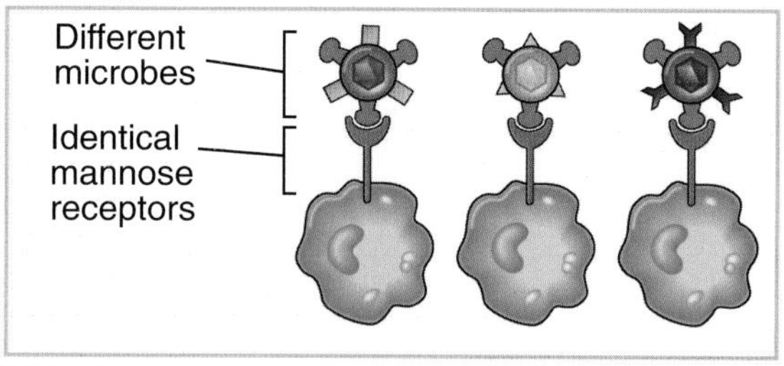 Different microbes Identical mannose receptors	For structural detail of microbial molecules (antigens); may recognize nonmicrobial antigens 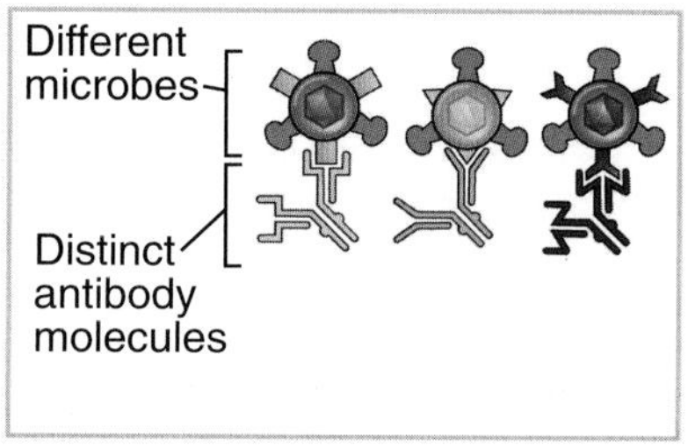 Different microbes Distinct antibody molecules
Receptors	Encoded in germline; limited diversity ("pattern recognition receptors") 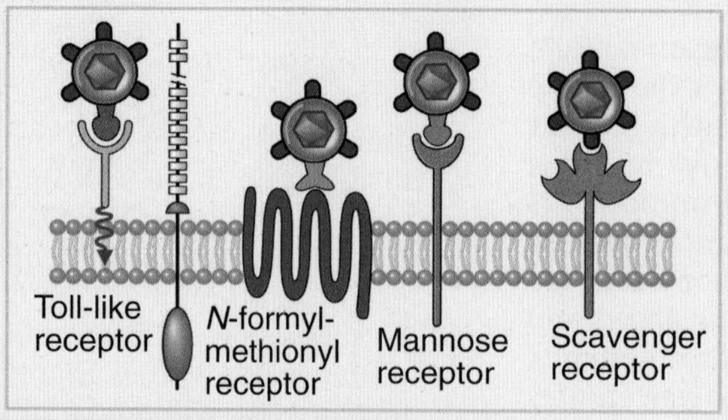 Toll-like receptor *N*-formyl-methionyl receptor Mannose receptor Scavenger receptor	Encoded by genes produced by somatic recombination of gene segments; greater diversity 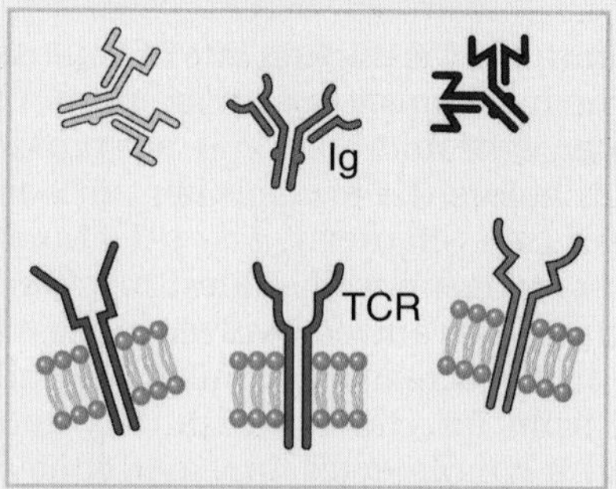 Ig TCR
Distribution of receptors	Nonclonal: identical receptors on all cells of the same lineage	Clonal: clones of lymphocytes with distinct specificities express different receptors
Discrimination between self and nonself	Yes; host cells are not recognized or they may express molecules that prevent innate immune reactions	Yes; based on selection against self-reactive lymphocytes; may be imperfect (giving rise to autoimmunity)

Table 2–2. Examples of Recognition Molecules of Innate Immunity and the Molecular Patterns of Microbes They Recognize

Cell-associated pattern recognition receptors	Location	Specific examples and their PAMP ligands
Toll-like receptors	Plasma membrane and endosomal membranes of dendritic cells, phagocytes, endothelial cells, and many other cell types	TLRs 1-9: Various bacterial and viral molecules (see Fig. 2–2)
C-type lectins	Plasma membranes of phagocytes	Mannose receptor: Microbial surface carbohydrates with terminal mannose and fructose
		Dectin: Glucans present in fungal cell walls
Scavenger receptors	Plasma membranes of phagocytes	CD36: microbial diacylglycerides
NLRs	Cytoplasm of phagocytes and other cells	Nod1, Nod2 and NALP3: bacterial peptidoglycans
N-formyl Met-Leu-Phe receptors	Plasma membranes of phagocytes	FPR and FPRL1: peptides containing *N*-formylmethionyl residues
Soluble recognition molecules	**Location**	**Specific examples and their PAMP ligands**
Pentraxins	Plasma	C reactive protein (CRP): Microbial phosphorylcholine and phosphatidylethanolamine
Collectins	Plasma	Mannose-binding lectin (MBL): Carbohydrates with terminal mannose and fructose
	Alveoli	Surfactant proteins SP-A and SP-D: Various microbial structures
Ficolins	Plasma	Ficolin: *N*-acetylglucosamine and lipoteichoic acid components of the cell walls of gram-positive bacteria

Abbreviations: TLR, Toll-like receptor; PAMP, pathogen-associated molecular pattern; NLR, Nod-like receptor

charides found in microbial but not in mammalian glycoproteins.

Because of this specificity for microbial structures, the innate immune system is able to distinguish self from nonself, but it does so very differently from the adaptive immune system. The mechanisms of innate immunity have evolved to recognize microbes (nonself) and not mammalian (self) molecules. In contrast, in the adaptive immune system, self/nonself discrimination is based not on inherited specificity for microbes but on the elimination or inactivation of lymphocytes specific for self antigens. In fact, the innate immune response is not known to react against self structures in healthy tissues and is thus even better at discriminating between self and nonself than the adaptive immune system is. As we shall see in Chapter 18, adaptive immune responses can occur against autologous antigens and result in autoimmune diseases, but this problem does not appear to happen with innate immunity.

- ***The innate immune system recognizes microbial products that are often essential for survival of the microbes.*** This host adaptation is important because it ensures that the targets of innate immunity cannot be discarded by microbes in an effort to evade recognition by the host. In contrast, as we shall see in Chapter 15, microbes may mutate or lose many of the antigens that are recognized by the adaptive immune system, thereby enabling the microbes to evade host defense without compromising their own survival. An example of a target of innate immunity that is essential for microbes is double-stranded viral RNA, which plays a critical role in the replication of certain viruses. Similarly, LPS and teichoic acid are structural components of bacterial cell walls that are required for bacterial survival and cannot be discarded.

- ***Pattern recognition molecules of the innate immune system include cell-associated pattern recognition***

receptors expressed on the surface of or inside various cell types, and soluble proteins in the blood and extracellular fluids (see Table 2–2). The cell-associated receptors may perform one or both of two major functions. First, they may transduce signals that activate antimicrobial and proinflammatory functions of the cells in which they are expressed. Second, they may facilitate uptake of the microbes into the cells. Soluble receptors are responsible for facilitating the clearance of microbes from blood and extracellular fluids by enhancing uptake into cells or by activating extracellular killing mechanisms. We will discuss these receptors and their functions in detail below.

- ***The pattern recognition receptors of the innate immune system are encoded in germline DNA.*** In contrast, T and B lymphocytes, the principal components of adaptive immunity, use somatic gene rearrangement to generate their antigen receptors (see Chapter 8). Because many fewer receptors can be encoded in the germline than can be generated through gene rearrangements, the innate immune system has a limited repertoire of specificities. It is estimated that the innate immune system can recognize about 10^3 molecular patterns of microbes. In contrast, the adaptive immune system is capable of recognizing 10^7 or more distinct antigens. Furthermore, whereas the adaptive immune system can distinguish between antigens of different microbes of the same class and even different antigens of one microbe, innate immunity can distinguish only classes of microbes.
- ***In addition to microbial products, the innate immune system can also recognize stressed or injured host cells.*** Stressed or injured cells often express molecules not found in abundance in healthy cells. These molecules, including heat shock proteins, certain class I major histocompatibility complex (MHC)-like molecules, and altered membrane phospholipids, are recognized by various innate immune system receptors. Cells that are directly infected or are in the vicinity of other infected cells may increase the expression of these molecules. In this way, innate immunity can contribute to the elimination of cells harboring microbes, even if microbial products are not exposed on the cell surface.

With this general introduction to innate immunity, we proceed to a discussion of the major classes of pattern recognition receptors and then the individual components of innate immunity and their functions in host defense.

Cellular Pattern Recognition Receptors

A wide variety of cell types express pattern recognition receptors and therefore participate in innate immune responses. These include neutrophils, macrophages, dendritic cells, and endothelial cells, which we will discuss later in this chapter. In addition, epithelial cells, lymphocytes, and other cell types also express pattern recognition receptors. These cell-associated pattern recognition receptors are present on the cell surface, in endosomal vesicles, and in the cytoplasm, ready to recognize microbes in any of these locations (Fig. 2–1). Pattern recognition receptors are linked to intracellular signal transduction pathways that activate various cellular responses, including the production of molecules that promote inflammation and defend against microbes. The major classes of these receptors are discussed next.

Toll-like Receptors (TLRs)

The TLRs are an evolutionarily conserved family of pattern recognition receptors expressed on many cell types, which play essential roles in innate immune responses to microbes (Fig. 2–2 and Box 2–1). Toll was originally identified as a *Drosophila* gene involved in establishing the dorsal-ventral axis during embryogenesis of the fly, but subsequently it was discovered that the Toll protein also mediated antimicrobial responses. There are eleven different human TLRs, named TLR 1 to 11. All these receptors contain a Toll/IL-1 receptor (TIR) homology domain in their cytoplasmic region, which is

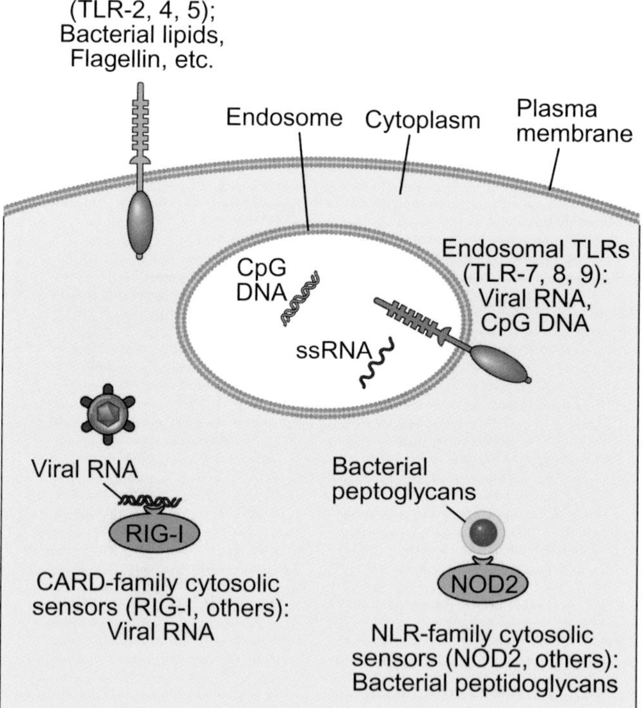

FIGURE 2–1 Cellular locations of pattern recognition molecules of the innate immune system. Some pattern recognition molecules of the TLR family (see Fig. 2–7), such as TLRs 2, 4, and 5, are expressed on the cell surface, where they may bind extracellular pathogen-associated molecular patterns. Other TLRs are expressed on endosomal membranes, such as TLRs 3, 7, 8, and 9, all of which can recognize nucleic acids of microbes that have been phagocytosed by cells. Cells also contain cytoplasmic sensors of microbial infection (discussed later in the chapter), including the NLR family of proteins, which recognize bacterial peptidoglycans, and a subset of CARD family of proteins, which bind viral RNA.

Box 2–1 ▪ IN DEPTH: TOLL-LIKE RECEPTOR STRUCTURE AND SIGNALING PATHWAYS

TLRs are membrane signaling receptors that play essential roles in innate defense against microbes. TLR genes have been highly conserved during evolution, and are found in *Caenorhabditis elegans, Drosophila,* and mammals. There are 12 mammalian TLR genes (11 expressed in humans), all of which are type I integral membrane glycoproteins that contain leucine-rich repeats flanked by characteristic cysteine-rich motifs in their extracellular regions and a cytoplasmic TIR homology domain (see Figure). TIR domains are also found in the cytoplasmic

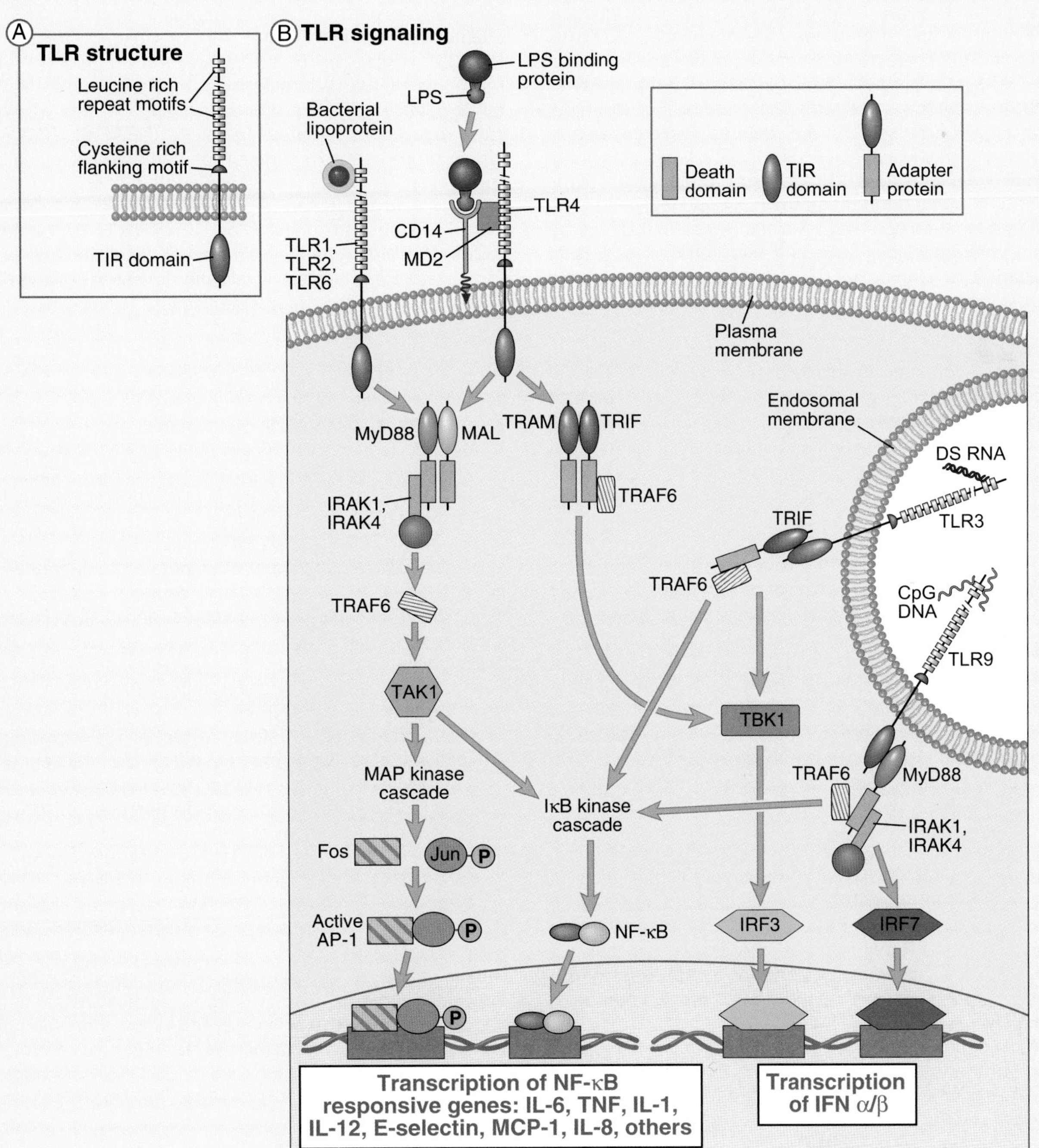

Continued on following page

Box 2–1 ▪ IN DEPTH: TOLL-LIKE RECEPTOR STRUCTURE AND SIGNALING PATHWAYS (Continued)

tails of the receptors for the cytokines IL-1 and IL-18, and similar signaling pathways are engaged by TLRs, IL-1, and IL-18.

The TLR binding sites for microbial ligands are being studied by x-ray crystallography and mutational analyses. To date, the structural basis for the different TLR specificities remains unknown. TLR signaling requires dimerization of TLR proteins in the cell membrane, which sometimes involves homodimerization of two identical TLR proteins and sometimes heterodimerization of two different TLR proteins. The repertoire of specificities of the TLR system is apparently extended by the ability of TLRs to heterodimerize with one another. For example, dimers of TLR2 and TLR6 are required for responses to peptidoglycan. Specificities of the TLRs are also influenced by various non-TLR accessory molecules. This is most thoroughly understood for TLR4 and its ligand LPS. LPS first binds to soluble LPS-binding protein (LBP) in the blood or extracellular fluid, and this complex serves to facilitate LPS binding to CD14, which exists as both a soluble plasma protein and a glycophosphatidylinositol-linked membrane protein on most cells except endothelium. Once LPS binds to CD14, LBP dissociates, and the LPS-CD14 complex physically associates with TLR4. An additional extracellular accessory protein called MD2 also binds to the complex with CD14. LPS, CD14, and MD2 are all required for efficient LPS-induced signaling, but it is not yet clear if direct physical interaction of LPS with TLR4 is necessary. Different combinations of accessory molecules in TLR complexes may serve to broaden the range of microbial products that can induce innate immune responses. For example, both CD14 and MD2 are associated with complexes of other TLRs (e.g., TLR2).

The details of TLR signaling are the focus of active investigation, and new information continues to change our understanding of the pathways; the following discussion is an overview of current knowledge. Ligand-induced TLR dimerization permits the binding of cytoplasmic adapter proteins to the TLR cytoplasmic tails, via homotypic interactions of TIR domains found in both the TLR and the adapter protein. Four of these adapters are MyD88, Mal (MyD88 adapter-like)/TIRAP (TIR domain-containing adapter protein), Trif (TIR-domain-containing adapter inducing interferon-β), and TRAM (Trif-related adapter molecule). Different combinations of the adapters are used by different TLRs, as discussed below, which is the basis for common and unique downstream effects of the TLRs. In all cases, the adapter proteins are crucial for the assembly of signaling complexes, which include protein kinases (usually IRAK family members) and TRAF.

A major downstream effect of TLR signaling is the activation of the transcription factor NF-κB, which is required for expression of many genes related to innate immunity and inflammation. In resting cells, functional NF-κB dimers are present in an inactive state in the cytoplasm, bound to inhibitory proteins called IκBs. The activation of NF-κB is initiated by the signal-induced degradation of IκB proteins by an enzymatic complex called IκB kinase (IKK). The same TLRs that lead to NF-κB activation often also lead to activation of another transcription factor called AP-1. NF-κB and AP-1 activation by TLRs involves a signal transduction pathway that is dependent on the MyD88 adapter protein (see Figure). All TLRs except TLR3 bind MyD88, which, in most cases, then interacts with members of the IL-1 receptor-associated kinase **(IRAK)** family, and the IRAK proteins interact with and activate TNF receptor–associated factor 6 **(TRAF-6).** TRAF-6, which promotes ubiquitination of downstream signaling molecules, activates TGF-β-activated kinase 1 (TAK1), which in turn initiates the mitogen activated protein (MAP) kinase and inhibitor of NF-κB (IκB) kinase cascades. The MAP kinase and the IκB kinase cascades lead to activation and nuclear localization of the AP-1 and NF-κB transcription factors, respectively.

TLR4, which responds to bacterial LPS (see Box 15–1, Chapter 15), engages at least two different signaling pathways, each of which utilizes a different pair of TIR family adapter proteins. In one pathway, MyD88 and Mal/TIRAP are recruited and lead to NF-κB activation via IRAK, TRAF-6, and TAK1. In a second pathway, TRAM and Trif are recruited and lead to activation of interferon response factor-3 (IRF-3), via TBK1. IRF-3 is a transcription factor that enhances expression of type 1 interferon genes (IFN-α and IFN-β). Therefore, TLR4 signaling can also result in expression of a wide variety of inflammatory and antiviral genes.

TLR9, which recognizes bacterial and viral unmethylated CpG DNA within endosomes, recruits MyD88, leading to activation of IRF7, a transcription factor that, like IRF3, induces type I interferon gene expression. TLR9 signaling also activates NF-κB.

A second major downstream effect of TLR signaling is the activation of IRF-3 and -7, which are transcription factors required for expression of type I interferon genes (IFN-α and IFN-β). TLR3, the endosomal receptor for viral double-stranded RNA, activates IRF-3. TLR3 does not bind MyD88, but utilizes the TRIF adapter protein, which activates TBK1 (TRAF family member associated NF-κB activator binding kinase). TRIF then activates the transcription factor IRF-3, which stimulates expression of type I interferon genes. The type I interferons are cytokines that block viral replication in cells. Therefore, molecular patterns that are produced by viruses (e.g., double-stranded RNA) engage TLRs that stimulate the transcription of antiviral cytokines. TRAF6 is also recruited to the signaling complex induced by TLR3 ligands, leading to NF-κB activation.

essential for signaling (see Box 2–1). The major cell types on which TLRs are expressed include macrophages, dendritic cells, neutrophils, mucosal epithelial cells, and endothelial cells.

Mammalian TLRs are involved in responses to widely divergent types of molecules that are commonly expressed by microbial but not mammalian cells (see Fig. 2–2). TLRs are found on the cell surface and on intracellular membranes, and are thus able to recognize microbes in different cellular locations. Some of the microbial products that stimulate TLR signals include gram-negative bacterial LPS, gram-positive bacterial peptidoglycan, bacterial lipoproteins, lipoteichoic acid, lipoarabinomannan, zymosan, the bacterial flagellar protein flagellin, respiratory syncytial virus fusion protein, unmethylated CpG motifs, double-stranded RNA, and single-stranded RNA. TLRs 3, 7, 8, and 9 are mainly expressed inside cells on endoplasmic reticulum (ER) and endosomal membranes, where they detect microbial nucleic acids (see Fig. 2–2). Although the nucleic acid ligands recognized by these TLRs are not all uniquely produced by microbes, the nucleic acids made by host cells are not normally in the endosomal locations of these TLRs. In other words, TLRs 3, 7, 8, and 9

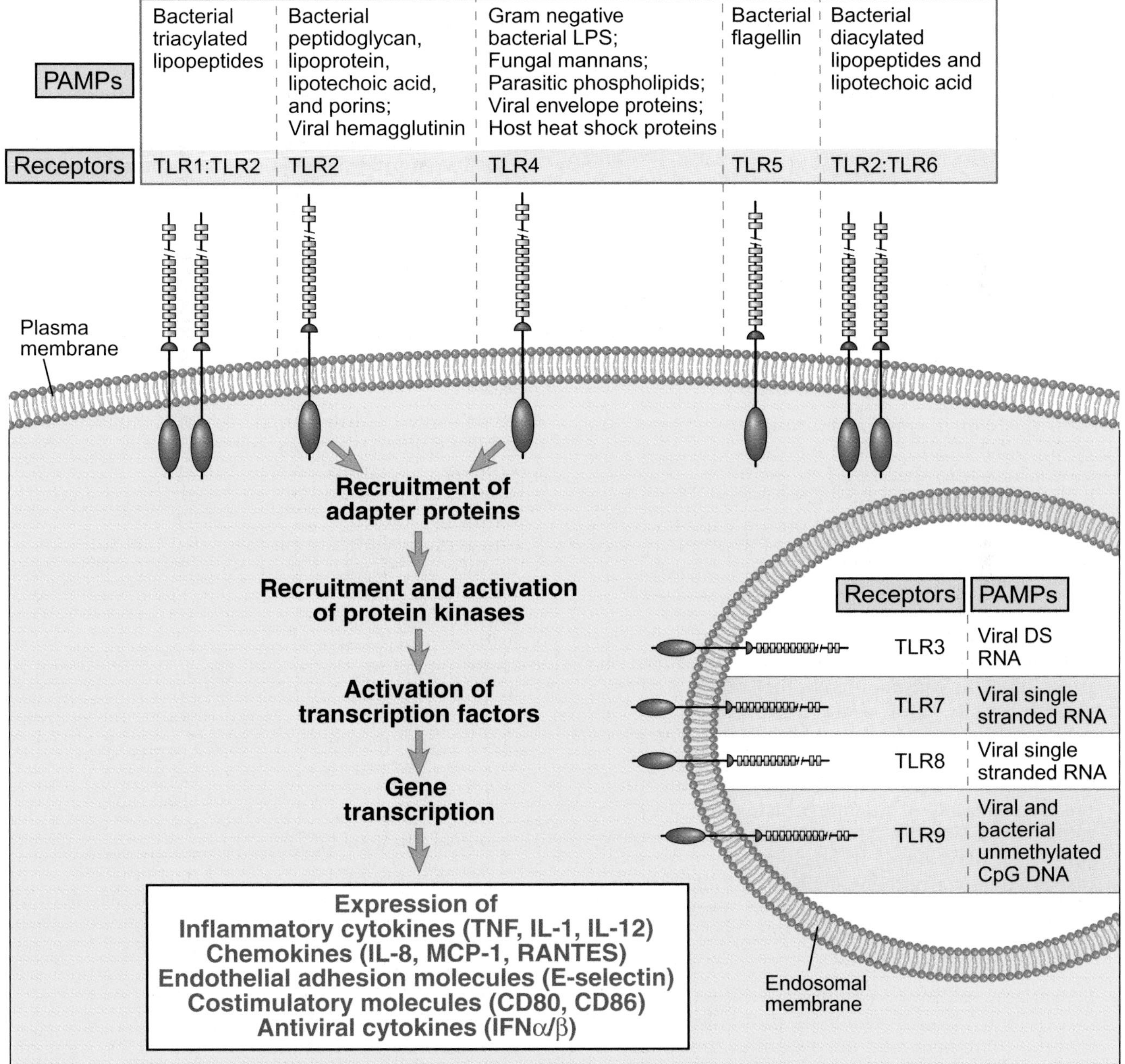

FIGURE 2–2 Mammalian TLRs: specificities, basic signaling mechanisms, and cellular responses. Ligands for TLRs are shown together with dimers of the TLRs that specially bind them. Note that some TLRs are expressed in endosomes and some on the cell surface (see Fig. 2–7). The basic steps in TLR signaling, illustrated only for TLR2 and TLR4, are applicable to all TLRs. Further details about the signaling pathways are described in Box 2–1.

distinguish self from foreign substances based on cellular location of the ligands they bind. In addition to TLRs, there are other intracellular pattern recognition receptors, located in the cytoplasm, that we will discuss later.

Several signaling pathways link TLR recognition of microbial ligands with activation of transcription factors, resulting in expression of genes important for innate immune responses (see Box 2–1). These signaling pathways are initiated by ligand binding to the TLR at the cell surface or in the ER or endosomes, leading to dimerization of the TLR proteins. TLR dimerization is followed by recruitment of TIR domain–containing adapter proteins, which facilitate the recruitment and activation of various protein kinases, leading to the activation of different transcription factors. The major transcription factors that are activated by TLR signaling pathways are nuclear factor κB (NF-κB), AP-1, IRF-3, and IRF-7. NF-κB and/or AP-1 stimulate the expression of genes encoding many of the molecules in the innate immune response, which we will discuss later in the chapter, including inflammatory cytokines (e.g. TNF and IL-1), chemokines (e.g. CCL2), and endothelial adhesion molecules (e.g. E-selectin). IRF-3 and IRF-7 promote expression of interferon (IFN)-α/β genes, important for innate immune responses to viruses. The use of different adapter proteins by different TLRs provides some variability in the type of cellular response that is stimulated by distinct microbial products.

Other Pattern Recognition Receptors

Several types of plasma membrane and cytoplasmic receptors other than TLRs are expressed on various cell types and recognize microbial molecules (see Table 2–2 and Fig. 2–1). Some of these receptors transmit activating signals, similar to TLRs, that promote inflammatory responses and enhance killing of microbes. Other receptors mainly participate in the uptake of microbes into phagocytes, as we will discuss in detail later.

- **C-type lectins** are a large family of calcium-dependent carbohydrate-binding molecules expressed on the plasma membranes of macrophages, dendritic cells, and other leukocytes. There are several types of C-type lectins with different specificities, and only partially understood functions. Some of these lectins recognize carbohydrate structures found on the cell walls of microorganisms but not mammalian cells. The best known is the **mannose receptor,** which plays a role in phagocytosis of microbes, discussed later. Another C-type lectin called Dectin1, which binds β-1,3- and β-1,6-linked glucans present in fungal cell walls, generates signals that intersect with TLR signaling pathways.
- **Scavenger receptors** comprise a structurally and functionally diverse group of molecules with the common characteristic of mediating the uptake of oxidized lipoproteins into cells. Some of the major scavenger receptors that are expressed on phagocytes are CD36, CD68, and SRB1. Scavenger receptors play pathologic roles in the generation of cholesterol-laden foam cells in atherosclerosis; they also recognize and mediate the uptake of microbes into phagocytes as part of innate immune responses.
- ***N*-formyl Met-Leu-Phe receptors,** including FPR and FPRL1, recognize short peptides containing *N*-formylmethionyl residues. FPR and FPRL1 are expressed by neutrophils and macrophages, respectively. Because all bacterial proteins and few mammalian proteins (only those synthesized within mitochondria) are initiated by *N*-formylmethionine, FPR and FPRL1 allow phagocytes to detect and respond to bacterial proteins. The ligands that bind these receptors are some of the first identified and most potent chemoattractants for leukocytes. FPR and FPRL1 belong to the seven-transmembrane, guanosine triphosphate (GTP)-binding (G) protein–coupled receptor superfamily. Like chemokine receptors, these receptors initiate intracellular responses through associated trimeric G proteins. In a resting cell, the receptor-associated G proteins form a stable inactive complex containing guanosine diphosphate (GDP) bound to Gα subunits. Occupancy of the receptor by ligand results in an exchange of GTP for GDP. The GTP-bound form of the G protein activates numerous cellular enzymes, including an isoform of phosphatidylinositol-specific phospholipase C that functions to increase intracellular calcium and activate protein kinase C. The G proteins also stimulate cytoskeletal changes, resulting in increased cell motility.
- **NLRs (NACHT-LRRs)** are a family of cytoplasmic molecules, defined by the presence of certain conserved domain structures, which serve as intracellular sensors of bacterial infection. Several members of this family are known to bind specific ligands inside cells and initiate signaling cascades that activate inflammatory responses. One subset of the NLRs is called Nods (**N**ucleotide-binding **o**ligomerization **d**omain), and another subfamily is called NALPs (**NA**CHT-, **L**RR- and **p**yrin domain-containing proteins). Three NLRs, including Nod1, Nod2, and NALP3, recognize derivatives of peptidoglycan, a common component of bacterial cell walls. After recognizing peptidoglycan, they recruit the protein kinase RICK, which links to downstream signaling pathways that lead to activation of NF-κB and AP-1, and production of cytokines and other mediators of innate immunity. It is likely that NLRs bind other microbial products as well.
- **Caspase activation and recruitment domain (CARD)–containing proteins**, including retinoic acid inducible gene-I (RIG-I) and melanoma differentiation–associated gene 5 (MDA5), are cytoplasmic receptors that bind viral RNA. Via their CARD domains, RIG-I and MDA5 engage signaling cascades that involve TBK1, similar to the TLR3 signaling pathway discussed earlier. Ultimately these pathways activate the IRF-3 and NF-κB transcription factors, which stimulate the expression of antiviral type I interferons.

Table 2–3. Components of Innate Immunity

Components	Principal Functions
Barriers	
Epithelial layers	Prevent microbial entry
Defensins/cathelicidin	Microbial killing
Intraepithelial lymphocytes	Microbial killing
Circulating effector cells	
Neutrophils	Early phagocytosis and killing of microbes
Macrophages	Efficient phagocytosis and killing of microbes, secretion of cytokines that stimulate inflammation
NK cells	Lysis of infected cells, activation of macrophages
Circulating effector proteins	
Complement	Killing of microbes, opsonization of microbes, activation of leukocytes
Mannose-binding lectin (collectin)	Opsonization of microbes, activation of complement (lectin pathway)
C-reactive protein (pentraxin)	Opsonization of microbes, activation of complement
Cytokines	
TNF, IL-1, chemokines	Inflammation
IFN-α, -β	Resistance to viral infection
IFN-γ	Macrophage activation
IL-12	IFN-γ production by NK cells and T cells
IL-15	Proliferation of NK cells
IL-10, TGF-β	Control of inflammation

Abbreviations: IFN, interferon; IL, interleukin; NK, natural killer; TGF-β, transforming growth factor-β, TNF, tumor necrosis factor

Components of the Innate Immune System

The innate immune system consists of epithelial barriers, circulating and tissue cells, and plasma proteins (Table 2–3). The principal effector cells of innate immunity are neutrophils, mononuclear phagocytes, and natural killer (NK) cells. These cells attack microbes that have breached epithelial barriers and entered into tissues or the circulation. Each of these cell types plays a distinct role in the response to microbes. Some of the cells of innate immunity, notably macrophages and NK cells, secrete cytokines that activate phagocytes and stimulate the cellular reaction of innate immunity, called **inflammation.** Inflammation consists of recruitment of leukocytes and extravasation of several plasma proteins into a site of infection, and activation of the leukocytes and proteins to eliminate the infectious agent. As we shall see later, inflammation can also injure normal tissues. If microbes enter the circulation, they are combated by various plasma proteins. The major circulating proteins of innate immunity are the proteins of the complement system and other plasma proteins that recognize microbial structures, such as mannose-binding lectin. In the following sections, we describe the properties and functions of each of these components of innate immunity.

Epithelial Barriers

Intact epithelial surfaces form physical barriers between microbes in the external environment and host tissue (Fig. 2–3). The three main interfaces between the environment and the host are the skin and the mucosal surfaces of the gastrointestinal and respiratory tracts. All three are protected by continuous epithelia that prevent the entry of microbes, and loss of integrity of these epithelia commonly predisposes to infection.

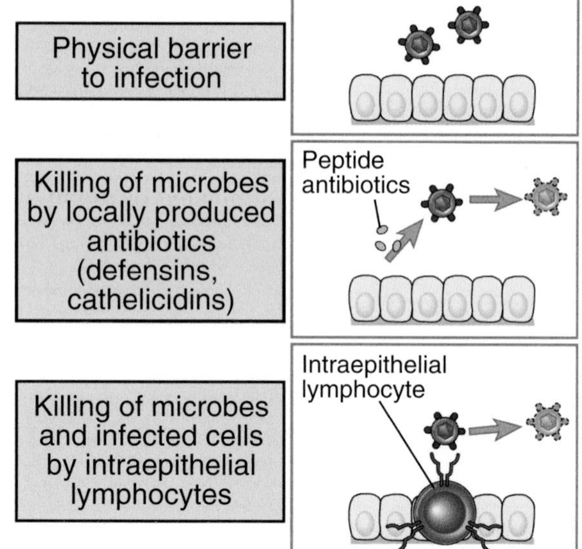

FIGURE 2–3 Epithelial barriers. Epithelia at the portals of entry of microbes provide physical barriers, produce antimicrobial substances, and harbor intraepithelial lymphocytes that are believed to kill microbes and infected cells.

Epithelia, as well as some leukocytes, produce peptides that have antimicrobial properties. Two structurally distinct families of antimicrobial peptides are the defensins and the cathelicidins. **Defensins** are small cationic peptides, 29 to 34 amino acids long, that contain three intrachain disulfide bonds. Three families of defensins, named α, β, and Φ, are distinguished by the location of these bonds. Defensins are produced by epithelial cells of mucosal surfaces and by granule-containing leukocytes, including neutrophils, NK cells, and cytotoxic T lymphocytes. The set of defensin molecules produced differs between different cell types. A major producer of α defensins are Paneth cells within the crypts of the small bowel. Paneth cell defensins are sometimes called crypticidins and serve to limit the amount of microbes in the lumen. Defensins are also produced elsewhere in the bowel, in respiratory mucosal cells, and in the skin. Some defensins are constitutively produced by some cell types, but their secretion may be enhanced by cytokines or microbial products. In other cells, defensins are produced in responses to cytokines and microbial products. The protective actions of the defensins include both direct toxicity to microbes, including bacteria and fungi, and the activation of cells involved in the inflammatory response to microbes. The mechanisms of direct microbicidal effects are poorly understood.

Cathelicidins are expressed by neutrophils and various barrier epithelia, including skin, gastrointestinal mucosal cells, and respiratory mucosal cells. An 18-kD two-domain precursor cathelicidin protein is transcribed and is proteolytically cleaved into two peptides, each with protective functions. Both precursor synthesis and proteolytic cleavage may be stimulated by inflammatory cytokines and microbial products. The C-terminal fragment, called LL-37 because it has two leucine residues at its N terminus, has multiple functions that serve to protect against infections. These include direct toxicity to a broad range of microorganisms, and the activation of various responses in leukocytes and other cell types that promote eradication of microbes. In addition, LL-37 can bind and neutralize LPS, which is a toxic component of the outer wall of gram-negative bacteria that is discussed later in this chapter. The other fragment of the cleaved cathelicidin precursor may also have antimicrobial activities, but these are less well defined.

Barrier epithelia and serosal cavities contain certain types of lymphocytes, including intraepithelial T lymphocytes and the B-1 subset of B cells, respectively, which recognize and respond to commonly encountered microbes. As we will discuss in greater detail in later chapters, most T and B lymphocytes are components of the adaptive immune system and are characterized by a highly diverse repertoire of specificities for different antigens. The diversity of antigen receptors is generated by somatic recombination of germline DNA segments and modification of nucleotide sequences at the junctions between the recombined segments, yielding unique antigen receptor genes in each lymphocyte clone (see Chapter 8). However, certain subsets of T and B lymphocytes have very little diversity, because the same DNA segments are recombined in each clone and there is little or no modification of junctional sequences. It appears that these T and B cell subsets recognize structures commonly expressed by many different or commonly encountered microbial species; in other words, they recognize PAMPs. Although these T and B cells are lymphocytes with antigen receptors like other T or B cells, and they perform similar effector functions as do other lymphocytes, the nature of their specificities places them in a special category of lymphocytes that is akin more to effector cells of innate immunity than to cells of adaptive immunity. Intraepithelial T lymphocytes are present in the epidermis of the skin and in mucosal epithelia (see Chapter 3). Various subsets of intraepithelial lymphocytes are present in different proportions, depending on species and tissue location. These subsets are distinguished mainly by the type of T cell antigen receptors (TCRs) they express. Some intraepithelial T lymphocytes express the conventional αβ form of TCR, which is present on most T cells in lymphoid tissues. Other T cells in epithelia express a form of antigen receptor called the γδ receptor that may recognize peptide and nonpeptide antigens. Intraepithelial lymphocytes may function in host defense by secreting cytokines, activating phagocytes, and killing infected cells. The peritoneal cavity contains a population of B lymphocytes, called B-1 cells, whose antigen receptors are immunoglobulin molecules, as in other B lymphocytes, but have limited diversity, like the antigen receptors of intraepithelial T lymphocytes. Many B-1 cells produce immunoglobulin M (IgM) antibodies specific for polysaccharide and lipid antigens, such as phosphorylcholine and LPS, that are shared by many types of bacteria. In fact, normal individuals have circulating antibodies against such bacteria, most of which are present in the intestines, without any evidence of infection. These antibodies are called natural antibodies and they are largely the product of B-1 cells.

Natural antibodies serve as a preformed defense mechanism against microbes that succeed in penetrating epithelial barriers.

A third population of cells present under many epithelia and in serosal cavities are **mast cells.** Mast cells respond directly to microbial products by secreting cytokines and lipid mediators that promote inflammation. We will return to a discussion of mast cells in Chapter 19.

Phagocytes and Inflammatory Responses

The most numerous effector cells of the innate immune system are bone marrow–derived cells that circulate in the blood and migrate into tissues. These include cells of the myeloid lineage, including neutrophils, mononuclear phagocytes, and dendritic cells, which we will discuss in this section, and cells of the lymphocyte lineage, including natural killer cells, which will be described later, as well as γδ T cells and B-1 B cells, which were described above.

Phagocytes, including neutrophils and macrophages, are cells whose primary function is to identify, ingest, and destroy microbes. The functional responses of phagocytes in host defense consist of sequential steps: active recruitment of the cells to the sites of infection, recognition of microbes, ingestion of the microbes by the process of phagocytosis, and destruction of ingested microbes. In addition, phagocytes produce cytokines that serve many important roles in innate and adaptive immune responses and tissue repair. These effector functions of phagocytes are important not only in innate immunity, but also in the effector phases of adaptive immune responses. For example, as we will discuss in Chapter 13, in T cell–mediated immunity, antigen-stimulated T cells can activate macrophages to become more efficient at killing phagocytosed microbes. In humoral immunity, antibodies coat, or opsonize, microbes and promote the phagocytosis of the microbes through macrophage surface receptors for antibodies (see Chapter 14). These are examples that illustrate two ways by which adaptive immunity works by enhancing the anti-microbial activities of a cell type of innate immunity (the macrophage). In the following discussion, we will describe the phagocytes that are important in innate immunity.

Neutrophils

Neutrophils, also called polymorphonuclear leukocytes, are the most abundant population of circulating white blood cells and mediate the earliest phases of inflammatory responses. Neutrophils circulate as spherical cells about 12 to 15 μm in diameter with numerous membranous projections. The nucleus of a neutrophil is segmented into three to five connected lobules, hence the synonym *polymorphonuclear leukocyte* (Fig. 2–4). The cytoplasm contains granules of two types. The majority, called specific granules, are filled with enzymes such as lysozyme, collagenase, and elastase. These granules do not stain strongly with either basic or acidic dyes (hematoxylin and eosin, respectively), which distinguishes neutrophil granules from those of basophils and eosinophils, respectively. The remainder of the granules of neutrophils, called azurophilic granules, are lysosomes containing enzymes and other microbicidal substances, including defensins and cathelicidins. Neutrophils are produced in the bone marrow and arise from a common lineage with mononuclear phagocytes. Production of neutrophils is stimulated by granulocyte colony-stimulating factor (G-CSF). An adult human produces more than 1×10^{11} neutrophils per day, each of which circulates in the blood for only about 6 hours. Neutrophils may migrate to sites of infection within a few hours after the entry of microbes. If a circulating neutrophil is not recruited into a site of inflammation within this period, it undergoes apoptosis and is usually phagocytosed by resident macrophages in the liver or spleen. Even after entering tissues, neutrophils function for a few hours and then die.

Mononuclear Phagocytes

The mononuclear phagocyte system consists of cells that have a common lineage whose primary function is phagocytosis, and that play central roles in innate and adaptive immunity. The cells of the mononuclear phagocyte system originate in the bone marrow, circulate in the blood, and mature and become activated in various tissues (Fig. 2–5). The first cell type that enters the peripheral blood after leaving the marrow is incompletely differentiated and is called the **monocyte.** Monocytes are 10 to 15 μm in diameter, and they have bean-shaped nuclei and finely granular cytoplasm containing lysosomes, phagocytic vacuoles, and cytoskeletal filaments (Fig. 2–6). Once they enter tissues, these cells mature and become **macrophages.** Macrophages may assume different morphologic forms after activation by external stimuli, such as microbes. Some develop abundant cytoplasm and are called epithelioid cells because of their resemblance to epithelial cells of the skin. Activated macrophages can fuse to form multinucleate giant cells. Macrophages in different tissues have been given special names to designate specific locations. For instance, in the central nervous system, they are called microglial cells; when lining the vascular sinusoids of the liver, they are called Kupffer cells; in pulmonary airways, they are called alveolar macrophages;

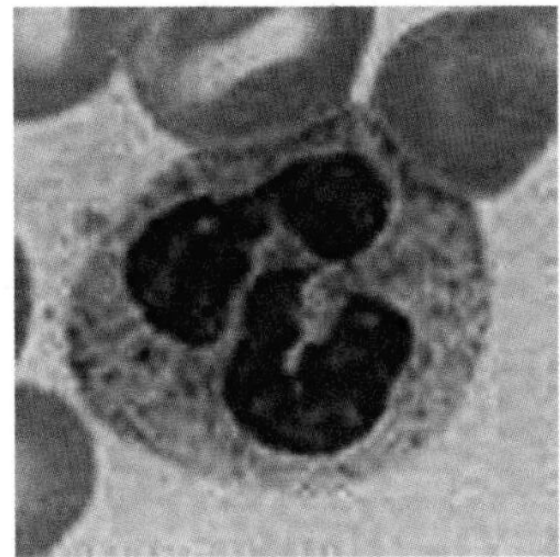

FIGURE 2–4 Morphology of neutrophils. The light micrograph of a blood neutrophil shows the multilobed nucleus, because of which these cells are also called polymorphonuclear leukocytes, and the faint cytoplasmic granules.

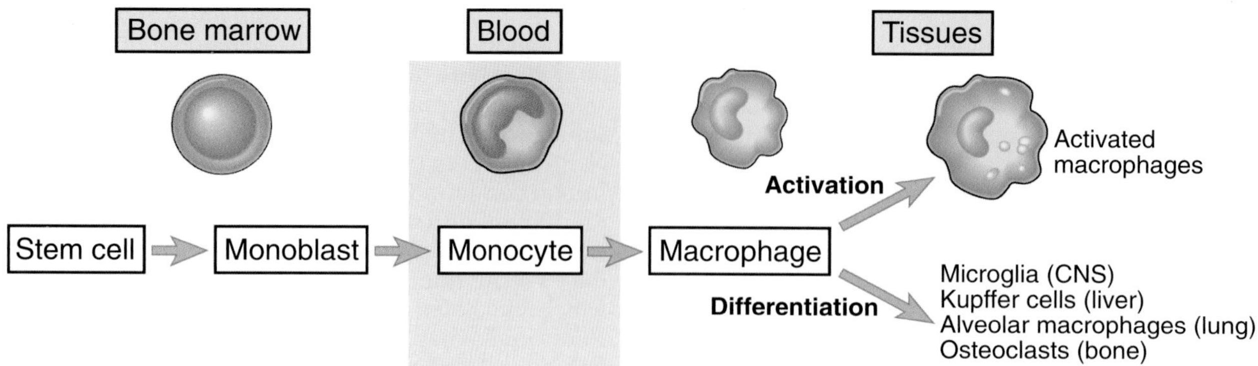

FIGURE 2–5 Maturation of mononuclear phagocytes. Mononuclear phagocytes develop in the bone marrow, circulate in the blood as monocytes, and are resident in all tissues of the body as macrophages. They may differentiate into specialized forms in particular tissues. CNS, central nervous system.

and multinucleate phagocytes in bone are called osteoclasts.

Macrophage-like cells are phylogenetically the oldest mediators of innate immunity. *Drosophila* responds to infection by surrounding microbes with "hemocytes," which are similar to macrophages, and these cells phagocytose the microbes and wall off the infection by inducing coagulation of the surrounding hemolymph. Similar phagocyte-like cells have been identified even in plants.

Macrophages typically respond to microbes nearly as rapidly as neutrophils do, but macrophages survive much longer at sites of inflammation. Unlike neutrophils, macrophages are not terminally differentiated and can undergo cell division at an inflammatory site. Therefore, macrophages are the dominant effector cells of the later stages of the innate immune response, 1 or 2 days after infection.

Dendritic Cells

Dendritic cells play important roles in innate responses to infections and in linking innate and adaptive immune responses. They have long membranous projections and phagocytic capabilities, and are widely distributed in lymphoid tissues, mucosal epithelium, and organ parenchyma. Dendritic cells are derived from bone-marrow precursors, and most are related in lineage to mononuclear phagocytes. They express pattern recognition receptors and respond to microbes by secreting cytokines. One subpopulation of dendritic cells, called plasmacytoid dendritic cells, are specialized early cellular responders to viral infection. They recognize endocytosed viruses and produce type I interferons, which have potent antiviral activities (see Chapter 12). Dendritic cells serve a critical function in adaptive immune responses by capturing and displaying microbial antigens to T lymphocytes. We will discuss dendritic cells in this context in Chapter 6.

Recruitment of Leukocytes to Sites of Infection

Neutrophils and monocytes are recruited from the blood to sites of infection by binding to adhesion molecules on endothelial cells and by chemoattractants produced in response to the infection. In the absence of infection, these leukocytes circulate in the blood and do not migrate into tissues. Their recruitment to sites of infection is a multistep process involving adherence of the circulating leukocytes to the luminal surface of endothe-

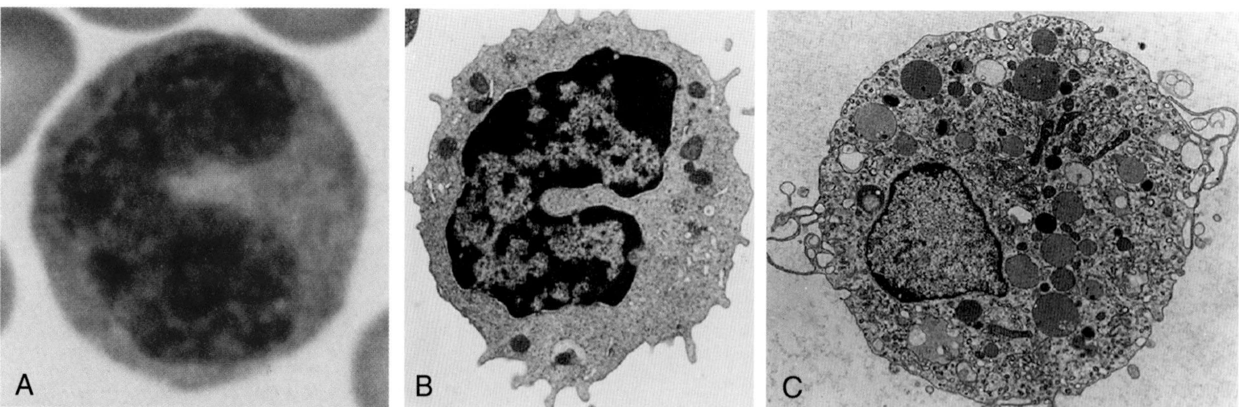

FIGURE 2–6 Morphology of mononuclear phagocytes. A. Light micrograph of a monocyte in a peripheral blood smear. B. Electron micrograph of a peripheral blood monocyte. (Courtesy of Dr. Noel Weidner, Department of Pathology, University of California, San Diego.) C. Electron micrograph of an activated tissue macrophage showing numerous phagocytic vacuoles and cytoplasmic organelles. (From Fawcett DW. Bloom & Fawcett's Textbook of Histology, 12th ed. Chapman & Hall, 1994. With kind permission of Springer Science and Business Media.)

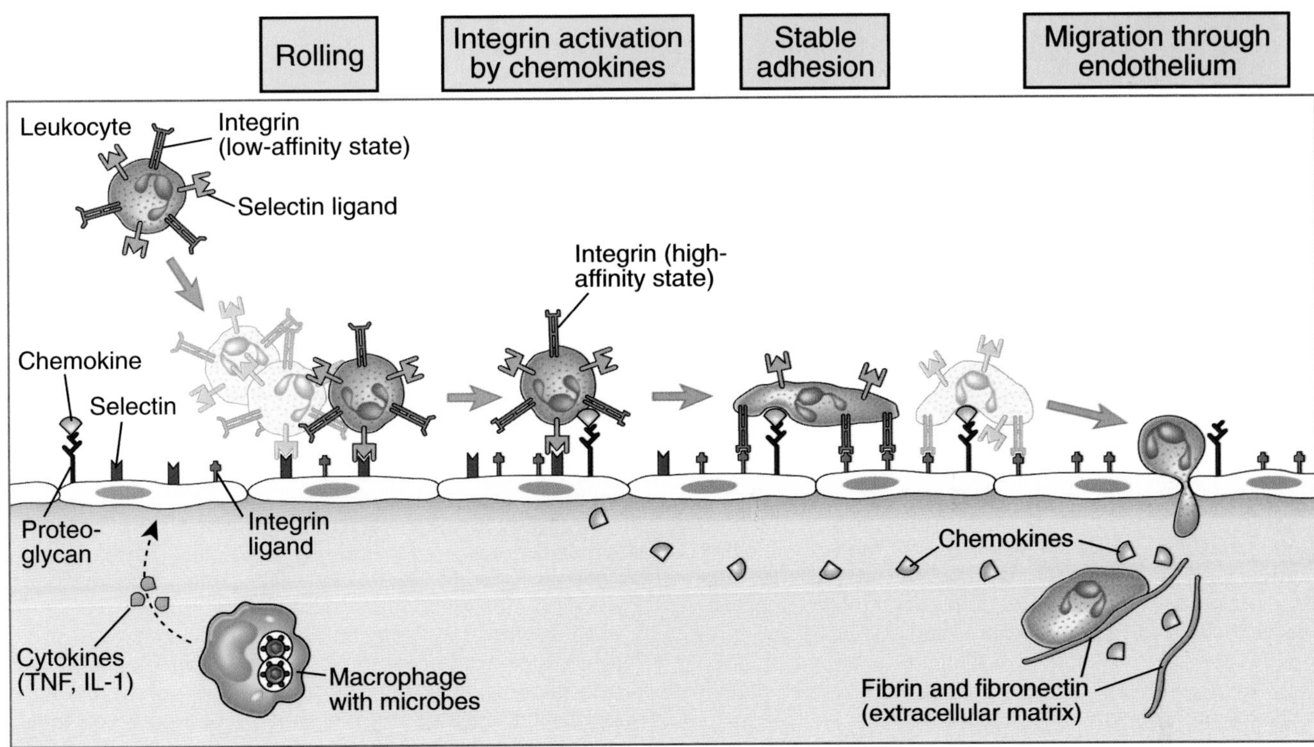

FIGURE 2–7 Recruitment of leukocytes. At sites of infection, macrophages that have encountered microbes produce cytokines (such as TNF and IL-1) that activate the endothelial cells of nearby venules to produce selectins, ligands for integrins, and chemokines. Selectins mediate weak tethering and rolling of blood leukocytes, such as neutrophils on the endothelium; integrins mediate firm adhesion of neutrophils; and chemokines increase the affinity of neutrophil integrins and stimulate the migration of the cells through the endothelium to the site of infection. Blood neutrophils, monocytes, and activated T lymphocytes use essentially the same mechanisms to migrate to sites of infection.

lial cells in postcapillary venules and migration through the vessel wall (Fig. 2–7). Each step is orchestrated by several different types of molecules.

1. ***Selectin-mediated rolling of leukocytes on endothelium.*** In response to microbes and cytokines produced by cells (e.g. macrophages) that encounter the microbes, endothelial cells lining postcapillary venules at the site of infection rapidly increase surface expression of proteins called **selectins** (Box 2–2). Cytokines are discussed in more detail in Chapter 12; the most important ones for activating the endothelium are tumor necrosis factor (TNF) and interleukin-1 (IL-1). The two types of selectins expressed by endothelial cells are P-selectin, which is stored in cytoplasmic granules and is rapidly redistributed to the surface in response to microbial products and cytokines, and E-selectin, which is synthesized in response to IL-1 and TNF as well as microbial products, and is expressed on the cell surface within 1 to 2 hours. A third selectin, called L-selectin (CD62L), is expressed on lymphocytes and other leukocytes. It serves as a homing receptor for naive T lymphocytes and dendritic cells to lymph nodes, mediating the binding of T cells to high endothelial venules (see Chapter 3). On neutrophils, it serves to bind these cells to endothelial cells that are activated by cytokines (TNF, IL-1, and IFN-γ) found at sites of inflammation. Leukocytes express L-selectin and the carbohydrate ligands for P- and E-selectins at the tips of their microvilli, facilitating interactions with molecules on the endothelial cell surface. Selectin–selectin ligand interactions are of low-affinity (K_d ~100 mm) with a fast off-rate, and they are easily disrupted by the shear force of the flowing blood. As a result, the leukocytes repetitively detach and bind again and thus roll along the endothelial surface. This slowing of leukocytes on the endothelium allows the next set of stimuli to act on the leukocytes.
2. ***Chemokine-mediated increase in affinity of integrins.*** Chemokines are small polypeptide cytokines produced by tissue macrophages, endothelial cells, and several other types of cells in response to microbial products and IL-1 and TNF, cytokines that are associated with infections. The major function of chemokines is to stimulate chemotaxis of cells ("chemokines" is a contraction of "chemoattractant cytokines"). The chemokines produced at an infection site are transported to the luminal surface of the endothelial cells of post capillary-venules, where they are bound by heparan sulfate glycosaminoglycans, and are displayed at high concentrations. At this location the chemokines bind to specific chemokine receptors on the surface of the rolling leukocytes. Leukocytes express a family of adhesion molecules called **integrins** (Box 2–3), which are in a low-affinity

Box 2–2 ■ IN DEPTH: SELECTINS AND SELECTIN LIGANDS

The selectin family of molecules consists of three separate but closely related proteins that mediate adhesion of leukocytes to endothelial cells (see Table). One member of this family of adhesion molecules is expressed on leukocytes, and the other two members are expressed on endothelial cells, but all three participate in the process of leukocyte-endothelium attachment. Each of the selectin molecules is a single-chain transmembrane glycoprotein with a similar modular structure. The amino terminus, expressed extracellularly, is related to mammalian carbohydrate-binding proteins known as C-type lectins. Like other C-type lectins, ligand binding by selectins is calcium dependent (hence the name C-type). The lectin domain is followed by domains homologous to those found in epidermal growth factors and others found in proteins of the complement system, and then a hydrophobic transmembrane region and a short cytoplasmic carboxy-terminal region. The genes for the three selectins are located in tandem on chromosome 1 in both mice and humans. The differences among the three selectins serve to confer differences both in binding specificity and in tissue expression. However, all three selectins mediate rapid low-affinity attachment of leukocytes to endothelium, an early and important step in leukocyte homing.

L-selectin (CD62L) is expressed on lymphocytes and other leukocytes. It serves as a homing receptor for naive T lymphocytes and dendritic cells to lymph nodes, mediating the binding of T cells to HEVs (see Chapter 3). On neutrophils, it serves to bind these cells to endothelial cells that are activated by cytokines (TNF-α, IL-1, and IFN-γ) found at sites of inflammation. L-selectin is located on the tips of microvillus projections of leukocytes, facilitating its interaction with ligands on endothelium.

At least three endothelial cell ligands can bind L-selectin: glycan-bearing cell adhesion molecule-1 (GlyCAM-1), a secreted proteoglycan found on HEVs of lymph node; MadCAM-1, expressed on endothelial cells in gut-associated lymphoid tissues; and CD34, a proteoglycan on endothelial cells (and bone marrow cells).

E-selectin, also known as endothelial leukocyte adhesion molecule-1 (ELAM-1) or CD62E, is expressed exclusively by cytokine-activated endothelial cells, hence the designation E. E-selectin recognizes complex sialylated carbohydrate groups related to the Lewis X or Lewis A family found on various surface proteins of granulocytes, monocytes, and some previously activated effector and memory T cells. E-selectin is important in migration of leukocytes, including neutrophils and of effector and memory T cells to some peripheral sites of inflammation. On a subset of T cells, the carbohydrate ligand for E-selectin is called CLA-1; this molecule mediates homing of the T cells to the skin.

P-selectin (CD62P) was first identified in the secretory granules of platelets, hence the designation P. It has since been found in secretory granules of endothelial cells, which are called Weibel-Palade bodies. When endothelial cells or platelets are stimulated, P-selectin is translocated within minutes to the cell surface as part of the exocytic secretory process. On reaching the endothelial cell surface, P-selectin mediates binding of neutrophils, T lymphocytes, and monocytes. In mice, P-selectin expression is regulated by cytokines, similar to the regulation of E-selectin. The carbohydrate ligands recognized by P-selectin are similar to those recognized by E-selectin. A protein called P-selectin glycoprotein ligand-1 (PSGL-1) is posttranslationally modified in leukocytes to express functional ligands for P-selectin. This modification involves both sulfation and fucosylation.

The synthesis of selectin ligands is regulated in different ways in different leukocytes, reflecting variations in the expression of glycosyl transferase enzymes that attach carbohydrates to the protein backbone of the ligands. For example, naive T cells express virtually no E- and P-selectin ligands, and T_H1 cells express significantly more than do T_H2 cells.

The physiologic roles of selectins have been demonstrated by studies of gene knockout mice. L-selectin-deficient mice have small, poorly formed lymph nodes and defective induction of T cell-dependent immune responses and inflammatory reactions. Mice lacking either E-selectin or P-selectin have only mild defects in leukocyte recruitment, suggesting that these two molecules are functionally redundant. Double knockout mice lacking both E-selectin and P-selectin have significantly impaired leukocyte recruitment and increased susceptibility to infections. Similarly, mice lacking the glycosyltransferase enzymes, such as fucosyltransferase-VII, which are required to synthesize the carbohydrate ligands that bind to selectins, have marked defects in T cell migration and cell-mediated immune responses. Humans who lack one of the enzymes needed to express the carbohydrate ligands for E-selectin and P-selectin on neutrophils have similar problems, resulting in a syndrome called type 2 leukocyte adhesion deficiency (LAD-2) (see Chapter 20).

Selectin	Size	Distribution	Ligand
L-selectin (CD62L)	90-110 kD (variation due to glycosylation)	Leukocytes (high expression on naive T cells, low expression on activated effector and memory cells)	Sialyl-Lewis X on GlyCAM-1, CD34, MadCAM-1, others
E-selectin (CD62E)	110 kD	Endothelium activated by cytokines (TNF, IL-1)	Sialyl-Lewis X (e.g., CLA-1) on various glycoproteins
P-selectin (CD62P)	140 kD	Storage granules and surface of endothelium and platelets	Sialyl-Lewis X on PSGL-1 and other glycoproteins

Abbreviations: CLA-1, cutaneous lymphocyte antigen-1; GlyCAM-1, glycan-bearing cell adhesion molecule-1; IL-1, interleukin-1; MadCAM-1, mucosal addressin cell adhesion molecule-1; PSGL-1, P-selectin glycoprotein ligand-1; TNF, tumor necrosis factor

Box 2–3 ▪ IN DEPTH: INTEGRINS

The adhesion of cells to other cells or to extracellular matrices is a basic component of cell migration and recognition and underlies many biologic processes, including embryogenesis, tissue repair, and immune and inflammatory responses. It is therefore not surprising that many different genes have evolved that encode proteins with specific adhesive functions. The integrin superfamily consists of about 30 structurally homologous proteins that promote cell-cell or cell-matrix interactions (see Table). The name of this family of proteins derives from the idea that they coordinate (i.e., "integrate") signals generated when they bind extracellular ligands with cytoskeleton-dependent motility, shape change, and phagocytic responses.

All integrins are heterodimeric cell surface proteins composed of two noncovalently linked polypeptide chains, α and β. The α chain varies in size from 120 to 200 kD, and the β chain varies from 90 to 110 kD. The amino terminus of each chain forms a globular head that contributes to interchain linking and to ligand binding. These globular heads contain divalent cation-binding domains, which are essential for integrin receptor function. Stalks extend from the globular heads to the plasma membrane, followed by transmembrane segments and cytoplasmic tails, which are usually less than 50 amino acid residues long. The extracellular domains of the two chains bind to various ligands, including extracellular matrix glycoproteins, activated complement components, and proteins on the surfaces of other cells. Several integrins bind to Arg-Gly-Asp (RGD) sequences in fibronectin and vitronectin molecules. The cytoplasmic domains of the integrins interact with cytoskeletal components (including vinculin, talin, actin, α-actinin, and tropomyosin).

Integrins are classified into several subfamilies based on the β chains in the heterodimers; the major members of these subfamilies are listed in the table.

The β_1-containing integrins are also called VLA molecules, referring to "very late antigens", because $\alpha_1\beta_1$ and $\alpha_2\beta_1$ were shown to be expressed on T cells 2 to 4 weeks after repetitive stimulation *in vitro.* In fact, other VLA integrins, including VLA-4, are constitutively expressed on some T cells and rapidly induced on others. The β_1 integrins are also called CD49a-fCD29, CD49a-f referring to different α chains (α_1 to α_6) and CD29 referring to the common β_1 subunit. Most of the β_1 integrins are widely expressed on leukocytes and nonhematopoietic cells and mediate attachment of cells to extracellular matrix ligands, such as fibronectin (VLA-4 and VLA-5) and laminin (VLA-6). VLA-4 ($\alpha_4\beta_1$ or CD49dCD29) is expressed only on leukocytes and can mediate attachment of these cells to endothelium by interacting with VCAM-1. VLA-4 is one of the principal surface proteins that mediate homing of lymphocytes and other leukocytes to endothelium at peripheral sites of inflammation.

The β_2 integrins, also known as the LFA-1 family, were identified by monoclonal antibodies that blocked adhesion-dependent lymphocyte functions such as killing of target cells by CTLs. LFA-1 plays an important role in the adhesion of lymphocytes with other cells, such as APCs and vascular endothelium. This family is also called CD11a-cCD18, CD11 referring to different α chains and CD18 to the common β_2 subunit. LFA-1 itself is termed CD11aCD18. Other members of the family include CD11bCD18 (Mac-1 or CR3) and CD11cCD18 (p150,95 or CR4), both of which have the same β subunit as LFA-1. CD11bCD18 and CD11cCD18 both mediate leukocyte attachment to endothelial cells and transmigration. One ligand for LFA-1 (CD11aCD18) is ICAM-1 (CD54), a membrane glycoprotein expressed on a variety of hematopoietic and nonhematopoietic cells, including B and T cells, dendritic cells, macrophages, fibroblasts, keratinocytes, and endothelial cells. Two other ligands for LFA-1 are ICAM-2, which is expressed on endothelial cells, and ICAM-3, which is expressed on lymphocytes. ICAM-1, -2, and -3 are members of the Ig superfamily. CD11bCD18 also functions as a fibrinogen receptor and as a complement receptor on phagocytic cells, binding particles opsonized with a product of complement activation called the inactivated C3b (iC3b) fragment (Chapter 14). An autosomal-recessive inherited deficiency in LFA-1, Mac-1, and p150,95 proteins, called type 1 leukocyte adhesion deficiency (LAD-1), has been identified in a few families and is characterized by recurrent bacterial and fungal infections, lack of polymorphonuclear leukocyte accumulations at sites of infection, and profound defects in adherence-dependent lymphocyte functions. The disease is a result of mutations in the CD18 gene, which encodes the β chain of LFA-1 subfamily molecules.

An important feature of integrins is their ability to respond to intracellular signals by rapidly increasing their avidity for their ligands. This is referred to as "activation," and occurs in response to signals generated from chemokine binding to chemokine receptors, and in lymphocytes by intracellular signals generated when antigen binds to antigen receptors. The process of changes in the binding functions of the extracellular domain of integrins induced by intracellular signals is called "inside-out signaling." Chemokine- and antigen-receptor–induced inside-out signaling involves several different guanosine triphosphatase–regulated pathways, eventually leading to the association of RAP family molecules and cytoskeletal-interacting proteins with the cytoplasmic tails of the integrin proteins. The resulting avidity changes are a consequence of clustering of the integrins in the leukocyte membrane, which increases the effective valency of ligand binding, and conformational changes in the extracellular domains that enhance affinity of binding. In the low affinity state, the stalks of the extracellular domains of each integrin subunit appear to be bent over, and the ligand-binding globular heads are close to the membrane. In response to alterations in the cytoplasmic tail, the stalks extend in switch-blade fashion, bringing the globular heads away from the membrane to a position where they more effectively interact with their ligands.

Upon ligand binding integrins also deliver stimulatory signals to cells on which they are expressed. The mechanism of signaling involves tyrosine phosphorylation of

Continued on following page

Box 2–3 ▪ IN DEPTH: INTEGRINS (Continued)

Subunits		Name	Major Ligands	Functions
β_1	α_1	VLA-1 (CD49aCD29)	Collagens	Cell-matrix adhesion
	α_2	VLA-2 (CD49bCD29)	Collagens	Cell-matrix adhesion
	α_3	VLA-3 (CD49cCD29)	Laminin	Cell-matrix adhesion
	α_4	VLA-4 (CD49dCD29)	VCAM-1, MadCAM-1	Cell-matrix adhesion; homing; T cell costimulation?
	α_5	VLA-5 (CD49eCD29)	Fibronectin	Cell-matrix adhesion
	α_6	VLA-6 (CD49fCD29)	Laminin	Cell-matrix adhesion
	α_7	CD49gCD29	Laminin	Cell-matrix adhesion
	α_8	CD51CD29	Fibronectin	Cell-matrix adhesion
	α_v	CD51CD29	Fibronectin	Cell-matrix adhesion
β_2	α_L	CD11aCD18 (LFA-1)	ICAM-1, ICAM-2, ICAM-3	Leukocyte adhesion to endothelium; T cell–APC adhesion; T cell costimulation?
	α_M	CD11bCD18 (MAC-1, CR3)	iC3b, fibronectin, Factor X, ICAM-1	Leukocyte adhesion and phagocytosis; cell-matrix adhesion
	α_x	CD11cCD18 (p150, 95; CR4)	iC3b; fibronectin	Leukocyte adhesion and phagocytosis; cell-matrix adhesion
	α_d	CD11dCD18	VCAM-1, ICAM-3	Leukocyte adhesion to endothelium
β_3	α_{IIb}	GPIIb/IIIa (CD41CD61)	Fibrinogen, von Willebrand factor, thrombospondin	Platelet adhesion and aggregation
	α_V	Vitronectin receptor (CD51CD61)	Fibronectin, vitronectin, von Willebrand factor, thrombospondin	Cell-matrix adhesion
β_4	α_6	CD49fCD104	Laminin	Cell-matrix adhesion
β_5	α_v		Vitronectin	Cell-matrix adhesion
β_6	α_v		Fibronectin	Cell-matrix adhesion
β_7	α_4	LPAM-1	VCAM-1, MadCAM-1	Lymphocyte homing to mucosal lymphoid tissues
	α_E	HML-1	E-cadherin	Retention of intraepithelial T cells

Abbreviations: APC, antigen-presenting cell; iC3b, C3b inactivated; ICAM, intercellular adhesion molecule; LFA, leukocyte function-associated antigen; MadCAM-1, mucosal addressin cell adhesion molecule 1; VCAM-1, vascular cell adhesion molecule 1.
Adapted from Hynes RO. Integrins: versatility, modulation, and signaling in cell adhesion. Cell 69:11–25, 1992. © Cell Press.

different substrates, inositol lipid turnover, elevated cytoplasmic calcium, and activation of guanosine triphosphate– binding proteins and the mitogen activated protein (MAP) kinase cascade. The functional consequences of these integrin-mediated signals vary with cell type. In epithelial cells, integrins cooperate with growth factor receptors to deliver anchorage-dependent mitotic signals. In phagocytes, integrin signals are linked to cytoskeleton reorganization required for motility and phagocytosis, reactive oxygen species generation, inflammatory gene expression, and apoptosis. In T lymphocytes, ICAM-1 binding to β_2 integrins may provide costimulatory signals that enhance cytokine gene expression, although this activity of integrins is probably less important than their role in cell-cell adhesion.

state in unactivated cells and ineffective in mediating adhesion interactions. Two consequences of chemokine receptor signaling are enhanced affinity of leukocyte integrins for their ligands, and membrane clustering of the integrins, resulting in increased avidity of integrin-mediated binding of the leukocytes to the endothelial surface.

3. ***Stable integrin-mediated adhesion of leukocytes to endothelium.*** In parallel with the activation of integrins and their conversion to the high-affinity state, cytokines (TNF and IL-1) also enhance endothelial expression of integrin ligands, mainly vascular cell adhesion molecule-1 (VCAM-1, the ligand for the VLA-4 integrin) and intercellular adhesion molecule-1 (ICAM-1, the ligand for the LFA-1 and Mac-1 integrins) (see Box 2–3). The net result of these changes is that the leukocytes attach firmly to the endothelium, their cytoskeleton is reorganized, and they spread out on the endothelial surface.
4. ***Transmigration of leukocytes through the endothelium.*** Chemokines then act on the adherent leukocytes and stimulate the cells to migrate through interendothelial spaces along the chemical concentration gradient (i.e., toward the infection site). Other proteins expressed on the leukocytes and endothelial cells, notably CD31, play a role in this migration through the endothelium. The leukocytes presumably produce enzymes that enable them to pass through the vessel wall, and they ultimately accumulate in the extravascular tissue around the infectious microbes.

Leukocyte accumulation in tissues is a major component of **inflammation.** It is typically elicited by microbes, but it may be seen in response to a variety of noninfectious stimuli as well. There is some specificity in this process of leukocyte migration based on the expression of distinct combinations of adhesion molecule and chemokine receptors on neutrophils versus monocytes. For example, neutrophil migration relies mainly on LFA-1–ICAM-1 interactions in combination with the chemokines receptors CXCR1 and CXCR2 binding the chemokines CXCL8, while monocytes mainly utilize VLA-4–VCAM-1 interactions together with the chemokine CCL2 binding to the chemokine receptor CCR2. Temporally distinct patterns of expression of adhesion molecules and chemokines at infectious sites typically result in early neutrophil recruitment (hours to days) followed later by monocyte recruitment (days to weeks). As we will see in Chapter 3, yet other combinations of adhesion molecules and chemokines control the migration of lymphocytes into lymphoid and nonlymphoid tissues.

Phagocytosis of Microbes

Neutrophils and macrophages ingest bound microbes into vesicles by the process of phagocytosis (Fig. 2–8).

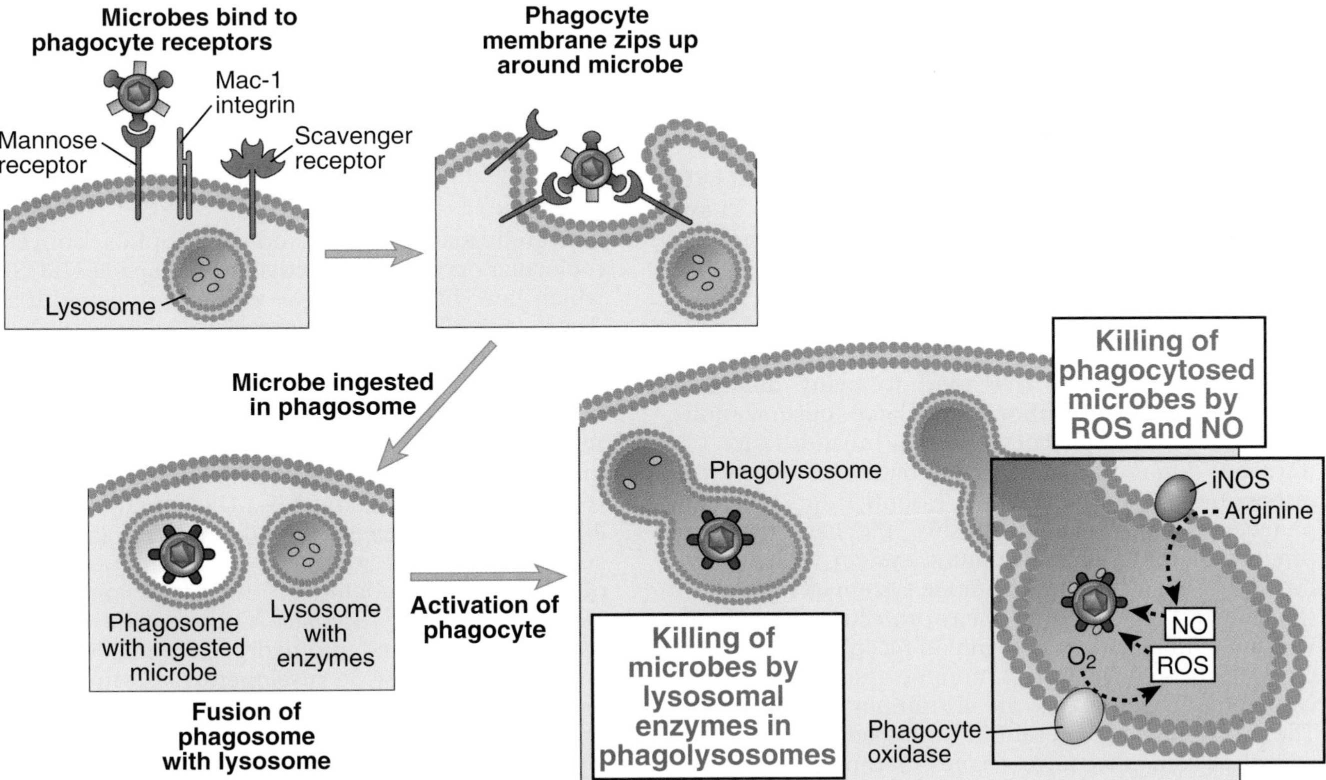

FIGURE 2–8 Phagocytosis and intracellular destruction of microbes. Microbes may be ingested by different membrane receptors of phagocytes; some directly bind microbes, and others bind opsonized microbes. (Note that the Mac-1 integrin binds microbes opsonized with complement proteins, not shown.) The microbes are internalized into phagosomes, which fuse with lysosomes to form phagolysosomes, where the microbes are killed by reactive oxygen and nitrogen intermediates and proteolytic enzymes. NO, nitric oxide; ROS, reactive oxygen species.

Phagocytosis is an active, energy-dependent process of engulfment of large particles (>0.5 μm in diameter). Microbial killing takes place in the vesicles formed by phagocytosis, and in this way, the mechanisms of killing, which could potentially injure the phagocyte, are isolated from the rest of the cell.

The first step in phagocytosis is the recognition of the microbe by the phagocyte. Neutrophils and macrophages are constantly exposed to normal cells, which they ignore, but will specifically ingest various microbes and particles. This specificity is due to the fact that neutrophils and macrophages express receptors that specifically recognize microbes, and these receptors are functionally linked to the mechanisms of phagocytosis. Some of these receptors are pattern recognition receptors, including C-type lectins and scavenger receptors, as we discussed previously. Pattern recognition receptors can contribute to phagocytosis only of organisms that express particular molecular patterns, such as mannose. Another group of receptors on phagocytes recognize certain host proteins that coat microbes. These proteins are called **opsonins,** and include antibodies, complement proteins, and lectins. The process of coating a microbe to target it for phagocytosis is called **opsonization.**

Phagocytes have high-affinity receptors that specially bind to antibody molecules, complement proteins, and lectins; these receptors are critical for phagocytosis of many different microbes. One of the most efficient systems for opsonizing microbes is coating them with antibodies. Antibody molecules have antigen-binding sites at one end, and the other end, called the Fc region, the antibody interacts with effector cells and molecules of the innate immune system. There are several types of antibodies, which we will discuss in detail in Chapters 4 and 14. Phagocytes express high-affinity Fc receptors called FcγRI specific for one type of antibody called IgG (see Chapter 14). Thus, if an individual responds to an infection by making IgG antibodies against microbial antigens, the IgG molecules bind to these antigens, the Fc ends of the bound antibodies can interact with FcγRI on phagocytes, and the end result is efficient phagocytosis of the microbes. Because many different antibodies may be produced that bind to many different microbial products, antibody-mediated opsonization contributes to the phagocytosis of a broader range of microbes than do pattern recognition receptors. Although IgG antibodies are essential for efficient phagocytosis of many organisms, they are really a product of the adaptive immune system (B lymphocytes) that engages innate immune system effector cells (phagocytes) to perform their protective functions. Various soluble pattern recognition receptors and effector molecules of the innate immune system, including complement and lectins, are also important opsonins. These opsonins are present in the blood, they bind to microbes, and phagocytes express receptors for these opsonins. We will discuss these soluble effectors of the innate immune system later in this chapter.

Once a microbe or particle binds to receptors on a phagocyte, the plasma membrane in the region of the receptors begins to redistribute, and extends a cup-shaped projection around the microbe. When the protruding membrane cup extends beyond the diameter of the particle, the top of the cup closes over, or "zips up," and pinches off the interior of the cup to form an "inside-out" intracellular vesicle (see Fig. 2–8). This vesicle, called a phagosome, contains the ingested foreign particle, and it breaks away from the plasma membrane. The cell surface receptors also deliver activating signals that stimulate the microbicidal activities of phagocytes. Phagocytosed microbes are destroyed, as described next; at the same time, peptides are generated from microbial proteins and presented to T lymphocytes to initiate adaptive immune responses (see Chapter 6).

Killing of Phagocytosed Microbes

Activated neutrophils and macrophages kill phagocytosed microbes by the action of microbicidal molecules in phagolysosomes (see Fig. 2–8). Several receptors that recognize microbes, including TLRs, G protein–coupled receptors, antibody Fc and complement C3 receptors, and receptors for cytokines, mainly IFN-γ, function cooperatively to activate phagocytes to kill ingested microbes. Fusion of phagocytic vacuoles (phagosomes) with lysosomes results in the formation of phagolysosomes, where most of the microbicidal mechanisms are concentrated; these mechanisms are described next.

- Activated neutrophils and macrophages produce several proteolytic **enzymes** in the phagolysosomes, which function to destroy microbes. One of the important enzymes in neutrophils is elastase, a broad-spectrum serine protease known to be required for killing many types of bacteria. Another important enzyme is cathepsin G. Mouse gene knockout studies have confirmed the essential requirement for these enzymes in phagocyte killing of bacteria.
- Activated macrophages and neutrophils convert molecular oxygen into **reactive oxygen species** (ROS), which are highly reactive oxidizing agents that destroy microbes (and other cells). The primary free radical–generating system is the phagocyte oxidase system. Phagocyte oxidase is a multisubunit enzyme that is assembled in activated phagocytes mainly in the phagolysosomal membrane. Phagocyte oxidase is induced and activated by many stimuli, including IFN-γ and signals from TLRs. The function of this enzyme is to reduce molecular oxygen into ROS such as superoxide radicals, with the reduced form of nicotinamide adenine dinucleotide phosphate (NADPH) acting as a cofactor. Superoxide is enzymatically dismutated into hydrogen peroxide, which is used by the enzyme myeloperoxidase to convert normally unreactive halide ions into reactive hypohalous acids that are toxic for bacteria. The process by which ROS are produced is called the respiratory burst. Although the generation of toxic ROS is commonly viewed as the major function of phagocyte oxidase, another function of the enzyme is to produce conditions within phagocytic vacuoles that are nec-

essary for the activity of the proteolytic enzymes discussed earlier. The oxidase acts as an electron pump, generating an electrochemical gradient across the vacuole membrane, which is compensated for by movement of ions into the vacuole. The result is an increase in pH and osmolarity inside the vacuole, which are necessary for elastase and cathepsin G activity. A disease called **chronic granulomatous disease** is caused by an inherited deficiency of one of the components of phagocyte oxidase; this deficiency compromises the capacity of neutrophils to kill certain species of gram-positive bacteria (see Chapter 20).

- In addition to ROS, macrophages produce reactive nitrogen intermediates, mainly **nitric oxide (NO),** by the action of an enzyme called inducible nitric oxide synthase (iNOS). iNOS is a cytosolic enzyme that is absent in resting macrophages but can be induced in response to microbial products that activate TLRs, especially in combination with IFN-γ. iNOS catalyzes the conversion of arginine to citrulline, and freely diffusible nitric oxide gas is released. Within phagolysosomes, nitric oxide may combine with hydrogen peroxide or superoxide, generated by phagocyte oxidase, to produce highly reactive peroxynitrite radicals that can kill microbes. The cooperative and redundant function of ROS and nitric oxide is demonstrated by the finding that knockout mice lacking both iNOS and phagocyte oxidase are more susceptible to bacterial infections than single phagocyte oxidase or iNOS knockout animals are.

When neutrophils and macrophages are strongly activated, they can injure normal host tissues by release of lysosomal enzymes, ROS, and NO. The microbicidal products of these cells do not distinguish between self tissues and microbes. As a result, if these products enter the extracellular environment, they are capable of causing tissue injury.

Other Functions of Activated Macrophages

In addition to killing phagocytosed microbes, macrophages serve many other functions in defense against infections (Fig. 2–9). Many of these functions are mediated by cytokines that will be described in more detail in Chapter 12 as the cytokines of innate immunity. We have already referred to the role of TNF, IL-1, and chemokines in inducing inflammatory reactions to microbes. In addition to these cytokines, macrophages produce IL-12, which stimulates NK cells and T cells to produce IFN-γ. High concentrations of LPS induce a systemic disease characterized by disseminated coagulation, vascular collapse, and metabolic abnormalities, all of which are pathologic effects of high levels of cytokines secreted by LPS-activated macrophages (see Box 15–1, Chapter 15). Activated macrophages also

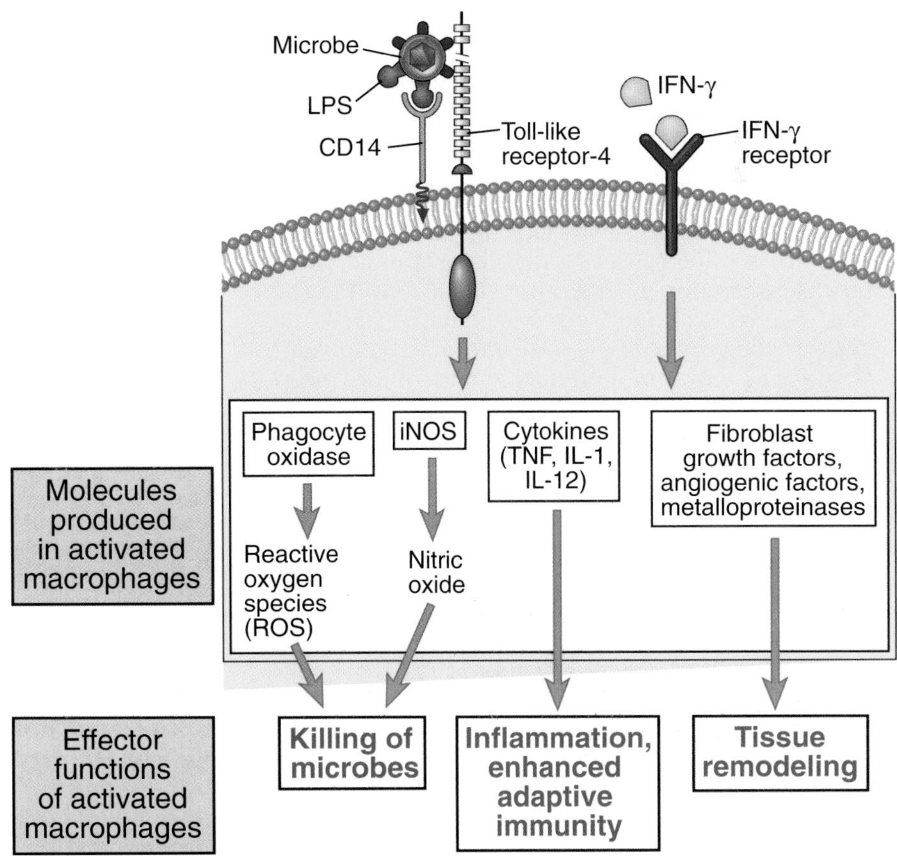

FIGURE 2–9 Effector functions of macrophages. Macrophages are activated by microbial products such as LPS and by NK cell-derived IFN-γ (described later in the chapter). The process of macrophage activation leads to the activation of transcription factors, the transcription of various genes, and the synthesis of proteins that mediate the functions of these cells. In adaptive cell-mediated immunity, macrophages are activated by stimuli from T lymphocytes (CD40 ligand and IFN-γ) and respond in essentially the same way (see Chapter 13, Fig. 13–14).

produce growth factors for fibroblasts and endothelial cells that participate in the remodeling of tissues after infections and injury. The role of macrophages, in cell-mediated immunity is described in Chapter 13.

Natural Killer (NK) Cells

NK cells are a lineage of cells related to lymphocytes that recognize infected and/or stressed cells and respond by directly killing these cells and by secreting inflammatory cytokines. NK cells constitute 5% to 20% of the mononuclear cells in the blood and spleen and are rare in other lymphoid organs. The term *natural killer* derives from the fact that if these cells are isolated from the blood or spleen, they kill various target cells without a need for additional activation. (In contrast, $CD8^+$ T lymphocytes need to be activated before they differentiate into cytotoxic T lymphocytes [CTLs] with the ability to kill targets.) In addition to killing infected cells directly, NK cells are a major source of IFN-γ, which activates macrophages to kill ingested microbes. NK cells are derived from bone marrow precursors and appear as large lymphocytes with numerous cytoplasmic granules, because of which they are sometimes called large granular lymphocytes. By surface phenotype and lineage, NK cells are neither T nor B lymphocytes, and they do not express somatically rearranged, clonally distributed antigen receptors like immunoglobulin or T cell receptors. Their target cells using germline DNA–encoded receptors, discussed below.

Recognition of Infected and Stressed Cells by Natural Killer Cells

NK cell activation is regulated by a balance between signals that are generated from activating receptors and inhibitory receptors (Fig. 2–10). There are several families of these receptors, which are described in detail in Box 2–4. Most of these receptors are complexes of ligand-binding subunits, which recognize molecules on the surface of other cells, and signaling subunits, which transduce activating or inhibitory signals into the cell. When an NK cell interacts with another cell, the outcome is determined by an integration of signals generated from an array of inhibitory and activating receptors that may be simultaneously expressed by the NK cell and simultaneously interact with ligands on the other cell. In general, activating signals must be blocked by inhibitory signals in order to prevent NK cell activation and attack of normal cells. Many of these receptors on NK cells recognize class I MHC molecules or proteins that are structurally homologous to class I MHC molecules. Class I MHC molecules display peptides derived from cytoplasmic proteins, including microbial proteins, on the cell surface for recognition by $CD8^+$ T cells. We will describe the structure and function of MHC molecules in relation to T cell antigen recognition in more detail in Chapters 5 and 6. For now, it is important to understand that NK cells use fundamentally different types of receptors than do T cells to recognize class I or class I–like MHC molecules.

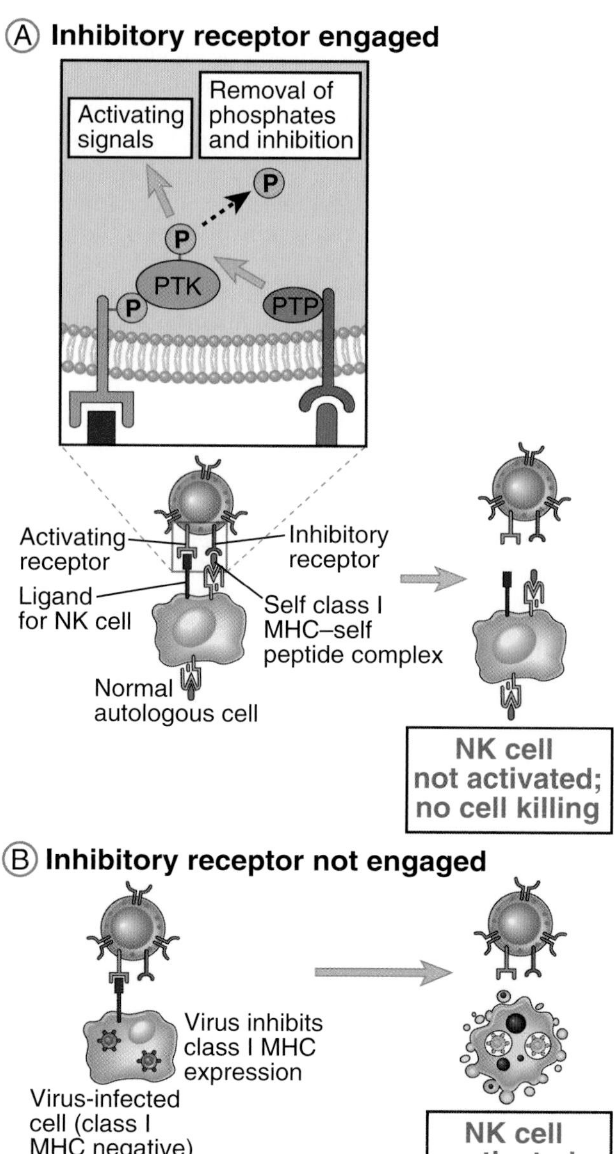

FIGURE 2–10 Activating and inhibitory receptors of NK cells. A. Activating receptors of NK cells recognize ligands on target cells and activate protein tyrosine kinase (PTK), whose activity is inhibited by inhibitory receptors that recognize class I MHC molecules and activate protein tyrosine phosphatase (PTP). NK cells do not efficiently kill class I MHC-expressing healthy cells. B. If a virus infection or other stress inhibits class I MHC expression on infected cells, and induces expression of additional activating ligands, the NK cell inhibitory receptor is not engaged and the activating receptor functions unopposed to trigger responses of NK cells, such as killing of target cells and cytokine secretion.

Activating receptors on NK cells recognize a heterogeneous group of ligands that are expressed on cells that have undergone stress, cells that are infected with viruses or other intracellular microbes, or cells that are malignantly transformed. One of the better studied activating receptors is called NKG2D (see Box 2–4), which binds a family of structurally related class I MHC-like proteins that are found on virally infected cells and

Box 2–4 ▪ IN DEPTH: INHIBITORY AND ACTIVATING RECEPTORS OF NATURAL KILLER CELLS

NK cells recognize and kill infected or malignantly transformed cells, but they do not usually harm normal cells. This ability to distinguish potentially dangerous targets from healthy self is dependent on the expression of both inhibitory and activating receptors. Inhibitory receptors on NK cells recognize class I MHC molecules, which are constitutively expressed on most healthy cells in the body but are often not expressed by cells infected with virus or cancer cells. Activating receptors on NK cells may recognize structures that are present on both NK- susceptible target cells and normal cells, but the influence of the inhibitory pathways dominates when class I MHC is recognized. In some cases, if the ligands for the activating receptors are newly induced or up-regulated in infected or transformed cells, the increased density of these ligands permits the activating receptors to overcome the action of the inhibitory receptors, thereby enabling the NK cell to kill cells expressing class I MHC. Some activating receptors recognize class I MHC-like molecules that are expressed only on stressed or transformed cells. Different families of NK cell receptors exist, and many of these receptors have evolved recently, as indicated by their absence in rodents and their structural divergence between chimpanzees and humans. The following discussion focuses on the properties of human NK cell inhibitory and activating receptors, with only brief consideration of murine NK receptors.

INHIBITORY RECEPTORS Inhibitory NK receptors fall into three main families (see Figure). A common feature of members of all three families is the presence of **immunoreceptor tyrosine-based inhibition motifs (ITIMs)** in their cytoplasmic tails. The signaling functions of ITIMs are discussed below. The first family to be discovered is named the KIR (killer cell Ig-like receptor) family because its members contain two or three extracellular Ig-like domains. The KIRs recognize different alleles of HLA-A, -B, and -C molecules. Structural and binding studies indicate that the sequence of the peptides bound to the MHC molecules is important for KIR recognition of MHC molecules. HLA class I molecule binding to KIRs is characterized by very fast on-rates and off-rates, which would be consistent with the ability of NK cells to rapidly "test" for the presence of MHC expression on many cells in a short time. Furthermore, the inhibitory signals generated in an NK cell by KIR recognition of an MHC molecule are not long lived, and the same NK cell can quickly go on to kill an MHC-negative target cell. Some members of the KIR family have short cytoplasmic tails without ITIMs, and these function as activating receptors, as discussed in more detail below. Mice do not express KIRs, but instead use the Ly49 family of C-type lectin proteins, which have similar class I MHC specificities and ITIMs in their cytoplasmic tails.

A second family of inhibitory receptors consists of Ig-like transcripts (ILTs) (also named LIR or CD85), which also contain Ig-like domains. One member of this family, ILT-2, has a broad specificity for many class I MHC alleles and contains four ITIMs in its cytoplasmic tail. Interestingly, cytomegalovirus encodes a molecule called UL18 that is homologous to human class I MHC and that can bind to ILT-2. This may represent a decoy mechanism by which the virus engages an inhibitory receptor and protects its cellular host from NK cell–mediated killing.

The third NK inhibitory receptor family consists of heterodimers composed of the C-type lectin NKG2A covalently bound to CD94. NKG2A has two ITIMs in its cytoplasmic tail. The CD94/NKG2A receptors bind HLA-E, a nonclassical MHC class I molecule. Stable expression of HLA-E on the surface of cells depends on the binding of signal peptides derived from HLA-A, -B, -C, or -G. Therefore, the CD94/NKG2A inhibitory receptors perform a surveillance function for the absence of HLA-E, classical class I MHC, and HLA-G molecules. As is the case for the KIR receptors, some CD94/NKG2 receptors do not have cytoplasmic ITIM motifs, and these function as NK-activating receptors, as discussed below.

The ITIMs in the cytoplasmic tails of inhibitory receptors are essential for the signaling functions of these molecules. ITIMs recruit phosphatase enzymes that counteract the effect of kinases in the signaling cascades initiated by activating receptors. ITIMs are composed of the sequence Ile/Val/Leu/Ser-x-Tyr-x-x-Leu/Val, where x denotes any amino acid, and are present in several different inhibitory receptors in the immune system. Upon binding class I MHC molecules to the extracellular regions of NK inhibitory receptors, the tyrosine residue in the ITIMs of the cytoplasmic tails are phosphorylated, and then phosphatases are recruited, including the protein-tyrosine phosphatases SHP (SH2-containing protein-tyrosine phosphatase)-1 and SHP-2, or the phospholipid-phosphatase SHIP (SH2-containing inositol polyphosphate 5-phosphatase). SHP-1 and SHP-2 remove phosphates from several signaling proteins, whereas SHIP degrades phosphatidylinositol-3,4,5-trisphosphate (PI-3,4,5-P3). The end result is reduced signaling by activating receptors, which are coupled to kinases that add phosphates to several intracellular substrates.

ACTIVATING RECEPTORS The activating receptors on NK cells include several structurally distinct groups of molecules, and only some of the ligands they bind are known. CD16, one of the first activating receptors identified on NK cells, is a low-affinity IgG Fc receptor that associates with FcεRIγ and ζ proteins and is responsible for NK cell–mediated antibody-dependent cellular cytotoxicity. A more recently discovered group of human NK-activating receptors, called natural cytotoxicity receptors, includes NKp46, NKp30, and NKp44. These are members of the Ig superfamily. NKp46 and NKp30 associate with FcεRIγ and ζ proteins, and NKp44 associates with DAP12. Although their ligands are not yet known, antibody-blocking studies suggest that they play a dominant role in NK-mediated killing of various tumor target cells. Ligand binding to activating NK cell receptors leads to cytokine production, enhanced migration to sites of infection, and killing activity against the ligand-bearing target cells.

A common feature of NK cell activating receptors is the presence of noncovalently linked subunits (e.g.,

Continued on following page

Box 2–4 ▪ IN DEPTH: INHIBITORY AND ACTIVATING RECEPTORS OF NATURAL KILLER CELLS (Continued)

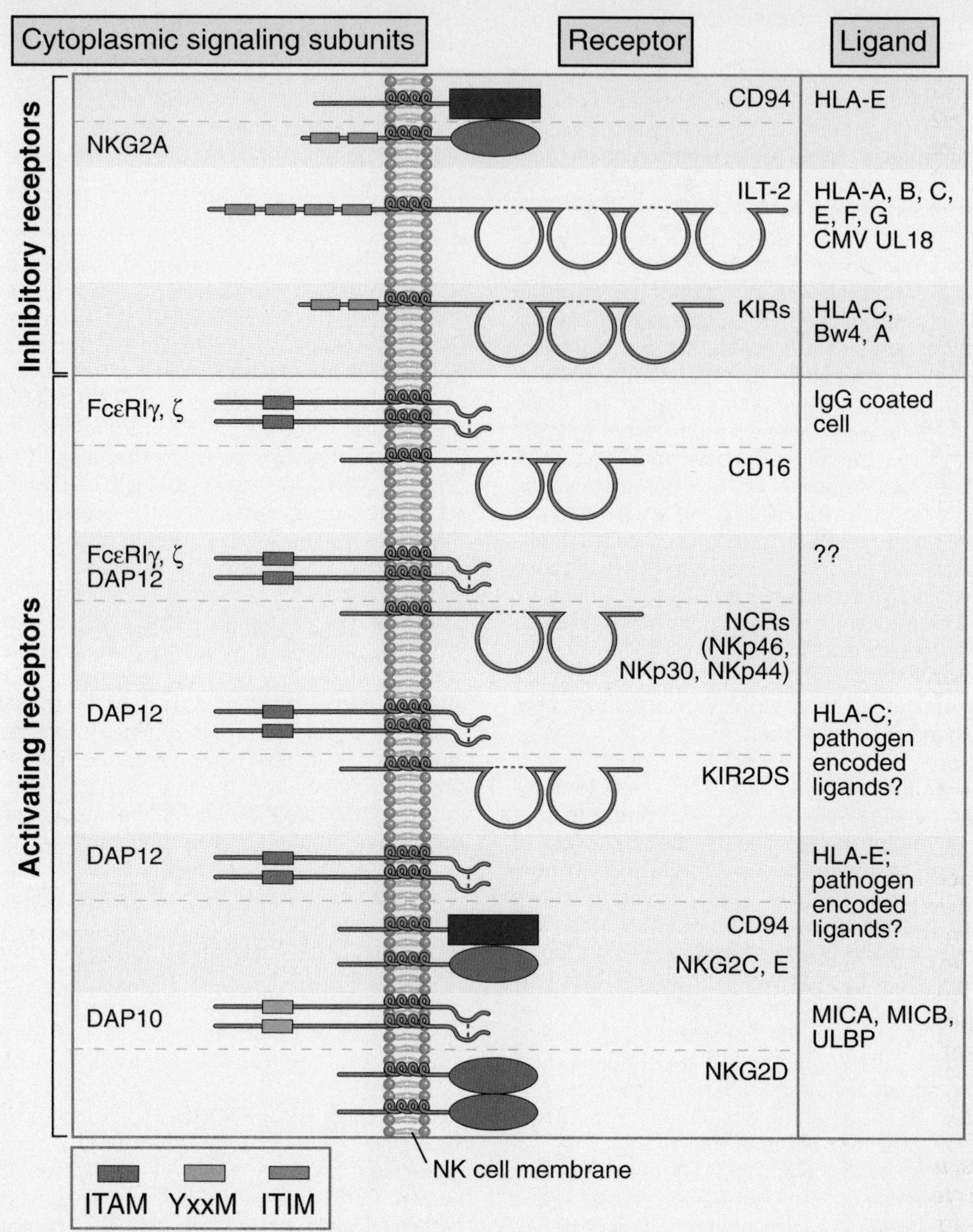

Examples of inhibitory and activating NK cell receptors and their ligands. CD16 and the natural cytotoxic receptors (NCRs) associate with ζ chain homodimers, FcRγ homodimers, or ζ-FcRγ heterodimers. There are multiple different KIRs, with varying ligand specificities.

FcεRIγ, ζ, and DAP12 proteins), whose cytoplasmic tails recruit kinases involved in signaling. CD16 and some other activating receptors associate with subunits that contain **immunoreceptor tyrosine-based activation motifs (ITAMs)** in their cytoplasmic tails. ITAMs are composed of a conserved sequence of amino acids, including two Tyr-x-x-Leu/Ile elements (where x is any amino acid) separated by six to eight amino acid residues. Upon ligand binding to the extracellular portion of these receptors, the tyrosine residues in the ITAMs become phosphorylated by cytoplasmic Src family kinases, and the phosphorylated ITAMs then bind other protein tyrosine kinases, such as Syk and ZAP-70, which act on additional substrates in a signaling cascade. These signaling events

Continued on following page

are very similar to those that occur in T and B lymphocytes after antigen recognition, and we will discuss them in more detail in Chapters 8 and 9. The NKG2D receptor (which is only distantly related to NKG2A or NKG2C) associates with a signaling subunit named DAP10, which has a Tyr-x-x-Met motif in its cytoplasmic domain. Upon phosphorylation, this motif binds phosphatidylinositol-3 kinase (PI3K) and Grb2, which initiates a different signaling cascade from that initiated by ITAM phosphorylation.

As mentioned, some members of the KIR and CD94/NKG2 families of MHC-specific receptors do not contain ITIMs but rather associate with ITAM-bearing accessory molecules (such as DAP12) and deliver activating signals to NK cells. These include KIR2DS, KIR3DS, and CD94/NKG2C. Some of these receptors are known to recognize normal class I MHC molecules, and it is not clear why these potentially dangerous receptors exist on NK cells. These activating receptors bind class I MHC molecules with lower affinities than the structurally related inhibitory receptors, and it is possible that the activating receptors actually bind MHC-related molecules specifically associated with pathological conditions.

NKG2D, which is expressed on NK cells, as well as on T cells, recognizes the MICA, MICB, and ULBP molecules in humans and the RAE-1, MULT1, and H60 molecules in mice. All these NKG2D ligands have domains homologous to class I MHC α and β domains, but do not display peptides or associate with β_2-microglobulin. These NKG2 ligands are not abundantly expressed on normal cells but are up-regulated by stress or DNA damage and are often found on tumor cells and virus-infected cells. Thus, NK cells may use these receptors to eliminate stressed (injured) host cells and tumor cells.

Most of the activating receptors on NK cells are also expressed on certain subsets of T cells, including γδT cells and CD8$^+$ T cells. However, the expression of these receptors on T cells is induced only after T cell activation by antigen, while expression of the receptor on NK cells is constitutive. This highlights an important distinction between innate and adaptive immunity—the effector cells of innate immunity, such as NK cells, are fully differentiated and ready to respond immediately to infections, while adaptive immune effector cells are generated from naive precursors only after antigen exposure.

tumor cells. Experimental evidence in mice has shown that NKG2 ligands are important for controlling viral infections and growth of tumors. Another type of activating receptor on NK cells, called CD16 (FcγRIIIa), is a low-affinity receptor for the Fc portions of IgG1 and IgG3 antibodies. As a result of this recognition, NK cells kill target cells that have been coated with antibody molecules. This process, called antibody-dependent cell-mediated cytotoxicity, will be described in more detail in Chapter 14 when we consider the effector mechanisms of humoral immunity. Kinase-dependent signaling cascades are initiated when activating receptors on NK cells bind their ligands, rapidly leading to cytotoxic activity against the target cells bearing the ligands and the production of cytokines. These signaling pathways are similar to those in T lymphocytes (see Chapter 9).

The inhibitory receptors on NK cells bind to class I MHC molecules, which are normally expressed on most healthy, uninfected cells. The binding of these inhibitory receptors to their ligands triggers phosphatase-dependent signaling cascades, which counteract the effect of kinases in the signaling cascades initiated by activating receptors. Because of specificity of inhibitory receptors for self-class I MHC, normal host cells are protected from NK-mediated killing. Infection of the host cells, especially by some viruses, often leads to reduced expression of class I MHC molecules, and therefore the ligands for the inhibitory NK cell receptors are lost. As a result, the NK cells are released from their normal state of inhibition. At the same time, ligands for activating receptors are expressed, and thus the infected cells are killed. This unusual specificity of the NK cell inhibitory receptors for normal class I MHC allows the innate immune system to attack virally infected cells that might be invisible to T cells, which require MHC expression for recognition. The largest group of NK inhibitory receptors are the killer cell immunoglobulin-like receptors (KIRs). These are members of the immunoglobulin superfamily, and they bind a variety of class I MHC molecules that otherwise function to present peptide antigens to CD8$^+$ T cells (see Box 2–4). A second important NK inhibitory receptor is CD94/NKG2A, which is a dimer of C-type lectins and recognizes a class I MHC molecule called HLA-E. Interestingly, HLA-E displays peptides derived from other class I MHC molecules, so in essence, CD94/NKG2 is a surveillance receptor for several different class I MHC molecules. A third family of NK inhibitory receptors, called the leukocyte Ig-like receptors (LIRs), are also Ig superfamily members that bind class I MHC molecules, albeit with lower affinity than the KIRs, and are more highly expressed on B cells than on NK cells.

The expansion and activities of NK cells are also stimulated by cytokines, mainly IL-15 and IL-12. IL-15, which is produced by macrophages and many other cell types, is a growth factor for NK cells, and knockout mice lacking IL-15 or its receptor show a profound reduction in the number of NK cells. The macrophage-derived cytokine IL-12 is a powerful inducer of NK cell IFN-γ production and cytotoxic activity. IL-18 may augment these actions of IL-12. IL-12 and IL-18 also stimulate IFN-γ production by T cells (see Chapter 13) and are thus central participants in IFN-γ production and the subsequent IFN-γ-mediated activation of macrophages in both innate and adaptive immunity. The type I IFNs, IFN-α and IFN-β, also activate the cytotoxic potential of NK cells, perhaps by increasing the expression of IL-12 receptors and therefore responsiveness to IL-12. IL-15,

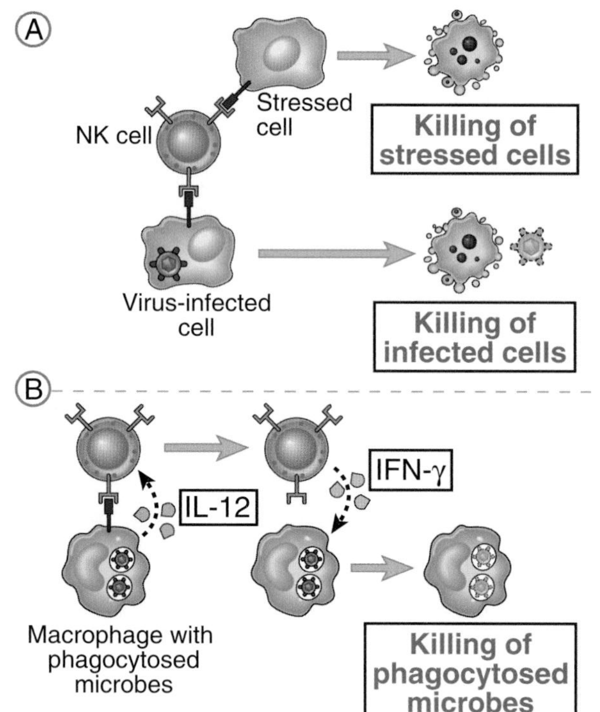

FIGURE 2–11 Functions of NK cells. A. NK cells recognize ligands on infected cells or cells undergoing other types of stress, and kill the host cells. In this way, NK cells eliminate reservoirs of infection as well as dysfunctional cells. B. NK cells respond to IL-12 produced by macrophages and secrete IFN-γ, which activates the macrophages to kill phagocytosed microbes.

IL-12, and type I IFNs are produced by macrophages in response to infection, and thus all three cytokines activate NK cells in innate immunity. High concentrations of IL-2 also stimulate the activities of NK cells, and culture in IL-2 is sometimes used to enhance NK cell killing.

Effector Functions of Natural Killer Cells

The effector functions of NK cells are to kill infected cells and to activate macrophages to destroy phagocytosed microbes (Fig. 2–11). The mechanism of NK cell–mediated cytotoxicity is essentially the same as that of CTLs (described in detail in Chapter 13). NK cells, like CTLs, have granules that contain proteins which mediate killing of target cells. When NK cells are activated, granule exocytosis releases these proteins adjacent to the target cells. One NK cell granule protein, called perforin, facilitates the entry of other granule proteins, called granzymes, into the cytoplasm of target cells. The granzymes are enzymes that initiate apoptosis of the target cells. By killing cells infected by viruses and intracellular bacteria, NK cells eliminate reservoirs of infection. Some tumors, especially those of hematopoietic origin, are targets of NK cells, perhaps because the tumor cells do not express normal levels or types of class I MHC molecules. NK cell–derived IFN-γ serves to activate macrophages, like IFN-γ produced by T cells, and increases the capacity of macrophages to kill phagocytosed bacteria (see Chapter 13).

NK cells play several important roles in defense against intracellular microbes. They kill virally infected cells before antigen-specific CTLs can become fully active, that is, during the first few days after viral infection. Early in the course of a viral infection, NK cells are expanded and activated by cytokines of innate immunity, such as IL-12 and IL-15, and they kill infected cells, especially those that display reduced levels of class I MHC molecules. In addition, the IFN-γ secreted by NK cells activates macrophages to destroy phagocytosed microbes. This IFN-γ-dependent NK cell–macrophage reaction can control an infection with intracellular bacteria such as *Listeria monocytogenes* for several days or weeks and thus allow time for T cell–mediated immunity to develop and eradicate the infection. Depletion of NK cells leads to increased susceptibility to infection by some viruses and intracellular bacteria. In mice lacking T cells, the NK cell response may be adequate to keep infection with such microbes in check for some time, but the animals eventually succumb in the absence of T cell–mediated immunity. NK cells may also kill infected cells that attempt to escape CTL-mediated immune attack by reducing expression of class I MHC molecules.

Because NK cells can kill certain tumor cells in vitro, it has also been proposed that NK cells serve to kill malignant clones in vivo.

Circulating Proteins of Innate Immunity

In addition to cell-associated molecules, several different soluble proteins found in plasma and extracellular fluids also recognize pathogen-associated molecular patterns and serve as effector molecules of the innate immune system. Other soluble molecules serve as opsonins, targeting microbes for phagocytosis by neutrophils or macrophages. The soluble pattern recognition proteins and associated effector molecules are sometimes called the humoral branch of innate immunity, analogous to the humoral branch of adaptive immunity mediated by antibodies. The major components of the humoral innate immune system are the complement system, the collectins, the pentraxins, and the ficolins.

The Complement System

The complement system consists of several plasma proteins that are activated by microbes and promote destruction of the microbes and inflammation. Recognition of microbes by complement occurs in three ways (Fig. 2–12). The classical pathway, so called because it was discovered first, uses a plasma protein called C1 to detect IgM, IgG1, or IgG3 antibodies bound to the surface of a microbe or other structure. The alternative pathway, which was discovered later but is

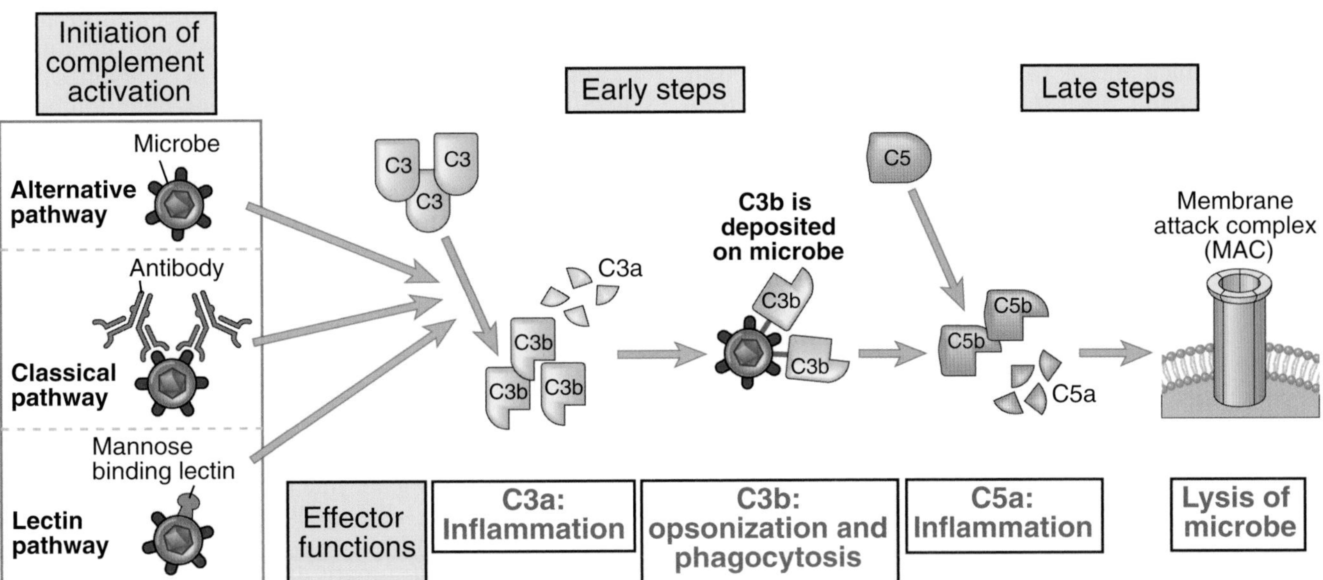

FIGURE 2–12 Pathways of complement activation. The activation of the complement system may be initiated by three distinct pathways, all of which lead to the production of C3b (the early steps). C3b initiates the late steps of complement activation, culminating in the production of peptides that stimulate inflammation (C5a) and polymerized C9, which forms the membrane attack complex, so called because it creates holes in plasma membranes. The principal functions of major proteins produced at different steps are shown. The activation, functions, and regulation of the complement system are discussed in much more detail in Chapter 14.

phylogenetically older than the classical pathway, is triggered by direct recognition of certain microbial surface structures and is thus a component of innate immunity. The lectin pathway is triggered by a plasma protein called mannose-binding lectin (MBL), which recognizes terminal mannose residues on microbial glycoproteins and glycolipids. MBL bound to microbes activates one of the proteins of the classical pathway, in the absence of antibody, by the action of an associated serine protease.

Recognition of microbes by any of these pathways results in sequential recruitment and assembly of additional complement proteins into protease complexes. The central protein of the complement system, C3, is cleaved, and its larger C3b fragment is deposited on the microbial surface where complement is activated. C3b becomes covalently attached to the microbes and serves as an opsonin to promote phagocytosis of the microbes. A smaller fragment, C3a, is released and stimulates inflammation by acting as a chemoattractant for neutrophils. C3b binds other complement proteins to form a protease that cleaves a protein called C5, generating a secreted peptide (C5a) and a larger fragment (C5b) that remains attached to the microbial cell membranes. C5a stimulates the influx of neutrophils to the site of infection as well as the vascular component of acute inflammation. C5b initiates the formation of a complex of the complement proteins C6, C7, C8, and C9, which are assembled into a membrane pore that causes lysis of the cells where complement is activated. Mammalian cells express several regulatory proteins that block complement activation and thus prevent injury to normal host cells. The complement system will be discussed in more detail in Chapter 14.

Pentraxins

Several plasma proteins that recognize microbial structures and participate in innate immunity belong to the **pentraxin** family, which is a phylogenetically old group of structurally homologous pentameric proteins. Prominent members of this family include the short pentraxins **C-reactive protein (CRP)** and **serum amyloid P (SAP)** and the long pentraxin **PTX3.** Plasma concentrations of CRP are very low in healthy individuals, but can increase up to 1000-fold during infections and in response to other inflammatory stimuli. The increased levels of CRP are a result of increased synthesis by the liver induced by the cytokines IL-6 and IL-1, which are produced by phagocytes as part of the innate immune response. Liver synthesis and plasma levels of several other proteins, including SAP and others unrelated to the pentraxins, also increase in response to IL-1 and IL-6, and as a group these plasma proteins are called **acute-phase reactants.** Both CRP and SAP bind to several different species of bacteria and fungi. The molecular ligands recognized by CRP and SAP include phosphorylcholine and phosphatidylethanolamine, respectively, which are phospholipid headgroups found on bacterial membranes and on apoptotic cells, but are not exposed on the surface of healthy eukaryotic cells. CRP functions as an opsonin by binding C1q and interacting with phagocyte C1q receptors or by binding directly to IgG Fc receptors. CRP may also contribute to complement activation through its attachment to C1q and activation of the classical pathway. PTX3 is produced by several cell types, including dendritic cells, endothelial cells, and macrophages, in response to TLR ligand and the innate immune system cytokine TNF, but it is not an acute-phase reactant. PTX3 binds to several ligands, including C1q, apoptotic cells, and certain microorganisms. Studies with knockout mice reveal that PTX3 provides protection against some microbes, including the fungus *Aspergillus fumigatus*.

Collectins and Ficolins

The **collectins** are a family of proteins that contain a collagen-like tail connected by a neck region to a calcium-dependent (C-type) lectin head. Three members of this family serve as soluble pattern recognition molecules in the innate immune system; these include MBL and pulmonary surfactant proteins SP-A and SP-D.

Mannose-binding lectin, which was mentioned earlier in relation to the complement system, is a plasma protein that functions as an opsonin. Plasma MBL, like the macrophage mannose receptor, binds carbohydrates with terminal mannose and fucose, which are typically found in microbial cell surface glycoproteins and glycolipids. Thus, MBL is a soluble pattern recognition receptor that binds to microbial but not mammalian cells. MBL is a hexamer that is structurally similar to the C1q component of the complement system. MBL binds to a macrophage surface receptor that is called the C1q receptor because it also binds C1q. This receptor mediates the phagocytosis of microbes that are opsonized by MBL. Moreover, MBL can activate the complement system, as discussed earlier. The gene encoding MBL is polymorphic, and certain alleles are associated with impaired hexamer formation and reduced blood levels. Low MBL levels are associated with increased susceptibility to a variety of infections, especially in combination with other immunodeficiency states.

Surfactant protein-A (**SP-A**) and surfactant-D (**SP-D**) are collectins with lipophilic surfactant properties shared by other surfactants, and are found in the alveoli of the lungs. Their major functions appear to be as modulators of innate immune responses in the lung. They bind to various microorganisms and act as opsonins, facilitating ingestion by alveolar macrophages. SP-A and SP-D can directly inhibit bacterial growth, and they also interact with and activate macrophages. SP-A– and SP-D–deficient mice have impaired abilities to resist a variety of pulmonary infections.

Ficolins are plasma proteins that are structurally similar to collectins, possessing a collagen-like domain, but instead of a C-type lectin domain, they have a fibrinogen-type carbohydrate recognition domain. Ficolins have been shown to bind several species of bacteria, opsonizing them and activating complement in a manner similar to that of MBL. The molecular ligands of the ficolins include *N*-acetylglucosamine and the lipoteichoic acid component of the cell walls of gram-positive bacteria.

Cytokines of the Innate Immune System

The cytokines of innate immunity recruit and activate leukocytes and produce systemic alterations, including increases in the synthesis of effector cells and proteins that potentiate antimicrobial responses. In innate immunity, the principal sources of cytokines are macrophages, neutrophils, and NK cells, but endothelial cells and some epithelial cells such as keratinocytes produce many of the same proteins. As in adaptive immunity, cytokines serve to communicate information among inflammatory cells and between inflammatory cells and responsive tissue cells, such as vascular endothelial cells.

The cytokines of innate immunity will be described further in Chapter 12. They include cytokines that control viral infections, namely, IFN-α and IFN-β; cytokines that mediate inflammation, namely, TNF, IL-1, and chemokines; cytokines that stimulate the proliferation and activity of NK cells, namely, IL-15 and IL-2; cytokines that activate macrophages, especially NK cell–derived IFN-γ; and cytokines that serve to limit macrophage activation, especially IL-10. In addition, some cytokines of innate immunity, such as IL-6, increase bone marrow production of neutrophils and the synthesis of various proteins involved in host defense, such as CRP.

Role of Innate Immunity in Stimulating Adaptive Immune Responses

The innate immune response provides signals that function in concert with antigen to stimulate the proliferation and differentiation of antigen-specific T and B lymphocytes. As the innate immune response is providing the initial defense, it also sets in motion the adaptive immune response. The activation of lymphocytes requires two distinct signals, the first being antigen and the second being components of innate immune responses to microbes or injured cells (Fig. 2–13). This idea is called the two-signal hypothesis for lymphocyte activation. The requirement for antigen (so-called signal 1) ensures that the ensuing immune response is specific. The requirement for additional stimuli triggered by microbes or innate immune reactions to microbes (signal 2) ensures that adaptive immune responses are induced when there is a dangerous infection and not when lymphocytes recognize harmless antigens, including self antigens. The molecules produced during innate immune reactions that function as second signals for lymphocyte activation include costimulators (for T cells), cytokines (for both T and B cells), and complement breakdown products (for B cells). We will return to the nature of second signals for lymphocyte activation in Chapters 9 and 10.

The second signals generated during innate immune responses to different microbes not only enhance the magnitude of the subsequent adaptive immune response but also influence the nature of the adaptive response. A major function of T cell–mediated immunity is to activate macrophages to kill intracellular microbes. Infectious agents that engage TLRs will tend to stimulate T cell–mediated immune responses. This is because TLR

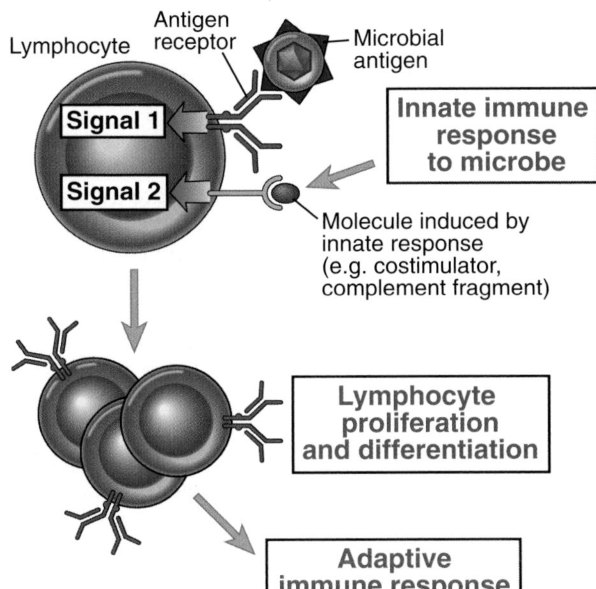

FIGURE 2–13 Stimulation of adaptive immunity by innate immune responses. Antigen recognition by lymphocytes provides signal 1 for the activation of the lymphocytes, and molecules induced on host cells during innate immune responses to microbes provide signal 2. In this illustration, the lymphocytes are B cells, but the same principles apply to T lymphocytes. The nature of second signals differs for B and T cells and is described in later chapters.

signaling enhances the ability of antigen-presenting cells to induce the differentiation of T cells into effector cells called T_H1 cells. T_H1 cells produce the cytokine IFN-γ, which can activate macrophages to kill microbes that might otherwise survive within phagocytic vesicles. T_H1 cells and cell-mediated immunity are discussed in detail in Chapter 13. In contrast, many extracellular microbes that enter the blood activate the alternative complement pathway, which in turn enhances the production of antibodies by B lymphocytes. This humoral immune response serves to eliminate extracellular microbes. The role of complement in enhancing B cell activation is discussed in Chapter 14.

The role of innate immunity in stimulating adaptive immune responses is the basis of the action of **adjuvants,** which are substances that need to be administered together with protein antigens to elicit maximal T cell–dependent immune responses (see Chapter 6). Adjuvants are useful in experimental immunology and in clinical vaccines. Many adjuvants in experimental use are microbial products, such as killed mycobacteria and LPS, that engage TLRs and elicit strong innate immune responses at the site of antigen entry.

SUMMARY

- The innate immune system provides the first line of host defense against microbes. The mechanisms of innate immunity exist before exposure to microbes. The components of the innate immune system include epithelial barriers, leukocytes (neutrophils, macrophages, and NK cells), circulating effector proteins (complement, collectins, pentraxins), and cytokines (e.g., TNF, IL-1, chemokines, IL-2, type I IFNs, and IFN-γ).

- The innate immune system uses cell-associated pattern recognition receptors to recognize structures called pathogen-associated molecular patterns (PAMPs), which are shared by microbes, are not present on mammalian cells, and are often essential for survival of the microbes, thus limiting the capacity of microbes to evade detection by mutating or losing expression of these molecules. TLRs are the most important family of pattern recognition receptors, recognizing a wide variety of ligands, including microbial nucleic acids, sugars, glycolipids, and proteins.

- Neutrophils and macrophages are phagocytes that kill ingested microbes by producing ROS, nitric oxide, and enzymes in phagolysosomes. Macrophages also produce cytokines that stimulate inflammation and promote tissue remodeling at sites of infection. Phagocytes recognize and respond to microbial products by several different types of receptors, including TLRs, C-type lectins, scavenger receptors, and *N*-formyl Met-Leu-Phe receptors.

- Neutrophils and monocytes (the precursors of tissue macrophages) migrate from blood into inflammatory sites during innate immune responses. Cytokines, including IL-1 and TNF, produced at these sites in response to microbial products induce the expression of adhesion molecules on the endothelial cells of local venules. These adhesion molecules mediate the attachment of the circulating leukocytes to the vessel wall. The process of leukocyte migration involves sequential steps, starting with low affinity leukocyte binding to and rolling along the endothelia surface (mediated by endothelial selectins and leukocyte selectin ligands). Next, the leukocytes become firmly bound, via interactions of leukocyte integrins binding to Ig-superfamily ligands on the endothelium. Intergrin binding is strengthened by chemokines, produced at the site of infection, which bind to receptors on the leukocytes. Chemokines also stimulate directed migration of the leukocytes through the vessel wall into the site of infection.

- NK cells are lymphocytes that defend against intracellular microbes by killing infected cells and providing a source of the macrophage-activating cytokine IFN-γ. NK cell recognition of infected cells is regulated by a combination of activating and inhibitory receptors. Inhibitory receptors recognize class I MHC molecules, because of which NK cells do not kill normal host cells but do kill cells in which class I MHC expression is reduced, such as virus-infected cells.

- The complement system is activated by microbes, and products of complement activation promote phagocytosis and killing of microbes and stimulate inflammation.

- The innate immune system includes other soluble pattern recognition and effector molecules found in the plasma, including pentraxins (e.g., CRP), collectins (e.g., MBL), and ficolins. These molecules bind microbial ligands and enhance clearance by complement-dependent and -independent mechanisms.

- Different cytokines of innate immunity recruit and activate leukocytes (e.g., TNF, IL-1, chemokines), enhance the microbicidal activities of phagocytes (IFN-γ), and stimulate NK cell and T cell responses (IL-2). In severe infections, excess systemic cytokine production is harmful and may even cause death of the host.

- Molecules produced during innate immune responses stimulate adaptive immunity and influence the nature of adaptive immune responses. Macrophages activated by microbes and by IFN-γ produce costimulators that enhance T cell activation and IL-2, which stimulates IFN-γ production by T cells and the development of IFN-γ-producing effector T cells. Complement fragments generated by the alternative pathway provide second signals for B cell activation and antibody production.

Selected Readings

Akira S, and K Takeda. Toll-like receptor signalling. Nature Reviews Immunology 4:499–511, 2004.

Akira S, S Uematsu, and O Takeuchi. Pathogen recognition and innate immunity. Cell 124:783–801, 2006.

Bulet P, R Stocklin, and L Menin. Anti-microbial peptides: from invertebrates to vertebrates. Immunological Reviews 198: 169–184, 2004.

Chen G, MH Shaw, YG Kim, and G Nuñez. Nod-like receptors: role in innate immunity and inflammatory disease. Annual Review of Pathology 4:365–398, 2008.

Dommett R, M Zilbauer, JT George, and M Bajaj-Elliott. Innate immune defence in the human gastrointestinal tract. Molecular Immunology 42:903–912, 2005.

Fujita T, M Matsushita, and Y Endo. The lectin-complement pathway—its role in innate immunity and evolution. Immunological Reviews 198:185–202, 2004.

Garlanda C, B Bottazzi, A Bastone, and A Mantovani. Pentraxins at the crossroads between innate immunity, inflammation, matrix deposition and female fertility. Annual Review of Immunology 23:337–366, 2004.

Hotchkiss RS, and IE Karl. The pathophysiology and treatment of sepsis. New England Journal of Medicine 348:138–150, 2003.

Inohara N, M Chamaillard, C McDonald, and G Nunez. NOD-LRR proteins: role in host-microbial interactions and inflammatory disease. Annual Review of Biochemistry 74:355–383, 2005.

Janeway CA, and R Medzhitov. Innate immune recognition. Annual Review of Immunology 20:197–216, 2002.

Kawai T and S Akira. Innate immune recognition of viral infection. Nature Immunology 7:131–137, 2006.

Klotman ME and TL Chang. Defensins in innate antiviral immunity. Nature Reviews Immunology 6:447–456, 2006.

Kopp E, and R Medzhitov. Recognition of microbial infection by Toll-like receptors. Current Opinion in Immunology 15:396–401, 2003.

Krieg A. CpG motifs in bacterial DNA and their immune effects. Annual Review of Immunology 20:709–760, 2002.

Lanier LL. NK cell recognition. Annual Review of Immunology 23:225–274, 2005.

Lehrer RI, and T Ganz. Defensins of vertebrate animals. Current Opinion in Immunology 14:96–102, 2002.

Ley K, Laudanna C, Cybulsky MI, Nourshargh S. Getting to the site of inflammation: the leukocyte adhesion cascade updated. Nature Reviews Immunology 7:678–689, 2007.

Meylan E, J Tschopp, and M Karin. Intracellular pattern recognition receptors in the host response. Nature 442:39–44, 2006.

Nauseef WM. How human neutrophils kill and degrade microbes: an integrated view. Immunological Reviews 219:88–102, 2007.

Pichlmair A, and C Reis e Sousa. Innate recognition of viruses. Immunity 27:370–383, 2007.

Segal AW. How neutrophils kill microbes. Annual Review of Immunology 23:197–223, 2005.

Selsted ME, and AJ Ouellette. Mammalian defensins in the antimicrobial immune response. Nature Immunology 6:551–557, 2005.

Strober W, PJ Murray, A Kitani, and T Watanabe. Signalling pathways and molecular interactions of NOD1 and NOD2. Nature Reviews Immunology 6:9–20, 2006.

Takeda K, T Kaisho, and S Akira. Toll-like receptors. Annual Review of Immunology 21:335–376, 2003.

Trinchieri G, and A Sher. Cooperation of Toll-like receptor signals in innate immune defence. Nature Reviews Immunology 7:179–190, 2007.

Underhill DM, and A Ozinsky. Phagocytosis of microbes: complexity in action. Annual Review of Immunology 20: 825–852, 2002.

Van de Wetering JK, LMG van Golde, and JJ Batenburg. Collectins: players of the innate immune system. European Journal of Biochemistry 271:229–249, 2004.

Vivier E, E Tomasello, M Baratin, T Walzer, and S Ugolini. Functions of natural killer cells. Nature Immunology 9:503–511, 2008.

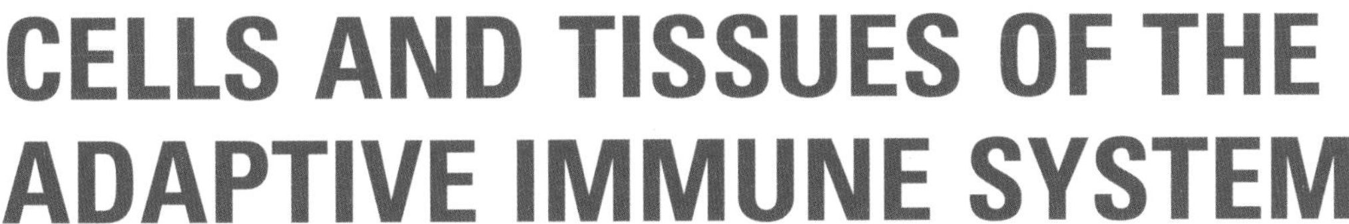

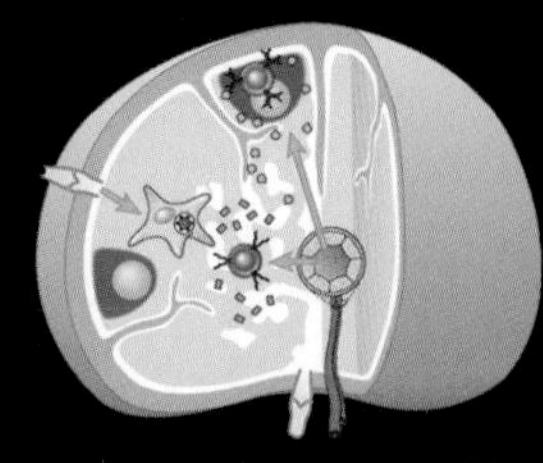

CELLS AND TISSUES OF THE ADAPTIVE IMMUNE SYSTEM

The cells of the adaptive immune system are normally present as circulating cells in the blood and lymph, as anatomically defined collections in lymphoid organs, and as scattered cells in virtually all tissues. The anatomic organization of these cells and their ability to circulate and exchange among blood, lymph, and tissues are of critical importance for the generation of immune responses. The immune system faces numerous challenges to generate effective protective responses against infectious pathogens. First, the system must be able to respond to small numbers of many different microbes that may be introduced at any site in the body. Second, very few naive lymphocytes specifically recognize and respond to any one antigen. Third, the effector mechanisms of the immune system (antibodies and effector T cells) may have to locate and destroy microbes at sites that are distant from the site of initial infection. The ability of the immune system to meet these challenges and to perform its protective functions optimally is dependent on several properties of its cells and tissues.

- ***Specialized tissues, called peripheral lymphoid organs, function to concentrate antigens that are introduced through the common portals of entry (skin and gastrointestinal and respiratory tracts).*** The capture of antigen and its transport to lymphoid organs are the first steps in adaptive immune responses. Antigens that are transported to lymphoid organs are displayed by antigen-presenting cells (APCs) for recognition by specific lymphocytes.
- ***Naive lymphocytes (lymphocytes that have not previously encountered antigens) migrate through these peripheral lymphoid organs, where they recognize antigens and initiate immune responses.*** The anatomy of lymphoid organs promotes cell-cell interactions that are required for the antigen recognition and activation phases of adaptive immune responses. Effector and memory lymphocytes develop from the progeny of antigen-stimulated naive cells.
- ***Effector and memory lymphocytes circulate in the blood, home to peripheral sites of antigen entry, and are efficiently retained at these sites.*** This ensures that

immunity is systemic (i.e., that protective mechanisms can act anywhere in the body).

Adaptive immune responses develop through a series of steps, in each of which the special properties of immune cells and tissues play critical roles. The key phases of these responses and the roles of different cells and tissues are illustrated schematically in Fig. 3–1. This chapter describes the cells, tissues, and organs of the adaptive immune system and concludes with a discussion of the traffic patterns of lymphocytes throughout the body.

CELLS OF THE ADAPTIVE IMMUNE SYSTEM

The cells that are involved in adaptive immune responses are antigen-specific lymphocytes, APCs that display antigens and activate lymphocytes, and effector cells that function to eliminate antigens. These cell types were introduced in Chapter 1. Here we describe the morphology and functional characteristics of lymphocytes and APCs and then explain how these cells are organized in lymphoid tissues. The numbers of some of these cell types in the blood are listed in Table 3–1.

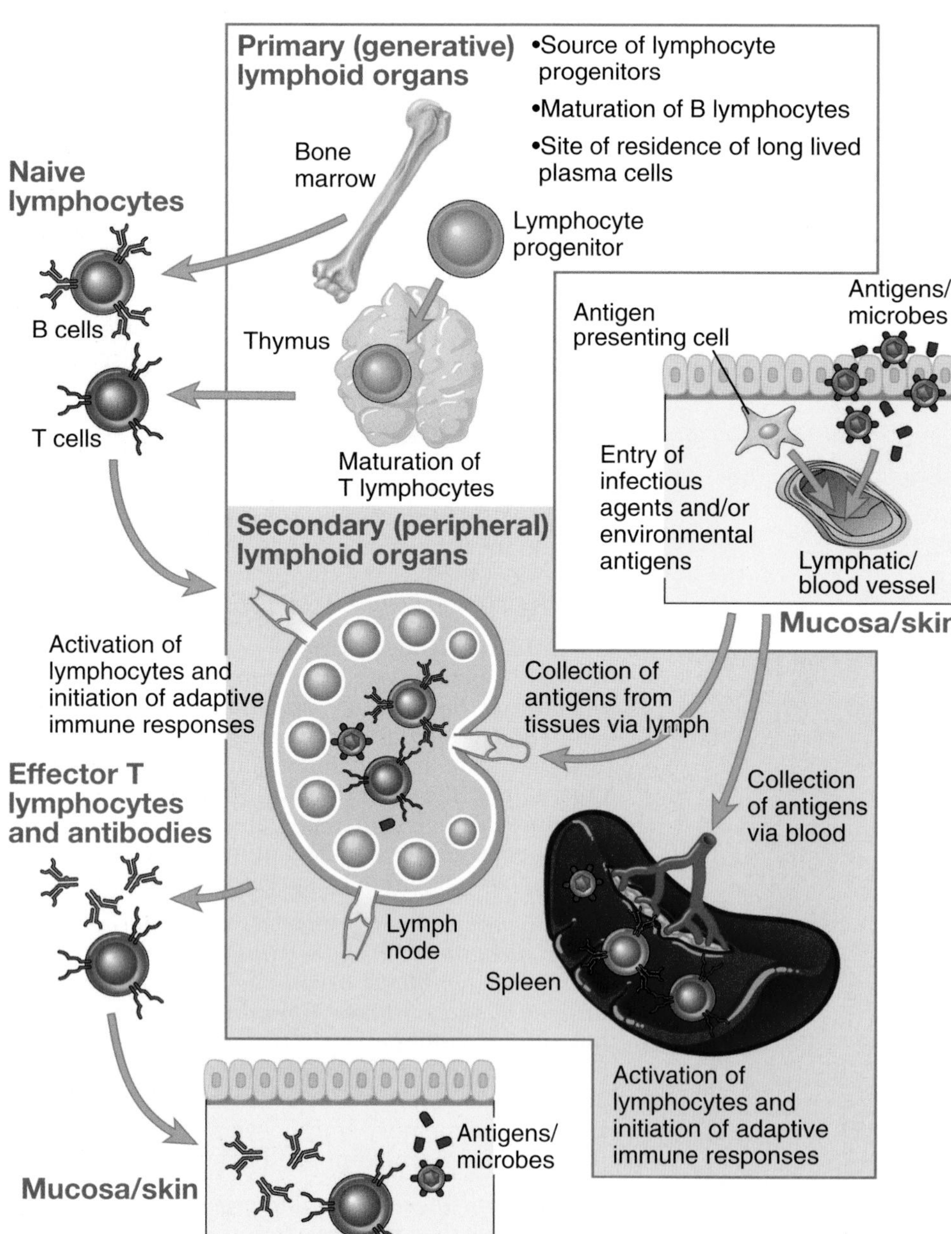

FIGURE 3–1 Overview of lymphocyte generation and immune responses in vivo. Lymphocytes mature in the bone marrow (B cells) and thymus (T cells), and enter secondary (peripheral) lymphoid organs as "naive" lymphocytes. Antigens are captured from their site of entry by dendritic cells and concentrated in lymph nodes, where they activate naive lymphocytes that migrate to the nodes through blood vessels. Effector and memory T cells develop in the nodes and enter the circulation, from which they may migrate to peripheral tissues. Antibodies are produced in lymphoid organs and enter the circulation, from which they may locate antigens at any site. Memory cells also enter the circulation and may reside in lymphoid organs and other tissues. This illustration depicts the key events in an immune response to a protein antigen in a lymph node; responses in other peripheral lymphoid organs are similar.

Table 3–1. Normal Blood Cell Counts

	Mean number per microliter	Normal range
White blood cells (leukocytes)	7400	4500–11,000
Neutrophils	4400	1800–7700
Eosinophils	200	0–450
Basophils	40	0–200
Lymphocytes	2500	1000–4800
Monocytes	300	0–800

Although these cells are found in the blood, their responses to antigens are localized to lymphoid and other tissues and are generally not reflected in changes in the total numbers of circulating leukocytes. The cells involved in innate immunity were described in detail in Chapter 2.

Lymphocytes

Lymphocytes are the only cells in the body capable of specifically recognizing and distinguishing different antigenic determinants and are responsible for the two defining characteristics of the adaptive immune response, specificity and memory. Several lines of evidence have established the role of lymphocytes as the cells that mediate adaptive immunity.

- Protective immunity to microbes can be adoptively transferred from immunized to naive individuals only by lymphocytes or their secreted products.
- Some congenital and acquired immunodeficiencies are associated with reduction of lymphocytes in the peripheral circulation and in lymphoid tissues. Furthermore, depletion of lymphocytes with drugs, irradiation, and cell type-specific antibodies, and by targeted gene disruptions in mice, leads to impaired adaptive immune responses.
- Stimulation of lymphocytes by antigens in culture leads to responses in vitro that show many of the characteristics of immune responses induced under more physiologic conditions in vivo.
- Most important, specific receptors for antigens are produced by lymphocytes but not by any other types of cells.

Subsets of Lymphocytes

Lymphocytes consist of distinct subsets that are different in their functions and protein products but are morphologically very similar (Table 3–2). This heterogeneity of lymphocytes was introduced in Chapter 1 (see Fig. 1–5). **B lymphocytes**, the cells that produce antibodies, were so called because in birds they were found to mature in an organ called the bursa of Fabricius. In mammals, no anatomic equivalent of the bursa exists, and the early stages of B cell maturation occur in the bone marrow. Thus, "B" lymphocytes refers to bursa-derived lymphocytes or bone marrow–derived lymphocytes. **T lymphocytes**, the mediators of cellular immunity, were named because their precursors, which arise in the bone marrow, migrate to and mature in the thymus; "T" lymphocytes refers to thymus-derived lymphocytes. B and T lymphocytes each consist of subsets with distinct phenotypic and functional characteristics. The major subsets of B cells are follicular B cells, marginal zone B cells, and B-1 B cells, each of which is found in distinct anatomic locations within lymphoid tissues. The two major T cell subsets are helper T lymphocytes and cytotoxic T lymphocytes (CTLs), which express an antigen receptor called the αβ receptor. $CD4^+$ regulatory T cells are now recognized as a third unique subset of T cells expressing the αβ receptor. Another population of T cells called **γδ T cells** expresses a similar but structurally distinct type of antigen receptor. The different functions of these classes of B and T cells will be discussed in later chapters.

B and T lymphocytes have clonally distributed antigen receptors, meaning that there are many clones of these cells with different antigen specificities, and all the members of each clone express antigen receptors of the same specificity that are different from the receptors of other clones. The genes encoding the antigen receptors of B and T lymphocytes are formed by recombinations of DNA segments during the maturation of these cells. There is a random aspect to these somatic recombination events, which results in the generation of millions of different receptor genes and a highly diverse repertoire of antigen specificities among different clones of lymphocytes (see Chapter 8). Some subsets of lymphocytes, including γδ T cells, marginal zone B cells, and B-1 B cells, are restricted in their use of DNA segments that contribute to their antigen receptor genes, and the repertoires of these lymphocyte subsets are very limited.

In addition to B and T cells, there exist other populations of cells that are called lymphocytes based on morphology and certain functional and molecular criteria, but which are not readily categorized as T or B cells. **Natural killer (NK) cells,** which were described in Chapter 2, have similar effector functions as CTLs, but their receptors are distinct from B or T cell antigen receptors and are not encoded by somatically recombined genes. **NKT cells** are a numerically small population of lymphocytes that share characteristic of both NK cells and T cells. They express αβ antigen receptors that are encoded by somatically recombined genes, but like γδ T cells and B-1 B cells, they lack diversity. NKT cells, γδ T cells, and B-1 B cells may all be considered as part of both adaptive and innate immune systems.

Membrane proteins may be used as phenotypic markers to distinguish functionally distinct populations of lymphocytes (see Table 3–2). For instance, most

Table 3–2. Lymphocyte Classes

Class	Functions	Antigen receptor and specificity	Selected markers	Percent of total lymphocytes (human)		
				Blood	Lymph node	Spleen
αβ T lymphocytes						
CD4+ helper T lymphocytes	B cell differentiation (humoral immunity) Macrophage activation (cell-mediated immunity)	αβ heterodimers Diverse specificities for peptide-class II MHC complexes	$CD3^+$, $CD4^+$, $CD8^-$	50–60*	50–60	50–60
CD8+ cytotoxic T lymphocytes	Killing of cell infected with microbes, killing of tumor cells	αβ heterodimers Diverse specificities for peptide-class I MHC complexes	$CD3^+$, $CD4^-$, $CD8^+$	20–25	15–20	10–15
Regulatory T cells	Suppress function of other T cells (regulation of immune responses, maintenance of self-tolerance)	αβ heterodimers	$CD3^+$, $CD4^+$, $CD25^+$ (Most common, but other phenotypes as well)	Rare	10	10
γδ T lymphocytes	Helper and cytotoxic functions (innate immunity)	γδ heterodimers Limited specificities for peptide and nonpeptide antigens	$CD3^+$, CD4, and CD8 variable			
B lymphocytes	Antibody production (humoral immunity)	Surface antibody Diverse specificities for all types of molecules	Fc receptors; class II MHC; CD19; CD21	10–15	20–25	40–45
Natural killer cells	Killing of virus-infected or damaged cells (innate immunity)	Various activating and inhibitory receptors Limited specificities for MHC or MHC-like molecules	CD16 (Fc receptor for IgG)	10	Rare	10
NKT cells	Suppress or activate innate and adaptive immune responses	αβ heterodimers (Limited specificity for glycolipid-CD1 complexes)	CD16 (Fc receptor for IgG); CD3	10	Rare	10

*In most cases, the ratio of $CD4^+CD8^-$ to $CD8^+CD4^-$ cells is about 2:1.
Abbreviations: IgG, immunoglobulin G; MHC, major histocompatibility complex

helper T cells express a surface protein called CD4, and most CTLs express a different surface protein called CD8. Antibodies that are specific for such markers, labeled with probes that can be detected by various methods, are often used to identify and isolate various lymphocyte populations. (Techniques for detecting labeled antibodies are described in Appendix III.) Many of the surface proteins that were initially recognized as phenotypic markers for various lymphocyte subpopulations have turned out, on further analysis, to play important roles in the activation and functions of these cells. The accepted nomenclature for lymphocyte markers uses the CD number designation. CD stands for "cluster of differentiation," a historical term referring to a cluster (or collection) of monoclonal antibodies that are specific for a particular marker of lymphocyte differentiation. The CD system provides a uniform way to identify cell surface molecules on lymphocytes, APCs, and many other cell types in the immune system (Box 3–1). Examples of some CD proteins are mentioned in Table 3–2, and the biochemistry and functions of the most important ones are described in later chapters. A current list of CD markers for leukocytes that are mentioned in the book is provided in Appendix II.

Box 3–1 ■ IN DEPTH: LYMPHOCYTE MARKERS AND THE CD NOMENCLATURE SYSTEM

From the time that functionally distinct classes of lymphocytes were recognized, immunologists have attempted to develop methods for distinguishing them. The basic approach was to produce antibodies that would selectively recognize different subpopulations. This was initially done by raising alloantibodies (i.e., antibodies that might recognize allelic forms of cell surface proteins) by immunizing inbred strains of mice with lymphocytes from other strains. Such techniques were successful and led to the development of antibodies that reacted with murine T cells (anti-Thy1 antibodies) and even against functionally different subsets of T lymphocytes (anti-Lyt1 and anti-Lyt2 antibodies). The limitations of this approach are obvious, however, because it is useful only for cell surface proteins that exist in different allelic forms. The advent of hybridoma technology gave such analyses a tremendous boost, with the production of monoclonal antibodies that reacted specifically and selectively with defined populations of lymphocytes, first in humans and subsequently in many other species. (Alloantibodies and monoclonal antibodies are described in Chapter 4.)

Functionally distinct classes of lymphocytes express distinct types of cell surface proteins. Immunologists often rely on monoclonal antibody probes to detect these surface molecules. The cell surface molecules recognized by monoclonal antibodies are called "antigens" because antibodies can be raised against them, or "markers," because they identify and discriminate between ("mark") different cell populations. These markers can be grouped into several categories; some are specific for cells of a particular lineage or maturational pathway, and the expression of others varies according to the state of activation or differentiation of the same cells. Biochemical analyses of cell surface proteins recognized by different monoclonal antibodies demonstrated that these antibodies, in many instances, recognized the equivalent protein in different species. In the past, considerable confusion was created because these surface markers were initially named according to the antibodies that reacted with them. To resolve this, a uniform nomenclature system was adopted, initially for human leukocytes. According to this system, a surface marker that identifies a particular lineage or differentiation stage, that has a defined structure, and that is recognized by a group ("cluster") of monoclonal antibodies is called a member of a cluster of differentiation (CD). Thus, all leukocyte surface antigens whose structures are defined are given a CD designation (e.g., CD1, CD2). Although this nomenclature was originally used for human leukocyte markers, it is now common practice to refer to homologous molecules in other species and on cells other than leukocytes by the same CD designation. Newly developed monoclonal antibodies are periodically exchanged among laboratories, and the antigens recognized are assigned to existing CD structures or introduced as new "workshop" candidates (CDw).

The classification of lymphocytes by CD antigen expression is now widely used in clinical medicine and experimental immunology. For instance, most helper T lymphocytes are $CD3^+CD4^+CD8^-$, and most CTLs are $CD3^+CD4^-CD8^+$. This has allowed immunologists to identify the cells participating in various immune responses, isolate them, and individually analyze their specificities, response patterns, and effector functions. Such antibodies have also been used to define specific alterations in particular subsets of lymphocytes that might be occurring in various diseases. For example, the declining number of blood $CD4^+$ T cells is often used to follow the progression of disease and response to treatment in human immunodeficiency virus–infected patients. Further investigations of the effects of monoclonal antibodies on lymphocyte function have shown that these surface proteins are not merely phenotypic markers but are themselves involved in a variety of lymphocyte responses. The two most frequent functions attributed to various CD molecules are (1) promotion of cell-cell interactions and adhesion and (2) transduction of signals that lead to lymphocyte activation. Examples of both types of functions are described throughout this book.

Development of Lymphocytes

Like all blood cells after birth, lymphocytes arise from stem cells in the bone marrow.

- The origin of lymphocytes from bone marrow progenitors was first demonstrated by experiments with radiation-induced bone marrow chimeras. Lymphocytes and their precursors are radiosensitive and are killed by high doses of γ-irradiation. If a mouse of one inbred strain is irradiated and then injected with bone marrow cells, or small numbers of hematopoietic stem cells (HSCs), of another strain that can be distinguished from the host, all the lymphocytes that develop subsequently are derived from the bone marrow cells or HSCs of the donor. Such approaches have proved useful for examining the maturation of lymphocytes and other blood cells (see Chapter 8).

All lymphocytes go through complex maturation stages during which they express antigen receptors and acquire the functional and phenotypic characteristics of mature cells (Fig. 3–2). B lymphocytes partially mature in the bone marrow, enter the circulation, and populate the peripheral lymphoid organs where they complete their maturation. T lymphocytes mature completely in the thymus, then enter the circulation and populate peripheral lymphoid tissues. We will discuss these processes of B and T lymphocyte maturation in much more detail in Chapter 8. These mature B and T cells are called **naive lymphocytes.** Upon activation by antigen,

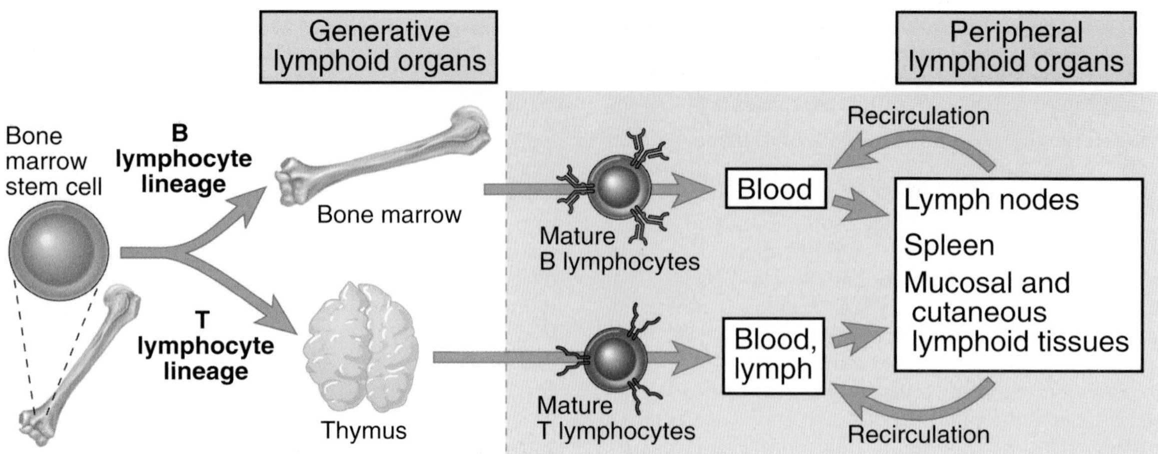

FIGURE 3–2 Maturation of lymphocytes. Mature lymphocytes develop from bone marrow stem cells in the generative lymphoid organs, and immune responses to foreign antigens occur in the peripheral lymphoid tissues.

lymphocytes go through sequential changes in phenotype and functional capacity.

Populations of Lymphocytes Distinguished by History of Antigen Exposure

In adaptive immune responses, naive lymphocytes that emerge from the bone marrow or thymus migrate into secondary lymphoid organs, where they are activated by antigens to proliferate and differentiate into effector and memory cells, some of which then migrate into tissues (Fig. 3–3). The activation of lymphocytes follows a series of sequential steps, beginning with the synthesis of new proteins, such as cytokine receptors and cytokines, which are required for many of the subsequent changes. The naive cells then undergo proliferation, resulting in increased size of the antigen-specific clones, a process that is called clonal expansion. In some infections, the numbers of microbe-specific T cells may increase more than 50,000-fold, and the numbers of specific B cells may increase more than 5000-fold. This rapid clonal expansion of microbe-specific lymphocytes is needed to keep pace with the ability of microbes to rapidly replicate and expand in numbers. Concomitant with clonal expansion, antigen-stimulated lymphocytes differentiate into effector cells, whose function is to eliminate the antigen. Some of the progeny of antigen-stimulated B and T lymphocytes differentiate into long-lived memory cells, whose function is to mediate rapid and enhanced (i.e., secondary) responses to subsequent exposures to antigens. Therefore, distinct populations of lymphocytes (naive, effector, memory) are always present in various sites throughout the body, and these populations can be distinguished by several functional and phenotypic criteria (Table 3–3). The details of lymphocyte activation and differentiation, as well as the functions of each of these populations, will be addressed later in this book. Here we will summarize the phenotypic characteristics of each population.

Naive Lymphocytes. Naive lymphocytes are mature T or B cell emigrants from generative lymphoid organs that have never encountered foreign antigen. They will die after 1 to 3 months if they do not recognize antigens. Naive and memory lymphocytes, discussed below, are both called resting lymphocytes, because they are not actively dividing, nor are they performing effector functions. Naive (and memory) B and T lymphocytes cannot be readily distinguished morphologically, and are both often called small lymphocytes when observed in blood smears or by flow cytometry (see Appendix III). A small lymphocyte is 8 to 10 μm in diameter and has a large nucleus with dense heterochromatin and a thin rim of cytoplasm that contains a few mitochondria, ribosomes, and lysosomes, but no visible specialized organelles (Fig. 3–4). Before antigenic stimulation, naive lymphocytes are in a state of rest, or in the G_0 stage of the cell cycle. In response to stimulation, they enter the G_1 stage of the cell cycle before going on to divide. Activated lymphocytes are larger (10 to 12 μm in diameter), have more cytoplasm and organelles and increased amounts of cytoplasmic RNA, and are called large lymphocytes, or lymphoblasts (see Fig. 3–4).

The survival of naive lymphocytes depends on engagement of antigen receptors, presumably by self antigens, and on cytokines. It is postulated that naive lymphocytes recognize various self antigens "weakly"—enough to generate survival signals, but without triggering the stronger signals that are needed to initiate clonal expansion and differentiation into effector cells.

- The need for antigen receptor expression to maintain the pool of naive lymphocytes in peripheral lymphoid organs has been demonstrated by studies in mice in which the immunoglobulin (Ig) genes that encode the antigen receptors of B cells were knocked out after the B cells had matured, or the antigen receptors of T cells were knocked out in mature T cells. (The method used is called the cre-lox technique and is described

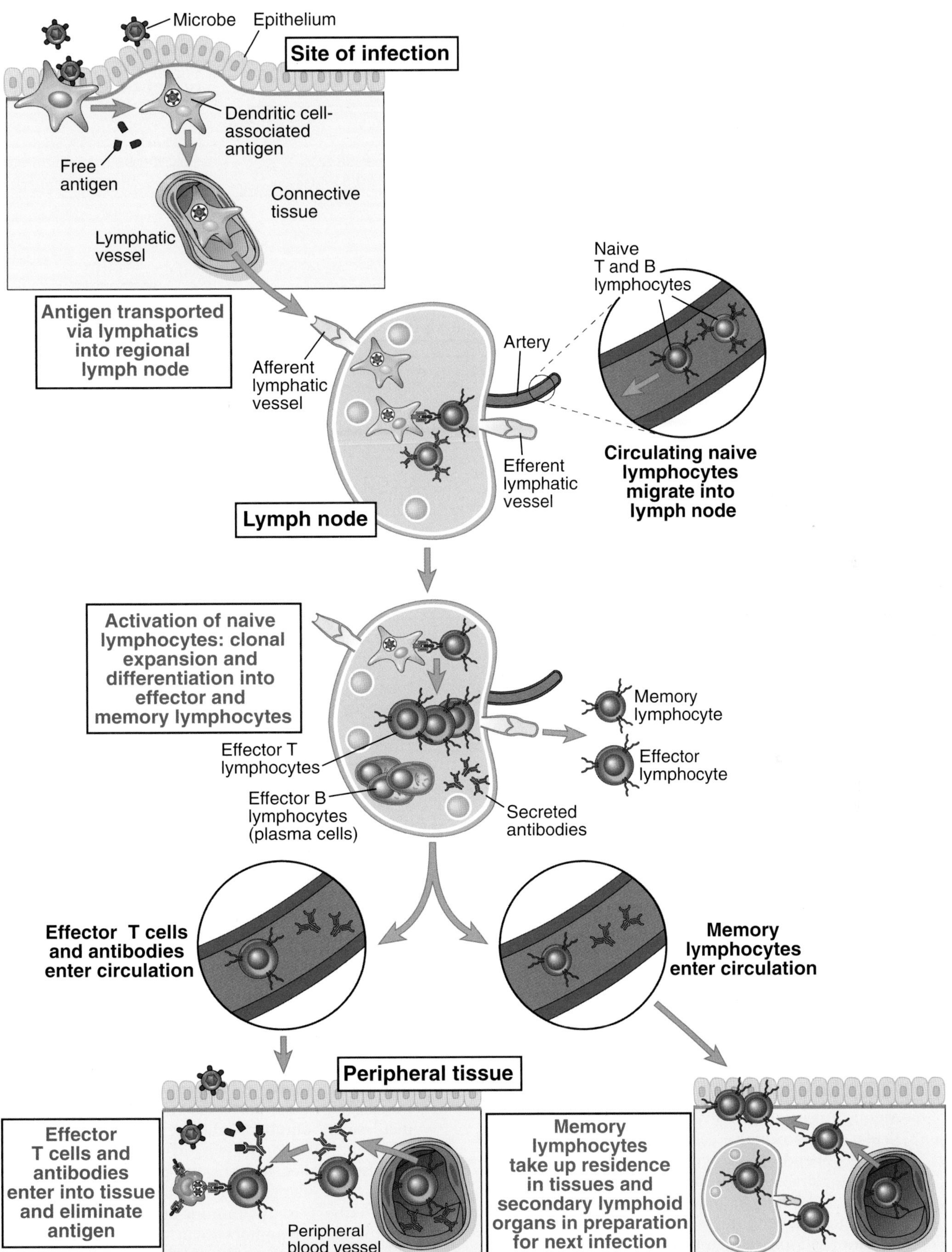

FIGURE 3–3 The anatomy of lymphocyte activation. Naive T cells emerging from the thymus and naive B cells emerging from the bone marrow migrate into secondary lymphoid organs, including lymph nodes and spleen. In these locations, they are activated by antigens, and differentiation into effector and memory lymphocytes. Some effector and memory lymphocytes migrate into peripheral tissue sites of infection.

Table 3–3. Characteristics of Naive, Effector, and Memory Lymphocytes

	Naive lymphocytes	Activated or effector lymphocytes	Memory lymphocytes
T lymphocytes			
Migration	Preferentially to peripheral lymphoid tissues	Preferentially to inflamed tissues	Preferentially to inflamed tissues, mucosal tissues
Frequency of cells responsive to particular antigen	Very low	High	Low
Effector functions	None	Cytokine secretion; cytotoxic activity	None
Cell cycling	No	Yes	+/–
Surface protein expression			
High-affinity IL-2 receptor	Low	High	Low
Peripheral lymph node homing receptor (L-selectin, CD62L)	High	Low	Low or variable
Adhesion molecules: integrins, CD44	Low	High	High
Chemokine receptor: CCR7	High	Low	Variable
Major CD45 isoform (humans only)	CD45RA	CD45RO	CD45RO; variable
Morphology	Small; scant cytoplasm	Large; more cytoplasm	Small
B lymphocytes			
Membrane immunoglobulin (Ig) isotype	IgM and IgD	Frequently IgG, IgA, IgE	Frequently IgG, IgA, IgE
Affinity of Ig produced	Relatively low	Increases during immune response	Relatively high
Effector function	None	Antibody secretion	None
Morphology	Small; scant cytoplasm	Large; more cytoplasm; some are plasma cells	Small
Chemokine receptor: CXCR5	High	Low	?
CD27	Low	High	High

Abbreviations: IL-2, interleukin-2

in Appendix III.) Mature naive lymphocytes that lost their antigen receprs died within 2 or 3 weeks.

- Among T cells, there is evidence that survival of particular clones of naive cells in peripheral lymphoid organs depends on recognition of the same ligands that the clones saw during their maturation in the thymus. In Chapter 8, we will discuss the process of T cell maturation and the selection of T cells by recognition of self antigens in the thymus. This selection process ensures that the cells that mature are capable of surviving in peripheral tissues by recognizing the selecting self antigens.

- If naive lymphocytes are transferred into a mouse that does not have any lymphocytes of its own, the transferred lymphocytes begin to proliferate and increase in number until they reach roughly the numbers of lymphocytes in normal mice. This process is called homeostatic proliferation because it serves to maintain homeostasis (a steady state of cell numbers) in the immune system. This proliferation of naive lymphocytes in the absence of overt exposure to antigen is triggered by the recognition of self antigens.

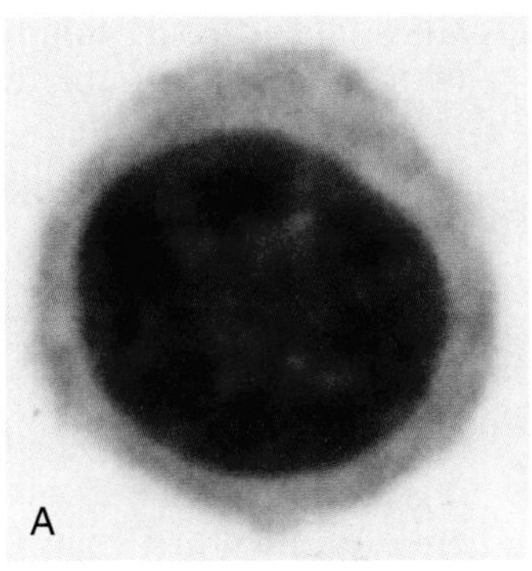

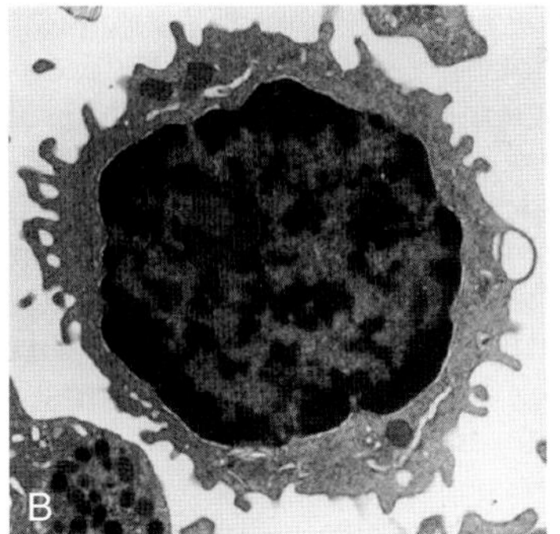

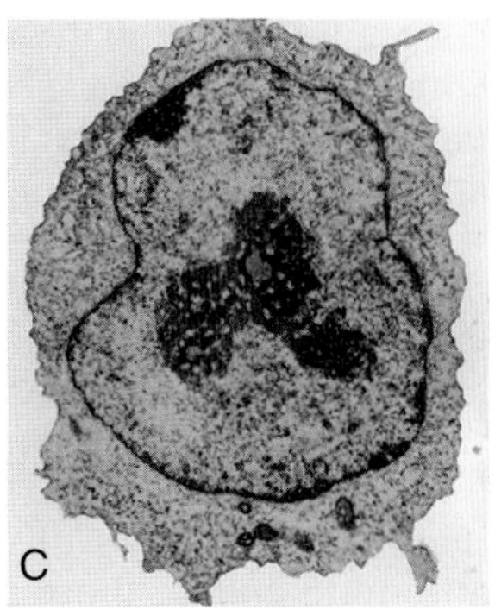

FIGURE 3–4 Morphology of lymphocytes. A. Light micrograph of a lymphocyte in a peripheral blood smear. B. Electron micrograph of a small lymphocyte. (Courtesy of Dr. Noel Weidner, Department of Pathology, University of California, San Diego.) C. Electron micrograph of a large lymphocyte (lymphoblast). (From Fawcett DW. Bloom & Fawcett's Textbook of Histology, 12th ed. Chapman & Hall, 1994. With kind permission of Springer Science and Business Media.)

Secreted proteins called cytokines are also essential for the survival of naive lymphocytes, and naive T and B cells constitutively express receptors for these cytokines. Among these cytokines are interleukin-7 (IL-7), which promotes survival and, perhaps, low-level cycling of naive T cells, and B cell activating factor (BAFF), which is required for naive B cell survival. Naive lymphocytes also express surface proteins that are involved in directing migration into lymph nodes, as we will discuss in detail later in this chapter.

Effector Cells. After naive lymphocytes are activated, they become larger and proliferate, and are called lymphoblasts. Some of these cells differentiate into effector lymphocytes have the ability to produce molecules capable of eliminating foreign antigens; effector lymphocytes include helper T cells, CTLs, and antibody-secreting B cells. Helper T cells, which are usually $CD4^+$, express surface molecules such as CD40 ligand (CD154) and secrete cytokines that interact with macrophages and B lymphocytes, leading to their activation. Differentiated CTLs contain cytoplasmic granules containing proteins that kill virus-infected and tumor cells. Both $CD4^+$ and $CD8^+$ effector T cells usually express surface proteins indicative of recent activation, including CD25 (a component of the receptor for the T cell growth factor IL-2), and class II major histocompatability complex (MHC) molecules (in humans, but not mice). A subset of $CD4^+$ T cells called regulatory T cells, which are distinct from and suppress effector T cells, constitutively express CD25 (discussed in Chapter 11). The majority of differentiated effector T lymphocytes are short lived and not self-renewing.

Many antibody-secreting B cells are morphologically identifiable as **plasma cells.** They have characteristic nuclei, abundant cytoplasm containing dense, rough endoplasmic reticulum that is the site where antibodies (and other secreted and membrane proteins) are synthesized, and distinct perinuclear Golgi complexes where antibody molecules are converted to their final forms and packaged for secretion (Fig. 3–5). It is estimated that half or more of the messenger RNA in plasma cells codes for antibody proteins. Plasma cells develop in lymphoid organs and at sites of immune responses and often migrate to the bone marrow, where some of them may survive for long periods after the immune response is induced and even after the antigen is eliminated.

Memory Cells. Memory cells may survive in a functionally quiescent or slowly cycling state for many years after the antigen is eliminated. They can be identified by their expression of surface proteins that distinguish them from naive and recently activated effector lymphocytes, although it is still not clear which of these surface proteins are definitive markers of memory populations (see Table 3–3). Memory B lymphocytes express certain classes (isotypes) of membrane Ig, such as IgG, IgE, or IgA, as a result of isotype switching, whereas naive B cells express only IgM and IgD (see Chapters 4 and 10). In humans, CD27 expression is a good marker for memory B cells. Memory T cells, like naive but not effector T cells, express high levels of IL-7 receptors. Memory T cells also express surface molecules that promote their migration into sites of infection anywhere in the body (discussed later in the chapter). In humans, most naive T cells express a 200-kD isoform of a surface molecule called CD45 that contains a segment encoded by an exon designated A. This CD45 isoform can be recognized by antibodies specific for the A-encoded segment and is therefore called CD45RA (for "restricted A"). In contrast, most activated and memory T cells express a 180-kD isoform of CD45 in which the A exon RNA has been spliced out; this isoform is called CD45RO. However, this way of distinguishing naive from memory T cells is not perfect, and interconversion between $CD45RA^+$ and $CD45RO^+$ populations has been documented. Memory T

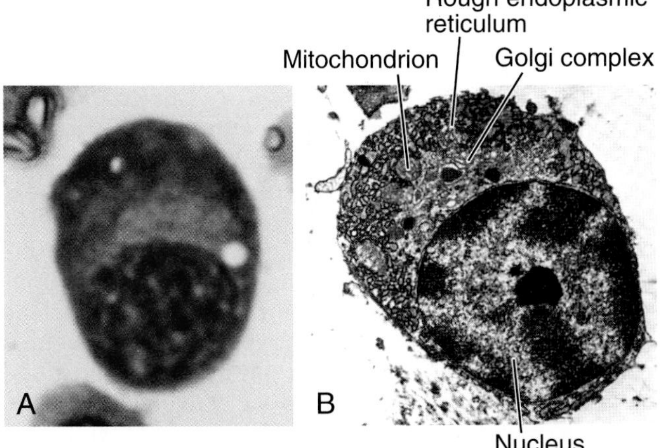

FIGURE 3–5 Morphology of plasma cells. A. Light micrograph of a plasma cell in tissue. B. Electron micrograph of a plasma cell. (Courtesy of Dr. Noel Weidner, Department of Pathology, University of California, San Diego, California.)

cells appear to be heterogeneous in many respects. Some, called central memory T cells, migrate preferentially to lymph nodes, where they provide a pool of antigen-specific lymphocytes that can rapidly be activated to proliferate and differentiate into effector cells if the antigen is reintroduced. Others, called effector memory cells, reside in mucosal tissues or circulate in the blood, from where they may be recruited to any site of infection and mount rapid effector responses that serve to eliminate the antigen. The migration of memory T cells is discussed later in this chapter, and more details about the generation of memory cells, and the signals for their maintenance, are discussed in Chapters 10 and 13.

Antigen-Presenting Cells

APCs are cell populations that are specialized to capture microbial and other antigens, display them to lymphocytes, and provide signals that stimulate the proliferation and differentiation of the lymphocytes. By convention, *APC* usually refers to a cell that displays antigens to T lymphocytes. The major type of APC that is involved in initiating T cell responses is the dendritic cell. Macrophages present antigens to T cells during cell-mediated immune responses, and B lymphocytes function as APCs for helper T cells during humoral immune responses. A specialized cell type called the follicular dendritic cell (FDC) displays antigens to B lymphocytes during particular phases of humoral immune responses. APCs link responses of the innate immune system to responses of the adaptive immune system, and therefore they may be considered as components of both systems. In addition to the introduction presented here, APC function will be described in more detail in Chapter 6.

Dendritic Cells

Dendritic cells play important roles in innate immunity to microbes and in antigen capture and the induction of T lymphocyte responses to protein antigens. Dendritic cells arise from bone marrow precursors, mostly of the monocyte lineage, and are found in many organs, including epithelial barrier tissues, where they are poised to capture foreign antigens and transport these antigens to peripheral lymphoid organs. They have long cytoplasmic projections, which effectively increases their surface area, and they actively sample and internalize components of the extracellular tissue environment by pinocytosis and phagocytosis. In addition, dendritic cells express various surface receptors, such as Toll-like receptors (see Chapter 2), that recognize pathogen-associated molecular patterns and transduce activating signals into the cell. Once activated, dendritic cells become mobile and migrate to regional lymphoid tissues, where they participate in presenting peptides derived from internalized protein antigens to T lymphocytes. These activated dendritic cells also express molecules, called costimulators, which function in concert with antigen to stimulate T cells.

Mononuclear Phagocytes

Mononuclear phagocytes function as APCs in T cell–mediated adaptive immune responses. We introduced mononuclear phagocytes (monocytes and macrophages) in the context of innate immune responses in Chapter 2. Macrophages containing ingested microbes display microbial antigens to differentiated effector T cells. The effector T cells then activate the macrophages to kill the microbes. This process is a major mechanism of cell-mediated immunity against intracellular microbes (see Chapter 13).

Mononuclear phagocytes are also important effector cells in both innate and adaptive immunity. Their effector functions in innate immunity are to phagocytose microbes and to produce cytokines that recruit and activate other inflammatory cells (see Chapter 2). Macrophages serve numerous roles in the effector phases of adaptive immune responses. As mentioned above, in cell-mediated immunity, antigen-stimulated T cells activate macrophages to destroy phagocytosed microbes. In humoral immunity, antibodies coat, or opsonize, microbes and promote the phagocytosis of the microbes through macrophage surface receptors for antibodies (see Chapter 14).

Follicular Dendritic Cells (FDC)

FDCs are cells with membranous projections, which are present intermingled in specialized collections of activated B cells, called germinal centers, found in the lymphoid follicles of the lymph nodes, spleen, and mucosal lymphoid tissues. FDCs are not derived from precursors in the bone marrow and are unrelated to the dendritic cells that present antigens to T lymphocytes. FDCs trap antigens complexed to antibodies or complement products and display these antigens on their surfaces for recognition by B lymphocytes. This is important for the selection of activated B lymphocytes whose antigen receptors bind the displayed antigens with high affinity (see Chapter 10).

Anatomy and Functions of Lymphoid Tissues

To optimize the cellular interactions necessary for the recognition and activation phases of specific immune responses, lymphocytes and APCs are localized and concentrated in anatomically defined tissues or organs, which are also the sites where foreign antigens are transported and concentrated. Such anatomic compartmentalization is not fixed because, as we will discuss later in this chapter, many lymphocytes recirculate and constantly exchange between the circulation and the tissues.

Lymphoid tissues are classified as generative organs, also called primary lymphoid organs, where lympho-

cytes first express antigen receptors and attain phenotypic and functional maturity, and as peripheral organs, also called secondary lymphoid organs, where lymphocyte responses to foreign antigens are initiated and develop (see Fig. 3–2). Included in the generative lymphoid organs of adult mammals are the bone marrow, where all the lymphocytes arise and B cells mature, and the thymus, where T cells mature and reach a stage of functional competence. The peripheral lymphoid organs and tissues include the lymph nodes, spleen, cutaneous immune system, and mucosal immune system. In addition, poorly defined aggregates of lymphocytes are found in connective tissue and in virtually all organs except the central nervous system.

Bone Marrow

The bone marrow is the site of generation of all circulating blood cells in the adult, including immature lymphocytes, and is the site of early events in B cell maturation. During fetal development, the generation of all blood cells, called **hematopoiesis** (Fig. 3–6), occurs initially in blood islands of the yolk sac and the para-aortic mesenchyme and later in the liver and spleen. This function is taken over gradually by the bone marrow and increasingly by the marrow of the flat bones so that, by puberty, hematopoiesis occurs mostly in the sternum, vertebrae, iliac bones, and ribs. The red marrow that is found in these bones consists of a sponge-like reticular framework located between long trabeculae. The spaces in this framework are filled with fat cells, stromal fibroblasts, and precursors of blood cells. These precursors mature and exit through the dense network of vascular sinuses to enter the vascular circulation. When the bone marrow is injured or when an exceptional demand for production of new blood cells occurs, the liver and spleen can be recruited as sites of extramedullary hematopoiesis.

All the blood cells originate from a common **hematopoietic stem cell** that becomes committed to differentiate along particular lineages (i.e., erythroid, megakaryocytic, granulocytic, monocytic, and lymphocytic) (see Fig. 3–6). Stem cells lack the markers of differentiated blood cells and instead express two proteins called CD34 and stem cell antigen-1 (Sca-1). These markers are used to identify and enrich stem cells from suspensions of bone marrow or peripheral blood cells for transplantation to reconstitute the hematopoietic system. The proliferation and maturation of precursor cells in the bone marrow are stimulated by cytokines. Many of these cytokines are called colony-stimulating factors because they were originally assayed by their ability to stimulate the growth and development of various leukocytic or erythroid colonies from marrow cells. These molecules are discussed in Chapter 12. Hematopoietic cytokines are produced by stromal cells and macrophages in the bone marrow, thus providing the local environment for hematopoiesis. They are also produced by antigen-stimulated T lymphocytes and

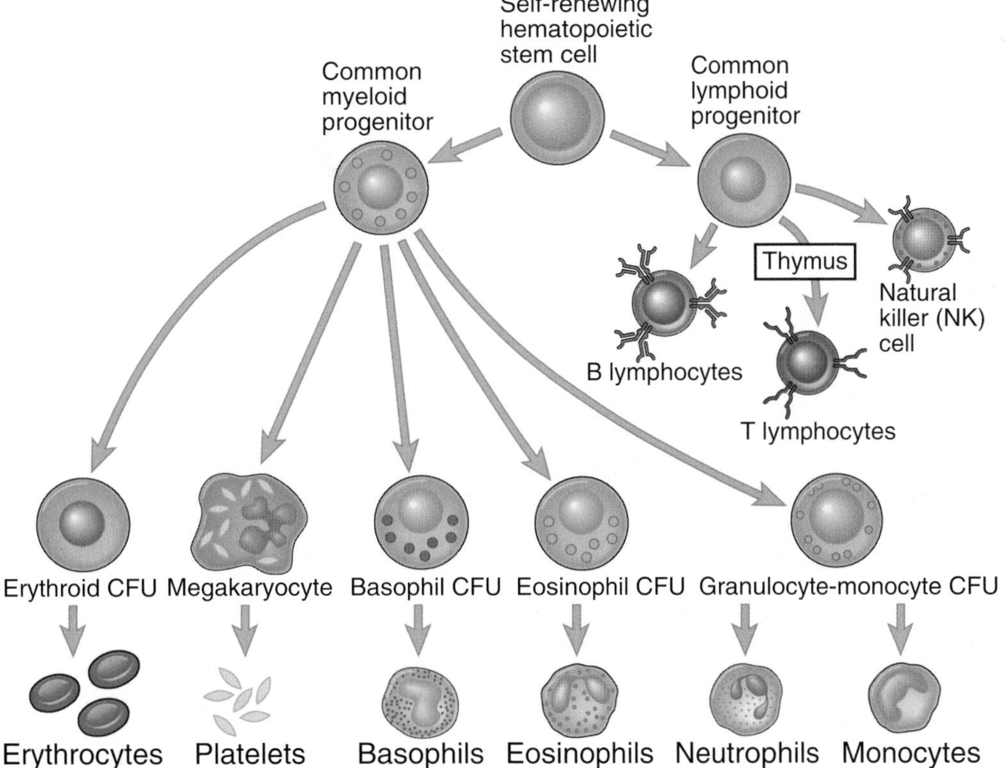

FIGURE 3–6 Hematopoiesis. The development of the different lineages of blood cells is depicted in this "hematopoietic tree." The roles of cytokines in hematopoiesis are illustrated in Chapter 12, Figure 12–15. CFU, colony-forming unit.

cytokine-activated or microbe-activated macrophages, providing a mechanism for replenishing leukocytes that may be consumed during immune and inflammatory reactions.

In addition to self-renewing stem cells and their differentiating progeny, the marrow contains numerous antibody-secreting plasma cells. These plasma cells are generated in peripheral lymphoid tissues as a consequence of antigenic stimulation of B cells and then migrate to the marrow, where they may live and continue to produce antibodies for many years. Some long-lived memory T lymphocytes also migrate to and may reside in the bone marrow.

Thymus

The thymus is the site of T cell maturation. The thymus is a bilobed organ situated in the anterior mediastinum. Each lobe is divided into multiple lobules by fibrous septa, and each lobule consists of an outer cortex and an inner medulla (Fig. 3–7). The cortex contains a dense collection of T lymphocytes, and the lighter-staining medulla is more sparsely populated with lymphocytes. Scattered throughout the thymus are nonlymphoid epithelial cells, which have abundant cytoplasm, as well as bone marrow–derived macrophages and dendritic cells. In the medulla are structures called Hassall's corpuscles, which are composed of tightly packed whorls of epithelial cells that may be remnants of degenerating cells. The thymus has a rich vascular supply and efferent lymphatic vessels that drain into mediastinal lymph nodes. The thymus is derived from invaginations of the ectoderm in the developing neck and chest of the embryo, forming structures called branchial clefts. Humans with DiGeorge syndrome suffer from T cell deficiency because of mutations in genes required for thymus development. In the "nude" mouse strain, which has been widely used in immunology research, a mutation in the gene encoding a transcription factor causes a failure of differentiation of certain types of epithelial cells that are required for normal development of the thymus and hair follicles. Consequently, these mice lack T cells and hair (see Chapter 20).

The lymphocytes in the thymus, also called **thymocytes,** are T lymphocytes at various stages of maturation. In general, the most immature cells of the T cell lineage enter the thymic cortex through the blood vessels. Maturation begins in the cortex, and as thymocytes mature, they migrate toward the medulla, so that the medulla contains mostly mature T cells. Only mature T cells exit the thymus and enter the blood and peripheral lymphoid tissues. The details of thymocyte maturation are described in Chapter 8.

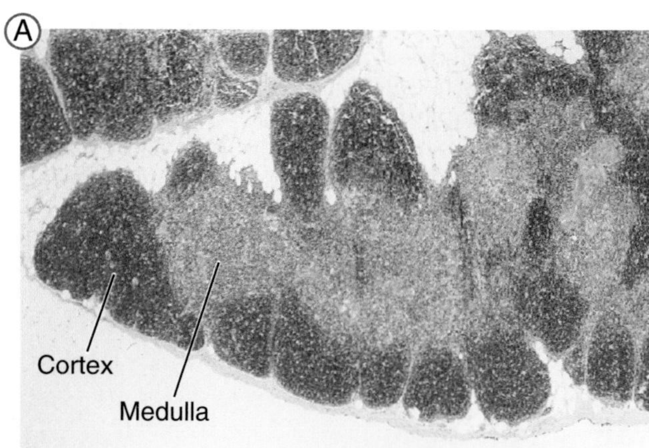

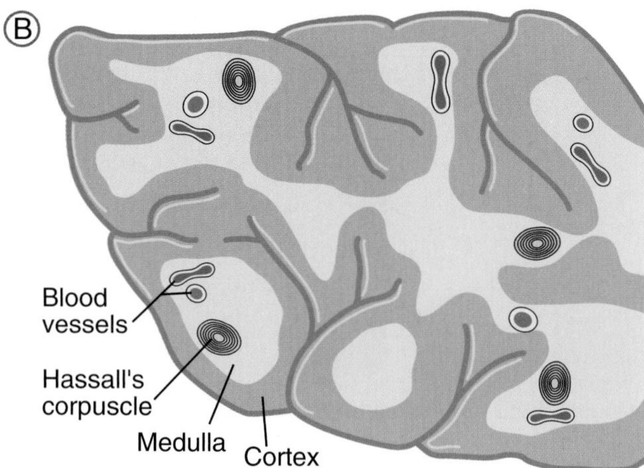

FIGURE 3–7 Morphology of the thymus. A. Light micrograph of a lobe of the thymus showing the cortex and medulla. The blue-stained cells are developing T cells called thymocytes. (Courtesy of Dr. James Gulizia, Department of Pathology, Brigham and Women's Hospital, Boston.) B. Schematic diagram of the thymus illustrating a portion of a lobe divided into multiple lobules by fibrous trabeculae.

Lymph Nodes and the Lymphatic System

Antigens are transported to lymph nodes mainly in lymphatic vessels. The skin, epithelia, and parenchymal organs contain numerous lymphatic capillaries that absorb and drain fluid from spaces between tissue cells (made of plasma filtrate) (Fig. 3–8). The absorbed interstitial fluid, called **lymph,** flows through the lymphatic capillaries into convergent, ever larger lymphatic vessels. These vessels merge into afferent lymph vessels that drain into the subcapsular sinuses of lymph nodes. Lymphatic vessels that carry lymph into a lymph node are referred to as afferent, and vessels that drain the lymph from the node are called efferent. Because lymph nodes are connected in series along the lymphatics, an efferent lymphatic exiting one node may serve as the afferent vessel for another. The efferent lymph vessel at the end of a lymph node chain joins other lymph vessels, eventually culminating into one large lymphatic vessel called the thoracic duct. Lymph from the thoracic duct is emptied into the superior vena cava, thus returning the fluid to the blood stream. About 2 L of lymph are normally returned to the circulation each day, and disruption of the lymphatic system may lead to rapid tissue swelling.

The function of collecting antigens from their portals of entry and delivering them to lymph nodes is performed largely by the lymphatic system. Microbes enter

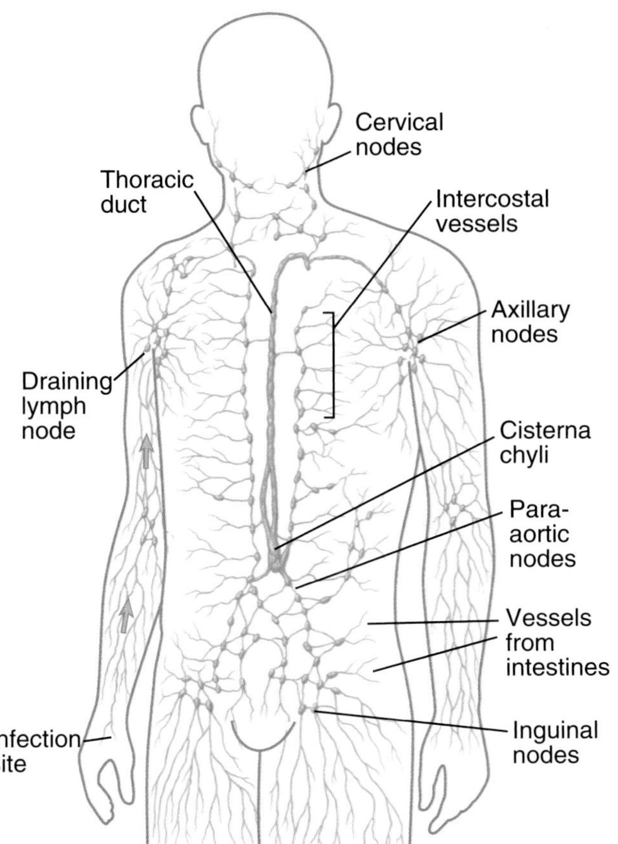

FIGURE 3–8 The lymphatic system. The major lymphatic vessels and collections of lymph nodes are illustrated. Antigens are captured from a site of infection, and the draining lymph node to which these antigens are transported and where the immune response is initiated.

the body most often through the skin and the gastrointestinal and respiratory tracts. All these tissues are lined by epithelia that contain dendritic cells, and all are drained by lymphatic vessels. The dendritic cells capture some microbial antigens and enter lymphatic vessels. Other antigens enter the lymphatics in cell-free form. In addition, soluble inflammatory mediators, such as chemokines, produced at sites of infection enter the lymphatics. The lymph nodes are interposed along lymphatic vessels and act as filters that sample the lymph before it reaches the blood. In this way, antigens captured from the portals of entry are transported to lymph nodes, and molecular signals of inflammation are also delivered to the draining lymph nodes.

Lymph enters a lymph node via an afferent lymphatic vessel into the subcapsular sinus, and tissue-derived dendritic cells within the lymph then leave the sinus and enter the paracortex. In this new location, the dendritic cells can present antigens derived from the tissue to naive T cells and initiate adaptive immune responses (see Chapter 6). The mechanisms by which the dendritic cells gain access to the paracortex are not well understood. Some of the lymph from the subcapsular sinus is channeled through specialized conduits that run through the paracortical T cell zone toward specialized vessels called high endothelial venules (HEV) (see Fig. 3–9B). These conduits are organized around collagen-containing reticular fibers and are delimited by basement membrane–like matrix molecules and a sheath of specialized cells called fibroblastic reticular cells. Dendritic cells that are resident in the lymph node are also closely associated with the conduits. The conduit system serves several functions. It provides a direct route for delivery of lymph-borne chemokines that are produced in inflamed tissues, such as CCL2, to the HEV, where they contribute to the regulation of leukocyte recruitment into the lymph node. The specialized lining of the conduit serves as a selective filtration barrier, allowing only some molecules of particular size or chemical properties to enter the T cell zones of the node. The resident dendritic cells lining the conduits sample cell-free protein antigens transported through the conduits, so that these antigens may be processed and presented to T cells in the adjacent paracortex.

Adaptive immune responses to antigens that enter through epithelia or are found in tissues are initiated in lymph nodes. Lymph nodes are small nodular organs situated along lymphatic channels throughout the body. A lymph node consists of an outer cortex and an inner medulla. As described earlier, each lymph node is surrounded by a fibrous capsule that is pierced by numerous afferent lymphatics, which empty the lymph into a subcapsular or marginal sinus (Fig. 3–9). The lymph percolates through the cortex into the medullary sinus and leaves the node through the efferent lymphatic vessel in the hilum. Beneath the subcapsular sinus, the outer cortex contains aggregates of cells called follicles. Some follicles contain central areas called **germinal centers,** which stain lightly with commonly used histologic stains. Follicles without germinal centers are called primary follicles, and those with germinal centers are secondary follicles. The cortex around the follicles is called the parafollicular cortex or paracortex, and is organized into cords, which are regions containing reticular fibers, lymphocytes, dendritic cells, and mononuclear phagocytes, arranged around lymphatic and vascular sinusoids. Lymphocytes and APCs in these cords are often found near one another, but there is significant movement of these cells relative to one another. Internal to the cortex is the medulla, consisting of medullary cords separated by a labyrinthine arrangement of sinuses that drain into fibroblastic reticular cell conduits, and eventually into a main medullary sinus. These medullary cords are populated by macrophages and plasma cells. Blood is delivered to a lymph node by an artery that enters through the hilum and branches into capillaries in the outer cortex, and it leaves the node by a single vein that exits through the hilum.

Different classes of lymphocytes are sequestered in distinct regions of the cortex of lymph nodes (Fig. 3–10). Follicles are the B cell zones of lymph nodes. Primary follicles contain mostly mature, naive B lymphocytes. Germinal centers develop in response to antigenic stimulation. They are sites of remarkable B cell proliferation, selection of B cells producing high-affinity antibodies, and generation of memory B cells. The processes of

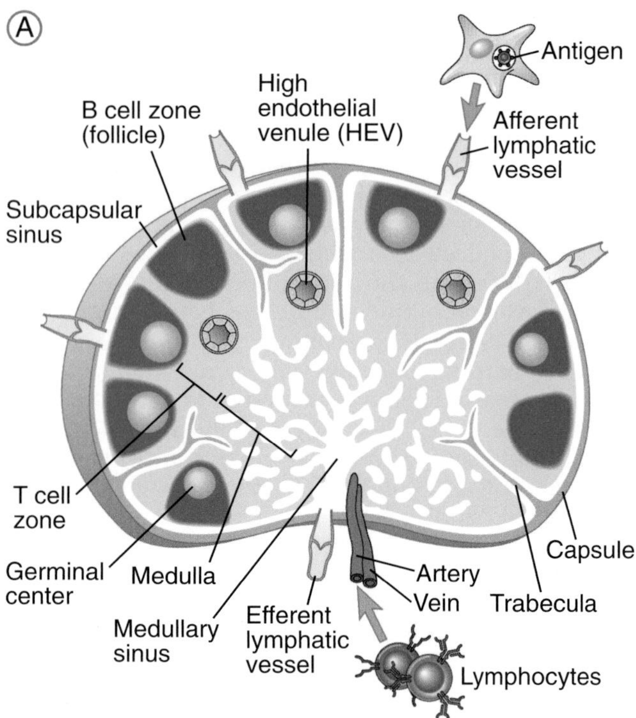

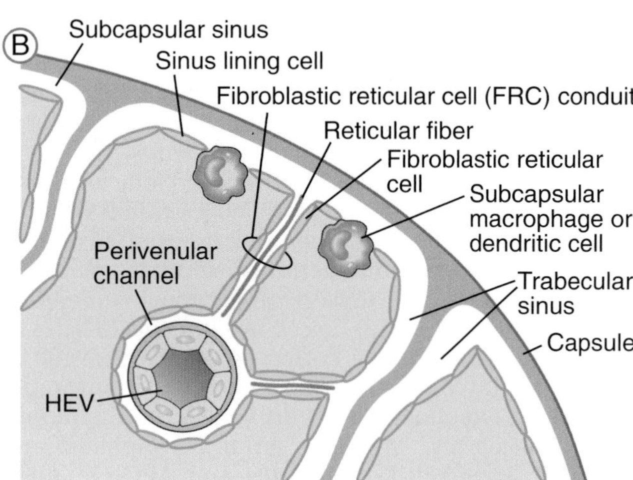

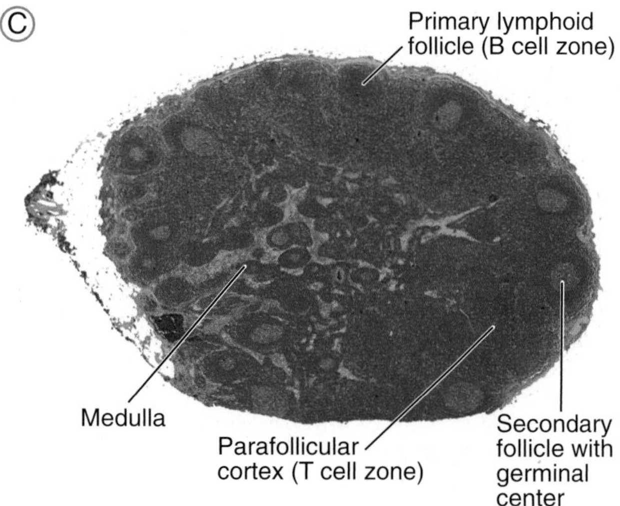

FDCs interdigitate to form a dense reticular network in the germinal centers. The T lymphocytes are located mainly beneath and more centrally to the follicles, in the paracortical cords. Most (~70%) of these T cells are $CD4^+$ helper T cells, intermingled with relatively sparse $CD8^+$ cells. These proportions can change dramatically during the course of an infection. For example, during a viral infection, there may be a marked increase in $CD8^+$ T cells. Dendritic cells are also concentrated in the paracortex of the lymph nodes.

The anatomic segregation of different classes of lymphocytes in distinct areas of the node is dependent on cytokines (see Fig. 3–10). Naive T and B lymphocytes enter the node through an artery. These cells leave the circulation and enter the stroma of the node through specialized vessels called high endothelial venules (HEVs, described in more detail later), which are located in the center of the cortical cords. The naive T cells express a receptor called CCR7 that binds the CCL19 and CCL21 chemokines produced in the T cell zones of the lymph node. **Chemokines** (chemoattractant cytokines) include a large family of 8- to 10-kDa proteins that are involved in a wide variety of cell motility functions in development, maintenance of tissue architecture, and immune and inflammatory responses. Chemokines exert their biologic effects by binding to chemokine receptors, which are cell surface, G protein–linked receptors that are linked to various signal transduction pathways. The general properties of chemokines and chemokine receptors are discussed in detail in Chapter 12. CCL 19 and CCL21 attract the naive T cells into the T cell zone. Dendritic cells also express CCR7, and this is why they migrate to the same area of the node as do naive T cells (see Chapter 6). Naive B cells express another chemokine receptor, CXCR5, which recognizes a chemokine CXCL13 produced only in follicles. Thus, B cells are attracted into the follicles, which are the B cell zones of lymph nodes. Another cytokine, called lymphotoxin, plays a role in stimulating CXCL13 production, especially in the follicles. The functions of various cytokines in directing the movement of lymphocytes in lymphoid organs and in the formation of these organs have been established by numerous studies in mice.

- Knockout mice lacking the membrane form of the cytokine lymphotoxin (LTβ) or the LTβ receptor show

FIGURE 3–9 Morphology of a lymph node. A. Schematic diagram of a lymph node illustrating the T cell–rich and B cell–rich zones and the routes of entry of lymphocytes and antigen (shown captured by a dendritic cell). B. Schematic of the microanatomy of a lymph node depicting the route of lymph drainage from the subcapsular sinus, through fibroreticular cell conduits, to the perivenular channel around the HEV. C. Light micrograph of a lymph node illustrating the T cell and B cell zones. (Courtesy of Dr. James Gulizia, Department of Pathology, Brigham and Women's Hospital, Boston, Massachusetts.)

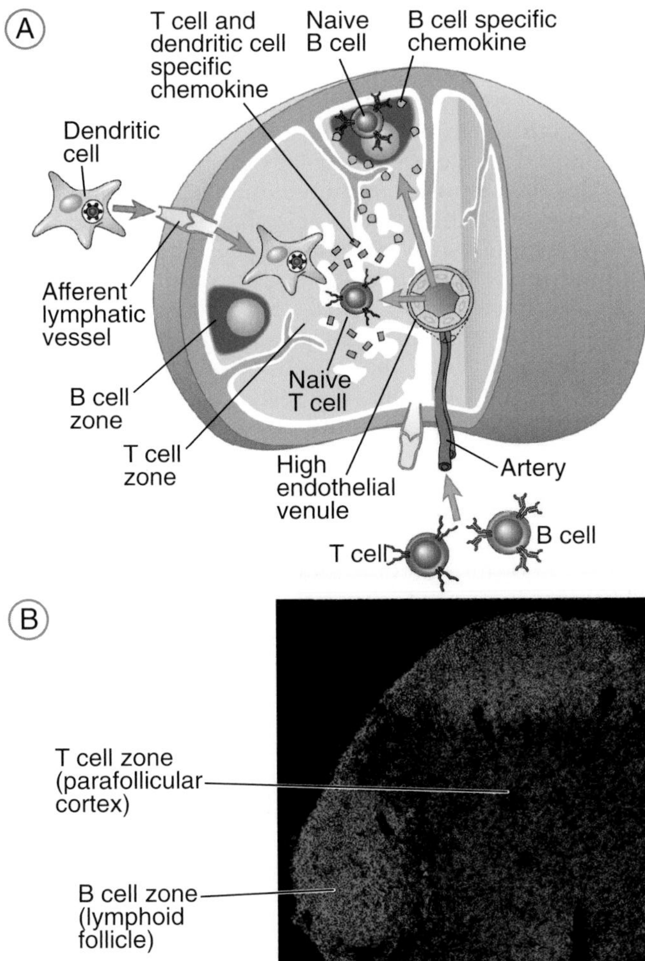

FIGURE 3–10 Segregation of B cells and T cells in a lymph node. A. The schematic diagram illustrates the path by which naive T and B lymphocytes migrate to different areas of a lymph node. The lymphocytes enter through an artery and reach an HEV, shown in cross-section, from where naive lymphocytes are drawn to different areas of the node by chemokines that are produced in these areas and bind selectively to either cell type. Also shown is the migration of dendritic cells, which pick up antigens from the sites of antigen entry, enter through afferent lymphatic vessels, and migrate to the T cell–rich areas of the node. B. In this section of a lymph node, the B lymphocytes, located in the follicles, are stained green; the T cells, in the parafollicular cortex, are red. The method used to stain these cells is called immunofluorescence (see Appendix III for details). (Courtesy of Drs. Kathryn Pape and Jennifer Walter, University of Minnesota School of Medicine, Minneapolis.) The anatomic segregation of T and B cells is also seen in the spleen (see Fig. 3–11).

absence of peripheral lymph nodes and a marked disorganization of the architecture of the spleen, with loss of the segregation of B and T cells.

- Overexpression of lymphotoxin or tumor necrosis factor (TNF) in an organ, either as a transgene in experimental animals or in response to chronic inflammation in humans, can lead to the formation in that organ of lymph node–like structures that contain B cell follicles with FDCs and interfollicular T cell–rich areas containing mature dendritic cells.
- CXCR5 knockout mice lack B cell zones in lymph nodes and spleen. Similarly, CCR7 knockout mice lack T cell zones.

The anatomic segregation of T and B cells ensures that each lymphocyte population is in close contact with the appropriate APCs (i.e., T cells with dendritic cells and B cells with FDCs). Furthermore, because of this precise segregation, B and T lymphocyte populations are kept apart until it is time for them to interact in a functional way. As we will see in Chapter 10, after stimulation by antigens, T and B cells lose their anatomic constraints and begin to migrate toward one another. Activated T cells may either migrate toward follicles to help B cells or exit the node and enter the circulation, whereas activated B cells migrate into germinal centers and, following differentiation into plasma cells, they may home to the bone marrow.

Spleen

The spleen is the major site of immune responses to blood-borne antigens. The spleen, an organ weighing about 150 g in adults, is located in the left upper quadrant of the abdomen. It is supplied by a single splenic artery, which pierces the capsule at the hilum and divides into progressively smaller branches that remain surrounded by protective and supporting fibrous trabeculae (Fig. 3–11). The lymphocyte-rich regions of the spleen, called the white pulp, are organized around branches of these arteries, called central arteries. The architecture of the white pulp is analogous to the organization of lymph nodes, with segregated T cell and B cell zones. In mouse spleen, the central arteries are surrounded by cuffs of lymphocytes, most of which are T cells. Because of their anatomic location, morphologists call these areas **periarteriolar lymphoid sheaths.** Several smaller branches of each central arteriole pass through the periarteriolar lymphoid sheaths and drain into a vascular sinus known as the **marginal sinus.** B cell–rich follicles occupy the space between the marginal sinus and the periarteriolar sheath. Outside the marginal sinus is a distinct region called the **marginal zone,** which forms the outer boundary of the white pulp and is populated by B cells and specialized macrophages. The B cells in the marginal zone are functionally distinct from follicular B cells and are known as marginal zone B cells. The architecture of the white pulp is more complex in humans than in mice, with both inner and outer marginal zones, and a perifollicular zone. The segregation of T lymphocytes in the periarteriolar lymphoid sheaths, and B cells in follicles and marginal zones, is a highly regulated process, dependent on the production of different cytokines and chemokines by the stromal cells in these different areas, analogous to the case for lymph nodes. The chemokine CXCL13 and its receptor CXCR5 are required for B cell migration into the follicles, and CCL19 and CCL21 and their receptor CCR7 are required for naive T cell migration into the periarteriolar sheath. The production of these chemokines by non-lymphoid stromal cells is stimulated by the cytokine lymphotoxin.

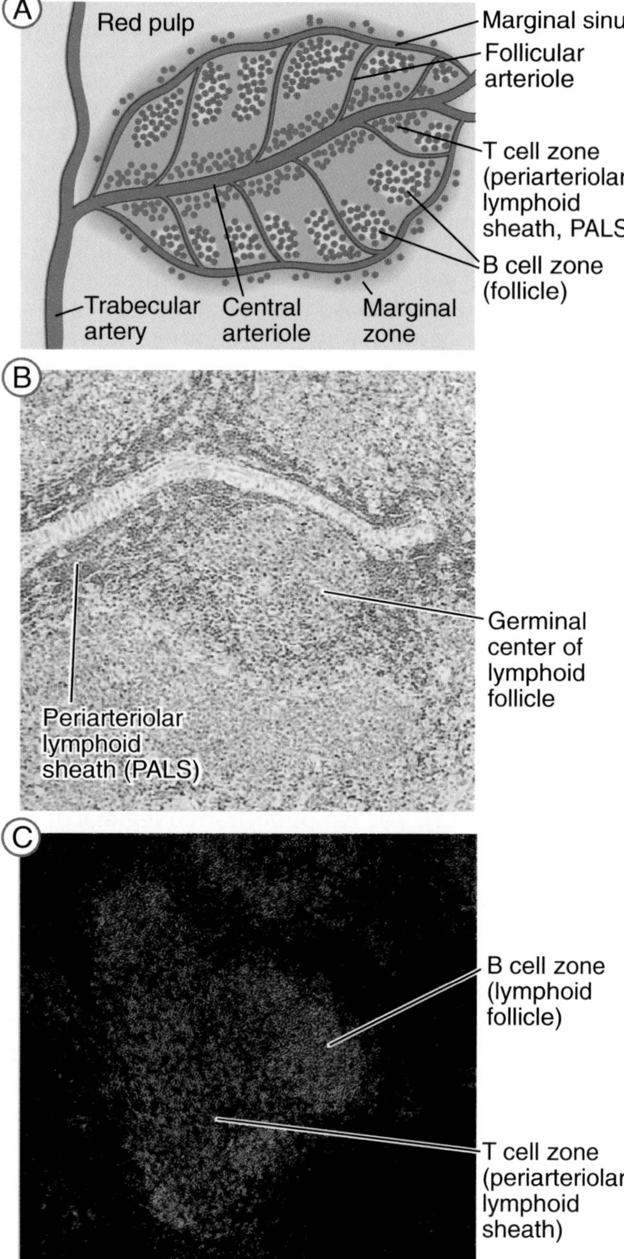

FIGURE 3–11 Morphology of the spleen. A. Schematic diagram of the spleen illustrating T cell and B cell zones, which make up the white pulp. B. Photomicrograph of a section of human spleen showing a trabecular artery with adjacent periarteriolar lymphoid sheath and a lymphoid follicle with a germinal center. Surrounding these areas is the red pulp, rich in vascular sinusoids. C. Immunohistochemical demonstration of T cell and B cell zones in the spleen, shown in a cross-section of the region around an arteriole. T cells in the periarteriolar lymphoid sheath are stained red, and B cells in the follicle are stained green. (Courtesy of Drs. Kathryn Pape and Jennifer Walter, University of Minnesota School of Medicine, Minneapolis, Minnesota.)

The function of the white pulp is to promote adaptive immune responses to blood-borne antigens. These antigens are delivered into the marginal sinus by circulating dendritic cells, or are sampled by the macrophages in the marginal zone. The anatomic arrangements of the APCs, B cells, and T cells promotes the interactions required for the efficient development of humoral immune responses, as will be discussed in Chapter 10.

The spleen is also an important filter for the blood. Some of the arteriolar branches of the splenic artery ultimately end in extensive vascular sinusoids, distinct from the marginal sinuses, scattered among which are large numbers of erythrocytes, macrophages, dendritic cells, sparse lymphocytes, and plasma cells; these constitute the **red pulp.** The sinusoids end in venules that drain into the splenic vein, which carries blood out of the spleen and into the portal circulation. Red pulp macrophages clear the blood of microbes, and of damaged red blood cells. The spleen is the major site for the phagocytosis of antibody-coated (opsonized) microbes. Individuals lacking a spleen are highly susceptible to infections with encapsulated bacteria such as pneumococci and meningococci because such organisms are normally cleared by opsonization and phagocytosis, and this function is defective in the absence of the spleen.

Cutaneous Immune System

The skin contains a specialized cutaneous immune system consisting of lymphocytes and APCs. The skin is the largest organ in the body and is an important physical barrier between an organism and its external environment. In addition, the skin is an active participant in host defense, with the ability to generate and support local immune and inflammatory reactions. Many foreign antigens gain entry into the body through the skin, and this tissue is the site of many immune responses.

The principal cell populations within the epidermis are keratinocytes, melanocytes, epidermal Langerhans cells, and intraepithelial T cells (Fig. 3–12). Keratinocytes produce several cytokines that may contribute to innate immune reactions and cutaneous inflammation. Langerhans cells, located in the suprabasal portion of the epidermis, are the immature dendritic cells of the cutaneous immune system. Langerhans cells form an almost continuous meshwork that enables them to capture antigens that enter through the skin. When Langerhans cells encounter microbes, they are activated by engagement of Toll-like receptors (Chapter 2). The cells lose their adhesiveness for the epidermis, enter lymphatic vessels, begin to express the CCR7 chemokine receptor, and migrate to the T cell zones of draining lymph nodes in response to chemokines produced in that location. The Langerhans cells also mature into efficient APCs. This process is described in more detail in Chapter 6.

Intraepidermal lymphocytes constitute only about 2% of skin-associated lymphocytes (the rest reside in the dermis), and the majority are $CD8^+$ T cells. Intraepidermal T cells may express a more restricted set of antigen receptors than do T lymphocytes in most extracutaneous tissues. In mice (and some other species), many intraepidermal lymphocytes are T cells that express an

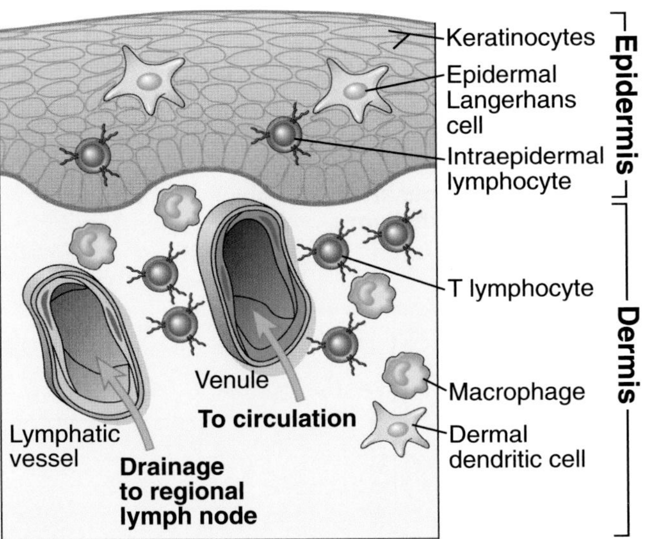

FIGURE 3–12 Cellular components of the cutaneous immune system. The major components of the cutaneous immune system shown in this schematic diagram include keratinocytes, Langerhans cells, and intraepidermal lymphocytes, all located in the epidermis, and T lymphocytes and macrophages, located in the dermis.

uncommon type of T cell antigen receptor (TCR) formed by γ and δ chains instead of the usual α and β chains of the antigen receptors of CD4$^+$ and CD8$^+$ T cells (see Chapter 7). As we shall discuss shortly, this is also true of intraepithelial lymphocytes in the intestine, raising the possibility that γδ T cells, at least in some species, may be uniquely committed to recognizing microbes that are commonly encountered at epithelial surfaces. However, neither the specificity nor the function of this T cell subpopulation is clearly defined.

The dermis, which is composed of connective tissue, contains T lymphocytes (both CD4$^+$ and CD8$^+$ cells), predominantly in a perivascular location, and scattered macrophages. This is essentially similar to connective tissues in other organs. The T cells usually express phenotypic markers typical of activated or memory cells. It is not clear whether these cells reside permanently within the dermis or are merely in transit between blood and lymphatic capillaries as part of memory T cell recirculation (described later).

Mucosal Immune System

The mucosal surfaces of the gastrointestinal and respiratory tracts are colonized by lymphocytes and APCs that are involved in immune responses to ingested and inhaled antigens. Like the skin, these mucosal epithelia are barriers between the internal and external environments and are therefore an important site of entry of microbes. Much of our knowledge of mucosal immunity is based on studies of the gastrointestinal tract, and this is emphasized in the discussion that follows. In comparison, little is known about immune responses in the respiratory mucosa, even though the airways are a major portal of antigen entry. It is likely, however, that the features of immune responses are similar in all mucosal lymphoid tissues.

In the mucosa of the gastrointestinal tract, lymphocytes are found in large numbers in three main regions: within the epithelial layer, scattered throughout the lamina propria, and in organized collections in the lamina propria, including **Peyer's patches** (Fig. 3–13). Cells at each site have distinct phenotypic and functional characteristics. The majority of intraepithelial lymphocytes are T cells. In humans, most of these are CD8$^+$ cells. In mice, about 50% of intraepithelial lymphocytes express the γδ form of the TCR, similar to intraepidermal lymphocytes in the skin. In humans, only about 10% of intraepithelial lymphocytes are γδ cells, but this proportion is still higher than the proportions of γδ cells found among T cells in other tissues. Both the αβ and the γδ TCR-expressing intraepithelial lymphocytes show limited diversity of antigen receptors. All these findings support the idea that mucosal intraepithelial lymphocytes have a limited range of specificity, distinct from that of most T cells and this restricted repertoire may have evolved to recognize commonly encountered intraluminal antigens.

The intestinal lamina propria contains a mixed population of cells. These include T lymphocytes, most of which are CD4$^+$ and have the phenotype of activated cells. It is likely that T cells initially recognize and respond to antigens in mesenteric lymph nodes draining the intestine and migrate back to the intestine to populate the lamina propria. This is similar to the postulated origin of T cells in the dermis of the skin. The lamina propria also contains large numbers of activated B lymphocytes and plasma cells as well as macrophages, dendritic cells, eosinophils, and mast cells.

In addition to scattered lymphocytes, the mucosal immune system contains organized lymphoid tissues, the most prominent of which are the Peyer's patches of the small intestine. Like lymphoid follicles in the spleen and lymph nodes, the central regions of these mucosal follicles are B cell–rich areas that often contain germinal centers. Peyer's patches also contain small numbers of CD4$^+$ T cells, mainly in the interfollicular regions. In adult mice, 50% to 70% of Peyer's patch lymphocytes are B cells, and 10% to 30% are T cells. Some of the epithelial cells overlying Peyer's patches are specialized M (membranous) cells. M cells lack microvilli, are actively pinocytic, and transport macromolecules from the intestinal lumen into subepithelial tissue by a mechanism of transepithelial transport known as transcytosis. They are thought to play an important role in delivering antigens to Peyer's patches. Follicles similar to Peyer's patches are abundant in the appendix and are found in smaller numbers in much of the gastrointestinal and respiratory tracts. Pharyngeal tonsils are also mucosal lymphoid follicles analogous to Peyer's patches. Because of the vast size of the mucosal tissues, a large portion of the body's lymphocytes are normally present in these tissues.

Immune responses to oral antigens differ in some fundamental respects from responses to antigens encountered at other sites. The two most striking differences are the high levels of IgA antibody production associated with mucosal tissues (see Chapter 14) and the tendency of oral immunization with protein antigens

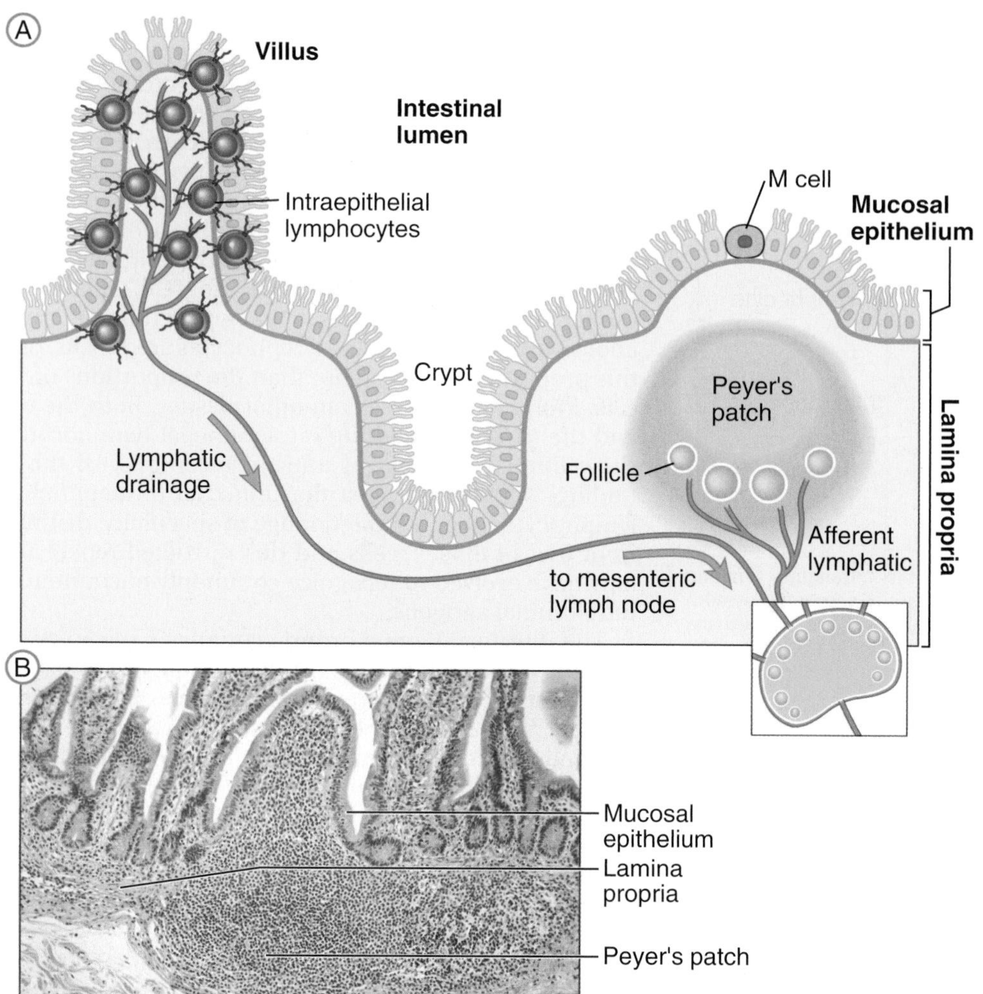

FIGURE 3–13 The mucosal immune system. A. Schematic diagram of the cellular components of the mucosal immune system in the intestine. B. Photomicrograph of mucosal lymphoid tissue in the human intestine. Similar aggregates of lymphoid tissue are found throughout the gastrointestinal tract and the respiratory tract.

to induce T cell tolerance rather than activation (see Chapter 11).

Pathways and Mechanisms of Lymphocyte Recirculation and Homing

Lymphocytes are continuously moving through the blood stream, lymphatics, secondary lymphoid tissues, and peripheral nonlymphoid tissues, and functionally distinct populations of lymphocytes show different trafficking patterns through these sites (Fig. 3–14). Naive lymphocytes will move from the blood stream into lymph nodes, and via lymphatics back into the blood stream many times, until they encounter an antigen they recognize within a lymph node. This traffic pattern of naive lymphocytes, called **lymphocyte recirculation,** enables the limited number of naive lymphocytes that are specific for a particular foreign antigen to search for that antigen throughout the body. Lymphocytes that have reacted to that antigen and differentiated into effector and memory cells within secondary lymphoid tissues may move back into the blood stream and then migrate into sites of infection and/or inflammation in peripheral (nonlymphoid) tissues. Some effector lymphocyte subsets will preferentially migrate into a particular tissue, such as skin or gut. The process by which particular populations of lymphocytes selectively enter lymph nodes or some tissues but not others is called lymphocyte **homing.** The existence of different homing patterns ensures that different subsets of lymphocytes are delivered to the tissue microenvironments where they are required for adaptive immune responses and not, wastefully, to places where they would serve no purpose. In the following section, we describe the mechanisms and pathways of lymphocyte recirculation and homing. Our discussion emphasizes T cells because much more is known about their movement through tissues than is known about B cell recirculation.

The mechanisms of lymphocyte migration out of blood vessels into the extravascular sites in lymph nodes or peripheral tissues are fundamentally similar to the mechanisms of migration of other leukocytes into inflammatory sites, described in Chapter 2. The adhesion molecules involved include selectins, integrins, and members of the Ig superfamily. The adhesion molecules expressed on lymphocytes are often called

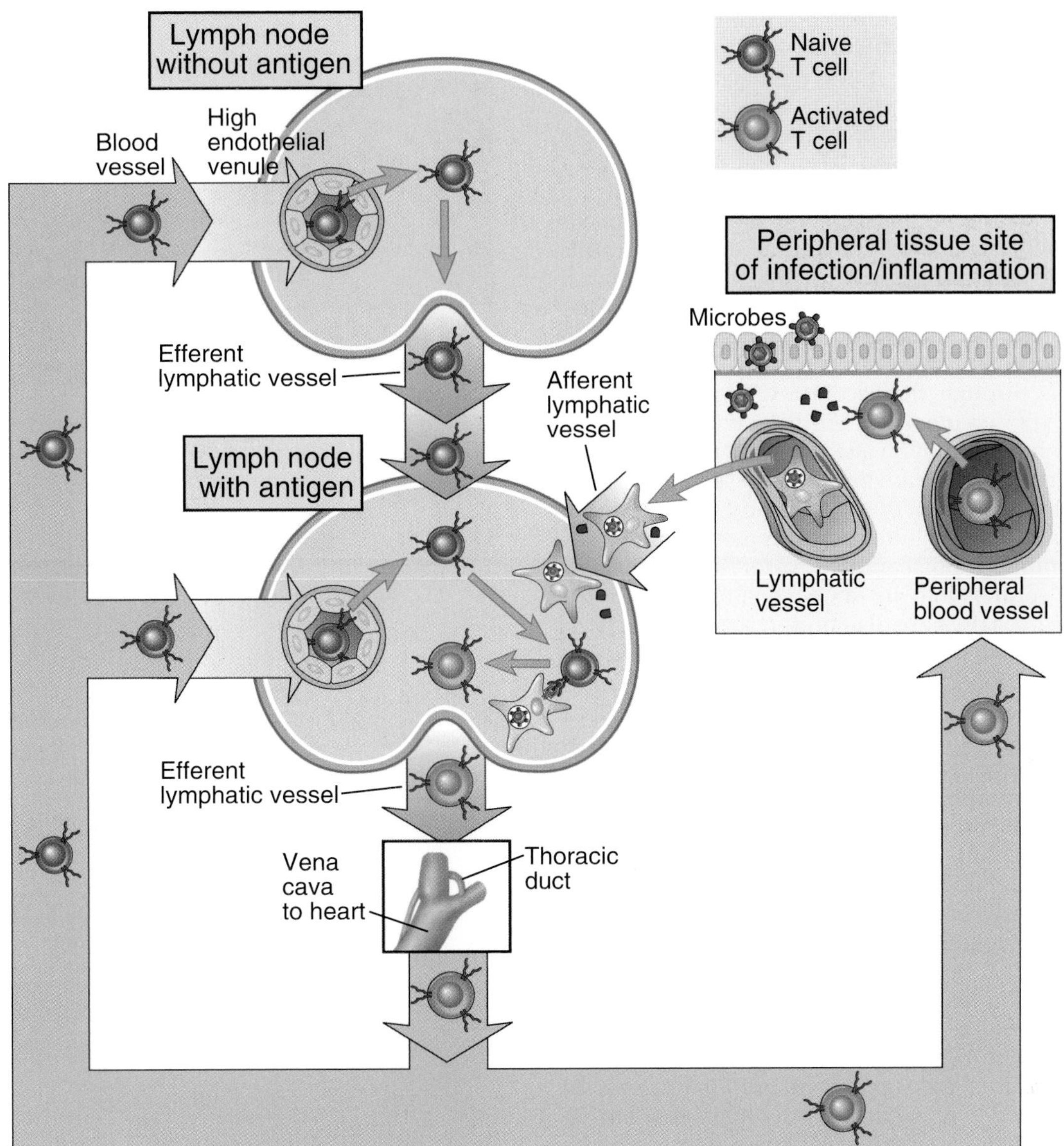

FIGURE 3–14 Pathways of T lymphocyte recirculation. Naive T cells preferentially leave the blood and enter lymph nodes across the HEVs. Dendritic cells bearing antigen enter the lymph node through lymphatic vessels. If the T cells recognize antigen, they are activated, and they return to the circulation through the efferent lymphatics and the thoracic duct, which empties into the superior vena cava, then into the heart, and ultimately into the arterial circulation. Effector and memory T cells preferentially leave the blood and enter peripheral tissues through venules at sites of inflammation. Recirculation through peripheral lymphoid organs other than lymph nodes is not shown.

homing receptors, and the adhesion molecules that the homing receptors bind to on the endothelial cells are often called addressins. Chemokines influence lymphocyte adhesion to endothelial cells and various aspects of movement of the lymphocytes through the vessel wall and in the extravascular space. Chemokines involved in lymphocyte traffic are produced constitutively in secondary lymphoid organs and inducibly at sites of infection. Adhesion to and detachment from extracellular matrix components within tissues determine how long lymphocytes are retained at a particular extravascular site before they return through the lymphatics to the blood.

Recirculation of Naive T Lymphocytes Between Blood and Secondary Lymphoid Organs

Specific homing of naive T cells to lymph nodes and mucosal lymphoid tissues occurs through specialized postcapillary venules and involves several different adhesion molecules and chemokines. The homing mechanisms are very efficient, resulting in a net flux of lymphocytes through lymph nodes of up to 25×10^9 cells each day (i.e., each lymphocyte goes through a node once a day on the average). Peripheral tissue inflammation causes a significant increase in T cell influx into lymph nodes draining the site of inflammation, while egress of the T cells into efferent lymphatics is transiently reduced. The mechanism of this transient retention involves innate immune system cytokines interferon-α and -β, which inhibit the function of sphingosine 1-phosphate receptor-1 (S1P1), described later. The net result is a rapid increase in the number of naive T cells that are retained in a lymph node draining a site of infection or inflammation. Antigens are concentrated in the secondary lymphoid organs, including lymph nodes, mucosal lymphoid tissues, and spleen, where they are presented by mature dendritic cells, the APCs that are best able to initiate responses of naive T cells. Thus, movement of naive T cells through the secondary lymphoid organs maximizes the chances of specific encounter with antigen and initiation of an adaptive immune response.

Naive T lymphocytes are delivered to secondary lymphoid tissues via arterial blood flow, and they leave the circulation and migrate into the stroma of lymph nodes through modified postcapillary venules called **high endothelial venules** that are lined by plump endothelial cells (Fig. 3–15). HEVs are also present in mucosal lymphoid tissues, such as Peyer's patches in the gut, but not in the spleen. HEVs display certain adhesion molecules and chemokines on their surfaces, discussed below, which support the selective homing of only certain populations of lymphocytes. The development and maintenance of the morphologic and molecular phenotype of HEVs depend on soluble factors present in lymph. In addition, certain cytokines, such as lymphotoxin, are required for HEV development. In fact, HEVs may develop in extralymphoid sites of chronic inflammation where such cytokines are produced for prolonged periods of time.

Migration of naive T cells out of the blood into lymph node parenchyma is a multi-step process consisting of selectin-mediated rolling of the cells, integrin-mediated firm adhesion, and transmigration through the vessel wall. This sequence of events for T lymphocyte homing is similar to migration of other leukocytes into peripheral inflamed tissues discussed in Chapter 2. Different selectins and integrins are involved in the migration of naive and activated lymphocytes to different tissues (Fig. 3–16). The rolling of naive T cells on HEVs in peripheral lymphoid organs is mediated by L-selectin on the lymphocytes binding to its peripheral node addressin (PNAd) on HEVs. (Selectins are described in Box 2–2, Chapter 2.) The carbohydrate groups that bind L-selectin may be attached to different sialomucins on the endothelium in different tissues. For example, on lymph node HEVs, the PNAd is displayed by two sialomucins, called GlyCAM-1 (glycan-bearing cell adhesion molecule-1) and CD34. In Peyer's patches in the intestinal wall, the L-selectin ligand is a molecule called MadCAM-1 (mucosal addressin cell adhesion molecule-1). The subsequent firm adhesion of the T cells to the HEVs is mediated by integrins, mainly LFA-1 and VLA-4 (see Box 2–3, Chapter 2). The affinity of the integrins is rapidly increased by two chemokines, called CCL19 and CCL21, which are produced mainly in lymphoid tissues. CCL19 is constitutively produced by HEV and is bound to glycosaminoglycans on the cell surface for display to rolling

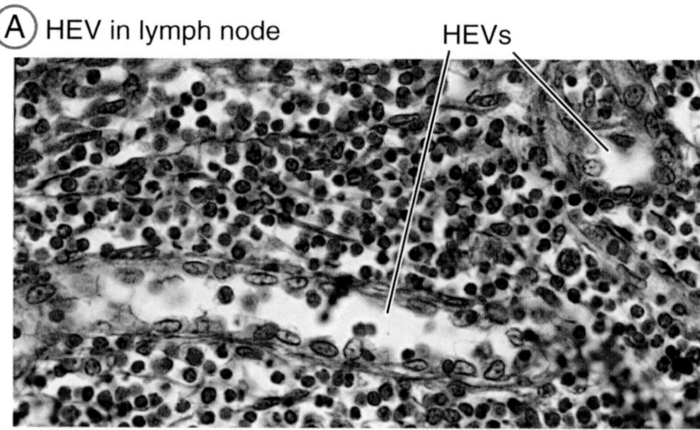

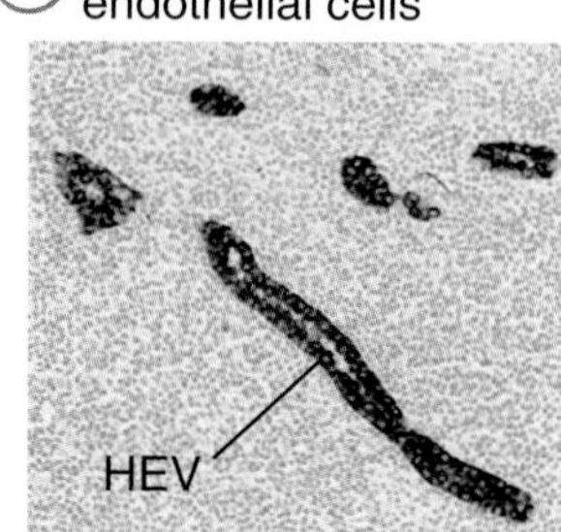

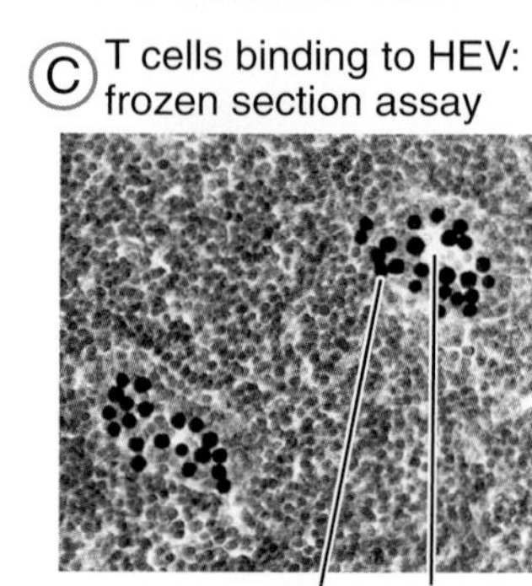

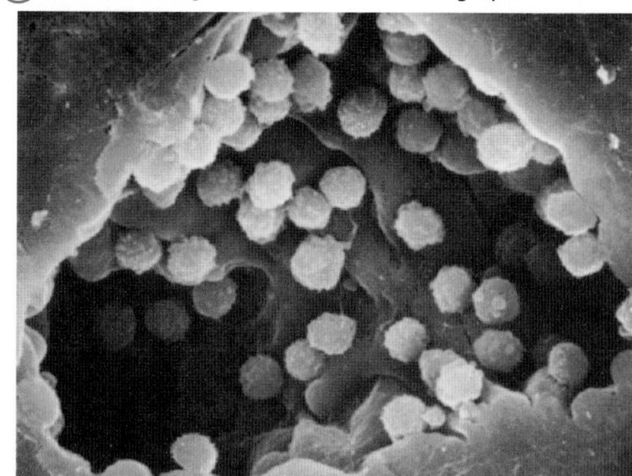

FIGURE 3–15 High endothelial venules. A. Light micrograph of an HEV in a lymph node illustrating the tall endothelial cells. (Courtesy of Dr. Steve Rosen, Department of Anatomy, University of California, San Francisco.) B. Expression of L-selectin ligand on HEVs, stained with a specific antibody by the immunoperoxidase technique. (The location of the antibody is revealed by a brown reaction product of peroxidase, which is coupled to the antibody; see Appendix III for details.) The HEVs are abundant in the T cell zone of the lymph node. (Courtesy of Drs. Steve Rosen and Akio Kikuta, Department of Anatomy, University of California, San Francisco.) C. A binding assay in which lymphocytes are incubated with frozen sections of a lymph node. The lymphocytes (stained dark blue) bind selectively to HEVs. (Courtesy of Dr. Steve Rosen, Department of Anatomy, University of California, San Francisco.) D. Scanning electron micrograph of an HEV with lymphocytes attached to the luminal surface of the endothelial cells. (Courtesy of J. Emerson and T. Yednock, University of California San Francisco School of Medicine, San Francisco. From Rosen SD, and LM Stoolman. Potential role of cell surface lectin in lymphocyte recirculation. *In* Olden K, and J Parent (eds). Vertebrate Lectins. Van Nostrand Reinhold, New York, 1987.)

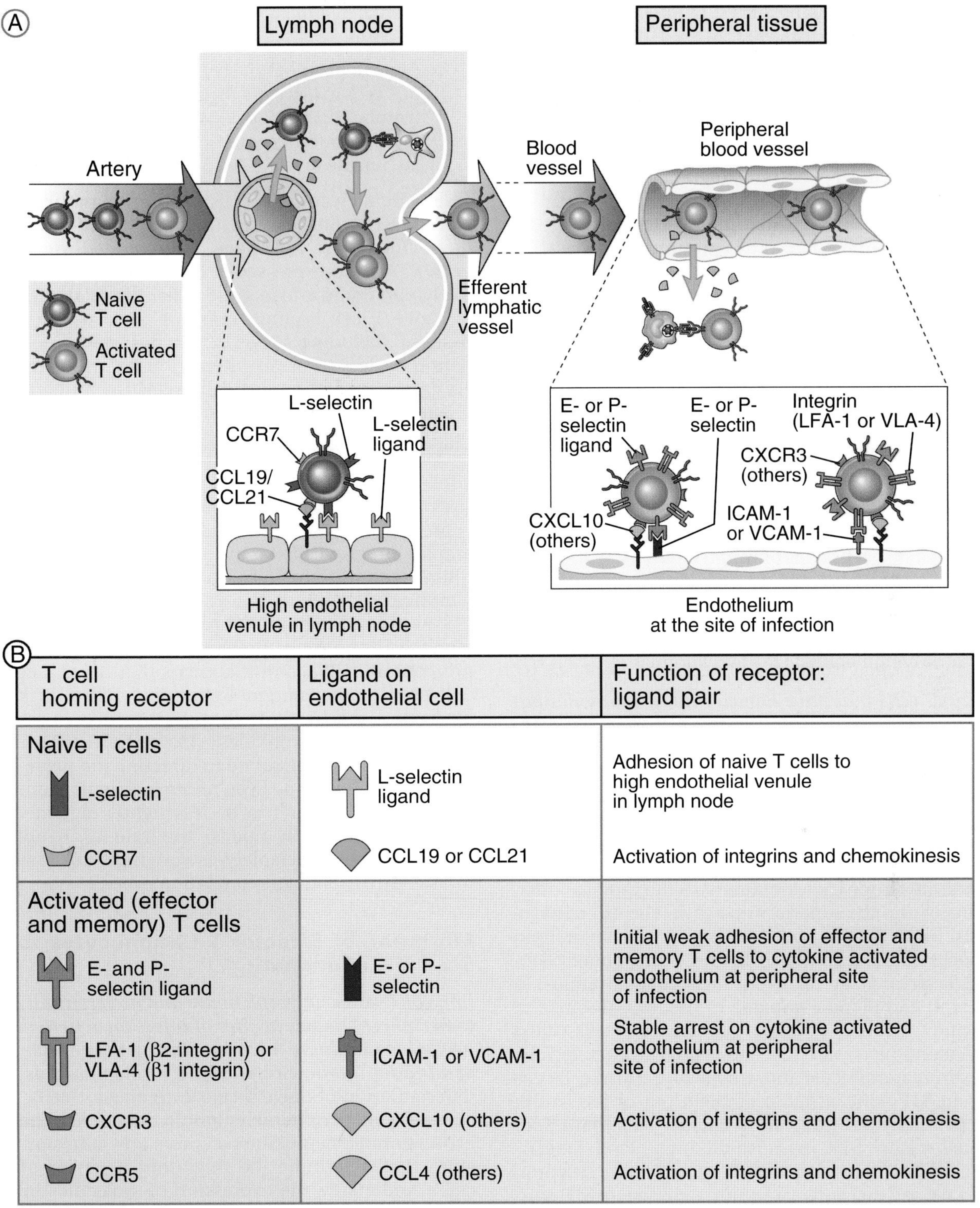

T cell homing receptor	Ligand on endothelial cell	Function of receptor: ligand pair
Naive T cells		
L-selectin	L-selectin ligand	Adhesion of naive T cells to high endothelial venule in lymph node
CCR7	CCL19 or CCL21	Activation of integrins and chemokinesis
Activated (effector and memory) T cells		
E- and P- selectin ligand	E- or P- selectin	Initial weak adhesion of effector and memory T cells to cytokine activated endothelium at peripheral site of infection
LFA-1 (β2-integrin) or VLA-4 (β1 integrin)	ICAM-1 or VCAM-1	Stable arrest on cytokine activated endothelium at peripheral site of infection
CXCR3	CXCL10 (others)	Activation of integrins and chemokinesis
CCR5	CCL4 (others)	Activation of integrins and chemokinesis

FIGURE 3–16 Migration of naive and effector T lymphocytes. A. Naive T lymphocytes home to lymph nodes as a result of L-selectin binding to its ligand on HEVs, which are present only in lymph nodes, and as a result of binding chemokines (CCL19 and CCL21) displayed on the surface of the HEV. Activated T lymphocytes, including effector cells, home to sites of infection in peripheral tissues, and this migration is mediated by E- and P-selectins and integrins, and chemokines that are produced at sites of infection. Additional chemokines and chemokine receptors, besides the ones shown, are involved in effector/memory T cell migration. B. The adhesion molecules, chemokines, and chemokine receptors involved in naive and effector/memory T cell migration are described.

lymphocytes. CCL21 is produced by other cell types in the lymph node and displayed by the HEV in the same fashion as CCL19. Both these chemokines bind to the chemokine receptor called CCR7, which is highly expressed on naive lymphocytes. This interaction of the chemokines with CCR7 ensures that naive T cells increase integrin avidity and are able to adhere firmly to HEVs. The final step of transmigration of the firmly attached lymphocytes through the vessel wall occurs in response to the same CCR7-binding chemokines produced in the lymph node, and is presumably assisted by surface molecules such as CD31 on the lymphocytes and the endothelial cells.

The important role for L-selectin and chemokines in naive T cell homing to secondary lymphoid tissues is supported by many different experimental observations.

- Lymphocytes from L-selectin knockout mice do not bind to peripheral lymph node HEVs, and the mice have a marked reduction in the number of lymphocytes in peripheral lymph nodes.
- Studies indicate that CCL19 and CCL21, the two chemokines that bind to CCR7 on T cells, are produced in T cell zones of lymph nodes.
- There are very few naive T cells in the lymph nodes of mice with genetic deficiencies in CCL19 and CCL21, or CCR7, but the B cell and memory T cell content of these lymph nodes is relatively normal.

Naive T cells that have homed into lymph nodes but fail to recognize antigen and become activated will eventually return to the blood stream. This return to the blood completes one recirculation loop, and provides the naive T cells another chance to seek out the antigens they can recognize in other lymph nodes. The major route of reentry into the blood is through the efferent lymphatics, perhaps via other lymph nodes in the same chain, and then via the lymphatic vasculature to the thoracic duct, and finally into the superior vena cava. The exit of naive T cells from lymph nodes is dependent on a lipid chemoattractant called **sphingosine 1-phosphate** (S1P), which is present at relatively high concentrations in the lymph and blood compared to tissues. S1P binds to a specific G protein–coupled receptor on T cells called S1P1 (mentioned earlier), and signals generated by S1P1 stimulate directed movement of the naive T cells along an S1P concentration gradient out of the lymph node parenchyma. Circulating naive T cells have very little cell surface S1P1 because the high blood concentration of S1P causes internalization of the receptor. Once a naive T cell enters a lymph node, where S1P concentrations are low, it may take several hours for surface S1P1 to be re-expressed. This allows time for the naive T cell to interact with APCs before it is directed out of the node toward the S1P gradient. S1P and the S1P1 receptor are also required for mature naive T cell egress from the thymus.

- A drug called FTY720 functionally inactivates S1P1, blocks T cell egress from lymphoid organs, and acts as a potent immunosuppressive drug for experimental treatment of graft rejections and autoimmune diseases.
- Genetic ablation of S1P1 in mice results in a failure of T cells to leave the thymus and populate secondary lymphoid organs. If T cells lacking this receptor are injected into mice, the cells enter lymph nodes but are unable to exit.

Following activation, T cells transiently reduce expression of S1P1 and stay in the lymph nodes for a few days. Once these cells have differentiated into effector cells, S1P1 is re-expressed and the cells are able to leave the lymph nodes and migrate to peripheral tissues.

Naive T cell homing into gut-associated lymphoid tissues, including Peyer's patches and mesenteric lymph nodes, relies on interactions of the T cells with HEVs, which are mediated by selectins, integrins, and chemokines. One particular feature of naive T cell homing to the gut is the contribution of an Ig superfamily molecule called MadCAM-1 (mucosal addressin cell adhesion molecule-1) that is expressed on HEVs in these sites but not typically elsewhere in the body. Naive T cells express two ligands that bind to MadCAM-1, L-selectin and an integrin called $\alpha4\beta7$, and both contribute to the rolling step of naive T cell homing into gut-associated lymphoid tissues.

Naive T cell migration into the spleen is not as finely regulated as homing into lymph nodes. The spleen does not contain HEVs, and it appears that naive T cells are delivered to the marginal zone and red pulp sinuses by passive mechanisms that do not involve selectins, integrins, or chemokines. However, CCR7-binding chemokines do participate in directing the naive T cells into the white pulp. Even though splenic homing of naive T cells appears to be less tightly regulated than homing into lymph nodes, the rate of lymphocyte passage through the spleen is very high, about half the total body lymphocyte population every 24 hours.

Migration of Effector T Lymphocytes to Sites of Inflammation

Effector T cells exit lymph nodes and preferentially home to peripheral tissues at sites of infection, where they are needed to eliminate microbes during the effector phase of adaptive immune responses. A fundamental aspect of differentiation of naive T cells into effector cells, which occurs in the peripheral lymphoid organs, is a change in expression of chemokine receptors and adhesion molecules that determine the migratory behavior of these cells. Predictably, the expression of molecules involved in naive T cell homing into lymph nodes, including L-selectin and CCR7, decreases shortly after antigen-induced activation of the naive T cells. As a result, the effector cells that develop are no longer constrained to stay in the node. L-selectin and CCR7 may be re-expressed later, allowing for some homing of circulating effector T cells back into lymph nodes. The egress of activated lymphocytes from lymph nodes is also actively driven by the S1P-S1P1 receptor pathway (discussed earlier).

Effector T cell migration into inflammatory sites is dependent on a multistep sequence of events at the blood-endothelial interface, similar to the processes described for migration of other leukocytes in Chapter 2 and for naive T cells in this chapter. Homing to these sites involves adhesion to, and transmigration through, the endothelial lining of postcapillary venules in the infected tissue. Effector T cells express adhesion molecules and chemokine receptors, which bind ligands typically present on endothelial cells at peripheral inflammatory sites. The ligands include endothelial adhesion molecules and chemokines whose expression is induced as part of the innate immune response to infections. The adhesion molecules and cytokines that control the migration of effector T cells to inflammatory sites are described in Chapter 13.

Some effector cells have a propensity to migrate to particular tissues. This selective migration capacity is acquired during the differentiation of the T cells. By enabling different subsets of effector cells to migrate to different sites, the adaptive immune system directs cells with specialized effector functions to the locations where they are best suited to deal with particular types of infections. The clearest examples of populations of effector T cells that specifically home to different tissues are skin-homing and gut-homing T cells. Skin-homing effector T cells express a carbohydrate ligand for E-selectin called CLA-1 (for cutaneous lymphocyte antigen-1), and the CCR4 and CCR10 chemokine receptors, which bind CCL17 and CCL27, chemokines that are commonly expressed in inflamed skin. Gut-homing effector T cells express the $\alpha4\beta7$ integrin, which binds to MadCam-1 on gut endothelial cells, and CCR9, which binds to CCL25, a chemokine expressed in inflamed bowel. Remarkably, these distinct migratory phenotypes of skin- and gut-homing effector T cells may be induced by distinct signals delivered to naive T cells at the time of antigen presentation by DCs in either subcutaneous lymph nodes or gut associated lymphoid tissues, respectively. Although the molecular basis for this imprinting of migratory phenotype is not known, there is evidence that DCs in Peyer's patches produce retinoic acid, which promotes the expression of $\alpha4\beta7$ and CCR9 by responding T cells. A different subset of T cells that is found within the intestinal epithelium express an integrin called CD103 ($\alpha E\beta7$) that can bind to E-cadherin molecules on epithelial cells, allowing T cells to maintain residence as intraepithelial lymphocytes. Another example of heterogeneity of the migratory phenotpye of effector T cells are subsets of $CD4^+$ effector T cells, called Th1 and Th2 cells; these are discussed in detail in Chapter 13.

Memory T Cell Migration

Memory T cells are heterogeneous in their patterns of expression of adhesion molecules and chemokine receptors and in their propensity to migrate to different tissues. Subsets of memory cells arise from the same clones of T cells that give rise to skin- and gut-homing effector cells described above, and these memory cells likely retain the homing properties of their corresponding effector cell brethren. Because we have only imperfect ways of identifying memory T cells, the distinction between effector and memory T cells in experimental studies is often not precise. Two subsets of memory T cells described earlier in this chapter, namely, central memory and effector memory T cells, were initially defined based on differences in CCR7 and L-selectin expression. Central memory T cells were defined as human $CD45RO^+$ blood T cells that express high levels of CCR7 and L-selectin, while effector memory T cells were defined as $CD45RO^+$ blood T cells that express low levels of CCR7 and L-selectin but express other chemokine receptors that bind inflammatory chemokines. These phenotypes suggest that central memory T cells home to secondary lymphoid organs, while effector memory T cells home to peripheral tissues. Although central and effector memory T cell populations can also be detected in mice, experimental homing studies have indicated that CCR7 expression is an imperfect marker to distinguish central and effector memory T cells. Nonetheless, it is clear that some memory T cells either remain in, or tend to home to, secondary lymphoid organs, while others migrate into peripheral tissues, especially mucosal tissues. In general, the peripheral tissue homing effector memory T cells respond to antigenic stimulation by rapidly producing effector cytokines, while the lymphoid tissue based central memory cells tend to proliferate more (providing a pool of cells for recall responses), and provide helper functions for B cells.

Homing of B Lymphocytes

B cells utilize the same basic mechanisms as do naive T cells to home to secondary lymphoid tissues throughout the body, which enhances their likelihood of responding to microbial antigens in different sites. Immature B cells leave the bone marrow via the blood and enter the red pulp of the spleen from open-ended arterioles at the perimeter of the white pulp. Once in the spleen, the immature B cells mature either into follicular B cells or marginal zone B cells. As the follicular B cells mature they migrate, in an integrin-dependent manner, into the white pulp in response to a chemokine called CXCL13, which binds to the chemokine receptor CXCR5, and, to a lesser extent, in response to CCL19 and CCL21, which bind to CCR7. Once the maturation is completed within the splenic white pulp, naive follicular B cells will re-enter the circulation and home to lymph nodes and mucosal lymphoid tissues. Homing of naive B cells from the blood into lymph nodes involves tethering/rolling interactions on HEV, chemokine activation of integrins, and stable arrest, as described earlier for naive T cells. Naive B cells express L-selectin, CCR7, and LFA1, which bind to PNAd, CCL19 and CCL21, and ICAM-1, respectively, on lymph node HEVs. In addition, naive B cells express another chemokine receptor called CXCR4, which binds the chemokine CXCL12, and this interaction also plays a significant role in naive B cell integrin activation and homing into lymph nodes. Once naive B cells enter the stroma of secondary lymphoid organs, they migrate into follicles, the site where they may encounter antigen and become activated. This migration of naive B cells into follicles is mediated by CXCL13, which is produced in follicles. Homing of naive B cells into Peyer's patches involves CXCR5, and the integrin α4β7, which binds to MadCAM1. During the course of B cell responses to protein antigens, B cells and helper T cells must directly interact, and this involves highly regulated movements of both B and T cells within the secondary lymphoid organs. These local migratory events, and the chemokines that orchestrate them, will be discussed in detail in Chapter 10. Presumably, naive B cells that have entered secondary lymphoid tissues but do not become activated by antigen reenter the circulation, like naive T cells do, but how this process is controlled is not clear.

Subsets of B cells committed to expressing particular types of antibodies migrate from secondary lymphoid organs into specific tissues. As we will describe in later chapters, different populations of activated B cells may secrete different types of antibodies, called isotypes, each of which performs a distinct set of effector functions. Many antibody-producing plasma cells migrate to the bone marrow, where they secrete antibodies for long periods of time. Most bone marrow–homing plasma cells produce IgG antibodies, which are then distributed throughout the body via the blood stream. B cells within mucosal associated lymphoid tissues usually become committed to expressing the IgA isotype of antibody, and these committed cells may home specifically to epithelial-lined mucosal tissues. This homing pattern combined with the local differentiation within mucosa of B cells into IgA-secreting plasma cells serve to optimize IgA responses to mucosal infections, because IgA is efficiently excreted into the lumen of mucosal epithelial-lined tissues, such as the gut and respiratory tree. The mechanisms by which different B cell populations migrate to different tissues are, not surprisingly, similar to the mechanisms we described for tissue-specific migration of effector T cells, and depend on expression of distinct combinations of adhesion molecules and chemokine receptors on each B cell subset. For example, bone marrow–homing IgG-secreting plasma cells express VLA-4 and CXCR4, which bind respectively to VCAM-1 and CXCL12 expressed on bone marrow sinusoidal endothelial cells. In contrast, mucosal-homing IgA-secreting plasma cells express α4β7, CCR9, and CCR10, which bind respectively to MadCAM-1, CCL25, and CCL28, expressed on mucosal endothelial cells. IgG-secreting B cells are also recruited to chronic inflammatory sites in various tissues, and this pattern of homing can be attributed to CXCR3 and VLA-4 on these B cells binding to VCAM-1 , CXCL9, and CXCL10, which are often found on the endothelial surface at sites of chronic inflammation.

SUMMARY

- The anatomic organization of the cells and tissues of the immune system is of critical importance for the generation of immune responses. This organization permits the small number of lymphocytes specific for any one antigen to locate and respond effectively to that antigen regardless of where in the body the antigen is introduced.
- The adaptive immune response depends on antigen-specific lymphocytes, APCs required for lymphocyte activation, and effector cells that eliminate antigens.
- B and T lymphocytes express highly diverse and specific antigen receptors and are the cells responsible for the specificity and memory of adaptive immune responses. NK cells are a distinct class of lymphocytes that do not express highly diverse antigen receptors and whose functions are largely in innate immunity. Many surface molecules are differentially expressed on different subsets of lymphocytes, as well as on other leukocytes, and these are named according to the CD nomenclature.
- Both B and T lymphocytes arise from a common precursor in the bone marrow. B cell development proceeds in the bone marrow, whereas T cell precursors migrate to and mature in the thymus. After maturing, B and T cells leave the bone marrow and thymus, enter the circulation, and populate peripheral lymphoid organs.
- Naive B and T cells are mature lymphocytes that have not been stimulated by antigen. When they encounter antigen, they differentiate into effector lymphocytes that have functions in protective immune responses. Effector B lymphocytes are antibody-secreting plasma cells. Effector T cells include cytokine-secreting $CD4^+$ helper T cells and $CD8^+$ CTLs.
- Some of the progeny of antigen-activated B and T lymphocytes differentiate into memory cells that survive for long periods in a quiescent state. These memory cells are responsible for the rapid and enhanced responses to subsequent exposures to antigen.
- APCs function to display antigens for recognition by lymphocytes and to promote the activation of lymphocytes. APCs include dendritic cells, mononuclear phagocytes, and FDCs.
- The organs of the immune system may be divided into the generative organs (bone marrow and thymus), where lymphocytes mature, and the

peripheral organs (lymph nodes and spleen), where naive lymphocytes are activated by antigens.

- Bone marrow contains the stem cells for all blood cells, including lymphocytes, and is the site of maturation of all of these cell types except T cells, which mature in the thymus.

- The lymph nodes are the sites where B and T cells respond to antigens that are collected by the lymph from peripheral tissues. The spleen is the organ in which lymphocytes respond to blood-borne antigens. Both lymph nodes and spleen are organized into B cell zones (the follicles) and T cell zones. The T cell areas are also the sites of residence of mature dendritic cells, which are APCs specialized for the activation of naive T cells. FDCs reside in the B cell areas and serve to activate B cells during humoral immune responses to protein antigens. The development of secondary lymphoid tissue architecture depends on cytokines.

- The cutaneous immune system consists of specialized collections of APCs and lymphocytes adapted to respond to environmental antigens encountered in the skin. A network of immature dendritic cells called Langerhans cells, present in the epidermis of the skin, serves to trap antigens and then transport them to draining lymph nodes. The mucosal immune system includes specialized collections of lymphocytes and APCs organized to optimize encounters with environmental antigens introduced through the respiratory and gastrointestinal tracts.

- Lymphocyte recirculation is the process by which lymphocytes continuously move between sites throughout the body through blood and lymphatic vessels, and it is critical for the initiation and effector phases of immune responses.

- Naive T cells normally recirculate among the various peripheral lymphoid organs, increasing the likelihood of encounter with antigen displayed by APCs such as mature dendritic cells. Effector T cells more typically are recruited to peripheral sites of inflammation where microbial antigens are located. Memory T cells may enter either lymphoid organs or peripheral tissues.

- Different populations of lymphocytes exhibit distinct patterns of homing. Naive T cells migrate preferentially to lymph nodes; this process is mediated by binding of L-selectin on the T cells to peripheral lymph node addressin on HEVs in lymph nodes and by the CCR7 receptor on T cells that binds to chemokines produced in lymph nodes. The effector and memory T cells that are generated by antigen stimulation of naive T cells exit the lymph node. They have decreased L-selectin and CCR7 expression but increased expression of integrins and E-selectin and P-selectin ligands, and these molecules mediate binding to endothelium at peripheral inflammatory sites. Effector and memory lymphocytes also express receptors for chemokines that are produced in peripheral tissues.

Selected Readings

Bromley SK, TR Mempel, and AD Luster. Orchestrating the orchestrators: chemokines in control of T cell traffic. Nature Immunology 9:970–980, 2008.

Cyster JG. Chemokines, sphingosine-1-phosphate, and cell migration in secondary lymphoid organs. Annual Review of Immunology 23:127–159, 2005.

Drayton DL, S Liao, RW Mcunzer, and NH Ruddle. Lymphoid organ development: from ontogeny to neogenesis. Nature Immunology 7:344–353, 2006.

Harty JT, and VP Badovinac. Shaping and reshaping CD8+ T-cell memory. Nature Reviews Immunology 8:107–119, 2008.

Johansson-Lindbom B, and WW Agace. Generation of gut-homing T cells and their localization to the small intestinal mucosa. Immunolgical Reviews 215:226–242, 2007.

Kupper TS, and RC Fuhlbrigge. Immune surveillance in the skin: mechanisms and clinical consequences. Nature Reviews Immunology 4:211–222, 2004.

Marrack P, and J Kappler. Control of T cell viability. Annual Review of Immunology 22:765–787, 2004.

Mebius RE, and G Kraal. Structure and function of the spleen. Nature Reviews Immunology 5:606–616, 2005.

Nagler-Anderson C. Man the barrier! Strategic defences in the intestinal mucosa. Nature Reviews Immunology 1:59–67, 2001.

Sallusto F, and M Baggiolini. Chemokines and leukocyte traffic. Nature Immunology 9:949–952, 2008.

Schluns KS, and L Lefrancois. Cytokine control of memory T-cell development and survival. Nature Reviews Immunology 3:269–279, 2003.

Serbina NV, T Jia, TM Hohl, and EG Pamer. Monocyte-mediated defense against microbial pathogens. Annual Review of Immunology 26:421–452, 2008.

Sigmundsdottir H, and EC Butcher. Environmental cues, dendritic cells and the programming of tissue-selective lymphocyte trafficking. Nature Immunology 9:981–987, 2008.

Sprent J, JH Cho, O Boyman, and CD Surh. T cell homeostasis. Immunology and Cell Biology 86:312–319, 2008.

Von Andrian UH, and CR Mackay. T cell function and migration: two sides of the same coin. New England Journal of Medicine 343:1020–1034, 2000.

Von Andrian UH, and TR Mempel. Homing and cellular traffic in lymph nodes. Nature Reviews Immunology 3:867–878, 2003.

Section II

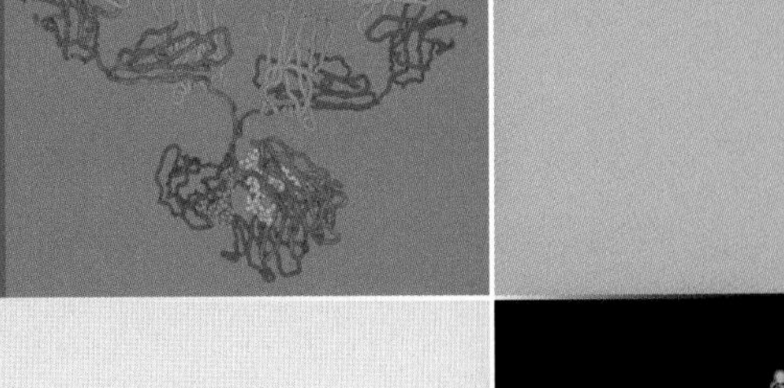

Recognition of Antigens

Adaptive immune responses are initiated by the specific recognition of antigens by lymphocytes. This section is devoted to a discussion of the cellular and molecular basis of antigen recognition and the specificities of B and T lymphocytes.

We begin with antibodies, which are the antigen receptors and effector molecules of B lymphocytes, because our understanding of the structural basis of antigen recognition has evolved from studies of these molecules. Chapter 4 describes the structure of antibodies and how these proteins recognize antigens.

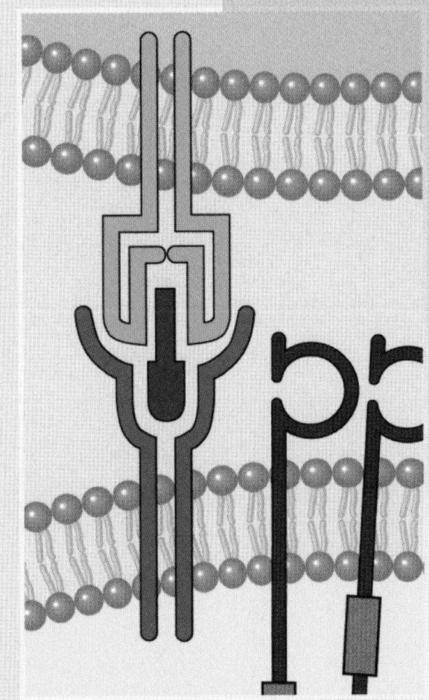

The next three chapters consider antigen recognition by T lymphocytes, which play a central role in all immune responses to protein antigens. In Chapter 5, we describe the genetics and biochemistry of the major histocompatibility complex (MHC), whose products are integral components of the ligands that T cells specifically recognize. Chapter 6 discusses the association of foreign peptide antigens with MHC molecules and the cell biology and physiologic significance of antigen presentation. Chapter 7 deals with the T cell antigen receptor and the other T cell membrane molecules that are involved in the recognition of antigens and the responses of the T cells.

Chapter 4

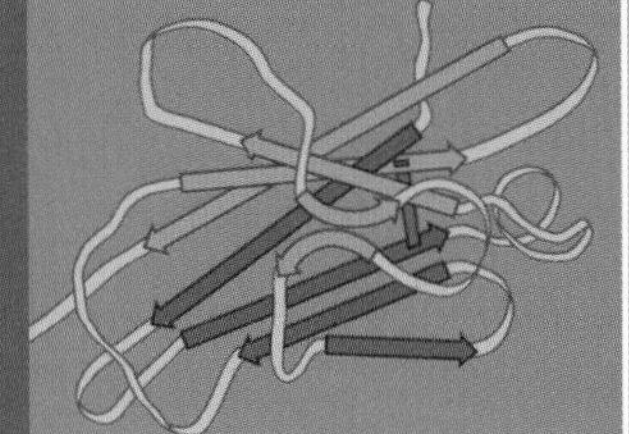

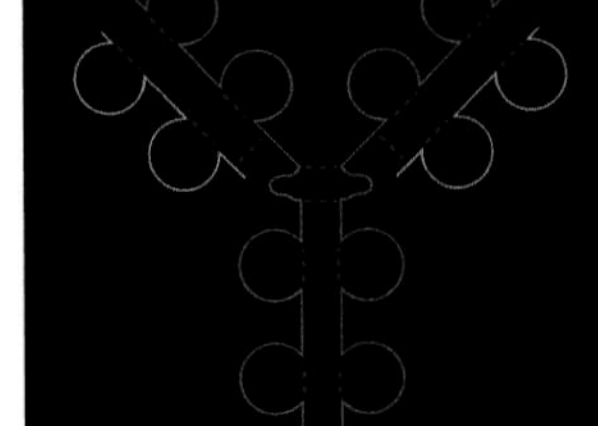

ANTIBODIES AND ANTIGENS

Antibodies are circulating proteins that are produced in vertebrates in response to exposure to foreign structures known as antigens. Antibodies are incredibly diverse and specific in their ability to recognize foreign shapes, and are the primary mediators of humoral immunity against all classes of microbes. One of the earliest experimental demonstrations of adaptive immunity was the finding by von Behring and Kitasato in 1890 that chemically inactivated toxins could induce protective immunity when injected into experimental animals, and that protection could be transferred to other susceptible animals by injecting serum from their immune counterparts. Based on this discovery, life-threatening human diphtheria infections were successfully treated by the administration of serum from horses immunized with a chemically modified form of the diphtheria toxin. The family of circulating proteins that mediate these protective responses were initially called antitoxins. When it was appreciated that similar proteins could be generated against many substances, not just toxins, these proteins were given the general name "antibodies." The substances that generated or were recognized by antibodies were then called **antigens**. Antibodies, major histocompatibility complex (MHC) molecules (see Chapter 5), and T cell antigen receptors (see Chapter 7) are the three classes of molecules used in adaptive immunity to recognize antigens (Table 4–1). Of these three, antibodies bind the widest range of antigenic structures, show the greatest ability to discriminate between different antigens, and bind antigens with the greatest strength. Antibodies represent the first of the three types of antigen-binding molecules to be discovered and characterized. Therefore, we begin our discussion of how the immune system specifically recognizes antigens by describing the structure and the antigen-binding properties of antibodies.

Antibodies can exist in two forms: membrane-bound antibodies on the surface of B lymphocytes function as receptors for antigen, and secreted antibodies that reside in the circulation, tissues, and mucosal sites bind antigens, neutralize toxins, and prevent the entry and spread of pathogens. The recognition of antigen by membrane-bound antibodies on specific naive B cells activates these lymphocytes and initiates a humoral immune response. Antibodies are also produced in a secreted form by antigen-stimulated B cells. In the effector phase of humoral immunity, these secreted antibodies bind to antigens and trigger several effector mechanisms that eliminate the antigens. The elimination of antigen often requires interaction of antibody with other components of the immune system, includ-

Table 4–1. Features of Antigen Binding by the Antigen-Recognizing Molecules of the Immune System

Feature	Antigen binding molecule		
	Immunoglobulin (Ig)	T cell receptor (TCR)	MHC molecules*
Antigen binding site	Made up of three CDRs in V_H and three CDRs in V_L	Made up of three CDRs in V_α and three CDRs in V_β	Peptide-binding cleft made of $\alpha 1$ and $\alpha 2$ (class I) or $\alpha 1$ and $\beta 1$ (class II)
Nature of antigen that may be bound	Macromolecules (proteins, lipids, polysaccharides) and small chemicals	Peptide-MHC complexes	Peptides
Nature of antigenic determinants recognized	Linear and conformational determinants of various macromolecules and chemicals	Linear determinants of peptides; only 2 or 3 amino acid residues of a peptide bound to an MHC molecule	Linear determinants of peptides; only some amino acid residues of a peptide
Affinity of antigen binding	K_d 10^{-7} – 10^{-11} M; average affinity of Igs increases during immune response	K_d 10^{-5} – 10^{-7} M	K_d 10^{-6} – 10^{-9} M; extremely stable binding

*The structures and functions of MHC and TCR molecules are discussed in Chapters 5 and 7, respectively.
Abbreviations: CDR, complementarity-determining region; K_d, dissociation constant; MHC, major histocompatibility complex; V_H, variable domain of heavy chain Ig; V_L, variable domain of light chain Ig

ing molecules such as complement proteins and cells that include phagocytes and eosinophils. Antibody-mediated effector functions include neutralization of microbes or toxic microbial products; activation of the complement system; opsonization of pathogens for enhanced phagocytosis; antibody-dependent cell-mediated cytotoxicity, by which antibodies target microbes for lysis by cells of the innate immune system; and immediate hypersensitivity, in which antibodies trigger mast cell activation. These effector functions of antibodies are described in detail in Chapter 14. In this chapter, we discuss the structural features of antibodies that underlie their antigen recognition and effector functions.

Natural Distribution and Production of Antibodies

Antibodies are distributed in biologic fluids throughout the body and are found on the surface of a limited number of cell types. B lymphocytes are the only cells that synthesize antibody molecules. These cells initially express an integral membrane form of the antibody molecule on the cell surface where it functions as the B cell antigen receptor. After exposure to an antigen, much of the initial antibody response occurs in lymphoid tissues, mainly the spleen, lymph nodes, and mucosal lymphoid tissues, but long-lived antibody-producing plasma cells may persist in other tissues, especially in the bone marrow (see Chapter 10). Secreted forms of antibodies accumulate in the plasma (the fluid portion of the blood), in mucosal secretions, and in the interstitial fluid of tissues. Secreted antibodies often attach to the surface of other immune effector cells, such as mononuclear phagocytes, natural killer (NK) cells, and mast cells, which have specific receptors for binding antibody molecules (see Chapter 14).

When blood or plasma forms a clot, antibodies remain in the residual fluid, called **serum.** Any serum sample that contains detectable antibody molecules that bind to a particular antigen is commonly called an **antiserum.** (The study of antibodies and their reactions with antigens is therefore classically called **serology.**) The concentration of antibody molecules in serum specific for a particular antigen is often estimated by determining how many serial dilutions of the serum can be made before binding can no longer be observed; sera with a high concentration of antibody molecules specific for a particular antigen are said to have a "high titer."

A healthy 70-kg adult human produces about 2g–3g of antibodies every day. Almost two thirds of this is an antibody called IgA, which is produced by activated B cells and plasma cells in the walls of the gastrointestinal and respiratory tracts and actively transported into the lumens. The large amount of IgA produced reflects the large surface areas of these organs. Antibodies that enter the circulation have limited half-lives. The most common type of antibody, called IgG, is primarily found in the serum (though IgG antibodies can also be transported to mucosal sites) and has a half-life of about 3 weeks.

MOLECULAR STRUCTURE OF ANTIBODIES

An understanding of the structure of antibodies has provided important insights regarding antibody function. The analysis of antibody structure also paved the way to the eventual characterization of the genetic organization of antigen receptor genes in both B and T cells, and the elucidation of the mechanisms of immune diversity, issues that will be considered in depth in Chapter 8.

Early studies of antibody structure relied on antibodies purified from the blood of individuals immunized with various antigens. It was not possible, using this approach, to define antibody structure precisely because serum contains a mixture of different antibodies produced by many clones of B lymphocytes that may respond to different portions (epitopes) of an antigen (so-called polyclonal antibodies). A major breakthrough providing antibodies whose structures could be elucidated was the discovery that patients with multiple myeloma, a monoclonal tumor of antibody-producing plasma cells, often have large amounts of biochemically identical antibody molecules (produced by the neoplastic clone) in their blood and urine. Immunologists found that these antibodies could be purified to homogeneity and analyzed. The recognition that myeloma cells make monoclonal immunoglobulins led to an extremely powerful technique for producing monoclonal antibodies, described by Georges Köhler and Cesar Milstein in 1975. They developed a method for immortalizing individual antibody-secreting cells from an immunized animal by producing "hybridomas," each of which secreted individual **monoclonal antibodies** of predetermined specificity. These antibodies have proved to be of tremendous importance in most avenues of biologic research, and have many practical applications in clinical diagnosis and therapy (Box 4–1).

Box 4–1 ▪ IN DEPTH: MONOCLONAL ANTIBODIES

The ability to produce virtually unlimited quantities of identical antibody molecules specific for a particular antigenic determinant has revolutionized immunology and has had a far-reaching impact on research in diverse fields as well as on clinical medicine. The first method for producing homogeneous or monoclonal antibodies of known specificity was described by Georges Köhler and Cesar Milstein in 1975, and this approach remains the most common one used today to generate such antibodies. This technique is based on the fact that each B lymphocyte produces antibody of a single specificity. Because normal B lymphocytes cannot grow indefinitely, it is necessary to immortalize B cells that produce a specific antibody. This is achieved by cell fusion, or somatic cell hybridization, between a normal antibody-producing B cell and a myeloma cell, followed by selection of fused cells that secrete antibody of the desired specificity derived from the normal B cell. Such fusion-derived immortalized antibody-producing cell lines are called **hybridomas,** and the antibodies they produce are **monoclonal antibodies.**

The technique of producing hybridomas requires cultured myeloma cell lines that will grow in normal culture medium but not in a defined "selection" medium because they lack functional genes required for DNA synthesis in this selection medium. Fusing normal cells to these defective myeloma fusion partners provides the necessary genes from the normal cells, so that only the somatic cell hybrids will grow in the selection medium. Moreover, the uncontrolled growth property of the myeloma cell makes such hybrids immortal. Myeloma cell lines that can be used as fusion partners are created by inducing defects in nucleotide synthesis pathways. Normal animal cells synthesize purine nucleotides and thymidylate, both precursors of DNA, by a *de novo* pathway requiring tetrahydrofolate. Antifolate drugs, such as aminopterin, block activation of tetrahydrofolate, thereby inhibiting the synthesis of purines and therefore preventing DNA synthesis by the *de novo* pathway. Aminopterin-treated cells can use a salvage pathway in which purine is synthesized from exogenously supplied hypoxanthine by the enzyme hypoxanthine-guanine phosphoribosyltransferase (HGPRT), and thymidylate is synthesized from thymidine by the enzyme thymidine kinase (TK). Therefore, cells grow in the presence of aminopterin only if the culture medium is also supplemented with hypoxanthine and thymidine (called HAT medium). Myeloma cell lines can be made defective in HGPRT or TK by mutagenesis followed by selection in media containing substrates for these enzymes that yield lethal products. Only HGPRT- or TK-deficient cells will survive under these selection conditions. Such HGPRT- or TK-negative myeloma cells cannot use the salvage pathway and will therefore die in HAT medium. If normal B cells are fused to HGPRT- or TK-negative cells, the B cells provide the necessary enzymes so that the hybrids synthesize DNA and grow in HAT medium.

To produce a monoclonal antibody specific for a defined antigen, a mouse or rat is immunized with that

Continued on following page

Box 4–1 ▪ IN DEPTH: MONOCLONAL ANTIBODIES (Continued)

antigen, and B cells are isolated from the spleen or lymph nodes of the animal. These B cells are then fused with an appropriate immortalized cell line. Myeloma lines are the best fusion partners for B cells because like cells tend to fuse and give rise to stable hybrids more efficiently than unlike cells. In current practice, the myeloma lines that are used do not produce their own Ig, and cell fusion is achieved with polyethylene glycol. Hybrids are selected for growth in HAT medium; under these conditions, unfused HGPRT- or TK-negative myeloma cells die

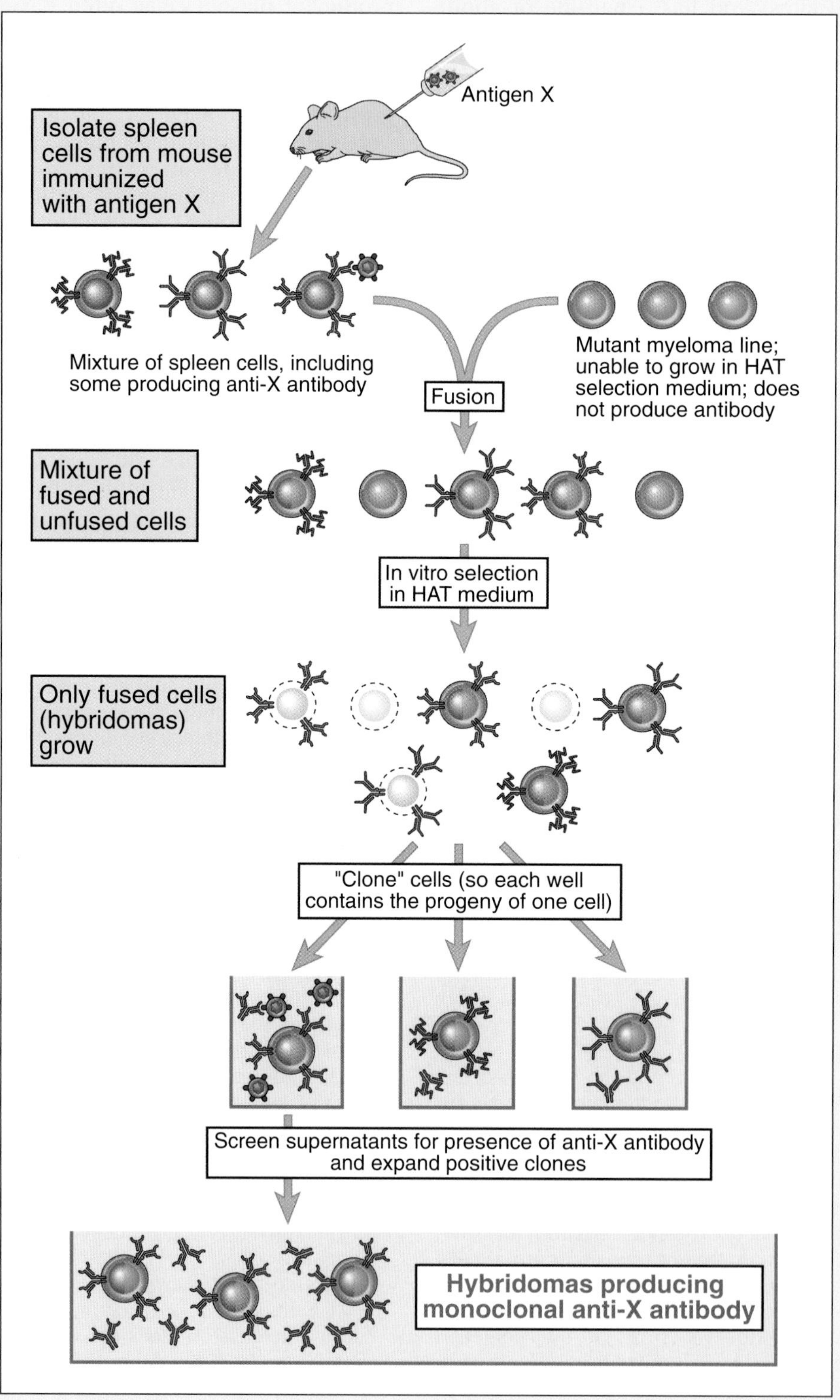

Antigen X
Isolate spleen cells from mouse immunized with antigen X
Mixture of spleen cells, including some producing anti-X antibody
Fusion
Mutant myeloma line; unable to grow in HAT selection medium; does not produce antibody
Mixture of fused and unfused cells
In vitro selection in HAT medium
Only fused cells (hybridomas) grow
"Clone" cells (so each well contains the progeny of one cell)
Screen supernatants for presence of anti-X antibody and expand positive clones
Hybridomas producing monoclonal anti-X antibody

Continued on following page

because they cannot use the salvage pathway, and unfused B cells cannot survive for more than 1 to 2 weeks because they are not immortalized, so that only hybrids will grow (see Figure). The fused cells are cultured at a concentration at which each culture well is expected initially to contain only one hybridoma cell. The culture supernatant from each well in which growing cells are detected is then tested for the presence of antibody reactive with the antigen used for immunization. The screening method depends on the antigen being used. For soluble antigens, the usual technique is radioimmunoassay or enzyme-linked immunosorbent assay; for cell surface antigens, a variety of assays for antibody binding to viable cells can be used (see Appendix III: Laboratory Methods Using Antibodies). Once positive wells (i.e., wells containing hybridomas producing the desired antibody) are identified, the cells are cloned in semisolid agar or by limiting dilution, and clones producing the antibody are isolated by another round of screening. These cloned hybridomas produce monoclonal antibodies of a desired specificity. Hybridomas can be grown in large volumes or as ascitic tumors in syngeneic mice to produce large quantities of monoclonal antibodies.

Some of the common applications of hybridomas and monoclonal antibodies include the following:

- Identification of phenotypic markers unique to particular cell types. The basis for the modern classification of lymphocytes and other leukocytes is the binding of population-specific monoclonal antibodies. These have been used to define clusters of differentiation (CD markers) for various cell types (see Chapter 3).
- Immunodiagnosis. The diagnosis of many infectious and systemic diseases relies on the detection of particular antigens or antibodies in the circulation or in tissues by use of monoclonal antibodies in immunoassays.
- Tumor diagnosis. Tumor-specific monoclonal antibodies are used for detection of tumors by imaging techniques.
- Therapy. A number of monoclonal antibodies are used therapeutically today. Some examples include the use of antibodies against tumor necrosis factor in the therapy of rheumatoid arthritis, antibodies against CD20 for the treatment of B cell leukemias, antibodies against the type 2 epidermal growth factor receptor in patients with breast cancer, antibodies against vascular endothelial growth factor, a promoter of angiogenesis, in patients with colon cancer, and so on.
- Functional analysis of cell surface and secreted molecules. In immunologic research, monoclonal antibodies that bind to cell surface molecules and either stimulate or inhibit particular cellular functions are invaluable tools for defining the functions of surface molecules, including receptors for antigens. Antibodies that bind and neutralize cytokines are routinely used for detecting the presence and functional roles of these protein hormones in vitro and in vivo.

At present, hybridomas are most often produced by fusing HAT-sensitive mouse myelomas with B cells from immunized mice, rats, or hamsters. Attempts are being made to generate human monoclonal antibodies, primarily for administration to patients, by developing human myeloma lines as fusion partners. However, it is a general rule that the stability of hybrids is low if cells from species that are far apart in evolution are fused, and for this reason human B cells do not form hybridomas with mouse myeloma lines at high efficiency.

Genetic engineering techniques are used to expand the usefulness of monoclonal antibodies. The complementary DNAs (cDNAs) that encode the polypeptide chains of a monoclonal antibody can be isolated from a hybridoma, and these genes can be manipulated in vitro. As we shall discuss later in this chapter, only small portions of the antibody molecule are responsible for binding to antigen; the remainder of the antibody molecule can be thought of as a "framework." This structural organization allows the DNA segments encoding the antigen-binding sites from a murine monoclonal antibody to be "stitched" into a cDNA encoding a human myeloma protein, creating a hybrid gene. When expressed, the resultant hybrid protein, which retains antigen specificity, is referred to as a humanized antibody. Humanized antibodies are far less likely to appear "foreign" in humans and to induce anti-antibody responses (see Box 4–3) that limit the usefulness of murine monoclonal antibodies when they are administered to patients.

Genetic engineering is also being used to create monoclonal antibody–like molecules of defined specificity without the need for producing hybridomas. One approach, called "phage display," uses random collections of cDNAs encoding just the antigen-binding regions of antibodies. These cDNAs are generated from messenger RNA isolated from the spleens of immunized mice, and amplified by polymerase chain reaction technology. The cDNAs are then cloned into bacteriophages to form phage display libraries. Although the antigen-binding regions of antibodies are formed from two different polypeptide chains, synthetic antigen-binding sites can be created by expressing fusion proteins in which sequences from the two chains are covalently joined in a tandem array. Such fusion proteins can be expressed on the surfaces of the bacteriophages, and pools of phage can be tested for their ability to bind to a particular antigen. The virus that binds to the antigen presumably contains cDNA encoding the desired synthetic antigen-binding site. The cDNA is isolated from that virus and linked with DNA encoding the non-antigen-binding parts of a generic antibody molecule. The final construct can then be transfected into a suitable cell type, expressed in soluble form, purified, and used. The advantage of phage display technology lies in the fact that the number of binding sites that can be screened for the desired specificity is three to four orders of magnitude greater than the practical limit of hybridomas that can be screened.

The availability of homogeneous populations of antibodies and immortalized antibody-producing plasma cells (myelomas and hybridomas) permitted the complete amino acid sequence determination and molecular cloning of individual antibody molecules. The ready availability of monoclonal immunoglobulins culminated in the x-ray crystallographic determinations of the three-dimensional structure of several antibody molecules and of antibodies bound to antigens.

General Features of Antibody Structure

Plasma or serum proteins are traditionally separated by solubility characteristics into albumins and globulins and may be further separated by migration in an electric field, a process called electrophoresis. Most antibodies are found in the third fastest migrating group of globulins, named **gamma globulins** for the third letter of the Greek alphabet. Another common name for antibody is **immunoglobulin (Ig),** referring to the immunity-conferring portion of the gamma globulin fraction. The terms *immunoglobulin* and *antibody* are used interchangeably throughout this book.

All antibody molecules share the same basic structural characteristics but display remarkable variability in the regions that bind antigens. This variability of the antigen-binding regions accounts for the capacity of different antibodies to bind a tremendous number of structurally diverse antigens. There are believed to be a million or more different antibody molecules in every

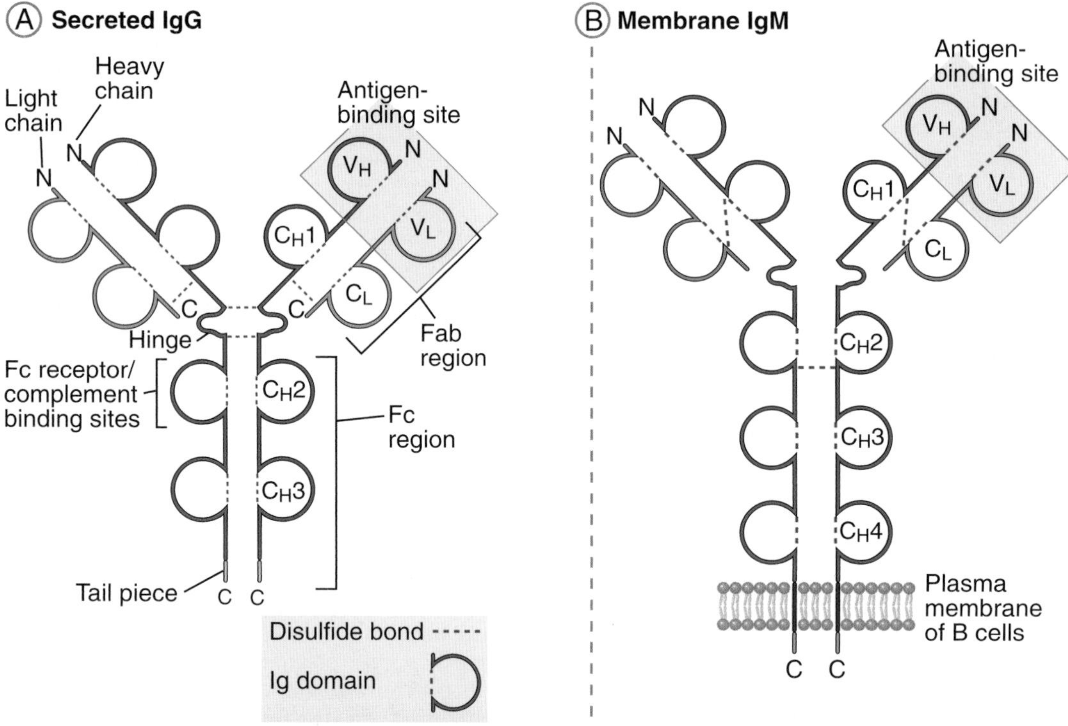

FIGURE 4–1 Structure of an antibody molecule. A. Schematic diagram of a secreted IgG molecule. The antigen-binding sites are formed by the juxtaposition of V_L and V_H domains. The heavy chain C regions end in tail pieces. The locations of complement- and Fc receptor-binding sites within the heavy chain constant regions are approximations. B. Schematic diagram of a membrane-bound IgM molecule on the surface of a B lymphocyte. The IgM molecule has one more C_H domain than IgG, and the membrane form of the antibody has C-terminal transmembrane and cytoplasmic portions that anchor the molecule in the plasma membrane. C. Structure of a human IgG molecule as revealed by x-ray crystallography. In this ribbon diagram of a secreted IgG molecule, the heavy chains are colored blue and red, and the light chains are colored green; carbohydrates are shown in gray. (Courtesy of Dr. Alex McPherson, University of California, Irvine.)

individual (theoretically the antibody repertoire may include more than 10^9 different antibodies), each with unique amino acid sequences in their antigen-combining sites. The effector functions and common physicochemical properties of antibodies are associated with the non-antigen-binding portions, which exhibit relatively few variations among different antibodies.

An antibody molecule has a symmetric core structure composed of two identical light chains and two identical heavy chains (see Fig. 4–1). Both the light chains and the heavy chains contain a series of repeating, homologous units, each about 110 amino acid residues in length, that fold independently in a globular motif that is called an **Ig domain.** An Ig domain contains two layers of β-pleated sheet, each layer composed of three to five strands of antiparallel polypeptide chain (Fig. 4–2). The two layers are held together by a disulfide bridge, and adjacent strands of each β-sheet are connected by short loops. It is the amino acids in some of these loops that are critical for antigen recognition, as discussed below. Many other proteins of importance in the immune system contain domains that use the same folding motif and have amino acid sequences that are similar to Ig amino acid sequences. All molecules that contain this type of domain are said to belong to the **Ig superfamily,** and all the gene segments encoding the Ig domains of these molecules are believed to have evolved from one ancestral gene (Box 4–2).

Both heavy chains and light chains consist of amino-terminal variable (V) regions that participate in antigen recognition and carboxy-terminal constant (C) regions; the C regions of the heavy chains mediate effector functions. In the heavy chains, the V region is composed of one Ig domain and the C region is composed of three or four Ig domains. Each light chain is made up of one V region Ig domain and one C region Ig domain. Variable regions are so named because they contain regions of variability in amino acid sequence that distinguish the antibodies made by one clone of B cells from the antibodies made by other clones. The V region of one heavy chain (V_H) is juxtaposed with the V region of one light chain (V_L) to form an antigen-binding site (see Fig. 4–1). Because the core structural unit of each antibody molecule contains two heavy chains and two light chains, it has two antigen-binding sites. The C region domains are separate from the antigen-binding site and do not participate in antigen recognition. The heavy chain C regions interact with other effector molecules and cells of the immune system and therefore mediate most of the biologic functions of antibodies. In addition, the carboxy-terminal ends of one form of the heavy chains anchor membrane-bound antibodies in the plasma membranes of B lymphocytes. The C regions of light chains do not participate in effector functions and are not directly attached to cell membranes.

Each light chain is about 24 kD, and each heavy chain is 55 to 70 kD. Heavy and light chains are covalently linked by disulfide bonds formed between cysteine residues in the carboxyl terminus of the light chain and the C_H1 domain of the heavy chain. Noncovalent inter-

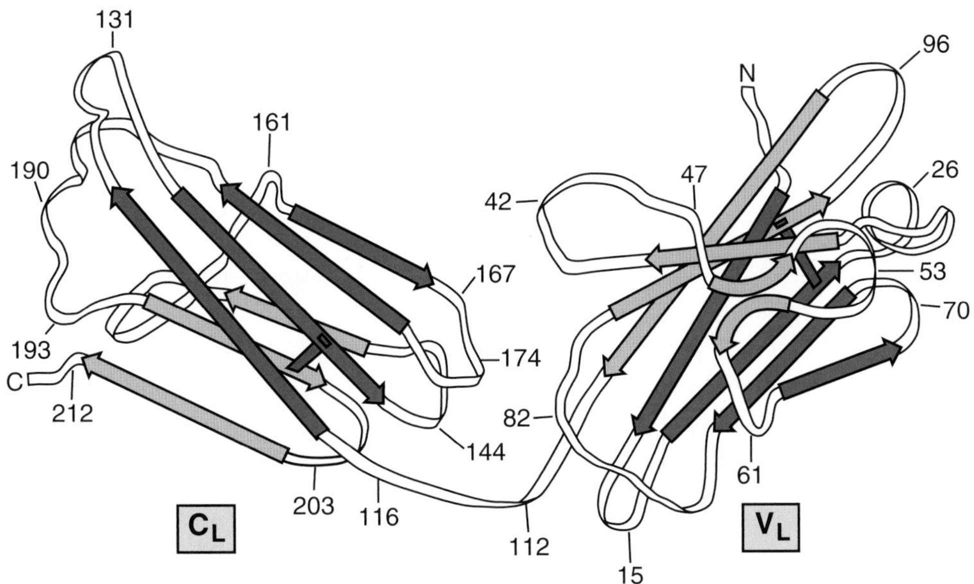

FIGURE 4–2 Structure of an antibody light chain. The secondary and tertiary structures of a human Ig light chain are shown schematically. The V and C regions each independently fold into Ig domains. Each domain is composed of two antiparallel arrays of β-strands represented by the flat arrows, colored yellow and red, respectively, to form two β-pleated sheets. In the C domain, there are three and four β-strands in the two sheets. In the V domain, which is about 16 amino acid residues longer than the C domain, the two sheets are composed of five and four strands. The dark blue bars are intrachain disulfide bonds, and the numbers indicate the positions of amino acid residues counting from the amino (N) terminus. Similar Ig C and V domain structures are found in the extracellular portions of many other membrane proteins in the immune system, as discussed in Box 4–2. (Adapted with permission from Edmundson AB, KR Ely, EE Abola, M Schiffer, and N Panagiotopoulos. Rotational allomerism and divergent evolution of domains in immunoglobulin light chains. Biochemistry 14:3953–3961, 1975. Copyright 1975 American Chemical Society.)

Box 4–2 ▪ IN DEPTH: THE IMMUNOGLOBULIN SUPERFAMILY

Many of the cell surface and soluble molecules that mediate recognition, adhesion, or binding functions in the vertebrate immune system share partial amino acid sequence homology and tertiary structural features that were originally identified in Ig heavy and light chains. In addition, the same features are found in many molecules outside the immune system that also perform similar functions. These diverse proteins are members of the **Ig superfamily** (sometimes called the Ig supergene family). A superfamily is broadly defined as a group of proteins that share a certain degree of sequence homology, usually at least 15%. The conserved sequences shared by superfamily members often contribute to the formation of compact tertiary structures referred to as domains,

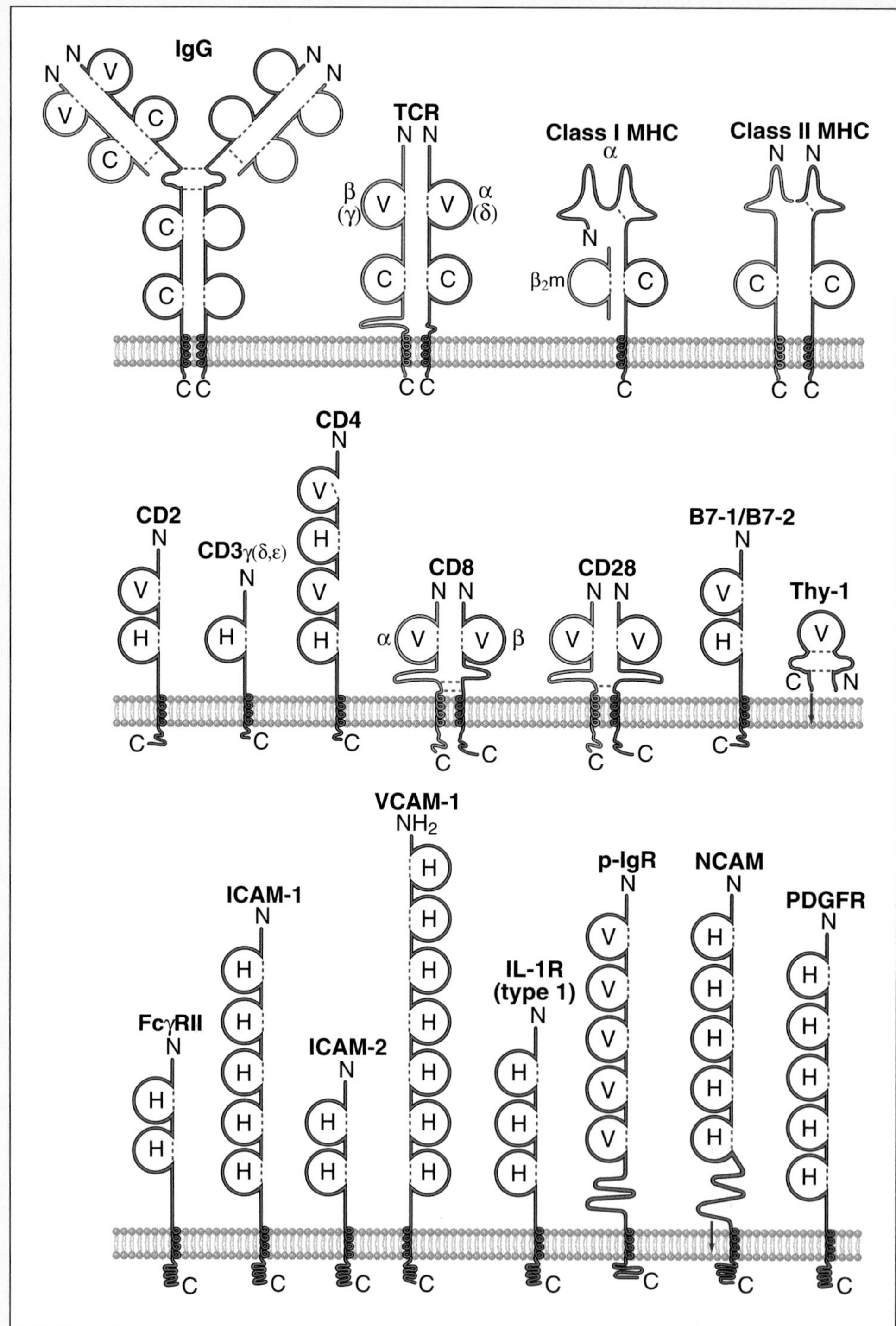

Continued on following page

Box 4–2 ■ IN DEPTH: THE IMMUNOGLOBULIN SUPERFAMILY (Continued)

and most often the entire sequence of a domain characteristic of a particular superfamily is encoded by a single exon. Members of a superfamily are likely to be derived from a common precursor gene by divergent evolution, and multidomain proteins may belong to more than one superfamily. The criterion for inclusion of a protein in the Ig superfamily is the presence of one or more Ig domains (also called Ig homology units), which are regions of 70 to 110 amino acid residues homologous to either Ig variable (V) or Ig constant (C) domains. The Ig domain contains conserved residues that permit the polypeptide to assume a globular tertiary structure called an antibody (or Ig) fold, composed of a sandwich arrangement of two β-sheets, each made up of three to five antiparallel β-strands of 5 to 10 amino acid residues. This sandwich-like structure is stabilized by hydrophobic amino acid residues on the β-strands pointing inward, which alternate with hydrophilic residues pointing out. Because the inward-pointing residues are essential for the stability of the tertiary structure, they are the major contributors to the regions that are conserved between Ig superfamily members. In addition, there are usually conserved cysteine residues that contribute to the formation of an intrachain disulfide-bonded loop of 55 to 75 amino acids (~90 kD). Ig domains are classified as V-like or C-like on the basis of closest homology to either Ig V or Ig C domains. V domains are formed from a longer polypeptide than are C domains and contain two extra β-strands within the β-sheet sandwich. A third type of Ig domain, called C2 or H, has a length similar to C domains but has sequences typical of both V and C domains.

Using several criteria of evolutionary relatedness, such as primary sequence, intron-exon structure, and ability to undergo DNA rearrangements, molecular biologists have postulated a scheme, or family tree, depicting the evolution of members of the Ig superfamily. In this scheme, an early event was the duplication of a gene for a primordial surface receptor followed by divergence of V and C exons. Modern members of the superfamily contain different numbers of V or C domains. The early divergence is reflected by the lack of significant sequence homology in Ig and TCR V and C units, although they share similar tertiary structures. A second early event in the evolution of this family was the acquisition of the ability to undergo DNA recombination, which has remained a unique feature of the antigen receptor gene members of the family.

Most identified members of the Ig superfamily (see Figure) are integral plasma membrane proteins with Ig domains in the extracellular portions, transmembrane domains composed of hydrophobic amino acids, and widely divergent cytoplasmic tails, usually with no intrinsic enzymatic activity. There are exceptions to these generalizations. For example, the platelet-derived growth factor receptors have cytoplasmic tails with tyrosine kinase activity, and the Thy-1 molecule has no cytoplasmic tail but, rather, is anchored to the membrane by a phosphatidylinositol linkage.

One recurrent characteristic of the Ig superfamily members is that interactions between Ig domains on different polypeptide chains are essential for the functions of the molecules. These interactions can be homophilic, occurring between identical domains on opposing polypeptide chains of a multimeric protein, as in the case of $C_H:C_H$ pairing to form functional Fc regions of Ig molecules. Alternatively, they can be heterophilic, as occurs in the case of $V_H:V_L$ or $V_\beta:V_\alpha$ pairing to form the antigen-binding sites of Ig or TCR molecules, respectively. Heterophilic interactions can also occur between Ig domains on entirely distinct molecules expressed on the surfaces of different cells. Such interactions provide adhesive forces that stabilize cell-cell interactions and initiate signals resulting from such interactions. For example, the presentation of an antigen to a helper T cell by an antigen-presenting cell involves heterophilic intercellular Ig domain interactions between several Ig superfamily molecules, including CD4:class II MHC and CD28:B7 (see Chapter 7). Numerous Ig superfamily members have been identified on cells of the developing and mature nervous system, consistent with the functional importance of highly regulated cell-cell interactions in these sites.

actions between the V_L and V_H domains and between the C_L and C_H1 domains may also contribute to the association of heavy and light chains. The two heavy chains of each antibody molecule are also covalently linked by disulfide bonds. In IgG antibodies, the first class of antibodies to be structurally analyzed, these bonds are formed between cysteine residues in the C_H2 regions, close to the region known as the hinge (see below). In other isotypes, the disulfide bonds may be in different locations. Noncovalent interactions (e.g., between the third C_H domains [C_H3]) may also contribute to heavy chain pairing.

The associations between the chains of antibody molecules and the functions of different regions of antibodies were first deduced from experiments done by Rodney Porter in which rabbit IgG was cleaved by proteolytic enzymes into fragments with distinct structural and functional properties. In IgG molecules, the hinge between the C_H1 and C_H2 domains of the heavy chain is the region most susceptible to proteolytic cleavage. If rabbit IgG is treated with the enzyme papain under conditions of limited proteolysis, the enzyme acts on the hinge region and cleaves the IgG into three separate pieces (Fig. 4–3). Two of the pieces are identical to each other and consist of the complete light chain (V_L and C_L) associated with a V_H-C_H1 fragment of the heavy chain. These fragments retain the ability to bind antigen because each contains paired V_L and V_H domains, and

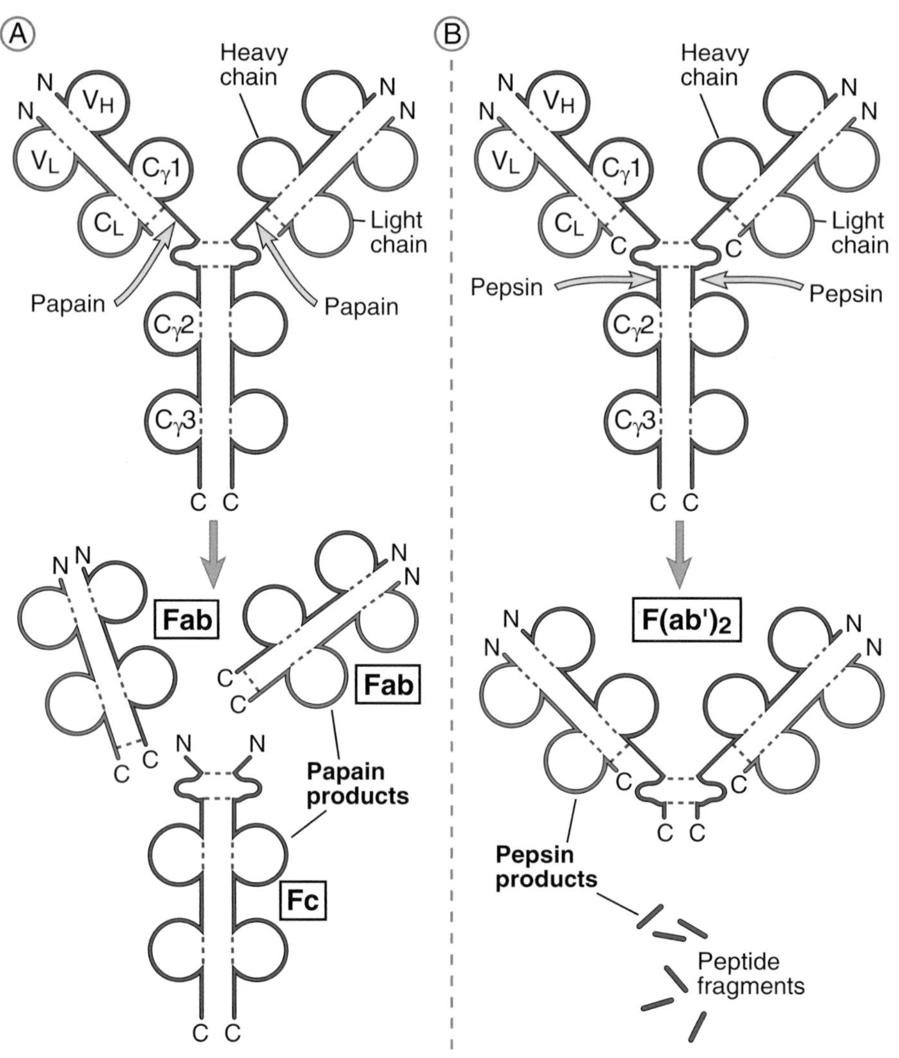

FIGURE 4–3 Proteolytic fragments of an IgG molecule. IgG molecules are cleaved by the enzymes papain (A) and pepsin (B) at the sites indicated by arrows. Papain digestion allows separation of two antigen-binding regions (the Fab fragments) from the portion of the IgG molecule that binds to complement and Fc receptors (the Fc fragment). Pepsin generates a single bivalent antigen-binding fragment, F(ab′)$_2$.

they are called Fab (fragment, antigen binding). The third piece is composed of two identical, disulfide-linked peptides containing the heavy chain C_H2 and C_H3 domains. This piece of IgG has a propensity to self-associate and to crystallize into a lattice and is therefore called Fc (fragment, crystallizable). When pepsin (instead of papain) is used to cleave rabbit IgG under limiting conditions, proteolysis occurs distal to the hinge region, generating an F(ab′)$_2$ antigen-binding fragment of IgG with the hinge and the interchain disulfide bonds intact (see Fig. 4–3).

The results of limited papain or pepsin proteolysis of other isotypes besides IgG, or of IgGs of species other than the rabbit, do not always recapitulate the studies with rabbit IgG. However, the basic organization of the Ig molecule that Porter deduced from his experiments is common to all Ig molecules of all isotypes and of all species. In fact, these proteolysis experiments provided the first evidence that the antigen recognition functions and the effector functions of Ig molecules are spatially segregated.

Structural Features of Variable Regions and Their Relationship to Antigen Binding

Most of the sequence differences among different antibodies are confined to three short stretches in the V region of the heavy chain and to three stretches in the V region of the light chain. These diverse stretches are known as **hypervariable segments**, and they correspond to three protruding loops connecting adjacent strands of the β-sheets that make up the V domains of Ig heavy and light chain proteins (Fig. 4–4). The hypervariable regions are each about 10 amino acid residues long, and they are held in place by more conserved framework sequences that make up the Ig domain of the V region. The genetic mechanisms leading to amino acid variability are discussed in Chapter 8. In an antibody molecule, the three hypervariable regions of a V_L domain and the three hypervariable regions of a V_H domain are brought together to form an antigen-binding surface. Because these sequences form a surface that is complementary

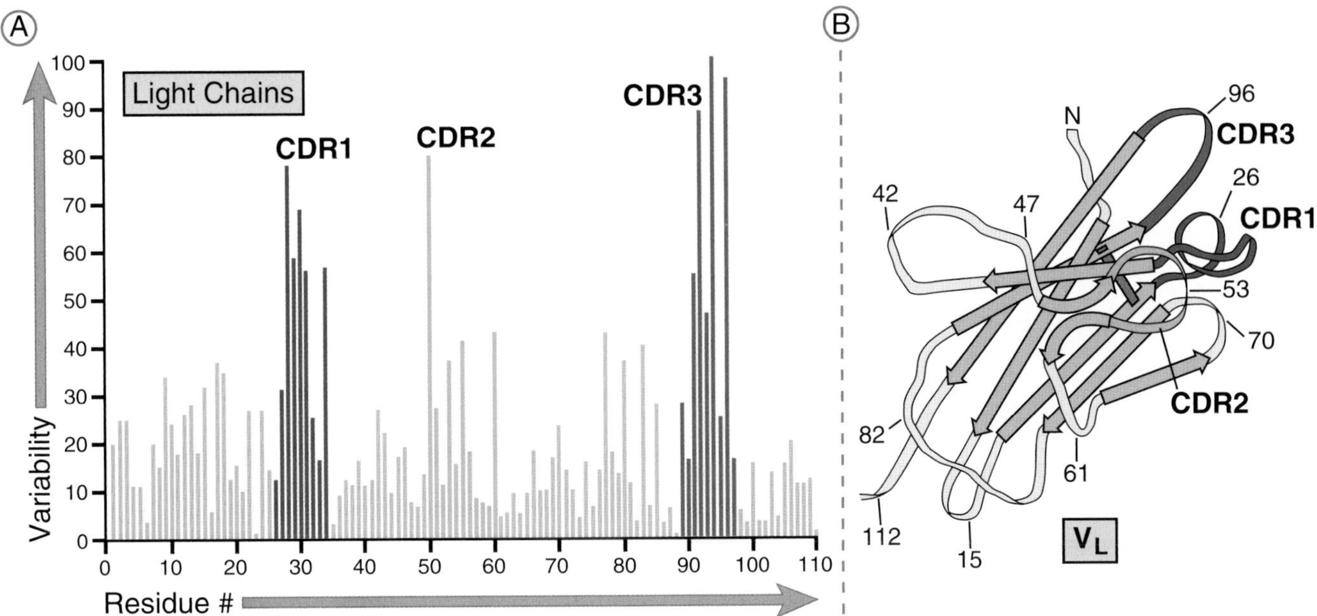

FIGURE 4–4 Hypervariable regions in Ig molecules. A. Kabat-Wu plot of amino acid variability in Ig molecules. The histograms depict the extent of variability defined as the number of differences in each amino acid residue among various independently sequenced Ig light chains, plotted against amino acid residue number, measured from the amino terminus. This method of analysis, developed by Elvin Kabat and Tai Te Wu, indicates that the most variable residues are clustered in three "hypervariable" regions, colored in blue, yellow, and red, corresponding to CDR1, CDR2, and CDR3, respectively. Three hypervariable regions are also present in heavy chains. (Courtesy of Dr. E.A. Kabat, Department of Microbiology, Columbia University College of Physicians and Surgeons, New York.) B. Three-dimensional view of the hypervariable CDR loops in a light chain V domain. The V region of a light chain is shown with CDR1, CDR2, and CDR3 loops, colored in blue, yellow, and red, respectively. These loops correspond to the hypervariable regions in the variability plot in A. Heavy chain hypervariable regions (not shown) are also located in three loops, and all six loops are juxtaposed in the antibody molecule to form the antigen-binding surface (see Fig. 4–5).

to the three-dimensional structure of the bound antigen, the hypervariable regions are also called **complementarity-determining regions (CDRs)**. Proceeding from either the V_L or the V_H amino terminus, these regions are called CDR1, CDR2, and CDR3 (see Fig. 4–4). The CDR3s of both the V_H segment and the V_L segment are the most variable of the CDRs. As we will discuss in Chapter 8, there are special genetic mechanisms for generating more sequence diversity in CDR3 than in CDR1 and CDR2. Crystallographic analyses of antibodies reveal that the CDRs form extended loops that are exposed on the surface of the antibody and are thus available to interact with antigen (see Fig. 4–4). Sequence differences among the CDRs of different antibody molecules contribute to distinct interaction surfaces and, therefore, specificities of individual antibodies. The ability of a V region to fold into an Ig domain is mostly determined by the conserved sequences of the framework regions adjacent to the CDRs. Confining the sequence variability to three short stretches allows the basic structure of all antibodies to be maintained despite the variability among different antibodies.

Antigen binding by antibody molecules is primarily a function of the hypervariable regions of V_H and V_L. Crystallographic analyses of antigen-antibody complexes show that the amino acid residues of the hypervariable regions form multiple contacts with bound antigen (Fig. 4–5). The most extensive contact is with the third hypervariable region (CDR3), which is also the most variable of the three CDRs. However, antigen binding is not solely a function of the CDRs, and framework residues may also contact the antigen. Moreover, in the binding of some antigens, one or more of the CDRs may be outside the region of contact with antigen, thus not participating in antigen binding.

Structural Features of Constant Regions and Their Relationship to Effector Functions

Antibody molecules can be divided into distinct classes and subclasses on the basis of differences in the structure of their heavy chain C regions. The classes of antibody molecules are also called **isotypes** and are named IgA, IgD, IgE, IgG, and IgM (Table 4–2). In humans, IgA and IgG isotypes can be further subdivided into closely related subclasses, or subtypes, called IgA1 and IgA2, and IgG1, IgG2, IgG3, and IgG4. (Mice, which are often used in the study of immune responses, differ in that the IgG isotype is divided into the IgG1, IgG2a, IgG2b, and IgG3 subclasses.) The heavy chain C regions of all antibody molecules of one isotype or subtype have essentially the same amino acid sequence. This sequence is different in antibodies of other isotypes or subtypes. Heavy chains are designated by the letter of the Greek alphabet corresponding to the isotype of the antibody:

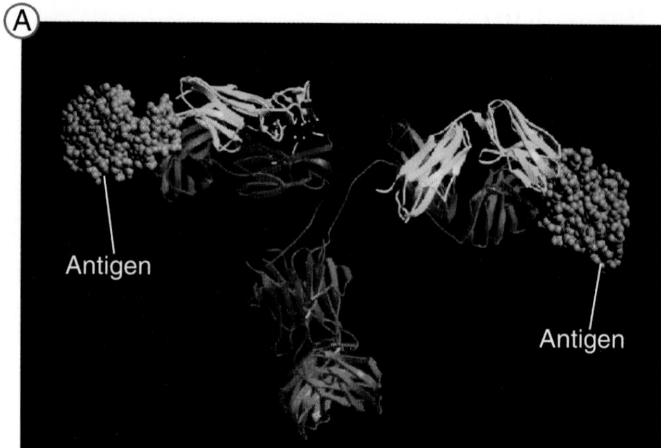

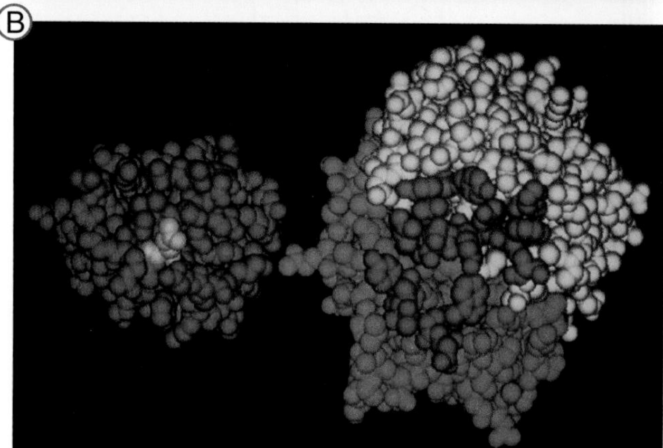

FIGURE 4–5 Binding of an antigen by an antibody. A. This model of a globular protein antigen (hen egg lysozyme) bound to an antibody molecule shows how the antigen-binding site can accommodate soluble macromolecules in their native (folded) conformation. The heavy chains of the antibody are colored red, the light chains are yellow, and the antigen is colored blue. (Courtesy of Dr. Dan Vaughn, Cold Spring Harbor Laboratory, Cold Spring Harbor, New York.) B. A view of the interacting surfaces of hen egg lysozyme (in green) and an Fab fragment of a monoclonal anti-hen egg lysozyme antibody (V_H in blue and V_L in yellow) is provided. The residues of hen egg lysozyme and of the Fab fragment that interact with one another are shown in red. A critical glutamine residue on lysozyme (in magenta) fits into a "cleft" in the antibody. (This figure is based on Figure 3B and reprinted with permission from Amit AG, RA Mariuzza, SE Phillips, and RJ Poljak. Three dimensional structure of an antigen antibody complex at 2.8A resolution. Science 233, 747–753, 1986. Copyright 1986 AAAS.)

IgA1 contains α1 heavy chains; IgA2, α2; IgD, δ; IgE, ε; IgG1, γ1; IgG2, γ2; IgG3, γ3; IgG4, γ4; and IgM, μ. In human IgM and IgE antibodies, the C regions contain four tandem Ig domains. The C regions of IgG, IgA, and IgD contain only three Ig domains. These domains are designated C_H and numbered sequentially from amino terminus to carboxyl terminus (e.g., C_H1, C_H2, and so on). In each isotype, these regions may be designated more specifically (e.g., $C_\gamma 1$, $C_\gamma 2$ in IgG). Antibodies can act as antigens when introduced into foreign hosts, eliciting the production of anti-antibodies (Box 4–3). By immunizing an animal of one species with Ig of another species, it is possible to produce anti-antibodies specific for one Ig class or subclass, and such antibodies are routinely used in the clinical and experimental analyses of humoral immune responses.

Different isotypes and subtypes of antibodies perform different effector functions. The reason for this is that most of the effector functions of antibodies are mediated by the binding of heavy chain C regions to Fc receptors on different cells, such as phagocytes, NK cells, and mast cells, and to plasma proteins, such as complement proteins. Antibody isotypes and subtypes differ in their C regions and therefore in what they bind to and what effector functions they perform. The effector functions mediated by each antibody isotype are listed in Table 4–2 and are discussed in more detail later in this chapter and in Chapter 14.

Antibody molecules are flexible, permitting them to bind to different arrays of antigens. Every antibody contains at least two antigen-binding sites, each formed by a pair of V_H and V_L domains. Many Ig molecules can orient these binding sites so that two antigen molecules on a planar (e.g., cell) surface may be engaged at once (Fig. 4–6). This flexibility is conferred, in large part, by a **hinge region** located between C_H1 and C_H2 in certain isotypes. The hinge region varies in length from 10 to more than 60 amino acid residues in different isotypes. Portions of this sequence assume a random and flexible conformation, permitting molecular motion between the C_H1 and C_H2 domains. Some of the greatest differences between the constant regions of the IgG subclasses are concentrated in the hinge. This leads to different overall shapes of the IgG subtypes. In addition, some flexibility of antibody molecules is due to the ability of each V_H domain to rotate with respect to the adjacent C_H1 domain.

There are two classes, or isotypes, of light chains, called κ and λ, which are distinguished by their carboxy-terminal constant (C) regions. An antibody molecule has either two κ light chains or two λ light chains, but never one of each. In humans, about 60% of antibody molecules have κ light chains, and about 40% have λ light

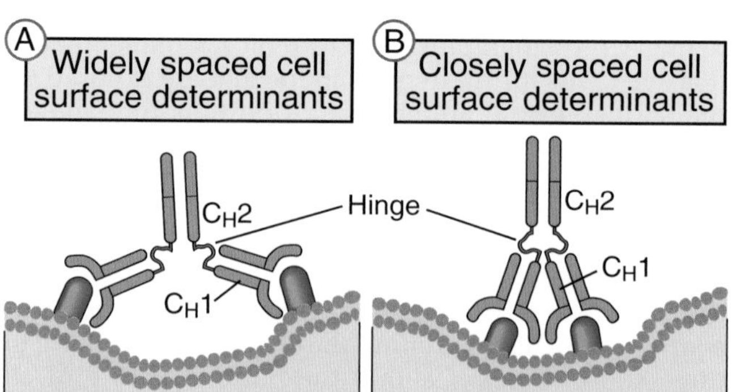

FIGURE 4–6 Flexibility of antibody molecules. The two antigen-binding sites of an Ig monomer can simultaneously bind to two determinants separated by varying distances. In A, an Ig molecule is depicted binding to two widely spaced determinants on a cell surface, and in B, the same antibody is binding to two determinants that are close together. This flexibility is mainly due to the hinge regions located between the C_H1 and C_H2 domains, which permit independent movement of antigen-binding sites relative to the rest of the molecule.

Table 4–2. Human Antibody Isotypes

Isotype of antibody	Subtypes	H chain	Serum concentr. (mg/mL)	Serum half-life (days)	Secreted form	Functions
IgA	IgA1,2	α(1 or 2)	3.5	6	**IgA (dimer)** Monomer, dimer, trimer 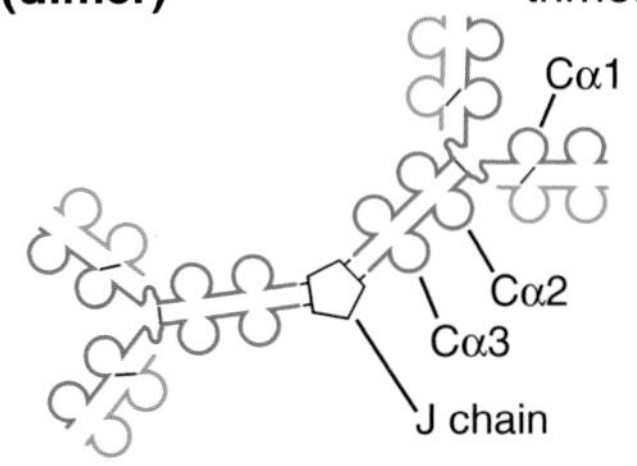 Cα1 Cα2 Cα3 J chain	Mucosal immunity
IgD	None	δ	Trace	3	None	Naive B cell antigen receptor
IgE	None	ε	0.05	2	**IgE** Monomer 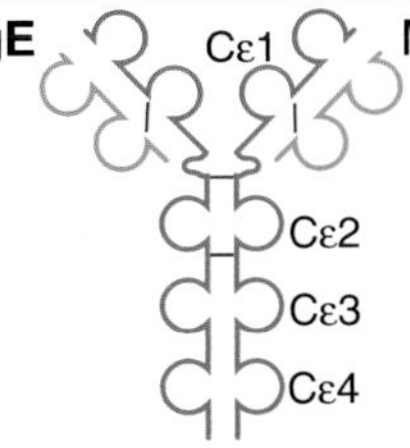 Cε1 Cε2 Cε3 Cε4	Defense against helminthic parasites, immediate hypersensitivity
IgG	IgG1-4	γ(1,2,3 or 4)	13.5	23	**IgG1** Monomer 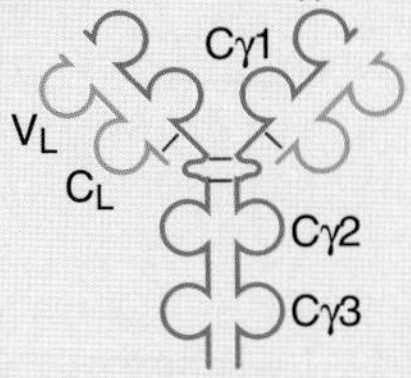 V_H Cγ1 V_L C_L Cγ2 Cγ3	Opsonization, complement activation, antibody-dependent cell-mediated cytotoxicity, neonatal immunity, feedback inhibition of B cells
IgM	None	μ	1.5	5	**IgM** Pentamers, hexamers 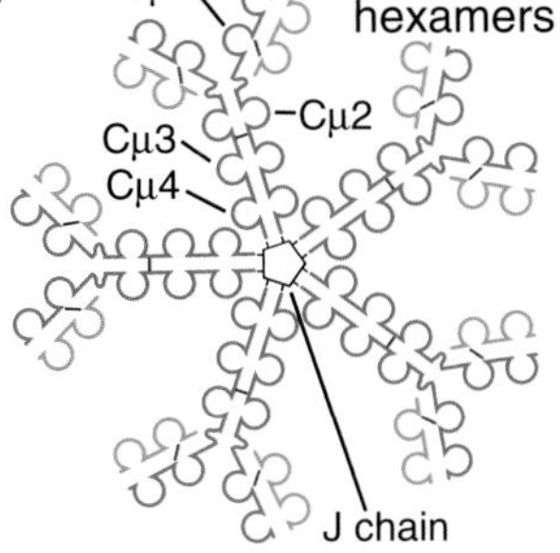 Cμ1 Cμ2 Cμ3 Cμ4 J chain	Naive B cell antigen receptor, complement activation

The effector functions of antibodies are discussed in detail in Chapter 14.

chains. Marked changes in this ratio can occur in patients with monoclonal B cell tumors because the neoplastic clone produces antibody molecules with the same light chain. In fact, the ratio of κ-bearing cells to λ-bearing cells is often used clinically in the diagnosis of B cell lymphomas. In mice, κ-containing antibodies are about 10 times more abundant than λ-containing antibodies. Unlike in heavy chain isotypes, there are no known differences in function between κ-containing antibodies and λ-containing antibodies.

Secreted and membrane-associated antibodies differ in the amino acid sequence of the carboxy-terminal end of the heavy chain C region. In the secreted form, found in blood and other extracellular fluids, the carboxy-terminal portion is hydrophilic. The membrane-bound form of antibody contains a carboxy-terminal stretch that includes a hydrophobic α-helical transmembrane anchor region followed by an intracellular juxtamembrane positively charged stretch that helps anchor the protein in the membrane (Fig. 4–7). In membrane IgM

Box 4–3 ▪ IN DEPTH: ANTI-Ig ANTIBODIES: ALLOTYPES AND IDIOTYPES

Antibody molecules are proteins and can therefore be immunogenic. Immunologists have exploited this fact to produce antibodies specific for Ig molecules that can be used as reagents to analyze the structure and function of the Ig molecules. To obtain an anti-antibody response, it is necessary that the Ig molecules used to immunize an animal be recognized in whole or in part as foreign. The simplest approach is to immunize an animal of one species (e.g., rabbit) with Ig molecules of a second species (e.g., mouse). Populations of antibodies generated by such cross-species immunizations are largely specific for epitopes present in the constant (C) regions of light or heavy chains. Antisera generated in this way can be used to define the isotype of an antibody.

When an animal is immunized with Ig molecules derived from another animal of the same species, the immune response is confined to epitopes of the immunizing Ig that are absent or uncommon on the Ig molecules of the responder animal. Two types of determinants have been defined by this approach. First, determinants may be formed by minor structural differences (polymorphisms) in amino acid sequences located in the conserved portions of Ig molecules, called **allotopes.** All antibody molecules that share a particular allotope are said to belong to the same **allotype.** In simple terms, an allotype is the protein product of a distinct allelic form of an Ig gene. Different individuals in a species may inherit two different forms of any Ig gene. Most allotopes are located in the C regions of light or heavy chains, but some are found in the framework portions of V regions. Allotypic differences have been important in the study of Ig genetics. For example, allotypes detected by anti-Ig antibodies were initially used to locate the position of Ig genes by linkage analysis. In addition, the remarkable observation that, in homozygous animals, all the heavy chains of a particular isotype (e.g., IgM) share the same allotype even though the V regions of these antibodies have different amino acid sequences provided the first evidence that the C regions of all Ig molecules of a particular isotype are encoded by a single gene segment that is separate from the gene segments encoding V regions. As is discussed in Chapter 8, we now know that this surprising conclusion is correct.

The second type of determinant on antibody molecules that can be recognized as foreign by other animals of the same species is that formed by the hypervariable regions of the Ig variable domains. When a homogeneous population of antibody molecules (e.g., a myeloma protein, or a monoclonal antibody) is used as an immunogen, antibodies are produced that react with the unique hypervariable loops of that antibody. These determinants are recognized as foreign because they are usually present in very small quantities in any given animal (i.e., at too low a level to induce self-tolerance). The unique determinants of individual antibody molecules are called **idiotopes,** and all antibody molecules that share an idiotope are said to belong to the same **idiotype.** As is discussed in Chapter 8, hypervariable sequences that form idiotopes arise both from inherited germline diversity and from somatic events. Idiotopes may be involved in regulation of B cell functions. The theory of lymphocyte regulation through idiotopes of antigen receptors, called the network hypothesis, is mentioned in Chapter 11.

In addition to experimentally elicited anti-Ig antibodies, immunologists have been interested in naturally occurring antibodies reactive with self Ig molecules. Anti-Ig antibodies are particularly prevalent in an autoimmune disease called rheumatoid arthritis (see Chapter 18), in which setting they are known as rheumatoid factor. Rheumatoid factor is usually an IgM antibody that reacts with the constant regions of self IgG. The significance of rheumatoid factor in the pathogenesis of rheumatoid arthritis is unknown.

Patients treated with mouse monoclonal antibodies may make antibodies against the mouse Ig, called a human anti-mouse antibody (HAMA) response. These anti-Ig antibodies eliminate the injected monoclonal antibody. Humanized antibodies have been developed to circumvent this problem, but even humanized antibodies contain hypervariable regions derived from the original monoclonal antibody, and these can elicit a response in treated patients.

and IgD molecules, the cytoplasmic portion of the heavy chain is short, only three amino acid residues in length; in membrane IgG and IgE molecules, it is somewhat longer, up to 30 amino acid residues in length, but this includes the positively charged three–amino acid juxtamembrane sequence.

Secreted IgG and IgE, and all membrane Ig molecules, regardless of isotype, are monomeric with respect to the basic antibody structural unit (i.e., they contain two heavy chains and two light chains). In contrast, the secreted forms of IgM and IgA form multimeric complexes in which two or more of the four-chain core antibody structural units are covalently joined. IgM may be secreted as pentamers and hexamers of the core four-chain structure, while IgA is often secreted as an Ig dimer. These complexes are formed by interactions between regions, called tail pieces, that are located at the carboxy-terminal ends of the secreted forms of μ and α heavy chains (see Table 4–2). Multimeric IgM and IgA molecules also contain an additional 15-kD polypeptide called the joining (J) chain, which is disulfide bonded to the tail pieces and serves to stabilize the multimeric complexes, and to transport multimers across epithelia from the basolateral to the luminal end.

Synthesis, Assembly, and Expression of Ig Molecules

Ig heavy and light chains, like most secreted and membrane proteins, are synthesized on membrane-bound ribosomes in the rough endoplasmic reticulum. The protein is translocated into the endoplasmic reticulum,

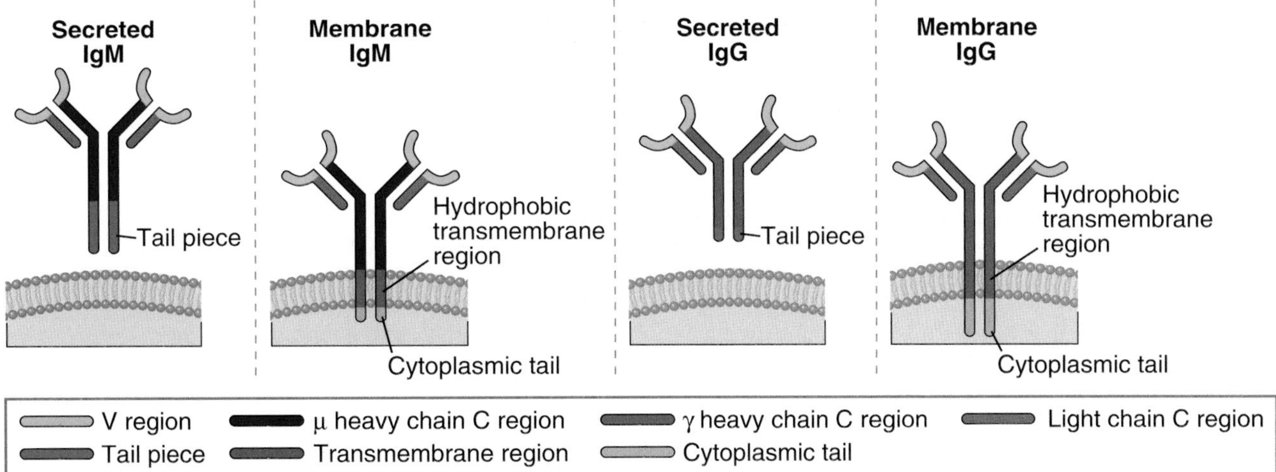

FIGURE 4–7 Membrane and secreted forms of Ig heavy chains. The membrane forms of the Ig heavy chains, but not the secreted forms, contain transmembrane regions made up of hydrophobic amino acid residues and cytoplasmic domains that differ significantly among the different isotypes. The cytoplasmic portion of the membrane form of the μ chain contains only 3 residues, whereas the cytoplasmic region of IgG heavy chains contains 20–30 residues. The secreted forms of the antibodies end in C-terminal tail pieces, which also differ among isotypes: μ has a long tail piece (21 residues) that is involved in pentamer formation, whereas IgGs have a short tail piece (3 residues).

and Ig heavy chains are N-glycosylated during the translocation process. The proper folding of Ig heavy chains and their assembly with light chains are regulated by proteins resident in the endoplasmic reticulum called chaperones. These proteins, which include calnexin and a molecule called BiP (binding protein), bind to newly synthesized Ig polypeptides and ensure that they are retained or targeted for degradation unless they become properly folded and assembled into Ig molecules. The covalent association of heavy and light chains, stabilized by the formation of disulfide bonds, also occurs in the endoplasmic reticulum. After assembly, the Ig molecules are released from the chaperones and directed into the cisternae of the Golgi complex, where carbohydrates are modified, and the antibodies are then transported to the plasma membrane in vesicles. Antibodies of the membrane form are anchored in the plasma membrane and the secreted form is transported out of the cell. Other proteins that bind to Ig are coordinately regulated. For instance, secreted IgA and IgM antibodies are maintained as multimers by the attached J chains. In plasma cells, transcription of Ig heavy and light chain genes is accompanied by coordinate J chain gene transcription and biosynthesis.

The maturation of B cells from bone marrow progenitors is accompanied by specific changes in Ig gene expression, resulting in the production of Ig molecules in different forms (Fig. 4–8). The earliest cell in the B lymphocyte lineage that produces Ig polypeptides, called the pre-B cell, synthesizes the membrane form of the μ heavy chain. These μ chains associate with proteins called surrogate light chains to form the pre-B cell receptor, and a small proportion of the synthesized pre-B cell receptor is expressed on the cell surface. Immature and mature B cells produce κ or λ light chains, which associate with μ proteins to form IgM molecules. Mature B cells express membrane forms of IgM and IgD (the μ and δ heavy chains associated with κ or λ light chains). These membrane Ig receptors serve as cell surface receptors that recognize antigens and initiate the process of B cell activation. The pre-B cell receptor and the B cell antigen receptor are noncovalently associated with two other integral membrane proteins, Igα and Igβ, which serve signaling functions and are essential for surface expression of IgM and IgD. The molecular and cellular events in B cell maturation underlying these changes in antibody expression are discussed in detail in Chapter 8.

When mature B lymphocytes are activated by antigens and other stimuli, the cells differentiate into antibody-secreting cells. This process is also accompanied by changes in the pattern of Ig production. One such change is the enhanced production of the secreted form of Ig as opposed to the membrane form. This alteration occurs at the level of posttranscriptional processing and will be discussed in Chapter 10. The second change is the expression of Ig heavy chain isotypes other than IgM and IgD. This process, called heavy chain isotype (or class) switching, is described later in this chapter and in more detail in Chapter 10, when we discuss B cell activation.

ANTIBODY BINDING OF ANTIGENS

Features of Biologic Antigens

An **antigen** is any substance that may be specifically bound by an antibody molecule or T cell receptor. Antibodies can recognize as antigens almost every kind of biologic molecule, including simple intermediary metabolites, sugars, lipids, autacoids, and hormones, as well as macromolecules such as complex carbohydrates, phospholipids, nucleic acids, and proteins. This is in contrast to T cells, which mainly recognize peptides (see Chapter 6).

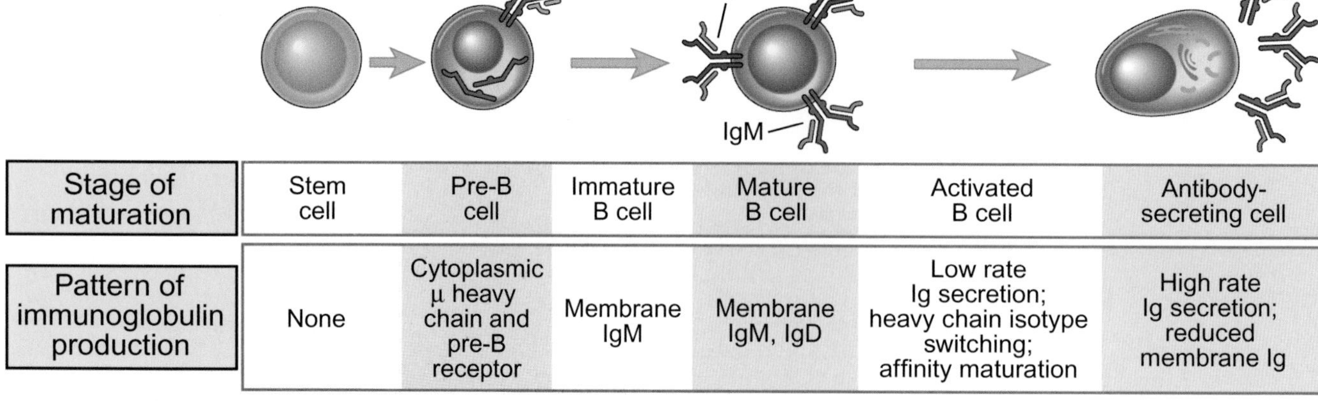

IgD
IgM
Stage of maturation
Stem cell
Pre-B cell
Immature B cell
Mature B cell
Activated B cell
Antibody-secreting cell
Pattern of immunoglobulin production
None
Cytoplasmic μ heavy chain and pre-B receptor
Membrane IgM
Membrane IgM, IgD
Low rate Ig secretion; heavy chain isotype switching; affinity maturation
High rate Ig secretion; reduced membrane Ig

FIGURE 4–8 Ig expression during B lymphocyte maturation. Stages in B lymphocyte maturation are shown with associated changes in the production of Ig heavy and light chains. IgM heavy chains are shown in red, IgD heavy chains in blue, and light chains in green. The molecular events accompanying these changes are discussed in Chapters 8 and 10.

Although all antigens are recognized by specific lymphocytes or by antibodies, only some antigens are capable of activating lymphocytes. Molecules that stimulate immune responses are called **immunogens.** Only macromolecules are capable of stimulating B lymphocytes to initiate humoral immune responses, because B cell activation requires either the bringing together (cross-linking) of multiple antigen receptors, or requires protein antigens to elicit T cell help. Small chemicals, such as dinitrophenol, may bind to antibodies, and are therefore antigens, but cannot activate B cells on their own (i.e., they are not immunogenic). To generate antibodies specific for such small chemicals, immunologists commonly attach them to a protein before immunization. In these cases, the small chemical is called a **hapten,** and the protein to which it is conjugated is called a **carrier.** The hapten-carrier complex, unlike free hapten, can act as an immunogen (see Chapter 10). A second approach to make a hapten immunogenic is to render it multivalent, as discussed below, often by attaching a number of hapten molecules to a single molecule of a polysaccharide.

Macromolecules, such as proteins, polysaccharides, and nucleic acids, are usually much bigger than the antigen-binding region of an antibody molecule (see Fig. 4–5). Therefore, any antibody binds to only a portion of the macromolecule, which is called a **determinant** or an **epitope.** These two words are synonymous and are used interchangeably throughout this book. Macromolecules typically contain multiple determinants, some of which may be repeated, and each of which, by definition, can be bound by an antibody. The presence of multiple identical determinants in an antigen is referred to as **polyvalency** or **multivalency.** Most globular proteins do not contain multiple identical epitopes and are not polyvalent, unless they are in aggregates. In the case of polysaccharides and nucleic acids, many identical epitopes may be regularly spaced, and the molecules are said to be polyvalent. Cell surfaces, including microbes, often display polyvalent arrays of protein or carbohydrate antigenic determinants. Polyvalent antigens can induce clustering of the B cell receptor and thus initiate the process of B cell activation.

The spatial arrangement of different epitopes on a single protein molecule may influence the binding of antibodies in several ways. When determinants are well separated, two or more antibody molecules can be bound to the same protein antigen without influencing each other; such determinants are said to be nonoverlapping. When two determinants are close to one another, the binding of antibody to the first determinant may cause steric interference with the binding of antibody to the second; such determinants are said to be overlapping. In rarer cases, binding of one antibody may cause a conformational change in the structure of the antigen, positively or negatively influencing the binding of a second antibody at another site on the protein by means other than steric hindrance. Such interactions are called allosteric effects.

Any available shape or surface on a molecule that may be recognized by an antibody constitutes an antigenic determinant or epitope. Antigenic determinants may be delineated on any type of compound, including but not restricted to carbohydrates, proteins, lipids, and nucleic acids. In the case of proteins, the formation of some determinants depends only on the primary structure, and the formation of other determinants reflects tertiary structure (Fig. 4–9). Epitopes formed by several adjacent amino acid residues are called **linear determinants.** The antigen-binding site of an antibody can usually accommodate a linear determinant made up of about six amino acids. If linear determinants appear on the external surface or in a region of extended conformation in the native folded protein, they may be accessible to antibodies. More often, linear determinants may be inaccessible in the native conformation and appear only when the protein is denatured. In contrast, **conformational determinants** are formed by amino acid residues that are not in a sequence but become spatially juxtaposed in the folded protein. Antibodies specific for certain linear determinants and antibodies specific for conformational determinants can be used to ascertain

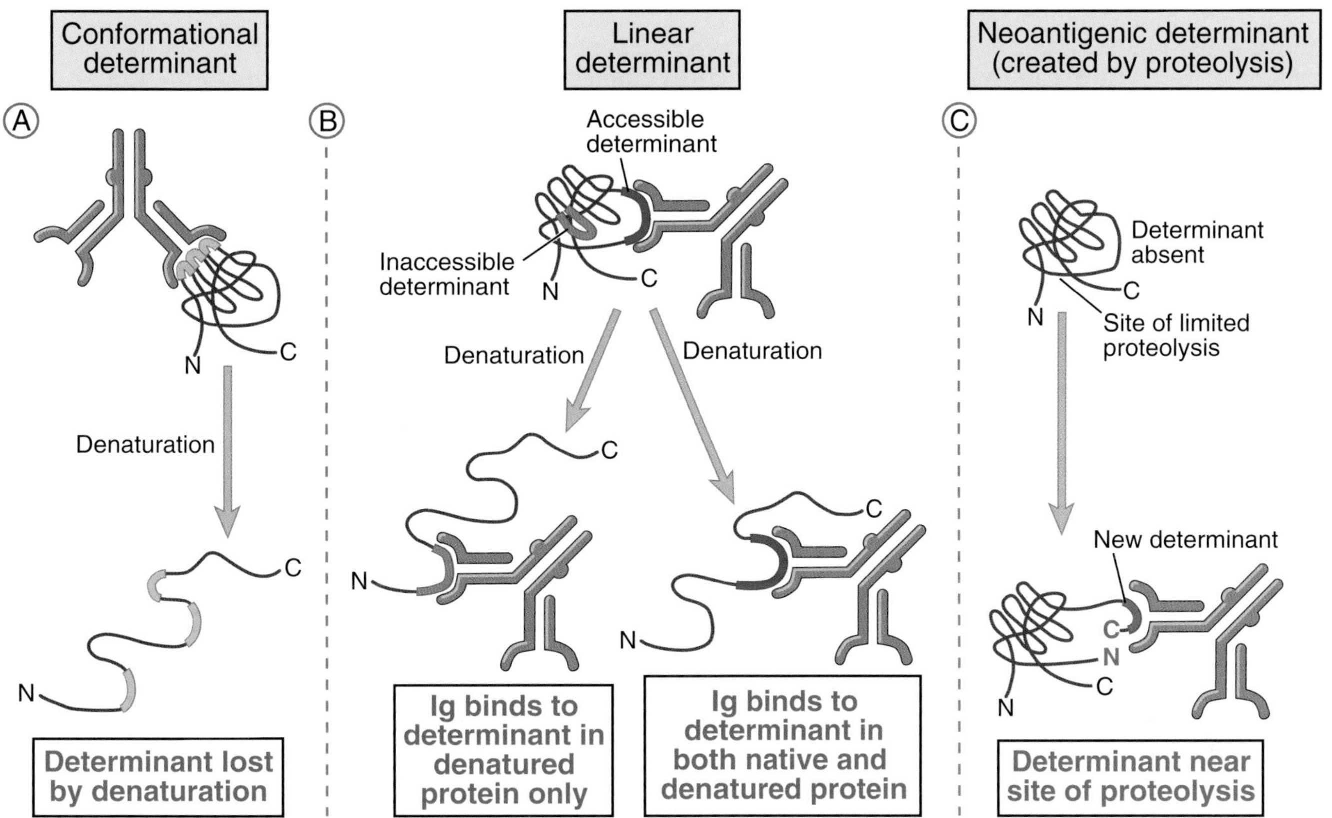

FIGURE 4–9 The nature of antigenic determinants. Antigenic determinants (shown in orange, red, and blue) may depend on protein folding (conformation) as well as on primary structure. Some determinants are accessible in native proteins and are lost on denaturation (A), whereas others are exposed only on protein unfolding (B). Neodeterminants arise from postsynthetic modifications such as peptide bond cleavage (C).

whether a protein is denatured or in its native conformation, respectively. Proteins may be subjected to modifications such as glycosylation, phosphorylation, or proteolysis. These modifications, by altering the structure of the protein, can produce new epitopes. Such epitopes are called **neoantigenic determinants,** and they too may be recognized by specific antibodies.

Structural and Chemical Basis of Antigen Binding

The antigen-binding sites of most antibodies are planar surfaces that can accommodate conformational epitopes of macromolecules, allowing the antibodies to bind large macromolecules (see Fig. 4–5). As is discussed in Chapter 5, this is a key difference between the antigen-binding sites of antibody molecules and those of certain other antigen-binding molecules of the immune system, namely, MHC molecules, which contain antigen-binding clefts that bind small peptides but not native globular proteins (see Table 4–1). In some instances, such as antibodies specific for small carbohydrates, the antigen is bound in a cleft between V_L and V_H domains.

The recognition of antigen by antibody involves noncovalent, reversible binding. Various types of noncovalent interactions may contribute to antibody binding of antigen, including electrostatic forces, hydrogen bonds, van der Waals forces, and hydrophobic interactions. The relative importance of each of these depends on the structures of the binding site of the individual antibody and of the antigenic determinant. The strength of the binding between a single combining site of an antibody and an epitope of an antigen is called the **affinity** of the antibody. The affinity is commonly represented by a dissociation constant (K_d), which indicates how easy it is to separate an antigen-antibody complex into its constituents. A smaller K_d indicates a stronger or higher-affinity interaction because a lower concentration of antigen and of antibody is required for complex formation. The K_d of antibodies produced in typical humoral immune responses usually varies from about 10^{-7} M to 10^{-11} M. Serum from an immunized individual will contain a mixture of antibodies with different affinities for the antigen, depending primarily on the amino acid sequences of the CDRs.

Because the hinge region of antibodies gives them flexibility, a single antibody may attach to a single multivalent antigen by more than one binding site. For IgG or IgE, this attachment can involve, at most, two binding sites, one on each Fab. For pentameric IgM, however, a single antibody may bind at up to 10 different sites (Fig. 4–10). Polyvalent antigens will have more than one copy of a particular determinant. Although the affinity of any one antigen-binding site will be the same for each epitope of a polyvalent antigen, the strength of attachment of the antibody to the antigen must take into account binding of all the sites to all the available epitopes. This overall strength of attachment is called the **avidity** and is much greater than the affinity of any one antigen-binding site. Thus, a low-affinity IgM molecule can still bind tightly to a polyvalent antigen because many low-affinity interactions (up to 10 per IgM molecule) can produce a single high-avidity interaction.

Polyvalent antigens are important from the viewpoint of B cell activation, as discussed earlier. Polyvalent interactions between antigen and antibody are also of biologic significance because many effector functions of antibodies are triggered optimally when two or more antibody molecules are brought close together by binding to a polyvalent antigen. If a polyvalent antigen is mixed with a specific antibody in a test tube, the two interact to form immune complexes (Fig. 4–11). At the correct concentration, called a zone of equivalence, antibody and antigen form an extensively cross-linked network of attached molecules such that most or all of the antigen and antibody molecules are complexed into large masses. Immune complexes may be dissociated into smaller aggregates either by increasing the concentration of antigen so that free antigen molecules will displace antigen bound to the antibody (zone of antigen excess) or by increasing antibody so that free antibody molecules will displace bound antibody from antigen determinants (zone of antibody excess). If a zone of equivalence is reached in vivo, large immune complexes can form in the circulation. Immune complexes that are trapped or formed in tissues can initiate an inflammatory reaction, resulting in immune complex diseases (see Chapter 18).

STRUCTURE-FUNCTION RELATIONSHIPS IN ANTIBODY MOLECULES

Many structural features of antibodies are critical for their ability to recognize antigens and for their effector functions. In the following section, we summarize how the structure of antibodies contributes to their functions.

Features Related to Antigen Recognition

Antibodies are able to specifically recognize a wide variety of antigens with varying affinities. All the features of antigen recognition reflect the properties of antibody V regions.

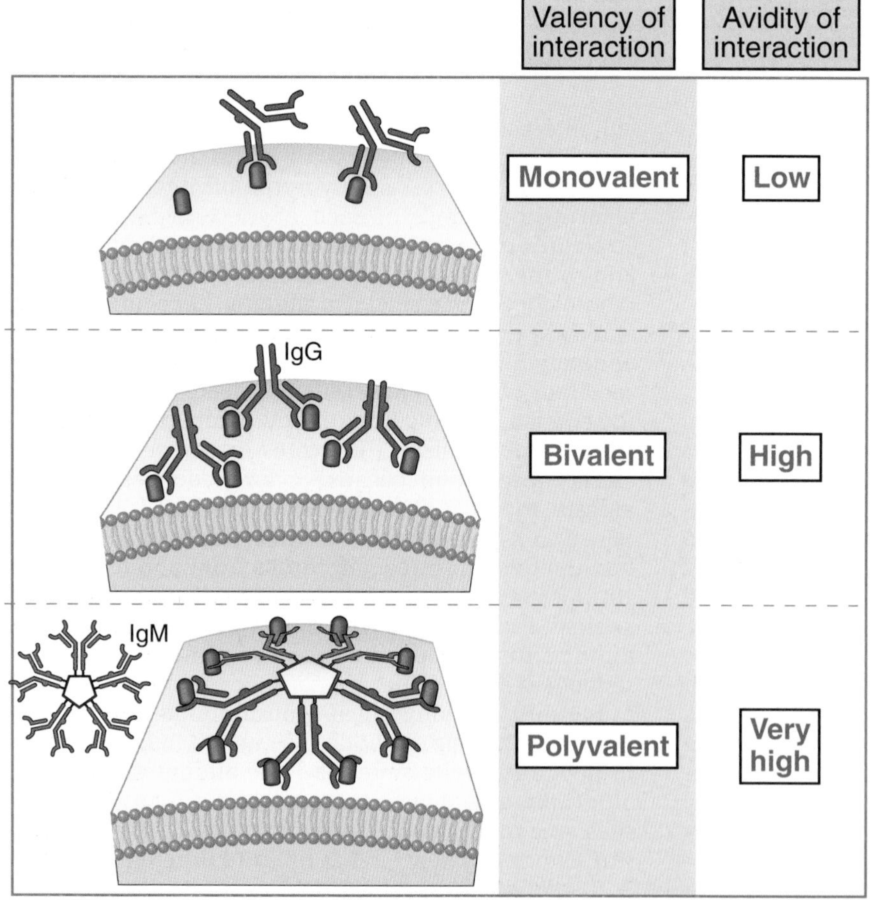

FIGURE 4–10 Valency and avidity of antibody-antigen interactions. Monovalent antigens, or epitopes spaced far apart on cell surfaces, will interact with a single binding site of one antibody molecule. Although the affinity of this interaction may be high, the overall avidity may be relatively low. When repeated determinants on a cell surface are close enough, both the antigen-binding sites of a single IgG molecule can bind, leading to a higher-avidity bivalent interaction. The hinge region of the IgG molecule accommodates the shape change needed for simultaneous engagement of both binding sites. IgM molecules have 10 identical antigen-binding sites that can theoretically bind simultaneously with 10 repeating determinants on a cell surface, resulting in a polyvalent, high-avidity interaction.

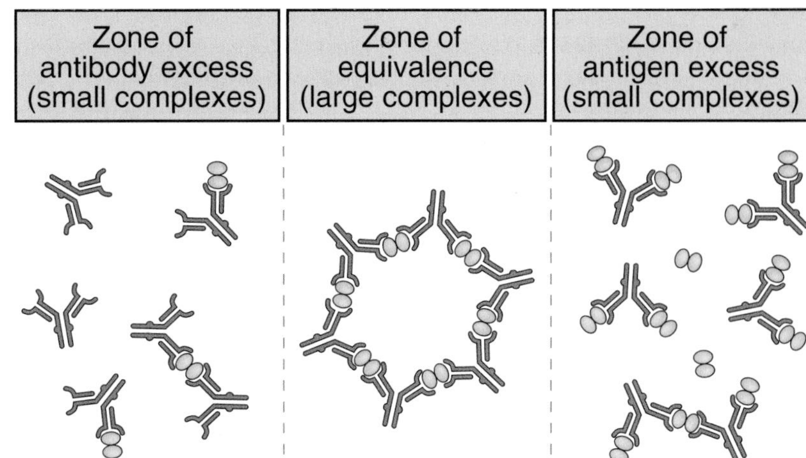

FIGURE 4–11 Antigen-antibody complexes. The sizes of antigen-antibody (immune) complexes are a function of the relative concentrations of antigen and antibody. Large complexes are formed at concentrations of multivalent antigens and antibodies that are termed the zone of equivalence; the complexes are smaller in relative antigen or antibody excess.

Specificity

Antibodies can be remarkably specific for antigens, distinguishing between small differences in chemical structure. Classic experiments performed by Karl Landsteiner in the 1930s demonstrated that antibodies made in response to an aminobenzene hapten with a meta-substituted sulfonate group would bind strongly to this hapten but weakly or not at all to ortho- or para-substituted isomers. These antigens are structurally similar and differ only in the location of the sulfonate group on the benzene ring.

The fine specificity of antibodies applies to the recognition of all classes of molecules. For example, antibodies can distinguish between two linear protein determinants differing by only a single conservative amino acid substitution that has little effect on secondary structure. Because the biochemical constituents of all living organisms are fundamentally similar, this high degree of specificity is necessary so that antibodies generated in response to the antigens of one microbe usually do not react with structurally similar self molecules or with the antigens of other microbes. However, some antibodies produced against one antigen may bind to a different but structurally related antigen. This is referred to as a **cross-reaction.** Antibodies that are produced in response to a microbial antigen sometimes cross-react with self antigens, and this may be the basis of certain immunologic diseases (see Chapter 18).

Diversity

As we discussed earlier in this chapter, an individual is capable of making a tremendous number of structurally distinct antibodies, perhaps up to 10^9, each with a distinct specificity. The ability of antibodies in any individual to specifically bind a large number of different antigens is a reflection of antibody **diversity,** and the total collection of antibodies with different specificities represents the **antibody repertoire.** The genetic mechanisms that generate such a large antibody repertoire occur exclusively in lymphocytes. They are based on the random recombination of a limited set of inherited germline DNA sequences into functional genes that encode the V regions of heavy and light chains as well as on the addition of nucleotide sequences during the recombination process. These mechanisms are discussed in detail in Chapter 8. The millions of resulting variations in structure are concentrated in the hypervariable regions of both heavy and light chains and thereby determine specificity for antigens.

Affinity Maturation

The ability of antibodies to neutralize toxins and infectious microbes is dependent on tight binding of the antibodies. As we have discussed, tight binding is achieved by high-affinity and high-avidity interactions. A mechanism for the generation of high-affinity antibodies involves subtle changes in the structure of the V regions of antibodies during T cell–dependent humoral immune responses to protein antigens. These changes come about by a process of **somatic mutation** in antigen-stimulated B lymphocytes that generates new V domain structures, some of which bind the antigen with greater affinity than did the original V domains (Fig. 4–12). Those B cells producing higher-affinity antibodies preferentially bind to the antigen and, as a result of selection, become the dominant B cells with each subsequent exposure to the antigen. This process, called **affinity maturation,** results in an increase in the average binding affinity of antibodies for an antigen as a humoral immune response evolves. Thus, an antibody produced during a primary immune response to a protein antigen often has a K_d in the range of 10^{-7} to 10^{-9} M; in secondary responses, the affinity increases, with a K_d of 10^{-11} M or even less. The mechanisms of somatic mutation and affinity maturation are discussed in Chapter 10.

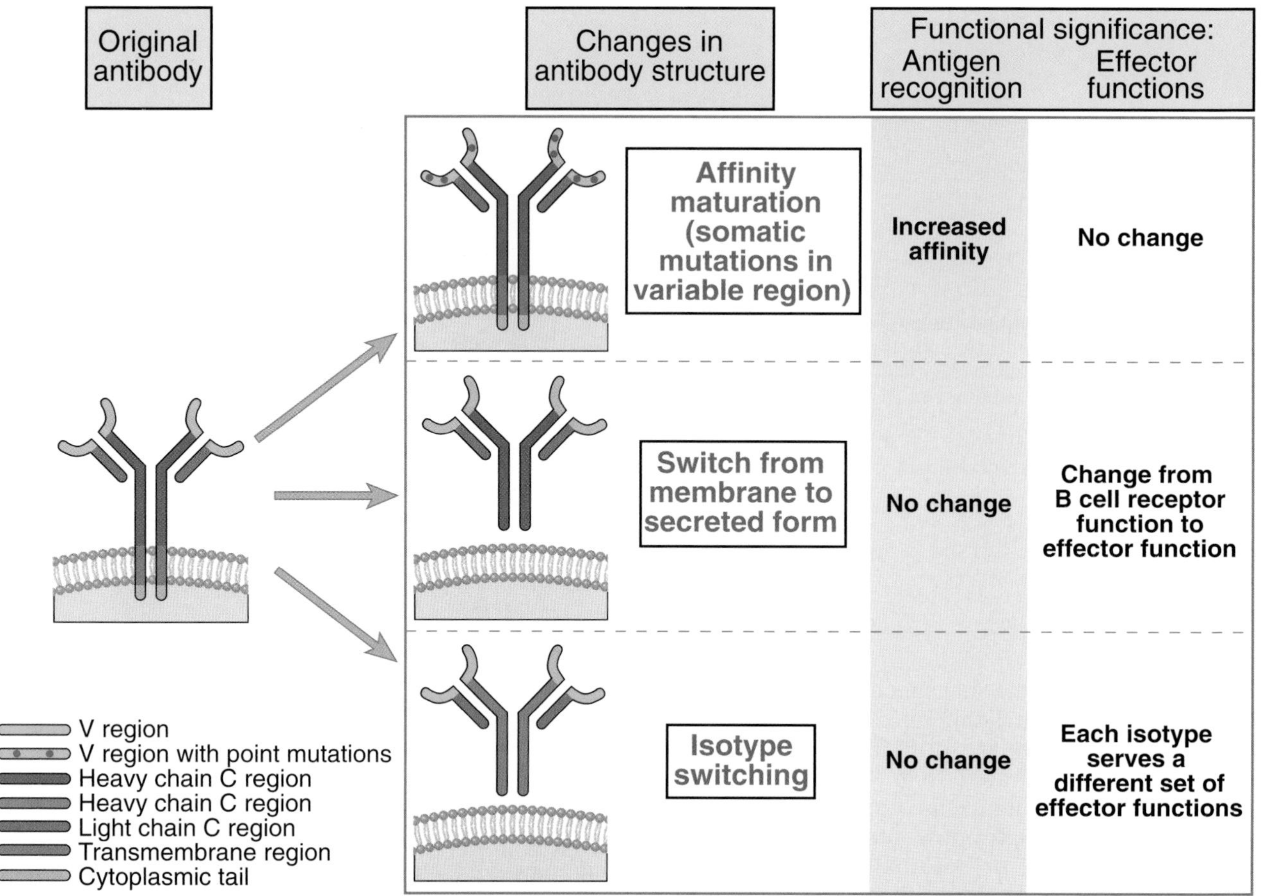

FIGURE 4–12 Changes in antibody structure during humoral immune responses. The illustration depicts the changes in the structure of antibodies that may be produced by the progeny of activated B cells (one clone) and the related changes in function. During affinity maturation, mutations in the V region (indicated by red dots) lead to changes in fine specificity without changes in C region–dependent effector functions. Activated B cells may shift production from largely membrane-bound antibodies containing transmembrane and cytoplasmic regions to secreted antibodies. Secreted antibodies may or may not show V gene mutations (i.e., secretion of antibodies occurs before and after affinity maturation). In isotype switching, the C regions change (indicated by color change from blue to orange) without changes in the antigen-binding V region. Isotype switching is seen in membrane-bound and secreted antibodies. The molecular basis for these changes is discussed in Chapter 10.

Features Related to Effector Functions

Many of the effector functions of immunoglobulins are mediated by the Fc portions of the molecules, and antibody isotypes that differ in these Fc regions perform distinct functions. We have mentioned previously that the effector functions of antibodies require the binding of heavy chain C regions, which make up the Fc portions, to other cells and plasma proteins. For example, IgG coats microbes and targets them for phagocytosis by neutrophils and macrophages. This occurs because the antigen-complexed IgG molecule is able to bind, through its Fc region, to γ heavy chain–specific Fc receptors (FcRs) that are expressed on neutrophils and macrophages. In contrast, IgE binds to mast cells and triggers their degranulation because mast cells express IgE-specific FcRs. Another Fc-dependent effector mechanism of humoral immunity is activation of the classical pathway of the complement system. The system generates inflammatory mediators and promotes microbial phagocytosis and lysis. It is initiated by the binding of a complement protein called C1q to the Fc portions of antigen-complexed IgG or IgM. The FcR- and complement-binding sites of antibodies are found within the heavy chain C domains of the different isotypes (see Fig. 4–1). The structure and functions of FcRs and complement proteins are discussed in detail in Chapter 14.

The effector functions of antibodies are initiated only by antibodies that have bound antigens and not by free Ig. The reason that only antibodies with bound antigens activate effector mechanisms is that two or more adjacent antibody Fc portions are needed to bind to and trigger various effector systems, such as complement proteins and FcRs of phagocytes (see Chapter 14). This requirement for adjacent antibody molecules ensures that the effector functions are targeted specifically toward eliminating antigens that are recognized by the antibody and that circulating free antibodies do not wastefully trigger effector responses.

Changes in the isotypes of antibodies during humoral immune responses influence how and where the responses work to eradicate antigen. After stimulation by an antigen, a single clone of B cells may produce antibodies with different isotypes yet identical V domains, and therefore identical antigen specificity. Naive B cells, for example, simultaneously produce IgM and IgD that function as membrane receptors for antigens. When these B cells are activated by an antigen such as a microbe, they may undergo a process called **isotype switching** in which the type of C_H region, and therefore the antibody isotype, produced by the B cell changes, but the V regions and the specificity do not (see Fig. 4–12). As a result of isotype switching, different progeny of the original IgM- and IgD-expressing B cell may produce isotypes and subtypes that are best able to eliminate the antigen. For example, the antibody response to many bacteria and viruses is dominated by IgG antibodies, which promote phagocytosis of the microbes, and the response to helminths consists mainly of IgE, which aids in the destruction of the parasites. The mechanisms and functional significance of isotype switching are discussed in Chapter 10.

The heavy chain C regions of antibodies also determine the tissue distribution of antibody molecules. As we mentioned earlier, after B cells are activated, they gradually lose expression of the membrane-bound antibody and express more of it as a secreted protein (see Fig. 4–12). IgA can be secreted efficiently through mucosal epithelia and is the major class of antibody in mucosal secretions and milk. Neonates are protected from infections by IgG antibodies they acquire from their mothers during gestation and early after birth. This transfer of maternal IgG is mediated by a special type of Fc receptor that is expressed in the placenta (through which antibodies enter the fetal circulation) and in the intestine. This receptor also protects IgG molecules from intracellular degradation and thus contributes to the long half-life of this antibody isotype.

SUMMARY

- Antibodies, or immunoglobulins, are a family of structurally related glycoproteins produced in membrane-bound or secreted form by B lymphocytes. Membrane-bound antibodies serve as receptors that mediate the antigen-triggered activation of B cells. Secreted antibodies function as mediators of specific humoral immunity by engaging various effector mechanisms that serve to eliminate the bound antigens.

- The antigen-binding regions of antibody molecules are highly variable, and any one individual has the potential to produce up to 10^9 different antibodies, each with distinct antigen specificity.

- All antibodies have a common symmetric core structure of two identical covalently linked heavy chains and two identical light chains, each linked to one of the heavy chains. Each chain consists of two or more independently folded Ig domains of about 110 amino acids containing conserved sequences and intrachain disulfide bonds.

- The N-terminal domains of heavy and light chains form the V regions of antibody molecules, which differ among antibodies of different specificities. The V regions of heavy and light chains each contain three separate hypervariable regions of about 10 amino acids that are spatially assembled to form the antigen-combining site of the antibody molecule.

- Antibodies are classified into different isotypes and subtypes on the basis of differences in the heavy chain C regions, which consist of three or four Ig C domains, and these classes and subclasses have different functional properties. The antibody classes are called IgM, IgD, IgG, IgE, and IgA. Both light chains of a single Ig molecule are of the same light chain isotype, either κ or λ, which differ in their single C domains.

- Most of the effector functions of antibodies are mediated by the C regions of the heavy chains, but these functions are triggered by binding of antigens to the spatially distant combining site in the V region.

- Antigens are substances specifically bound by antibodies or T lymphocyte antigen receptors. Antigens that bind to antibodies are a wide variety of biologic molecules, including sugars, lipids, carbohydrates, proteins, and nucleic acids. This is in contrast to T cell antigen receptors, which recognize only peptide antigens.

- Macromolecular antigens contain multiple epitopes, or determinants, each of which may be recognized by an antibody. Linear epitopes of protein antigens consist of a sequence of adjacent amino acids, and conformational determinants are formed by folding of a polypeptide chain.

- The affinity of the interaction between the combining site of a single antibody molecule and a single epitope is generally measured as a K_d. Polyvalent antigens contain multiple identical epitopes to which identical antibody molecules can bind. Antibodies can bind to two or, in the case of IgM, up to 10 identical epitopes simultaneously, leading to enhanced avidity of the antibody-antigen interaction. The relative concentrations of polyvalent antigens and antibodies may favor the formation of immune complexes that may deposit in tissues and cause damage.

- Antibody binding to antigen can be highly specific, distinguishing small differences in chemical structures, but cross-reactions may also occur in which two or more antigens may be bound by the same antibody.

- Several changes in the structure of antibodies made by one clone of B cells may occur in the course of an immune response. B cells initially produce only membrane-bound Ig, but in activated B cells and plasma cells, synthesis is induced of soluble Ig with the same antigen-binding specificity as the original membrane-bound Ig receptor. Changes in the use of C region gene segments without changes in V regions are the basis of isotype switching, which leads to changes in effector function without a change in specificity. Point mutations in the V regions of an antibody specific for an antigen lead to increased affinity for that antigen (affinity maturation).

Selected Readings

Fagarasan S. Evolution, development, mechanism and function of IgA in the gut. Current Opinion in Immunology 20:170–177, 2008.

Harris LJ, SB Larsen, and A McPherson. Comparison of intact antibody structures and the implications for effector functions. Advances in Immunology 72:191–208, 1999.

Köhler G, and C Milstein. Continuous cultures of fused cells secreting antibody of predefined specificity. Nature 256: 495–497, 1975.

Law M, and L Hengartner. Antibodies against viruses: passive and active immunization. Current Opinion in Immunology 20:486–492, 2008.

Lonberg N. Fully human antibodies from transgenic mouse and phage display platforms. Current Opinion in Immunology 20:450–459, 2008.

Schaedel O, and Y Reiter. Antibodies and their fragments as anti-cancer agents. Current Pharmaceutical Design 12:363–378, 2006.

Stanfield RL, and IA Wilson. Structural studies of human HIV-1 V3 antibodies. Human Antibodies 14:73–80, 2005.

Chapter 5

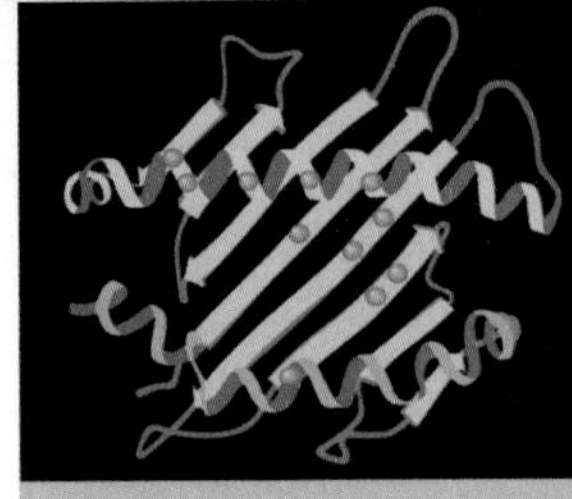

THE MAJOR HISTOCOMPATIBILITY COMPLEX

The principal functions of T lymphocytes are defense against intracellular microbes and activation of other cells, such as macrophages and B lymphocytes. All these functions require that T lymphocytes interact with other cells, which may be infected host cells, dendritic cells, macrophages, and B lymphocytes. The antigen receptors of T cells can only recognize antigens that are displayed on other cells. This specificity of T lymphocytes is in contrast to that of B lymphocytes and their secreted products, antibodies, which can recognize soluble antigens as well as cell-associated antigens. The task of displaying cell-associated antigens for recognition by T cells is performed by specialized proteins that are encoded by genes in a locus called the **major histocompatibility complex** (MHC). The MHC was discovered as an extended locus containing highly polymorphic genes that determine the outcome of tissue transplants. We now know that the physiologic function of MHC molecules is the presentation of peptides to T cells. In fact, MHC molecules are integral components of the ligands that most T cells recognize because the antigen receptors of T cells are actually specific for complexes of foreign peptide antigens and self MHC molecules (schematically illustrated in Fig. 5–1). There are two main types of MHC gene products, called **class I MHC molecules** and **class II MHC molecules,** which sample different pools of protein antigens, cytosolic (most commonly endogenously synthesized) antigens, and extracellular antigens endocytosed into vesicles, respectively. Class I MHC molecules present peptides to $CD8^+$ cytotoxic T lymphocytes (CTLs), and class II MHC molecules to $CD4^+$ helper T cells. Thus, knowledge of the structure and biosynthesis of MHC molecules and the association of peptide antigens with MHC molecules is fundamental to understanding how T cells recognize antigens.

We begin our discussion of antigen recognition by T cells with a description of the structure of MHC molecules, the biochemistry of peptide binding to MHC molecules, and the genetics of the MHC. In Chapter 6, we will discuss in more detail the presentation of antigens to T lymphocytes, the roles of class I and class II MHC molecules in this process, and the physiologic significance of MHC-associated antigen presentation. The structure of T cell antigen receptors is described in Chapter 7. The role of MHC molecules in graft rejection is described in Chapter 16. The terminology and

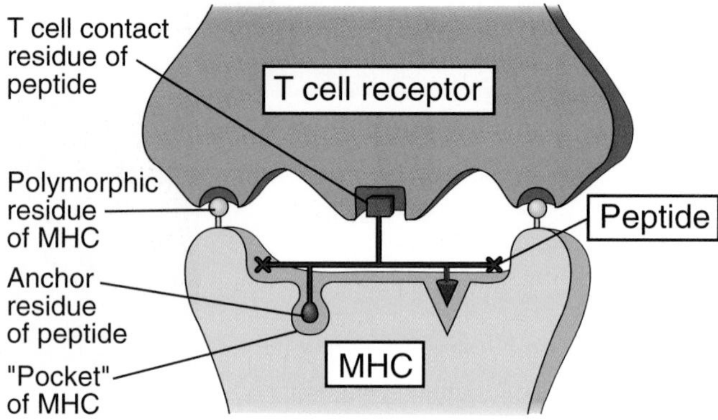

FIGURE 5–1 T cell recognition of a peptide-MHC complex. This schematic illustration shows an MHC molecule binding and displaying a peptide and a T cell receptor recognizing two polymorphic residues of the MHC molecule and one residue of the peptide. Details of the interactions of peptides, MHC molecules, and T cell receptors are described in Chapters 5, 6, and 7.

genetics of the MHC are best understood from a historical perspective, and we begin with a description of how the MHC was discovered.

DISCOVERY OF THE MHC AND ITS ROLE IN IMMUNE RESPONSES

Discovery of the Mouse MHC

The MHC was discovered as the genetic locus whose products are responsible for rapid rejection of tissue grafts exchanged between inbred strains of mice. Key to understanding this discovery is the concept of genetic polymorphism. Some genes are represented by only one normal nucleic acid sequence in all the members of a species (except for relatively rare mutations); such genes are said to be nonpolymorphic, and the normal, or wild-type, gene sequence is usually present on both chromosomes of a pair in every member of the species. By contrast, alternate forms, or variants, of other genes are present at stable frequencies in different members of the population. Such genes are said to be polymorphic, and each common variant of a polymorphic gene is called an allele. For polymorphic genes, an individual can have the same allele at that genetic locus on both chromosomes of the pair and would be said to be homozygous, or an individual can have two different alleles, one on each chromosome, and would be termed heterozygous.

In the 1940s, George Snell and his colleagues used genetic techniques to analyze the rejection of transplanted tumors and other tissues grafted between strains of laboratory mice. To do this, it was necessary to first produce inbred mouse strains by repetitive mating of siblings. After about 20 generations, every member of an inbred strain has identical nucleic acid sequences at all locations on all chromosomes. In other words, inbred mice are homozygous at every genetic locus, and every mouse of an inbred strain is genetically identical (**syngeneic**) to every other mouse of the same strain. In the case of polymorphic genes, each inbred strain, because it is homozygous, expresses a single allele from the original population. Different strains may express different alleles and are said to be **allogeneic** to one another.

When a tissue or an organ, such as a patch of skin, is grafted from one animal to another, two possible outcomes may ensue. In some cases, the grafted skin survives and functions as normal skin. In other cases, the immune system destroys the graft, a process called **rejection.** (We will discuss graft rejection in more detail in Chapter 16.) Skin grafting experiments showed that grafts exchanged between animals of one inbred strain are accepted, whereas grafts exchanged between animals of different inbred strains (or between outbred animals) are rejected (Fig. 5–2A). Therefore, the recognition of a graft as self or foreign is an inherited trait. The genes responsible for causing a grafted tissue to be perceived as similar to or different from one's own tissues were called **histocompatibility genes** (genes that determine tissue compatibility between individuals), and the differences between self and foreign were attributed to polymorphisms among different histocompatibility gene alleles.

The tools of genetics, namely, breeding and analysis of the offspring, were then applied to identify the relevant genes (Box 5–1). The critical strategy in this effort was the breeding of congenic mouse strains; in two congenic strains, the mice are identical at all loci except the one at which they are selected to be different. Analyses of congenic mice that were selected for their ability to reject grafts from one another indicated that a single genetic region is primarily responsible for rapid graft rejection, and this region was called the major histocompatibility locus. The particular locus that was identified in mice by Snell's group was linked to a gene on chromosome 17 encoding a blood group antigen called antigen II, and therefore this region was named histocompatibility-2, or simply H-2. Initially, this locus was thought to contain a single gene that controlled tissue compatibility. However, occasional recombination events occurred within the H-2 locus during interbreeding of different strains, indicating that it actually contained several different but closely linked genes, each involved in graft rejection. The genetic region that controlled graft rejection and contained several linked genes was named the major histocompatibility complex. Genes that determine the fate of grafted tissues are present in all mammalian species, are homologous to the *H-2* genes first identified in mice, and are all called MHC genes (Fig. 5–3). Other genes that contribute to graft rejection to a lesser degree are called minor histocompatibility genes; we will return to these in Chapter 16, when we discuss transplantation immunology. The nomenclature of mouse MHC genes is described in Box 5–1.

MHC genes control immune responsiveness to protein antigens. For almost 20 years after the MHC was discovered, its only documented role was in graft rejection. This was a puzzle to immunologists because transplantation is not a normal phenomenon, and there was no obvious reason why a set of genes should be preserved

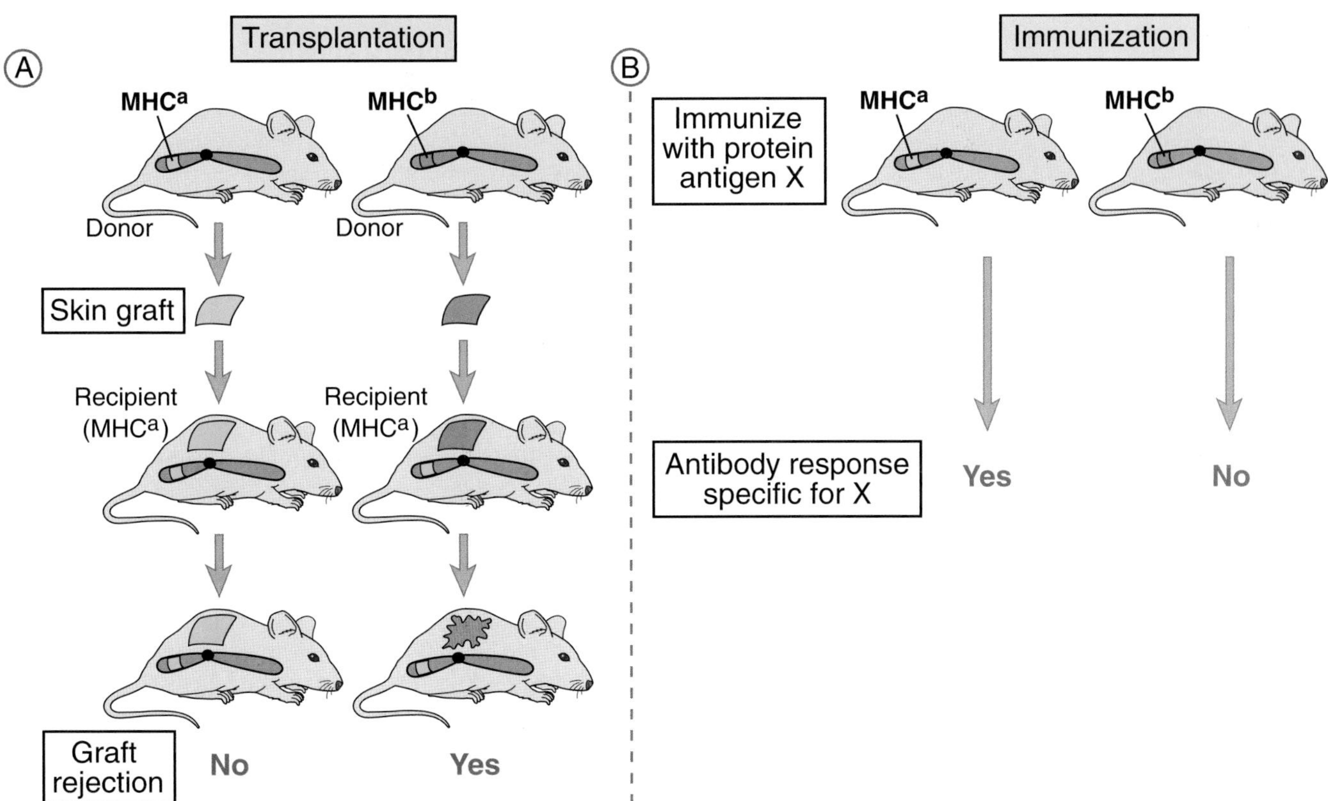

FIGURE 5–2 MHC genes control graft rejection and immune responses. The two strains of mice shown are identical except for their MHC alleles (referred to as a and b). These strains reject skin grafts from each other (A) and respond differently to immunization with a model protein antigen (usually a simple polypeptide) (B).

through evolution if the only function of the genes was to control the rejection of foreign tissue grafts. In the 1960s and 1970s, it was discovered that MHC genes are of fundamental importance for all immune responses to protein antigens. Baruj Benacerraf, Hugh McDevitt, and their colleagues found that inbred strains of guinea pigs and mice differed in their ability to make antibodies against simple synthetic polypeptides, and responsiveness was inherited as a dominant mendelian trait (Fig. 5–2B). The relevant genes were called **immune response (Ir) genes,** and they were all found to map to the MHC. We now know that Ir genes are, in fact, MHC genes that

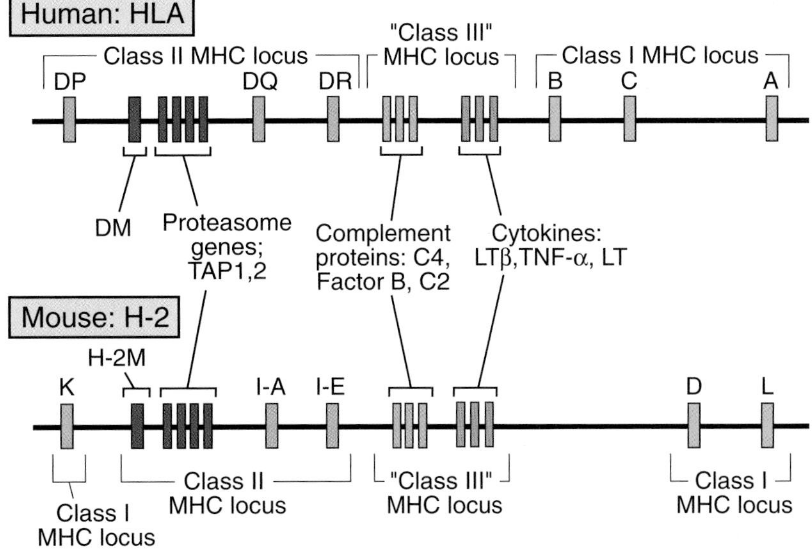

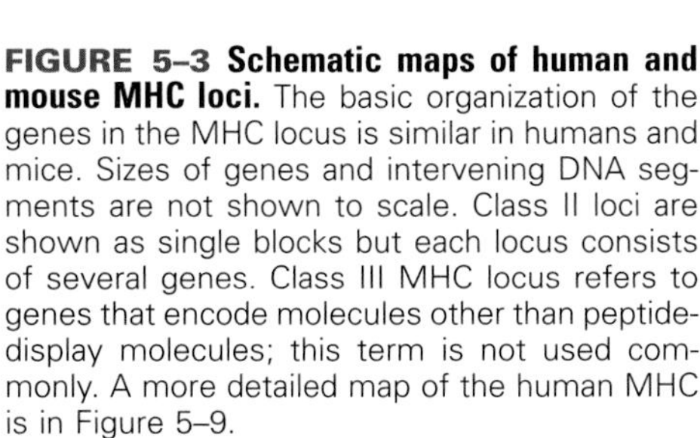
FIGURE 5–3 Schematic maps of human and mouse MHC loci. The basic organization of the genes in the MHC locus is similar in humans and mice. Sizes of genes and intervening DNA segments are not shown to scale. Class II loci are shown as single blocks but each locus consists of several genes. Class III MHC locus refers to genes that encode molecules other than peptide-display molecules; this term is not used commonly. A more detailed map of the human MHC is in Figure 5–9.

Box 5–1 ▪ IN DEPTH: IDENTIFICATION AND NOMENCLATURE OF MHC GENES IN MICE

Our knowledge of the organization of the MHC locus is in large part the result of mouse breeding studies. A key development in these studies was the creation of congenic mouse strains that differ only in the genes responsible for graft rejection. Mice of a congenic strain are identical to the parent strain at every genetic locus except the one for which they are selected to differ. The strategy for deriving congenic mice is based on breeding and selection for a particular trait. In their original experiments, Snell and colleagues used acceptance or rejection of transplantable tumors as their assay for histocompatibility, but this is more easily done with skin grafts. For instance, a cross between inbred strains A and B generates (A × B)F_1 offspring (F_1 for first filial generation). The offspring are repeatedly backcrossed to parental strain A, and at each stage the mice that are selected for breeding are those that accept a skin graft from strain B. By this method, one can generate mice that are genetically identical to strain A except that they have the MHC locus of strain B. In other words, mice with the strain B MHC do not recognize strain B tissues as foreign and will accept strain B grafts, even though all other genetic loci are from strain A. Such mice are said to be congenic to strain A and to have the "B MHC on an A background." Such congenic strains have been used to study the function of the MHC genes and to produce antibodies against MHC-encoded proteins.

In mice, the MHC alleles of particular inbred strains are designated by lowercase letters (e.g., *a*, *b*, *c*). The individual genes within the MHC are named for the MHC type of mouse strain in which they were first identified. The two independent MHC loci known to be most important for graft rejection in mice encode class I MHC molecules and are called *H-2K* and *H-2D*. The *K* gene was first discovered in a strain whose MHC had been designated k, and the *D* gene was first discovered in a strain whose MHC had been designated d. In the parlance of mouse geneticists, the allele of the *H-2K* gene in a strain with the k-type MHC is called K^k (pronounced K of k), whereas the allele of the *H-2K* gene in a strain of MHC d is called K^d (K of d). A third locus similar to K and D was discovered later and called L.

Several other genes were subsequently mapped to the region between the *K* and *D* genes responsible for skin rejection. For example, *S* genes were found that coded for polymorphic serum proteins, now known to be components of the complement system. Most important, the polymorphic Ir genes described in the text were assigned to a region within the MHC called *I* (the letter, not the Roman numeral). The *I* region, in turn, was further subdivided into *I-A* and *I-E* subregions on the basis of recombination events during breeding between congenic strains. The *I* region was also found to code for certain cell surface antigens against which antibodies could be produced by interstrain immunizations. These antigens were called I region–associated molecules, or Ia molecules, and are the murine class II MHC molecules. The genes of the *I-A* and *I-E* loci, which were discovered as Ir genes, code for Ia antigens, which are called I-A and I-E molecules, respectively. The I-A molecule found in the inbred mouse strain with the K^k and D^k alleles is called I-A^k (pronounced I A of k). Similar terminology is used for I-E molecules. Analysis of the mouse class II region revealed some surprises that were not anticipated by classical genetics. For instance, the *I-A* subregion, originally defined by recombinations during interbreeding of inbred strains, codes for the α and β chains of the I-A molecule as well as for the highly polymorphic β chain of the I-E molecule. The *I-E* subregion identified from breeding codes only for the less polymorphic α chain of the I-E molecule.

The nomenclature of the HLA locus takes into account the enormous polymorphism identified by serologic and molecular methods. Thus, individual alleles may be called HLA-A*0201, referring to the 01 subtype of HLA-A2, or HLA-DRB1*0401, referring to the 01 subtype of the HLA-DRB4 allele, and so on.

encode MHC molecules that differ in their ability to bind and display peptides derived from various protein antigens. Responder strains inherit MHC alleles whose products do bind such peptides, forming peptide-MHC complexes that can be recognized by helper T cells. These T cells then help B cells to produce antibodies. Nonresponder strains express MHC molecules that are not capable of binding peptides derived from the polypeptide antigen, and therefore these strains cannot generate helper T cells or antibodies specific for the antigen.

The first explanation for the role of MHC molecules in T cell antigen recognition came with the discovery of the phenomenon of **MHC restriction** of T cells, which we will describe in Chapter 6 when we consider the characteristics of the ligands that T cells recognize.

Discovery of the Human MHC

Human MHC molecules are called human leukocyte antigens (HLA) and are equivalent to the H-2 molecules of mice. The kinds of experiments used to discover and define MHC genes in mice, requiring inbreeding, obviously cannot be performed in humans. However, the development of blood transfusion and especially organ transplantation as methods of treatment in clinical medicine provided a strong impetus to detect and define genes that control rejection reactions in humans. Jean Dausset, Jan van Rood, and their colleagues first showed that individuals who reject kidneys or have transfusion reactions to white blood cells often contain circulating antibodies reactive with antigens on the white blood cells of the blood or organ donor. Sera that react against the cells of other, allogeneic individuals are called **alloantisera** and are said to contain **alloantibodies,** whose molecular targets are called **alloantigens.** It was presumed that these alloantigens are the products of polymorphic genes that distinguish foreign tissues from self tissues. Panels of alloantisera were collected from alloantigen-immunized donors, including multiparous women (who are immunized by paternal alloantigens expressed by the fetus during pregnancy), actively immunized volunteers, and transfusion or transplant recipients. These sera were compared for their ability to bind to and lyse lymphocytes from different donors. Efforts at international workshops, involving exchanges of reagents among laboratories, led to the identification of several polymorphic genetic loci, clustered together in a single locus on chromosome 6, whose products are recognized by alloantibodies. Because these alloantigens are expressed on human leukocytes, they were called **human leukocyte antigens (HLAs).** Family studies were then used to construct the map of the HLA locus (see Fig. 5–3). The first three genes defined by serologic approaches were called *HLA-A, HLA-B,* and *HLA-C.*

The use of antibodies to study alloantigenic differences between donors and recipients was complemented by the mixed leukocyte reaction (MLR), a test for T cell recognition of allogeneic cells. The MLR is also an *in vitro* model for allograft rejection and will be discussed more fully in the context of transplantation (see Chapter 16). It was found that T lymphocytes from one individual would proliferate in response to leukocytes of another individual, and this assay was used to map the genes that elicited allogeneic T cell reactions. The first gene to be identified from these studies of cellular responses mapped to a region adjacent to the serologically defined HLA locus and was therefore called *HLA-D.* The protein encoded by the *HLA-D* locus was later detected by alloantibodies and was called the HLA-D-related, or HLA-DR, molecule. Two additional genes that mapped adjacent to *HLA-D* were found to encode proteins structurally similar to HLA-DR and also were found to contribute to MLRs; these genes were called *HLA-DQ* and *HLA-DP,* with Q and P chosen for their proximity in the alphabet to R.

We now know that differences in HLA alleles between individuals are important determinants of the rejection of grafts from one individual to another (see Chapter 16). Thus, the HLA locus of humans is functionally equivalent to the H-2 locus of mice defined by transplantation experiments. As we shall see later, MHC molecules in all mammals have essentially the same structure and function.

The accepted nomenclature of MHC genes and their encoded proteins is based on sequence and structural homologies and is applicable to all vertebrate species (see Fig. 5–3). The genes identified as determinants of graft rejection in mice (*H-2K, H-2D,* and *H-2L*) are homologous to the serologically defined human HLA genes (*HLA-A, HLA-B,* and *HLA-C*), and all of these are grouped as **class I MHC genes.** The Ir genes of mice (*I-A* and *I-E*) are homologous to the human genes identified by lymphocyte responses in the MLR (*HLA-DR, HLA-DP,* and *HLA-DQ*) and are grouped as **class II MHC genes.** There are many other genes contained within the MHC; we will return to these later in this chapter.

Properties of MHC Genes

Several important characteristics of MHC genes and their products were deduced from classical genetic and biochemical analyses done in mice and humans.

- ***The two types of polymorphic MHC genes, namely, the class I and class II MHC genes, encode two groups of structurally distinct but homologous proteins.*** Class I MHC molecules present peptides to and are recognized by $CD8^+$ T cells, and class II MHC molecules present peptides to $CD4^+$ T cells.
- ***MHC genes are the most polymorphic genes present in the genome.*** The studies of the mouse MHC were accomplished with a limited number of inbred and congenic strains. Although it was appreciated that mouse MHC genes were polymorphic, only about 20 alleles of each MHC gene were identified in the available inbred strains of mice. The human serologic studies were conducted on outbred human populations. A remarkable feature to emerge from the studies of the human MHC genes is the unprecedented and unanticipated extent of their polymorphism. For some HLA loci (HLA-B), as many as 250 alleles have been identified by serologic assays. Molecular sequencing has shown that a single serologically defined HLA allele may actually consist of multiple variants that differ slightly. Therefore, the polymorphism is even greater than that predicted from serologic studies.
- ***MHC genes are codominantly expressed in each individual.*** In other words, for a given MHC gene, each individual expresses the alleles that are inherited from each of the two parents. For the individual, this maximizes the number of MHC molecules available to bind peptides for presentation to T cells.

The set of MHC alleles present on each chromosome is called an **MHC haplotype.** In humans, each HLA allele is given a numerical designation. For instance, an HLA haplotype of an individual could be HLA-A2, HLA-B5, HLA-DR3, and so on. All heterozygous individuals, of course, have two HLA haplotypes. In mice, each H-2 allele is given a letter designation. Inbred mice, being homozygous, have a single haplotype. Thus, the haplotype of an H-2^d mouse is H-$2K^d$ I-A^d I-E^d D^d L^d. In humans, certain HLA alleles at different loci are inherited together more frequently than would be predicted by random assortment, a phenomenon called linkage disequilibrium.

The discoveries of the phenomena of MHC-linked immune responsiveness and MHC restriction (see Chapter 6) led to the conclusion that MHC genes control not only graft rejection but also immune responses to all protein antigens. These breakthroughs moved the study of the MHC to the forefront of immunology research.

STRUCTURE OF MHC MOLECULES

The elucidation of the biochemistry of MHC molecules has been one of the most important accomplishments of modern immunology. The key advance in this field was the solution of the crystal structures for the extracellular portions of human class I and class II molecules by Don Wiley, Jack Strominger, and their colleagues. Subsequently, many MHC molecules with bound peptides have been crystallized and analyzed in detail. On the basis of this knowledge, we now understand how MHC molecules function to display peptides.

In this section of the chapter, we first summarize the biochemical features that are common to class I and class II MHC molecules and that are most important for the function of these molecules. We then describe the structures of class I and class II proteins, pointing out their important similarities and differences (Table 5–1).

Properties of MHC Molecules

All MHC molecules share certain structural characteristics that are critical for their role in peptide display and antigen recognition by T lymphocytes.

- ***Each MHC molecule consists of an extracellular peptide-binding cleft, or groove, followed by immunoglobulin (Ig)-like domains and transmembrane and cytoplasmic domains.*** As we shall see later, class I molecules are composed of one polypeptide chain encoded in the MHC and a second, non-MHC-encoded chain, whereas class II molecules are made up of two MHC-encoded polypeptide chains. Despite this difference, the overall three-dimensional structures of class I and class II molecules are similar.
- ***The polymorphic amino acid residues of MHC molecules are located in and adjacent to the peptide-binding cleft.*** This cleft is formed by the folding of the amino termini of the MHC-encoded proteins and is composed of paired α-helices resting on a floor made up of an eight-stranded β-pleated sheet. The polymorphic residues, which are the amino acids that vary among different MHC alleles, are located in and around this cleft. This portion of the MHC molecule binds peptides for display to T cells, and the antigen receptors of T cells interact with the displayed peptide and with the α-helices of the MHC molecules (see Fig. 5–1). Because of amino acid variability in this region, different MHC molecules bind and display different peptides and are recognized specifically by the antigen receptors of different T cells. We will return to a discussion of peptide binding by MHC molecules later in this chapter.
- ***The nonpolymorphic Ig-like domains of MHC molecules contain binding sites for the T cell molecules CD4 and CD8.*** CD4 and CD8 are expressed on distinct subpopulations of mature T lymphocytes and participate, together with antigen receptors, in the recognition of antigen; that is, CD4 and CD8 are T cell "coreceptors" (see Chapter 7). CD4 binds selectively to class II MHC molecules, and CD8 binds to class I molecules. This is why $CD4^+$ T cells recognize only peptides displayed by class II molecules, and $CD8^+$ T cells recognize peptides presented by class I molecules. Most $CD4^+$ T cells function as helper cells, and most $CD8^+$ cells are CTLs.

Class I MHC Molecules

Class I molecules consist of two noncovalently linked polypeptide chains: an MHC–encoded 44–47 kD **α chain** (or heavy chain) and a non-MHC–encoded 12 kD subunit called **β_2-microglobulin** (Fig. 5–4). Each α chain is oriented so that about three quarters of the complete polypeptide extends into the extracellular milieu, a short

Table 5–1. Features of Class I and Class II MHC Molecules

Feature	Class I MHC	Class II MHC
Polypeptide chains	α (44–47 kD) β_2-Microglobulin (12 kD)	α (32–34 kD) β (29–32 kD)
Locations of polymorphic residues	α1 and α2 domains	α1 and β1 domains
Binding site for T cell coreceptor	α3 region binds CD8	β2 region binds CD4
Size of peptide-binding cleft	Accommodates peptides of 8-11 residues	Accommodates peptides of 10-30 residues or more
Nomenclature		
Human	HLA-A, HLA-B, HLA-C	HLA-DR, HLA-DQ, HLA-DP
Mouse	H-2K, H-2D, H-2L	I-A, I-E

Abbreviations: HLA, human leukocyte antigen; MHC, major histocompatibility complex

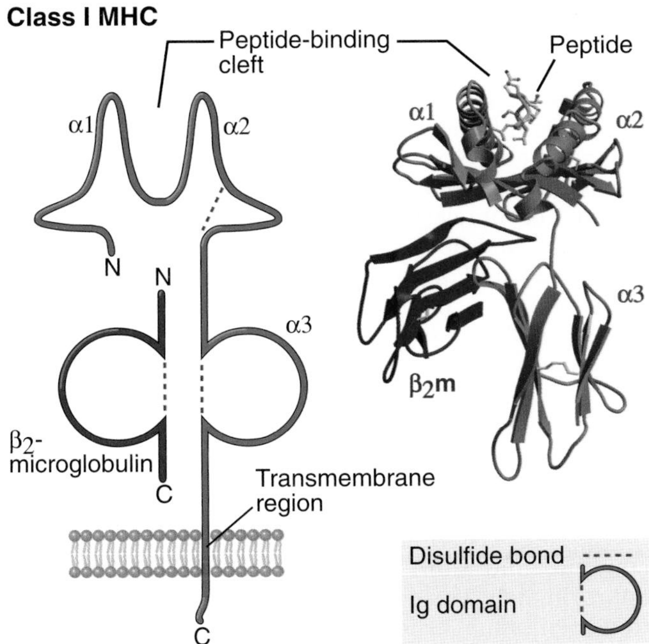

FIGURE 5–4 Structure of a class I MHC molecule. The schematic diagram *(left)* illustrates the different regions of the MHC molecule (not drawn to scale). Class I molecules are composed of a polymorphic α chain noncovalently attached to the nonpolymorphic β_2-microglobulin (β2m). The α chain is glycosylated; carbohydrate residues are not shown. The ribbon diagram *(right)* shows the structure of the extracellular portion of the HLA-B27 molecule with a bound peptide, resolved by x-ray crystallography. (Courtesy of Dr. P. Bjorkman, California Institute of Technology, Pasadena, California.)

hydrophobic segment spans the cell membrane, and the carboxy-terminal residues are located in the cytoplasm. The amino-terminal (N-terminal) α1 and α2 segments of the α chain, each approximately 90 residues long, interact to form a platform of an eight-stranded, antiparallel β-pleated sheet supporting two parallel strands of α-helix. This forms the peptide-binding cleft of class I molecules. Its size is large enough (~25Å × 10Å × 11Å) to bind peptides of 8 to 11 amino acids in a flexible, extended conformation. The ends of the class I peptide-binding cleft are closed so that larger peptides cannot be accommodated. Therefore, native globular proteins have to be "processed" to generate fragments that are small enough to bind to MHC molecules and to be recognized by T cells (see Chapter 6). The polymorphic residues of class I molecules are confined to the α1 and α2 domains, where they contribute to variations among different class I alleles in peptide binding and T cell recognition (Fig. 5–5). The α3 segment of the α chain folds into an Ig domain whose amino acid sequence is conserved among all class I molecules. This segment contains the binding site for CD8. At the carboxy-terminal end of the α3 segment is a stretch of approximately 25 hydrophobic amino acids that traverses the lipid bilayer of the plasma membrane. Immediately following this are approximately 30 residues located in the cytoplasm, included in which is a cluster of basic amino acids that interact with phospholipid head groups of the inner leaflet of the lipid bilayer and anchor the MHC molecule in the plasma membrane.

The light chain of class I molecules, which is encoded by a gene outside the MHC, is called β_2-microglobulin for its electrophoretic mobility (β_2), size (micro), and solubility (globulin). β_2-microglobulin interacts noncovalently with the α3 domain of the α chain. Like the α3 segment, β_2-microglobulin is structurally homologous to an Ig domain and is invariant among all class I molecules.

The fully assembled class I molecule is a heterotrimer consisting of an α chain, β_2-microglobulin, and a bound

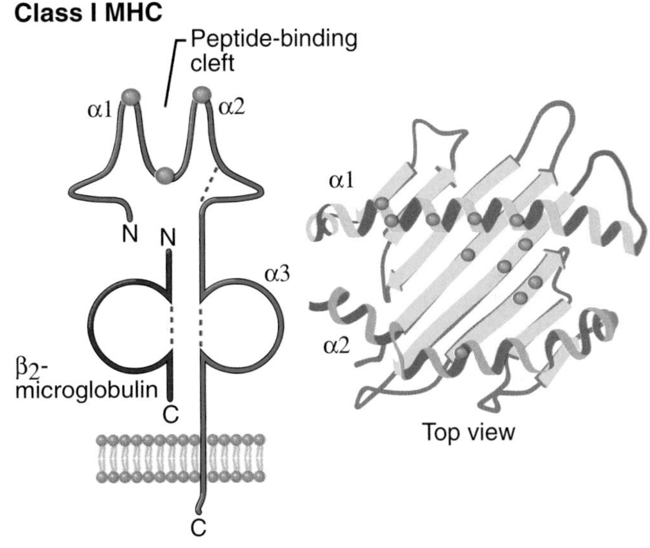

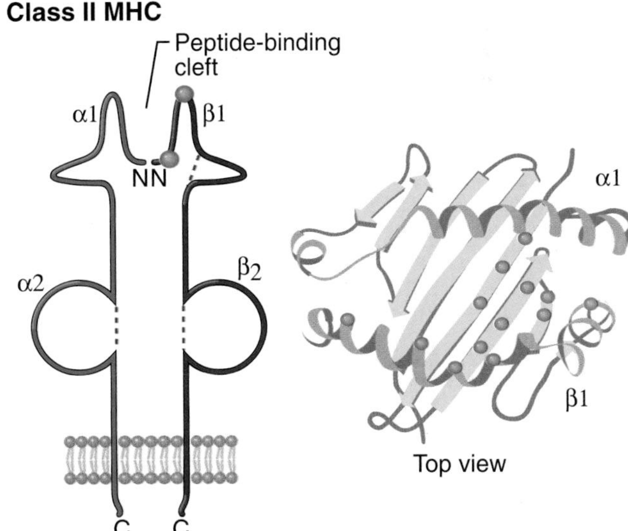

FIGURE 5–5 Polymorphic residues of MHC molecules. The polymorphic residues of class I and class II MHC molecules (shown as red circles) are located in the peptide-binding clefts and the α-helices around the clefts. In the class II molecule shown (HLA-DR), essentially all the polymorphism is in the β chain. However, other class II molecules in humans and mice show varying degrees of polymorphism in the α chain and usually much more in the β chain. (Courtesy of Dr. J. McCluskey, University of Melbourne, Parkville, Australia.)

antigenic peptide, and stable expression of class I molecules on cell surfaces requires the presence of all three components of the heterotrimer. The reason for this is that the interaction of the α chain with β_2-microglobulin is stabilized by binding of peptide antigens to the cleft formed by the α1 and α2 segments, and conversely, the binding of peptide is strengthened by the interaction of β_2-microglobulin with the α chain. Because antigenic peptides are needed to stabilize the MHC molecules, only useful peptide-loaded MHC molecules are expressed on cell surfaces. The process of assembly of stable peptide-loaded class I molecules will be detailed in Chapter 6.

Most individuals are heterozygous for MHC genes and therefore express six different class I molecules on every cell, containing α chains encoded by the two inherited alleles of *HLA-A, HLA-B,* and *HLA-C* genes.

Class II MHC Molecules

Class II MHC molecules are composed of two noncovalently associated polypeptide chains, a 32 to 34 kD α chain and a 29 to 32 kD β chain (Fig. 5–6). Unlike class I molecules, the genes encoding both chains of class II molecules are polymorphic.

The amino-terminal α1 and β1 segments of the class II chains interact to form the peptide-binding cleft, which is structurally similar to the cleft of class I molecules. Four strands of the floor of the cleft and one of the α-helical walls are formed by the α1 segment, and the other four strands of the floor and the second wall are formed by the β1 segment. The polymorphic residues are located in the α1 and β1 segments, in and around the peptide-binding cleft, as in class I molecules (see Fig. 5–5). In human class II molecules, most of the polymorphism is in the β chain. In class II molecules, the ends of the peptide-binding cleft are open, so that peptides of 30 residues or more can fit.

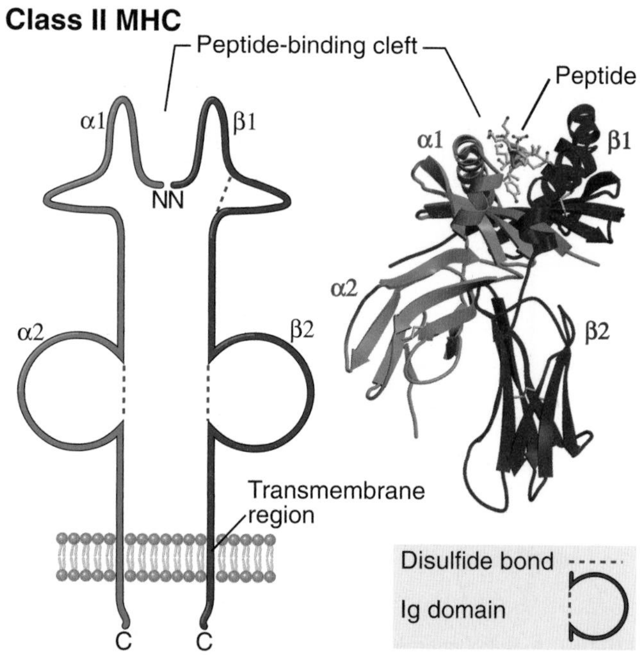

FIGURE 5–6 Structure of a class II MHC molecule. The schematic diagram *(left)* illustrates the different regions of the MHC molecule (not drawn to scale). Class II molecules are composed of a polymorphic α chain noncovalently attached to a polymorphic β chain. Both chains are glycosylated; carbohydrate residues are not shown. The ribbon diagram *(right)* shows the structure of the extracellular portion of the HLA-DR1 molecule with a bound peptide, resolved by x-ray crystallography. (Courtesy of Dr. P. Bjorkman, California Institute of Technology, Pasadena, California.)

The α2 and β2 segments of class II molecules, like class I α3 and β_2-microglobulin, are folded into Ig domains and are nonpolymorphic among various alleles of a particular class II gene. The β2 segment of class II molecules contains the binding site for CD4, similar to the binding site for CD8 in the α3 segment of the class I heavy chain. In general, α chains of one class II MHC locus (e.g., DR) most often pair with β chains of the same locus and less commonly with β chains of other loci (e.g., DQ, DP).

The carboxy-terminal ends of the α2 and β2 segments continue into short connecting regions followed by approximately 25–amino acid stretches of hydrophobic transmembrane residues. In both chains, the transmembrane regions end with clusters of basic amino acid residues, followed by short, hydrophilic cytoplasmic tails.

The fully assembled class II molecule is a heterotrimer consisting of an α chain, a β chain, and a bound antigenic peptide, and stable expression of class II molecules on cell surfaces requires the presence of all three components of the heterotrimer. As in class I molecules, this ensures that the MHC molecules that end up on the cell surface are the molecules that are serving their normal function of peptide display.

Humans inherit, from each parent, one DPB1 and one DPA1 gene encoding, respectively, the β and α chains of an HLA-DP molecule; one DQA1 and one DQB1 gene; and one DRA1 gene, a DRB1 gene, and a separate duplicated DRB gene that may encode the alleles DRB3, 4, or 5. Thus, each heterozygous individual inherits six or eight class II MHC alleles, three or four from each parent (one set each of DP and DQ, and one or two of DR). Typically, there is not much recombination between genes of different loci (i.e., DRα with DQβ, and so on), and each haplotype tends to be inherited as a single unit. However, because some haplotypes contain extra DRB loci that produce β chains that assemble with DRα, and some DQα molecules encoded on one chromosome can associate with DQβ molecules encoded from the other chromosome, the total number of expressed class II molecules may be considerably more than 6.

Binding of Peptides to MHC Molecules

With the realization that MHC molecules are the peptide display molecules of the adaptive immune system, considerable effort has been devoted to elucidating the molecular basis of peptide-MHC interactions and the characteristics of peptides that allow them to bind to MHC molecules. These issues are important not only for understanding the biology of T cell antigen recognition but also for defining the properties of a protein that make it immunogenic. All proteins that are immunogenic in an individual must generate peptides that can bind to the MHC molecules of that individual. Information about peptide-MHC interactions may be used to design vaccines, by inserting MHC-binding amino acid sequences into antigens used for immunization. In the section that follows, we summarize the key features of the interactions between peptides and class I or class II MHC molecules.

Several analytical methods have been used to study peptide-MHC interactions:

- The earliest studies relied on functional assays of helper T cells and CTLs responding to antigen-presenting cells that were incubated with different peptides. By determining which types of peptides derived from complex protein antigens could activate T cells from animals immunized with these antigens, it was possible to define the features of peptides that allowed them to be presented by antigen-presenting cells.
- After MHC molecules were purified, it was possible to study their interactions with radioactively or fluorescently labeled peptides in solution by methods such as equilibrium dialysis and gel filtration to quantitate bound and free peptides.
- The nature of MHC-binding peptides generated from intact proteins has been analyzed by exposing antigen-presenting cells to a protein antigen for various times, purifying the MHC molecules from these cells by affinity chromatography, and eluting the bound peptides for amino acid sequencing by mass spectroscopy. The same approach may be used to define the endogenous peptides that are displayed by antigen-presenting cells isolated from animals or humans.
- X-ray crystallographic analysis of peptide-MHC complexes has provided valuable information about how peptides sit in the clefts of MHC molecules and about the residues of each that participate in this binding.

On the basis of such studies, we now understand the physicochemical characteristics of peptide-MHC interactions in considerable detail. It has also become apparent that the binding of peptides to MHC molecules is fundamentally different from the binding of antigens to the antigen receptors of B and T lymphocytes (see Chapter 4, Table 4–1).

Characteristics of Peptide-MHC Interactions

MHC molecules show a broad specificity for peptide binding, in contrast to the fine specificity of antigen recognition of the antigen receptors of T lymphocytes. There are several important features of the interactions of MHC molecules and antigenic peptides.

- ***Each class I or class II MHC molecule has a single peptide-binding cleft that binds one peptide at a time, but each MHC molecule can bind many different peptides.*** This ability of any MHC molecule to bind many different peptides was established by several lines of experimental evidence.
  - If a T cell specific for one peptide is stimulated by antigen-presenting cells presenting that peptide, the response is inhibited by the addition of an excess of other, structurally similar peptides (Fig. 5–7). In these experiments, the MHC molecule bound different peptides, but the T cell recognized only one of these peptides presented by the MHC molecule.
  - Direct binding studies with purified MHC molecules in solution definitively established that a single MHC molecule can bind multiple different peptides (albeit only one at a time) and that multiple peptides compete with one another for binding to the single binding site of each MHC molecule.
  - The analyses of peptides eluted from MHC molecules purified from antigen-presenting cells showed that many different peptides can be eluted from any one type of MHC molecule.

The solution of the crystal structures of class I and class II MHC molecules confirmed the presence of a single peptide-binding cleft in these molecules (see Figs. 5–4 and 5–6). It is not surprising that a single MHC molecule can bind multiple peptides because each individual contains only a few different MHC molecules (6 class I and as many as 10 to 20 class II molecules in a heterozygous individual), and these must be able to present peptides from the enormous number of protein antigens that one is likely to encounter.

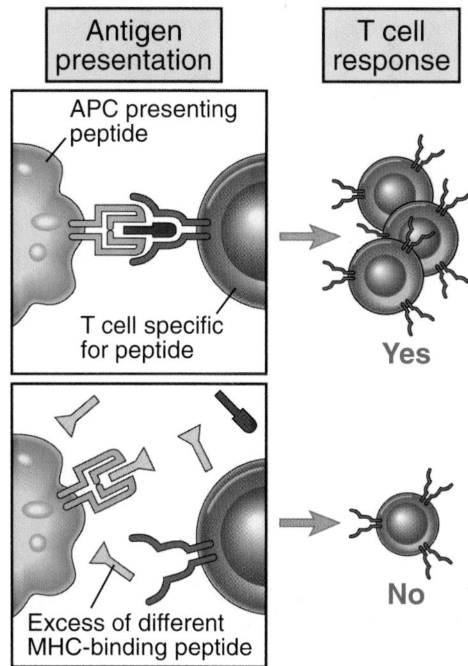

FIGURE 5–7 Antigen competition for T cells. A T cell recognizes a peptide presented by one MHC molecule. An excess of a different peptide that binds to the same MHC molecule competitively inhibits presentation of the peptide that the T cell recognizes. APC, antigen-presenting cell.

- ***The peptides that bind to MHC molecules share structural features that promote this interaction.*** One of these features is the size of the peptide—class I molecules can accommodate peptides that are 8 to 11 residues long, and class II molecules bind peptides that may be 10 to 30 residues long or longer, the optimal length being 12 to 16 residues. In addition, peptides that bind to a particular allelic form of an MHC molecule contain amino acid residues that allow complementary interactions between the peptide and that allelic MHC molecule. The residues of a peptide that bind to MHC molecules are distinct from those that are recognized by T cells.
- ***The association of antigenic peptides and MHC molecules is a saturable interaction with a very slow off-rate.*** In a cell, several chaperones and enzymes facilitate the binding of peptides to MHC molecules (see Chapter 6). Once formed, most peptide-MHC complexes are stable, and kinetic dissociation constants are indicative of long half-lives that range from hours to many days. This extraordinarily slow off-rate of peptide dissociation from MHC molecules allows peptide-MHC complexes to persist long enough on the surfaces of antigen-presenting cells that the antigen can be found by T cells. This feature of antigen display enables the few T cells that are specific for the antigen to locate the antigen as the cells circulate through tissues, and thus to generate effective immune responses against the antigen.
- ***The MHC molecules of an individual do not discriminate between foreign peptides (e.g., those derived from microbial proteins) and peptides derived from the proteins of that individual (self antigens).*** Thus, MHC molecules display both self peptides and foreign peptides, and T cells survey these displayed peptides for the presence of foreign antigens. This process is central to the surveillance function of T cells. However, the inability of MHC molecules to discriminate between self antigens and foreign antigens raises two questions. First, because MHC molecules are continuously exposed to, and presumably occupied by, abundant self peptides, how can their peptide-binding sites ever be available to bind and display foreign peptides, which are likely to be relatively rare? Second, if self peptides are constantly being presented, why do individuals not develop autoimmune reactions? The answers to these questions lie in the cell biology of MHC biosynthesis and assembly, in the specificity of T cells, and in the exquisite sensitivity of these cells to small amounts of peptide-MHC complexes. We will return to these questions in more detail in Chapter 6.

Structural Basis of Peptide Binding to MHC Molecules

The binding of peptides to MHC molecules is a noncovalent interaction mediated by residues both in the peptides and in the clefts of the MHC molecules. Protein antigens are proteolytically cleaved in antigen-presenting cells to generate the peptides that will be bound and displayed by MHC molecules (see Chapter 6). These peptides bind to the clefts of MHC molecules in an extended conformation. Once bound, the peptides and their associated water molecules fill the clefts, making extensive contacts with the amino acid residues that form the β-strands of the floor and the α-helices of the walls of the cleft (Fig. 5–8). In most MHC molecules, the β-strands in the floor of the cleft contain "pockets." The amino acid residues of a peptide may contain side chains that fit into these pockets and bind to complementary amino acids in the MHC molecule, often through hydrophobic interactions. Such residues of the peptide are called anchor residues because they contribute most of the favorable interactions of the binding (i.e., they anchor the peptide in the cleft of the MHC molecule). The anchor residues of peptides may be located in the middle or at the ends of the peptide. Each MHC-binding peptide usually contains only one or two anchor residues, and this presumably allows greater variability in the other residues of the peptide, which are the residues that are recognized by specific T cells. Not all peptides use anchor residues to bind to MHC molecules, especially to class II molecules. Specific interactions of peptides with the α-helical sides of the MHC cleft also contribute to peptide binding by forming hydrogen bonds or charge interactions (salt bridges). Class I–binding peptides usually contain hydrophobic or basic amino acids at their carboxyl termini that also contribute to the interaction.

Because many of the residues in and around the peptide-binding cleft of MHC molecules are polymorphic (i.e., they differ among various MHC alleles), different alleles favor the binding of different peptides. This is the structural basis of the function of MHC genes as "immune response genes"; only animals that express MHC alleles that can bind a particular peptide and display it to T cells can respond to that peptide.

The antigen receptors of T cells recognize both the antigenic peptide and the MHC molecules, with the peptide being responsible for the fine specificity of antigen recognition and the MHC residues accounting for the MHC restriction of the T cells. A portion of the bound peptide is exposed from the open top of the cleft of the MHC molecule, and the amino acid side chains of this portion of the peptide are recognized by the antigen receptors of specific T cells. The same T cell receptor also interacts with polymorphic residues of the α-helices of the MHC molecule itself (see Fig. 5–1). Predictably, variations in either the peptide antigen or the peptide-binding cleft of the MHC molecule will alter presentation of that peptide or its recognition by T cells. In fact, one can enhance the immunogenicity of a peptide by incorporating into it a residue that strengthens its binding to commonly inherited MHC molecules in a population.

- By introducing mutations in an immunogenic peptide, it is possible to identify residues involved in binding to MHC molecules and those that are critical for T cell recognition. This approach has been applied to many peptide antigens, using T cells to measure responses to these peptides (see Fig. 5–8C).

The realization that the polymorphic residues of MHC molecules determine the specificity of peptide binding and T cell antigen recognition has led to the question of why MHC genes are polymorphic. One possibility is that the presence of multiple MHC alleles in a population provides an evolutionary advantage because it will ensure that virtually all peptides derived from microbial antigens will be recognized by the immune system of at least some individuals. At the population level, this will increase the range of microbial peptides that may be presented to T cells and reduce the likelihood that a single pathogen can evade host defenses in all the individuals in a given species.

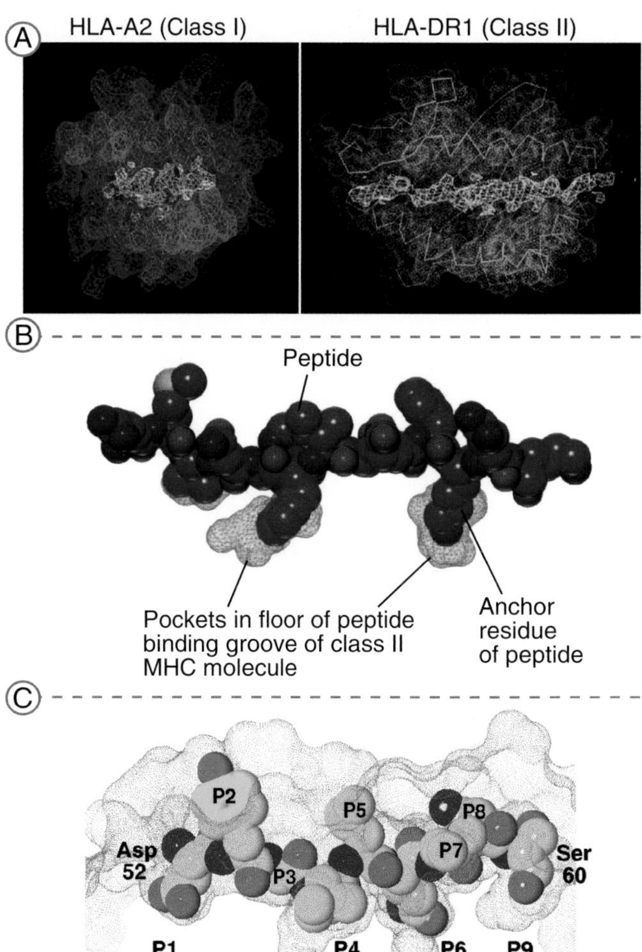

FIGURE 5–8 Peptide binding to MHC molecules. A. These top views of the crystal structures of MHC molecules show how peptides lie in the peptide-binding clefts. The class I molecule shown is HLA-A2, and the class II molecule is HLA-DR1. The cleft of the class I molecule is closed, whereas that of the class II molecule is open. As a result, class II molecules accommodate longer peptides than do class I molecules. (Reprinted with permission of Macmillan Publishers Ltd. from Bjorkman PJ, MA Saper, B Samraoui, WS Bennett, JL Strominger, and DC Wiley. Structure of the human class I histocompatibility antigen HLA-A2. Nature 329:506–512, 1987; and Brown J et al. Three-dimensional structure of the human class II histocompatibility antigen HLA-DR1. Nature 364:33–39, 1993.) B. The side view of a cut-out of a peptide bound to a class II MHC molecule shows how anchor residues of the peptide hold it in the pockets in the cleft of the MHC molecule. (From Scott CA, PA Peterson, L Teyton, and IA Wilson. Crystal structures of two I-A^d-peptide complexes reveal that high affinity can be achieved without large anchor residues. Immunity 8:319–329, 1998. Copyright 1998, with permission from Elsevier Science.) C. Different residues of a peptide bind to MHC molecules and are recognized by T cells. The immunodominant epitope of the protein hen egg lysozyme (HEL) in H-2^k mice is a peptide composed of residues 52–62. The ribbon diagram modeled after crystal structures shows the surface of the peptide-binding cleft of the I-A^k class II molecule and the bound HEL peptide with amino acid residues (P1–P9) indicated as spheres. Mutational analysis of the peptide has shown that the residues involved in binding to MHC molecules are P1 (Asp52), P4 (Ile55), P6 (Gln57), P7 (Ile 58), and P9 (Ser60); these are the residues that project down and fit into the peptide-binding cleft. The residues involved in recognition by T cells are P2 (Tyr53), P5 (Leu56), and P8 (Asn59); these residues project upward and are available to T cells. (From Fremont DH, D Monnale, CA Nelson, WA Hendrickson, and ER Unanue. Crystal structure of I-A in complex with a dominant epitope of lysozyme. Immunity 8:305–317, 1998. Copyright 1998, with permission from Elsevier Science.)

Genomic Organization of the MHC

In humans, the MHC is located on the short arm of chromosome 6, and β_2-microglobulin is encoded by a gene on chromosome 15. The human MHC occupies a large segment of DNA, extending about 3500 kilobases (kb). (For comparison, a large human gene may extend up to 50 to 100 kb, and the size of the entire genome of the bacterium *Escherichia coli* is approximately 4500 kb.) In classical genetic terms, the MHC locus extends about 4 centimorgans, meaning that crossovers within the MHC occur with a frequency of about 4% at each meiosis. A molecular map of the human MHC is shown in Figure 5–9.

Many of the proteins involved in the processing of protein antigens and the presentation of peptides to T cells are encoded by genes located within the MHC. In other words, this genetic locus contains much of the information needed for the machinery of antigen presentation. The class I genes, *HLA-A*, *HLA-B*, and *HLA-C*, are in the most telomeric portion of the HLA locus, and the class II genes are the most centromeric in the HLA locus. Within the class II locus are genes that encode several proteins that play critical roles in antigen processing. One of these proteins, called the transporter associated with antigen processing (TAP), is a heterodimer that transports peptides from the cytosol into the endoplasmic reticulum, where the peptides can associate with newly synthesized class I molecules. The two subunits of the TAP dimer are encoded by two genes within the class II region. Other genes in this cluster encode subunits of a cytosolic protease complex, called the proteasome, that degrades cytosolic proteins into peptides that are subsequently presented by class I MHC molecules. Another pair of genes, called *HLA-DMA* and *HLA-DMB*, encodes a nonpolymorphic heterodimeric class II–like molecule, called HLA-DM (or H-2M in mice), that is involved in peptide binding to class II molecules. The functions of these proteins in antigen presentation are discussed in Chapter 6.

Between the class I and class II gene clusters are genes that code for several components of the complement system; for three structurally related cytokines, tumor

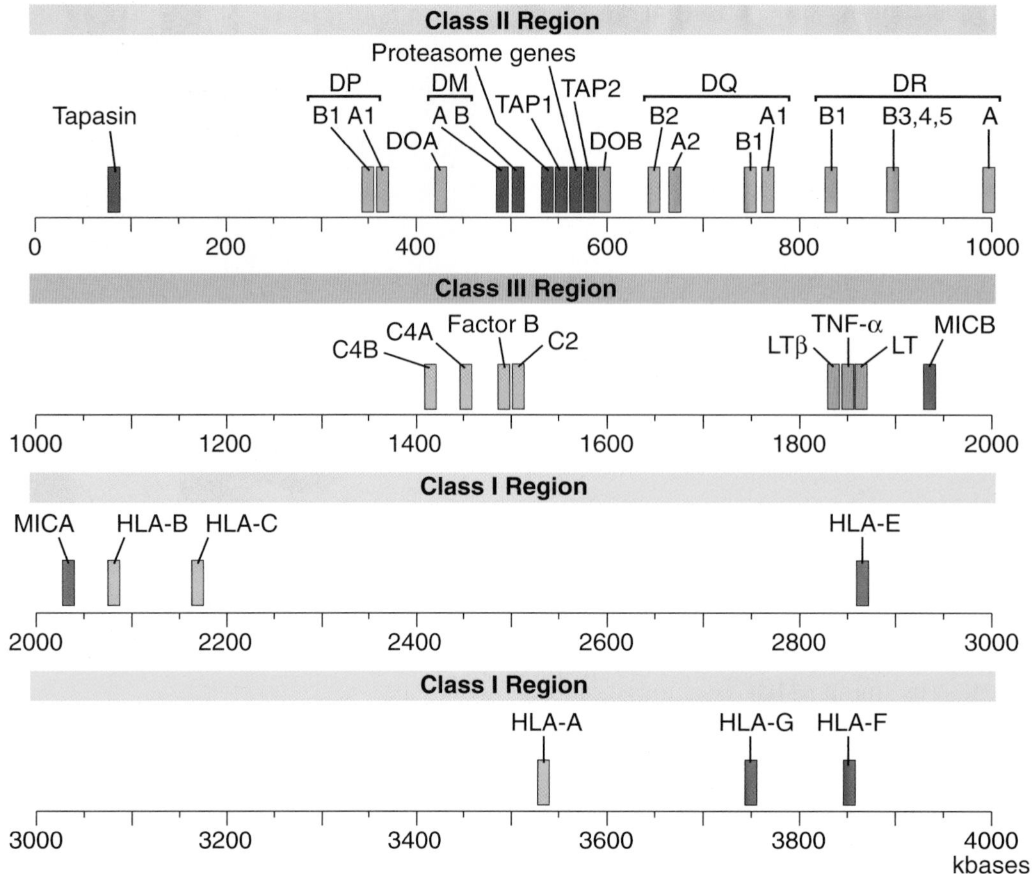

FIGURE 5–9 Map of the human MHC. This map is simplified to exclude many genes that are of unknown function. HLA-E, HLA-F, and HLA-G, and the MIC genes are class I–like molecules, many of whose products are recognized by NK cells; C4, C2, and factor B genes encode complement proteins; tapasin, DM, DO, TAP, and proteasome encode proteins involved in antigen processing; LTA, B, and TNF encode cytokines. Many pseudogenes and genes whose roles in immune responses are not established are located in the HLA complex but are not shown.

necrosis factor (TNF), lymphotoxin-α (LT-α), and LT-β; and for some heat shock proteins. The genes within the MHC that encode these diverse proteins have been called class III MHC genes. Between *HLA-C* and *HLA-A*, and telomeric to *HLA-A*, are many genes that are called class I–like because they resemble class I genes but exhibit little or no polymorphism. Some of these encode proteins that are expressed in association with β_2-microglobulin and are called class IB molecules, to distinguish them from the classical polymorphic class I molecules. Among the class IB molecules is HLA-G, which may play a role in antigen recognition by natural killer (NK) cells, and HLA-H, which appears to be involved in iron metabolism and has no known function in the immune system. Many of the class I–like sequences are pseudogenes. The functions of most of these class I–like genes and pseudogenes are not known. One role may be that during evolution, these DNA sequences serve as repositories of coding sequences that are used for generating polymorphic sequences in conventional class I and class II MHC molecules by the process of gene conversion. In this process, a portion of the sequence of one gene is replaced with a portion of another gene without a reciprocal recombination event. Gene conversion is a more efficient mechanism than point mutation for producing genetic variation without loss of function because several changes can be introduced at once, and amino acids necessary for maintaining protein structure can remain unchanged if identical amino acids at those positions are encoded by both of the genes involved in the conversion event. It is clear from population studies that the extraordinary polymorphism of MHC molecules has been generated by gene conversion and not by point mutations.

The mouse MHC, located on chromosome 17, occupies about 2000 kb of DNA, and the genes are organized in an order slightly different from the human MHC gene. One of the mouse class I genes *(H-2K)* is centromeric to the class II region, but the other class I genes and the nonpolymorphic class IB genes are telomeric to the class II region. As in the human, β_2-microglobulin is encoded not by the MHC but by a gene located on a separate chromosome (chromosome 2).

There are β_2-microglobulin-associated proteins other than class I MHC molecules that may serve important functions in the immune system. These include the neonatal Fc receptor (see Chapter 14), and the CD1 molecules, which are involved in presenting lipid and other nonpeptide antigens to unusual populations of T cells. These proteins are homologous to the class I MHC α chain but are encoded outside the MHC, on different chromosomes.

EXPRESSION OF MHC MOLECULES

Because MHC molecules are required to present antigens to T lymphocytes, the expression of these proteins in a cell determines whether foreign (e.g., microbial) antigens in that cell will be recognized by T cells. There are several important features of the expression of MHC molecules.

- ***Class I molecules are constitutively expressed on virtually all nucleated cells, whereas class II molecules are normally expressed on only dendritic cells, B lymphocytes, macrophages, and a few other cell types.*** This pattern of MHC expression is linked to the functions of class I–restricted and class II–restricted T cells. The effector function of class I–restricted CD8$^+$ T cells is to kill cells infected with intracellular microbes, such as viruses. Because viruses can infect virtually any nucleated cell, the ligands that CD8$^+$ T cells recognize need to be displayed on all nucleated cells. The expression of class I MHC molecules on nucleated cells serves precisely this purpose, providing a display system for viral antigens. In contrast, class II–restricted CD4$^+$ helper T lymphocytes have a set of functions that require recognizing antigen presented by a more limited number of cell types. In particular, naive CD4$^+$ T cells need to recognize antigens that are presented by dendritic cells in peripheral lymphoid organs. Differentiated CD4$^+$ helper T lymphocytes function mainly to activate (or help) macrophages to eliminate extracellular microbes that have been phagocytosed and to activate B lymphocytes to make antibodies that also eliminate extracellular microbes. Class II molecules are expressed mainly on these cell types and provide a system for displaying peptides derived from extracellular microbes and proteins.
- ***The expression of MHC molecules is increased by cytokines produced during both innate and adaptive immune responses*** (Fig. 5–10). On most cell types, the interferons IFN-α, IFN-β, and IFN-γ increase the level of expression of class I molecules, and TNF and LT can have the same effect. (The properties and biologic activities of cytokines are discussed in Chapter 12.) The interferons are produced during the early innate immune response to many viruses (see Chapter 2), and TNF and LT are produced in response to many microbial infections. Thus, innate immune responses to microbes increase the expression of the MHC molecules that display microbial antigens to microbe-specific T cells. This is one of the mechanisms by which innate immunity stimulates adaptive immune responses.

The expression of class II molecules is also regulated by cytokines and other signals in different cells. IFN-γ is the principal cytokine involved in stimulating expression of class II molecules in antigen-presenting cells such as dendritic cells and macrophages (see Fig. 5–10). The IFN-γ may be produced by NK cells during innate immune reactions, and by antigen-activated T cells during adaptive immune reactions. The ability of IFN-γ to increase class II expression on antigen-presenting cells is an amplification mechanism in adaptive immunity. In dendritic cells, the expression of class II molecules also increases in response to signals from Toll-like receptors responding to microbial components, thus promoting the display of microbial antigens (Chapter 6). B lymphocytes constitutively express class II molecules and can increase expression in response to antigen recognition and cytokines produced by helper T cells, thus enhancing antigen presentation to helper cells (Chapter 10). Vascular endothelial cells, like macrophages, increase class II expression in response to IFN-γ; the significance of this phenomenon is unclear. Most nonimmune cell types express few, if any, class II MHC molecules unless exposed to high levels of IFN-γ. These cells are unlikely to present antigens to CD4$^+$ T cells except in unusual circum-

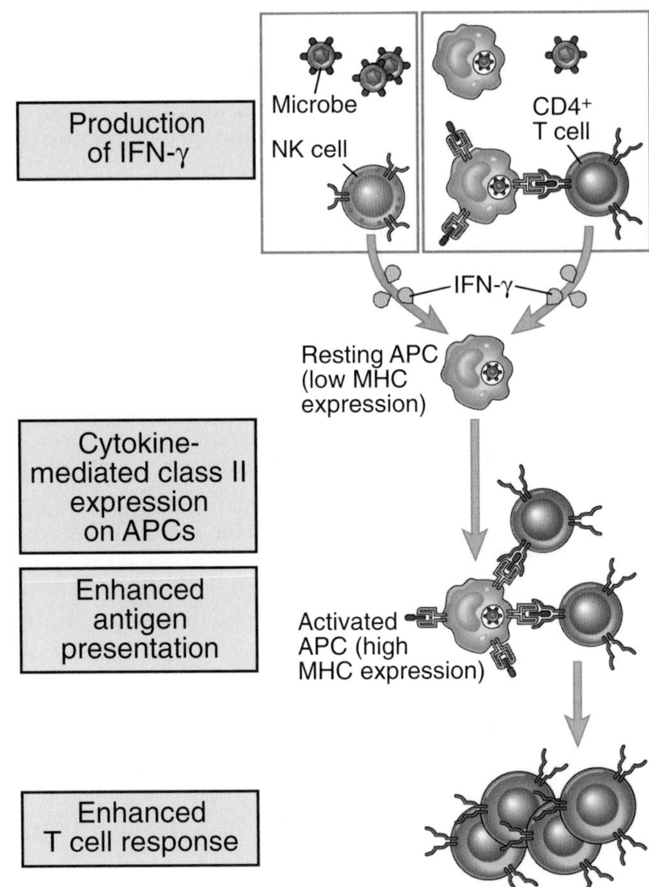

FIGURE 5–10 Enhancement of class II MHC expression by IFN-γ. IFN-γ, produced by NK cells and other cell types during innate immune reactions to microbes, or by T cells during adaptive immune reactions, stimulates class II MHC expression on antigen-presenting cells (APCs) and thus enhances the activation of CD4$^+$ T cells. IFN-γ has a similar effect on the expression of class I MHC molecules and the activation of CD8$^+$ T cells.

stances. Some cells, such as neurons, never appear to express class II molecules. Human, but not mouse, T cells express class II molecules after activation; however, no cytokine has been identified in this response, and its functional significance is unknown.

- ***The rate of transcription is the major determinant of the level of MHC molecule synthesis and expression on the cell surface.*** Cytokines enhance MHC expression by stimulating the rate of transcription of class I and class II genes in a wide variety of cell types. These effects are mediated by the binding of cytokine-activated transcription factors to regulatory DNA sequences in the promoter regions of MHC genes. Several transcription factors may be assembled and bind a protein called the class II transcription activator (CIITA), and the entire complex binds to the class II promoter and promotes efficient transcription. By keeping the complex of transcription factors together, CIITA functions as a master regulator of class II gene expression. CIITA is synthesized in response to IFN-γ, explaining how this cytokine can increase expression of class II MHC molecules. Mutations in several of these transcription factors have been identified as the cause of human immunodeficiency diseases associated with defective expression of MHC molecules. The best studied of these disorders is the **bare lymphocyte syndrome** (see Chapter 20). Knockout mice lacking CIITA also show an absence of class II expression on dendritic cells and B lymphocytes and an inability of IFN-γ to induce class II on macrophages.

The expression of many of the proteins involved in antigen processing and presentation is coordinately regulated. For instance, IFN-γ increases the transcription not only of class I and class II genes but also of β_2-microglobulin, of the genes that encode two of the subunits of the proteasome, and of the genes encoding the subunits of the TAP heterodimer.

SUMMARY

- The MHC is a large genetic region coding for class I and class II MHC molecules as well as for other proteins. MHC genes are highly polymorphic, with more than 250 alleles for some of these genes in the population.

- The function of MHC-encoded class I and class II molecules is to bind peptide antigens and display them for recognition by antigen-specific T lymphocytes. Peptide antigens associated with class I molecules are recognized by $CD8^+$ CTLs, whereas class II–associated peptide antigens are recognized by $CD4^+$ (mostly helper) T cells. MHC molecules were originally recognized for their role in triggering T cell responses that caused the rejection of transplanted tissue.

- Class I MHC molecules are composed of an α (or heavy) chain in a noncovalent complex with a nonpolymorphic polypeptide called β_2-microglobulin. The class II molecules contain two MHC-encoded polymorphic chains, an α chain and a β chain. Both classes of MHC molecules are structurally similar and consist of an extracellular peptide-binding cleft, a nonpolymorphic Ig-like region, a transmembrane region, and a cytoplasmic region. The peptide-binding cleft of MHC molecules has α-helical sides and an eight-stranded antiparallel β-pleated sheet floor. The peptide-binding cleft of class I molecules is formed by the α1 and α2 segments of the α chain, and that of class II molecules by the α1 and β1 segments of the two chains. The Ig-like domains of class I and class II molecules contain the binding sites for the T cell coreceptors CD8 and CD4, respectively.

- MHC molecules bind only one peptide at a time, and all the peptides that bind to a particular MHC molecule share common structural motifs. Peptide binding is saturable, and the off-rate is very slow, so that complexes, once formed, persist for a sufficiently long time to be recognized by T cells. Every MHC molecule has a broad specificity for peptides and can bind multiple peptides that have common structural features, such as anchor residues.

- The peptide-binding cleft of class I molecules can accommodate peptides that are 8 to 11 amino acid residues long, whereas the cleft of class II molecules allows larger peptides (up to 30 amino acid residues in length or more) to bind. The polymorphic residues of MHC molecules are localized to the peptide-binding domain. Some polymorphic MHC residues determine the binding specificities for peptides by forming structures, called pockets, that interact with complementary residues of the bound peptide, called anchor residues. Other polymorphic MHC residues and some residues of the peptide are not involved in binding to MHC molecules but instead form the structure recognized by T cells.

- In addition to the polymorphic class I and class II genes, the MHC contains genes encoding complement proteins, cytokines, nonpolymorphic class I–like molecules, and several proteins involved in antigen processing.

- Class I molecules are expressed on all nucleated cells, whereas class II molecules are expressed mainly on specialized antigen-presenting cells, such as dendritic cells, macrophages, and B lymphocytes, and a few other cell types, including endothelial cells and thymic epithelial cells. The expression of MHC gene products is enhanced by inflammatory and immune stimuli, particularly cytokines like IFN-γ, which stimulate the transcription of MHC genes.

Selected Readings

Bjorkman PJ, MA Saper, B Samraoui, WS Bennett, JL Strominger, and DC Wiley. Structure of the human class I histocompatibility antigen HLA-A2. Nature 329:506–512, 1987.

Horton R, L Wilming, V Rand, et al. Gene map of the extended human MHC. Nature Reviews Genetics 5:889–899, 2004.

Kelley J, L Walter, and J Trowsdale. Comparative genomics of major histocompatibility complexes. Immunogenetics 56: 683–695, 2005.

Klein J, and A Sato. The HLA system. New England Journal of Medicine 343:702–709 and 782–786, 2000.

Mach B. The bare lymphocyte syndrome and the regulation of MHC expression. Annual Review of Immunology 19:331–373, 2001.

Madden DR. The three dimensional structure of peptide-MHC complexes. Annual Review of Immunology 13:587–622, 1995.

Marrack P, JP Scott-Browne, S Dai, L Gapin, and JW Kappler. Evolutionarily conserved amino acids that control TCR-MHC interaction. Annual Review of Immunology 26:171–203, 2008.

Mazza C, and B Malissen. What guides MHC-restricted TCR recognition? Seminars in Immunology 19:225–235, 2007.

Reith W, S Leibundgut-Landmann, and JM Waldburger. Regulation of MHC class II gene expression by the class II transactivator. Nature Reviews Immunology 5:793–806, 2005.

Chapter 6

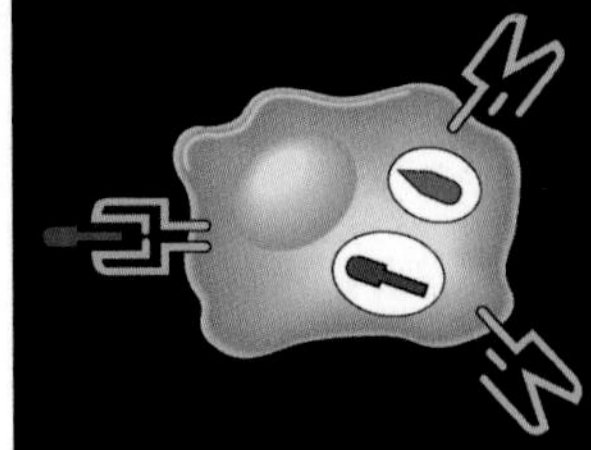

ANTIGEN PROCESSING AND PRESENTATION TO T LYMPHOCYTES

T lymphocytes play central roles in all adaptive immune responses against protein antigens. In cell-mediated immunity, $CD4^+$ T cells activate macrophages to destroy phagocytosed microbes, and $CD8^+$ T cells kill cells infected with intracellular microbes. In humoral immunity, $CD4^+$ helper T cells interact with B lymphocytes and stimulate the proliferation and differentiation of these B cells. Both the induction phase and the effector phase of T cell responses are triggered by the specific recognition of antigen. In Chapter 5, we introduced the concept that T cells recognize peptide fragments that are derived from protein antigens and are bound to cell surface molecules encoded by genes of the major histocompatibility complex (MHC) (see Fig. 5–1). The cells that display MHC-associated peptides are called **antigen-presenting cells** (APCs). Certain APCs present antigens to naive T cells during the recognition phase of immune responses to initiate these responses, and some APCs present antigens to differentiated T cells during the effector phase to trigger the mechanisms that eliminate the antigens. In Chapter 5, we focused on the structures and functions of MHC molecules. In this chapter, we continue the discussion of the ligands that T cells recognize by focusing on the generation of peptide-MHC complexes on APCs. Specifically, we describe the characteristics of the APCs that form and display these peptide-MHC complexes and how protein antigens are converted by APCs to peptides that associate with MHC molecules. We then discuss the importance of MHC-restricted antigen presentation in adaptive immunity. Finally, we briefly describe how lipid antigens are presented to rare populations of T lymphocytes.

PROPERTIES OF ANTIGENS RECOGNIZED BY T LYMPHOCYTES

Our current understanding of T cell antigen recognition is the culmination of a vast amount of research that began with studies of the nature of antigens that stimulate cell-mediated immunity. The early studies showed that the physicochemical forms of antigens that are recognized by T cells are different from those recognized by B lymphocytes and antibodies, and this knowledge led to the discovery of the role of the MHC in T cell antigen recognition. Several features of antigen recognition are unique to T lymphocytes (Table 6–1).

- ***Most T lymphocytes recognize only peptides,*** whereas B cells can recognize peptides, proteins, nucleic acids, polysaccharides, lipids, and small chemicals. As a result, T cell–mediated immune responses are usually induced by protein antigens (the natural source of foreign peptides), whereas humoral immune responses are seen with protein and nonprotein antigens. Some T cells are specific for small chemical haptens such as dinitrophenol, urushiol of poison ivy, and β lactams of penicillin antibiotics. In these situations, it is likely that the haptens bind to self proteins and that hapten-conjugated peptides are recognized by T cells.
- ***T cells are specific for amino acid sequences of peptides.*** In contrast, B cells recognize conformational determinants of antigens, even proteins, in their native tertiary (folded) configuration. The antigen receptors of T cells recognize very few residues even within a single peptide, and different T cells can distinguish peptides that differ even at single amino acid residues. We will return to the structural basis of this remarkable fine specificity of T cells in Chapter 7.
- ***T cells recognize and respond to foreign peptide antigens only when the antigens are attached to the surfaces of APCs,*** whereas B cells and secreted antibodies bind soluble antigens in body fluids as well as exposed cell surface antigens. This is because T cells can recognize only peptides bound to and displayed by MHC molecules, and MHC molecules are integral membrane proteins expressed on APCs. The properties and functions of APCs are discussed later in this chapter.
- ***T cells from any one individual recognize foreign peptide antigens only when these peptides are bound to and displayed by the MHC molecules of that individual.*** This feature of antigen recognition by T cells, called **self MHC restriction,** can be demonstrated in experimental situations in which T lymphocytes from one individual are mixed with APCs from another individual.
    - The first demonstration of MHC restriction came from the studies of Rolf Zinkernagel and Peter Doherty, who examined the recognition of virus-infected cells by virus-specific cytotoxic T lymphocytes (CTLs) in inbred mice. If a mouse is infected with a virus, $CD8^+$ CTLs specific for the virus develop in the animal. These CTLs recognize and kill virus-infected cells only if the infected cells express alleles of MHC molecules that are expressed in the animal in which the CTLs were generated (Fig. 6–1). By use of MHC congenic strains of mice, it was shown that the CTLs and the infected target cell must be derived from mice that share a class I MHC allele. Thus, the recognition of antigens by $CD8^+$ CTLs is restricted by self class I MHC alleles. Essentially similar experiments demonstrated that responses of $CD4^+$ helper T lymphocytes to antigens are self class II MHC restricted.

The self MHC restriction of T cells is a consequence of selection processes during T cell maturation in

Table 6–1. Features of T Cell Antigen Recognition

Features of antigens recognized by T cells	Explanation
Most T cells recognize peptides and no other molecules	Only peptides bind to MHC molecules
T cells recognize cell-associated and not soluble antigens	MHC molecules are membrane proteins that display stably bound peptides on cell surfaces
$CD4^+$ and $CD8^+$ T cells preferentially recognize antigens sampled from the vesicular and cytosolic pools, respectively	Pathways of assembly of MHC molecules ensure that class II molecules display peptides that are derived from extracellular proteins and taken up into vesicles in APCs, and class I molecules present peptides from cytosolic proteins; CD4 and CD8 bind to nonpolymorphic regions of class II and class I MHC molecules, respectively

Abbreviations: APC, antigen-presenting cell; MHC, major histocompatibility complex

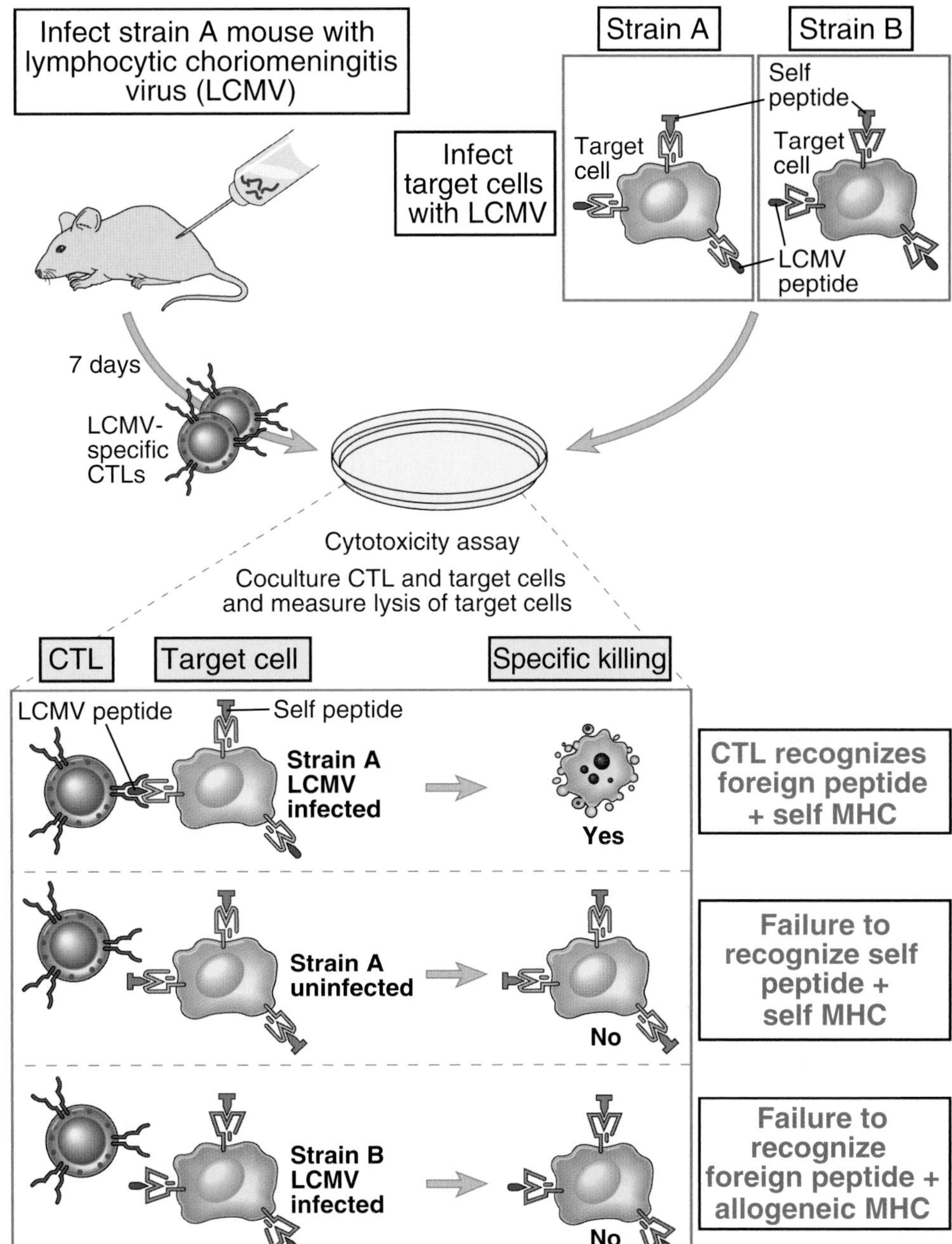

FIGURE 6–1 MHC restriction of cytotoxic T lymphocytes. Virus-specific cytotoxic T lymphocytes (CTLs) generated from virus-infected strain A mice kill only syngeneic (strain A) target cells infected with that virus. The CTLs do not kill uninfected strain A targets (which express self peptides but not viral peptides) or infected strain B targets (which express different MHC alleles than does strain A). By use of congenic mouse strains that differ only at class I MHC loci, it has been proved that recognition of antigen by $CD8^+$ CTLs is self class I MHC restricted.

the thymus. During this process of maturation, the T cells that express antigen receptors specific for peptides bound to self MHC are selected to survive, and the cells that do not "see" self MHC are allowed to die (see Chapter 8). This process ensures that the T cells that attain maturity are the useful ones because they will be able to recognize antigens displayed by the individual's MHC molecules. The discovery of self MHC restriction provided the definitive evidence that T cells see not only protein antigens but also polymorphic residues of MHC molecules, which are the residues that distinguish self from foreign MHC. Thus, MHC molecules display peptides for recognition by T lymphocytes and are also integral components of the ligands that T cells recognize. Although T cells are self MHC restricted, they recognize foreign MHC molecules present in tissue grafts and reject these grafts. The basis of this cross-reaction against foreign MHC molecules will be described in Chapter 16.

- ***$CD4^+$ helper T cells recognize peptides bound to class II MHC molecules, whereas $CD8^+$ T cells recognize peptides bound to class I MHC molecules.*** Stated differently, $CD4^+$ T cells are class II MHC restricted, and $CD8^+$ T cells are class I MHC restricted. The reason for this segregation is that CD4 binds directly to class II MHC molecules and CD8 to class I molecules (see Chapter 5). We will return to the role of CD4 and CD8 in determining the class I or class II MHC restriction patterns of T cells in Chapter 7.

- ***$CD4^+$ class II–restricted T cells recognize peptides derived mainly from extracellular proteins that are internalized into the vesicles of APCs, whereas $CD8^+$ T cells recognize peptides derived from cytosolic, usually endogenously synthesized, proteins.*** The reason for this is that vesicular proteins enter the class II peptide loading and presentation pathway, and cytosolic proteins enter the class I pathway. The mechanisms and physiologic significance of this segregation are major themes of this chapter.
- In addition to MHC-associated presentation of peptides, there is another antigen presentation system that is specialized to present lipid antigens. The class I–like nonpolymorphic molecule CD1 is expressed on a variety of APCs and epithelia, and it presents lipid antigens to unusual populations of T cells that are not MHC-restricted. Studies with culture-derived cloned lines of T cells indicate that a variety of cells can recognize lipid antigens presented by CD1; these include $CD4^+$, $CD8^+$, and $CD4^-CD8^-$ T cells expressing the $\alpha\beta$ T cell receptor (TCR) as well as $\gamma\delta$ T cells. There has been much interest in a small subset of T cells that express markers of NK cells. These are called NK-T cells, and they recognize CD1-associated lipids and glycolipids, including some produced by bacteria. In this chapter, we discuss mainly the presentation of peptide antigens by class I and class II MHC molecules to $CD8^+$ and $CD4^+$ T lymphocytes.

ANTIGEN-PRESENTING CELLS

All the functions of T lymphocytes depend on their interactions with other cells. For this reason, a great deal of effort has been devoted to defining how cell-associated antigens are displayed to T lymphocytes. In this section of the chapter, we describe the APCs that are involved in activating T cells, and the functions of these APCs in immune responses to protein antigens.

Discovery of Antigen-Presenting Cells and Their Role in Immune Responses

The responses of antigen-specific T lymphocytes to protein antigens require the participation of antigen-presenting cells (APCs), which capture and display the antigens to T cells. This conclusion is based on several lines of experimental evidence.

- T cells present in the blood, spleen, or lymph nodes of individuals immunized with a protein antigen can be activated by exposure to that antigen in tissue culture. If contaminating dendritic cells, macrophages, and B cells are removed from the cultures, the purified T lymphocytes do not respond to the antigen, and responsiveness can be restored by adding back dendritic cells, macrophages, or B lymphocytes (Fig. 6–2). Such experimental approaches are commonly used to determine which cell types are able to function as APCs for the activation of T lymphocytes.
- If an antigen is taken up by dendritic cells or macrophages in vitro and then injected into mice, the amount of cell-associated antigen required to induce a response is 1000 times less than the amount of the same antigen required when administered by itself in a cell-free form. In other words, cell-associated proteins are much more immunogenic than are soluble proteins on a molar basis. The explanation for this finding is that the immunogenic form of the antigen is the APC-associated form, and only a small fraction of injected free antigen ends up associated with APCs *in vivo*. This concept is now being exploited to immunize patients with cancer against their tumors by growing APCs (specifically, dendritic cells) from these patients, incubating the APCs with tumor antigens, and injecting them back into the patients as a cellular vaccine.

APCs serve two important functions in the activation of T cells. First, APCs convert protein antigens to peptides, and they display peptide-MHC complexes for recognition by the T cells. The conversion of native proteins to MHC-associated peptide fragments by APCs is called **antigen processing** and is discussed later in this chapter. Second, some APCs provide stimuli to the T cell beyond those initiated by recognition of peptide-MHC complexes by the T cell antigen receptor. These stimuli, referred to as **costimulators,** are required for the full responses of the T cells, especially naive $CD4^+$ cells. The nature and mode of action of costimulators are discussed further in Chapter 9.

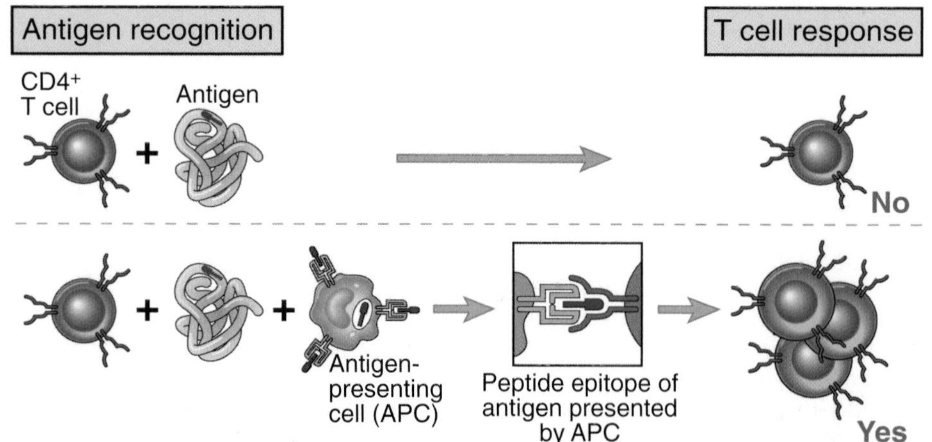

FIGURE 6–2 Antigen-presenting cells are required for T cell activation. Purified $CD4^+$ T cells do not respond to a protein antigen by itself but do respond to the antigen in the presence of antigen-presenting cells (APCs). The function of the APCs is to display peptides derived from the antigen to T cells. APCs also express costimulators that are important for T cell activation; these are not shown.

The antigen-presenting function of APCs is enhanced by exposure to microbial products. Dendritic cells and macrophages express Toll-like receptors (Chapter 2) that respond to microbes by increasing expression of MHC molecules and costimulators, by improving the efficiency of antigen presentation, and by activating the APCs to produce cytokines, which stimulate T cell responses. In addition, dendritic cells and macrophages that are activated by microbes express chemokine receptors that stimulate their migration to sites of infection, further amplifying antigen presentation and T cell activation. To induce a T cell response to a protein antigen in a vaccine or experimentally, the antigen must be administered with substances called **adjuvants.** Adjuvants are either products of microbes, such as killed mycobacteria (used experimentally), or they mimic microbes and stimulate T cell responses by the same mechanisms as do microbial products. It is not possible to use most microbial adjuvants in humans because of the pathologic inflammation that microbial products elicit. Some adjuvants that are used in humans, such as alum, are especially good at stimulating antibody responses but are less potent T cell stimulators. Attempts are ongoing to develop effective adjuvants for clinical use, mainly to maximize the immunogenicity of vaccines. Protein antigens administered in aqueous form, without adjuvants, either fail to induce T cell responses or induce a state of unresponsiveness, called tolerance (see Chapter 11).

Different cell types function as APCs to activate naive and previously differentiated effector T cells (Fig. 6–3 and Table 6–2). Dendritic cells are the most effective APCs for activating naive $CD4^+$ and $CD8^+$ T cells, and therefore for initiating T cell responses. Macrophages present antigens to differentiated (effector) $CD4^+$ T cells in the effector phase of cell-mediated immunity, and B lymphocytes present antigens to helper T cells during humoral immune responses. Dendritic cells, macrophages, and B lymphocytes express class II MHC molecules and costimulators, and are, therefore, capable of activating $CD4^+$ T lymphocytes. For this reason, these three cell types have been called professional APCs; however, this term is sometimes used to refer only to dendritic cells because this is the only cell type whose principal function is to capture and present antigens, and the only APC capable of initiating T cell responses.

Antigen Presentation to Naive T Lymphocytes: Role of Dendritic Cells in Initiating T Cell Responses

Dendritic cells are present in lymphoid organs, in the epithelia of the skin and gastrointestinal and respiratory tracts, and in the interstitium of most parenchymal organs. These cells are identified morphologically by their membranous or spinelike projections (Fig. 6–4). There are subsets of dendritic cells that may be distinguished by the expression of various cell surface markers and may play different roles in immune responses (Box 6–1). All dendritic cells are thought to arise from bone marrow precursors, and most, called myeloid dendritic cells, are related in lineage to mononuclear phagocytes. The prototypes of epithelial dendritic cells are the Langerhans cells of the epidermis. Because of their long

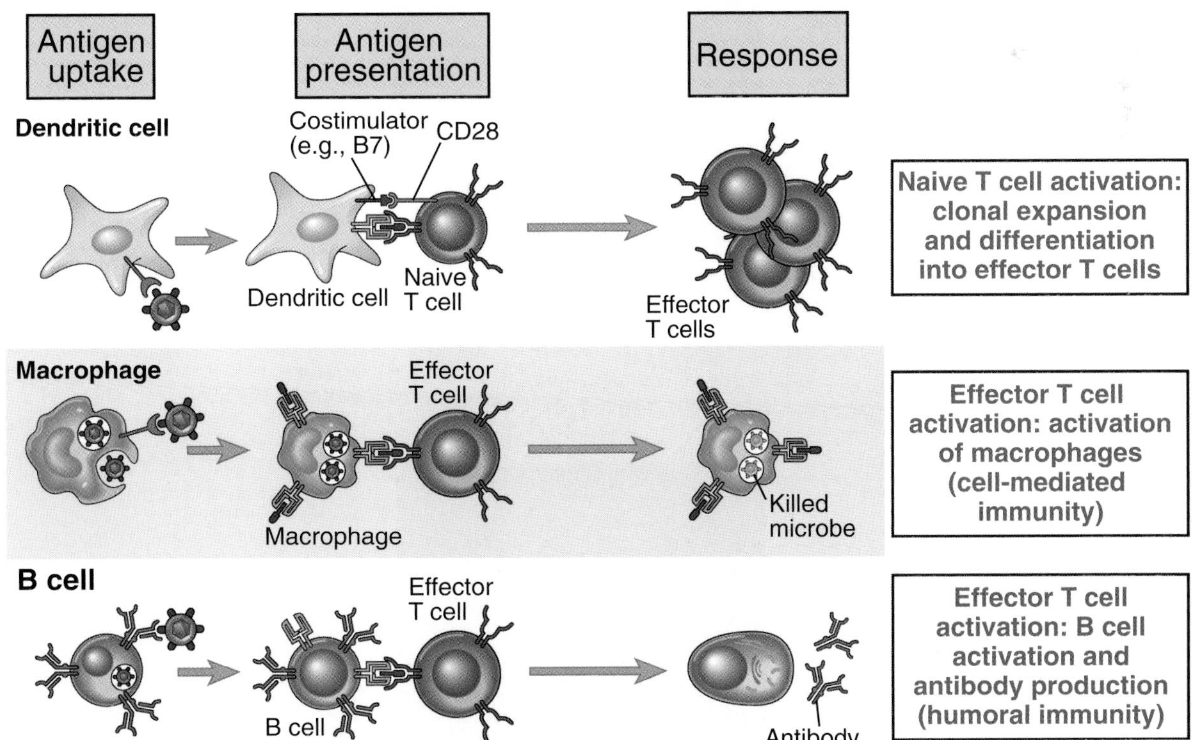

FIGURE 6–3 Functions of different antigen-presenting cells. The three major types of antigen-presenting cells for $CD4^+$ T cells function to display antigens at different stages and in different types of immune responses. Note that effector T cells activate macrophages and B lymphocytes by production of cytokines and by expressing surface molecules; these will be described in later chapters.

Table 6–2. Properties and Functions of Antigen-Presenting Cells

Cell type	Expression of		Principal function
	Class II MHC	Costimulators	
Dendritic cells	Constitutive; increases with maturation; increased by IFN-γ	Constitutive; increase with maturation; inducible by IFN-γ, CD40-CD40L interactions	Initiation of T cell responses to protein antigens (priming)
Macrophages	Low or negative; inducible by IFN-γ	Inducible by LPS, IFN-γ, CD40-CD40L interactions	Effector phase of cell-mediated immune responses
B lymphocytes	Constitutive; increased by IL-4	Induced by T cells (CD40-CD40L interactions), antigen receptor cross-linking	Antigen presentation to CD4+ helper T cells in humoral immune responses (cognate T cell-B cell interactions)
Vascular endothelial cells	Inducible by IFN-γ; constitutive in humans	Constitutive (inducible in mice)	May promote activation of antigen-specific T cells at site of antigen exposure
Various epithelial and mesenchymal cells	Inducible by IFN-γ	Probably none	No known physiologic function

Abbreviations: IFN-γ, interferon-γ; IL-4, interleukin-4; LPS, lipopolysaccharide

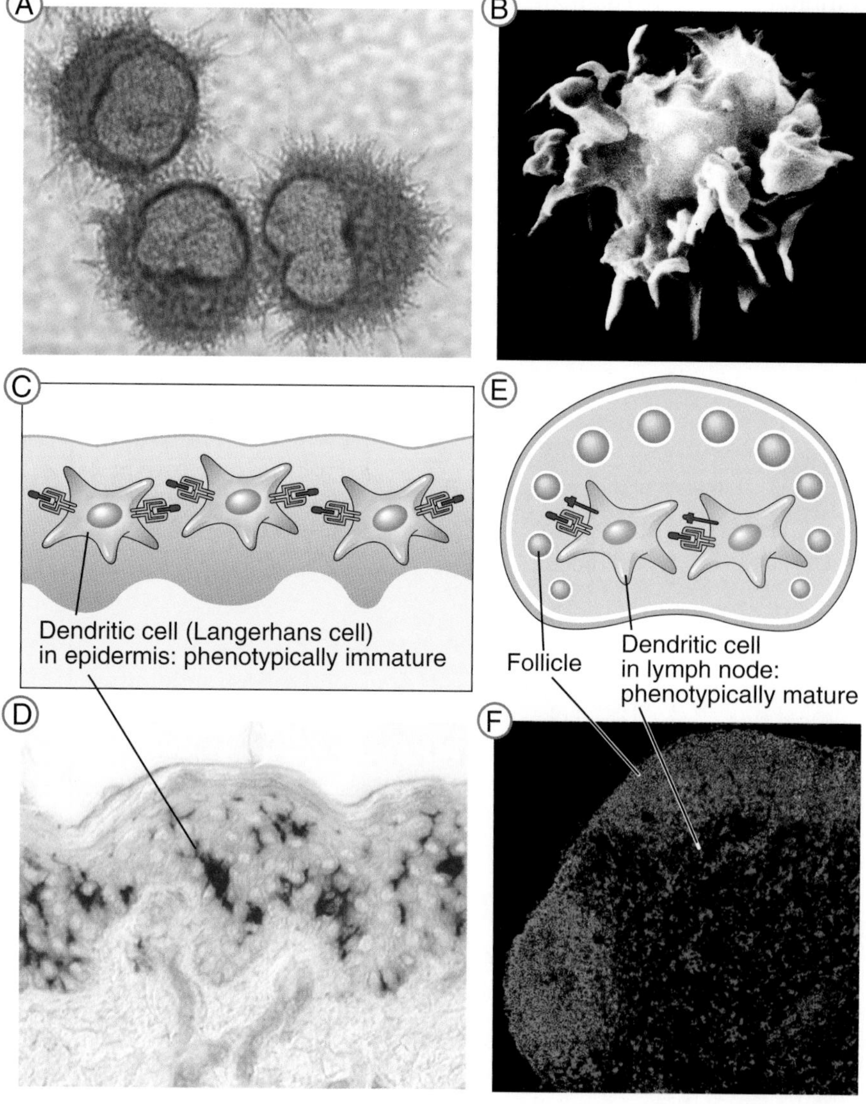

FIGURE 6–4 Dendritic cells. A. Light micrograph of cultured dendritic cells derived from bone marrow precursors. (Courtesy of Dr. Y-J Liu, M. D. Anderson Cancer Center, Houston, TX.) B. A scanning electron micrograph of a dendritic cell, showing the extensive membrane projections. (Courtesy of Dr. Y-J Liu, M. D. Anderson Cancer Center, Houston, TX.) C, D. Dendritic cells in the skin, illustrated schematically (C) and in a section of the skin stained with an antibody specific for Langerhans cells (which appear blue in this immunoenzyme stain) (D). (The micrograph of the skin is courtesy of Dr. Y-J Liu, M. D. Anderson Cancer Center, Houston, TX.) E, F. Dendritic cells in a lymph node, illustrated schematically (E) and in a section of a mouse lymph node stained with fluorescently labeled antibodies against B cells in follicles (green) and dendritic cells in the T cell zone (red) (F). (The micrograph is courtesy of Drs. Kathryn Pape and Jennifer Walter, University of Minnesota School of Medicine, Minneapolis.)

Box 6–1 ■ IN DEPTH: DENDRITIC CELL SUBSETS

Subpopulations of dendritic cells (DCs) have been described in humans and mice, based on distinct phenotypic characteristics and functional response patterns. The interest in defining these subsets is that they may serve distinct functions in innate immunity and in regulating T cell responses to foreign and self antigens. Most studies in mice are based on the isolation of DCs from lymphoid organs, whereas most of the studies on human DCs rely on culturing these cells from precursors in the blood. It is, therefore, often difficult to establish clear parallels across the species. The problem of defining the subsets is compounded by the plasticity of DC phenotypes and functions (i.e., the realization that the characteristics of the same DC population may change in different anatomic locations or in response to different external stimuli).

Despite these caveats, it is generally accepted that there are two main subsets of DCs, called myeloid DCs and plasmacytoid DCs. Myeloid DCs are the "classical" or "conventional" DCs that were first identified by their ability to stimulate strong T cell responses. They can be cultured from bone marrow or blood cells, including blood monocytes, and are the most numerous DC subset in lymphoid organs. It is believed that myeloid DCs enter the circulation from the bone marrow, and are capable of slow constitutive migration into tissues that serves to maintain the resident tissue population of DCs. Upon activation by encounter with microbes or cytokines, these tissue DCs mature and migrate into draining lymph nodes, where they initiate T cell responses. Tissue-derived conventional DCs are also sometimes classified into the Langerhans cell type, representing DCs in epithelia and in skin-draining lymph nodes, and the interstitial/dermal type, representing cells in most other tissues. Although these subpopulations of myeloid DCs can be distinguished by the expression of various surface markers, it may be that they are not distinct lineages but activation stages of a single lineage whose phenotype changes in response to different local environmental signals. Plasmacytoid DCs resemble plasma cells morphologically, and acquire the dendritic morphology only after activation. They are found in the blood as precursors, and in small numbers in lymphoid organs. A subset of myeloid DCs that expresses the T cell marker CD8 has been described in mice (but not found in humans) and called "lymphoid DCs" because of the suggestion that they develop from common lymphoid progenitors. However, $CD8^+$ DCs are now known to develop from myeloid precursors, and the term *lymphoid DC* is not generally used.

The major DC subsets have a number of distinguishing features that are summarized in the Table. It should, however, be pointed out that the heterogeneity of DCs may be substantially greater than what is described in the Table. It has also been widely believed that the function of epithelial DCs, such as Langerhans cells, is to capture the antigens of microbes that try to enter through epithelia and to transport these antigens to lymphoid organs. However, recent studies have shown that T cell responses to antigens administered through the skin can be elicited even in the absence of Langerhans cells, suggesting that dermal DCs may serve the same function and compensate for the absence of Langerhans cells.

DCs have also been divided into immature and mature populations. We have mentioned in the text that DCs located in epithelia are considered immature, and their major function is to capture antigens, whereas DCs that

Feature	Myeloid DCs CD8 negative	Plasmacytoid DCs	Myeloid DCs CD8 positive
Surface markers	CD11c-high, CD11b-high	CD11c-low, CD11b-negative, B220-high	$CD8\alpha^+$, CD11c-low/high, CD11b-negative
Growth factors for *in vitro* derivation	GM-CSF, Flt3-ligand	Flt3-ligand	Flt3-ligand?
Expression of Toll-like receptors (TLRs)	TLR-4, 5, 8 high	TLR-7, 9 high	TLR-3 high
Major cytokines produced	TNF, IL-6	Type I interferons	IL-12
Ability to cross-present	+/-	+/-	++
Postulated major functions	Induction of T cell responses against most antigens	Innate immunity and induction of T cell responses against viruses	Activation of $CD8^+$ T cells by cross-priming

Continued on following page

Box 6–1 ▪ IN DEPTH: DENDRITIC CELL SUBSETS (Continued)

have encountered microbes undergo maturation and function to present the antigens to T cells and to activate the T cells, particularly in lymphoid organs. It is worth noting that many DCs present in lymphoid organs and in nonlymphoid tissues appear to be in an immature functional state, i.e., able to capture antigens but unable to initiate T cell immunity. These DCs may be important for presenting self antigens to self-reactive T cells and thus for maintaining self-tolerance. Because the immature DC phenotype may be transient, and the cells rapidly mature upon isolation, it has proved difficult to use purified DCs to define the key features that mark the immature state, or that correlate with the tolerogenic potential of DCs. Instead, approaches have been developed to study the function of DCs *in situ,* by selectively targeting antigens to the cells either in the steady state or following administration of a maturation stimulus (see Chapter 11).

cytoplasmic processes, Langerhans cells occupy as much as 25% of the surface area of the epidermis, even though they constitute less than 1% of the cell population. Normally, epithelial and tissue dendritic cells are in a resting or "immature" state. These dendritic cells capture microbial protein antigens and transport the antigens to draining lymph nodes. In response to encounter with microbial components, the dendritic cells mature while they are migrating to lymph nodes and become extremely efficient at presenting antigens and stimulating naive T cells. Mature dendritic cells reside in the T cell zones of the lymph nodes, and in this location they display antigens to the T cells. These lymph node dendritic cells are called interdigitating dendritic cells or, simply, dendritic cells.

The responses of CD4$^+$ T cells are initiated in the peripheral lymphoid organs, to which protein antigens are transported after being collected from their portal of entry (Fig. 6–5). The common routes through which foreign antigens, such as microbes, enter a host are the skin and the epithelia of the gastrointestinal and respiratory systems. In addition, microbial antigens may be produced in any tissue that has been infected. The skin, mucosal epithelia, and parenchymal organs contain numerous lymphatic capillaries that drain lymph from these sites and into the regional lymph nodes. The lymph contains a sampling of all the soluble and cell-associated antigens present in these tissues. Lymph nodes that are interposed along lymphatic vessels act as filters that sample the lymph at numerous points before it reaches the blood (see Fig. 3–8, Chapter 3). Antigens that enter the blood stream may be similarly sampled by the spleen.

Dendritic cells that are resident in epithelia and tissues capture protein antigens and transport the antigens to draining lymph nodes (Fig. 6–6). Resting (immature) dendritic cells express membrane receptors that bind microbes, such as mannose receptors (see Chapter 2). Dendritic cells use these receptors to capture and endocytose microbial antigens, and begin to process the proteins into peptides capable of binding to MHC molecules. Dendritic cells also express Toll-like receptors that recognize microbial molecules and activate the cells to secrete cytokines and start their process of maturation. Dendritic cells that are activated by microbes and by locally produced cytokines, such as

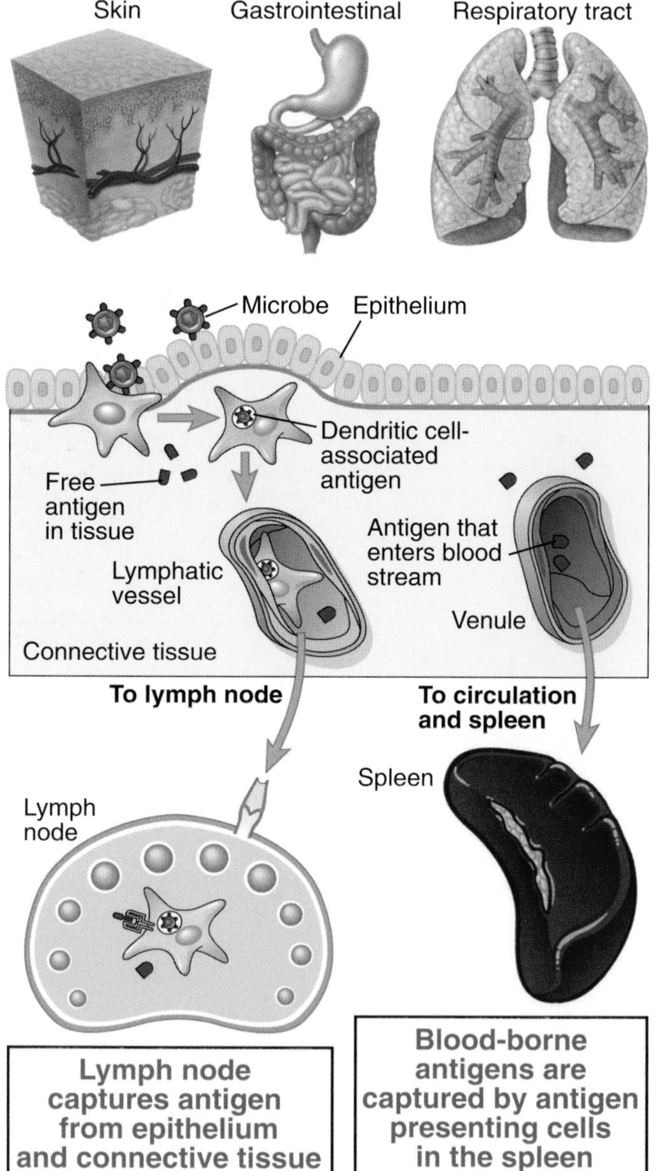

FIGURE 6–5 Routes of antigen entry. Microbial antigens commonly enter through the skin and gastrointestinal and respiratory tracts, where they are captured by dendritic cells and transported to regional lymph nodes. Antigens that enter the blood stream are captured by antigen-presenting cells in the spleen.

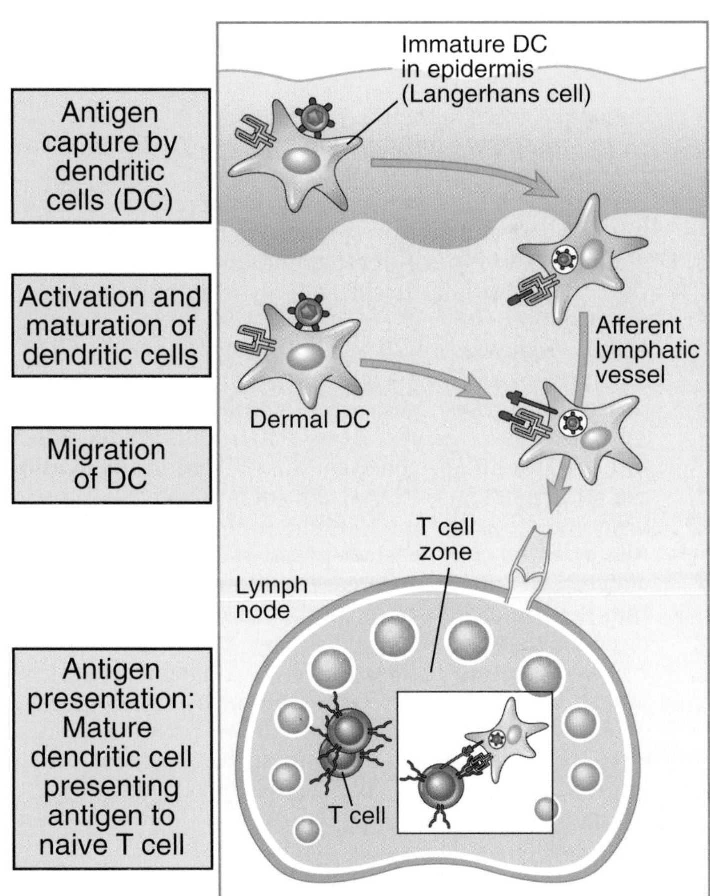

	Immature dendritic cell	Mature dendritic cell
Principal function	Antigen capture	Antigen presentation to T cells
Expression of Fc receptors, mannose receptors	++	–
Expression of molecules involved in T cell activation: B7, ICAM-1, IL-12	– or low	++
Class II MHC molecules		
Half-life	~10 hr	>100 hr
Number of surface molecules	~10^6	~7 x 10^6

FIGURE 6–6 Role of dendritic cells in antigen capture and presentation. Immature dendritic cells in the skin (Langerhans cells) or dermis (dermal DCs) capture antigens that enter through the epidermis and transport the antigens to regional lymph nodes. During this migration, the dendritic cells mature and become efficient antigen-presenting cells. The table summarizes some of the changes during dendritic cell maturation that are important in the functions of these cells.

tumor necrosis factor, lose their adhesiveness for epithelia and begin to express a chemokine receptor called CCR7 that is specific for chemokines produced in the T cell zones of lymph nodes. The chemokines attract the dendritic cells bearing microbial antigens into the T cell zones of the regional lymph nodes. (Recall that in Chapter 3 we mentioned that naive T cells also express CCR7, and this is why naive T cells migrate to the same regions of lymph nodes where antigen-bearing dendritic cells are concentrated.) Maturation also converts the dendritic cells from cells whose function is to capture antigen into cells that are able to display antigens to naive T cells and activate the lymphocytes. Mature dendritic cells express high levels of class II MHC molecules with bound peptides as well as costimulators required for T cell activation. This process of maturation can be reproduced in vitro by culturing bone marrow–derived immature dendritic cells with cytokines (such as tumor necrosis factor and granulocyte-macrophage colony-stimulating factor) and microbial products (such as endotoxin). Thus, by the time these cells become resident in lymph nodes, they have developed into potent APCs with the ability to activate T lymphocytes. Naive T cells that recirculate through lymph nodes encounter these APCs. T cells that are specific for the displayed peptide-MHC complexes are activated, and an immune response is initiated.

Several properties of dendritic cells make them the most effective APCs for initiating primary T cell responses. First, dendritic cells are strategically located at the common sites of entry of microbes and foreign antigens and in tissues that may be colonized by microbes. Second, dendritic cells express receptors that enable them to capture microbes and respond to microbes. Third, these cells migrate preferentially to the T cell zones of lymph nodes, through which naive T lymphocytes circulate, searching for foreign antigens. Fourth, mature dendritic cells express high levels of costimulators, which are needed to activate naive T lymphocytes.

Antigens may also be transported to lymph nodes in soluble form. When lymph enters a lymph node through an afferent lymphatic vessel, it percolates through the node. Here, the lymph-borne soluble antigens can be extracted from the fluid by resident dendritic cells and macrophages. B cells in the node may also recognize and internalize soluble antigens. Dendritic cells, macrophages, and B cells that have taken up protein antigens can then process and present these antigens to naive T cells and to effector T cells that have been generated by previous antigen stimulation. Thus, APC populations in lymph nodes accumulate and concentrate antigens and display them in a form that can be recognized by antigen-specific CD4$^+$ T lymphocytes.

The collection and concentration of foreign antigens in lymph nodes are supplemented by two other anatomic adaptations that serve similar functions. First, the mucosal surfaces of the gastrointestinal and respiratory systems, in addition to being drained by lymphatic capillaries, contain specialized collections of secondary lymphoid tissue that can directly sample the luminal contents of these organs for the presence of antigenic material. The best characterized of these mucosal lymphoid organs are Peyer's patches of the ileum and the pharyngeal tonsils. Second, the blood stream is monitored by APCs in the spleen for any antigens that reach the circulation. Such antigens may reach the blood either directly from the tissues or by way of the lymph from the thoracic duct.

Dendritic cells can ingest infected or tumor cells and present antigens from these cells to CD8$^+$ T lymphocytes. Dendritic cells are the best APCs for inducing the primary responses of CD8$^+$ T cells, but this poses a special problem because the antigens these lymphocytes recognize may be produced in any cell type, such as a virus-infected or tumor cell. Dendritic cells have the special ability to ingest virus-infected or tumor cells and present antigens from these cells on class I MHC molecules. This pathway of antigen presentation is contrary to the usual rule that antigens ingested into vesicles are displayed on class II MHC molecules, whereas class I MHC-associated peptides are derived from cytosolic proteins (discussed later). This process is called **cross-presentation**, or cross-priming, to indicate that one cell type (the dendritic cell) can present antigens from another cell (the virus-infected or tumor cell) and prime, or activate, T cells specific for these antigens. We will discuss the role of cross-presentation in the induction of CTL responses in Chapter 9.

B lymphocytes recognize soluble antigens as well as antigens displayed by dendritic cells. A specialized cell type called follicular dendritic cells, which are quite distinct from the dendritic cells mentioned earlier, present antigens to previously activated B lymphocytes in germinal centers (see Chapter 10).

Antigen Presentation to Differentiated Effector T Lymphocytes

In cell-mediated immune responses, macrophages present the antigens of phagocytosed microbes to effector T cells, which activate the macrophages to kill the microbes. This process is the central reaction of cell-mediated immunity and delayed type hypersensitivity (see Chapter 13). Circulating monocytes are able to migrate to any site of infection and inflammation, where they differentiate into macrophages and phagocytose and destroy microbes. CD4$^+$ T cells enhance the microbicidal activities of these macrophages. Most macrophages express low levels of class II MHC molecules and costimulators, and higher levels are induced by the cytokine interferon-γ (IFN-γ). This is a mechanism by which IFN-γ enhances antigen presentation and T cell activation (see Chapter 5, Fig. 5–10).

In humoral immune responses, B lymphocytes internalize soluble protein antigens and present processed peptides derived from these proteins to helper T cells. The antigen-presenting function of B cells is essential for helper T cell-dependent antibody production, a process that occurs mainly in lymphoid organs (see Chapter 10).

All nucleated cells can present class I MHC–associated peptides, derived from cytosolic protein antigens, to CD8$^+$ cytotoxic T lymphocytes because all nucleated cells express class I MHC molecules. Most foreign protein antigens that are present in the cytosol are endogenously synthesized, such as viral proteins in virus-infected cells and mutated proteins in tumor cells. All nucleated cells are susceptible to viral infections and cancer-causing mutations. Therefore, it is important that the immune system be able to recognize cytosolic antigens harbored in any cell type. Differentiated CD8$^+$ CTLs are able to recognize class I–associated peptides and to kill any antigen-expressing cell. The ubiquitous expression of class I molecules allows class I–restricted CTLs to recognize and eliminate any type of virus-infected or tumor cell. Phagocytosed microbes may also be recognized by CD8$^+$ CTLs because some of these microbes or their antigens may escape from phagocytic vesicles into the cytosol.

Vascular endothelial cells in humans express class II MHC molecules and may present antigens to blood T cells that have become adherent to the vessel wall. This may contribute to the recruitment and activation of T cells in cell-mediated immune reactions (see Chapter 13). Endothelial cells in grafts are also targets of T cells reacting against graft antigens (see Chapter 16). Various epithelial and mesenchymal cells may express class II MHC molecules in response to IFN-γ. The physiologic significance of antigen presentation by these cell populations is unclear. Because they generally do not express costimulators, it is unlikely that they play an important role in most T cell responses. Thymic epithelial cells constitutively express class II MHC molecules and play a critical role in presenting peptide-MHC complexes to maturing T cells in the thymus as part of the selection processes that shape the repertoire of T cell specificities (see Chapter 8).

Cell Biology of Antigen Processing

The pathways of antigen processing convert protein antigens derived from the extracellular space or the cytosol into peptides and load these peptides onto MHC molecules for display to T lymphocytes (Fig. 6–7). Our understanding of the cell biology of antigen processing has increased greatly since the 1980s with the discovery and characterization of the molecules and organelles that generate peptides from intact proteins and promote the assembly and peptide loading of MHC molecules.

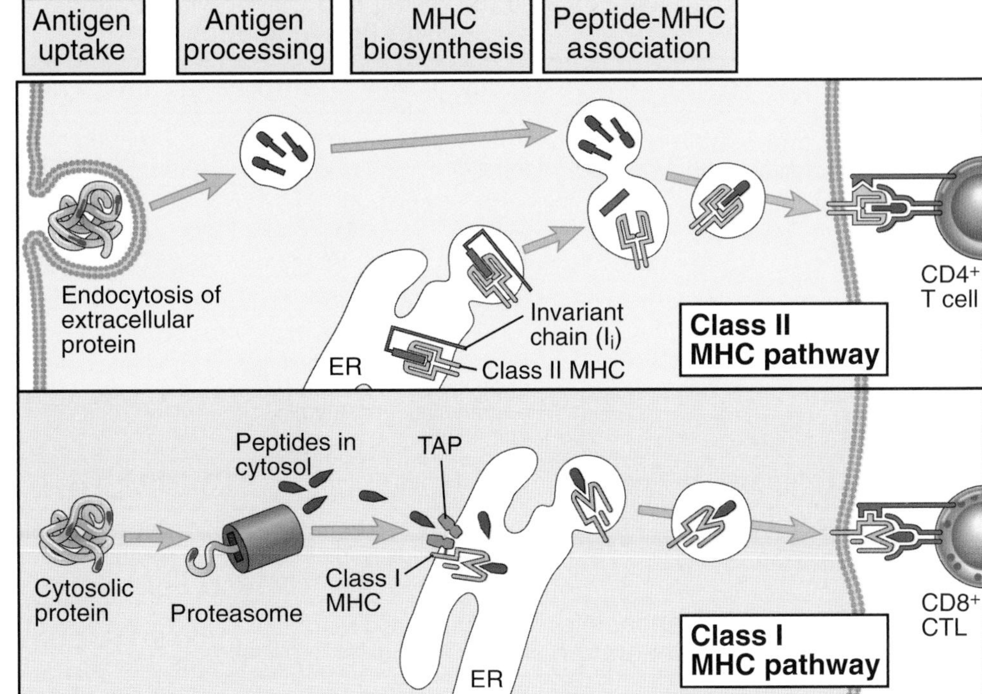

FIGURE 6–7 Pathways of antigen processing and presentation. In the class II MHC pathway *(top panel)*, extracellular protein antigens are endocytosed into vesicles, where the antigens are processed and the peptides bind to class II MHC molecules. In the class I MHC pathway *(bottom panel)*, protein antigens in the cytosol are processed by proteasomes, and peptides are transported into the ER, where they bind to class I MHC molecules. Details of these processing pathways are in Figures 6–9 and 6–13.

The pathways of antigen processing and presentation use subcellular organelles and enzymes that have generalized protein degradation and recycling functions that are not exclusively used for antigen display to the immune system. In other words, both class I and class II MHC antigen presentation pathways have evolved as adaptations of basic cellular functions. The cellular mechanisms of antigen processing are designed to generate peptides that have the structural characteristics required for associating with MHC molecules and to place these peptides in the same cellular location as the appropriate MHC molecules with available peptide-binding clefts. Peptide binding to MHC molecules occurs before cell surface expression and is an integral component of the biosynthesis and assembly of MHC molecules. In fact, peptide association is required for the stable assembly and surface expression of both class I and class II MHC molecules.

Protein antigens present in acidic vesicular compartments of APCs generate class II–associated peptides, whereas antigens present in the cytosol generate class I–associated peptides. The different fates of vesicular and cytosolic antigens are due to the segregated pathways of biosynthesis and assembly of class I and class II MHC molecules (see Fig. 6–7 and Table 6–3).

- This fundamental difference between vesicular and cytosolic antigens has been demonstrated experimentally by analyzing the presentation of the same antigen introduced into APCs in different ways (Fig. 6–8). If a globular protein is added in soluble form to APCs and endocytosed into the vesicles of the APCs, it is subsequently presented as class II–associated peptides and is recognized by antigen-specific CD4⁺ T cells. In contrast, if the same protein antigen is produced in the cytoplasm of APCs as the product of a transfected gene (modified so it cannot enter the secretory pathway), or introduced directly into the cytoplasm of the APCs by osmotic shock, it is presented in the form of class I–associated peptides that are recognized by CD8⁺ T cells.

The major comparative features of the class I and class II MHC pathways of antigen presentation are summarized in Table 6–3. In the following sections, we describe these pathways individually in more detail.

Processing of Endocytosed Antigens for Class II MHC–Associated Presentation

The generation of class II MHC-associated peptides from endocytosed antigens involves the proteolytic degradation of internalized proteins in endocytic vesicles and the binding of peptides to class II MHC molecules in these vesicles. This sequence of events is illustrated in Figure 6–9, and the individual steps are described here.

1. UPTAKE OF EXTRACELLULAR PROTEINS INTO VESICULAR COMPARTMENTS OF APCs

Most class II–associated peptides are derived from protein antigens that are captured and internalized into endosomes by specialized APCs. The initial steps in the presentation of an extracellular protein antigen are the binding of the native antigen to an APC and the internalization of the antigen. Different APCs can bind protein antigens in several ways and with varying efficiencies and specificities. Dendritic cells and macrophages express a variety of surface receptors that

Table 6–3. Comparative Features of Class II and Class I MHC Pathways of Antigen Processing and Presentation

Feature	Class II MHC Pathway	Class I MHC pathway
Composition of stable peptide-MHC complex	Polymorphic α and β chains, peptide Peptide, α, β	Polymorphic α chain, β_2-microglobulin, peptide Peptide, α, β_2-microglobulin
Types of APCs	Dendritic cells, mononuclear phagocytes, B lymphocytes; endothelial cells, thymic epithelium	All nucleated cells
Responsive T cells	$CD4^+$ T cells	$CD8^+$ T cells
Source of protein antigens	Endosomal/lysosomal proteins (mostly internalized from extracellular environment)	Cytosolic proteins (mostly synthesized in the cell; may enter cytosol from phagosomes)
Enzymes responsible for peptide generation	Endosomal and lysosomal proteases (e.g., cathepsins)	Cytosolic proteasome
Site of peptide loading of MHC	Specialized vesicular compartment	Endoplasmic reticulum
Molecules involved in transport of peptides and loading of MHC molecules	Chaperones in ER; invariant chain in ER, Golgi and MIIC/CIIV; DM	Chaperones, TAP in ER

Abbreviations: APC, antigen-presenting cell; CIIV, class II vesicle; ER, endoplasmic reticulum; MHC, major histocompatibility complex; MIIC, MHC class II compartment; TAP, transporter associated with antigen processing

recognize structures shared by many microbes (see Chapter 2). Thus, these APCs bind and internalize microbes efficiently. Macrophages also express receptors for the Fc portions of antibodies and receptors for the complement protein C3b, which bind antigens with attached antibodies or complement proteins and enhance their internalization. Another example of specific receptors on APCs is the surface immunoglobulin on B cells, which, because of its high affinity for antigens, can effectively mediate the internalization of proteins present at very low concentrations in the extracellular fluid (see Chapter 10).

After their internalization, protein antigens become localized in intracellular membrane-bound vesicles called **endosomes.** Endosomes are vesicles with acidic pH that contain proteolytic enzymes. The endosomal pathway of intracellular protein traffic communicates with lysosomes, which are more dense membrane-bound enzyme-containing vesicles. A subset of class II MHC-rich late endosomes plays a special role in antigen processing and presentation by the class II pathway; this is described below. Particulate microbes are internalized into vesicles called **phagosomes,** which may fuse with lysosomes, producing vesicles called phagolysosomes or secondary lysosomes. Some microbes, such as mycobacteria and *Leishmania,* may survive and even replicate within phagosomes or endosomes, providing a persistent source of antigens in vesicular compartments.

2. PROCESSING OF INTERNALIZED PROTEINS IN ENDOSOMAL AND LYSOSOMAL VESICLES

Internalized proteins are degraded enzymatically in late endosomes and lysosomes to generate peptides that are able to bind to the peptide-binding clefts of class II MHC molecules. The degradation of protein antigens in vesicles is an active process mediated by proteases that have acidic pH optima.

- The processing of soluble proteins by macrophages (and other APCs) is inhibited by rendering the APCs metabolically inert by chemical fixation or by increasing the pH of intracellular acid vesicles with agents such as chloroquine (Fig. 6–10B).
- Several types of proteases are present in endosomes and lysosomes, and specific inhibitors of these enzymes block the presentation of protein antigens by APCs.

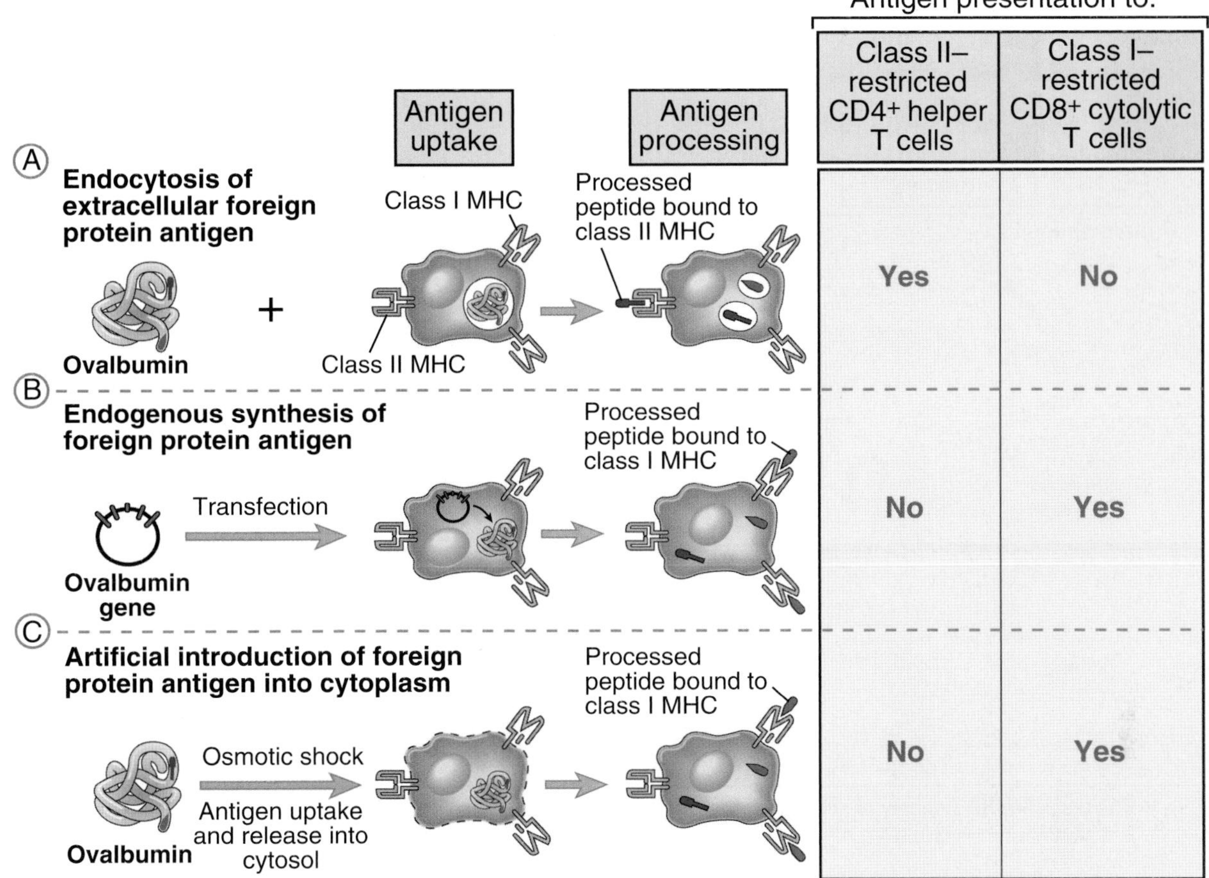

FIGURE 6–8 Presentation of extracellular and cytosolic antigens. When a model protein ovalbumin is added as an extracellular antigen to an antigen-presenting cell that expresses both class I and class II MHC molecules, ovalbumin-derived peptides are presented only in association with class II molecules (A). When ovalbumin is synthesized intracellularly as a result of transfection of its gene modified to lack the N-terminal signal sequences (B), or when it is introduced into the cytoplasm through membranes made leaky by osmotic shock (C), ovalbumin-derived peptides are presented in association with class I MHC molecules. The measured response of class II–restricted helper T cells is cytokine secretion, and the measured response of class I–restricted CTLs is killing of the antigen-presenting cells.

- The processed forms of most protein antigens that T cells recognize can be artificially generated by proteolysis in the test tube. APCs that are chemically fixed or treated with chloroquine before they have processed a protein antigen can effectively present predigested peptide fragments of that antigen, but not the intact protein, to specific T cells (Fig. 6–10C).

Many different enzymes may participate in the degradation of protein antigens in the endosomes. The most abundant proteases of endosomes are cathepsins, which are thiol and aspartyl proteases with broad substrate specificities. Cathepsins may play an important role in generating peptides for the class II pathway. Partially degraded or cleaved proteins bind to the open-ended clefts of class II MHC molecules and are then trimmed enzymatically to their final size.

Most class II MHC-binding peptides are derived from proteins internalized from the extracellular milieu and proteins from the secretory compartment that are normally degraded in lysosomes. Less often, cytoplasmic and membrane proteins may also enter the class II pathway. In some cases, this may result from the enzymatic digestion of cytoplasmic contents, referred to as autophagy. In this pathway, cytoplasmic proteins are trapped within endoplasmic reticulum (ER)-derived vesicles called autophagosomes; these vesicles fuse with lysosomes, and the cytoplasmic proteins are proteolytically degraded. The peptides generated by this route may be delivered to the same class II–bearing vesicular compartment as are peptides derived from extracellular and ingested antigens. Some peptides that associate with class II molecules are derived from membrane proteins, which may be recycled into the same endocytic pathway as extracellular proteins. Thus, even viruses, which replicate in the cytoplasm of infected cells, may produce cytoplasmic and membrane proteins that are degraded into peptides that enter the class II MHC pathway of antigen presentation. This may be a mechanism for the activation of viral antigen-specific $CD4^+$ helper T cells.

3. BIOSYNTHESIS AND TRANSPORT OF CLASS II MHC MOLECULES TO ENDOSOMES

Class II MHC molecules are synthesized in the ER and transported to endosomes with an associated protein called the invariant chain (I_i), which occupies the peptide-binding clefts of the newly synthesized class II molecules. The α and β chains of class II MHC molecules are coordinately synthesized and associate with each other in the ER. Nascent class II dimers are structurally unstable, and their folding and assembly are aided by

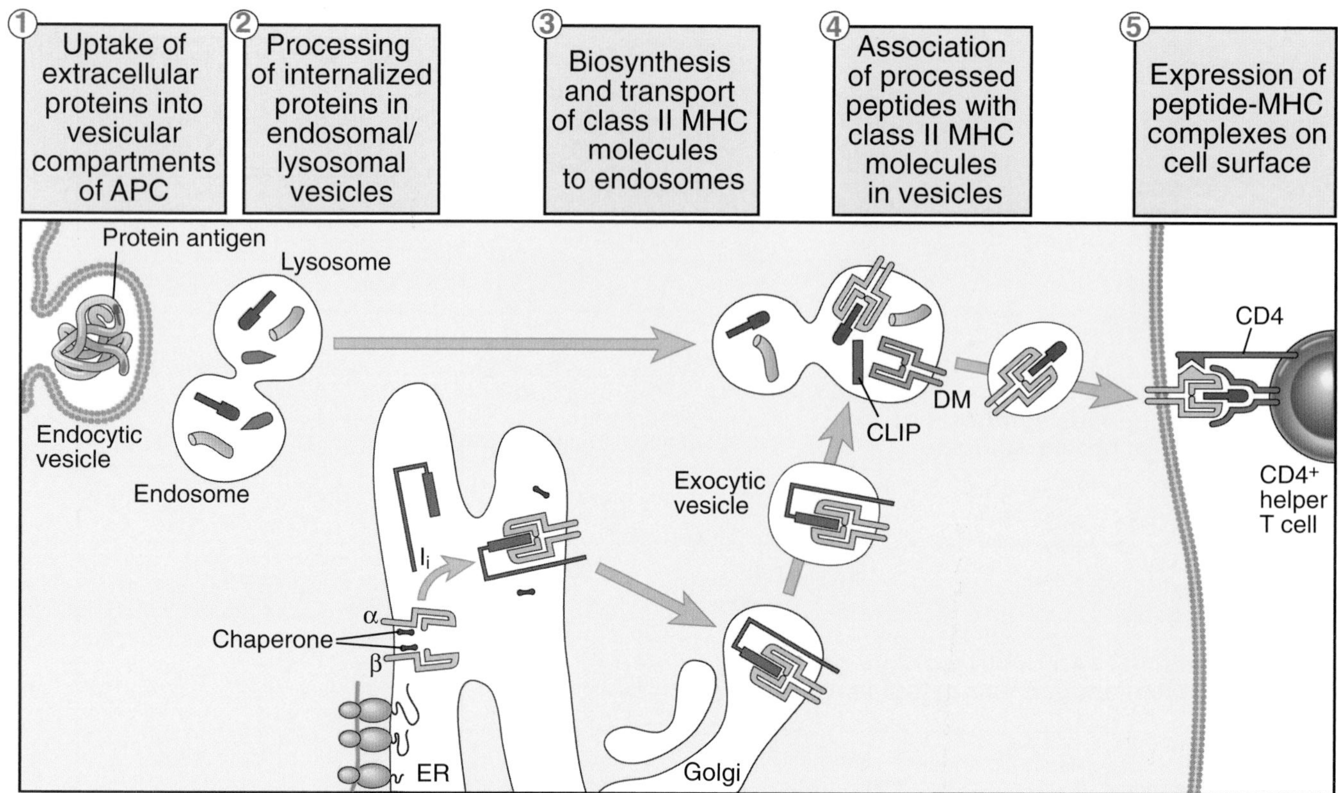

FIGURE 6–9 The class II MHC pathway of antigen presentation. The numbered stages in processing of extracellular antigens correspond to the stages described in the text. APC, antigen-presenting cell.

ER-resident chaperones, such as calnexin. The nonpolymorphic I_i also associates with the class II MHC αβ heterodimers in the ER. The I_i is a trimer composed of three 30-kD subunits, each of which binds one newly synthesized class II αβ heterodimer in a way that interferes with peptide loading of the cleft formed by the α and β chains (Fig. 6–11). As a result, class II MHC molecules cannot bind and present peptides they encounter in the ER, leaving such peptides to associate with class I molecules. The I_i also promotes folding and assembly of class II molecules and directs newly formed class II molecules to the late endosomes and lysosomes where internalized proteins have been proteolytically degraded into peptides. Unlike vesicles containing proteins destined for secretion or for the cell surface, vesicles containing class II MHC molecules emerge from the Golgi complex and are targeted to late endosomes and lysosomes. During their passage toward the cell surface, the exocytic vesicles transporting class II molecules out of the ER meet and fuse with the endocytic vesicles containing internalized and processed antigens. The net result of this sequence of events is that class II molecules enter the vesicles that also contain peptides generated by proteolysis of endocytosed proteins.

Immunoelectron microscopy and subcellular fractionation studies have defined a class II–rich subset of late endosomes that plays an important role in antigen presentation (Fig. 6–12). In macrophages and human B cells, it is called the MHC class II compartment, or MIIC. (In some mouse B cells, a similar organelle containing class II molecules has been identified and named the class II vesicle.) The MIIC has a characteristic multilamellar appearance by electron microscopy. Importantly, it contains all the components required for peptide–class II association, including the enzymes that degrade protein antigens, the class II molecules, the I_i (or invariant chain–derived peptides), and a molecule called human leukocyte antigen DM (HLA-DM), whose function is described below.

APCs from knockout mice lacking the I_i show defective presentation of some protein antigens but are still able to present class II–associated peptides derived from a wide variety of proteins. This result suggests that the importance of the I_i may vary according to the antigen being presented.

4. ASSOCIATION OF PROCESSED PEPTIDES WITH CLASS II MHC MOLECULES IN VESICLES

Within the MIIC, the I_i dissociates from class II MHC molecules by the combined action of proteolytic enzymes and the HLA-DM molecule, and antigenic peptides are then able to bind to the available peptide-binding clefts of the class II molecules (see Fig. 6–11). Because the I_i blocks access to the peptide-binding cleft of a class II MHC molecule, it must be removed before complexes of peptide and class II molecules can form. The same proteolytic enzymes, such as cathepsin S, that generate peptides from internalized proteins also act on the I_i, degrading it and leaving only a 24-amino acid remnant called class II–associated invariant chain peptide (CLIP).

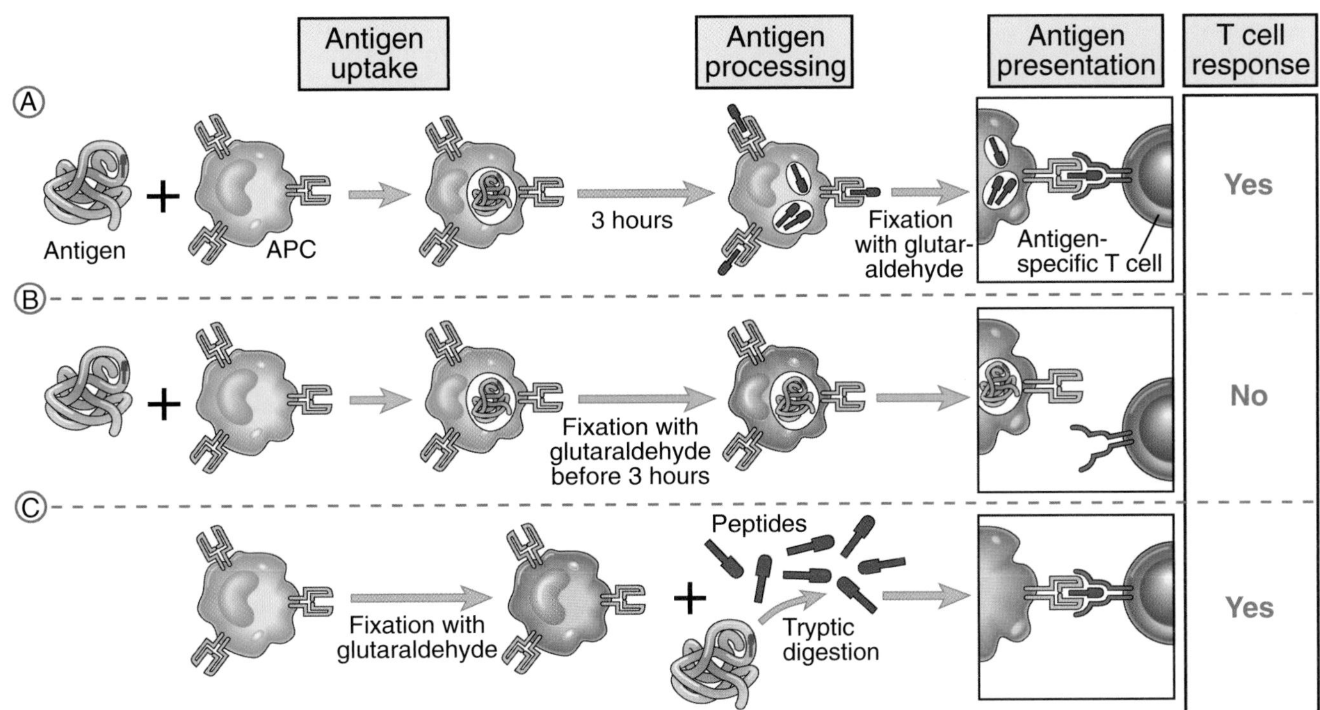

FIGURE 6–10 Antigen processing requires time and cellular metabolism and can be mimicked by *in vitro* proteolysis. If an antigen-presenting cell (APC) is allowed to process antigen and is then chemically fixed (rendered metabolically inert) 3 hours or more after antigen internalization, it is capable of presenting antigen to T cells (A). Antigen is not presented if APCs are fixed less than 3 hours after antigen uptake, implying that for this antigen and APC population, the minimum time needed for processing of the antigen is 3 hours (B). Fixed APCs bind and present proteolytic fragments of antigens to specific T cells (C). The artificial proteolysis therefore mimics physiologic antigen processing by APCs. Effective antigen presentation is assayed by measuring a T cell response, such as cytokine secretion. (Note that this type of experiment is done with populations of antigen-specific T cells, such as T cell hybridomas, which respond to processed antigens on fixed APCs, but that normal T cells require costimulators that may be destroyed by fixation. Also, the time required for antigen processing is 3 hours in this experiment, but it may be different with other antigens and APCs.)

X-ray crystallographic analysis has shown that CLIP sits in the peptide-binding cleft in the same way that other peptides bind to class II MHC molecules. Therefore, removal of CLIP is required before the cleft becomes accessible to peptides produced from extracellular proteins. This is accomplished by the action of a molecule called HLA-DM (or H-2M in the mouse), which is encoded within the MHC, has a structure similar to that of class II MHC molecules, and colocalizes with class II molecules in the MIIC compartment. HLA-DM molecules differ from class II MHC molecules in several respects: they are not polymorphic, they do not associ-

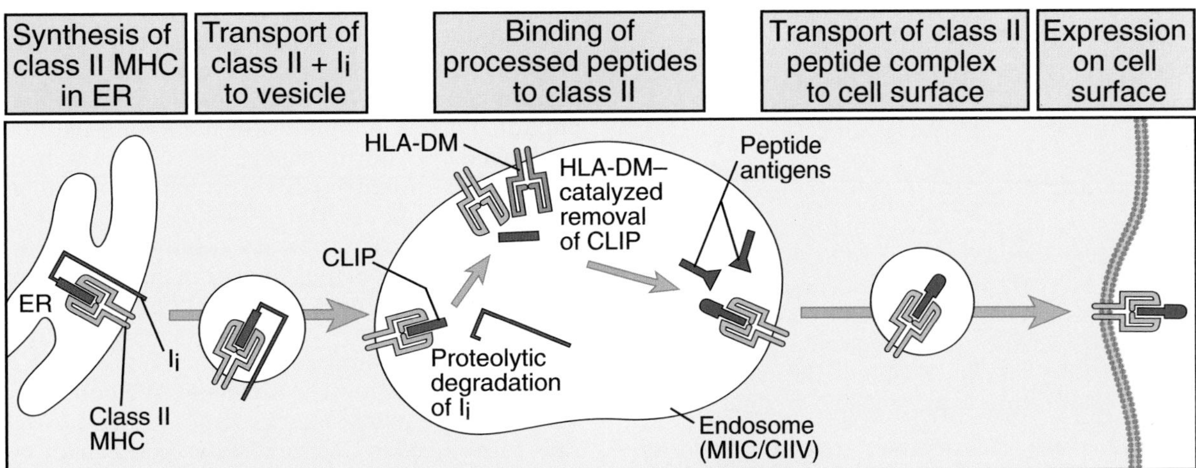

FIGURE 6–11 The functions of class II MHC-associated invariant chains and HLA-DM. Class II molecules with bound invariant chain, or CLIP, are transported into vesicles, where the CLIP is removed by the action of DM. Antigenic peptides generated in the vesicles are then able to bind to the class II molecules. Another class II–like protein, called HLA-DO, may regulate the DM-catalyzed removal of CLIP. CIIV, class II vesicle.

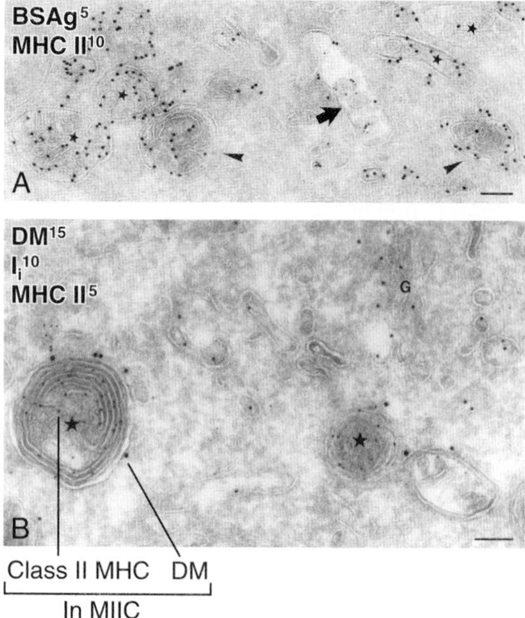

FIGURE 6–12 Morphology of class II MHC–rich endosomal vesicles. A. Immunoelectron micrograph of a B lymphocyte that has internalized bovine serum albumin into early endosomes (labeled with 5-nm gold particles, *arrow*) and contains class II MHC molecules (labeled with 10-nm gold particles) in MIICs *(arrowheads)*. The internalized albumin will reach the MIICs ultimately. (From Kleijmeer MJ, S Morkowski, JM Griffith, AY Rudensky, and HJ Geuze. Major histocompatibility complex class II compartments in human and mouse B lymphoblasts represent conventional endocytic compartments. Reproduced from The Journal of Cell Biology 139:639–649, 1997, by copyright permission of The Rockefeller University Press.) B. Immunoelectron micrograph of a B cell showing location of class II MHC molecules and DM in MIICs *(stars)* and invariant chain concentrated in the Golgi (G) complex. In this example, there is virtually no invariant chain detected in the MIIC, presumably because it has been cleaved to generate CLIP. (Courtesy of Drs. H. J. Geuze and M. Kleijmeer, Department of Cell Biology, Utrecht University, The Netherlands.)

ate with the I_i, and they are not expressed on the cell surface. HLA-DM acts as a peptide exchanger, facilitating the removal of CLIP and the addition of other peptides to class II MHC molecules.

- The critical role of HLA-DM is demonstrated by the finding that mutant cell lines that lack DM, and knockout mice that lack the homologous mouse protein H-2M, are defective in presenting peptides derived from extracellular proteins. When class II MHC molecules are isolated from these DM-mutant cell lines or from APCs from H-2M knockout mice, they are found to have CLIP almost exclusively occupying their peptide-binding clefts, consistent with a role for DM in removing CLIP. Transfection of the gene encoding DM into these mutant cell lines restores normal class II–associated antigen presentation.

Once CLIP is removed, peptides generated by proteolysis of internalized protein antigens are able to bind to class II MHC molecules. The HLA-DM molecule may accelerate the rate of peptide binding to class II molecules. Because the ends of the class II MHC peptide-binding cleft are open, large peptides or even unfolded whole proteins may bind and are then "trimmed" by proteolytic enzymes to the appropriate size for T cell recognition. As a result, the size of peptides eluted from cell surface class II MHC molecules is usually restricted to 10 to 30 amino acids. The peptides that are displayed by class II MHC molecules are mostly generated by this trimming step.

B lymphocytes, and perhaps other APCs, express another nonpolymorphic class II–like heterodimer called HLA-DO. Much of the DO in the cell is found in association with DM, suggesting that the DO molecule may regulate the efficiency of antigen presentation or the types of peptides that are generated in B cells. However, DO is not required for antigen processing, and its function remains poorly defined.

5. EXPRESSION OF PEPTIDE–CLASS II COMPLEXES ON THE APC SURFACE

Class II MHC molecules are stabilized by the bound peptides, and the stable peptide–class II complexes are delivered to the surface of the APC, where they are displayed for recognition by CD4⁺ T cells. The requirement for bound peptide to stabilize class II MHC molecules ensures that only properly loaded peptide–MHC complexes will survive long enough to get displayed on the cell surface. A similar phenomenon occurs in class I MHC assembly. Once expressed on the APC surface, the peptide–class II complexes are recognized by specific $CD4^+$ T cells, with the CD4 coreceptor playing an essential role by binding to nonpolymorphic regions of the class II molecule. The slow off-rate and therefore long half-life of peptide-MHC complexes increase the chance that a T cell specific for such a complex will make contact, bind, and be activated by that complex. Interestingly, while peptide-loaded class II molecules traffic from the late endosomes and lysosomes to the cell surface, other molecules involved in antigen presentation, such as DM, stay in the vesicles and are not expressed as membrane proteins. The mechanism of this selective traffic is unknown.

Very small numbers of peptide-MHC complexes are capable of activating specific T lymphocytes. Because APCs continuously present peptides derived from all the proteins they encounter, only a very small fraction of cell surface peptide-MHC complexes will contain the same peptide. Furthermore, most of the bound peptides will be derived from normal self proteins because there is no mechanism to distinguish self proteins from foreign proteins in the process that generates the peptide–MHC complexes. This is borne out by studies in which class II MHC molecules are purified from APCs from normal individuals and the bound peptides are eluted and sequenced; it is seen that most of these peptides are derived from self proteins.

The finding that MHC molecules are constantly displaying self peptides raises two important questions that were introduced in Chapter 5. First, how can a T cell recognize and be activated by any foreign antigen if normally all APCs are displaying mainly self peptide–MHC complexes? The answer is that T cells are remarkably sensitive and need to specifically recognize very few peptide-MHC complexes to be activated. It has been estimated that as few as 100 complexes of a particular peptide with a class II MHC molecule on the surface of an APC can initiate a specific T cell response. This represents less than 0.1% of the total number of class II molecules likely to be present on the surface of the APC. Thus, a newly introduced antigen may be processed into peptides that load enough MHC molecules of APCs to activate T cells specific for that antigen, even though most of the MHC molecules are occupied with self peptides. In fact, the ability of APCs to internalize, process, and present the heterogeneous mix of self proteins and foreign proteins ensures that the immune system will not miss transient or quantitatively small exposures to foreign antigens. Antigen recognition by a T cell may also trigger redistribution of MHC molecules on the APC toward the T cell, thus setting up a positive feedback loop that promotes recognition of the antigen.

Second, if individuals process their own proteins and present them in association with their own class II MHC molecules, why do we normally not develop immune responses against self proteins? The answer is that self peptide–MHC complexes are formed but do not induce autoimmunity because T cells specific for such complexes are killed or inactivated. Therefore, T cells cannot normally respond to self antigens (see Chapter 11).

Processing of Cytosolic Antigens for Class I MHC–Associated Presentation

Class I MHC-associated peptides are produced by the proteolytic degradation of cytosolic proteins, the transport of the generated peptides into the ER, and their binding to newly synthesized class I molecules. This sequence of events is illustrated in Figure 6–13, and the individual steps are described next.

1. SOURCES OF CYTOSOLIC ANTIGENS

The peptides that are presented bound to class I MHC molecules are derived from cytosolic proteins, most of which are endogenously synthesized in nucleated cells. Foreign antigens in the cytosol may be the products of viruses or other intracellular microbes that infect such cells. In tumor cells, various mutated or overexpressed genes may produce protein antigens that are recognized by class I–restricted CTLs (see Chapter 17). Peptides that are presented in association with class I molecules may also be derived from microbes and other particulate antigens that are internalized into phagosomes. Some microbes are able to damage phagosome membranes and create pores through which the microbes and their antigens enter the cytosol. For instance, pathogenic strains of *Listeria monocytogenes* produce a protein, called listeriolysin, which enables bacteria to escape from vesicles into the cytosol. (This escape is a mechanism that the bacteria have evolved to resist killing by the microbicidal mechanisms of phagocytes, most of which are limited to phagolysosomes.) Once the antigens of the phagocytosed microbes are in the cytosol, they are processed like other cytosolic antigens.

2. PROTEOLYTIC DEGRADATION OF CYTOSOLIC PROTEINS

The major mechanism for the generation of peptides from cytosolic protein antigens is proteolysis by the proteasome. The proteasome is a large multiprotein enzyme complex with a broad range of proteolytic activity that is found in the cytoplasm of most cells. A 700-kD form of

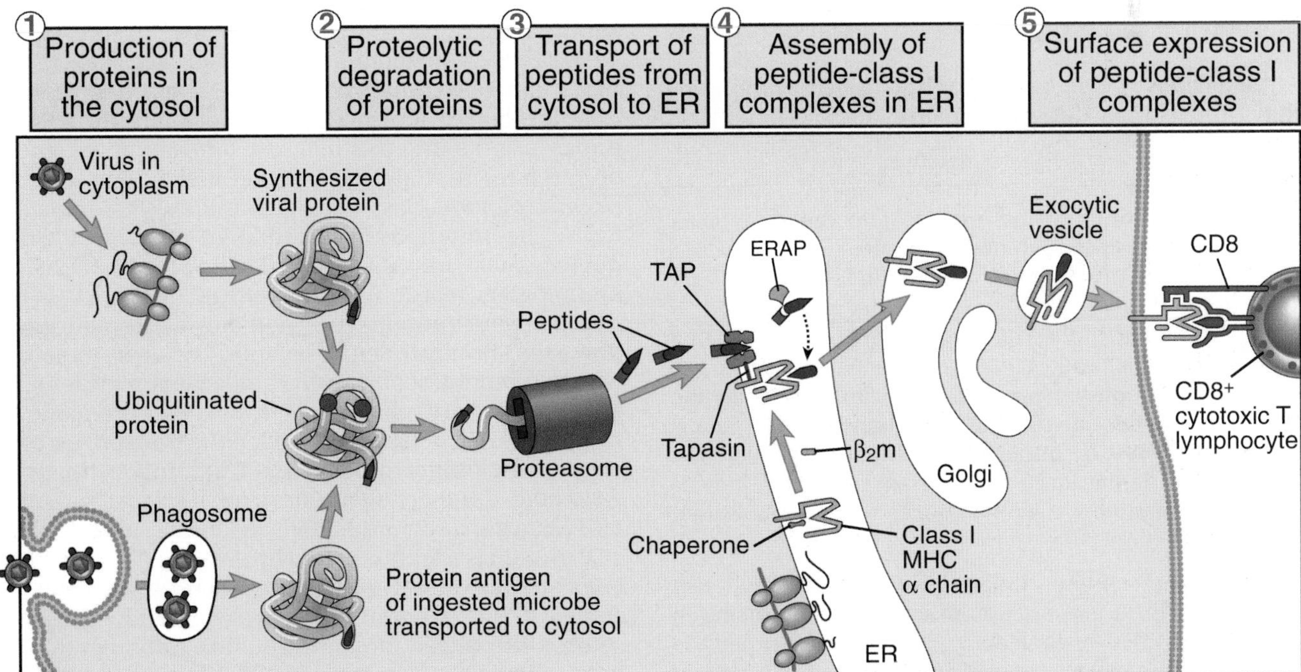

FIGURE 6–13 The class I MHC pathway of antigen presentation. The numbered stages in the processing of cytosolic proteins correspond to the stages described in the text. β_2m, β_2-microglobulin.

proteasome appears as a cylinder composed of a stacked array of two inner and two outer rings, each ring being composed of seven subunits. Three of the seven subunits are the catalytic sites for proteolysis. A larger, 1500-kD proteasome is likely to be most important for generating class I–binding peptides and is composed of the 700-kD structure plus several additional subunits that regulate proteolytic activity. Two catalytic subunits present in many 1500-kD proteasomes, called LMP-2 and LMP-7, are encoded by genes in the MHC, and are particularly important for generating class I–binding peptides.

The proteasome performs a basic housekeeping function in cells by degrading many damaged or improperly folded proteins. These proteins are targeted for proteasomal degradation by covalent linkage of several copies of a small polypeptide called ubiquitin. Ubiquitinated proteins are recognized by the proteasomal cap, and are then unfolded, the ubiquitin is removed, and the proteins are "threaded" through proteasomes. The proteasome has broad substrate specificity and can generate a wide variety of peptides from cytosolic proteins (but usually does not degrade proteins completely into single amino acids). Interestingly, in cells treated with the cytokine IFN-γ, there is increased transcription and synthesis of LMP-2 and LMP-7, and these proteins replace two of the subunits of the proteasome. This results in a change in the substrate specificity of the proteasome so that the peptides produced are 6 to 30 residues long and usually contain carboxy-terminal basic or hydrophobic amino acids. Both features are typical of peptides that are transported into the class I pathway and that bind to class I molecules (often after further trimming). This is one mechanism by which IFN-γ enhances antigen presentation, another mechanism being increased expression of MHC molecules (see Fig. 5–10, Chapter 5). Thus, proteasomes are excellent examples of organelles whose basic cellular function has been adapted for a specialized role in antigen presentation.

Many lines of evidence have conclusively established that proteasomal degradation of cytosolic proteins is required for entry into the class I antigen-processing pathway.

- Specific inhibitors of proteasomal function block presentation of a cytoplasmic protein to class I MHC-restricted T cells specific for a peptide epitope of that protein. However, if the peptide that is recognized by the CTLs is synthesized directly in the cytoplasm of a cell as the product of a transfected minigene, the peptide is presented and the cell can be killed by the CTLs. In this situation, presentation of the peptide is not blocked by inhibitors of proteasomal enzymes, indicating that once antigens are converted to cytosolic peptides, they no longer need proteasomal degradation.
- In some cell lines, inhibition of ubiquitination also inhibits the presentation of cytoplasmic proteins to class I MHC-restricted T cells specific for a peptide epitope of that protein. Conversely, modification of proteins by attachment of an N-terminal sequence that is recognized by ubiquitin-conjugating enzymes leads to enhanced ubiquitination and more rapid class I MHC-associated presentation of peptides derived from those proteins.
- Mice in which the genes encoding selected subunits of proteasomes (LMP-2 or LMP-7) are deleted show defects in the generation of CTLs against some viruses, presumably because of defective class I–associated presentation of viral antigens.

Thus, the proteolytic mechanisms that generate antigenic peptides that bind to class I MHC molecules are different from the mechanisms described earlier for peptide–class II MHC molecule associations. This is also evident from the observation that agents that raise endosomal and lysosomal pH, or directly inhibit endosomal proteases, block class II–restricted but not class I–restricted antigen presentation, whereas inhibitors of ubiquitination or proteasomes selectively block class I–restricted antigen presentation.

Some protein antigens apparently do not require ubiquitination or proteasomes to be presented by the class I MHC pathway. This may be because other, less well-defined mechanisms of cytoplasmic proteolysis exist. Some newly synthesized proteins are degraded in the ER. For example, the signal sequences of membrane and secreted proteins are usually cleaved by signal peptidase and degraded proteolytically soon after synthesis and translocation into the ER. This ER processing generates class I–binding peptides without a need for proteolysis in the cytosol.

3. TRANSPORT OF PEPTIDES FROM THE CYTOSOL TO THE ER

Peptides generated in the cytosol are translocated by a specialized transporter into the ER, where newly synthesized class I MHC molecules are available to bind the peptides. Because antigenic peptides for the class I pathway are generated in the cytosol, but class I MHC molecules are synthesized in the ER, a mechanism must exist for delivery of cytosolic peptides into the ER. The initial insights into this mechanism came from studies of cell lines that are defective in assembling and displaying peptide–class I MHC complexes on their surfaces. The mutations responsible for this defect turned out to involve two genes located within the MHC that are homologous to the ABC transporter family of genes, which encode proteins that mediate adenosine triphosphate (ATP)-dependent transport of low molecular weight compounds across cellular membranes. The genes in the MHC that belong to this family encode the two chains of a heterodimer called the **transporter associated with antigen processing** (TAP). (Interestingly, the *TAP1* and *TAP2* genes are next to the genes encoding LMP-2 and LMP-7 in the MHC, and the synthesis of the TAP protein is also stimulated by IFN-γ.) The TAP protein is located in the ER membrane, where it mediates the active, ATP-dependent transport of peptides from the cytosol into the ER lumen (Fig. 6–14). Although the TAP heterodimer has a broad range of specificities, it optimally transports peptides ranging from 6 to 30 amino

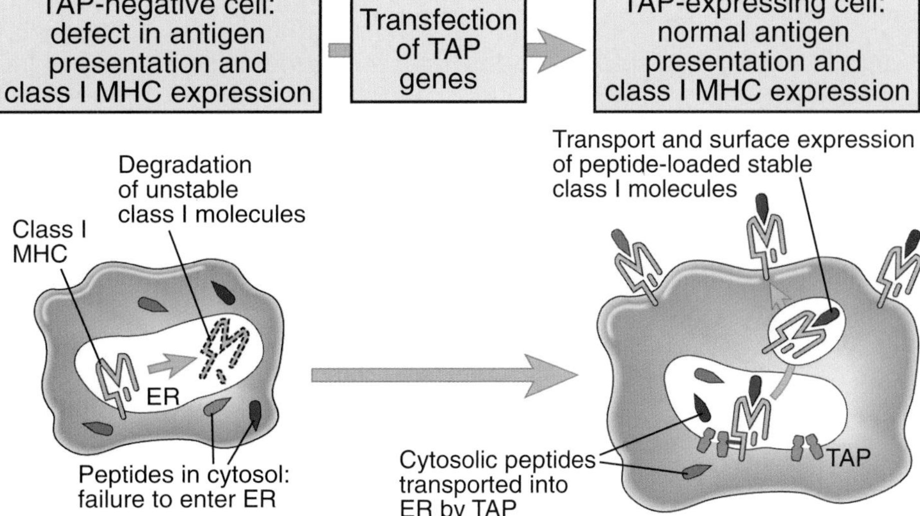

FIGURE 6–14 Role of TAP in class I MHC-associated antigen presentation. In a cell line lacking functional TAP, class I molecules are not efficiently loaded with peptides and are degraded, mostly in the ER. When a functional TAP gene is transfected into the cell line, normal assembly and expression of peptide-associated class I MHC molecules are restored. Note that the TAP dimer may be attached to class I molecules by a linker protein called tapasin, which is not shown in this and other illustrations.

acids long and containing carboxyl termini that are basic (in humans) or hydrophobic (in humans and mice). As mentioned before, these are the properties of peptides that are generated in the proteasome and are able to bind to MHC molecules.

- TAP-deficient cell lines, and mice in which the *TAP1* gene is deleted, show defects in class I MHC surface expression and cannot effectively present class I–associated antigens to T cells. The class I MHC molecules that do get expressed on the surface of TAP-deficient cells have bound peptides that are mostly derived from signal sequences of proteins destined for secretion or membrane expression. As mentioned before, these signal sequences may be degraded to peptides within the ER, without a requirement for TAP.
- Rare examples of human *TAP1* and *TAP2* gene mutations have been identified, and the patients carrying these mutant genes also show defective class I MHC-associated antigen presentation and increased susceptibility to infections with some bacteria.

On the luminal side of the ER membrane, the TAP protein is noncovalently attached to newly synthesized class I MHC molecules by a linker protein called tapasin. Thus, the class I molecule is strategically located at the site where it can receive peptides.

4. ASSEMBLY OF PEPTIDE–CLASS I MHC COMPLEXES IN THE ER

Peptides translocated into the ER bind to class I MHC molecules that are attached to the TAP dimer. The synthesis and assembly of class I molecules involve a multistep process in which peptide binding plays a key role. Class I α chains and β_2-microglobulin are synthesized in the ER. Appropriate folding of the nascent α chains is assisted by various ER chaperone proteins, such as calnexin and calreticulin. Within the ER, the newly formed "empty" class I dimers remain attached to the TAP complex by tapasin. After a peptide enters the ER via TAP, it is often trimmed to the appropriate size for MHC binding by the ER-resident aminopeptidase, ERAP. The peptide is then able to bind to the cleft of the adjacent class I molecule, after which the peptide–class I complex is released from tapasin, and it is able to exit the ER and be transported to the cell surface. In the absence of bound peptide, many of the newly formed α chain–β_2-microglobulin dimers are unstable, cannot be transported out of the ER efficiently, and are presumably degraded in the ER (see Fig. 6–14).

Peptides transported into the ER preferentially bind to class I, but not class II, MHC molecules, for two reasons. First, newly synthesized class I molecules are attached to the luminal aspect of the TAP complex, ready to receive peptides. Second, as mentioned previously, in the ER the peptide-binding clefts of newly synthesized class II molecules are blocked by the associated I_i.

5. SURFACE EXPRESSION OF PEPTIDE–CLASS I MHC COMPLEXES

Class I MHC molecules with bound peptides are structurally stable and are expressed on the cell surface. Stable peptide–class I MHC complexes that were produced in the ER move through the Golgi complex and are transported to the cell surface by exocytic vesicles. Once expressed on the cell surface, the peptide–class I complexes may be recognized by peptide antigen-specific $CD8^+$ T cells, with the CD8 coreceptor playing an essential role by binding to nonpolymorphic regions of the class I molecule. In later chapters, we will return to a discussion of the role of class I–restricted CTLs in protective immunity. Several viruses have evolved mechanisms that interfere with class I assembly and peptide loading, emphasizing the importance of this pathway for antiviral immunity (see Chapter 15).

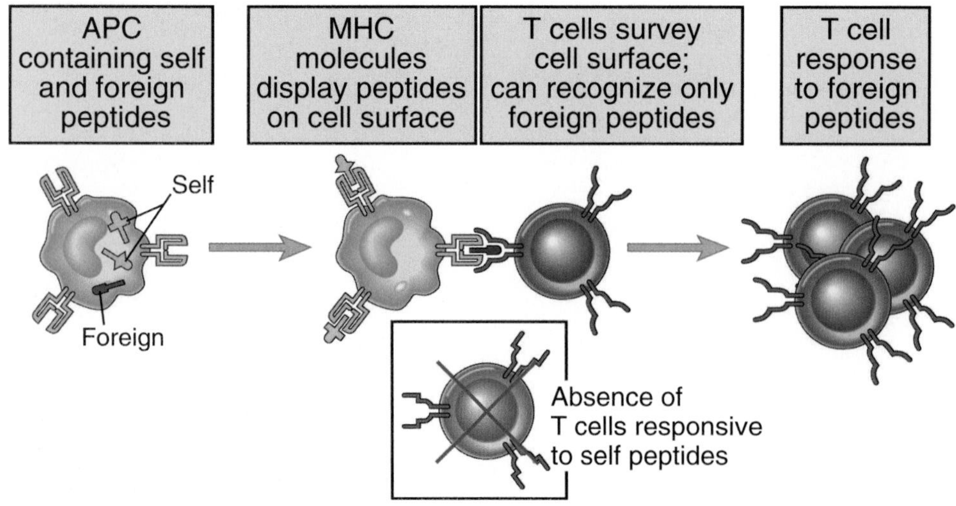

FIGURE 6–15 T cells survey antigen-presenting cells (APCs) for foreign peptides. APCs present self peptides and foreign peptides associated with MHC molecules, and T cells respond to the foreign peptides. In response to infections, APCs also express costimulators (not shown) that activate T cells specific for the microbial antigens. The figure shows that T cells specific for self antigens are not present; some self-reactive T cells may be present, but these are incapable of responding to the self antigens (see Chapter 11).

PHYSIOLOGIC SIGNIFICANCE OF MHC-ASSOCIATED ANTIGEN PRESENTATION

So far, we have discussed the specificity of $CD4^+$ and $CD8^+$ T lymphocytes for MHC-associated foreign protein antigens and the mechanisms by which complexes of peptides and MHC molecules are produced. In this section, we consider the importance of MHC-associated antigen presentation in the role that T cells play in protective immunity, the nature of T cell responses to different antigens, and the types of antigens that T cells recognize.

T Cell Surveillance for Foreign Antigens

The class I and class II pathways of antigen presentation sample available proteins for display to T cells. Most of these proteins are self proteins. Foreign proteins are relatively rare; these may be derived from infectious microbes, other foreign antigens that are introduced into the body, and tumors. T cells survey all the displayed peptides for the presence of these rare foreign peptides and respond to the foreign antigens (Fig. 6–15). Self peptides do not stimulate T cell responses, either because T cells with receptors for these peptides were deleted during their maturation in the thymus or the cells have been rendered inactive by recognition of the self antigens (see Chapter 11). MHC molecules sample both the extracellular space and the cytosol of nucleated cells, and this is important because microbes may reside in both locations. Even though peptides derived from foreign (e.g., microbial) antigens may not be abundant, these foreign antigens are recognized by the immune system because of the exquisite sensitivity of T cells. In addition, infectious microbes stimulate the expression of costimulators on APCs that enhance T cell responses, thus ensuring that T cells will be activated when microbes are present.

Nature of T Cell Responses

The expression and functions of MHC molecules determine how T cells respond to different types of antigens and mediate their effector functions.

- ***The presentation of vesicular versus cytosolic proteins by the class II or class I MHC pathways, respectively, determines which subsets of T cells will respond to antigens found in these two pools of proteins*** (Fig. 6–16). Extracellular antigens usually end up in endosomal vesicles and activate class II–restricted $CD4^+$ T cells because vesicular proteins are processed into class II–binding peptides. $CD4^+$ T cells function as helpers to stimulate effector mechanisms, such as antibodies and phagocytes, which serve to eliminate extracellular antigens. Conversely, endogenously synthesized antigens are present in the cytoplasmic pool of proteins, where they are inaccessible to antibodies and phagocytes. These cytosolic antigens enter the pathway for loading class I molecules and activate class I–restricted $CD8^+$ CTLs, which kill the cells producing the intracellular antigens. The expression of class I molecules in all nucleated cells ensures that peptides from virtually any intracellular protein may be displayed for recognition by $CD8^+$ T cells. Thus, antigens from microbes that reside in different cellular locations selectively stimulate the T cell responses that are most effective at eliminating that type of microbe. This is especially important because the antigen receptors of helper T cells and CTLs cannot distinguish between extracellular and intracellular microbes. By segregating peptides derived from these types of microbes, the MHC molecules guide these subsets of T cells to respond to the microbes that each subset can best combat.
- ***The unique specificity of T cells for cell-bound antigens is essential for the functions of T lymphocytes, which are largely mediated by interactions requiring***

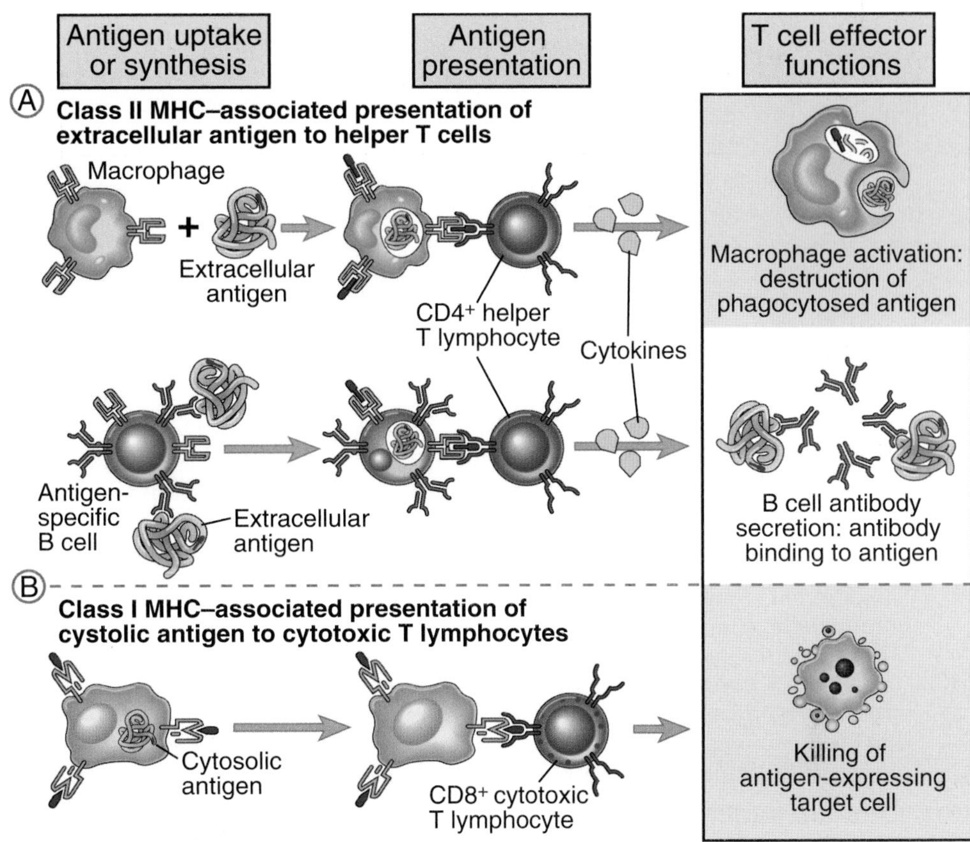

FIGURE 6–16 Presentation of extracellular and cytosolic antigens to different subsets of T cells. A. Extracellular antigens are presented by macrophages or B lymphocytes to CD4+ helper T lymphocytes, which activate the macrophages or B cells and eliminate the extracellular antigens. B. Cytosolic antigens are presented by nucleated cells to CD8+ CTLs, which kill (lyse) the antigen-expressing cells.

direct cell-cell contact and by cytokines that act at short distances. APCs not only present antigens to T lymphocytes but also are the targets of T cell effector functions (see Fig. 6–16). For instance, macrophages with phagocytosed microbes present microbial antigens to CD4+ T cells, and the T cells respond by activating the macrophages to destroy the microbes. B lymphocytes that have specifically bound and endocytosed a protein antigen present peptides derived from that antigen to helper T cells, and the T cells then stimulate the B lymphocytes to produce antibodies against the protein. B lymphocytes and macrophages are two of the principal cell types that express class II MHC genes, function as APCs for CD4+ helper T cells, and focus helper T cell effects to their immediate vicinity. Similarly, the presentation of class I–associated peptides allows CD8+ CTLs to detect and respond to antigens produced in any nucleated cell and to destroy these cells. We will return to a fuller discussion of these interactions of T cells with APCs when we discuss the effector functions of T cells in later chapters.

Immunogenicity of Protein Antigens

MHC molecules determine the immunogenicity of protein antigens in two related ways.

- The epitopes of complex proteins that elicit the strongest T cell responses are the peptides that are generated by proteolysis in APCs and bind most avidly to MHC molecules. If an individual is immunized with a multideterminant protein antigen, in many instances the majority of the responding T cells are specific for one or a few linear amino acid sequences of the antigen. These are called the **immunodominant epitopes** or determinants. The proteases involved in antigen processing produce a variety of peptides from natural proteins, and only some of these peptides possess the characteristics that enable them to bind to the MHC molecules present in each individual (Fig. 6–17).

  - In H-2^k mice immunized with the antigen hen egg lysozyme (HEL), a large proportion of the HEL-specific T cells are specific for one epitope formed by residues 52 to 62 of HEL in association with the I-A^k class II molecule. This is because the HEL(52–62) peptide binds to I-A^k better than do other HEL peptides. *In vitro*, if I-A^k–expressing APCs are incubated with HEL, up to 20% of the I-A^k molecules may get loaded with this one peptide. Thus, the HEL(52–62) peptide is the immunodominant epitope of HEL in H-2^k mice. This approach has been used to identify immunodominant epitopes of many other protein antigens. In inbred mice infected with a virus, such as the lymphocytic choriomeningitis virus, the virus-specific T cells that are activated may be specific for as few as two or three viral peptides recognized in association with one of the inherited class I alleles.

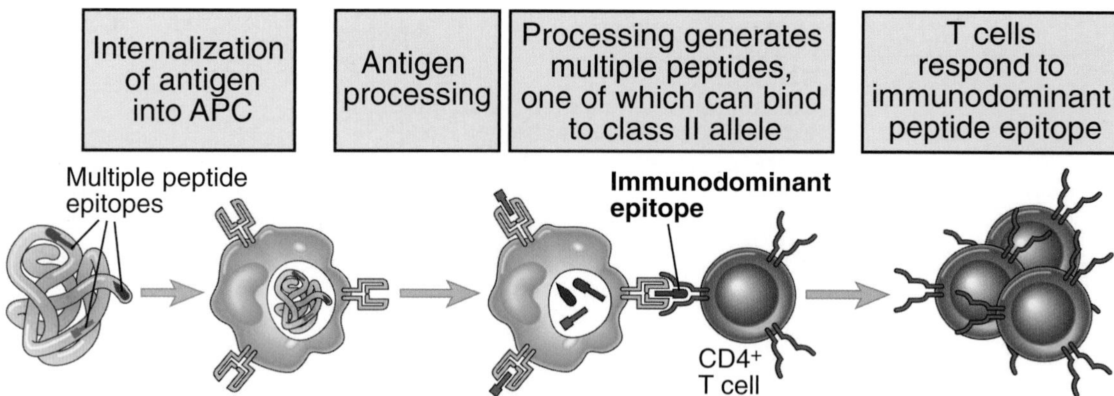

FIGURE 6–17 Immunodominance of peptides. Protein antigens are processed to generate multiple peptides; immunodominant peptides are the ones that bind best to the available class I and class II MHC molecules. The illustration shows an extracellular antigen generating a class II–binding peptide, but this also applies to peptides of cytosolic antigens that are presented by class I MHC molecules. APC, antigen-presenting cell.

Similarly, in humans infected with the human immunodeficiency virus, individual patients contain T cells that recognize a small number of viral epitopes. This phenomenon has been seen with many viruses and intracellular bacteria. These results imply that even complex microbes produce very few peptides capable of binding to any one allelic MHC molecule.

It is important to define the structural basis of immunodominance because this may permit the efficient manipulation of the immune system with synthetic peptides. An application of such knowledge is the design of vaccines. For example, a viral protein could be analyzed for the presence of amino acid sequences that would form typical immunodominant epitopes capable of binding to MHC molecules with high affinity. Synthetic peptides containing these epitopes may be effective vaccines for eliciting T cell responses against the viral peptide expressed on an infected cell. Conversely, some individuals do not respond to vaccines (such as hepatitis B virus surface antigen vaccine) presumably because their HLA molecules cannot bind and display the major peptides of the antigen.

- The expression of particular class II MHC alleles in an individual determines the ability of that individual to respond to particular antigens. The phenomenon of genetically controlled immune responsiveness was introduced in Chapter 5. We now know that the immune response (Ir) genes that control antibody responses are the class II MHC structural genes. They influence immune responsiveness because various allelic class II MHC molecules differ in their ability to bind different antigenic peptides and therefore to stimulate specific helper T cells.

  - H-2^k mice are responders to HEL(52–62), but H-2^d mice are nonresponders to this epitope. Equilibrium dialysis experiments have shown that HEL(52–62) binds to I-A^k but not to I-A^d molecules. X-ray crystallographic analysis of peptide-MHC complexes shows that the HEL(52–62) peptide binds tightly to the peptide-binding cleft of the I-A^k molecule (see Chapter 5, Fig. 5–8C). Modeling studies indicate that the HEL(52–62) peptide cannot bind tightly to the cleft of the I-A^d molecule (which has different amino acids in the binding cleft than does I-A^k). This explains why the H-2^d mouse is a nonresponder to this peptide. Similar results have been obtained with numerous other peptides.

These concepts of immunodominance and genetically controlled immune responsiveness are based largely on studies with simple peptide antigens and inbred homozygous strains of mice because in these cases, limited numbers of epitopes are presented by few MHC molecules, making the analyses simple. However, the same principles are also relevant to the understanding of responses to complex multideterminant protein antigens in outbred species. It is likely that most individuals will express at least one MHC molecule capable of binding at least one determinant of a complex protein, so that all individuals will be responders to such complex antigens. As we mentioned in Chapter 5, the need for every species to produce MHC molecules capable of binding many different peptides may be the evolutionary pressure for maintaining MHC polymorphism.

PRESENTATION OF LIPID ANTIGENS BY CD1 MOLECULES

An exception to the rule that T cells can see only peptides is the recognition of lipid and glycolipid antigens by a numerically rare population of T cells called NK-T cells. These lymphocytes have many unusual properties, including the expression of markers that are characteristic of both T cells and NK cells, and the limited diversity of their antigen receptors (see Chapter 8). NK-T cells recognize lipids and glycolipids displayed by the class I–like "non-classical" MHC molecule called

CD1. There are several CD1 proteins expressed in humans and mice. Although their intracellular traffic pathways differ in subtle ways, all the CD1 molecules bind and display lipids by a unique pathway. Newly synthesized CD1 molecules pick up cellular lipids and carry these to the cell surface. From here, the CD1-lipid complexes are endocytosed into endosomes or lysosomes, where lipids that have been ingested from the external environment are captured and the new CD1-lipid complexes are returned to the cell surface. Thus, CD1 molecules acquired endocytosed lipid antigens during recycling and present these antigens without apparent processing. The NK-T cells that recognize the lipid antigens may play a role in defense against microbes, especially mycobacteria (which are rich in lipid components).

SUMMARY

- T cells recognize antigens only in the form of peptides displayed by the products of self MHC genes on the surface of APCs. $CD4^+$ helper T lymphocytes recognize antigens in association with class II MHC gene products (class II MHC–restricted recognition), and $CD8^+$ CTLs recognize antigens in association with class I gene products (class I MHC–restricted recognition).

- Specialized APCs, such as dendritic cells, macrophages, and B lymphocytes, capture extracellular protein antigens, internalize and process them, and display class II–associated peptides to $CD4^+$ T cells. Dendritic cells are the most efficient APCs for initiating primary responses by activating naive T cells, and macrophages and B lymphocytes present antigens to differentiated helper T cells in the effector phase of cell-mediated immunity and in humoral immune responses, respectively. All nucleated cells can present class I–associated peptides, derived from cytosolic proteins such as viral and tumor antigens, to $CD8^+$ T cells.

- Antigen processing is the conversion of native proteins into MHC-associated peptides. This process consists of the introduction of exogenous protein antigens into vesicles of APCs or the synthesis of antigens in the cytosol, the proteolytic degradation of these proteins into peptides, the binding of peptides to MHC molecules, and the display of the peptide-MHC complexes on the APC surface for recognition by T cells. Thus, both extracellular and intracellular proteins are sampled by these antigen-processing pathways, and peptides derived from both normal self proteins and foreign proteins are displayed by MHC molecules for surveillance by T lymphocytes.

- For class II–associated antigen presentation, extracellular proteins are internalized into endosomes, where these proteins are proteolytically cleaved by enzymes that function at acidic pH. Newly synthesized class II MHC molecules associated with the I_i are transported from the ER to the endosomal vesicles. Here the I_i is proteolytically cleaved, and a small peptide remnant of the I_i, called CLIP, is removed from the peptide-binding cleft of the MHC molecule by the DM molecules. The peptides that were generated from extracellular proteins then bind to the available cleft of the class II MHC molecule, and the trimeric complex (class II MHC α and β chains and peptide) moves to and is displayed on the surface of the cell.

- For class I–associated antigen presentation, cytosolic proteins are proteolytically degraded in the proteasome, generating peptides with features that enable them to bind to class I molecules. These peptides are delivered from the cytoplasm to the ER by an ATP-dependent transporter called TAP. Newly synthesized class I MHC–β_2-microglobulin dimers in the ER are attached to the TAP complex and receive peptides transported into the ER. Stable complexes of class I MHC molecules with bound peptides move out of the ER, through the Golgi complex, to the cell surface.

- These pathways of MHC-restricted antigen presentation ensure that most of the body's cells are screened for the possible presence of foreign antigens. The pathways also ensure that proteins from extracellular microbes preferentially generate peptides bound to class II MHC molecules for recognition by $CD4^+$ helper T cells, which activate effector mechanisms that eliminate extracellular antigens. Conversely, proteins synthesized by intracellular (cytosolic) microbes generate peptides bound to class I MHC molecules for recognition by $CD8^+$ CTLs, which function to eliminate cells harboring intracellular infections. The immunogenicity of foreign protein antigens depends on the ability of antigen-processing pathways to generate peptides from these proteins that bind to self MHC molecules.

Selected Readings

Ackerman AL, and P Cresswell. Cellular mechanisms governing cross-presentation of exogenous antigens. Nature Immunology 5:678–684, 2004.

Antoniou AN, and SJ Powis. Pathogen evasion strategies for the major histocompatibility complex class I assembly pathway. Immunology 124:1–12, 2008.

Barral DC, and MB Brenner. CD1 antigen presentation: how it works. Nature Reviews Immunology 7:929–941, 2007.

Bousso P. T-cell activation by dendritic cells in the lymph node: lessons from the movies. Nature Reviews Immunology 8: 675–684, 2008.

Bryant PW, AM Lennon-Dumenil, E Fiebiger, C Lagaudriere-Gesbert, and HL Ploegh. Proteolysis and antigen presentation by MHC class II molecules. Advances in Immunology 80:71–114, 2002.

Chapman HA. Endosomal proteases in antigen presentation. Current Opinion in Immunology 18:78–84, 2006.

Germain RN, and MK Jenkins. In vivo antigen presentation. Current Opinion in Immunology 16:120–125, 2004.

Heath WR, and FR Carbone. Cross-presentation, dendritic cells, tolerance and immunity. Annual Review of Immunology 19:47–61, 2001.

Hewitt EW. The MHC class I antigen presentation pathway: strategies for viral immune evasion. Immunology 110: 163–169, 2003.

Honey K, and AY Rudensky. Lysosomal cysteine proteases regulate antigen presentation. Nature Reviews Immunology 3:472–482, 2003.

López-Bravo M, and C Ardavín. In vivo induction of immune responses to pathogens by conventional dendritic cells. Immunity 29:343–351, 2008.

Moser M. Dendritic cells in immunity and tolerance: do they display opposite functions? Immunity 19:5–8, 2003.

Purcell AW, and T Elliott. Molecular machinations of the MHC-I peptide loading complex. Current Opinion in Immunology 20:75–81, 2008.

Randolph GJ, V Angeli, and MA Swartz. Dendritic cell trafficking to lymph nodes through lymphatic vessels. Nature Reviews Immunology 5:617–628, 2005.

Reis e Sousa C. Dendritic cells in a mature age. Nature Reviews Immunology 6:476–483, 2006.

Rocha N, and J Neefjes. MHC class II molecules on the move for successful antigen presentation. EMBO Journal 27:1–5, 2008.

Rock KL, IA York, and AL Goldberg. Post-proteasomal antigen processing for major histocompatibility class I presentation. Nature Immunology 5:670–677, 2004.

Shortman K, and Y-J Liu. Mouse and human dendritic cell subtypes. Nature Reviews Immunology 2:151–161, 2003.

Stern LJ, I Potolicchio, and L Santambrogio. MHC Class II compartment subtypes: structure and function. Current Opinion in Immunology 18:64–69, 2006.

Trombetta ES, and I Mellman. Cell biology of antigen processing in vitro and in vivo. Annual Review of Immunology 23:975–1028, 2005.

Villadangos JA, and L Young. Antigen-presentation properties of plasmacytoid dendritic cells. Immunity 29:352–361, 2008.

Vyas JM, AG Van der Veen, and HL Ploegh. The known unknowns of antigen processing and presentation. Nature Reviews Immunology 8:607–618, 2008.

Watts C. The exogenous pathway for antigen presentation on major histocompatibility complex class II and CD1 molecules. Nature Immunology 5:685–692, 2004.

Yewdell JW, and JR Bennink. Immunodominance in major histocompatibility class I–restricted T lymphocyte responses. Annual Review of Immunology 17:51–88, 1999.

Yewdell JW, and SM Haeryfar. Understanding presentation of viral antigens to $CD8^+$ T cells in vivo: the key to rational vaccine design. Annual Review of Immunology 23:651–682, 2005.

Chapter 7

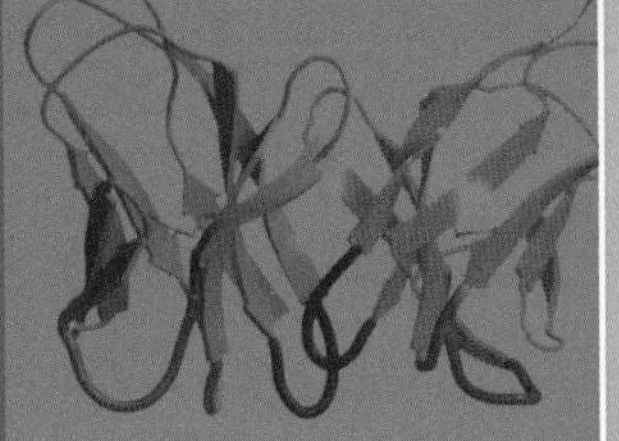

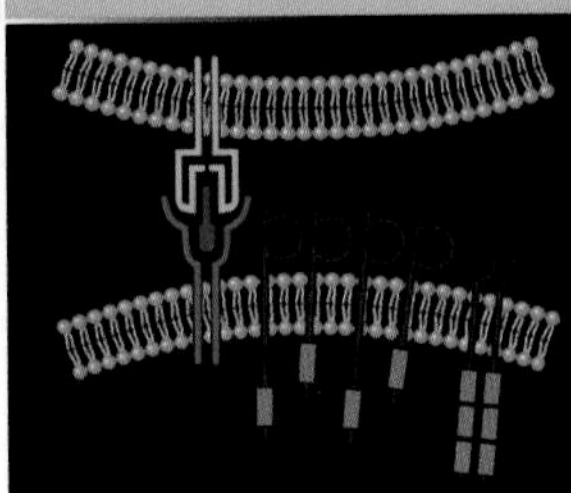

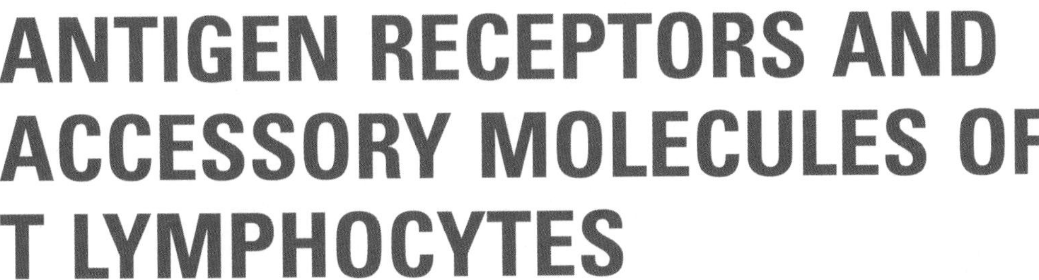

ANTIGEN RECEPTORS AND ACCESSORY MOLECULES OF T LYMPHOCYTES

T lymphocytes respond to peptide fragments of protein antigens that are displayed by antigen-presenting cells (APCs). The initiation of these responses requires specific antigen recognition by the T cells, stable adhesion of the T cells to the APCs, and the transduction of signals from the cell surface to the nucleus of T cells. Each of these events is mediated by distinct sets of molecules on the T cell surface (Fig. 7–1). In this chapter, we describe the cell surface molecules involved in T cell antigen recognition and signaling. The molecules involved in the adhesion of T cells to APCs have been described in Chapter 3.

T lymphocytes have a dual specificity: they recognize polymorphic residues of self major histocompatibility complex (MHC) molecules, which accounts for their MHC restriction, and they also recognize residues of peptide antigens displayed by these MHC molecules, which is responsible for their specificity. As we discussed in Chapters 5 and 6, MHC molecules and peptides form complexes on the surface of APCs. The receptor that recognizes these peptide-MHC complexes is called the **T cell receptor** (TCR). The TCR is a clonally distributed receptor, meaning that clones of T cells with different specificities express different TCRs. The biochemical signals that are triggered in T cells by antigen recognition are transduced not by the TCR itself but by invariant proteins called CD3 and ζ, which are noncovalently linked to the antigen receptor to form the **TCR complex.** Thus, in T cells, and, as we shall see in Chapter 10, in B cells as well, antigen recognition and signaling are segregated among two sets of molecules—a highly variable antigen receptor (the TCR in T cells and membrane immunoglobulin [Ig] in B cells) and invariant signaling proteins (CD3 and ζ chains in T cells and Igα and Igβ in B cells) (Fig. 7–2). The T cell receptor not only plays a role in activating mature T cells that encounter antigens, but this receptor and a related receptor called the pre-T

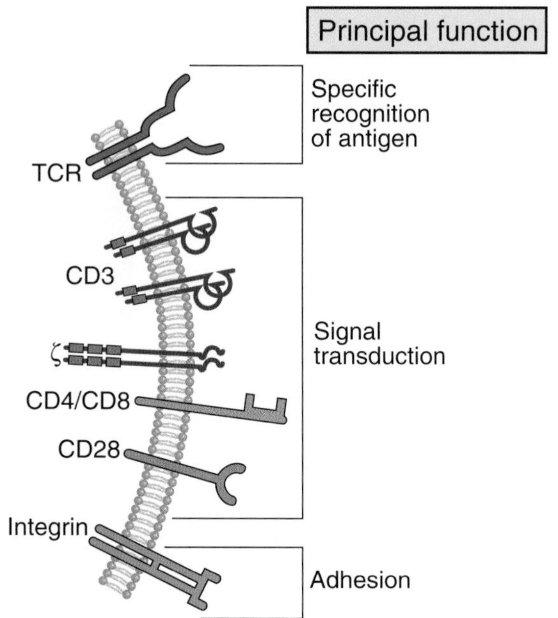

FIGURE 7–1 T cell receptors and accessory molecules. The principal T cell membrane proteins involved in antigen recognition and in responses to antigens are shown. The functions of these proteins fall into three groups: antigen recognition, signal transduction, and adhesion.

receptor (see Chapter 8) play important roles during the development of T cells.

T cells also express other membrane receptors that do not recognize antigen but participate in responses to antigens; these are collectively called **accessory molecules**. The physiologic role of some accessory molecules is to facilitate signaling by the TCR complex, while others provide "second signals" to fully activate T cells. Yet other accessory molecules function as adhesion molecules to stabilize the binding of T cells to APCs, thus allowing the TCR to be engaged by antigen long enough to transduce the necessary signals. Adhesion molecules also regulate the migration of T cells to the sites where they locate and respond to antigens, as discussed in Chapter 3. In addition to mediating firm attachment, most adhesion molecules initiate signaling and participate in the formation of "immunological synapses" between T cells and APCs (Chapter 9).

With this background, we proceed to describe the T cell membrane molecules that are required for antigen recognition and the initiation of functional responses. The maturation of T cells is discussed in Chapter 8, and the biology and biochemistry of T cell responses to antigen are discussed in Chapter 9.

αβ TCR FOR MHC-ASSOCIATED PEPTIDE ANTIGEN

The TCR was discovered in the early 1980s, around the same time that the structure of MHC-peptide complexes was being defined. A number of separate approaches were used to molecularly identify the TCR (Box 7–1). One approach depended on the identification of genes that were expressed only in T cells and that also could be shown to have undergone recombination specifically in these cells. The first gene thus identified was homologous to immunoglobulin genes. In another approach, clonal populations of T cells were generated and monoclonal antibodies that recognized specific clones were identified. These clonotype-specific antibodies identified the TCR. These early studies have culminated in the x-ray crystallographic analysis of TCRs and, most informatively, of trimolecular complexes of MHC molecules, bound peptides, and specific TCRs. As we shall see in the following section, on the basis of these analyses, we now understand the structural features of antigen recognition by the TCR precisely. The components of the TCR complex, in addition to the TCR itself, have been identified by biochemical studies and molecular cloning.

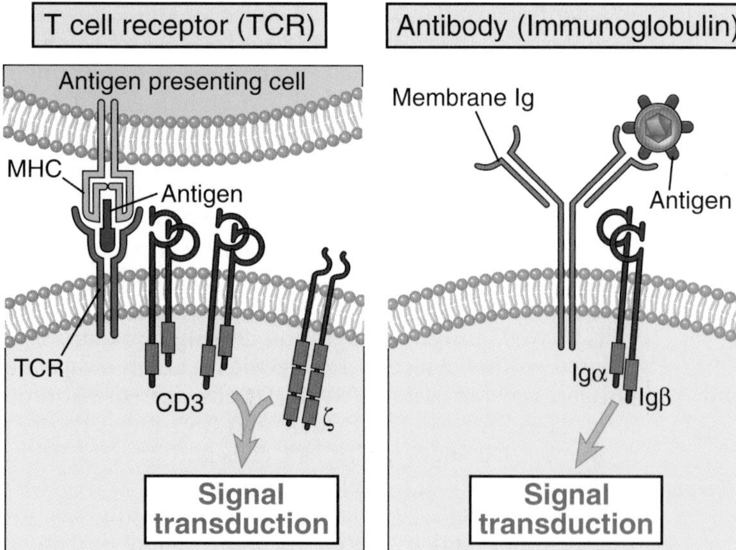

FIGURE 7–2 Antigen recognition and signaling functions of lymphocyte antigen receptors. The antigen recognition and signaling functions of antigen receptors are mediated by distinct proteins of the antigen receptor complex. When TCR or Ig molecules recognize antigens, signals are delivered to the lymphocytes by proteins associated with the antigen receptors. The antigen receptors and attached signaling proteins form the T and B cell receptor complexes. Note that single antigen receptors are shown recognizing antigens, but signaling requires the cross-linking of two or more receptors by binding to adjacent antigen molecules.

Box 7–1 ▪ IN DEPTH: IDENTIFICATION OF THE TCR

To identify TCRs for MHC-associated peptide antigens, it was necessary to develop monoclonal T cell populations in which all the cells express the same TCR. The first such populations to be used for studying TCR proteins were tumors derived from T lymphocytes. Subsequently, methods were developed for propagating monoclonal T cell populations *in vitro,* including T-T hybridomas and antigen-specific T cell clones. The earliest techniques for purifying TCR molecules for biochemical studies relied on producing antibodies specific for unique (idiotypic) determinants of the antigen receptors of a clonal T cell population. Antigen receptors were isolated by use of such antibodies, and limited amino acid sequencing of these receptor proteins suggested that the TCRs were structurally homologous to Ig molecules and contained highly variable regions that differed from one clone to another. However, the protein sequencing studies did not reveal the structure of the complete TCR.

The breakthrough came from attempts to clone the genes encoding TCRs, and this was accomplished before the structure of the proteins was fully defined. The strategy for the identification of TCR genes was based on the knowledge of Ig genes. Three criteria were chosen that needed to be fulfilled for genes to be considered TCR genes: (1) these genes would be uniquely expressed in T cells, (2) they would undergo somatic recombination during T cell development (as Ig genes do during B cell development; see Chapter 8), and (3) they would be homologous to Ig genes. One method that was used to identify TCR genes was subtractive hybridization, aimed at identifying T cell–specific genes. In this method, complementary DNA (cDNA) was prepared from T cell messenger RNA (mRNA) and hybridized to B cell mRNA. All the cDNAs that were common to T and B cells hybridized to the mRNA and were separated from non-hybridized cDNAs. The cDNAs that were left behind were unique to T cells. Some of the genes contained in this library of T cell–specific cDNAs were found to be homologous in sequence to Ig genes, and Southern blot hybridization showed that these genes had a different structure in non–T cells than in T cells. This difference in structure in lymphocytes compared to non-lymphocytes was a known characteristic of Ig genes (see Chapter 8) and suggested that the T cell genes that had been found encoded clonally distributed antigen receptors of T cells that underwent somatic rearrangement only in cells of the T lymphocyte lineage. Furthermore, the predicted amino acid sequences of the proteins encoded by these genes agreed with the partial sequences obtained from putative TCR proteins purified with TCR-specific anti-idiotypic antibodies. Other investigators discovered TCR genes among a library of T cell genes (without subtractive hybridization) based solely on the criteria mentioned before.

The molecular cloning of the TCR was a landmark achievement that came soon after the detailed structural analysis of MHC molecules and provided the structural basis for understanding how T cells recognize peptide-MHC complexes. The ability to express TCRs in ways that allowed them to be cleaved from cell membranes and solubilized was key to the crystallization of TCRs bound to peptide-MHC complexes. These advances have revolutionized our understanding of T cell antigen recognition and paved the way for many important techniques, including the expression of single TCRs of known specificities in transgenic animals. We will refer to such approaches for analyzing immune responses in later chapters.

Structure of the αβ TCR

The antigen receptor of MHC-restricted CD4⁺ helper T cells and CD8⁺ cytotoxic T lymphocytes (CTLs) is a heterodimer consisting of two transmembrane polypeptide chains, designated α and β, covalently linked to each other by a disulfide bridge (Fig. 7–3). (Another less common type of TCR, found on a small subset of T cells, is composed of γ and δ chains and is discussed later.) Each α chain and β chain consists of one Ig-like N-terminal variable (V) domain, one Ig-like constant (C) domain, a hydrophobic transmembrane region, and a short cytoplasmic region. Thus, the extracellular portion of the αβ heterodimer is structurally similar to the antigen-binding fragment (Fab) of an Ig molecule, which is made up of the V and C regions of a light chain and the V region and one C region of a heavy chain (see Chapter 4).

The V regions of the TCR α and β chains contain short stretches of amino acids where the variability between different TCRs is concentrated, and these form the hypervariable or complementarity-determining regions (CDRs). Three CDRs in the α chain are juxtaposed to three similar regions in the β chain to form the part of the TCR that specifically recognizes peptide-MHC complexes (described in the following section). The β chain V domain contains a fourth hypervariable region, which does not appear to participate in antigen recognition but is the binding site for microbial products called superantigens (see Chapter 15, Box 15–2). Each TCR chain, like Ig heavy and light chains, is encoded by multiple gene segments that undergo somatic rearrangements during the maturation of the T lymphocytes (see Chapter 8). In the α and β chains of the TCR, the third hypervariable regions are composed of sequences encoded by V and J (joining) gene segments (in the α chain) or V, D (diversity), and J segments (in the β chain). These CDR3 regions also contain junctional sequences that are encoded by added nucleotides, so-called N regions and P nucleotides (see Chapter 8). Therefore, most of the sequence variability in TCRs is concentrated in the CDR3 regions.

The C regions of both α and β chains continue into short hinge regions, which contain cysteine residues

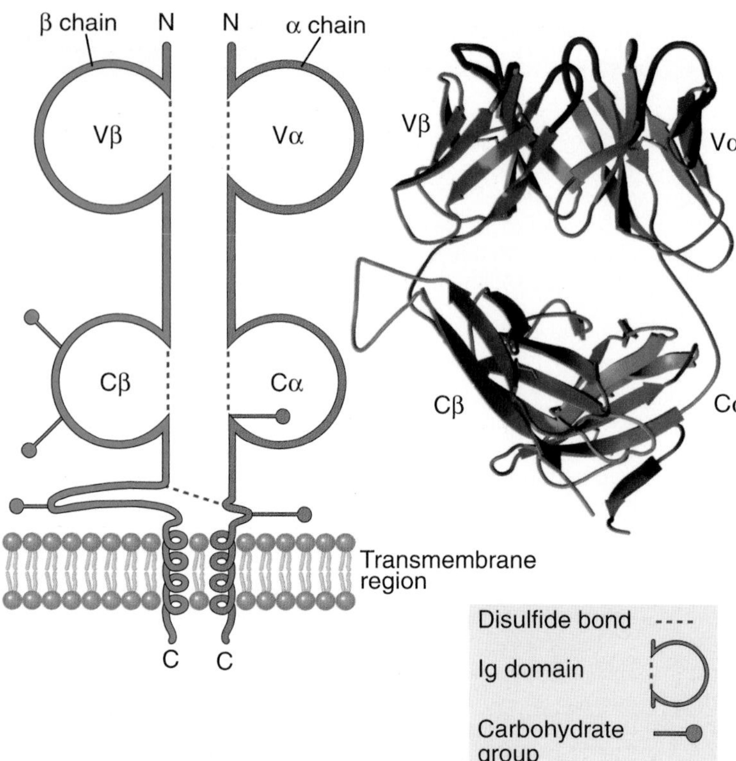

FIGURE 7–3 Structure of the T cell receptor. The schematic diagram of the αβ TCR *(left)* shows the domains of a typical TCR specific for a peptide-MHC complex. The antigen-binding portion of the TCR is formed by the V_α and V_β domains. The ribbon diagram *(right)* shows the structure of the extracellular portion of a TCR as revealed by x-ray crystallography. The hypervariable segment loops that form the peptide-MHC binding site are at the top. (Adapted from Bjorkman PJ. MHC restriction in three dimensions: a view of T cell receptor/ligand interactions. Cell 89:167–170, 1997. Copyright Cell Press.)

that contribute to a disulfide bond linking the two chains. The hinge is followed by hydrophobic transmembrane portions, an unusual feature of which is the presence of positively charged amino acid residues, including a lysine residue (in the α chain) or a lysine and an arginine residue (in the β chain). These residues interact with negatively charged residues present in the transmembrane portions of other polypeptides (CD3 and ζ) that are part of the TCR complex. Both α and β chains have carboxy-terminal cytoplasmic tails that are 5 to 12 amino acids long. Like membrane Ig on B cells, these cytoplasmic regions are too small to transduce signals, and specific molecules physically associated with the TCR serve the signal-transducing functions of this antigen receptor complex.

TCRs and Ig molecules are structurally similar, but there are also several significant differences between these two types of antigen receptors (Table 7–1). The TCR is not produced in a secreted form, and it does not perform effector functions on its own. Instead, on binding peptide-MHC complexes, the TCR complex initiates signals that activate the effector functions of T cells. Also, unlike antibodies, the TCR chains do not undergo changes in C region expression (i.e., isotype switching) or affinity maturation during T cell differentiation.

Role of the αβ TCR in the Recognition of MHC-Associated Peptide Antigen

The recognition of peptide-MHC complexes is mediated by the CDRs formed by both the α and β chains of the TCR. Several types of experiments have definitively established that both the α and β chains form a single heterodimeric receptor that is responsible for both the antigen (peptide) specificity and the MHC restriction of a T cell.

- Cloned lines of T cells with different peptide specificities and MHC restrictions differ in the sequences of the V regions of both α and β chains.
- TCR α and β genes can be isolated from a T cell clone of defined peptide and MHC specificity. When both these genes are expressed in other T cells by transfection, they confer on the recipient cell both the peptide specificity and the MHC restriction of the original clone from which they were isolated. Neither TCR chain alone is adequate for providing specific recognition of peptide-MHC complexes.
- To create transgenic mice expressing a TCR of a particular antigen specificity and MHC restriction, it is necessary to express both the α and β chains of the TCR as transgenes.

The antigen-binding site of the TCR is formed by the six CDRs of the α and β chains that are splayed out to form a surface for MHC-peptide recognition (Fig. 7–4). This interface resembles the antigen-binding surfaces of antibody molecules, which are formed by the V regions of the heavy and light chains (see Chapter 4, Fig. 4–5). In the TCR structures that have been analyzed in detail, the TCR contacts the peptide-MHC complex in a diagonal orientation, fitting between the

Table 7–1. Properties of Lymphocyte Antigen Receptors: T Cell Receptors and Immunoglobulins

	T cell receptor (TCR)	Immunoglobulin (Ig)
Components	α and β chains	Heavy and light chains
Number of Ig domains	One V domain and one C domain in each chain	Heavy chain; one V domain, three or four C domains Light chain; one V domain and one C domain
Number of CDRs	Three in each chain for antigen binding; fourth hypervariable region in β chain (of unknown function)	Three in each chain
Associated signaling molecules	CD3 and ζ	Igα and Igβ
Affinity for antigen (K_d)	10^{-5}–10^{-7} M	10^{-7}–10^{-11} M (secreted Ig)
Changes after cellular activation		
Production of secreted form	No	Yes
Isotype switching	No	Yes
Somatic mutations	No	Yes

Abbreviations: C, constant; CDR, complementarity-determining region; K_d, dissociation constant; V, variable.

high points of the MHC α-helices. In general, the CDR1 loops of the TCR α and β chains are positioned over the ends of the bound peptide, the CDR2 loops are over the helices of the MHC molecule, and the CDR3 loop is positioned over the center of the MHC-associated peptide. One surprising result of these structural analyses is that the side chains of only one or two amino acid residues of the MHC-bound peptide make contact with the TCR. This is structural proof for the remarkable ability of T cells to distinguish among diverse antigens on the basis of very few amino acid differences. Recall that mutational analyses of peptides

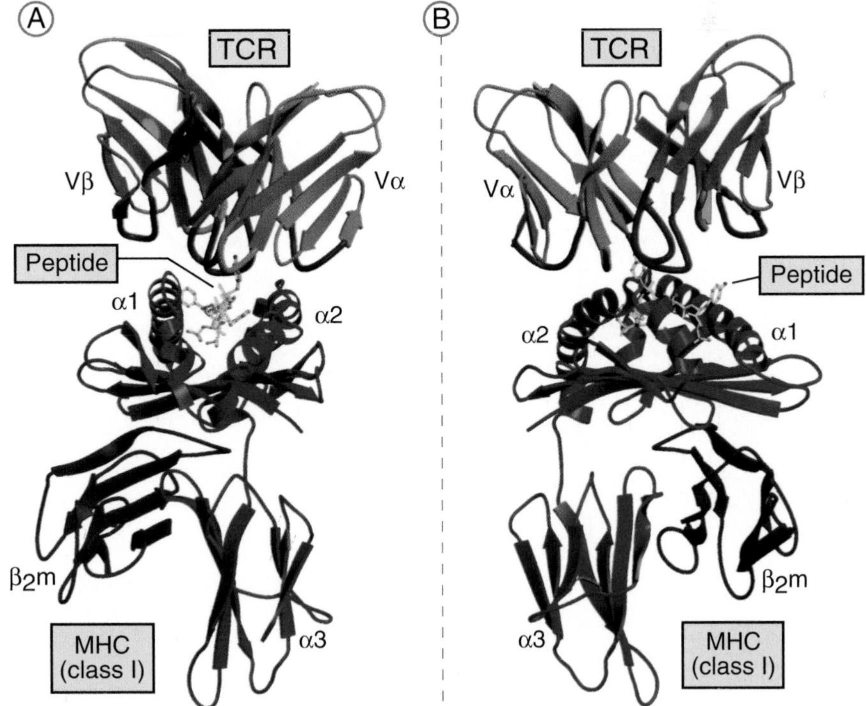

FIGURE 7–4 Binding of a TCR to a peptide-MHC complex. The V domains of a TCR are shown interacting with a human class I MHC molecule, HLA-A2, presenting a viral peptide (in yellow). A is a front view and B is a side view of the x-ray crystal structure of the trimolecular MHC-peptide–TCR complex. (From Bjorkman PJ. MHC restriction in three dimensions: a view of T cell receptor/ligand interactions. Cell 89:167–170, 1997. Copyright Cell Press.)

described in Chapter 5 also showed that very few residues of the peptide are responsible for the specificity of T cell antigen recognition (see Fig. 5–8C).

The affinity of the TCR for peptide-MHC complexes is low, much lower than that of most antibodies (see Chapter 4, Table 4–1). In the few T cells that have been analyzed in detail, the dissociation constant (K_d) of TCR interactions with peptide-MHC complexes varies from ~10^{-5} to ~10^{-7} M. This low affinity of specific antigen binding is the likely reason that adhesion molecules are needed to stabilize the binding of T cells to APCs, thus allowing biologic responses to be initiated. Signaling by the TCR complex appears to require prolonged or repeated engagement of peptide-MHC complexes, which is also promoted by stable adhesion between T cells and APCs. The TCR and accessory molecules in the T cell plasma membrane move coordinately with their ligands in the APC membrane to form a transient supramolecular structure that has been called the **immunological synapse.** The formation of this synapse regulates TCR-mediated signal transduction. We will return to a discussion of signal transduction by the TCR complex and the role of the synapse in Chapter 9.

CD3 and ζ Proteins of the TCR Complex

The CD3 and ζ proteins are noncovalently associated with the TCR αβ heterodimer, and when the TCR recognizes antigen, these associated proteins transduce the signals that lead to T cell activation. The components of the TCR complex are illustrated in Figure 7–5 and listed in Table 7–1. The CD3 molecule actually consists of three proteins that are designated CD3 γ, δ, and ε. The CD3 proteins and the ζ chain are identical in all T cells regardless of specificity, which is consistent with their role in signaling and not in antigen recognition.

Structure and Association of CD3 and ζ Proteins

The CD3 proteins were identified before the αβ heterodimer by the use of monoclonal antibodies raised against T cells, and the ζ chain was identified later by co-immunoprecipitation with αβ and CD3 proteins. The physical association of the αβ heterodimer, CD3, and ζ chains has been demonstrated in two ways.

- Antibodies against the TCR αβ heterodimer or any of the CD3 proteins coprecipitate the heterodimer and all the associated proteins from solubilized plasma membranes of T cells.
- When intact T cells are treated with either anti-CD3 or anti-TCR αβ antibodies, the entire TCR complex is endocytosed and disappears from the cell surface (i.e., all the proteins are comodulated).

The CD3 γ, δ, and ε proteins are homologous to each other. The N-terminal extracellular regions of γ, δ, and ε chains each contains a single Ig-like domain, and therefore these three proteins are members of the Ig superfamily. The transmembrane segments of all

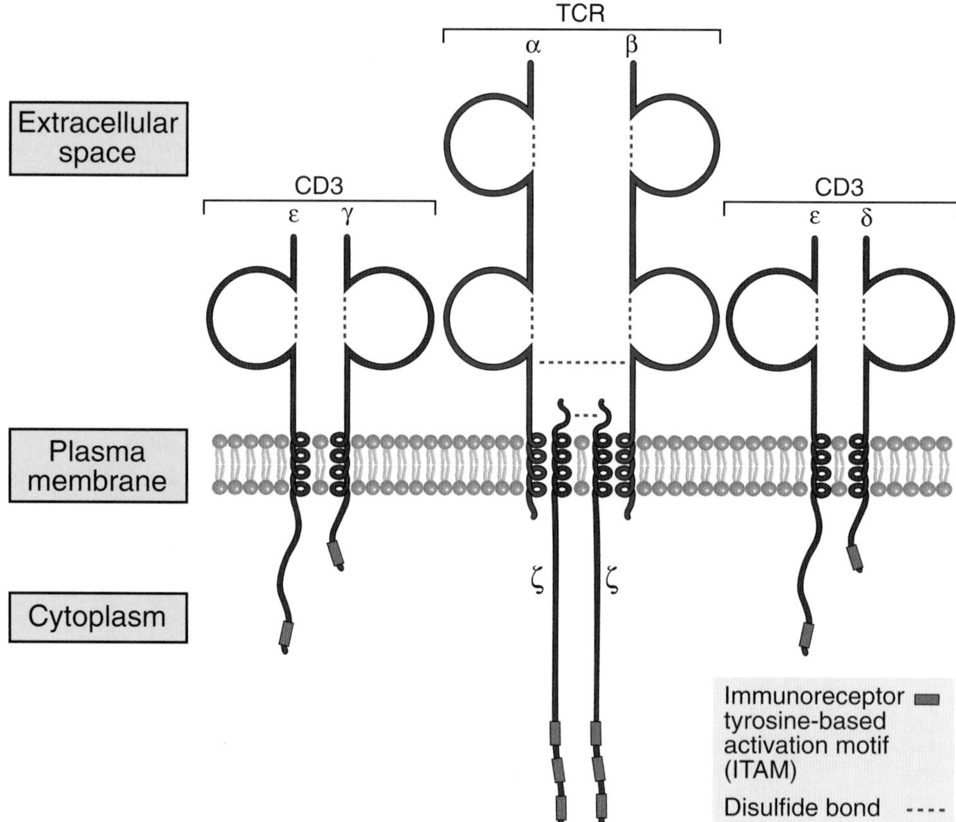

FIGURE 7–5 Components of the TCR complex. The TCR complex of MHC-restricted T cells consists of the αβ TCR noncovalently linked to the CD3 and ζ proteins. The association of these proteins with one another is mediated by charged residues in their transmembrane regions, which are not shown.

three CD3 chains contain a negatively charged aspartic acid residue, which binds to positively charged residues in the transmembrane domains of the TCR α and β chains. Each TCR complex contains one αβ dimer associated with one CD3 γε heterodimer, one CD3 δε heterodimer, and one disulfide-linked covalent ζζ homodimer.

The cytoplasmic domains of the CD3 γ, δ, and ε proteins range from 44 to 81 amino acid residues long, and each of these domains contains one copy of a conserved sequence motif important for signaling that is called the **immunoreceptor tyrosine-based activation motif** (ITAM). An ITAM contains two copies of the sequence tyrosine-X-X-leucine/isoleucine (in which X is an unspecified amino acid), separated by six to eight amino acid residues (i.e., YXXL/I$(X)_{6-8}$YXXL/I). ITAMs play a central role in signaling by the TCR complex. They are also found in the cytoplasmic tails of several other lymphocyte membrane proteins that are involved in signal transduction, including the ζ chain of the TCR complex, Igα and Igβ proteins associated with membrane Ig molecules of B cells (see Chapter 10, Fig. 10–3), and components of several Fc receptors (see Chapter 14, Box 14–1), and of the NKG2D activating receptor on natural killer (NK) cells.

The ζ chain has a short extracellular region of nine amino acids, a transmembrane region containing a negatively charged aspartic acid residue (similar to the CD3 chains), and a long cytoplasmic region (113 amino acids) that contains three ITAMs. It is normally expressed as a homodimer. The ζ chain is also associated with signaling receptors on lymphocytes other than T cells, such as the Fcγ receptor (FcγRIII) of NK cells.

The expression of the TCR complex requires synthesis of all its components. The need for all components of the complex to be present for expression was first established in cell lines (Fig. 7–6). During the maturation of T cells in the thymus, CD3 and ζ proteins are synthesized before the TCR α and β genes are expressed (see Chapter 8), but these proteins do not make their way to the plasma membrane, and are proteolytically degraded. Chaperones, such as calnexin, may retain individual members of the TCR complex in the endoplasmic reticulum (ER) before the complex is fully assembled. In mature T cells the entire TCR complex is assembled in the ER and transported to the cell surface. This sequence of events is essentially similar to the events that lead to expression of the B cell antigen receptor complex in B lymphocytes.

Functions of CD3 and ζ Proteins

The CD3 and ζ chains link antigen recognition by the TCR to the biochemical events that lead to the functional activation of T cells. Several lines of evidence support the critical role of these components of the TCR complex in signal transduction in T cells.

- Antibodies against CD3 proteins often stimulate T cell functional responses that are identical to antigen-induced responses. Unlike antigens, which stimulate only specific T cells, anti-CD3 antibodies bind to and stimulate all T cells, regardless of antigen specificity. Thus, anti-CD3 antibodies are polyclonal activators of T cells.
- The cytoplasmic tail of either the CD3ε or the ζ protein is sufficient to transduce the signals necessary for T cell activation in the absence of the other components of the TCR complex. This was shown by expressing, in certain T cell lines, genetically engineered chimeric molecules containing the cytoplasmic portion of CD3ε or the ζ chain fused to the extracellular and transmembrane domains of other

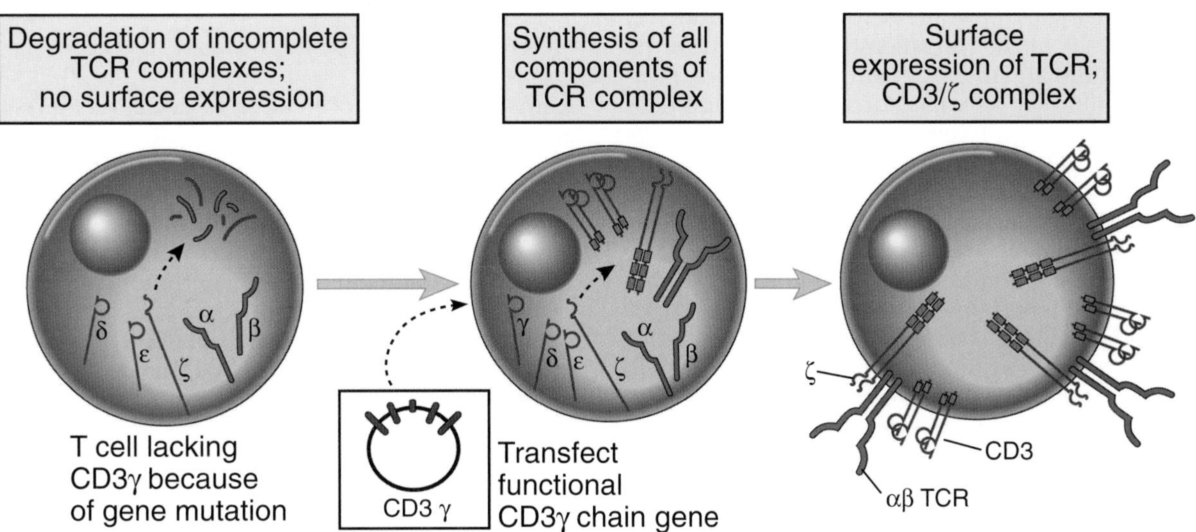

FIGURE 7–6 Assembly and surface expression of the TCR complex. In the absence of any one component (in this case, the CD3γ protein), the TCR complex is not assembled and all its proteins are degraded, presumably in proteasomes following retro-translocation from the endoplasmic reticulum. Introduction of the missing component by gene transfection allows the complex to be assembled and transported to the cell surface.

cell surface receptors for soluble ligands, such as the interleukin-2 (IL-2) receptor. Binding of the ligand (e.g., IL-2) to the chimeric receptors results in activation responses identical to those induced by stimulation through the normal TCR complex on the same T cells.

The earliest intracellular event that occurs in T cells after antigen recognition is the phosphorylation of tyrosine residues within the ITAMs in the cytoplasmic tails of the CD3 and ζ proteins by Src family kinases such as Lck or Fyn. Lck associates with the cytoplasmic tail of CD4 and CD8, and Fyn is physically linked to CD3. The phosphotyrosines in the ITAMs become docking sites for a tyrosine kinase with tandem Src homology 2 (SH2) domains. This kinase, called ZAP-70 (70-kD ζ-associated protein), is recruited to the ζ chain and triggers signal transduction pathways that ultimately lead to changes in gene expression in the T cells (discussed in Chapter 9).

ANTIGEN RECEPTORS OF γδ T CELLS

The γδ TCR is a second type of diverse, disulfide-linked heterodimer that is expressed on a small subset of αβ-negative T cells. This category of antigen receptor is also associated with CD3 and ζ proteins. (The γδ TCR should not be confused with the γ and δ components of the CD3 complex.) The TCR γ and δ chains consist of extracellular Ig-like V and C regions, short connecting or hinge regions, hydrophobic transmembrane segments, and short cytoplasmic tails, similar to the TCR α and β chains. The hinge regions contain cysteine residues involved in interchain disulfide linkages. The γδ heterodimer associates with the CD3 and ζ proteins in the same way as TCR αβ heterodimers do. The transmembrane regions of the TCR γ and δ chains, in a manner similar to the α and β chains, contain positively charged amino acid residues that interact with the negatively charged residues in the transmembrane regions of the CD3 polypeptides and of the ζ chain. Furthermore, TCR-induced signaling events typical of αβ-expressing T cells are also observed in γδ T cells. The majority of γδ T cells do not express CD4 or CD8. A number of biologic activities have been ascribed to γδ T cells that are also characteristic of αβ T cells, including secretion of cytokines and lysis of target cells.

T cells expressing the γδ TCR represent a lineage distinct from the more numerous αβ-expressing, MHC-restricted T lymphocytes. The percentages of γδ T cells vary widely in different tissues and species, but overall, less than 5% of all T cells express this form of TCR. Different subsets of γδ T cells may develop at distinct times during ontogeny, contain different V regions, and populate different tissues. For example, in mice, many skin γδ T cells develop in neonatal life and express one particular TCR with essentially no variability in the V region, whereas many of the γδ T cells in the vagina, uterus, and tongue appear later and express another TCR with a different V region. It is not known whether these subsets perform different functions, but the distinct V regions suggest that the subsets may be specific for different ligands. One intriguing feature of γδ T cells is their abundance in epithelial tissues of certain species. For example, more than 50% of lymphocytes in the small bowel mucosa of mice and chickens, called **intraepithelial lymphocytes,** are γδ T cells. In mouse skin, most of the intraepidermal T cells express the γδ receptor. Equivalent cell populations are not as abundant in humans; only about 10% of human intestinal intraepithelial T cells express the γδ TCR.

γδ T cells, along with NK-T cells (described below), B-1 B cells, and MZ B cells (see Chapters 8 and 10), may represent an important bridge between innate and adaptive immunity, functioning as lymphocytes that enhance the first line of defense against a range of pathogens. γδ T cells do not recognize MHC-associated peptide antigens and are not MHC restricted. Some γδ T cell clones recognize small phosphorylated molecules, alkyl amines, or lipids that are commonly found in mycobacteria and other microbes, and that may be presented by "nonclassical" class I MHC-like molecules. Other γδ T cells recognize protein or nonprotein antigens that do not require processing or any particular type of APCs for their presentation. Many γδ T cells are triggered by microbial heat shock proteins. The limited diversity of the γδ TCRs in many tissues suggests that the ligands for these receptors may be invariant and conserved. A working hypothesis for the specificity of γδ T cells is that they may recognize antigens that are frequently encountered at epithelial boundaries between the host and the external environment. Thus, they may initiate immune responses to a small number of common microbes at these sites, before the recruitment of antigen-specific αβ T cells. However, mice lacking γδ T cells, created by targeted disruption of the γ or δ TCR gene, have little or no immunodeficiency and only a modest increase in susceptibility to infections by some intracellular bacteria.

ANTIGEN RECEPTORS OF NK-T CELLS

A small population of T cells also expresses markers that are found on NK cells; these are called **NK-T cells.** The TCR α chains expressed by a subset of NK-T cells have limited diversity, and in humans these cells are characterized by a unique Vα24-Jα18 rearrangement. These invariant NK-T (iNK-T) cells also represent lymphocytes that bridge innate and adaptive immunity. Other NK-T cells exist that have quite diverse antigen receptors. All NK-T cell TCRs recognize lipids that are bound to class I MHC-like molecules called CD1 molecules. However, other cloned lines of αβ T cells that do not express NK-T markers but recognize CD1-associated lipid antigens have also been described and these cells may be $CD4^+$, $CD8^+$, or $CD4^-CD8^-$ αβ T cells. NK-T cells and other lipid antigen-specific T cells are capable of rapidly producing cytokines such as IL-4 and interferon (IFN)-γ after being triggered in a lipid- and CD1-dependent fashion. NK-T cells and other CD1-restricted T cells may mediate protective innate immune responses against some pathogens, and invariant NK-T cells may regulate adaptive immune responses primarily by secreting cytokines. The precise functions of these cells are still being elucidated.

Coreceptors and Costimulatory Receptors in T Cells

Other than the T cell receptor complex, many categories of molecules on the T-cell surface contribute in a major way to the activation and differentiation of T lymphocytes (Fig. 7–7). **Coreceptors** represent a category of membrane proteins that enhance TCR signaling; their name refers to the fact that they bind to MHC molecules, and thus recognize a part of the same ligands (peptide-MHC complexes) as do the antigen receptors. A group of proteins known as **costimulatory receptors** also deliver activating signals to T cells, but these proteins, in contrast to coreceptors, recognize molecules on APCs that are not part of the peptide-MHC complexes. Chemokine receptors and cytokine receptors are also of importance in T cell responses, and these molecules are discussed in Chapter 12.

CD4 and CD8: Coreceptors Involved in MHC-Restricted T Cell Activation

CD4 and CD8 are T cell proteins that bind to nonpolymorphic regions of MHC molecules and facilitate signaling by the TCR complex during T cell activation. Mature αβ T cells express either CD4 or CD8, but not both. CD4 and CD8 interact with class II and class I MHC molecules, respectively, when the antigen receptors of T cells specifically recognize peptide-MHC complexes on APCs (see Fig. 7–7). The major function of CD4 and CD8 is in signal transduction at the time of antigen recognition; they may also strengthen the binding of T cells to APCs. Because CD4 and CD8 participate together with the TCR in recognition of MHC molecules and in T cell activation, they are called coreceptors. About 65% of mature αβ-positive T cells in the blood and lymphoid tissues express CD4, and 35% express CD8.

Structure of CD4 and CD8

CD4 and CD8 are transmembrane glycoprotein members of the Ig superfamily, which mediate similar functions. CD4 is expressed as a monomer on the surface of peripheral T cells and thymocytes and is also present on mononuclear phagocytes and some dendritic cells. CD4 has four extracellular Ig-like domains, a hydrophobic transmembrane region, and a highly basic cytoplasmic tail 38 amino acids long (Fig. 7–8). The two N-terminal Ig-like domains of the CD4 protein bind to the nonpolymorphic β2 domain of the class II MHC molecule.

Most CD8 molecules exist as disulfide-linked heterodimers composed of two related chains called CD8α and CD8β (see Fig. 7–8). Both the α chain and the β chain have a single extracellular Ig domain, a hydrophobic transmembrane region, and a highly basic cytoplasmic tail about 25 amino acids long. The Ig domain of CD8 binds to the nonpolymorphic α3 domain of class I MHC molecules. Some T cells express CD8 αα homodimers, but this different form appears to function like the more common CD8 αβ heterodimers.

Functions of CD4 and CD8

The selective binding of CD4 to class II MHC molecules and of CD8 to class I MHC molecules ensures that CD4[+] T cells respond to class II–associated peptide antigens

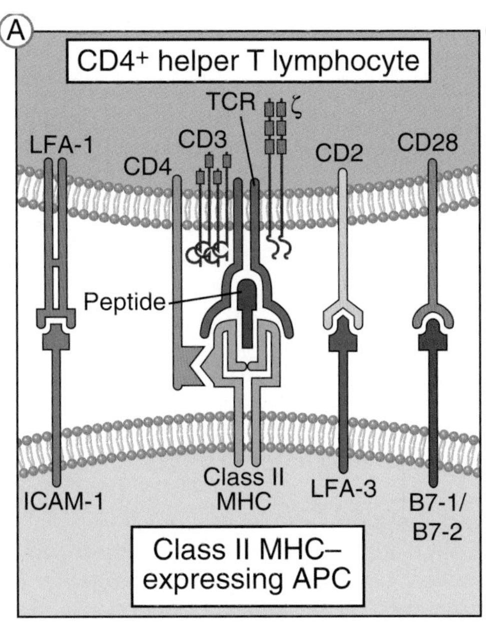

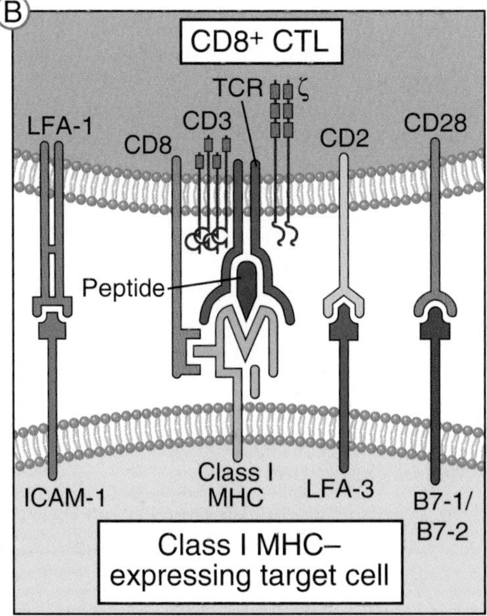

FIGURE 7–7 Accessory molecules of T lymphocytes. The interaction of a CD4[+] helper T cell with an APC (A), or of a CD8[+] CTL with a target cell (B), involves multiple T cell membrane proteins that recognize different ligands on the APC or target cell. Only selected accessory molecules and their ligands are illustrated. CD4 and CD8 are coreceptors. CD28 is the prototypical costimulatory receptor, and the LFA-1 integrin is an adhesion molecule that may also have signaling functions. APC, antigen-presenting cell.

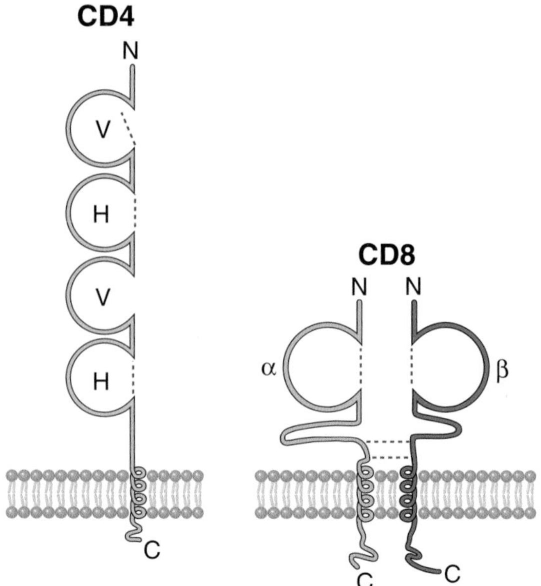

FIGURE 7–8 A schematic view of the structure of the CD4 and CD8 coreceptors. The CD4 protein is an integral membrane monomer consisting of four extracellular Ig domains, a transmembrane domain, and a cytoplasmic tail. The CD8 protein is either a disulfide-linked αβ integral membrane heterodimer or a disulfide linked αα homodimer (not shown). Each chain has a single extracellular Ig domain. The cytoplasmic portions of both CD4 and CD8 can associate with Lck (not shown).

and CD8⁺ T cells respond to class I–associated peptides. In Chapter 6, we described the processes by which class I and class II MHC molecules present peptides derived from intracellular (cytosolic) and extracellular (endocytosed) protein antigens, respectively. The segregation of CD4⁺ and CD8⁺ T cell responses to these different pools of antigens occurs because of the specificities of CD4 and CD8 for different classes of MHC molecules. CD4 binds to class II MHC molecules and is expressed on T cells whose TCRs recognize complexes of peptide and class II MHC molecules. Most CD4⁺ class II–restricted T cells are cytokine-producing helper cells and function in host defense against extracellular microbes that are ingested by macrophages or need to be recognized by antibodies in order to be cleared. CD8 binds to class I MHC molecules and is expressed on T cells whose TCRs recognize complexes of peptide and class I MHC molecules. Most CD8⁺ class I–restricted T cells are CTLs, which serve to eradicate infections by intracellular microbes that reside in the cytoplasm of infected cells. Some CD4⁺ T cells, especially in humans, function as CTLs, but even these are class II restricted. The physiologic importance of this segregation was discussed in Chapter 6 (see Fig. 6–17).

The essential roles of CD4 and CD8 in the functional responses of T cells have been demonstrated by many types of experiments.

- Antibodies specific for CD4 selectively block the stimulation of class II MHC–restricted T cells by antigen and APCs, and antibodies to CD8 selectively block killing of target cells by class I MHC–restricted CTLs.
- Formal proof of the obligatory function of these molecules came from gene transfection experiments. For example, if the TCR α and β genes are isolated from a CD4⁺ T cell clone and transfected into another T cell line that does not express CD4, the TCR-expressing transfected line will not respond to APCs bearing the relevant class II MHC–associated antigen. Responsiveness is restored if the CD4 gene is cotransfected along with the TCR genes. The same type of experiment has established the importance of CD8 in the responses of class I–restricted T cells.
- An APC lacking MHC molecules cannot present antigen to or activate T cells. The ability to activate T cells is restored by transfecting into the APC normal MHC molecules but not by transfecting MHC molecules in which the CD4-binding or CD8-binding nonpolymorphic domain is mutated.
- Knockout mice lacking CD4 or CD8 do not contain mature class II–restricted or class I–restricted T cells, respectively, because these coreceptors play essential roles in the maturation of T cells in the thymus (see Chapter 8).

CD4 and CD8 participate in the early signal transduction events that occur after T cell recognition of peptide-MHC complexes on APCs. These signal-transducing functions are mediated by a T cell–specific Src family tyrosine kinase called Lck that is noncovalently but tightly associated with the cytoplasmic tails of both CD4 and CD8. CD4/CD8-associated Lck is required for the maturation and activation of T cells, as demonstrated by studies with knockout mice and mutant cell lines.

- Disruption of the *lck* gene in mice leads to a block in T cell maturation, like the maturational arrest caused by deletion of CD4 and CD8 (see Chapter 8).
- In T cell lines or in knockout mice lacking CD4, normal T cell responses or maturation can be restored by reintroducing and expressing a wild-type CD4 gene but not by expressing a mutant form of CD4 that does not bind Lck.

When a T cell recognizes peptide-MHC complexes via its antigen receptor, simultaneous interaction of CD4 or CD8 with the MHC molecule brings the coreceptor and its associated Lck close to the TCR complex. Lck then phosphorylates tyrosine residues in the ITAMs of CD3 and ζ chains, thus initiating the T cell activation cascade (see Chapter 9). In addition to its physiologic roles, CD4 is a receptor for the human immunodeficiency virus (see Chapter 20).

Costimulatory and Inhibitory Receptors of the CD28 Family

CD28 is a membrane protein that transduces signals that function together with signals delivered by the TCR complex to activate naive T cells. A general property of naive T and B lymphocytes is that they need two distinct extracellular signals to initiate their proliferation and differentiation into effector cells. This two-signal concept was introduced in Chapter 1. The first signal is provided by antigen binding to the antigen receptor and is responsible for ensuring the specificity of the subsequent immune response. In the case of T cells, binding of peptide-MHC complexes to the TCR (and to the CD4 or CD8 coreceptor) provides signal 1. The second signal for T cell activation is provided by molecules that are collectively called **costimulators** (Fig. 7–9).

The best defined costimulators for T lymphocytes are a pair of related proteins, called B7–1 (CD80) and B7–2 (CD86), that are expressed on dendritic cells, macrophages, and B lymphocytes. These B7 costimulators on APCs are recognized by specific receptors on T cells. The first of these receptors for B7 to be discovered was the **CD28** molecule, which is expressed on more than 90% of CD4$^+$ T cells and on 50% of CD8$^+$ T cells in humans (and on all naive T cells in mice). CD28 is a disulfide-linked homodimer, each subunit of which has a single extracellular Ig domain. Binding of B7 molecules on APCs to CD28 delivers signals to the T cells that induce the expression of anti-apoptotic proteins, stimulate production of growth factors and other cytokines, and promote T cell proliferation and differentiation. Thus, ***CD28 is the principal costimulatory receptor for delivering second signals for T cell activation.*** A second receptor for B7 molecules was discovered later and called CTLA-4 (CD152). CTLA-4 is structurally homologous to CD28, but CTLA-4 is expressed on recently activated CD4$^+$ and CD8$^+$ T cells, and its function is to inhibit T cell activation by counteracting signals delivered by the TCR complex and CD28. Thus, CTLA-4 is involved in terminating T cell responses. How two receptors regulate responses in opposite ways even though they recognize the same B7 molecules on APCs is an intriguing question and an issue of active research.

Several other T cell surface molecules have recently been discovered that are homologous to CD28 and bind to ligands that are homologous to B7 molecules (see Chapter 9, Box 9–2). Some members of the CD28 family, such as CD28 itself and ICOS (inducible costimulator), provide activating signals, while others, such as CTLA-4 and PD-1, inhibit T cell responses. These costimulatory and inhibitory signals may serve different roles in various types of immune responses. We will discuss other members of the B7 family of ligands and the CD28 family of receptors, and the mechanisms and biologic significance of costimulation and inhibitory signals, in more detail in Chapter 9, when we describe the activation of T lymphocytes.

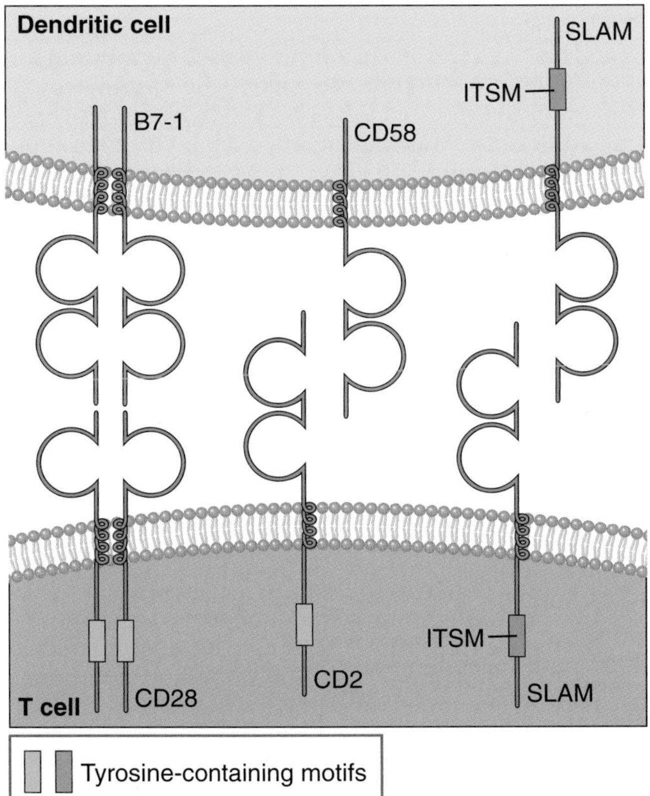

FIGURE 7–9 Selected costimulatory receptors of the CD28 and CD2 families and their ligands. The CD28 costimulatory receptor is a disulfide-linked homodimer on the T cell surface that binds to B7-1 on APCs or to B7-2 (not shown). The cytoplasmic tail of CD28 contains a tyrosine-based motif. CD2 and SLAM contain two extracellular Ig-like domains and their cytoplasmic tails also contain tyrosine-containing motifs. The tyrosine-based motif in the tail regions of SLAM and SLAM family members is called an ITSM, and binds to SAP or SAP-like proteins (not shown).

CD2 AND THE SLAM FAMILY OF COSTIMULATORY RECEPTORS

Although the best studied and most prominent family of costimulatory receptors on T cells is the CD28 family, other proteins also contribute to optimal T cell activation and differentiation. One important family of proteins that plays a role in the activation of T cells and NK cells is a group of proteins structurally related to a receptor called **CD2.** CD2 is a glycoprotein present on more than 90% of mature T cells, on 50% to 70% of thymocytes, and on NK cells. The molecule contains two extracellular Ig domains, a hydrophobic transmembrane region, and a long (116 amino acid residues) cytoplasmic tail. The principal ligand for CD2 in humans is a molecule called leukocyte function-associated antigen-3 (LFA-3, or CD58), also a member of the CD2 family. LFA-3 is expressed on a wide variety of hematopoietic and nonhematopoietic cells, either as an integral membrane protein or as a phosphatidyl inositol–anchored membrane molecule. In mice, the principal ligand for CD2 is CD48, which is also a member of the CD2 family and is distinct from but structurally similar to LFA-3.

CD2 is an example of an accessory molecule that functions both as an intercellular adhesion molecule and as a signal transducer.

- Some anti-CD2 antibodies increase cytokine secretion by and proliferation of human T cells cultured with anti-TCR/CD3 antibodies, indicating that CD2 signals can enhance TCR-triggered T cell responses.

- Some anti-CD2 antibodies block conjugate formation between T cells and other LFA-3–expressing cells, indicating that CD2 binding to LFA-3 also promotes cell-cell adhesion. Such antibodies inhibit both CTL activity and antigen-dependent helper T cell responses.
- Knockout mice lacking both CD28 and CD2 have more profound defects in T cell responses than do mice lacking either molecule alone. This indicates that CD28 and CD2 may compensate for each other, an example of the redundancy of accessory molecules of T cells.

On the basis of such findings, anti-CD2 antibodies are currently used in the therapy of psoriasis.

A distinct subgroup of the CD2 family of proteins is known as the **SLAM** (signaling lymphocytic activation molecule) family. SLAM, like all members of the CD2 family, is an integral membrane protein that contains two extracellular Ig domains and a relatively long cytoplasmic tail. The cytoplasmic tail of SLAM, but not of CD2, contains a specific tyrosine-based motif known as an immunoreceptor tyrosine-based switch motif (ITSM) that is distinct from the ITAM motif found on signaling proteins that are components of antigen receptor complexes, but is more like the ITIM (immune receptor tyrosine-based inhibitory motif) found in other inhibitory receptors. The Ig domains on SLAM are involved in homophilic interactions. SLAM on a T cell can interact with SLAM on a dendritic cell, and as a result the cytoplasmic tail of SLAM may deliver signals to T cells. The ITSM motif binds to an adapter called SAP (SLAM-associated protein) that contains an SH2 domain, and forms a bridge between SLAM and Fyn (a Src family kinase that is also linked to CD3). SLAM and other members of the SLAM family function as costimulatory receptors in T cells, NK cells, and some B cells. As we shall see in Chapter 20, mutations in SAP are the cause of a disease called the X-linked lymphoproliferative syndrome (XLP).

An important member of the SLAM family in NK cells, CD8 T cells, and $\gamma\delta$ T cells is called **2B4.** Unlike SLAM, 2B4 does not bind to other 2B4 molecules, but recognizes a known ligand for CD2 called CD48. Like SLAM, the cytoplasmic tail of 2B4 contains an ITSM motif, binds to the SAP adapter protein, and signals by recruiting Fyn. Defective 2B4 signaling may contribute in a major way to the immune deficit in XLP patients.

Other Accessory Molecules on T Cells

T lymphocytes express many other molecules that are involved in their activation, their migration, their effector functions, and their regulation. Not all fit into the categories of coreceptors, costimulators, and adhesion molecules. We consider a few other accessory proteins of T cells in this section.

CD44 is an acidic sulfated membrane glycoprotein expressed in several alternatively spliced and variably glycosylated forms on a variety of cell types, including mature T cells, thymocytes, B cells, granulocytes, macrophages, erythrocytes, and fibroblasts. Recently activated and memory T cells express higher levels of CD44 than do naive T cells. CD44 binds hyaluronate, and this property is responsible for the retention of T cells in extravascular tissues at sites of infection and for the binding of activated and memory T cells to endothelium at sites of inflammation and in mucosal tissues (see Chapter 13).

Activated $CD4^+$ T cells express a trimeric surface protein of the TNF family called **CD40 ligand** (CD40L or CD154), which binds to CD40 on B lymphocytes, macrophages, dendritic cells, and endothelial cells and activates these cells. Thus, CD40L is an important mediator of many of the effector functions of helper T cells, such as the stimulation of B cells to produce antibodies, the activation of dendritic cells during the initiation of cell-mediated immunity, and the activation of macrophages to destroy phagocytosed microbes. The role of CD40:CD40L interactions in humoral immune responses is discussed in Chapter 10 and in cell-mediated immunity in Chapter 13.

Activated T cells also express a trimeric ligand for the death receptor Fas (CD95). Engagement of Fas by **Fas ligand** on T cells results in apoptosis and is important for eliminating T cells that are repeatedly stimulated by antigens (see Chapter 11, Box 11–2). Fas ligand also provides one of the mechanisms by which CTLs kill their targets (see Chapter 13).

Activated T cells secrete cytokines, which function as growth and differentiation factors for the T cells and act on many other cell populations. Activated T cells also express receptors for many of these cytokines. We will discuss these effector molecules in later sections of the book when we describe the biologic responses and effector functions of T lymphocytes.

SUMMARY

- The functional responses of T cells are initiated by the recognition of peptide-MHC complexes on the surfaces of APCs. These responses require specific antigen recognition, stable adhesion between the T cells and APCs, and delivery of activating signals to the T cells. The various components of T cell responses to antigens are mediated by distinct sets of molecules expressed on the T cells.
- MHC-restricted T cells use clonally distributed TCRs to recognize peptide-MHC complexes on APCs. These TCRs are composed of two disulfide-linked polypeptide chains, called TCR α and β, that are homologous to the heavy and light chains of Ig

molecules. Each chain of the αβ TCR consists of a V region and a C region.

- The V segment of each TCR chain contains three hypervariable (complementarity-determining) regions, which form the portions of the receptor that recognize complexes of processed peptide antigens and MHC molecules. During T cell antigen recognition, the TCR makes contact with amino acid residues of the peptide as well as with polymorphic residues of the presenting self MHC molecules, accounting for the dual recognition of peptide and self MHC molecules.

- The γδ TCR is another clonally distributed heterodimer that is expressed on a small subset of αβ-negative T cells. These γδ T cells are not MHC restricted, and they recognize different forms of antigen than αβ T cells do, including lipids and some small molecules presented by nonpolymorphic MHC-like molecules.

- The αβ (and γδ) heterodimers are noncovalently associated with four invariant membrane proteins, three of which are components of CD3; the fourth is the ζ chain. The oligomeric assembly of the TCR, CD3, and ζ chain makes up the TCR complex. When the αβ TCR binds peptide-MHC complexes, the CD3 and ζ proteins transduce signals that initiate the process of T cell activation.

- In addition to expressing the TCR complex, T cells express several accessory molecules that are important in antigen-induced activation. Some of these molecules bind ligands on APCs or target cells and thereby provide stabilizing adhesive forces, and others transduce activating signals to the T cells.

- CD4 and CD8 are coreceptors expressed on mutually exclusive subsets of mature T cells that bind nonpolymorphic regions of class II and class I MHC molecules, respectively. CD4 is expressed on class II–restricted helper T cells, and CD8 is expressed on class I–restricted CTLs. When T cells recognize peptide-MHC complexes, CD4 and CD8 deliver signals that are critical for initiating T cell responses.

- CD28 is a receptor on T cells that binds to B7 costimulatory molecules expressed on professional APCs. CD28 delivers signals, often called signal 2, that are required in addition to TCR complex-generated signals (signal 1) for full T cell activation. A second receptor for B7, called CTLA-4, is induced after T cell activation and functions to inhibit responses.

- The CD2 family of receptors includes proteins such as CD2 and SLAM that provide additional activating signals to T cells.

Selected Readings

Bjorkman PJ. MHC restriction in three dimensions: a view of T cell receptor/ligand interactions. Cell 89:167–170, 1997.

Born WK, CL Reardon, and RL O'Brien. The function of gammadelta T cells in innate immunity. Current Opinion in Immunology 18:31–38, 2006.

Call ME, and KW Wucherpfennig. Common themes in the assembly and architecture of activating immune receptors. Nature Reviews Immunology 7:841–850, 2007.

Davis SJ, S Ikemizu, EJ Evans, L Fugger, TR Bakker, and PA van der Merwe. The nature of molecular recognition by T cells. Nature Immunology 4:217–224, 2003.

Hennecke J, and DC Wiley. T cell receptor-MHC interactions up close. Cell 104:1–4, 2001.

Kuhns MS, MM Davis, and KC Garcia. Deconstructing the form and function of the TCR/CD3 complex. Immunity 24:133–139, 2006.

Malissen B. An evolutionary and structural perspective on T cell antigen receptor function. Immunological Reviews 191:7–27, 2003.

Rudolph MG, RL Stanfield, and IA Wilson. How TCRs bind MHCs, peptides, and coreceptors. Annual Review of Immunology 24:419–466, 2006.

Veillette A. Immune regulation by SLAM family receptors and SAP related adaptors. Nature Reviews Immunology 6:56–66. 2006.

Wang JH, and EL Reinherz. Structural basis of T cell recognition of peptides bound to MHC molecules. Molecular Immunology 38:1039–1049, 2002.

Section III

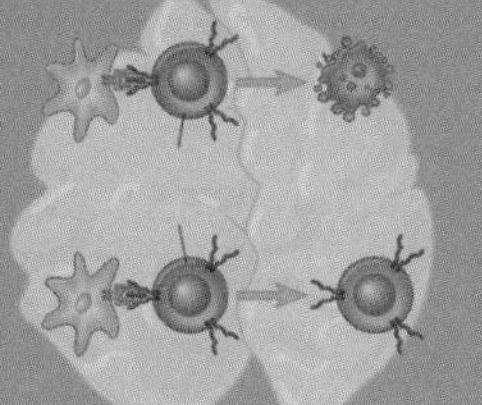

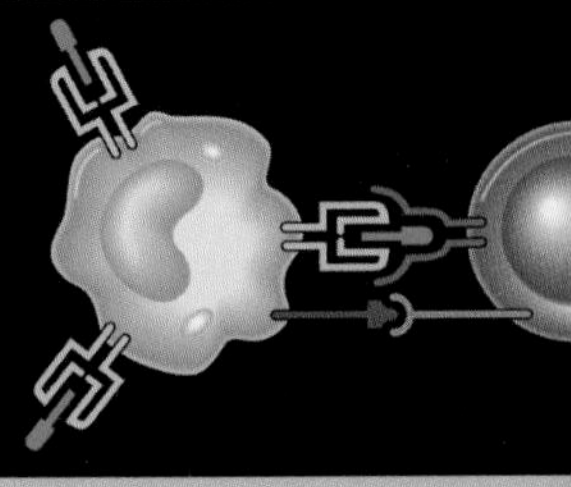

Maturation, Activation, and Regulation of Lymphocytes

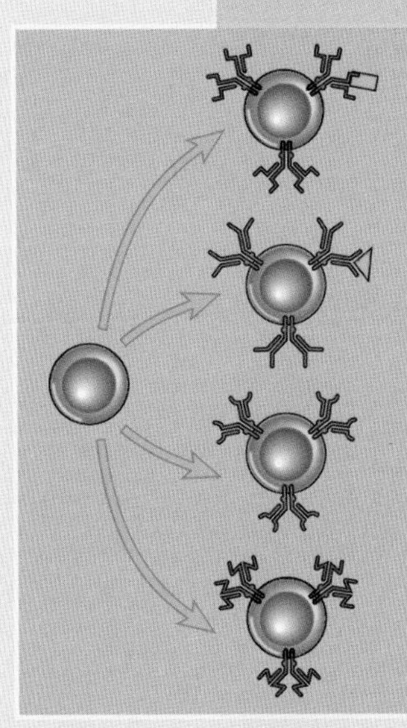

The activation of lymphocytes by foreign antigens is the central event in adaptive immune responses. Much of the science of immunology is devoted to studying the biology of B and T lymphocytes. In this section of the book, we focus on the generation of mature lymphocytes and the responses of these lymphocytes to antigen recognition.

Chapter 8 describes the development of B and T lymphocytes from uncommitted progenitors, with an emphasis on the molecular basis of the expression of antigen receptors and the generation of diverse lymphocyte repertoires. In Chapter 9, we discuss the biology and biochemistry of T lymphocyte activation. Chapter 10 deals with the activation of B lymphocytes and the mechanisms that lead to the production of antibodies against different types of antigens. In Chapter 11, we discuss the phenomenon of immunological tolerance and the mechanisms that control immune responses and maintain homeostasis in the immune system.

Chapter 8

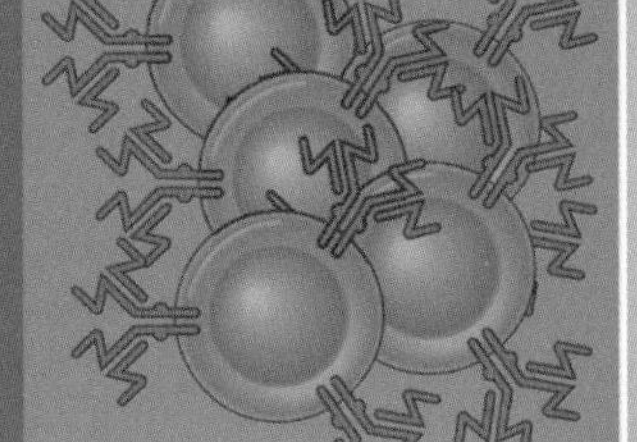

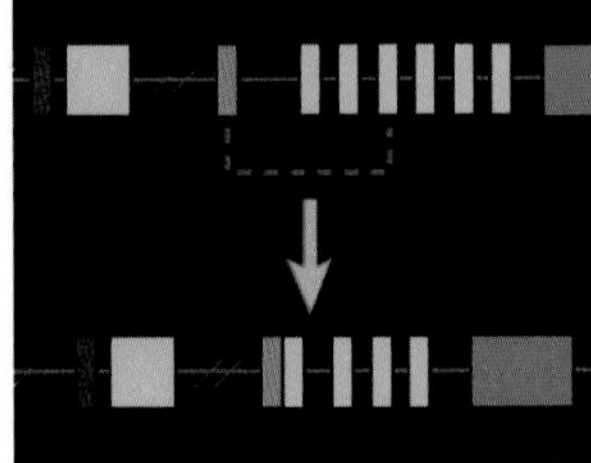

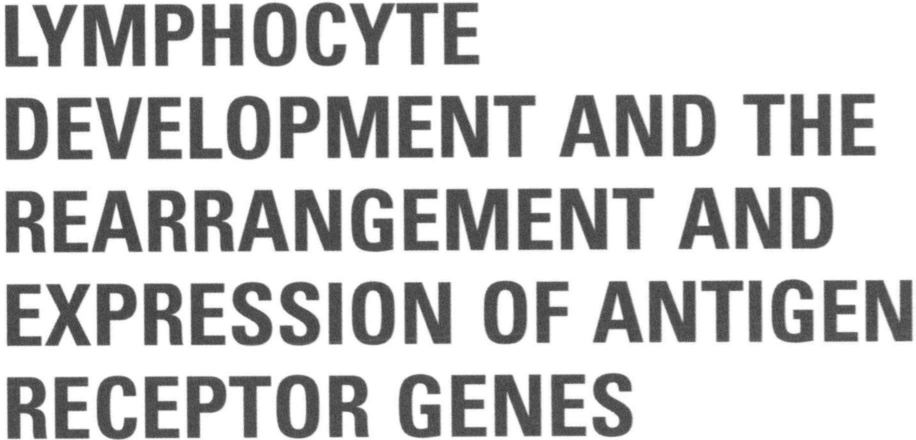

LYMPHOCYTE DEVELOPMENT AND THE REARRANGEMENT AND EXPRESSION OF ANTIGEN RECEPTOR GENES

Lymphocytes express highly diverse antigen receptors capable of recognizing a wide variety of foreign substances. This diversity is generated during the development of mature B and T lymphocytes from precursor cells that do not express antigen receptors and cannot recognize and respond to antigens. The process by which lymphocyte progenitors in central lymphoid organs such as the thymus and bone marrow differentiate into mature lymphocytes that populate peripheral lymphoid tissues is called **lymphocyte development** or **lymphocyte maturation.** The collection of antigen receptors, and therefore specificities, expressed by B and T lymphocytes makes up the **immune repertoire.** During maturation, specific cell surface receptors are triggered to initiate a program of sequential gene expression that commits developing cells to a B or a T cell fate, drives the proliferation of progenitors, and initiates the rearrangement of antigen receptor genes.

The rearrangement and expression of antigen receptor genes is a central feature of lymphocyte development, and very similar molecular and cellular events characterize the early development of B and T cells. We begin this chapter by considering the process of commitment to the B and T lymphocyte lineages and discuss some common principles of B and T cell development. This is followed by a description of the processes that are unique to the maturation of B cells and then of those unique to the development of cells of the T lymphocyte lineage.

Overview of Lymphocyte Development

The maturation of B and T lymphocytes involves a series of events that occur in the generative (central) lymphoid organs (Fig. 8–1):

- The **commitment** of progenitor cells to the B or T cell lineage
- A temporally ordered process of **rearrangement of antigen receptor genes** and expression of antigen receptor proteins
- **Selection events** that preserve cells that have produced correct antigen receptor proteins and eliminate potentially dangerous cells that strongly recognize self antigens. These developmental checkpoints ensure that only lymphocytes that express functional receptors with useful specificities will mature and enter the peripheral immune system.
- **Proliferation** of progenitors and immature committed cells at specific early stages of development, providing a large pool of cells that can generate useful lymphocytes
- **Differentiation of B and T cells into functionally and phenotypically distinct subpopulations.** B cells develop into follicular, marginal zone and B-1 B cells, and T cells develop into $CD4^+$ helper and $CD8^+$ cytotoxic T lymphocytes and γδ T cells (see Chapter 3). This differentiation into distinct classes provides the specialization that is characteristic of the adaptive immune system.

After the generation of a diverse lymphoid repertoire in central lymphoid organs, naive lymphocytes acquire the ability to re-circulate and subsequently move from one secondary lymphoid organ to the next in search of antigen.

Commitment to the B and T Cell Lineages

Pluripotent stem cells in the bone marrow (and fetal liver), generally referred to as hematopoietic stem cells (HSCs), give rise to all lineages of blood cells, including cells of the lymphocyte lineage. HSCs mature into common lymphoid progenitors (CLPs) that can give rise to B cells, T cells, NK cells, and some dendritic cells (Fig. 8–2). The maturation of B cells from progenitors committed to this lineage proceeds mostly in the bone marrow, and before birth, in the fetal liver. Fetal liver derived stem cells give rise mainly to a type of B cell called a B-1 B cell, whereas bone marrow derived HSCs give rise to the majority of circulating B cells (follicular B cells). Precursors of T lymphocytes leave the fetal liver before birth and the bone marrow later in life, and circulate to the thymus, where they complete their maturation. Most γδ T cells arise from fetal liver HSCs, and the majority of T cells, which are αβ T cells, develop from bone marrow derived HSCs. In general, less diverse B and T cells are generated early in fetal life. Despite their different anatomic locations, the early maturation events of both B and T lymphocytes are fundamentally similar.

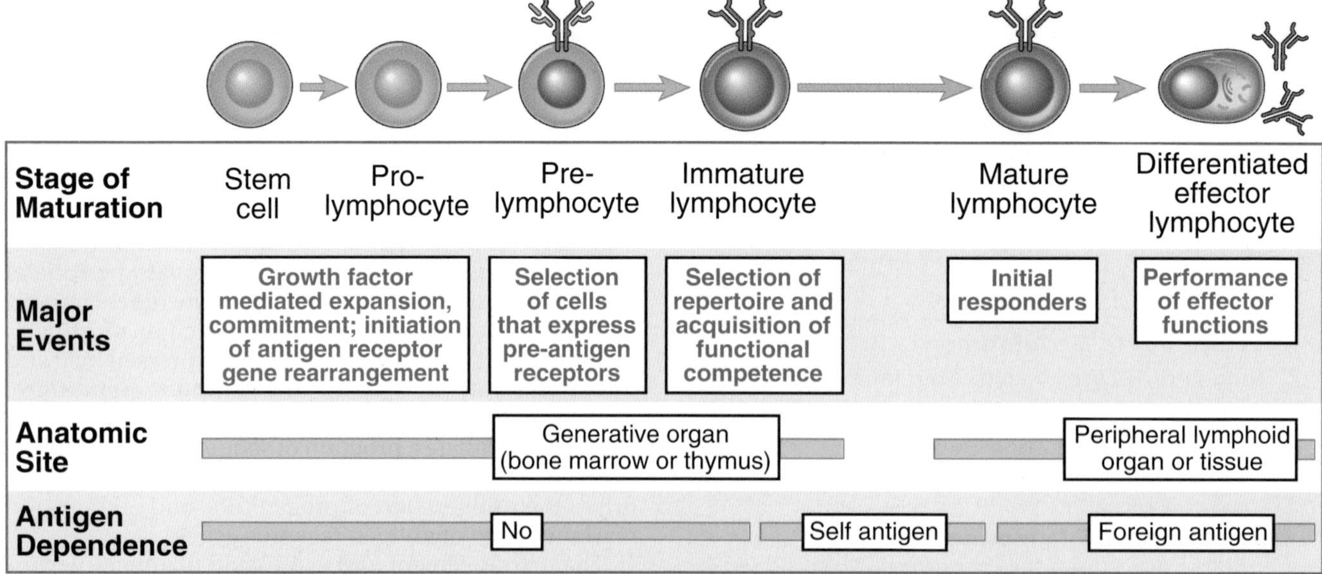

FIGURE 8–1 Stages of lymphocyte maturation. Development of both B and T lymphocytes involves the sequence of maturational stages shown. B cell maturation is illustrated, but the basic stages of T cell maturation are similar.

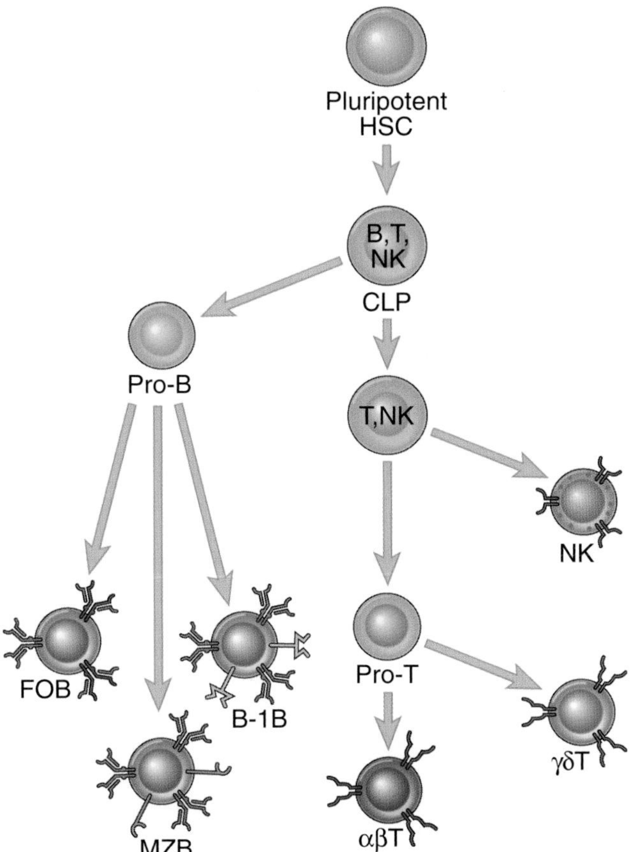

FIGURE 8–2 Pluripotent stem cells give rise to distinct B and T lineages. Hematopoietic stem cells (HSCs) give rise to distinct progenitors for various types of blood cells. One of these progenitor populations (shown here) is called a common lymphoid progenitor (CLP). CLPs give rise mainly to B and T cells but may also contribute to NK cells and some dendritic cells (not depicted here). Pro-B cells can eventually differentiate into follicular (FO) B cells, marginal zone (MZ) B cells, and B-1 B cells. Pro-T cells may commit to either the αβ or γδ T cell lineages.

Commitment to the B or T lineage depends on instructions received from the cell surface, followed by the induction of specific transcriptional regulators that drive a CLP to specifically assume a B cell or a T cell fate. The cell surface receptors and nuclear transcription factors that contribute to commitment will be described later in the chapter.

Early B and T cell development is characterized by the proliferation of progenitors, stimulated mainly by the cytokine interleukin-7(IL-7), resulting in marked increases in cell numbers. Proliferation ensures that a large enough pool of progenitor cells will be generated to eventually provide a highly diverse repertoire of antigen-specific lymphocytes. IL-7 is produced by stromal cells in the bone marrow and thymus. Mice with targeted mutations in either the IL-7 gene or the IL-7 receptor gene have profound deficiencies in mature T and B cells and little maturation of lymphocyte precursors beyond the earliest stages. Mutations in a chain of the IL-7 receptor, called the common γ chain because it is shared by several cytokine receptors, give rise to an immunodeficiency disorder in humans called X-linked severe combined immunodeficiency disease. This disease is characterized by a block mainly in T cell development, since human B cell progenitors proliferate in the absence of IL-7 signals (see Chapter 20). The proliferative activity in early lymphocyte development, driven mainly by IL-7, ceases before receptor gene rearrangement has been completed. Subsequent survival and proliferation of maturing lymphocytes are dependent on signals from the pre-B cell receptor and pre-T cell receptor. In fact, the greatest expansion of the B and T cell lineages occurs as a consequence of pre-antigen receptor signaling. This is an important checkpoint in development, because only cells that express functional receptors can proceed to the next stage.

Antigen Receptor Gene Rearrangement and Expression

The rearrangement of antigen receptor genes is the key event in lymphocyte development that drives the generation of a diverse repertoire. Antigen receptor gene products also provide signals that ensure the selective survival of lymphocytes with useful specificities. As we discussed in Chapters 4 and 7, each clone of B or T lymphocytes produces an antigen receptor with a unique antigen-binding structure. In any individual there may be 10^7 or more different B and T lymphocyte clones, each with a unique receptor. The ability of each individual to generate these enormously diverse lymphocyte repertoires has evolved in a way that does not require an equally large number of distinct antigen receptor genes; otherwise, a large proportion of the mammalian genome would be devoted to encoding immunoglobulin (Ig) and T cell receptor (TCR) molecules. Functional antigen receptor genes are produced in immature B cells in the bone marrow and in immature T cells in the thymus by a process of gene rearrangement, which is designed to generate a large number of variable region encoding exons using a relatively small fraction of the genome. In any given developing lymphocyte, one of many variable region gene segments is randomly selected and joined to a downstream DNA segment. This process involves the generation of site-specific double-strand breaks and the repair of these breaks by a mechanism known as nonhomologous end joining. The diversity of the lymphocyte repertoire is further enhanced by randomly adding and removing nucleotides during the joining of different gene segments. The DNA rearrangement events that lead to the production of antigen receptors are not dependent on, or influenced by, the presence of antigens. In other words, as the clonal selection hypothesis had proposed, antigen receptors are expressed before encounter with antigens. We will discuss the molecular details of antigen receptor gene rearrangement later in the chapter.

Selection Processes That Shape the B and T Lymphocyte Repertoires

Pre-antigen receptors and antigen receptors deliver signals to developing lymphocytes that are required

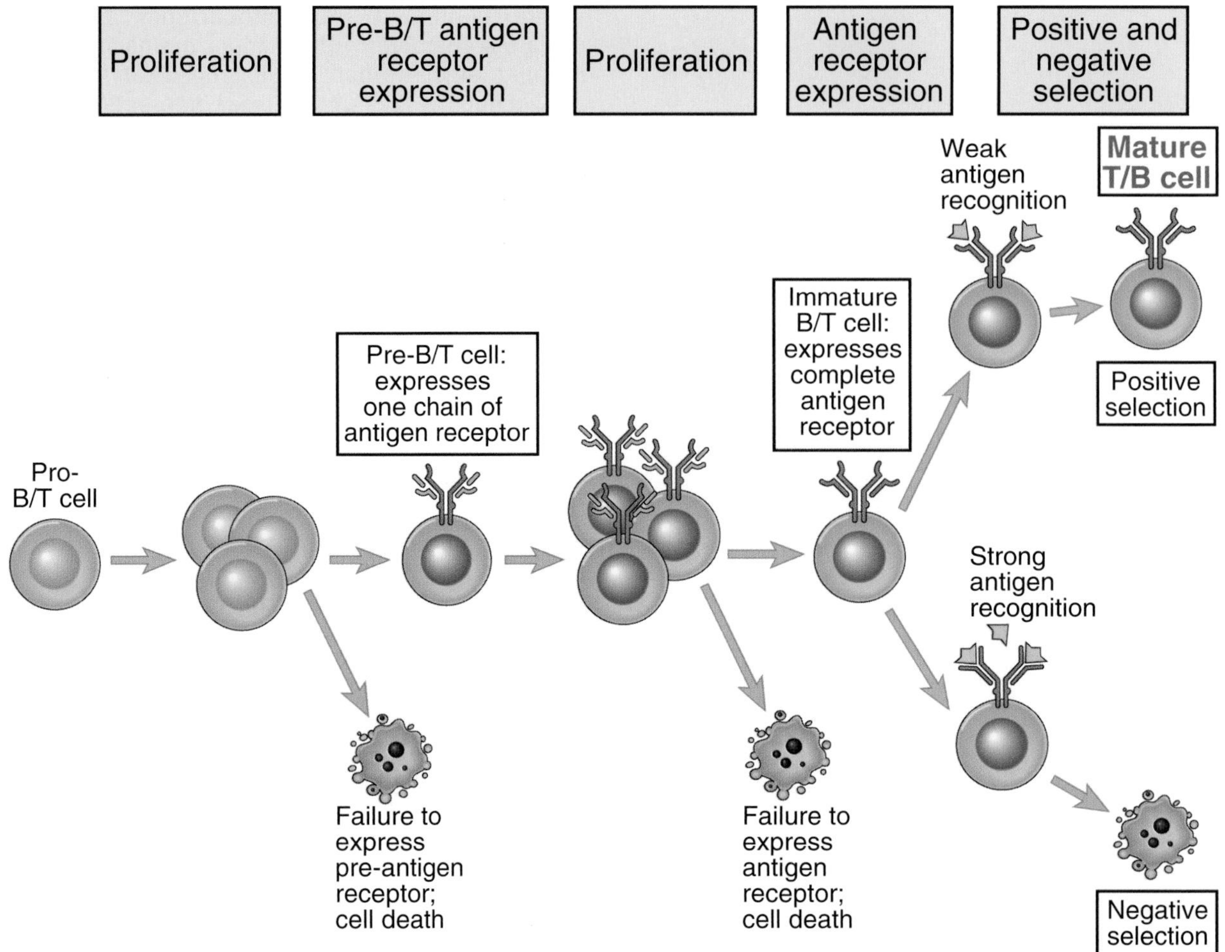

FIGURE 8–3 Checkpoints in lymphocyte maturation. During development, the lymphocytes that express receptors required for continued proliferation and maturation are selected to survive, and cells that do not express functional receptors die by apoptosis. Positive and negative selection further preserve cells with useful specificities. The presence of multiple checkpoints ensures that only cells with useful receptors complete their maturation.

for the survival of these cells and for their proliferation and continued maturation (Fig. 8–3). Immunoglobulin and T cell receptor gene rearrangement involves the random addition and removal of bases between gene segments being joined together in order to maximize diversity. Only about one in three developing B and T cells that rearranges an antigen receptor gene makes an in-frame rearrangement and is therefore capable of generating a proper full-length protein. In developing B cells, the first antigen receptor gene to be completely rearranged is the immunoglobulin heavy chain or IgH gene. In αβ T cells, the β chain of the TCR is rearranged first. Cells that successfully rearrange their Ig heavy chain genes express the Ig H chain protein and assemble a pre-antigen receptor known as the pre-B cell receptor. In an analogous fashion, developing T cells that make a productive TCR β chain gene rearrangement synthesize the TCR β chain protein and assemble a pre–antigen receptor known as the pre-TCR. In the absence of pre–antigen receptor expression, cells that make out-of-frame rearrangements at the Ig μ or TCR β chain loci undergo programmed cell death. It appears that assembled pre-BCR and pre-TCR complexes, in the absence of any known ligands, provide signals for survival, for proliferation, for the phenomenon of allelic exclusion discussed later, and for the further development of early B and T lineage cells.

Following the pre-antigen receptor checkpoint, lymphocytes develop further in central lymphoid organs and express the complete antigen receptor while they are still immature. At this immature stage, potentially harmful cells that avidly recognize self-structures may be eliminated or induced to alter their antigen receptors, and cells that express useful antigen receptors may be preserved (Fig. 8–4). The preservation of useful specificities involves a process called **positive selection.** In the T lineage, positive selection ensures the maturation of T cells whose receptors bind with low avidity (weakly) to self major histocompatibility complex (MHC) molecules. Mature T cells whose precursors were positively selected by self MHC molecules in the thymus are able to recognize foreign peptide antigens displayed by the same self MHC molecules on antigen-presenting cells in peripheral tissues. Positive selection provides survival

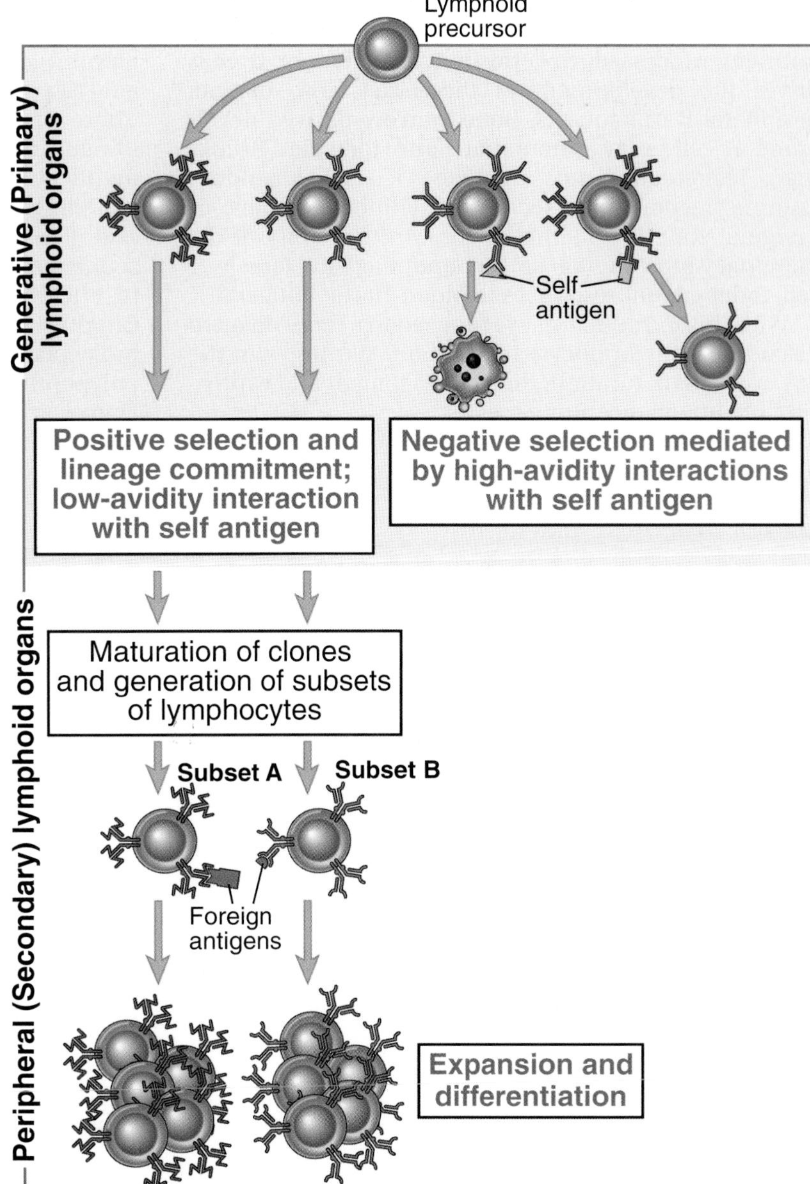

FIGURE 8–4 Selection processes in lymphocyte maturation. After immature clones of lymphocytes in generative lymphoid organs express antigen receptors, they are subject to both positive and negative selection processes. In positive selection, lymphocyte precursors with antigen receptors that bind some self ligand with low avidity are selected to survive and mature further. These positively selected lymphocytes enter peripheral lymphoid tissues, where they respond to foreign antigens. In negative selection, cells that bind antigens present within the generative organs, with high avidity, receive signals that either lead to cell death or induce further rearrangement of antigen receptor genes, a process known as receptor editing. As a result, the repertoire of mature lymphocytes lacks cells capable of responding to these self antigens. The diagram illustrates selection of B cells; the principles are the same for T lymphocytes, except that there is no receptor editing in the T lineage.

signals to both B and T lymphocytes that have properly rearranged both chains of their antigen receptors.

Negative selection is the process that eliminates or alters developing lymphocytes whose antigen receptors bind strongly to self antigens present in the generative lymphoid organs. Both developing B cells and developing T cells are susceptible to negative selection during a short period after antigen receptors are first expressed. Developing T cells with a high affinity for self-antigens are eliminated by apoptosis, a phenomenon known as **clonal deletion**. Strongly self-reactive immature B cells may be induced to make further Ig gene rearrangements and thus evade self-reactivity. This phenomenon is called **receptor editing.** Negative selection of developing lymphocytes is an important mechanism for maintaining tolerance to many self antigens; this is called central tolerance (see Chapter 11).

The Generation of Lymphocyte Subsets

Another important feature of lymphocyte development that appears to be mechanistically linked to positive selection is the generation of functionally distinct subsets in both the T and the B lineages (see Fig. 8–4). The process of positive selection provides lineage commitment signals to ensure that the $CD4^+$ and $CD8^+$ T lymphocyte subsets are properly matched to the appropriate class of MHC molecule the cells recognize. Precursors that express both CD4 and CD8 differentiate into either $CD4^+$ class II MHC-restricted T cells or $CD8^+$ class I MHC-restricted T cells. The $CD4^+$ cells that leave the thymus can be activated by antigens to differentiate into helper T cells whose effector functions are mediated by specific membrane proteins and by the production of cytokines. The $CD8^+$ cells can differentiate into cytotoxic T lymphocytes whose major effector function is to kill infected target cells. A similar lineage commitment process during positive selection of B cells drives the development of these cells into distinct peripheral B cell subsets. Bone marrow–derived developing B cells may differentiate into follicular B cells that recirculate and mediate T cell–dependent immune responses in secondary lymphoid organs, or marginal zone B cells that reside in the vicinity of the marginal sinus in the spleen and mediate largely T cell–independent responses to blood-borne antigens.

With this introduction, we proceed to a more detailed discussion of lymphocyte maturation, starting with the key event in maturation, the rearrangement and expression of antigen receptor genes.

Rearrangement of Antigen Receptor Genes in B and T Lymphocytes

The genes that encode diverse antigen receptors of B and T lymphocytes are generated by the rearrangement in individual lymphocytes of different variable (V) region gene segments with diversity (D) and/or joining (J) gene segments. A novel rearranged exon for each antigen receptor gene is generated by fusing a specific distant upstream V gene segment to a downstream segment on the same chromosome. This specialized process of site-specific gene rearrangement is called V(D)J recombination. (The terms *recombination* and *rearrangement* are used interchangeably.) Elucidation of the mechanisms of antigen receptor gene rearrangement, and therefore of the underlying basis for the generation of immune diversity, represents one of the landmark achievements of modern immunology.

The first insights into how millions of different antigen receptors could be generated from a limited amount of coding DNA in the genome came from analyses of the amino acid sequences of Ig molecules. These analyses showed that the polypeptide chains of many different antibodies of the same isotype shared identical sequences at their C-terminal ends (corresponding to the constant domains of antibody heavy and light chains) but differed considerably in the sequences at their N-terminal ends that correspond to the variable domains of immunoglobulins (see Chapter 4). Contrary to one of the central tenets of molecular genetics, enunciated as the "one gene—one polypeptide hypothesis" by Beadle and Tatum in 1941, Dreyer and Bennett postulated in 1965 that each antibody chain is actually encoded by at least two genes, one variable and the other constant, and that the two are physically combined at the level of DNA or of messenger RNA (mRNA) to eventually give rise to functional Ig proteins.

Formal proof of this hypothesis came more than a decade later when Susumu Tonegawa demonstrated that the structure of Ig genes in the cells of an antibody-producing tumor, called a myeloma or plasmacytoma, is different from that in embryonic tissues or in nonlymphoid tissues not committed to Ig production. These differences arise because during B cell development, there is a recombination of DNA sequences within the loci encoding Ig heavy and light chains. Furthermore, similar rearrangements occur during T cell development in the loci encoding the polypeptide chains of TCRs. Antigen receptor gene rearrangement is best understood by first describing the unrearranged, or germline, organization of Ig and TCR genes and then describing their rearrangement during lymphocyte maturation.

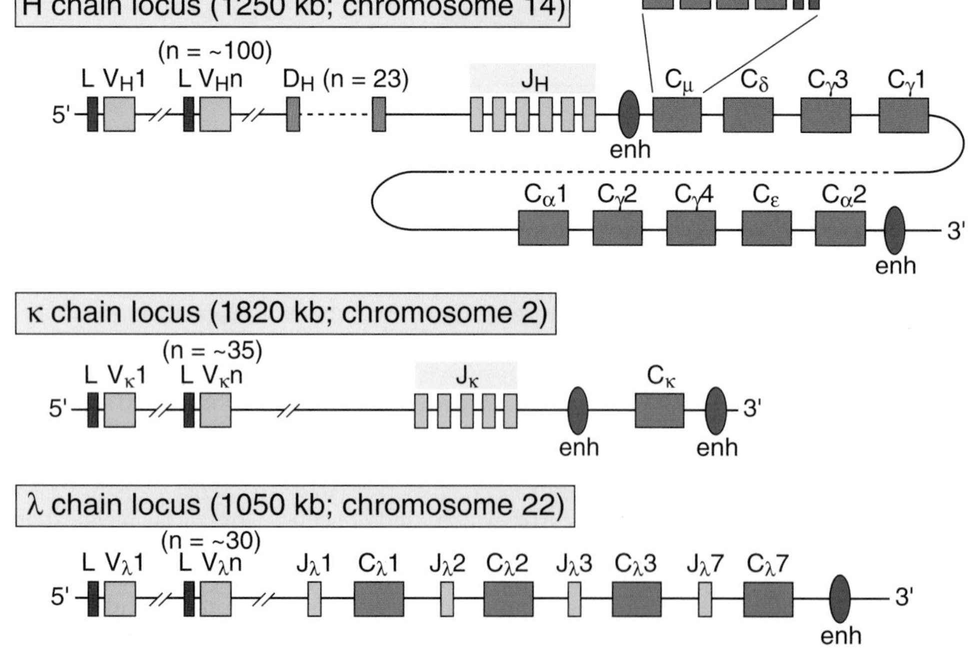

FIGURE 8–5 Germline organization of human Ig loci. The human heavy chain, κ light chain, and λ light chain loci are shown. Only functional genes are shown; pseudogenes have been omitted for simplicity. Exons and introns are not drawn to scale. Each C_H gene is shown as a single box but is composed of several exons, as illustrated for C_μ. Gene segments are indicated as follows: L, leader (often called signal sequence); V, variable; D, diversity; J, joining; C, constant; enh, enhancer.

Germline Organization of Ig and TCR Genes

The germline organizations of Ig and TCR genetic loci are fundamentally similar and are characterized by spatial segregation of sequences that must be joined together to produce functional genes coding for antigen receptor proteins. We first describe the Ig loci and then discuss the TCR loci in comparison.

Organization of Ig Gene Loci

Three separate loci encode, respectively, all the Ig heavy chains, the Ig κ light chain, and the Ig λ light chain. Each locus is on a different chromosome. The organization of human Ig genes is illustrated in Figure 8–5, and the relationship of gene segments after rearrangement to the domains of the Ig heavy and light chain proteins is shown in Figure 8–6A. Ig genes are organized in essentially the same way in all mammals, although their chromosomal locations and the number and sequence of different gene segments in each locus may vary. Each germline Ig locus is made up of multiple copies of at least two different types of gene segments, the V and J segments that lie upstream of constant (c) region exons. In addition, the Ig heavy chain locus has diversity (D) segments. Within each locus, the sets of each type of gene segment are separated from one another by stretches of noncoding DNA.

At the 5′ end of each of the Ig loci, there is a cluster of **V gene segments,** each V gene in the cluster being about 300 base pairs long. The numbers of V gene segments vary considerably among the different Ig loci and among different species. For example, there are about 35 V genes in the human κ light chain locus and about 100 functional genes in the human heavy chain locus, whereas the mouse λ light chain locus has only two V genes and the mouse heavy chain locus has more than 1000 V genes. The V gene segments for each locus are spaced over large stretches of DNA, up to 2000 kilobases long. Located 5′ of each V segment is a leader exon that encodes the 20 to 30 N-terminal residues of the translated protein. These residues are moderately hydrophobic and make up the leader (or signal) peptide. Signal sequences are found in all newly synthesized secreted and transmembrane proteins and are involved in guiding nascent polypeptides being generated on membrane-bound ribosomes into the lumen of the endoplasmic reticulum (ER). Here, the signal sequences are rapidly cleaved, and they are not present in the mature proteins. Upstream of each leader exon is a V gene promoter at which transcription can be initiated, but this occurs most efficiently, as discussed below, after rearrangement.

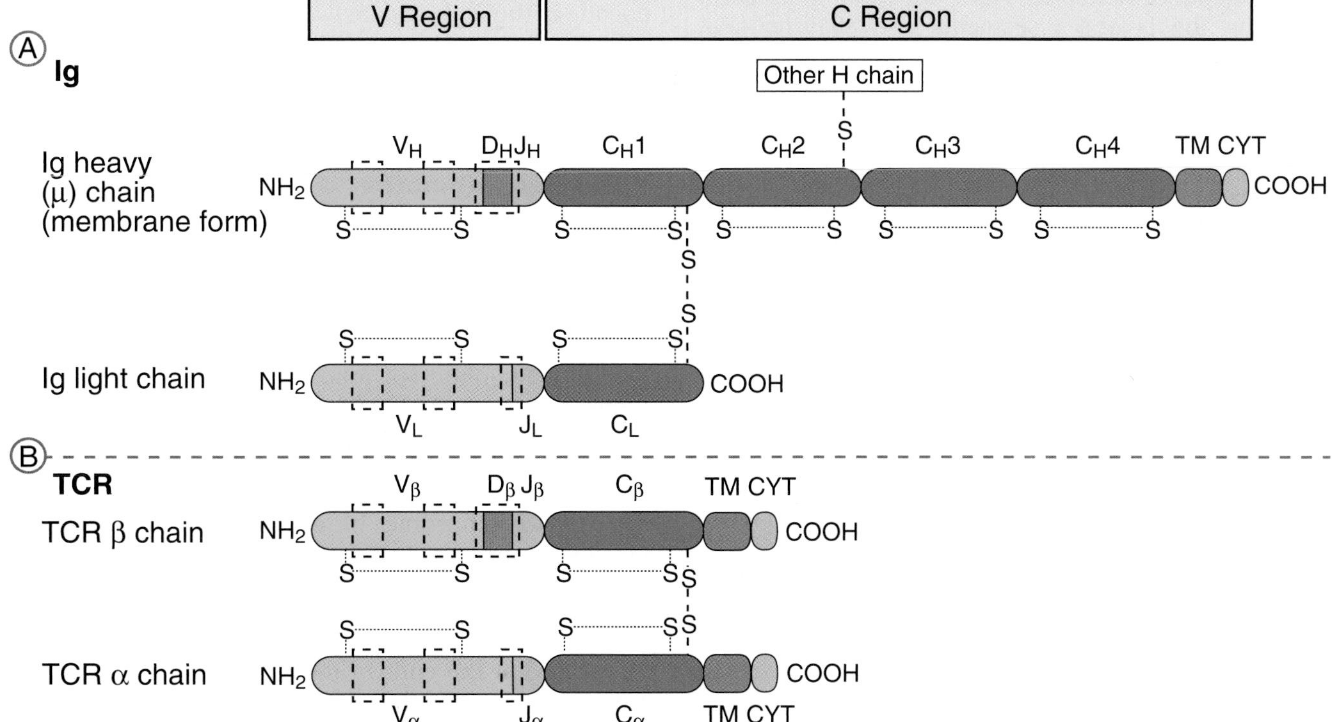

FIGURE 8–6 Domains of Ig and TCR proteins. The domains of Ig heavy and light chains are shown in A, and the domains of TCR α and β chains are shown in B. The relationships between the Ig and TCR gene segments and the domain structure of the antigen receptor polypeptide chains are indicated. The V and C regions of each polypeptide are encoded by different gene segments. The locations of intrachain and interchain disulfide bonds (S-S) are approximate. Areas in the dashed boxes are the hypervariable (complementarity-determining) regions. In the Ig μ chain and the TCR α and β chains, transmembrane (TM) and cytoplasmic (CYT) domains are encoded by separate exons.

At varying distances 3′ of the V genes are several **J segments** that are closely linked to downstream constant region exons. J segments are typically 30 to 50 base pairs long, separated by noncoding sequences. Between the V and J segments in the IgH locus there are additional segments know as D segments. In the human Ig heavy chain locus, 5′ of the entire array of C_H gene segments there is one cluster of 6 functional J segments and one cluster of more than 20 D segments. In the human κ chain locus, there is a cluster of five J segments 5′ of C_κ, and in the human λ locus, there is one J segment 5′ of each of the four functional C_λ genes.

Each Ig locus has a distinct arrangement and number of C region genes. In humans, the Ig κ light chain locus has a single C gene (C_κ) and the λ light chain locus has four functional C genes (C_λ). The Ig heavy chain locus has nine C genes (C_H), arranged in a tandem array, that encode the C regions of the nine different Ig isotypes and subtypes (see Chapter 4). The C_κ and C_λ genes are each composed of a single exon that encodes the entire C domain of the light chains. In contrast, each C_H gene is composed of five or six exons. Three or four exons (each similar in size to a V gene segment) encode the complete C region of each heavy chain isotype, and two smaller exons code for the carboxy-terminal ends of the membrane form of each Ig heavy chain, including the transmembrane and cytoplasmic domains of the heavy chains (see Fig. 8–6A).

In an Ig light chain protein (κ or λ), the V domain is encoded by the V and J gene segments, while in the Ig heavy chain protein, the V domain is encoded by the V, D, and J gene segments (see Fig. 8–6A). The VDJ junction including the D and J segments and all junctional residues in the case of IgH (and TCR β), or the VJ junction including the J segment and junctional sequences in the case of Ig light chains (or TCR α), make up the third hypervariable (also known as complementarity-determining) region (CDR3) of antibody molecules and TCRs. CDR1 and CDR2 are encoded in the germline on each V gene segment. The V and C domains of Ig (and TCR) molecules share structural features, including a tertiary structure called the Ig fold. As we discussed in Chapter 7, proteins that include this structure are members of the **Ig superfamily** (see Chapter 4, Box 4–2). On the basis of the tandem organization of V and C genes in each Ig or TCR locus, and the structural homologies between them, it is believed that these genes evolved from repeated duplication of a primordial gene. Each Ig domain of heavy and light chain proteins is encoded by a single exon.

Noncoding sequences in the Ig loci play important roles in recombination and gene expression. As we shall see later, sequences that dictate recombination of different gene segments are found adjacent to each coding segment in Ig genes. Also present are V gene promoters, and other cis-acting regulatory elements, such as locus control regions, enhancers, and silencers, which regulate gene expression at the level of transcription.

Organization of TCR Gene Loci

The genes encoding the TCR α chain, the TCR β chain, and the TCR γ chain map to three separate loci, and the TCR δ chain locus is contained within the TCR α locus (Fig. 8–7). Each germline TCR locus includes V, J, and C gene segments. In addition, TCR β and TCR δ loci also have D segments, like the Ig heavy chain locus. At the 5′ end of each of the TCR loci, there is a cluster of several **V gene segments,** arranged in a very similar way to the Ig V gene segments. Upstream of each TCR V gene is an exon that encodes a leader peptide, and upstream of each leader exon is a promoter for each V gene.

At varying distances 3′ of the TCR V genes are the **C region genes.** There are two C genes in each of the human TCR β (C_β) and TCR γ (C_γ) loci and only one C gene in each of the TCR α (C_α) and TCR δ (C_δ) loci. Each TCR C region gene is composed of four exons encoding the extracellular C region, a short hinge region, the transmembrane segment, and the cytoplasmic tail.

J segments are found immediately upstream of the C genes in all the TCR loci, and **D segments** are found only in the TCR β and TCR δ chain loci (which resemble the Ig heavy chain locus). Each human TCR C gene has its own associated 5′ cluster of J segments. In the TCR α or γ chains (analogous to Ig light chains), the V domain is encoded by the V and J exons, and in the TCR β and δ proteins, the V domain is encoded by the V, D, and J gene segments.

The relationship of the TCR gene segments and the corresponding portions of TCR proteins that they encode is shown in Figure 8–6B. As in Ig molecules, the TCR V and C domains assume an Ig fold tertiary structure, and thus the TCR is a member of the Ig superfamily of proteins.

V(D)J Recombination

The germline organization of Ig and TCR loci described in the preceding section exists in all cell types in the body. Germline genes cannot be transcribed into mRNA that gives rise to antigen receptor proteins. Functional antigen receptor genes are created only in developing B and T lymphocytes following DNA rearrangement events that bring randomly chosen V, (D), and J gene segments into contiguity. This recombinational process involves a number of sequential steps. Initially the chromatin must be opened in specific regions of the antigen receptor chromosome in order to make randomly selected gene segments accessible to the recombinational machinery. Recombination involves bringing together the appropriate gene segments across vast chromosomal distances. Double-strand breaks are then introduced at the ends of these segments, nucleotides are added or removed at the broken ends, and finally the processed ends are ligated to produce clonally unique but diverse antigen receptor genes that can be efficiently transcribed.

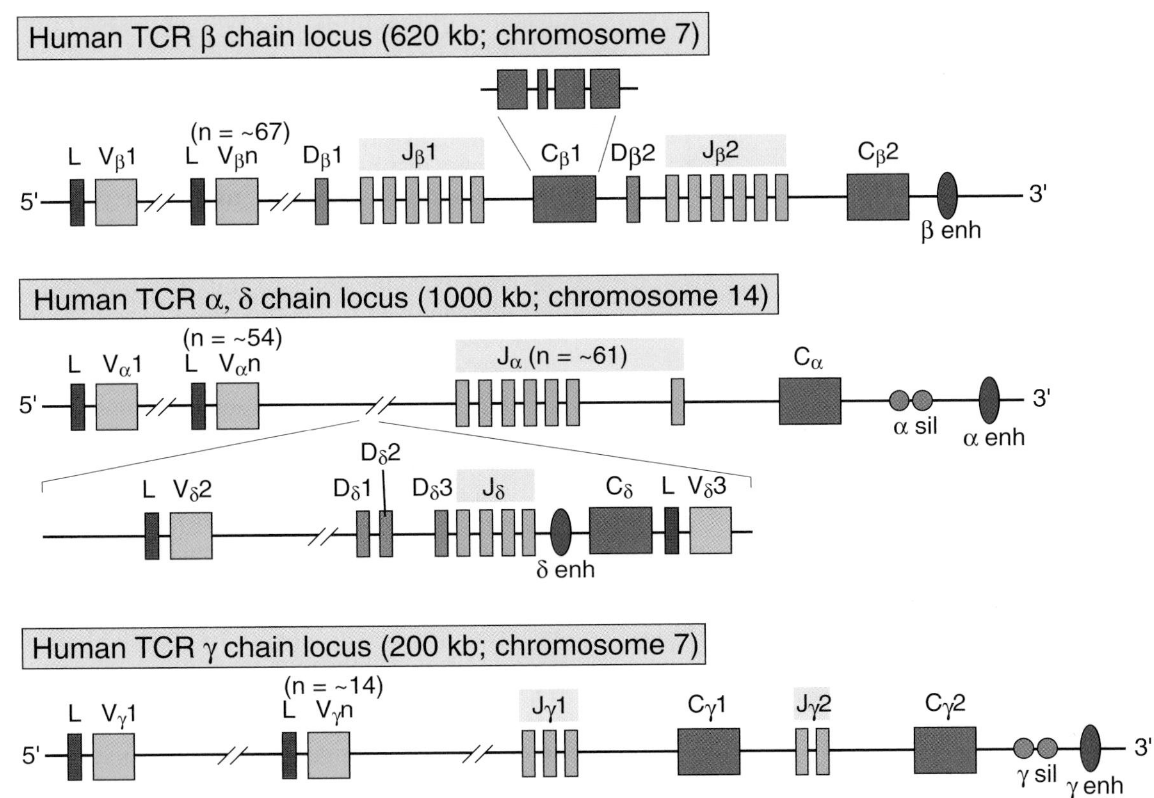

FIGURE 8–7 Germline organization of human TCR loci. The human TCR β, α, γ, and δ chain loci are shown, as indicated. Exons and introns are not drawn to scale, and nonfunctional pseudogenes are not shown. Each C gene is shown as a single box but is composed of several exons, as illustrated for C_β. Gene segments are indicated as follows: L, leader (usually called signal sequence); V, variable; D, diversity; J, joining; C, constant; enh, enhancer; sil, silencer (sequences that regulate TCR gene transcription).

- The recombination of antigen receptor genes can be demonstrated by a technique called Southern blot hybridization, which is used to examine the sizes of DNA fragments produced by restriction enzyme digestion of genomic DNA. By this method, it can be shown that the enzyme-generated DNA fragments containing Ig or TCR gene segments are a different size when the DNA is from cells that make antibodies or TCRs, respectively, than when the DNA is from cells that do not make these antigen receptors (Fig. 8–8). The explanation for these different sizes is that V and C regions of antigen receptor chains are encoded by different gene segments that are located far apart in embryonic and nonlymphoid cells and brought close together in cells committed to antibody or TCR synthesis (i.e., in B or T lymphocytes).

The process of V(D)J recombination at any Ig or TCR locus involves selecting one V gene, one J segment, and one D segment (when present) in each lymphocyte and rearranging these gene segments together to form a single V(D)J exon that will code for the variable region of an antigen receptor protein. The C regions lie downstream of the V(D)J exon separated by the same germline J-C intron in the rearranged DNA as well as in the primary RNA transcript. RNA splicing brings together the leader exon, the V(D)J exon, and the C region exons, forming an mRNA that can be translated on membrane-bound ribosomes to produce one of the chains of the antigen receptor. Different clones of lymphocytes use different combinations of V, D, and J gene segments at each relevant locus to generate functional receptor chains (Fig. 8–9). In addition, during V(D)J recombination, nucleotides are added to or removed from the junctions. As we will discuss in more detail later, these processes contribute to the tremendous diversity of antigen receptors. The details and unique features of the processes of Ig and TCR gene rearrangement will be described when we consider the maturation of B and T lymphocytes, respectively.

Mechanisms of V(D)J Recombination

Rearrangement of Ig and TCR genes represents a special kind of nonhomologous DNA recombination event, mediated by the coordinated activities of several enzymes, some of which are found only in developing lymphocytes while others are ubiquitous DNA double-strand break repair (DSBR) enzymes. Critical lymphocyte-specific factors that mediate V(D)J recombination recognize certain DNA sequences called **recombination signal sequences** (RSSs), located 3′ of each V gene segment, 5′ of each J segment, and flanking each D segment on both sides (Fig. 8–10A). The recombination signal sequences consist of a highly conserved stretch of 7 nucleotides, called the heptamer, usually CACAGTG, located adjacent to the coding sequence, followed by

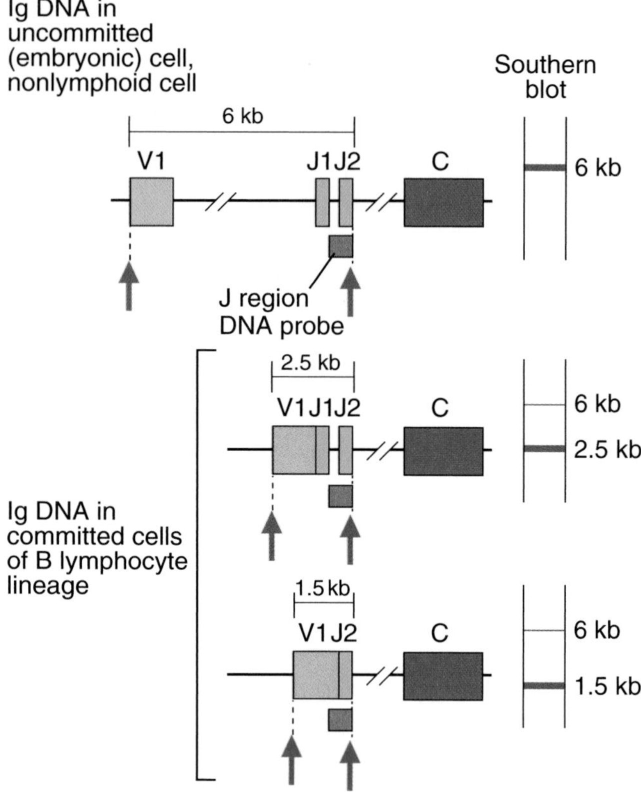

FIGURE 8–8 Antigen receptor gene rearrangements. Southern blot analysis of DNA from nonlymphoid cells and from two monoclonal populations of B lymphocyte lineage origin (e.g., B cell tumors) is shown in schematic fashion. The DNA is digested with a restriction enzyme, different-sized fragments are separated by electrophoresis, and the fragments are blotted onto a filter. The sites at which the restriction enzyme cleaves the DNA are indicated by arrows. The size of the fragments containing the J segment of the Ig κ light chain gene is determined by use of a radioactive probe that specifically binds to J segment DNA. In the hypothetical example shown, the size of the J segment containing DNA fragments from each of two B cells is smaller than that from non-B cell DNA. This indicates that the specific sites where the restriction enzyme cuts the DNA are in a different position in the genome of the B cells compared with the non-B cells. Thus, a rearrangement of the germline DNA sequence in the Ig κ locus has occurred in the B cells. Note that the fragment from the rearranged DNA may be larger or smaller than the fragment from the germline DNA, depending on the location of the sites where the restriction enzyme cuts the DNA.

a spacer of exactly 12 or 23 nonconserved nucleotides, followed by a highly conserved AT-rich stretch of 9 nucleotides, called the nonamer. The 12- and 23-nucleotide spacers roughly correspond to one or two turns of a DNA helix respectively, and they presumably bring two distinct heptamers into positions that are simultaneously accessible to the enzymes that catalyze the recombination process. A specific enzyme (described below) introduces double-strand breaks in the DNA, cleaving between the heptamer of the RSS and the adjacent V, D, or J coding sequence. In Ig light chain V-to-J recombination, for example, breaks will be made 3′ of a V segment and 5′ of a J segment. The intervening double-stranded DNA, containing signal ends (the ends that contain the heptamer and the rest of the RSS), is removed in the form of a circle, and this is accompanied by the joining of the V and J coding ends (Fig. 8–10B). Some V genes, especially in the Ig κ locus, are in the same orientation as the J segments, such that the RSSs linked to these V segments and J segments do not "face" each other. In these cases, the intervening DNA is inverted and the V and J exons are properly aligned and the fused RSSs are not deleted but retained in the chromosome (Fig. 8–10C). Most Ig and TCR gene rearrangements occur by deletion; rearrangement by inversion occurs in up to 50% of rearrangements in the Ig κ locus. Recombination occurs between two segments only if one of the segments is flanked by a 12-nucleotide spacer and the other is flanked by a 23-nucleotide spacer; this is called the 12/23 rule. A "one-turn" coding segment therefore always recombines with a "two-turn" segment. The type of the flanking RSSs (one turn or two turn) ensures that the appropriate gene segments will recombine. For example, in the Ig heavy chain locus, both V and J segments have 23-nucleotide spacers and therefore cannot join directly; D-to-J recombination occurs first, followed by V-to-DJ recombination, and this is possible because the D segments are flanked on both sides by 12-nucleotide spacers, allowing D-J and then V-DJ joining. The recombination signal sequences described here are unique to Ig and TCR genes. Therefore, V(D)J recombination is relevant for antigen receptor genes but not for other genes.

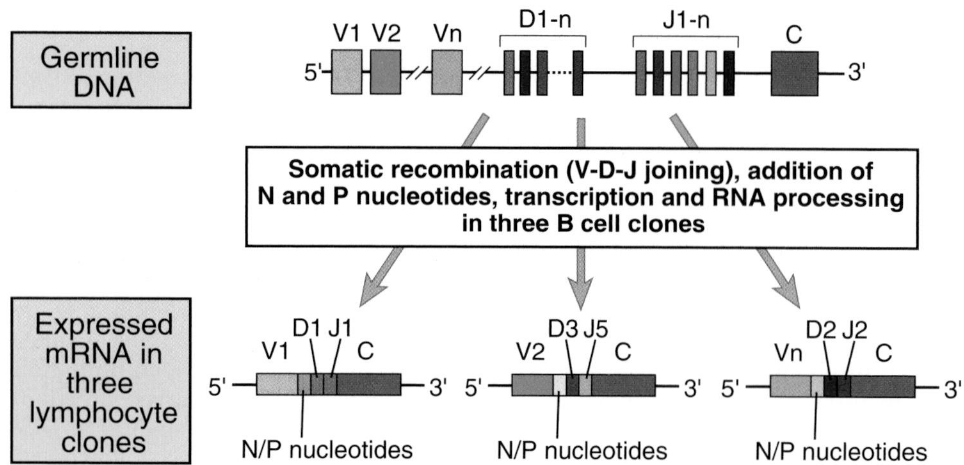

FIGURE 8–9 Diversity of antigen receptor genes. From the same germline DNA, it is possible to generate recombined DNA sequences and mRNAs that differ in their V-D-J junctions. In the example shown, three distinct antigen receptor mRNAs are produced from the same germline DNA by the use of different gene segments and the addition of nucleotides to the junctions.

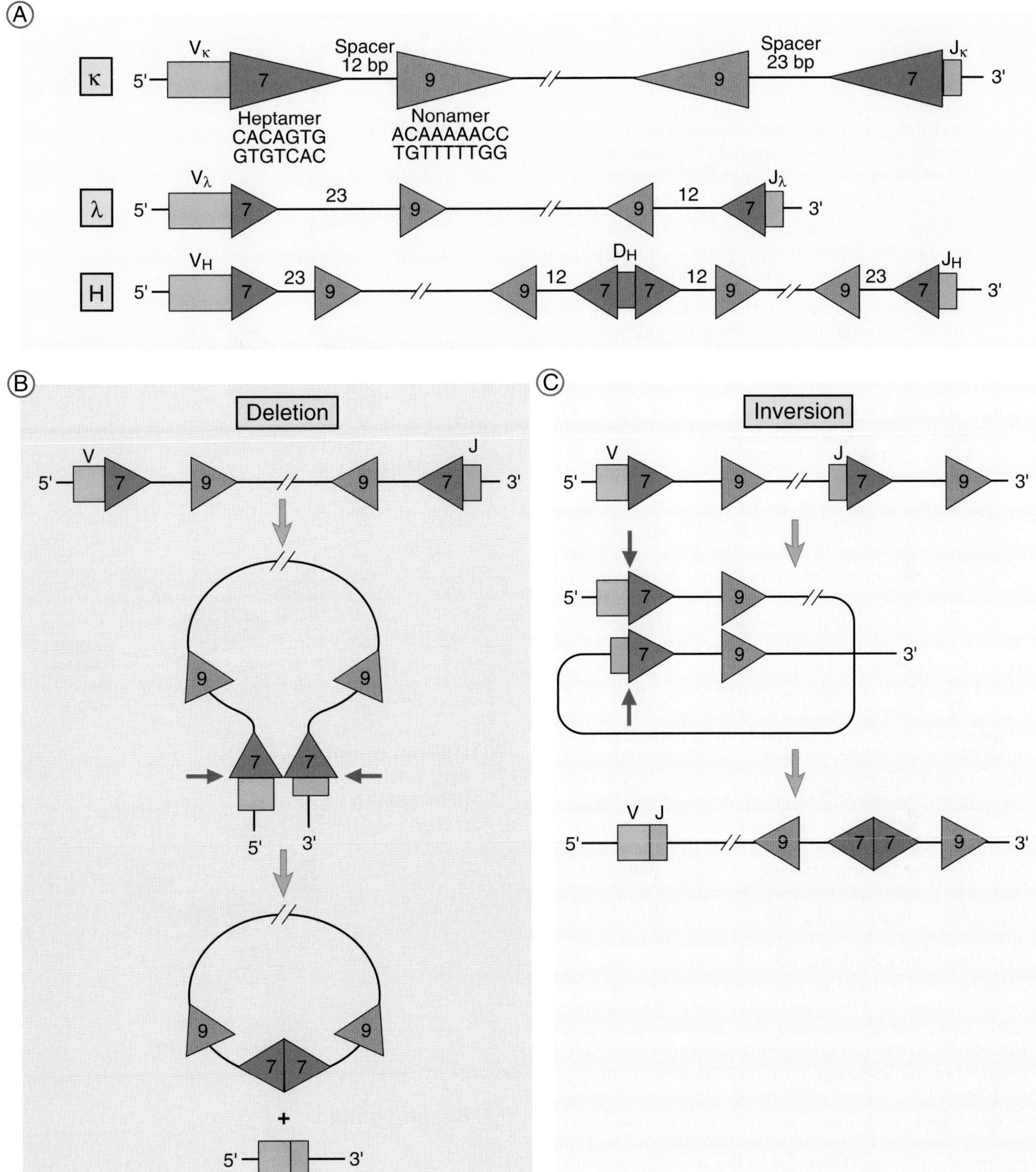

FIGURE 8–10 V(D)J recombination. The DNA sequences and mechanisms involved in recombination in the Ig gene loci are depicted. The same sequences and mechanisms apply to recombinations in the TCR loci. A. Conserved heptamer (7 bp) and nonamer (9 bp) sequences, separated by 12- or 23-bp spacers, are located adjacent to V and J exons (for κ and λ loci) or to V, D, and J exons (in the H chain locus). The V(D)J recombinase recognizes these recombination signal sequences and brings the exons together. B. Recombination of V and J exons may occur by deletion of intervening DNA and ligation of the V and J segments or, C, if the V gene is in the opposite orientation, by inversion of the DNA followed by ligation of adjacent gene segments. Red arrows indicate the sites where germline sequences are cleaved prior to their ligation to other Ig or TCR gene segments.

The process of V(D)J recombination can be divided into four distinct events that flow sequentially into each other (Fig. 8–11):

1. *Synapsis:* Portions of the antigen receptor chromosome are made accessible to the recombination machinery, and two selected coding segments and their adjacent RSSs are brought together by a chromosomal looping event and held in position for subsequent cleavage, processing, and joining.
2. *Cleavage:* Double-strand breaks are enzymatically generated at RSS–coding sequence junctions using machinery that is lymphoid specific.
3. *Coding end processing:* The broken coding ends (but not the signal/RSS ends) are modified by the addition or removal of bases, and thus greater diversity is generated.
4. *Joining:* The broken coding ends as well as the signal ends are brought together and ligated by a double-strand break repair process found in all cells that is called non-homolgous end joining.

Two proteins encoded by lymphoid-specific genes called ***recombination-activating gene 1*** and ***recombination-activating gene 2*** (*Rag-1* and *Rag-2*) form a tetrameric complex that plays a major role in V(D)J recombination. The Rag-1 protein, in a manner similar to a restriction endonuclease, recognizes the DNA sequence at the junction between a hepatamer and a coding segment, and cleaves it, but it is enzymatically active only when complexed with the Rag-2 protein. The Rag-1/Rag-2 complex is also known as the **V(D) J recombinase**. The Rag-2 protein may help link the Rag-1/Rag-2 tetramer to other proteins, including accessibility factors that bring these proteins to specific "open" receptor gene loci at specific times and in defined stages of lymphocyte development. Rag-1 and Rag-2 contribute to holding together gene segments during the process of chromosomal folding or synapsis. Rag-1 then makes a nick (on one strand) between the coding end and the heptamer. The released 3′OH of the coding end then attacks the other strand forming a covalent hairpin. The signal end (including the heptamer and the rest of the RSS) does not form a hairpin and is generated as a blunt double-stranded DNA terminus that undergoes no further processing. This double-stranded break results in a closed hairpin of one coding segment being held in apposition to the closed hairpin of the other coding end and two blunt signal ends being placed next to each other. Rag-1 and Rag-2, apart from generating the double-stranded breaks, also hold the hairpin ends and the blunt ends together prior to the modification of the coding ends and the process of ligation.

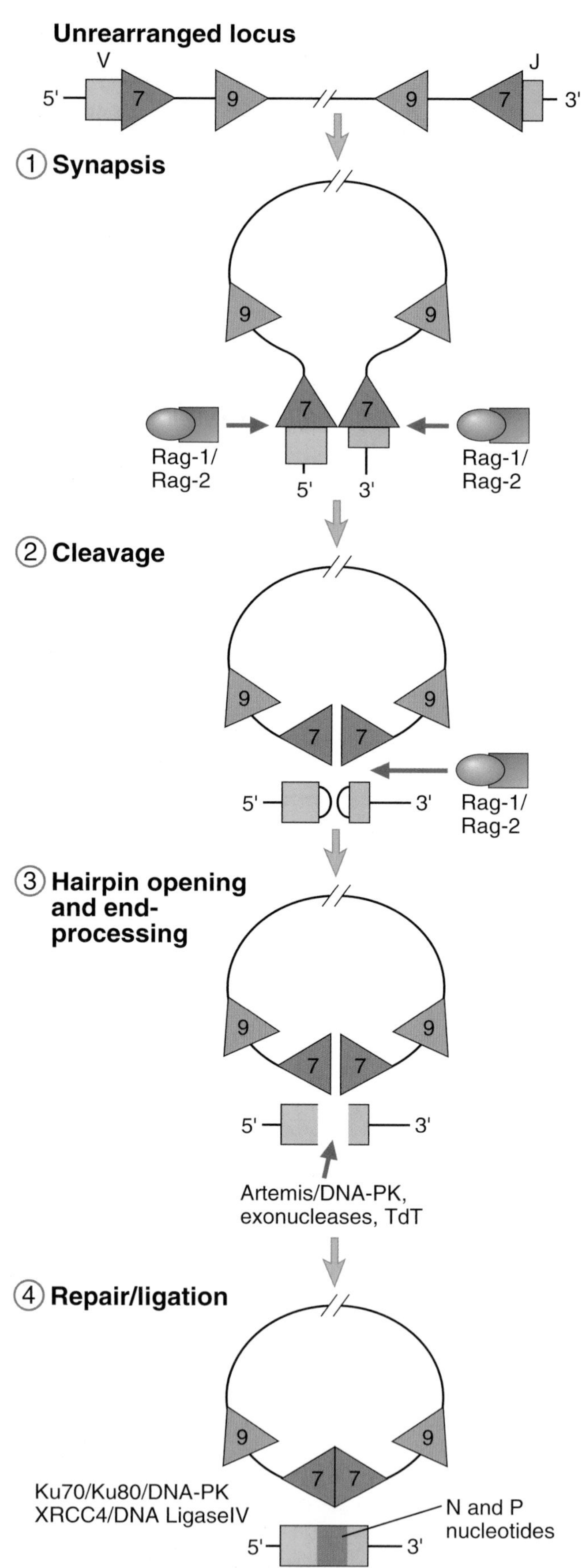

FIGURE 8–11 Sequential events during V(D)J recombination. Synapsis and cleavage of DNA at the heptamer/coding segment boundary is mediated by Rag-1 and Rag-2. The coding end hairpin is opened by the Artemis endonuclease and broken ends are repaired by the NHEJ machinery.

After the formation of double-stranded breaks, hairpins must be resolved (opened up) at the coding junctions, bases may be added to or removed from the coding ends to ensure even greater diversification, and then all the broken ends must be appropriately joined, coding end to coding end and signal end to signal end.

The importance of the *Rag* genes is illustrated by the finding that knockout mice lacking either *Rag1* or *Rag2* fail to produce Ig and TCR proteins and lack mature B and T lymphocytes. The Rag-1 and Rag-2 proteins exhibit several important properties. First, Rag-1 and Rag-2 are cell type specific, being produced only in cells of the B and T lymphocyte lineages. Second, the *Rag* genes are expressed only in immature lymphocytes. Therefore, V(D)J recombination is active in immature B and T lymphocytes but not in mature cells, explaining why Ig and TCR gene rearrangements do not continue in cells that express functional antigen receptors. Third, *Rag* genes are expressed mainly in the G_0 and G_1 stages of the cell cycle and are silenced in proliferating cells. It is thought that limiting DNA cleavage and recombination to nondividing cells minimizes the risk of generating inappropriate DNA breaks during DNA replication or during mitosis.

The same recombinase mediates rearrangement at both Ig and TCR loci. Because complete functional rearrangement of Ig genes normally occurs only in immature B cells and rearrangement of TCR genes normally occurs only in developing T cells, some other mechanism, other than the recombinase itself, must control the cell type specificity and the differentiation stage specificity of recombination. It is likely that the accessibility of the Ig and TCR loci to the recombinase is differentially regulated in developing B and T cells by several mechanisms, including alterations in chromatin structure, DNA methylation, and basal transcriptional activity in the unrearranged loci.

One other lymphoid-specific enzyme that functions downstream of the Rag proteins is terminal deoxynucleotidyl transferase (TdT), discussed below. All the other enzymes that are crucial for V(D)J recombination are involved in the process of non-homologous end joining that mediates double-strand break repair during V(D)J recombination. Their role in Ig and TCR gene recombination is to repair the double-stranded breaks introduced by the recombinase. Ku70 and Ku80 are DNA end binding proteins that bind to the breaks and recruit the catalytic subunit of DNA-dependent protein kinase (DNA-PK), a double-stranded DNA repair enzyme. This enzyme is defective in mice carrying the severe combined immunodeficiency *(scid)* mutation (see Chapter 20). Like *Rag*-deficient mice, *scid* mice fail to produce mature lymphocytes. DNA-PK phosphorylates and activates an enzyme called Artemis, which is an endonuclease that opens up the hairpins at the coding ends. In the absence of Artemis, hairpins cannot be opened and T and B cells cannot be generated. Mutations in *Artemis* result in the absence of T and B cells (Chapter 20). Ligation of the processed broken ends is mediated by DNA ligase IV.

One of the consequences of V(D)J recombination is that the process brings promoters located immediately 5′ of V genes in close proximity to downstream enhancers that are located in the J-C introns, and also 3′ of the C region genes (Fig. 8–12). These enhancers maximize the transcriptional activity of the V gene promoters and are thus important for high-level transcription of rearranged V genes in lymphocytes.

Because Ig and TCR genes are sites for multiple DNA recombination events in B and T cells, and because these sites become transcriptionally active after recombination, genes from other loci can be abnormally translocated to these loci and, as a result, may be aberrantly transcribed. In tumors of B and T lymphocytes, oncogenes are often translocated to Ig or TCR gene loci. Such chromosomal translocations are frequently accompanied by enhanced transcription of the oncogenes and are believed to be one of the factors causing the development of lymphoid tumors (Box 8–1).

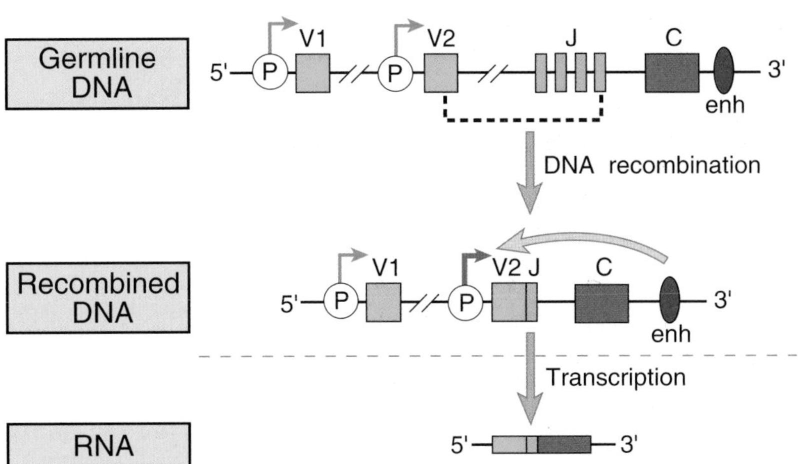

FIGURE 8–12 Transcriptional regulation of Ig genes. V-D-J recombination brings promoter sequences (shown as P) close to the enhancer (enh). The enhancer promotes transcription of the rearranged V gene (V2, whose active promoter is indicated by a bold green arrow).

Box 8–1 ▪ IN DEPTH: CHROMOSOMAL TRANSLOCATIONS IN TUMORS OF LYMPHOCYTES

Cytogeneticists first noted reciprocal chromosomal translocations in lymphomas and leukemias in the 1960s, but their significance remained unknown until almost 20 years later. At this time, sequencing of switch regions of IgH genes in two different B cell tumors bearing translocations, human Burkitt's lymphoma and murine plasmacytoma, revealed the presence of DNA segments that were not derived from Ig genes. The "foreign" DNA was identified as a portion of the *C-MYC* proto-oncogene, which normally resides on chromosome 8 in humans. Proto-oncogenes are normal cellular genes that often code for proteins involved in the regulation of cellular proliferation, differentiation, and survival, such as growth factors, receptors for growth factors, or transcription-activating factors. In normal cells, their function is tightly regulated. When these genes are altered by mutations, inappropriately expressed, or incorporated into and reintroduced in cells by retroviruses, they can exhibit either enhanced or aberrant activities and function as oncogenes. Dysfunction of oncogenes is one important mechanism leading to increased cellular growth and, ultimately, neoplastic transformation. The most common translocation in Burkitt's lymphoma is t(8;14), involving the Ig heavy chain locus on chromosome 14; less commonly, t(2;8) or t(8;22) translocations are found, involving the κ or λ light chain loci, respectively. In all cases of Burkitt's lymphoma, *C-MYC* is translocated from chromosome 8 to one of the Ig loci, producing the reciprocal 8;14, 2;8, or 8;22 translocations found in these tumors. The *C-MYC* gene product is a basic helix-loop-helix transcription factor, and translocation of the gene leads to its dysregulated expression. *C-MYC* function is still incompletely understood, but it activates the expression of a large number of genes that control metabolism, protein synthesis, and ribosome biogenesis, and thereby promotes cell growth and division.

Because antigen receptor genes normally undergo several genetic rearrangements during lymphocyte maturation, they are likely sites for accidental translocations of distant genes. DNA sequencing of antigen receptor genes involved in chromosomal translocations suggests that these mistakes occur at the time of attempted V(D)J rearrangement in pre-B and pre-T cells, during switch recombination in germinal center B cells, and possibly during the process of somatic hypermutation (also in germinal center B cells). Of interest, human lymphomas derived from germinal center B cells, which rely on regulated genomic instability to diversify their Ig genes, are common and often have chromosomal translocations involving the Ig genes. In contrast, tumors derived from mature T cells (which are genomically stable) are infrequent and only rarely have translocations involving the

Type of tumor	Chromosomal translocation	Genes involved in translocation
B Cell derived		
Burkitt's lymphoma	t(8;**14**)(q24.1;**q32.3**) most common	*C-MYC, IgH*
Acute lymphoblastic leukemia (pre-B-ALL)	t(12;**21**)(p13;q22) (25% of childhood cases)	*TEL1, AML1*
Pre-B-ALL; also chronic myelogenous leukemia	t(9;22)(q34;q11) (25% of adult ALL, 3% of childhood ALL)	*BCR, ABL* (Philadelphia chromosome)
Follicular lymphoma	t(**14**;18)(**q32.3**;q21.3)	*BCL-2, IgH*
Diffuse B cell lymphoma, large cell type	t(3;**14**)(q27;**q32.3**)	*BCL-6* (DNA-binding protein), *IgH*
Mantle cell lymphoma	t(11;**14**)(q13;**q32.3**)	*CCND1 (CYCLIN D1), IgH*
T Cell derived		
Pre-T cell acute lymphoblastic leukemia	t(1;**14**)(p32;**q11**) (5% of cases); del(1p32) (20% of cases)	*TAL1, TCRα; TAL1, SCL*
T cell lymphoma, anaplastic large cell type	t(2;5)(p23;q35)	*ALK* (tyrosine kinase), *NPM* (unknown function)

These are some examples of chromosomal translocations that have been molecularly cloned in human lymphoid tumors. Each translocation is indicated by the letter t. The first pair of numbers refers to the chromosomes involved, for example, (8;14), and the second pair to the bands of each chromosome, for example, (q24.1; q32.3). The normal chromosomal locations of antigen receptor genes (indicated in bold) are IgH, 14q32.3; Igκ, 2p12; Igλ, 22q11.2; TCRαδ, 14q11.2; TCRβ, 7q34; and TCRγ, 7p15.

Continued on following page

TCR genes. In some translocations associated with lymphoid tumors, DNA breakage near proto-oncogenes occurs at sites that resemble heptamer and nonamer sequences, suggesting that they are caused by an aberrant V(D)J recombinase activity. However, in most instances (and, more generally, in all translocations found in nonlymphoid tumors), such sequences are lacking and the cause of DNA breakage within or adjacent to proto-oncogenes is uncertain.

Since the discovery of *C-MYC* translocations in B cell lymphomas, the genes involved in translocations in many other lymphoid (and nonlymphoid) tumors have been identified (see Table). In most cases, these translocations result in dysregulation of transcription factors, cell survival proteins, or signal-transducing molecules such as kinases. One gene that has proved to be particularly important in acute pre-B cell and acute myeloid leukemias is *AML1,* a gene on chromosome 21 that encodes a member of the Runt family of transcription factors. About 25% of childhood acute pre-B cell lymphoblastic leukemias have a balanced (12;21) translocation that produces a fusion gene encoding the DNA-binding portion of AML1 and the dimerization domain of TEL1, a member of the Ets family of transcription factors. Similarly, about 20% of acute myelogenous leukemias have a balanced (8;21) translocation involving a different Ets-like transcription factor, ETO, and AML1. In both instances, the oncogenic AML1 fusion proteins appear to have "dominant negative" activity that inhibits normal AML1 function and results in a block in differentiation. This implies that the normal role of AML1 is to promote the terminal differentiation of blood cell progenitors, which is supported by the observation that *aml1* knockout mice die during embryogenesis because of a failure to produce blood cells. The most frequent chromosomal rearrangements in acute pre-T cell leukemias cause the inappropriate expression of *TAL1,* a gene encoding a basic helix-loop-helix transcription factor that appears to interfere with T cell differentiation. The Philadelphia chromosome, found in chronic myelogenous leukemia and some acute lymphoblastic leukemias, is created by a balanced t(9;22) translocation. This yields a *BCR/C-ABL* fusion gene that encodes a constitutively active tyrosine kinase. Diffuse large B cell lymphoma, the most common lymphoma of adults, is often associated with chromosomal translocations that dysregulate the expression of *BCL6,* which encodes a transcription factor that is required for germinal center B cell development. Inappropriate expression of BCL6 is believed to block B cell development beyond the germinal center stage and to inhibit the function of genes (such as *p53*) that respond to DNA damage. The (14;18) translocation found in greater than 85% of another common B cell lymphoma, follicular lymphoma, leads to overexpression of a survival gene, *BCL2,* and the prevention of programmed cell death.

This box was written with the assistance of Dr. Jon Aster, Department of Pathology, Brigham & Women's Hospital and Harvard Medical School, Boston.

Generation of Diversity in B and T Cells

The enormous diversity of the mature B and T cell repertoires is generated primarily by the rearrangement of Ig and TCR genes. Several genetic mechanisms contribute to this diversity, and the relative importance of each mechanism varies among the different antigen receptor loci (Table 8–1). Not discussed here is somatic hypermutation, a receptor diversification mechanism unique to the B cell lineage, which will be considered in Chapter 10.

- **Combinatorial diversity.** V(D)J recombination events involve multiple germline gene segments that may combine randomly, and different combinations produce different antigen receptors. The maximum possible number of combinations of these gene segments is the product of the numbers of V, J, and (if present) D gene segments at each antigen receptor locus. Therefore, the amount of combinatorial diversity that can be generated at each locus reflects the number of germline V, J, and D gene segments at that locus. After somatic recombination and expression of antigen receptor chains, combinatorial diversity is further enhanced by the juxtaposition of two different, randomly generated V regions (i.e., V_H and V_L in Ig molecules and V_α and V_β in TCR molecules). Therefore, the total combinatorial diversity is theoretically the product of the combinatorial diversity of each of the two associating chains. The actual degree of combinatorial diversity in the expressed Ig and TCR repertoires in any individual is likely to be considerably less than the theoretical maximum. This is because not all recombinations of gene segments are equally likely to occur, and not all pairings of Ig heavy and light chains or TCR α and β chains may form functional antigen receptors. Importantly, since the numbers of V, J, and D segments in each locus are limited (see Table 8–1), the maximum possible numbers of combinations are on the order of thousands. This is, of course, much less than the actual diversity of antigen receptors in mature lymphocytes.

- **Junctional diversity.** The largest contribution to the diversity of antigen receptors is made by the removal or addition of nucleotides between V and D, D and J, or V and J segments at the time of joining. These processes result in variability at the junctions of V, D, and J gene segments, called junctional diversity. One way this can occur is if endonucleases remove nucleotides from the germline sequences at the ends of the recombining gene segments. In addition, new nucleotide sequences, not present in the germline, may be added at junctions. Coding segments (e.g., V and J gene segments) that are cleaved by Rag-1 form hairpin loops whose ends are often

Table 8–1. Contributions of Different Mechanisms to the Generation of Diversity in Ig and TCR Genes

Mechanism	Immunoglobulin		TCR αβ		TCR γδ	
Mechanism	Heavy chain	κ	α	β	γ	δ
Variable (V) segments	85	35	54	67	14	20–30
Diversity (D) segments	27	0	0	2	0	3
D segments read in all three reading frames	Rare	—	—	Often	—	Often
N region diversification	V-D, D-J	None	V-J	V-D, D-J	V-J	V-D1, D1-D2, D1-J
Joining (J) segments	6	5	61	4	5	4
Total potential repertoire with junctional diversity	$\sim 10^{11}$		$\sim 10^{16}$		$\sim 10^{18}$	

The potential number of antigen receptors with junctional diversity is much greater than the number that can be generated only by combinations of V, D, and J gene segments. Note that although the upper limit on the numbers of Ig and TCR proteins that may be expressed is very large, it is estimated that each individual contains on the order of 10^7 clones of B and T cells with distinct specificities and receptors; in other words, only a fraction of the potential repertoire may actually be expressed.

cleaved asymmetrically by Artemis so that one DNA strand is longer than the other (Fig. 8–13). The shorter strand has to be extended with nucleotides complementary to the longer strand before the ligation of the two segments. The short lengths of added nucleotides are called P nucleotides, and their templated addition introduces new sequences at the V-D-J junctions. Another mechanism of junctional diversity is the random addition of up to 20 non-template-encoded nucleotides called N nucleotides (see Fig. 8–13). N

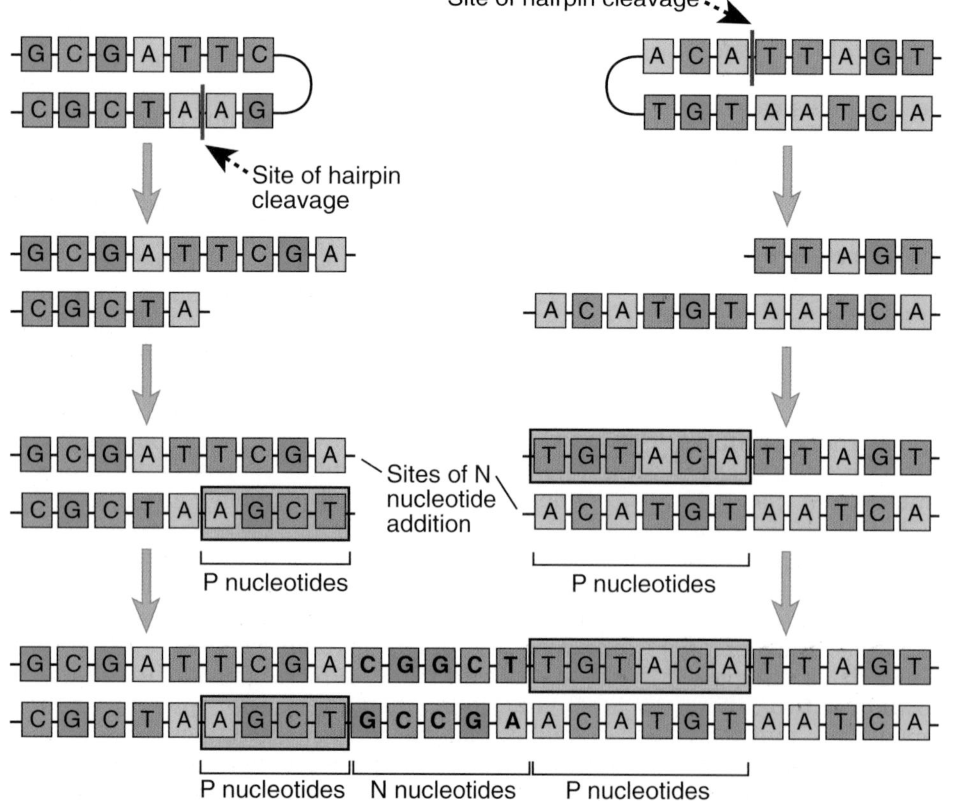

FIGURE 8–13 Junctional diversity. During the joining of different gene segments, addition or removal of nucleotides may lead to the generation of novel nucleotide and amino acid sequences at the junction. Nucleotides (P sequences) may be added to asymmetrically cleaved hairpins in a templated manner. Other nucleotides (N regions) may be added to the sites of VD, VJ, or DJ junctions in a nontemplated manner by the action of the enzyme TdT. These additions generate new sequences that are not present in the germline.

region diversification is more common in Ig heavy chains and in TCR β and γ chains than in Ig κ or λ chains. This addition of new nucleotides is mediated by the enzyme TdT (terminal deoxynucleotidyl transferase). In mice rendered deficient in TdT by gene knockout, the diversity of B and T cell repertoires is substantially less than in normal mice. The addition of P nucleotides and N nucleotides at the recombination sites may introduce frameshifts, theoretically generating termination codons in two of every three joining events. Such inefficiency is a price that is paid for generating diversity.

Because of junctional diversity, antibody and TCR molecules show the greatest variability at the junctions of V and C regions that form the third hypervariable region, or CDR3. The CDR3 regions of Ig and TCR molecules, which are formed at the sites of V(D)J recombination (see Fig. 8–6), are also the most important portions of these molecules for determining the specificity of antigen binding (see Chapters 4 and 7). In fact, because of junctional diversity, the numbers of different amino acid sequences that are present in the CDR3 regions of Ig and TCR molecules are much greater than the numbers that can be encoded by germline gene segments. Thus, the greatest diversity in antigen receptors is concentrated in the regions of the receptors that are the most important for antigen binding.

Although the theoretical limit of the number of Ig and TCR proteins that can be produced is enormous (see Table 8–1), the actual number of Ig and TCR genes expressed in each individual is probably only on the order of 10^7. This perhaps reflects the fact that most receptors, which are generated randomly, do not pass the selection processes needed for maturation.

A practical application of our knowledge of junctional diversity is the determination of the clonality of lymphoid tumors that have arisen from B or T cells. Because every lymphocyte clone expresses a unique antigen receptor CDR3 region, the sequence of nucleotides at the V(D)J recombination site serves as a specific marker for each clone. Thus, by sequencing the junctional regions of Ig or TCR genes in different B or T cell tumors, even from the same patient, one can establish whether these tumors arose from a single clone or independently from different clones. Furthermore, polymerase chain reaction–mediated amplification of these clone-specific sequences may be used as a sensitive detection method for small numbers of tumor cells in the blood or tissues.

Transcriptional Regulation of Early T and B Cell Development

As discussed earlier in this chapter, all lymphocytes develop from CLPs that in turn are derived from hematopoietic stem cells (see Fig. 8–2). CLPs in the bone marrow primarily give rise to B cells, and CLP-like cells that migrate to the thymus give rise to T cells. Commitment to the B and T lineages is orchestrated by different sets of transcription factors (Fig. 8–14). The Notch family of proteins are cell surface molecules that are proteolytically cleaved when they interact with specific ligands on neighboring cells. The cleaved intracellular portions of Notch proteins migrate to the nucleus and modulate the expression of specific target genes. Notch-1, a member of the Notch family, is activated in progenitor cells and collaborates with a transcription factor called GATA-3 to commit developing lymphocytes to the T lineage. These transcriptional regulators contribute to the induction of a number of genes that are required for the further development of αβ T cells. Downstream target genes include components of the pre-T cell receptor and of the machinery for V(D)J recombination. In B cells the EBF and E2A transcription factors contribute to the induction of another transcription factor called Pax-5, and these three nuclear proteins collaborate to induce the process of commitment to the B lineage by facilitating the expression of a number of genes. These genes include those encoding the Rag-1 and Rag-2 proteins, surrogate light chains, and the Igα and Igβ proteins that contribute to signaling via the pre-B cell receptor and the B cell receptor.

While gene expression during development is driven primarily by transcription factors, an additional level of regulation is mediated by micro RNAs. These endogenous non-coding RNAs fine-tune the process of lymphocyte development by regulating the translation and degradation of various target mRNAs.

B Lymphocyte Development

The principal events during the maturation of B lymphocytes are the rearrangement and expression of Ig genes in a precise order, selection and proliferation of developing B cells at the pre-antigen receptor checkpoint, and selection of the mature B cell repertoire. Before birth, B lymphocytes develop from committed precursors in the fetal liver; after birth, B cells are generated in the bone marrow. The majority of B lymphocytes arise from adult bone marrow progenitors that are initially Ig negative, develop into immature B cells that express membrane-bound IgM molecules, and then leave the bone marrow to mature further primarily in the spleen, where B cells of the follicular B cell lineage express IgM and IgD on the cell surface. It is in the spleen that these cells acquire the ability to recirculate and populate all peripheral lymphoid organs. Recirculating follicular B cells home to lymphoid follicles and have the ability to recognize foreign antigens and to respond to them. The development of a mature B cell from a lymphoid progenitor is estimated to take 2 to 3 days in humans.

Stages of B Lymphocyte Development

During their maturation, cells of the B lymphocyte lineage go through distinguishable stages, each characterized by distinct cell surface markers and a specific pattern of Ig gene expression (Fig. 8–15). The earliest bone marrow cell committed to the B cell lineage is called a **pro-B cell.** Pro-B cells do not produce Ig, but they can be distinguished from other immature cells by the expression of B lineage–restricted surface molecules such as CD19 and CD10. Rag proteins are first expressed

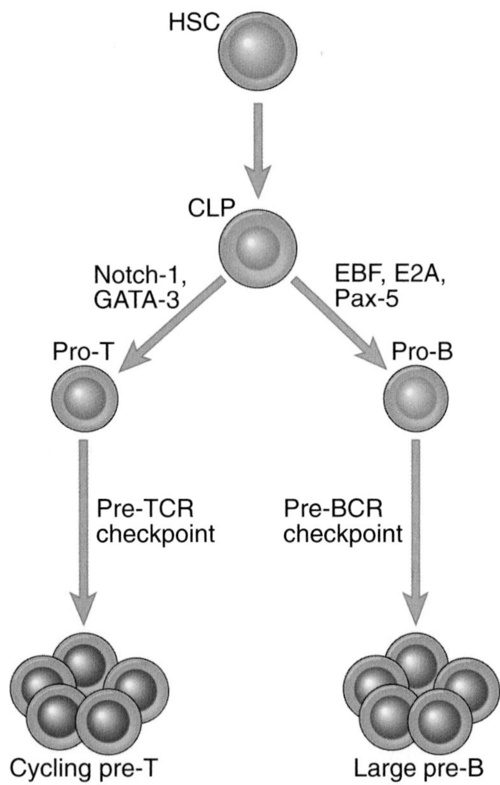

FIGURE 8–14 Specific transcriptional regulators drive commitment to the B and T lineages. Commitment to the T lineage depends on signals delivered by Notch-1, whose intracellular domain mediates transcriptional activation of T lineage genes in collaboration with other transcription factors such as GATA-3. Commitment to the B lineage is mediated initially by the EBF and E2A transcription factors, and subsequently by Pax-5. These transcription factors work together to induce the transcription of B cell–specific genes and of genes of the recombination machinery.

at this stage, and the first recombination of Ig genes occurs at the heavy chain locus. This recombination brings together one D and one J gene segment, with deletion of the intervening DNA (Fig. 8–16A). The D segments that are 5′ of the rearranged D segment, and the J segments that are 3′ of the rearranged J segment, are not affected by this recombination (e.g., D1 and J2 to J6 in Fig. 8–16A). After the D-J recombination event, one of the many 5′V genes is joined to the DJ unit, giving rise to a rearranged VDJ exon. At this stage, all V and D segments between the rearranged V and D genes are also deleted. V-to-DJ recombination at the Ig H chain locus occurs only in committed B lymphocyte precursors and is a critical event in Ig expression because only the rearranged V gene is subsequently transcribed. The TdT enzyme, which catalyzes the nontemplated addition of junctional N nucleotides, is expressed most abundantly during the pro-B stage when VDJ recombination occurs at the IgH locus, and levels of TdT decrease before light chain gene V-J recombination is complete. Therefore, junctional diversity attributed to N nucleotides is more abundant in rearranged heavy chain genes than in light chain genes. The heavy chain C region exons remain separated from the VDJ complex by DNA containing the distal J segments and the J-C intron. The rearranged Ig heavy chain gene is transcribed to produce a primary transcript that includes the rearranged VDJ complex and the Cμ exons. Multiple adenine nucleotides, called poly-A tails, are added to the 3′ end of the Cμ RNA after it is cleaved downstream of one of two consensus polyadenylation sites. The nuclear RNA undergoes splicing, an RNA processing event in which the introns are removed and exons joined together. In the case of the μ RNA, introns between the leader exon and the VDJ exon, between the VDJ exon and the first exon of the C_μ locus, and between each of the subsequent constant region exons of Cμ are removed, thus giving rise to a spliced mRNA for the μ heavy chain. If the mRNA is derived from an Ig locus at which rearrangement was productive (see below), translation of the rearranged μ heavy chain mRNA leads to synthesis of the μ protein.

In order for a rearrangement to be productive (in the correct reading frame), bases must be added or removed at junctions in multiples of three. This ensures that the rearranged Ig gene will be able to correctly encode an Ig protein. Approximately one in three pro-B cells make productive rearrangements at the IgH locus and can thus go on to synthesize the μ heavy chain protein. Only cells that make productive rearrangements survive and differentiate further. Once a productive Igμ rearrangement is made, a cell ceases to be called a pro-B cell and has differentiated into the pre-B stage. **Pre-B cells** are developing B lineage cells that express the Igμ protein but have yet to rearrange their light chain loci. The μ heavy chain associates with the λ5 and VpreB proteins, also called **surrogate light chains,** which are structurally homologous to κ and λ light chains but are invariant (i.e., they are identical in all pre-B cells) and are only synthesized in pro-B and pre-B cells (Fig. 8–17A). Complexes of μ, surrogate light chains, and signal transducing proteins called Igα and Igβ form the pre-antigen receptor of the B lineage, known as the **pre-B cell receptor** (pre-BCR). Igα and Igβ also form part of the B cell receptor in mature B cells (see Chapter 10). In cells that have made proper in-frame rearrangements at the IgH locus, the pre-BCR drives the pro-B to pre-B transition. This happens, as explained above, in approximately a third of pro-B cells that have completed VDJ rearrangement at the IgH locus, and pre-BCR signaling is responsible for the largest developmental expansion of B lineage cells in the bone marrow.

- The importance of pre-BCRs is illustrated by studies of knockout mice and rare cases of human deficiencies of these receptors. For instance, in mice, knockout of the gene encoding the μ chain or one of the surrogate light chains, called λ5, results in markedly reduced numbers of mature B cells. This suggests that the μ-λ5 complex delivers signals required for B cell maturation and that if either gene is disrupted, maturation does not proceed.

It is not known what the pre-BCR recognizes, but the consensus view at present is that this receptor functions in a ligand-independent manner, and when it

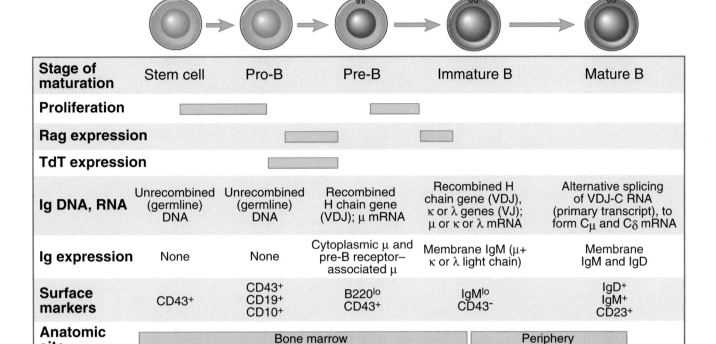

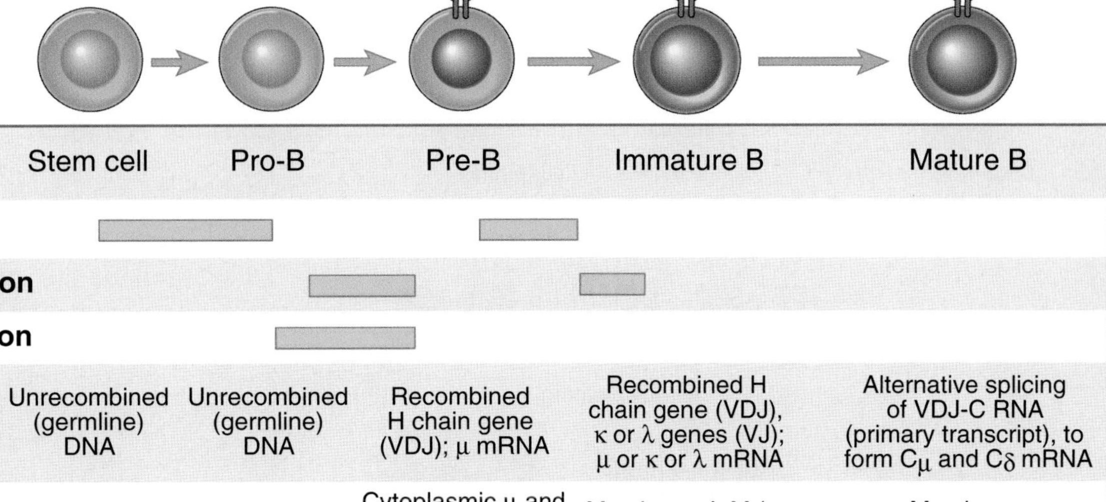

Stage of maturation	Stem cell	Pro-B	Pre-B	Immature B	Mature B
Proliferation					
Rag expression					
TdT expression					
Ig DNA, RNA	Unrecombined (germline) DNA	Unrecombined (germline) DNA	Recombined H chain gene (VDJ); μ mRNA	Recombined H chain gene (VDJ), κ or λ genes (VJ); μ or κ or λ mRNA	Alternative splicing of VDJ-C RNA (primary transcript), to form $C\mu$ and $C\delta$ mRNA
Ig expression	None	None	Cytoplasmic μ and pre-B receptor–associated μ	Membrane IgM (μ+ κ or λ light chain)	Membrane IgM and IgD
Surface markers	$CD43^+$	$CD43^+$ $CD19^+$ $CD10^+$	$B220^{lo}$ $CD43^+$	IgM^{lo} $CD43^-$	IgD^+ IgM^+ $CD23^+$
Anatomic site	Bone marrow	Bone marrow	Bone marrow	Periphery	Periphery
Response to antigen	None	None	None	Negative selection (deletion), receptor editing	Activation (proliferation and differentiation)

FIGURE 8–15 Stages of B cell maturation. Events corresponding to each stage of B cell maturation from a bone marrow stem cell to a mature B lymphocyte are illustrated. Several surface markers in addition to those shown have been used to define distinct stages of B cell maturation.

is assembled it is in the "on" conformation. Numerous signaling molecules linked to both the pre-BCR and the BCR are required for cells to successfully negotiate the pre-BCR-mediated checkpoint at the pro-B to pre-B cell transition. A kinase called Bruton's tyrosine kinase (Btk) is activated downstream of the pre-BCR and is required for delivering signals from this receptor that mediate survival, proliferation, and maturation at and beyond the pre-B cell stage. In humans, mutations in the ***BTK*** gene result in the disease called **X-linked agammaglobulinemia** (XLA), which is characterized by a failure of B cell maturation (see Chapter 20). In mice, mutations in *btk* result in a less severe B cell defect in a mouse strain called *Xid* (for X-linked immunodeficiency). The defect is less severe than in XLA because murine pre-B cells express a second Btk-like kinase called Tec that compensates for the defective Btk.

The pre-BCR regulates further rearrangement of Ig genes in two ways. First, if a μ protein is produced from the recombined heavy chain locus on one chromosome and forms a pre-BCR, this receptor signals to irreversibly inhibit rearrangement of the Ig heavy chain locus on the other chromosome. If the first rearrangement is nonproductive, the heavy chain allele on the other chromosome can complete VDJ rearrangement at the IgH locus. Thus, in any B cell clone, one heavy chain allele is productively rearranged and expressed, and the other is in the germline configuration or is nonproductively rearranged. As a result, an individual B cell can express Ig heavy chain proteins encoded by only one of the two inherited alleles. This phenomenon is called **allelic exclusion,** and it helps ensure that every B cell will express a single receptor, thus maintaining clonal specificity. If both alleles undergo nonproductive IgH gene rearrangements, the developing cell cannot produce Ig heavy chains, cannot generate a pre-BCR–dependent survival signal, and thus undergoes programmed cell death. This occurs frequently and in part explains why only a small fraction of the cells arising from B cell progenitors develop into mature B lymphocytes (see Fig. 8–3). Ig heavy chain allelic exclusion involves changes in chromatin structure in the heavy chain locus that limit accessibility to the V(D)J recombinase.

The second way the pre-BCR regulates V(D)J recombination is by stimulating light chain gene rearrangement. However, μ chain expression is not absolutely required for light chain gene recombination, as shown by the finding that knockout mice lacking the μ gene do initiate light chain gene rearrangements in some developing B cells (which, of course, cannot express func-

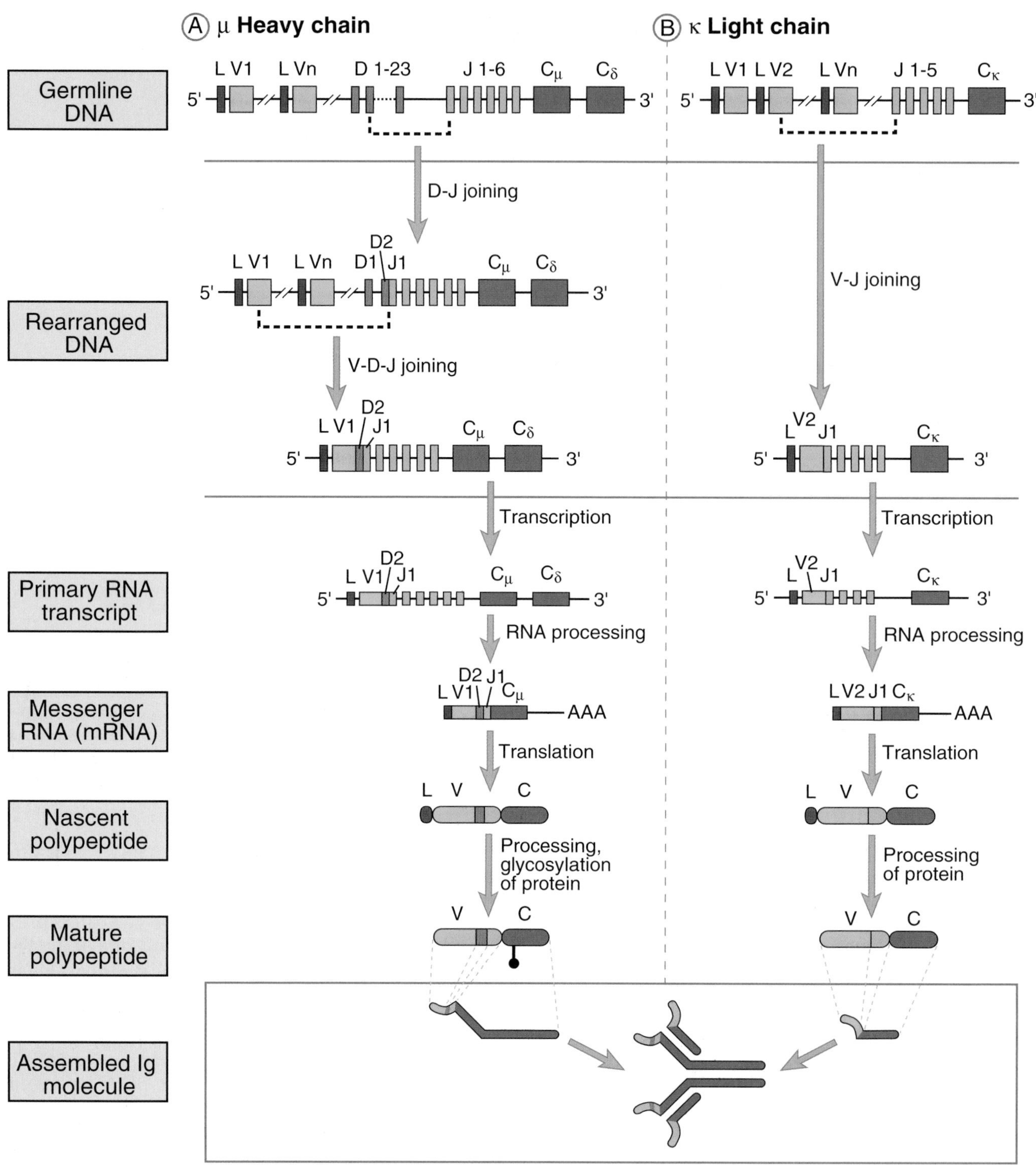

FIGURE 8–16 Ig heavy and light chain gene recombination and expression. The sequence of DNA recombination and gene expression events is shown for the Ig μ heavy chain (A) and the Ig κ light chain (B). In the example shown in A, the V region of the μ heavy chain is encoded by the exons V1, D2, and J1. In the example shown in B, the V region of the κ chain is encoded by the exons V1 and J1.

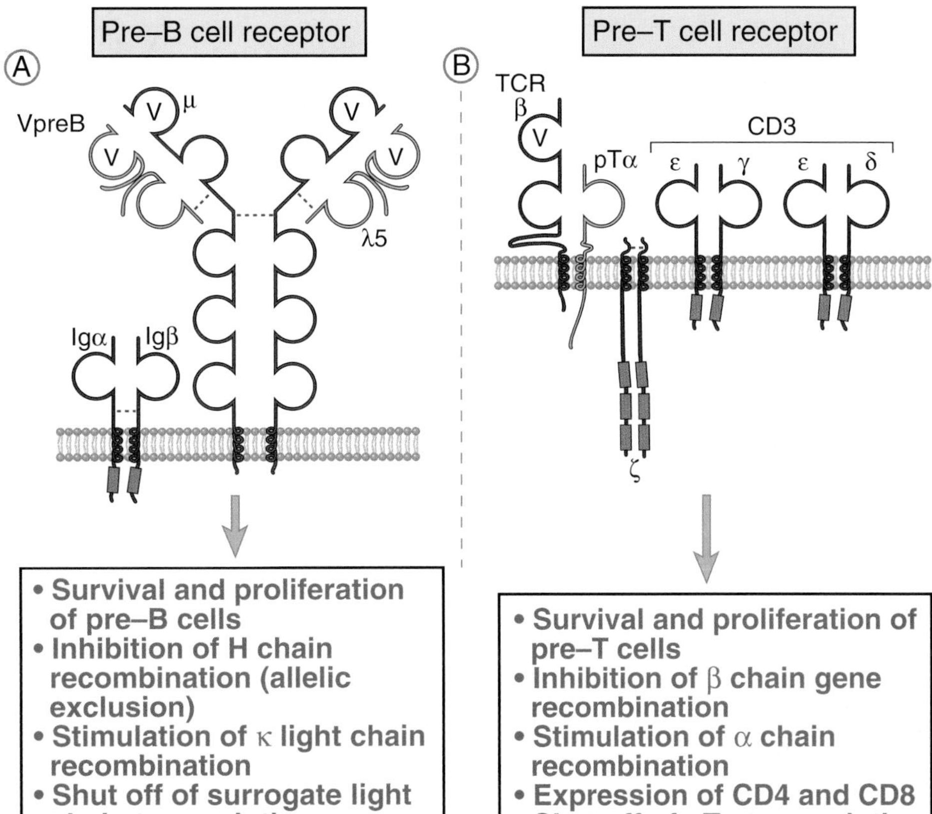

FIGURE 8–17 Pre-B cell and pre-T cell receptors. The pre-B cell receptor (A) and the pre-T cell receptor (B) are expressed during the pre-B and pre-T cell stages of maturation, respectively, and both receptors share similar structures and functions. The pre-B cell receptor is composed of the μ heavy chain and an invariant surrogate light chain. The surrogate light chain is composed of two proteins, the VpreB protein, which is homologous to a light chain V domain, and a λ5 protein that is covalently attached to the μ heavy chain by a disulfide bond. The pre-T cell receptor (B) is composed of the TCR β chain and the invariant pre-T α chain. The pre-B cell receptor is associated with the Igα and Igβ signaling molecules that are part of the BCR complex in mature B cells (see Chapter 9), and the pre-T cell receptor associates with the CD3 and ζ proteins that are part of the TCR complex in mature T cells (see Chapter 7).

tional antigen receptors and proceed to maturity). The pre-BCR also contributes to the inactivation of surrogate light chain gene expression as pre-B cells mature.

At the next stage in its maturation, each developing B cell also rearranges a κ or a λ light chain gene and produces a light chain protein, which associates with the previously synthesized μ chain to produce a complete IgM protein. The IgM-expressing B cell is called the **immature B cell.** DNA recombination in the κ or λ light chain locus occurs in a similar manner as in the Ig heavy chain locus (see Fig. 8–16B). There are no D segments in the light chain loci, and therefore recombination involves only the joining of one V segment to one J segment, forming a VJ exon. This VJ exon remains separated from the C region by an intron, and this separation is retained in the primary RNA transcript. Splicing of the primary transcript results in the removal of the intron between the VJ and C exons and generates an mRNA that is translated to produce the κ or λ protein. In the λ locus, alternative RNA splicing may lead to the use of any one of the four functional C_λ genes, but there is no known functional difference between the resulting types of λ light chains. The κ locus rearranges after heavy chain rearrangement and before λ gene rearrangement. Production of κ light chains inhibits rearrangement of the λ locus, and the λ locus will undergo recombination only if a κ light chain cannot be produced, or if induced to rearrange during the phenomenon of receptor editing described below, when a self-reactive previously rearranged light chain is deleted. Therefore, an individual B cell clone can produce only one of the two types of light chains during its life; this is called light chain isotype exclusion. As in the heavy chain locus, production of κ or λ is allelically excluded and is initiated from only one of the two parental chromosomes. Also, as for heavy chains, if one allele undergoes nonfunctional rearrangement, DNA recombination can occur on the other allele; however, if both alleles of both κ and λ chains are nonfunctional in a developing B cell, that cell dies.

The light chain that is produced complexes with the previously synthesized μ heavy chain, and the assembled IgM molecules are expressed on the cell surface in association with Igα and Igβ, where they function as specific receptors for antigens. Immature B cells do not proliferate and differentiate in response to antigens. In fact, their encounter in the bone marrow with high avidity antigens, such as multivalent self antigens, may lead to the induction of receptor editing, cell death, or functional unresponsiveness rather than activation. This property is important for the negative selection of B cells that are specific for self antigens present in the bone marrow (discussed later). Immature B cells leave the bone marrow and complete their maturation in the spleen before migrating to other peripheral lymphoid organs.

Distinct subsets of B cells develop from different progenitors (Fig. 8–18). Fetal liver-derived HSCs are the precursors of B-1 B cells, described below. Bone marrow-derived HSCs give rise to the majority of B cells, which are sometimes called B-2 B cells. These cells rapidly pass through two transitional stages and can commit to

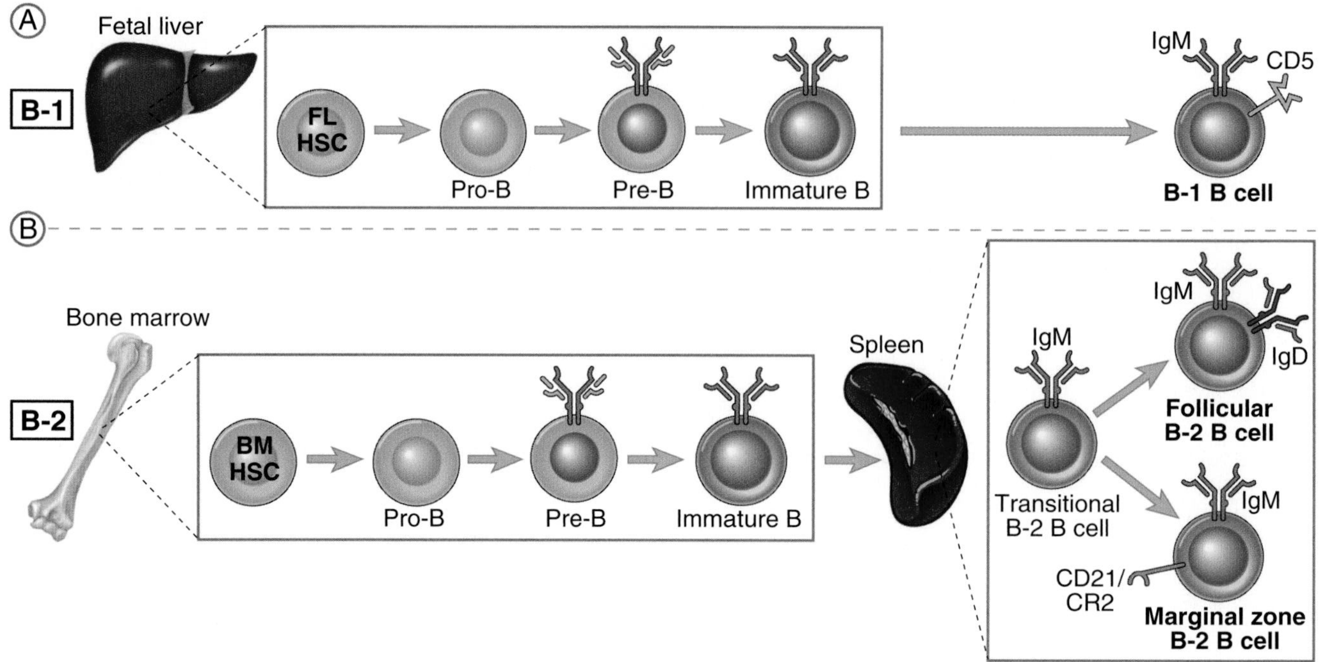

FIGURE 8–18 B lymphocyte subsets. A. Most B cells that develop from fetal liver–derived stem cells differentiate into the B-1 lineage. B. B lymphocytes that arise from bone marrow precursors after birth give rise to the B-2 lineage. Two major subsets of B lymphocytes are derived from B-2 B cell precursors. Follicular B cells are recirculating lymphocytes, while marginal zone B cells reside primarily in the spleen. These developmental pathways have been best defined in mice.

develop either into **marginal zone B cells,** also described below, or into **follicular B cells**. Most mature B cells are follicular B cells. They coexpress μ and δ heavy chains in association with the κ or λ light chain and therefore produce both membrane IgM and membrane IgD. Both classes of membrane Ig utilize the same VDJ exon and associate with identical light chains and therefore exhibit the same antigen specificity. Simultaneous expression in a single B cell of the same rearranged VDJ exon on two transcripts, one including C_μ exons and the other C_δ exons, is achieved by alternative RNA splicing (Fig. 8–19). A long primary RNA transcript is produced containing the rearranged VDJ unit as well as the C_μ and C_δ genes. If the introns are spliced out such that the VDJ exon is contiguous with C_μ exons, this results in the generation of a μ mRNA. If, however, the VDJ complex is not linked to C_μ exons but is spliced to C_δ exons, a δ mRNA is produced. Subsequent translation results in the synthesis of a complete μ or δ heavy chain protein. Thus, alternative splicing allows a B cell to simultaneously produce mature mRNAs and proteins of two different heavy chain isotypes. The precise mechanisms that regulate the choice of polyadenylation or splice acceptor sites by which the rearranged VDJ is joined to either C_μ or C_δ are poorly understood, as are the signals that determine when and why a B cell expresses both IgM and IgD rather than IgM alone. The coexpression of IgM and IgD is accompanied by the acquisition of functional competence and the ability to recirculate, and this is why follicular B cells are also called mature B cells. This correlation between expression of IgD and acquisition of functional competence has led to the suggestion that IgD is the essential activating receptor of mature B cells. However, there is no evidence for a functional difference between membrane IgM and membrane IgD. Moreover, knockout of the δ gene in mice does not have a significant impact on the maturation or antigen-induced responses of B cells. Follicular B cells are also often called recirculating B cells, since they migrate from one lymphoid organ to the next, residing in specialized niches known as B cell follicles. In these niches these B cells are maintained, in part, by signals delivered by a trophic ligand of the tumor necrosis factor (TNF) cytokine family called BAFF or BlyS (Chapter 10).

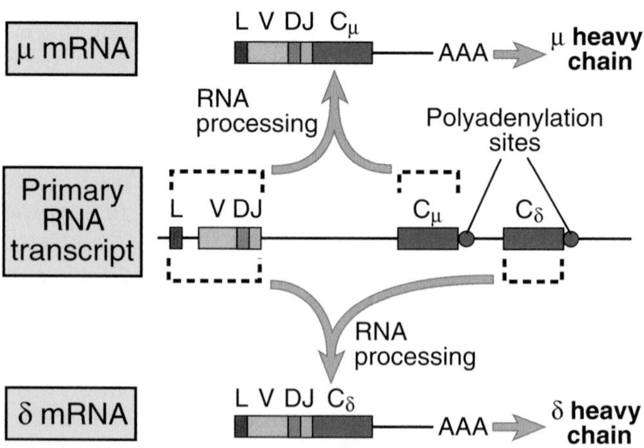

FIGURE 8–19 Coexpression of IgM and IgD. Alternative processing of a primary RNA transcript results in the formation of a μ or δ mRNA. Dashed lines indicate the H chain segments that are joined by RNA splicing.

Mature, naive B cells are responsive to antigens, and unless the cells encounter antigens that they recognize with high affinity and respond to, they die in a few months. In Chapter 10, we will discuss how these cells respond to antigens and how the pattern of Ig gene expression changes during antigen-induced B cell differentiation.

Selection of the Mature B Cell Repertoire

The repertoire of mature B cells is positively selected from the pool of immature B cells. As we shall see later, positive selection is well defined in T lymphocytes and is responsible for preserving self MHC–restricted $CD4^+$ and $CD8^+$ T cells from the much larger pool of unselected, immature T cells. There is no comparable restriction for B cell antigen recognition. Nevertheless, positive selection appears to be a general phenomenon geared to identifying lymphocytes that have completed their rearrangement program successfully and possibly facilitating lineage commitment to T or B cell subsets. It is believed that only B cells that express functional membrane Ig molecules receive constitutive BCR-derived survival signals. Self antigens appear to influence the strength of the BCR signal and thereby the subsequent choice of peripheral B cell lineage during B cell maturation.

Immature B cells that recognize self antigens with high avidity may be induced to change their specificities by a process called **receptor editing.** In this process, antigen recognition leads to reactivation of *Rag* genes, additional light chain V-J recombination events, and production of a new Ig light chain, allowing the cell to express a different B cell receptor that is not self-reactive. Receptor editing generally is targeted at self-reactive κ light chain genes. VJ_κ exons encoding the variable domains of autoreactive light chains are deleted and replaced by new VJ_κ exons or by λ light chain rearrangements. The new VJ_κ exon may be generated by the rearrangement of a V gene upstream of the original V gene that produced an autoreactive light chain, to a J segment downstream of the originally rearranged J segment. As many as 25% of mature B cells in mice show evidence of κ chain editing.

Immature B cells that express high-affinity receptors for self antigens and encounter these antigens in the bone marrow may also die or fail to mature further if they are not edited. Deletion is generally called **negative selection,** and it is partly responsible for maintaining B cell tolerance to self antigens that are present in the bone marrow (see Chapter 11). The antigens mediating negative selection—usually abundant or polyvalent (e.g., membrane-bound) self antigens—deliver strong signals to IgM-expressing immature B lymphocytes that happen to express receptors specific for these self antigens. Antigen recognition leads to apoptotic death of immature B cells, probably only when editing fails. Once the transition is made to the IgD^+IgM^+ mature B cell stage, antigen recognition leads to proliferation and differentiation, not to apoptosis or receptor editing. As a result, mature B cells that recognize antigens with high affinity in peripheral lymphoid tissues are activated, and this process leads to humoral immune responses (see Chapter 10).

B-1 and Marginal Zone Subsets of B Lymphocytes

A subset of B lymphocytes, called B-1 B cells, differs from the majority of B lymphocytes and develops in a unique manner. These cells develop from fetal liver-derived hematopoietic stem cells. Many B-1 cells express the CD5 (Ly-1) molecule. In the adult, large numbers of B-1 cells are found as a self-renewing population in the peritoneum and mucosal sites. B-1 cells develop earlier during ontogeny than do conventional B cells, and they express a relatively limited repertoire of V genes and exhibit far less junctional diversity than conventional B cells do (TdT is not expressed in the fetal liver). B-1 cells, as well as marginal zone B cells, spontaneously secrete IgM antibodies that often react with microbial polysaccharides and lipids. These antibodies are sometimes called **natural antibodies** because they are present in individuals without overt immunization, although it is possible that microbial flora in the gut are the source of antigens that stimulate their production. B-1 cells provide a source of rapid antibody production against microbes in particular sites, such as the peritoneum. At mucosal sites B-1 cells may differentiate into perhaps half the IgA-secreting cells in the lamina propria. B-1 cells are analogous to γδ T cells in that they both have limited antigen receptor repertoires, and they are both presumed to respond to commonly encountered microbial antigens early in immune responses.

Marginal zone B cells are located primarily in the vicinity of the marginal sinus in the spleen and are in some ways similar to B-1 cells in terms of their limited diversity, and their ability to respond to polysaccharide antigens and to generate natural antibodies. Marginal zone B cells express IgM and the surface marker CD21. They respond very rapidly to blood-borne microbes and differentiate into short-lived IgM-secreting plasma cells. Although they generally mediate T cell–independent immune responses to circulating pathogens, marginal zone B cells also appear capable of mediating some T cell–dependent immune responses.

MATURATION OF T LYMPHOCYTES

The maturation of T lymphocytes from committed progenitors involves the sequential rearrangement and expression of TCR genes, cell proliferation, antigen-induced selection, and the acquisition of functional capabilities (Fig. 8–20). In many ways, this is similar to B cell maturation. However, T cell maturation has some unique features that reflect the specificity of T lymphocytes for self MHC–associated peptide antigens and the need for a special microenvironment for selecting cells with this specificity.

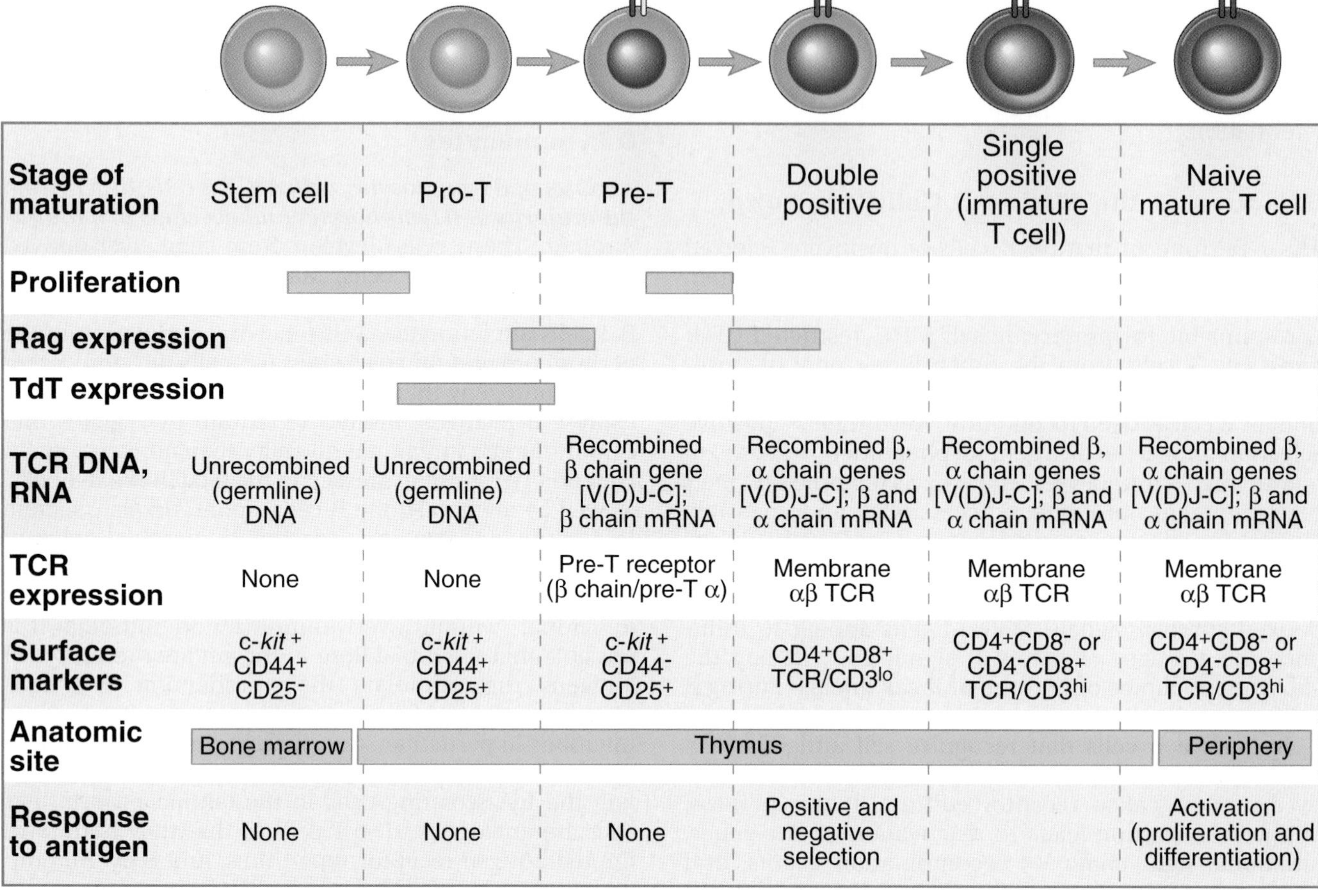

Stage of maturation	Stem cell	Pro-T	Pre-T	Double positive	Single positive (immature T cell)	Naive mature T cell
Proliferation						
Rag expression						
TdT expression						
TCR DNA, RNA	Unrecombined (germline) DNA	Unrecombined (germline) DNA	Recombined β chain gene [V(D)J-C]; β chain mRNA	Recombined β, α chain genes [V(D)J-C]; β and α chain mRNA	Recombined β, α chain genes [V(D)J-C]; β and α chain mRNA	Recombined β, α chain genes [V(D)J-C]; β and α chain mRNA
TCR expression	None	None	Pre-T receptor (β chain/pre-T α)	Membrane αβ TCR	Membrane αβ TCR	Membrane αβ TCR
Surface markers	c-*kit*$^+$ CD44$^+$ CD25$^-$	c-*kit*$^+$ CD44$^+$ CD25$^+$	c-*kit*$^+$ CD44$^-$ CD25$^+$	CD4$^+$CD8$^+$ TCR/CD3^{lo}	CD4$^+$CD8$^-$ or CD4$^-$CD8$^+$ TCR/CD3^{hi}	CD4$^+$CD8$^-$ or CD4$^-$CD8$^+$ TCR/CD3^{hi}
Anatomic site	Bone marrow	Thymus				Periphery
Response to antigen	None	None	None	Positive and negative selection		Activation (proliferation and differentiation)

FIGURE 8–20 Stages of T cell maturation. Events corresponding to each stage of T cell maturation from a bone marrow stem cell to a mature T lymphocyte are illustrated. Several surface markers in addition to those shown have been used to define distinct stages of T cell maturation.

Role of the Thymus in T Cell Maturation

The thymus is the major site of maturation of T cells. This function of the thymus was first suspected because of immunologic deficiencies associated with the lack of a thymus.

- If the thymus is removed from a neonatal mouse, this animal fails to develop mature T cells.
- The congenital absence of the thymus, as occurs in the DiGeorge syndrome in humans or in the nude mouse strain, is characterized by low numbers of mature T cells in the circulation and peripheral lymphoid tissues and severe deficiencies in T cell-mediated immunity (see Chapter 20).

The thymus involutes with age and is virtually undetectable in postpubertal humans, but some maturation of T cells continues throughout adult life, as indicated by the successful reconstitution of the immune system in adult recipients of bone marrow transplants. It may be that the remnant of the involuted thymus is adequate for some T cell maturation. Because memory T cells have a long life span (perhaps longer than 20 years in humans) and accumulate with age, the need to generate new T cells decreases as individuals age.

T lymphocytes originate from precursors that arise in the fetal liver and adult bone marrow and seed the thymus. In mice, immature lymphocytes are first detected in the thymus on the 11th day of the normal 21-day gestation. This corresponds to about week 7 or 8 of gestation in humans. Developing T cells in the thymus are called **thymocytes.** The most immature thymocytes do not express the TCR or CD4 and CD8 coreceptors (see Fig. 8–20). They are found in the subcapsular sinus and outer cortical region of the thymus. From here, the thymocytes migrate into and through the cortex, where most of the subsequent maturation events occur. It is in the cortex that the thymocytes first express γδ and αβ TCRs, and the αβ T cells begin to mature into CD4$^+$ class II MHC-restricted or CD8$^+$ class I MHC-restricted T cells. As these thymocytes undergo the final stages of maturation, they migrate from the cortex to the medulla and then exit the thymus through the circulation. In the following sections we discuss the maturation of αβ T cells; γδ T cells are discussed later in the chapter.

The thymic environment provides stimuli that are required for the proliferation and maturation of thymocytes. Many of these stimuli come from thymic cells other than the maturing T cells. These include thymic epithelial cells and bone marrow–derived macrophages and dendritic cells (see Chapter 3, Fig. 3–7). Within the cortex, the epithelial cells form a meshwork of long cytoplasmic processes, around which thymocytes must pass to reach the medulla. Epithelial cells are also present in the medulla. Bone marrow–derived dendritic cells are present at the corticomedullary junction and within the medulla, and macrophages are present primarily within the medulla. The migration of thymocytes through this anatomic arrangement allows physical interactions between the thymocytes and these other cells, which are necessary for the maturation of the T lymphocytes.

Two types of molecules produced by the nonlymphoid thymic cells are important for T cell maturation. The first are class I and class II MHC molecules, which are expressed on epithelial cells and dendritic cells in the thymus. The interactions of maturing thymocytes with these MHC molecules within the thymus are essential for the selection of the mature T cell repertoire, as we will discuss later. Second, thymic stromal cells, including epithelial cells, secrete cytokines and chemokines, which respectively stimulate the proliferation of immature T cells and orchestrate the cortical to medullary transit of developing αβ lineage thymocytes. The best defined of these cytokines is IL-7, which was mentioned earlier as a critical lymphopoietic growth factor. Chemokines such as CCL21 and CCL19, which are recognized by the CCR7 chemokine receptor on thymocytes, mediate the guided movement of developing T cells in the thymus.

The rates of cell proliferation and apoptotic death are extremely high in cortical thymocytes. A single precursor gives rise to many progeny, and 95% of these cells die by apoptosis before reaching the medulla. The cell death is due to a combination of failure to productively rearrange the TCR β chain gene and to thus negotiate the pre-TCR/β selection checkpoint described below, failure to be positively selected by MHC molecules in the thymus, and self antigen–induced negative selection (see Figs. 8–3 and 8–4). Cortical thymocytes are also sensitive to irradiation and glucocorticoids. *In vivo,* high doses of glucocorticoids induce apoptotic death of cortical thymocytes.

Stages of T Cell Maturation

During T cell maturation, there is a precise order in which TCR genes are rearranged and in which the TCR and CD4 and CD8 coreceptors are expressed (Figs. 8–20 and 8–21). In the mouse, surface expression of the γδ TCR occurs first, 3 to 4 days after precursor cells first arrive in the thymus, and the αβ TCR is expressed 2 or 3 days later. In human fetal thymuses, γδ T cell receptor expression begins at about 9 weeks of gestation, followed by expression of the αβ TCR at 10 weeks.

The most immature cortical thymocytes, which are recent arrivals from the bone marrow, contain TCR genes in their germline configuration and do not express TCR, CD3 or ζ chains, or CD4 or CD8; these cells are called **double-negative thymocytes.** This is also known as the **pro-T cell stage** of maturation. The majority (>90%) of the double-negative thymocytes will ultimately give rise to αβ TCR-expressing, MHC-restricted $CD4^+$ and $CD8^+$ T cells. Rag-1 and Rag-2 proteins are first expressed at this stage, and are required for the rearrangement of TCR genes. D_β-to-J_β rearrangements at the TCR β chain locus occur first; these involve either joining of the $D_\beta1$ gene segment to one of the six $J_\beta1$ segments or joining of the $D_\beta2$ segment to one of the six $J_\beta2$ segments (Fig. 8–22A). V_β-to-DJ_β rearrangements occur at the transition between the pro-T stage and the subsequent **pre-T stage** during αβ T cell development. The DNA sequences between the segments undergoing rearrangement, including D, J, and possibly $C_\beta1$ genes (if $D_\beta2$ and $J_\beta2$ segments are used), are deleted during this rearrangement process. The primary nuclear transcripts of the TCR β genes contain the intron between the recombined VDJ_β exon and the relevant C_β gene. Poly-A tails are added following cleavage of the primary transcript downstream of consensus polyadenylation sites located 3′ of the C_β region, and the sequences between the VDJ exon and C_β are spliced out to form a mature mRNA in which VDJ segments are juxtaposed to either of the two C_β genes (depending on which J segment was selected during the rearrangement process). Translation of this mRNA gives rise to a full-length C_β protein. The two C_β genes appear to be functionally interchangeable, and there is no evidence that an individual T cell ever switches from one C gene to another. Furthermore, the use of either C_β gene segment does not influence the function or specificity of the TCR. The promoters in the 5′ flanking regions of V_β genes function together with a powerful enhancer that is located 3′ of the $C_\beta2$ gene once V genes are brought close to the C gene by V(D)J recombination. This proximity of the promoter to the enhancer is responsible for high-level T cell–specific transcription of the rearranged TCR β chain gene.

If a productive (i.e., in-frame) rearrangement of the TCR β chain gene occurs in a given pro-T cell, the TCR β chain protein is expressed on the cell surface in association with an invariant protein called **pre-Tα** and with CD3 and ζ proteins to form the **pre-T cell receptor** (pre-TCR; see Fig. 8–17B). The pre-TCR mediates the selection of the roughly one-in-three developing pre-T cells that productively rearrange the β chain of the TCR (roughly two thirds of developing T cells add or remove bases at rearrangement junctions that are not multiples of three, and therefore these rearrangements fail to encode a TCR β protein). The function of the pre-TCR complex in T cell development is similar to that of the surrogate light chain–containing pre-BCR in B cell development. Signals from the pre-TCR mediate the survival of pre-T cells and contribute to the largest proliferative expansion during T cell development. Pre-TCR signals also initiate recombination at the TCR α chain locus and drive the transition from the double-negative to the double-positive stage of thymocyte development (discussed below). These signals also inhibit further rearrangement of the TCR β chain locus largely by limiting accessibility

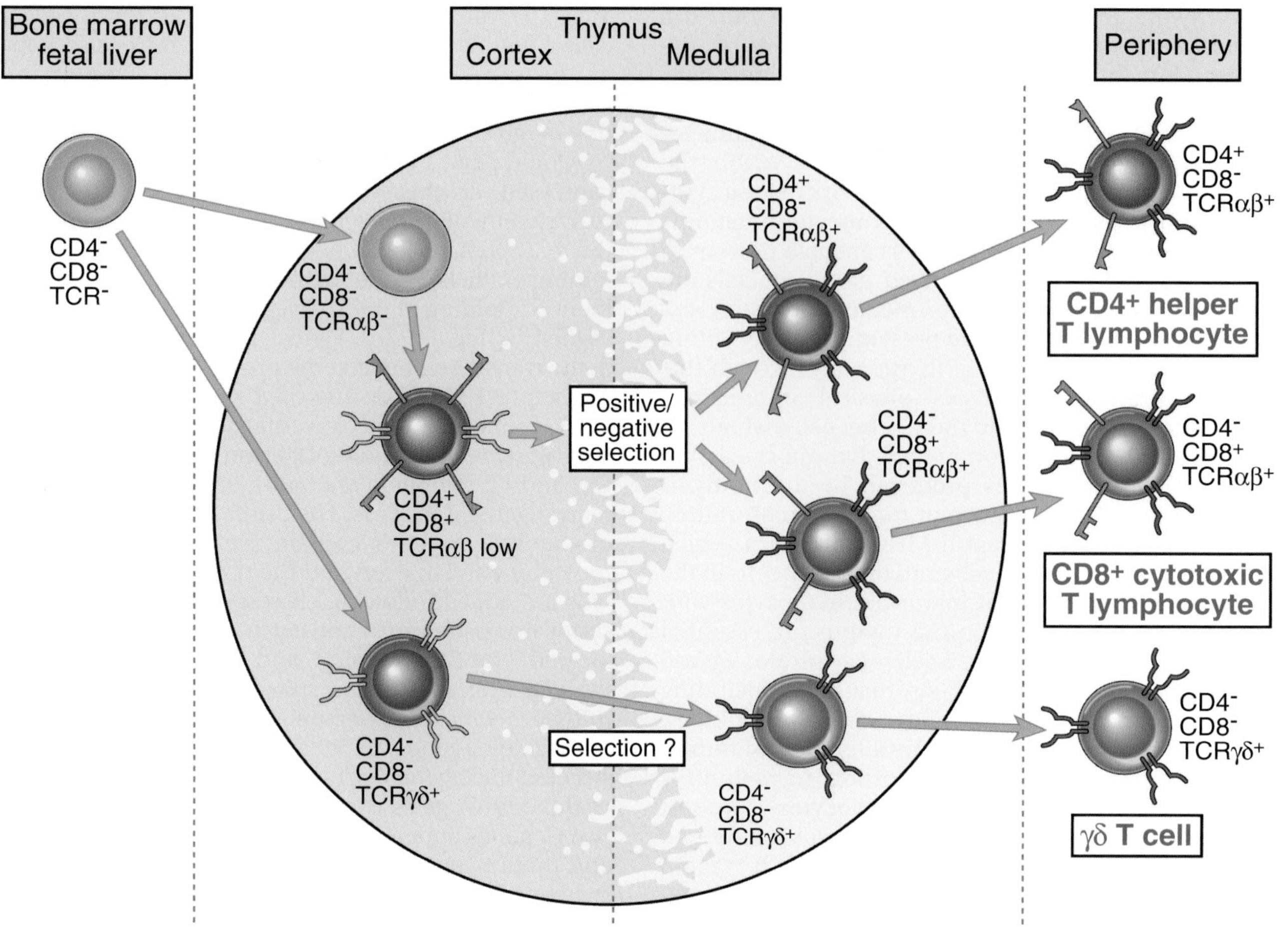

FIGURE 8–21 Maturation of T cells in the thymus. Precursors of T cells travel from the bone marrow through the blood to the thymus. In the thymic cortex, progenitors of αβ T cells express TCRs and CD4 and CD8 coreceptors. Selection processes eliminate self-reactive thymocytes and promote survival of thymocytes whose TCRs bind self MHC molecules with low affinity. Functional and phenotypic differentiation into $CD4^+CD8^-$ or $CD8^+CD4^-$ T cells occurs in the medulla, and mature T cells are released into the circulation. The γδ TCR-expressing T cells are also derived from bone marrow precursors and mature in the thymus as a separate lineage.

of the other allele to the recombination machinery. This results in β chain allelic exclusion (i.e., mature T cells express only one of the two inherited β chain alleles). As in pre-B cells, it is not known what, if any, ligand the pre-TCR recognizes. Pre-TCR signaling, like pre-BCR signaling, is generally believed to be initiated in a ligand-independent manner, dependent on the successful assembly of the pre-TCR complex. Pre-TCR signaling is mediated by a number of cytosolic kinases and adapter proteins that are known to also be linked to TCR signaling (Chapter 9). The essential function of the pre-TCR in T cell maturation has been demonstrated by numerous studies with genetically mutated mice.

- In Rag-1- or Rag-2-deficient mice, thymocytes cannot rearrange either α or β chain genes and fail to mature past the double-negative stage. If a functionally rearranged β chain gene is introduced into the Rag-deficient mice as a transgene, the expressed β chain associates with pre-Tα to form the pre-TCR, and maturation proceeds to the double-positive stage. An α chain transgene alone does not relieve the maturation block because the β chain is required for formation of the pre-TCR.
- Knockout mice lacking any component of the pre-TCR complex (i.e., the TCR β chain, pre-Tα, CD3, ζ, or Lck) show a block in the maturation of T cells at the double-negative stage.

At the next stage of T cell maturation, thymocytes express both CD4 and CD8 and are called **double-positive thymocytes.** Double-positive T cells also induce the expression of the CCR 7 chemokine receptor, which guides these cells from the cortex toward the medulla, where chemokines specific for this receptor are secreted by stromal cells. The expression of CD4 and CD8 is essential for subsequent selection events, discussed later. The rearrangement of the TCR α chain genes and the expression of TCR αβ heterodimers occur in the $CD4^+CD8^+$ double-positive population, just before or during migration of the thymocytes from the cortex to the medulla (see Figs. 8–20 and 8–21). A second wave of *Rag* gene expression late in the pre-T stage promotes TCR α gene recombination. Once α chain rearrangement commences, it proceeds for 3 or 4 days (in mice) until the expression of the *Rag-1* and *Rag-2* genes is turned off by signals from the αβ TCR during positive selection (discussed later). The steps involved in TCR α

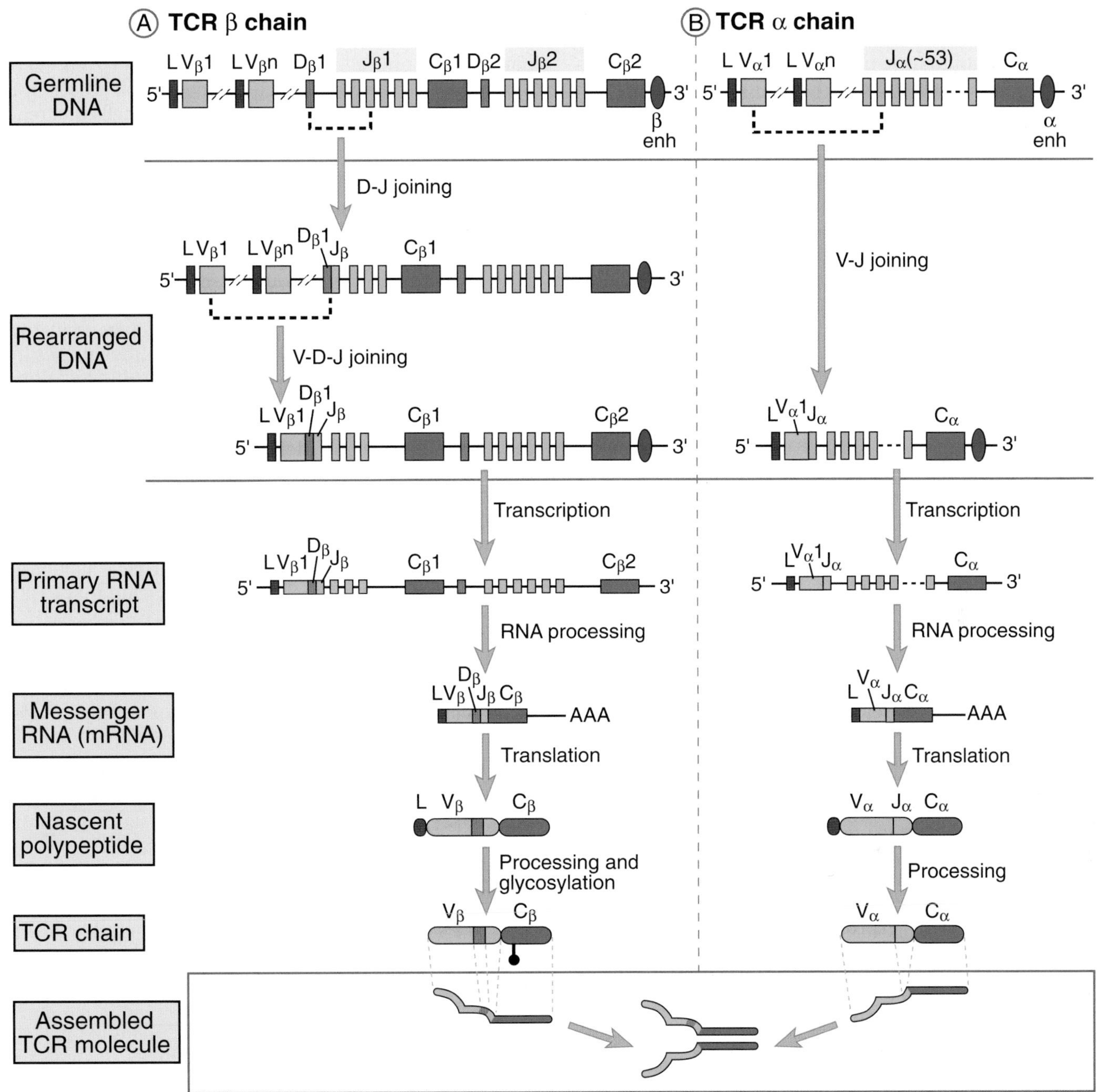

FIGURE 8–22 TCR α and β chain gene recombination and expression. The sequence of recombination and gene expression events is shown for the TCR β chain (A) and the TCR α chain (B). In the example shown in A, the variable (V) region of the rearranged TCR β chain includes the $V_{\beta}1$, and $D_{\beta}1$ gene segments, and the third J segment in the $J_{\beta}1$ cluster. The constant (C) region is encoded by the $C_{\beta}1$ exon. Note that at the TCRβ chain locus, rearrangement begins with D-to-J joining followed by V-to-DJ joining. 14 J_{β} segments have been identified in humans, and not all are shown in the figure. In the example shown in B, the V region of the TCR α chain includes the $V_{\alpha}1$ gene and the second J segment in the J_{α} cluster (this cluster is made up of at least 61 J_{α} segments in humans; not all are shown here).

chain gene rearrangement are broadly similar to those that occur during TCR β chain gene rearrangement (Fig. 8–22B). Because there are no D segments in the TCR α locus, rearrangement consists solely of the joining of V and J segments. The large number of J_{α} segments permits multiple attempts at productive V-J joining on each chromosome, thereby increasing the probability that a functional αβ TCR will be produced. In contrast to the TCR β chain locus, where production of the protein and formation of the pre-TCR suppress further rearrangement, there is little or no allelic exclusion in the α chain locus. Therefore, productive TCR α rearrangements may occur on both chromosomes, and if this happens, the T cell will express two α chains. In fact, up to 30% of mature peripheral T cells do express two different TCRs, with different α chains but the same β chain. The functional consequence of this dual receptor expression is unknown. Because only one TCR is required for positive selection, it is possible that the second TCR may not have any affinity for self MHC, and therefore it would have no function. Transcriptional regulation of the α chain gene occurs in a broadly similar manner to that of the β chain. There are promoters 5′ of each V_α gene that have low-level activity and are responsible for high-level T cell-specific transcription when brought close to an α chain enhancer located 3′ of the C_α gene. The inability to successfully rearrange the TCR α chain on either chromosome leads to a failure of positive selection (discussed below). The thymocyte that has failed to make a productive rearrangement will die by apoptosis.

TCR α gene expression early in the double-positive stage leads to the formation of the complete αβ TCR, which is expressed on the cell surface in association with CD3 and ζ proteins. The coordinate expression of CD3 and ζ proteins and the assembly of intact TCR complexes are required for surface expression. Rearrangement of the TCR α gene results in deletion of the TCR δ locus that lies between V segments (common to both α and δ loci) and J_α segments (see Fig. 8–7). As a result this T cell is no longer capable of becoming a γδ T cell. The expression of *Rag* genes and further TCR gene recombination cease after this stage of maturation. The first cells to express TCRs are in the thymic cortex, and expression is low compared with mature T cells. By virtue of their expression of complete TCR complexes, double-positive cells become responsive to antigens and are subjected to positive and negative selection.

Cells that successfully undergo these selection processes go on to mature into $CD4^+$ or $CD8^+$ T cells, which are called **single-positive thymocytes.** Thus, the stages of T cell maturation in the thymus can readily be distinguished by the expression of CD4 and CD8 (Fig. 8–23). This phenotypic maturation is accompanied by functional maturation. $CD4^+$ cells acquire the ability to produce cytokines in response to subsequent antigen stimulation and to express effector molecules (such as CD40 ligand) that "help" B lymphocytes and macrophages, whereas $CD8^+$ cells become capable of producing molecules that kill other cells. Mature single-positive thymocytes enter the thymic medulla and then leave the thymus to populate peripheral lymphoid tissues.

Selection Processes in the Maturation of MHC-Restricted αβ T Cells

The selection of developing T cells is dependent on recognition of antigen (peptide-MHC complexes) in the thymus and is responsible for preserving useful cells and eliminating potentially harmful ones (Fig. 8–24). The immature, or unselected, repertoire of T lymphocytes consists of cells whose receptors may recognize any peptide antigen (self or foreign) displayed by any MHC molecule (also self or foreign). In addition, receptors may be expressed that do not recognize any peptide-MHC molecule complex. In every individual, the only useful T cells are the ones specific for foreign peptides presented by that individual's MHC molecules, that is, self MHC molecules. (Recall that there are many alleles of MHC molecules in the population, and every individual inherits one allele of each MHC gene from each parent. These inherited alleles encode "self MHC" for that individual.) Also, in every individual, T cells that recognize self antigens with high avidity are potentially dangerous because such recognition may trigger autoimmunity. Selection processes act on the immature T cell repertoire to ensure that only the useful cells complete the process of maturation.

When double-positive thymocytes first express αβ TCRs, these receptors encounter self peptides (the only peptides normally present in the thymus) displayed by self MHC molecules (the only MHC molecules available to display peptides) mainly on thymic epithelial cells in the cortex, but also on dendritic cells in this location. **Positive selection** is the process in which thymocytes whose TCRs bind with low avidity (i.e., weakly) to self peptide–self MHC complexes are stimulated to survive (see Fig. 8–24A). Thymocytes whose receptors do not recognize self MHC molecules are permitted to die by a default pathway of apoptosis (see Fig. 8–24B). This ensures that the T cells that mature are self MHC restricted. Positive selection also fixes the class I or class II MHC restriction of T cell subsets, ensuring that $CD8^+$ T cells are specific for peptides displayed by class I MHC molecules and $CD4^+$ T cells for class II–associated peptides. **Negative selection** is the process in which thymocytes whose TCRs bind strongly to self peptide antigens in association with self MHC molecules are deleted (see

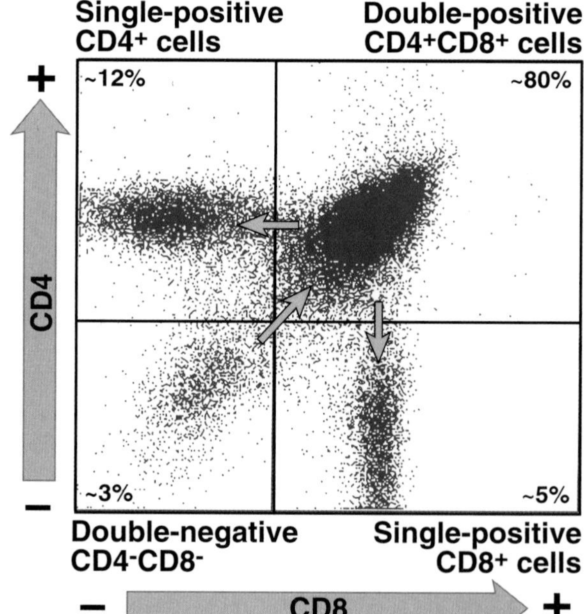

FIGURE 8–23 CD4 and CD8 expression on thymocytes. The maturation of thymocytes can be followed by changes in expression of the CD4 and CD8 coreceptors. A two-color flow cytometric analysis of thymocytes using anti-CD4 and anti-CD8 antibodies, each tagged with a different fluorochrome, is illustrated. The percentages of all thymocytes contributed by each major population are shown in the four quadrants. The least mature subset is the $CD4^-CD8^-$ (double-negative) cells. Arrows indicate the sequence of maturation.

Fig. 8–24C). This eliminates developing T cells that are strongly autoreactive against self antigens that are present at high concentrations in the thymus. The net result of these selection processes is that the repertoire of mature T cells that leaves the thymus is self MHC restricted and tolerant to many self antigens. In the following sections, we discuss the details of positive and negative selection.

Positive Selection of Thymocytes: Development of the Self MHC–Restricted T Cell Repertoire

Positive selection works by promoting the selective survival and expansion of thymocytes with self MHC–restricted TCRs (Fig. 8–24A). Double-positive thymocytes are produced without antigenic stimulation and begin to express αβ TCRs with randomly generated specificities. In the thymic cortex, these immature cells encounter epithelial cells that are displaying a variety of self peptides bound to class I and class II MHC molecules. If the TCR on a cell recognizes peptide-loaded class I MHC molecules, and at the same time CD8 interacts with the class I MHC molecules, that T cell receives signals that prevent its death and promote its continued maturation. To proceed along the maturation pathway, the T cell must continue to express the TCR and CD8 but can lose expression of CD4. The result is the development of a class I MHC-restricted $CD8^+$ T cell. An entirely analogous process leads to the development of class II MHC-restricted $CD4^+$ T cells. Any T cell that expresses a TCR that does not recognize a peptide-loaded MHC molecule in the thymus will die and be lost.

The essential roles of MHC molecules and TCR specificity in positive selection have been established by a variety of experiments.

- If a thymus from one inbred strain is transplanted into chimeric animals of another strain, the T cells that mature are restricted by the MHC type of the thymus. The transplanted thymuses may be irradiated or treated with cytotoxic drugs (such

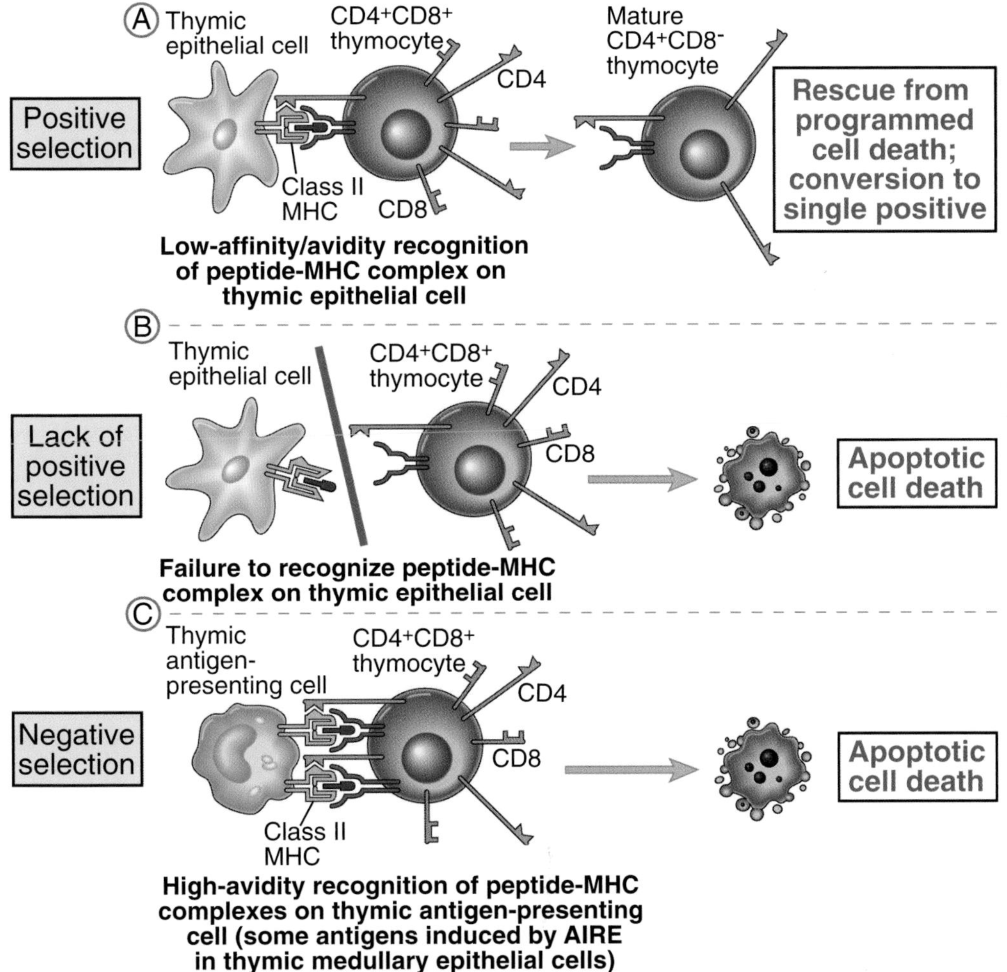

FIGURE 8–24 Selection processes in the thymus. A. Positive selection. If the thymocyte TCR engages in a low-affinity interaction with a self MHC molecule on a thymic epithelial cell, it is rescued from programmed cell death and continues to mature. B. Lack of positive selection. If the thymocyte TCR does not engage in any interactions with peptide-MHC molecule complexes on thymic epithelial cells, it will die by a default pathway of programmed cell death. C. Negative selection. If the thymocyte TCR binds peptide-MHC complexes on a thymic antigen-presenting cell with high affinity or avidity, it is induced to undergo apoptotic cell death.

as deoxyguanosine) to kill all resident bone marrow–derived macrophages, dendritic cells, and lymphoid cells, leaving only the resistant thymic epithelial cells. Again, mature T cells develop in these thymuses, and their ability to recognize antigen is restricted by MHC gene products expressed on the transplanted thymic epithelial cells and not necessarily by MHC gene products expressed on extrathymic cells. Therefore, the thymic epithelium is the critical host element for positive selection (i.e., the development of the MHC restriction patterns of T cells).

- If a transgenic αβ TCR with a known MHC restriction is expressed in a mouse strain that also expresses the MHC allele for which the TCR is specific, T cells will mature and populate peripheral lymphoid tissue. If the mouse is of another MHC haplotype and does not express the MHC molecule that the transgenic TCR recognizes, there are normal numbers of $CD4^+CD8^+$ thymocytes but very few mature transgenic TCR-expressing T cells (Fig. 8–25). This result demonstrates that double-positive thymocytes must express TCRs that can bind self MHC molecules to be positively selected. As we shall see later, the same experimental system has been used to study negative selection.

During the transition from double-positive to single-positive cells, thymocytes with class I–restricted TCRs become $CD8^+CD4^-$, and cells with class II–restricted TCRs become $CD4^+CD8^-$. CD4 and CD8 function as coreceptors with TCRs during positive selection and recognize the MHC molecules when the TCRs are recognizing peptide-MHC complexes. Signals from the TCR complex and the coreceptors function together to promote survival of thymocytes. This function of CD4 and CD8 is similar to their role in the activation of mature T cells (see Chapter 9). At this stage in maturation, there may be a random loss of either CD4 or CD8 gene, and only cells expressing the "correct" coreceptor (i.e., CD4 on a class II–restricted T cell or CD8 on a class I–restricted T cell) will continue to mature. It is also possible that the expression of the wrong coreceptor is actively suppressed, although how this is accomplished is unknown.

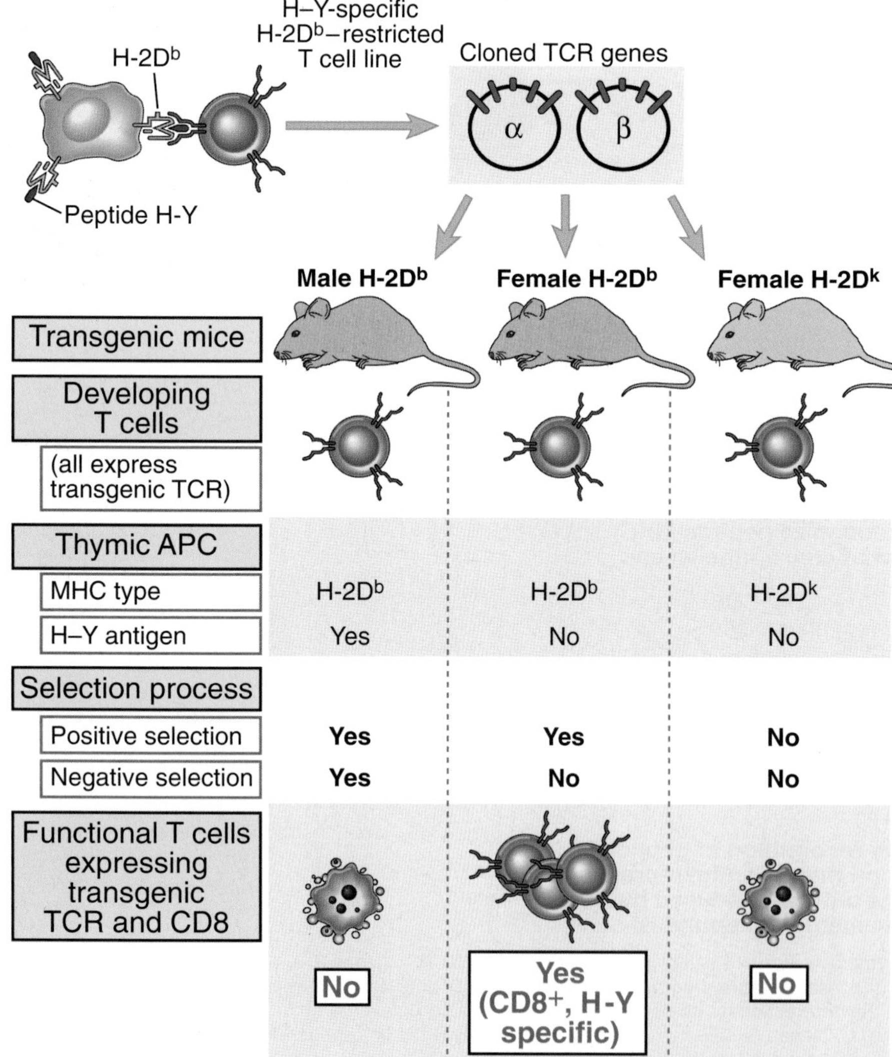

FIGURE 8–25 T cell maturation and selection in a TCR transgenic mouse model. In the experiment depicted, a transgenic mouse expresses a TCR specific for an H-2D^b-associated H-Y (male-specific) antigen, which is, in effect, a foreign antigen for a female mouse. In female mice expressing the D^b MHC allele, mature T cells expressing the transgenic TCR do develop because they are positively selected by the self MHC molecules. The T cells recognize self MHC, presumably weakly and with some self antigen (not H-Y). These T cells do not mature in male H-Y-expressing mice because they are negatively selected by strong H-Y antigen recognition in the thymus. Furthermore, mature T cells do not develop in female mice that express D^k but do not express the D^b allele because of a lack of positive selection of the D^b-restricted TCR-expressing T cells. APC, antigen-presenting cell.

- Knockout mice that lack class I MHC expression in thymic epithelial cells do not develop mature CD8⁺ T cells but do develop CD4⁺CD8⁺ thymocytes and mature CD4⁺ T cells. Conversely, class II MHC-deficient mice do not develop CD4⁺ T cells but do develop CD8⁺ cells. These results demonstrate that thymic epithelial cells must express class I or class II MHC molecules to positively select thymocytes to become CD8⁺ or CD4⁺ single-positive cells, respectively.
- In transgenic mice expressing a class II MHC-restricted TCR, the mature T cells that develop are almost exclusively CD4⁺, even though there are normal numbers of CD4⁺CD8⁺ thymocytes. Conversely, if the transgenic TCR is class I restricted, the T cells that mature are CD8⁺. Thus, the coreceptor and the MHC specificity of the TCR must match if a thymocyte is to develop into a mature T cell.

Peptides bound to MHC molecules on thymic epithelial cells play an essential role in positive selection. In Chapters 5 and 6, we described how cell surface class I and class II molecules always contain bound peptides. These MHC-associated peptides on thymic antigen-presenting cells probably serve two roles in positive selection—first, they promote stable cell surface expression of MHC molecules, and second, they may influence the specificities of the T cells that are selected. Obviously, the thymus cannot contain the foreign antigens to which an individual can respond. Therefore, foreign peptides cannot be involved in the positive selection of T cells that ultimately may recognize these peptides. Self peptides are required for positive selection, however, and exactly what role they play in this process has been the subject of numerous studies using a variety of experimental systems.

- To address the role of peptides in T cell selection, it was necessary to develop systems in which the array of peptides presented to developing thymocytes was limited and could be manipulated experimentally. For class I MHC-dependent positive selection, this was accomplished with use of TAP-1–deficient or β_2-microglobulin–deficient mice. In these mice, the class I molecules are not loaded with cytosolic peptides and are unstable, but they can readily be loaded with exogenously added peptides. If thymuses from such mice are cultured without added peptides, few mature T cells develop (Fig. 8–26). The addition of peptides dramatically increases the development of single-positive CD8⁺ T cells, indicating effective positive selection of thymocytes expressing class I MHC-restricted TCRs. A key finding in these experiments was that one or a few peptides induced the positive selection of a large repertoire of CD8⁺ T cells that could potentially recognize many different unrelated peptides. However, no single peptide was sufficient to generate a normal number (or repertoire) of mature T cells. Furthermore, complex mixtures of peptides induced the maturation of more CD8⁺ T cells than did single peptides. We do not know if the specificities of the T cells that mature are related to the peptides that induced their maturation.

The conclusion drawn from such experiments is that peptides bound to MHC molecules are required for positive selection of T cells and that some peptides are better than others in supporting this process. The finding that peptides differ in the repertoires of T cells they select suggests that specific antigen recognition, and not just MHC recognition, has some role in positive selec-

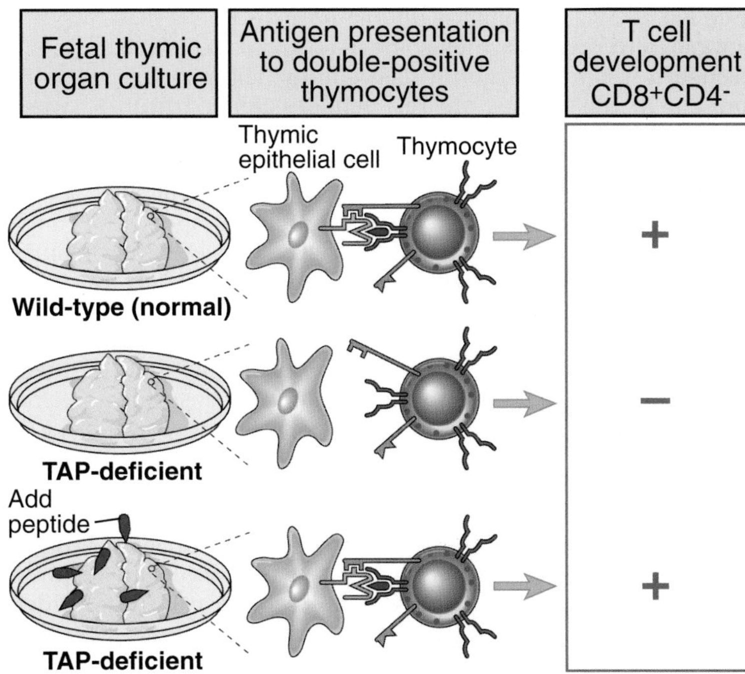

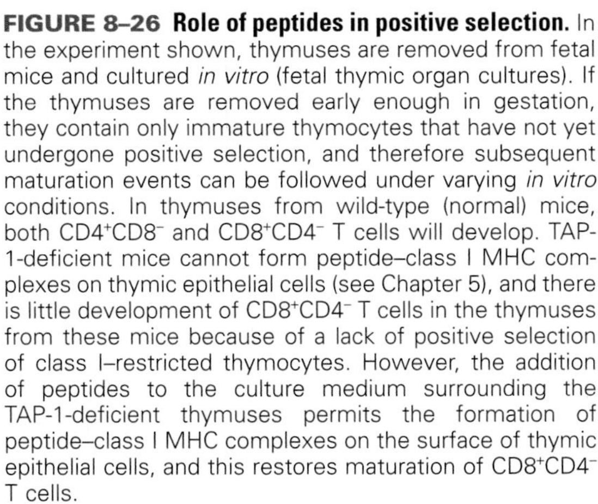

FIGURE 8–26 Role of peptides in positive selection. In the experiment shown, thymuses are removed from fetal mice and cultured *in vitro* (fetal thymic organ cultures). If the thymuses are removed early enough in gestation, they contain only immature thymocytes that have not yet undergone positive selection, and therefore subsequent maturation events can be followed under varying *in vitro* conditions. In thymuses from wild-type (normal) mice, both CD4⁺CD8⁻ and CD8⁺CD4⁻ T cells will develop. TAP-1-deficient mice cannot form peptide–class I MHC complexes on thymic epithelial cells (see Chapter 5), and there is little development of CD8⁺CD4⁻ T cells in the thymuses from these mice because of a lack of positive selection of class I–restricted thymocytes. However, the addition of peptides to the culture medium surrounding the TAP-1-deficient thymuses permits the formation of peptide–class I MHC complexes on the surface of thymic epithelial cells, and this restores maturation of CD8⁺CD4⁻ T cells.

tion. Weak, or low-avidity, recognition of peptides in the thymus protects immature T cells from a default pathway of apoptotic death and allows the cells to complete their maturation. We do not know what signals generated by weak antigen recognition protect immature T cells from death and how these signals differ from those generated by antigen recognition in mature, single-positive T cells. One consequence of self peptide–induced positive selection is that the T cells that mature have some capacity to recognize self peptides. We mentioned in Chapter 3 that the survival of naive lymphocytes before encounter with foreign antigens requires survival signals that are apparently generated by recognition of self antigens in peripheral lymphoid organs. The same self peptides that mediate positive selection of double-positive thymocytes in the thymus may be involved in keeping naive, mature (single-positive) T cells alive in peripheral organs, such as the lymph nodes and spleen.

This model of positive selection based on weak recognition of self antigens raises a fundamental question: How does positive selection driven by self antigens produce a repertoire of mature T cells specific for foreign antigens? The likely answer is that positive selection allows many different T cell clones to survive and differentiate, and many of these T cells that recognize self peptides with low affinity will, after maturing, fortuitously recognize foreign peptides with a high enough affinity to be activated and to generate immune responses. As we discuss next, strong recognition of self antigens in the thymus results in negative selection of developing T cells.

Negative Selection of Thymocytes: Central Tolerance

Negative selection of thymocytes works by inducing apoptotic death of cells whose receptors recognize peptide-MHC complexes in the thymus with high avidity (see Fig. 8–24C). Among the double-positive T cells that are generated in the thymus, some may express TCRs that recognize self antigens with high affinity. The peptides present in the thymus are self peptides derived from widely expressed protein antigens as well as from some proteins believed to be restricted to particular tissues (see below). In immature T cells, the consequence of high-avidity antigen recognition is the triggering of apoptosis, leading to death, or deletion, of the cells. Therefore, the immature thymocytes that express high-affinity receptors for self antigens in the thymus are eliminated, resulting in negative selection of the T cell repertoire. This process eliminates the potentially most harmful self-reactive T cells and is one of the mechanisms ensuring that the immune system does not respond to many self antigens, a property called self-tolerance. Tolerance induced in immature lymphocytes by recognition of self antigens in the generative (or central) lymphoid organs is also called **central tolerance**, to be contrasted with peripheral tolerance induced in mature lymphocytes by self antigens in peripheral tissues. We will discuss the mechanisms and physiologic importance of immunologic tolerance in more detail in Chapter 11.

Formal proof for deletion of T cell clones reactive with antigens in the thymus (also called clonal deletion) has come from several experimental approaches that allowed investigators to observe the effects of self antigen recognition by a large number of developing T cells.

- When TCR-transgenic mice are exposed to the peptide for which the TCR is specific, a large amount of cell death is induced in the thymus and a block occurs in the development of mature transgenic TCR-expressing T cells. In one such study, a transgenic mouse line was created that expressed a class I MHC-restricted TCR specific for the Y chromosome–encoded antigen H-Y, which is expressed by many cell types in male mice but not in female mice (see Fig. 8–25). Female mice with this transgenic TCR have normal numbers of thymocytes in the thymic medulla and large numbers of $CD8^+$ T cells in the periphery because they do not express the H-Y antigen that may induce negative selection. In contrast, male transgenic mice have few TCR-expressing, single-positive thymocytes in the medulla and few mature peripheral $CD8^+$ T cells because of deletion of the H-Y-specific thymocytes induced by H-Y antigen in the thymus.
- Similar deletion of immature T cells is seen if transgenic mice expressing a TCR specific for a known peptide antigen are bred with mice expressing that antigen or if the mice are injected with large doses of the antigen. This can also be mimicked *in vitro* by culturing intact thymuses from TCR-transgenic mice with high concentrations of the peptide for which the TCR is specific. In all these examples, there is a block of T cell maturation after the cortical double-positive stage, presumably because immature thymocytes express the transgenic TCR, recognize the antigen on thymic antigen-presenting cells, and are deleted before they can mature into single-positive cells.

The deletion of immature self-reactive T cells occurs when the TCR on a $CD4^+CD8^+$ thymocyte binds strongly to a self peptide presented by another thymic cell. Negative selection may occur both at the double-positive stage in the cortex and in newly generated single-positive T cells in the medulla. The thymic antigen presenting cells that mediate negative selection are primarily dendritic cells and thymic medullary epithelial cells, whereas cortical epithelial cells are especially (and perhaps uniquely) effective at inducing positive selection. Double-positive T cells are drawn to the thymic medulla by the CCR7 specific chemokines, CCL21 and CCL19. In the medulla, thymic medullary epithelial cells express a nuclear protein called **AIRE** (autoimmune regulator) that induces the expression of a number of tissue-specific genes in the thymus, thus making a host of tissue-specific peptides available for presentation in the thymus to double-positive and single-positive T cells during the process of negative selection. As will be discussed in Chapter 11, a mutation in the gene that encodes AIRE results in an autoimmune polyendocrine syndrome, underscoring the importance of AIRE in mediating central tolerance to tissue-specific antigens.

The key factor determining the choice between positive and negative selection is the strength of antigen recognition, with low-avidity recognition leading to positive selection and high-avidity recognition inducing negative selection. CD4 and CD8 molecules probably play a role in negative selection, as they do in positive selection, because these coreceptors participate in recognition of MHC molecules presenting self peptides. The cellular basis of negative selection in the thymus is the induction of death by apoptosis. Unlike the phenomenon of death by default (or neglect), which occurs in the absence of positive selection, in negative selection, active death-promoting signals are generated when the TCR of immature thymocytes binds with high affinity to antigen. The induction by TCR signaling of a pro-apoptotic protein called Bim probably plays a crucial role in the induction of mitochondrial leakiness and thymocyte apoptosis during negative selection (Chapter 11).

Recognition of self antigens in the thymus can also generate a population of regulatory T cells, which function to prevent autoimmune reactions (see Chapter 11). It is not clear how a self antigen causes deletion of some immature T cells and the development of regulatory T cells from other immature thymocytes of the same specificity.

γδ T Lymphocytes

TCR αβ- and γδ-expressing thymocytes are separate lineages with a common precursor. In fetal thymuses, the first TCR gene rearrangements involve the γ and δ loci. Recombination of TCR γ and δ loci proceeds in a fashion similar to that of other antigen receptor gene rearrangements, although the order of rearrangement appears to be less rigid than in other loci.

T cells that express functional γ and δ chains do not express αβ TCRs and vice versa. The independence of these lineages is indicated by several lines of evidence.

- Mature αβ-expressing T cells often contain out-of-frame rearrangements of δ genes, indicating that these cells could never have expressed γδ receptors.
- TCR δ gene knockout mice develop normal numbers of αβ T cells, and TCR β gene knockout mice develop normal numbers of γδ T cells.

The diversity of the γδ T cell repertoire is theoretically even greater than that of the αβ T cell repertoire, in part because the heptamer-nonamer recognition sequences adjacent to D segments permit D-to-D joining. Paradoxically, however, the actual diversity of expressed γδ TCRs is limited because only a few of the available V, D, and J segments are used in mature γδ T cells, for unknown reasons. This limited diversity is reminiscent of the limited diversity of the B-1 subset of B lymphocytes and is in keeping with the concept that γδ T cells serve as an early defense against a limited number of commonly encountered microbes at epithelial barriers.

NK-T Cells

In Chapter 7, we also mentioned another small subset of T cells known as NK-T cells, which are not MHC restricted and do not recognize peptides displayed by antigen-presenting cells. These NK-T cells express αβ TCRs that are CD1 restricted, and also bear a surface marker found on NK cells, hence their name. The TCRs of NK-T cells recognize lipid antigens bound to the groove of CD1 molecules. CD1 molecules are MHC class I–like molecules made up of a heavy chain and β_2-microglobulin. The heavy chain has a groove made up of hydrophobic residues that can bind and present lipid antigens. These lipid antigens may be derived from endocytosed microbes or they may be self lipids (see Chapter 6). A large number of CD1-restricted NK-T cells have an "invariant" T cell receptor resulting from a unique and stereotypic TCR α chain gene rearrangement event. NK-T cells secrete cytokines and participate in host defense, but may also be of relevance from a regulatory standpoint in the context of autoimmunity and allergy.

Developing αβ T cell expressing invariant TCRs may be positively selected in the thymic cortex at the double-positive stage by CD1 and self lipids presented on the surface of other cortical thymocytes. These selected NK-T cells do not express CCR7, and therefore do not migrate toward the medulla like other conventional αβ T cells. Instead, they receive instructions to exit the thymus and home to a number of peripheral sites, the most prominent being the liver.

SUMMARY

- B and T lymphocytes arise from a common bone marrow–derived precursor that becomes committed to the lymphocyte lineage. B cell maturation proceeds in the bone marrow, whereas early T cell progenitors migrate to and complete their maturation in the thymus. Early maturation is characterized by cell proliferation induced by cytokines, mainly IL-7, leading to marked increases in the numbers of immature lymphocytes.
- B and T cell maturation involves the somatic rearrangement of antigen receptor gene segments and the initial expression of Ig heavy chain proteins in B cell precursors and TCR β molecules in T cell precursors. The expression of pre-antigen receptors and antigen receptors is essential for survival and maturation of developing lymphocytes and for selection processes that lead to a diverse repertoire of useful antigen specificities.
- The antigen receptors of B and T cells are encoded by genes formed by the somatic rearrangement of a limited number of gene segments that are spatially segregated in the germline antigen receptor loci. There are separate loci encoding the Ig heavy chain, Ig κ light chain, Ig λ light chain, TCR β chain,

TCR α and δ chains, and TCR γ chain. These loci contain V, J, and, in the Ig heavy chain and TCR β and δ loci only, D gene segments. These segments lie upstream of exons encoding constant domains. Somatic rearrangement of both Ig and TCR loci involves the joining of D and J segments in the loci that contain D segments, followed by the joining of the V segment to the recombined DJ segments in these loci, or direct V-to-J joining in the other loci. This process of somatic gene recombination is mediated by a recombinase enzyme complex that includes the lymphocyte-specific components Rag-1 and Rag-2.

- The diversity of the antibody and TCR repertoires is generated by the combinatorial associations of multiple germline V, D, and J genes and junctional diversity generated by the addition or removal of random nucleotides at the sites of recombination. These mechanisms generate the most diversity at the junctions of the segments that form the third hypervariable regions of both antibody and TCR polypeptides.

- B cell maturation occurs in stages characterized by different patterns of Ig gene rearrangement and expression. In the earliest B cell precursors, called pro-B cells, Ig genes are initially in the germline configuration. At the pro-B to pre-B cell transition, V-D-J recombination is completed at the Ig H chain locus. A primary RNA transcript containing the VDJ complex and Ig C gene segments is produced, and the μ C region exons of the heavy chain RNA are spliced to the VDJ exon to generate a mature mRNA that is translated into the μ heavy chain protein. The pre-BCR is formed by pairing of the μ chain with nonvariable surrogate light chains and by association with the signaling molecules Igα and Igβ. This receptor delivers survival and proliferation signals and also signals to inhibit rearrangement on the other heavy chain allele (allelic exclusion). At the immature B cell stage, V-J recombination occurs in the κ and λ loci, and light chain proteins are expressed. Heavy and light chains are then assembled into intact IgM molecules and expressed on the cell surface. Immature B cells leave the bone marrow to populate peripheral lymphoid tissues, where they complete their maturation. At the mature B cell stage, synthesis of both μ and δ heavy chains occurs in the same B cells mediated by alternative splicing of primary heavy chain RNA transcripts, and membrane IgM and IgD are expressed.

- During B lymphocyte maturation, immature B cells that express high-affinity antigen receptors specific for self antigens present in the bone marrow are either induced to edit their receptor genes or these cells are eliminated.

- T cell maturation in the thymus also progresses in stages distinguished by expression of antigen receptor genes, CD4 and CD8 coreceptor molecules, and location in the thymus. The earliest T lineage immigrants to the thymus do not express TCRs or CD4 or CD8 molecules. The developing T cells within the thymus, called thymocytes, initially populate the outer cortex, where they undergo proliferation, rearrangement of TCR genes, and surface expression of CD3, TCR, CD4, and CD8 molecules. As the cells mature, they migrate from the cortex to the medulla.

- The least mature thymocytes, called pro-T cells, are $CD4^-CD8^-$ (double negative), and the TCR genes are in the germline configuration. At the pre-T stage, thymocytes remain double negative, but V-D-J recombination is completed at the TCR β chain locus. Primary β chain transcripts are expressed and processed to bring a C_β segment adjacent to the VDJ complex, and β chain polypeptides are produced. The β chain associates with the invariant pre-Tα protein to form a pre-TCR. The pre-TCR transduces signals that inhibit rearrangement on the other β chain allele (allelic exclusion) and promotes CD4 and CD8 expression and further proliferation of immature thymocytes. At the $CD4^+CD8^+$ (double-positive) stage of T cell development, V-J recombination occurs at the TCR α locus, α chain polypeptides are produced, and low levels of the TCR are expressed on the cell surface.

- Selection processes drive maturation of TCR-expressing, double-positive thymocytes and shape the T cell repertoire toward self MHC restriction and self-tolerance. Positive selection of $CD4^+CD8^+$ TCRαβ thymocytes requires low-avidity recognition of peptide-MHC complexes on thymic epithelial cells, leading to a rescue of the cells from programmed death. Negative selection of $CD4^+CD8^+$ TCRαβ double-positive thymocytes occurs when these cells recognize, with high avidity, antigens that are present in the thymus. This process is responsible for tolerance to many self antigens. Most of the cortical thymocytes do not survive these selection processes. As the surviving TCRαβ thymocytes mature, they move into the medulla and become either $CD4^+CD8^-$ or $CD8^+CD4^-$. Medullary thymocytes acquire the ability to differentiate into either helper or cytotoxic effector cells and finally emigrate to peripheral lymphoid tissues.

Selected Readings

Boehm T. Thymus development and function. Current Opinion in Immunology 20:178–184, 2008.

Busslinger M. Transcriptional control of early B cell development. Annual Review of Immunology 22:55–79, 2004.

Germain RN. T cell development and the CD4-CD8 lineage decision. Nature Reviews Immunology 2:309–322, 2002.

Hardy RR, and K Hayakawa. B cell development pathways. Annual Review of Immunology 19:595–622, 2001.

Hoefig KP, and V Heissmeyer. MicroRNAs grow up in the immune system. Current Opinion in Immunology 20:281–287, 2008.

Jenkinson EJ, WE Jenkinson, SW Rossi, and G Anderson. The thymus and T-cell commitment: the right choice for Notch? Nature Reviews Immunology 6:551–555, 2006.

Jung D, C Giallourakis, R Mostoslavsky, and FW Alt. Mechanism and control of V(D)J recombination at the immunoglobulin heavy chain locus. Annual Review of Immunology 24:541–570, 2006.

Kuppers R, and R Dalla-Favera. Mechanisms of chromosomal translocations in B cell lymphomas. Oncogene 20:5580–5594, 2001.

Kyewski B and L Klein. A central role for central tolerance. Annual Review of Immunology 24:571–606, 2006.

Lodish HF, B Zhou, G Liu, and CZ Chen. Micromanagement of the immune system by microRNAs. Nature Reviews Immunology 8:120–130, 2008.

Maillard I, T Fang, and WS Pear. Regulation of lymphoid development, differentiation, and function by the Notch pathway. Annual Review of Immunology 23:945–974, 2005.

Meffre E, R Casellas, and MC Nussenzweig. Antibody regulation of B cell development. Nature Immunology 1:379–385, 2000.

Nemazee D. Receptor editing in lymphocyte development and central tolerance. Nature Reviews Immunology 6:728–740, 2006.

Palmer E. Negative selection—clearing out the bad apples from the T cell repertoire. Nature Reviews Immunology 3:383–391, 2003.

Rodewald HR: Thymus organogenesis. Annual Review of Immunology 26:355–388, 2008.

Rolink AG, C Schaniel, J Andersson, and F Melchers. Selection events operating at various stages in B cell development. Current Opinion in Immunology 13:202–207, 2001.

Rothenberg EV, JE Moore, and MA Yui. Launching the T-cell-lineage developmental programme. Nature Reviews Immunology 8:9–21, 2008.

Schatz DG, and E Spanopoulou. Biochemistry of V(D)J recombination. Current Topics in Microbiology and Immunology 290:49–85, 2005.

Schlissel MS. Regulating antigen-receptor gene assembly. Nature Reviews Immunology 3:890–899, 2003.

Singer A, S Adoro, and JH Park. Lineage fate and intense debate: myths, models and mechanisms of CD4 versus CD8 lineage choice. Nature Reviews Immunology 8:788–801, 2008.

Singh H, KL Medina, and JM Pongubala. Contingent gene regulatory networks and B cell fate specification. Proceedings of the National Academy of Science U S A 102:4949–4953, 2005.

von Boehmer H, I Aifantis, F Gounari, O Azugui, L Haughn, I Apostolou, E Jaeckel, F Grassi, and L Klein. Thymic selection revisited: how essential is it? Immunological Reviews 191:62–78, 2003.

Xiao C and K Rajewsky. MicroRNA control in the immune system: Basic principles. Cell 136:26–36, 2009.

Chapter 9

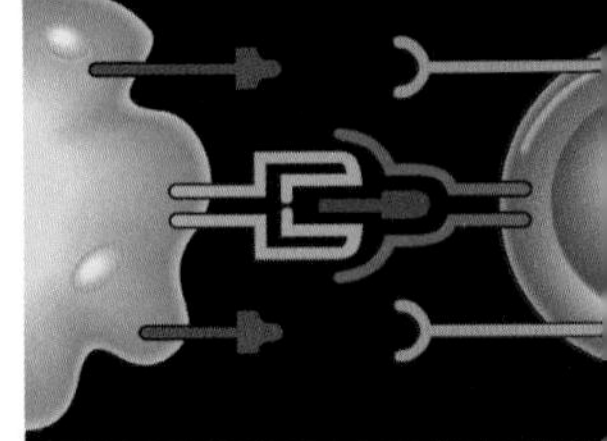

ACTIVATION OF T LYMPHOCYTES

The activation and effector phases of T cell–mediated adaptive immune responses are triggered by antigen recognition by T lymphocytes. In Chapter 6, we described the specificity of T cells for peptide fragments, derived from protein antigens, that are displayed bound to self major histocompatibility complex (MHC) molecules. In Chapter 7, we described the antigen receptors and accessory molecules of T cells that are involved in the activation of T cells by antigens. In this chapter, we describe the biological and biochemical basis of T cell activation by antigens and by additional signals provided by antigen-presenting cells (APCs). We begin with a brief overview of T cell activation, consider the biology of $CD4^+$ and $CD8^+$ T cell responses, discuss the role of costimulators in T cell activation, and then proceed to a discussion of the biochemical mechanisms of T cell receptor (TCR) signaling. Finally we discuss the regulation of T cell signaling by inhibitory receptors and by other molecules that attenuate signals emanating from the TCR, coreceptors, and costimulatory receptors.

OVERVIEW OF T LYMPHOCYTE ACTIVATION

Naive T lymphocytes home to secondary lymphoid organs, where they may encounter antigens presented by mature dendritic cells on class I or class II MHC molecules and thus become activated. This results in the expansion of the antigen-specific lymphocyte pool and the differentiation of these cells into effector and memory lymphocytes (Fig. 9–1). Protein antigens that cross epithelial barriers are captured by immature dendritic cells and transported to lymph nodes. Antigens that enter the circulation may be captured by dendritic cells in the blood and in the spleen. If these antigens are associated with "pathogen-associated molecular patterns," such as ligands for Toll-like receptors (see Chapter 2), the dendritic cells are activated and induced

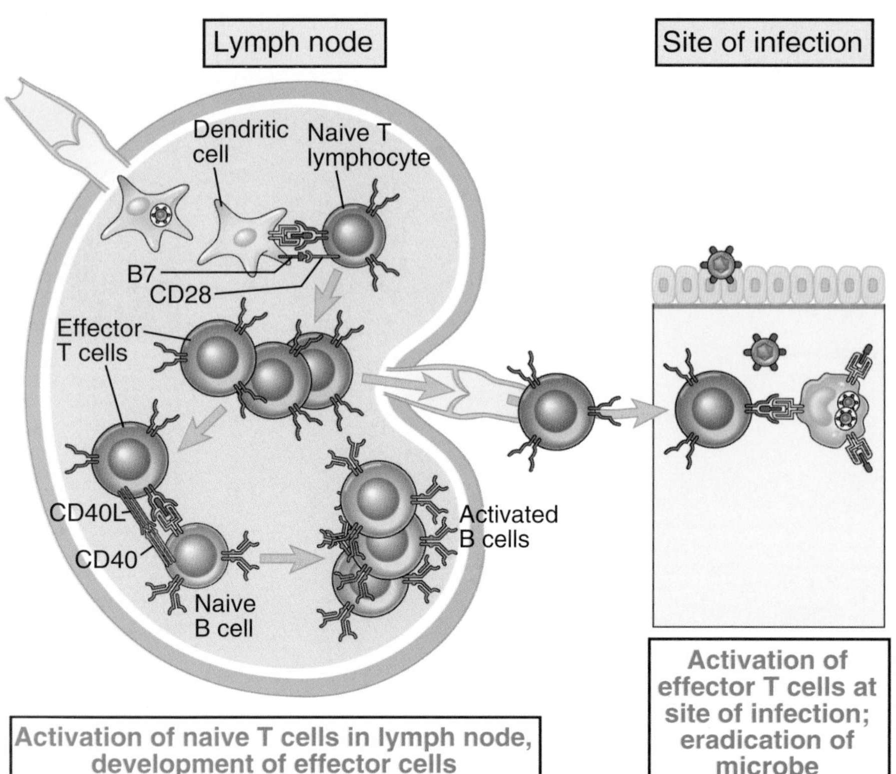

FIGURE 9–1 Activation of naive and effector T cells by antigen. Antigens that are transported by dendritic cells to lymph nodes are recognized by naive T lymphocytes that recirculate through these lymph nodes. The T cells are activated to differentiate into effector and memory cells, which may remain in the lymphoid organs or migrate to nonlymphoid tissues. At sites of infection, the effector cells are again activated by antigens and perform their various functions, such as macrophage activation.

to express costimulators such as B7 proteins on the cell surface. Dendritic cells that have encountered microbes and internalized their antigens begin to mature and migrate to the T cell zones of secondary lymphoid organs such as the lymph nodes. As discussed in Chapter 6, both naive T cells and dendritic cells are drawn to T cell zones by chemokines that activate the CCR7 chemokine receptor. When they reach these T cell areas, the dendritic cells present antigens on MHC molecules and also express costimulators that can provide second signals to naive T cells. When a naive T cell of the correct specificity recognizes antigen, in the form of peptide-MHC complexes, and receives signals via the interaction of B7 with costimulatory receptors on the T cell, that naive lymphocyte is activated. Antigen-stimulated T cells that have received both "signal one" through the antigen receptor and "second signals" via costimulatory receptors may be induced to secrete cytokines and to express cytokine receptors. The cytokine interleukin-2 (IL-2) provides autocrine signals to activated T cells, leading to expansion of antigen-specific clones. IL-2 and other cytokines produced by the T cells and by APCs also stimulate the differentiation of the T cells into effector and memory cells (Fig. 9–2). Some of these activated T cells leave the lymphoid organ where activation occurred and enter the circulation. Other activated $CD4^+$ T cells remain in the lymphoid organ, where they help B lymphocytes to differentiate into antibody-secreting plasma cells (Chapter 10).

Effector T cells recognize antigens in lymphoid organs or in peripheral nonlymphoid tissues and are activated to perform their effector functions (see Fig. 9–1). Effector T cells are able to migrate to any site of infection or inflammation. Here the cells again encounter the antigen for which they are specific and respond in ways that serve to eliminate the source of the antigen. Effector T cells of the $CD4^+$ helper subset express membrane molecules and secrete cytokines that activate (help) macrophages to kill phagocytosed microbes. Some $CD4^+$ helper T cells remain in lymphoid organs and help B cells to differentiate into cells that secrete antibodies that bind to the antigens. $CD8^+$ cytotoxic T lymphocytes (CTLs), the effector cells of the $CD8^+$ subset, kill infected cells and tumor cells that display class I MHC–associated antigens. We will return to the effector functions of T cells in Chapters 10 and 13. Memory T cells are an expanded population of T cells specific for antigen that can respond rapidly to subsequent encounter with the antigen and differentiate into effector cells that eliminate the antigen. In general, the activation of memory T cells depends only on the ligation of the TCR, and costimulatory "second signals" are not required at this stage of differentiation.

T cell responses decline after the antigen is eliminated by effector cells. This decline is important for returning the immune system to a state of rest, or homeostasis. T cell responses decline mainly because the majority of antigen-activated T cells die by apoptosis. The reason for this is that as the antigen is eliminated, lymphocytes are deprived of survival stimuli that are normally provided by the antigen and by the costimulators and cytokines produced during inflammatory reactions to the antigen. It is estimated that more than 95% of the antigen-specific $CD8^+$ T cells that arise by clonal

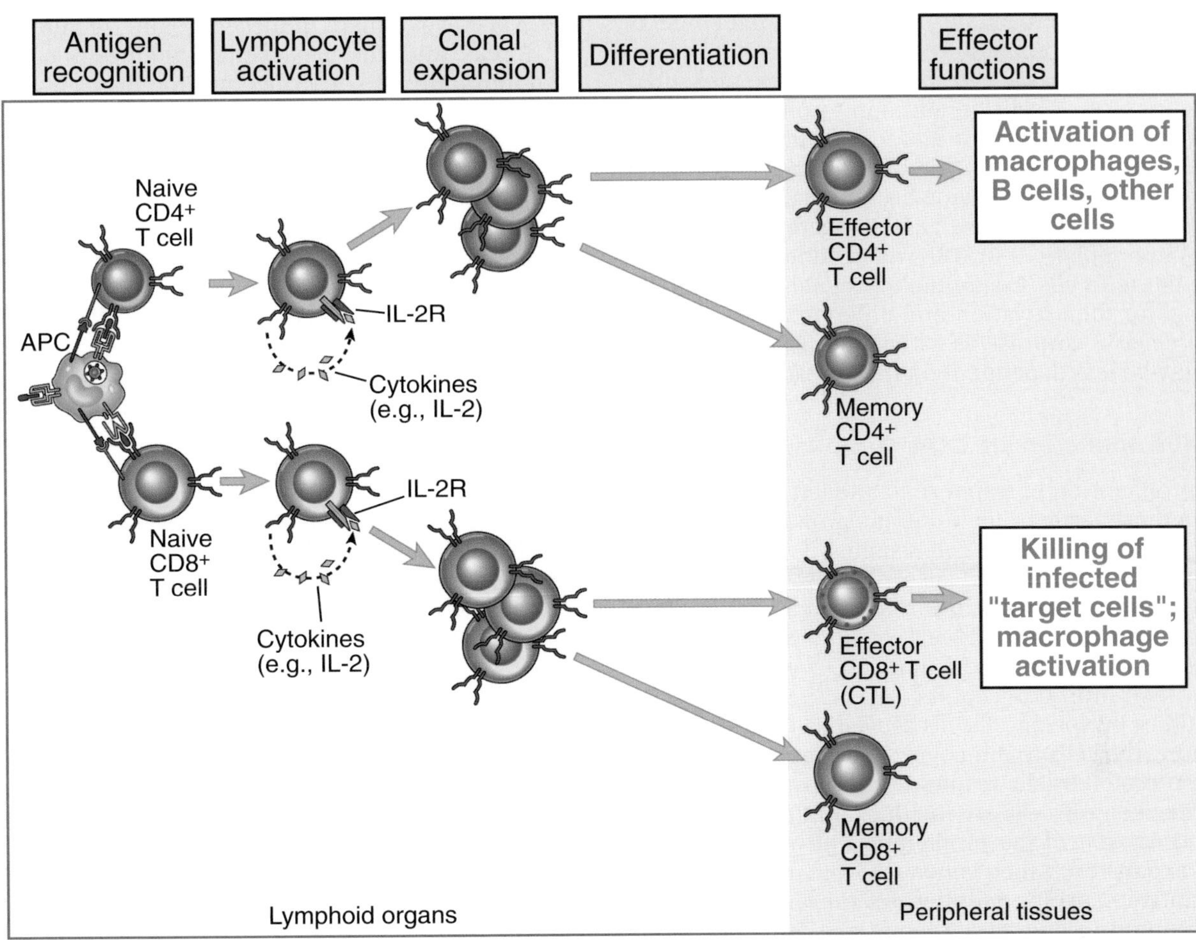

FIGURE 9–2 Phases of T cell responses. Antigen recognition by T cells induces cytokine (e.g., IL-2) secretion, clonal expansion as a result of IL-2-induced autocrine cell proliferation, and differentiation of the T cells into effector cells or memory cells. In the effector phase of the response, the effector CD4$^+$ T cells respond to antigen by producing cytokines that have several actions, such as the activation of macrophages and B lymphocytes, and CD8$^+$ CTLs respond by killing other cells. APC, antigen-presenting cell.

expansion die by apoptosis as the antigen is cleared. We will return to the mechanisms of homeostasis in the immune system in Chapter 11.

The sequence of events in the responses of CD4$^+$ and CD8$^+$ T cells are fundamentally similar (see Fig. 9–2). However, there are enough differences in the initiation and culmination of these responses that they are best discussed separately.

ACTIVATION OF CD4$^+$ T LYMPHOCYTES

The differentiation of naive CD4$^+$ T lymphocytes into effector cells of cell-mediated immunity (CMI) requires antigen recognition and costimulation. The initiation of cell-mediated immune responses requires that naive CD4$^+$ T cells and the antigens they recognize must be present in the same lymphoid tissue at the same time. This is accomplished by recirculation of naive T cells, which was described in Chapter 3, and by transport of antigens to lymphoid organs, described in Chapter 6. Naive T cells migrate from the blood into lymphoid organs, from one lymphoid organ to another, and back into the blood, until they encounter the antigen for which they express specific receptors. Antigen is delivered to lymph nodes by lymphatic drainage, and to the spleen by the blood. Dendritic cells play an important role in taking up antigens at sites of infection, and migrating through lymphatic vessels to draining lymph nodes. During their migration to the lymph nodes, dendritic cells mature and become efficient antigen presenting cells (APCs) (see Chapter 6, Fig. 6–5).

Activation of naive CD4$^+$ T cells requires antigen presentation by dendritic cells. Once in the lymph node, dendritic cells present peptides derived from the endocytosed protein antigens in association with class II MHC molecules to naive CD4$^+$ T cells. CD4$^+$ T cell–mediated immune reactions are elicited by protein antigens of extracellular microbes that are ingested by dendritic cells, or by soluble protein antigens that are administered with adjuvants, in the case of vaccinations, and taken up by dendritic cells. These microbial or soluble antigens are internalized into vesicles by the dendritic cells and presented in association with class II MHC molecules (see Chapter 6). Some chemicals introduced through the skin also elicit T cell reactions, called

contact sensitivity reactions. It is believed that contact-sensitizing chemicals bind to and modify self proteins, creating new antigenic determinants that are presented to $CD4^+$ or $CD8^+$ T cells. In addition to presenting antigens, dendritic cells respond to microbial structures by expressing high levels of costimulators, such as B7-1 and B7-2 proteins, which provide second signals for T cell activation (described below), and by secreting cytokines such as interleukin-12 (IL-12), which stimulate differentiation of the T cells. Costimulatory signals are generally essential for the activation and differentiation of naive $CD4^+$ T cells. In contrast, as we will discuss later, $CD8^+$ T cells may be less dependent on these costimulators.

Clonal Expansion of $CD4^+$ T Cells

T cell proliferation in response to antigen recognition is mediated primarily by an autocrine growth pathway, in which the responding T cell secretes its own growth-promoting cytokines and also expresses cell surface receptors for these cytokines. The principal autocrine growth factor for most T cells is IL-2 (see Fig. 12–9, Chapter 12). Both the production of IL-2 and the expression of high-affinity receptors for IL-2 require antigen recognition by specific T cells as well as costimulation. Therefore, the cells that recognize antigen produce IL-2 and also preferentially respond to it, ensuring that the antigen-specific T cells are the ones that proliferate the most. The result of the proliferation of naive T cells is **clonal expansion**, which generates from a small pool of naive antigen-specific lymphocytes the large number of cells required to eliminate the antigen. Before antigen exposure, the frequency of naive T cells specific for any antigen is 1 in 10^5 to 10^6 lymphocytes. After antigen exposure, the numbers of $CD4^+$ T cells specific for that antigen may increase to about 1 in 100 to 1000 cells. The magnitude of clonal expansion is even greater for $CD8^+$ T cells, as described below. These numbers rapidly decline as the antigen is eliminated, and after the immune response subsides, the surviving memory cells specific for the antigen number on the order of 1 in 10^4.

As the antigens are eliminated, many of the activated T cells die by apoptosis, thereby providing a homeostatic mechanism that returns the immune system to its basal state of rest after the infection is cleared (see Chapter 11). Some of the T cells that have proliferated differentiate into effector cells, and other progeny of the antigen-stimulated lymphocytes differentiate into memory cells, which are long-lived and poised to respond rapidly to antigen challenge.

Differentiation of $CD4^+$ T Cells

Effector cells of the CD4 lineage are characterized by their ability to express surface molecules that activate other cells (B lymphocytes, macrophages, and dendritic cells), and to secrete cytokines that are involved in the functions of these T cells. Whereas naive $CD4^+$ T cells produce mostly IL-2 upon activation, effector $CD4^+$ T cells are capable of producing a large number and variety of cytokines that have diverse biological activities. The development of these cytokine-secreting effector T cells, and the roles of the cytokines in cell-mediated immunity, are described in Chapter 13.

Activation of $CD8^+$ T Cells

The activation of naïve $CD8^+$ T cells also requires antigen recognition and second signals, but the nature of the second signals may be different from those for $CD4^+$ cells. To be stimulated to proliferate and differentiate into effector CTLs, naive $CD8^+$ T cells must recognize class I-associated peptide antigens and also encounter costimulators on APCs or signals provided by helper T cells.

Dendritic cells play an essential role in activating naïve $CD8^+$ T cells. $CD8^+$ T cell responses are elicited by microbial peptides that are present in the cytosol of infected cells and are displayed by class I MHC molecules. The microbes that produce cytosolic antigens are typically viruses, which express proteins in the cytoplasm of infected cells. $CD8^+$ T cells may respond to some phagocytosed bacteria and viruses if these microbes or their protein antigens are transported out of phagosomes into the cytosol. Examples of such microbes include the bacterium *Listeria monocytogenes*. Dendritic cells that express these cytosolic antigens are able to activate naive $CD8^+$ T cells, much like the way dendritic cells initiate $CD4^+$ T cell responses. However, the induction of a $CD8^+$ T cell response poses a special problem because the antigen these cells recognize may be produced in a cell type, such as a tissue cell that is infected by a virus or transformed, that is not a professional APC and is not capable of activating naive T cells. In order to initiate the response of $CD8^+$ T cells, the antigen has to access the class I MHC pathway of dendritic cells. Dendritic cells have a special ability to capture and ingest virus-infected or tumor cells, and present the viral or tumor antigens to naive $CD8^+$ T cells (Fig. 9–3). In this pathway, the ingested antigens are transported from vesicles to the cytosol, from where peptides enter the class I pathway. As we discussed in Chapter 6, most ingested proteins do not enter the cytosolic-class I pathway of antigen presentation. This permissiveness for protein traffic from endosomal vesicles to the cytosol is unique to dendritic cells. (At the same time, the dendritic cells can present class II MHC-associated peptides generated in the vesicles to $CD4^+$ helper T cells.) This process is called **cross-presentation**, or cross-priming, to indicate that one cell type (the dendritic cell) can present antigens from another cell (the virus-infected or tumor cell) and prime, or activate, T cells specific for these antigens.

The full activation of naïve $CD8^+$ T cells and their differentiation into functional CTLs may require the participation of $CD4^+$ helper cells. In other words, helper T cells can provide "second signals" for $CD8^+$ T cells. The requirement for helper cells may vary according to the type of antigen exposure. In the setting of a strong innate immune response to a microbe, if professional APCs are directly infected by the microbe, or if cross-presentation

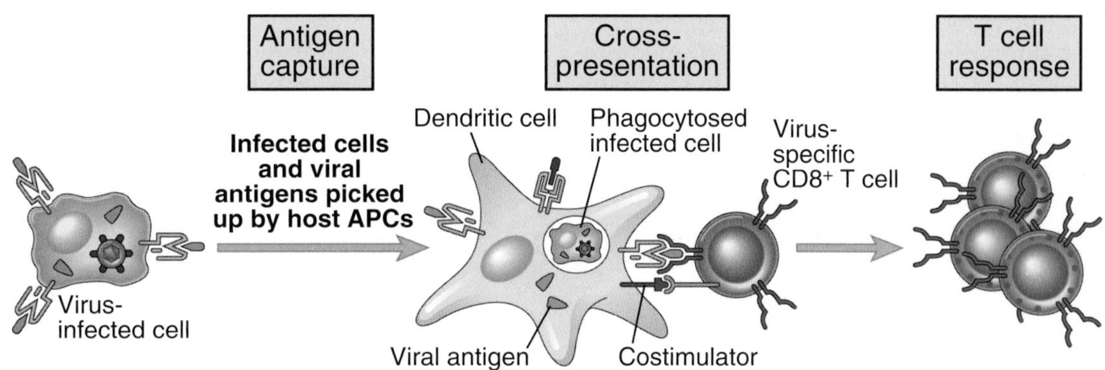

FIGURE 9–3 Cross-presentattion of antigens to CD8⁺ T cells. Cells infected with intracellular microbes, such as viruses, are ingested by dendritic cells, and the antigens of the infectious microbes are processed and presented in association with class I MHC molecules to $CD8^+$ T cells. Thus, dendritic cells are able to present endocytosed vesicular antigens by the class I pathway. Note that the same cross-presenting APC may display class II MHC-associated antigens from the microbe for recognition by $CD4^+$ helper T cells.

of microbial antigens is efficient, $CD4^+$ T cell help may not be required. $CD4^+$ helper T cells may be required for $CD8^+$ T cell responses to latent viral infections, organ transplants, and tumors, all of which tend to elicit weak innate immune reactions. The varying importance of $CD4^+$ T cells in the development of CTL responses is illustrated by studies with CD4 knockout mice, which lack helper T cells. In these mice some viral infections fail to generate effective CTLs and are not eradicated, while other viruses do stimulate effective CTL responses. A lack of $CD4^+$ T cell helper function is the accepted explanation for the defects in CTL generation seen in individuals infected with human immunodeficiency virus (HIV), which infects and eliminates only $CD4^+$ T cells.

Helper T cells may promote $CD8^+$ T cell activation by several mechanisms (Fig. 9–4). Helper T cells may secrete cytokines that stimulate the differentiation of

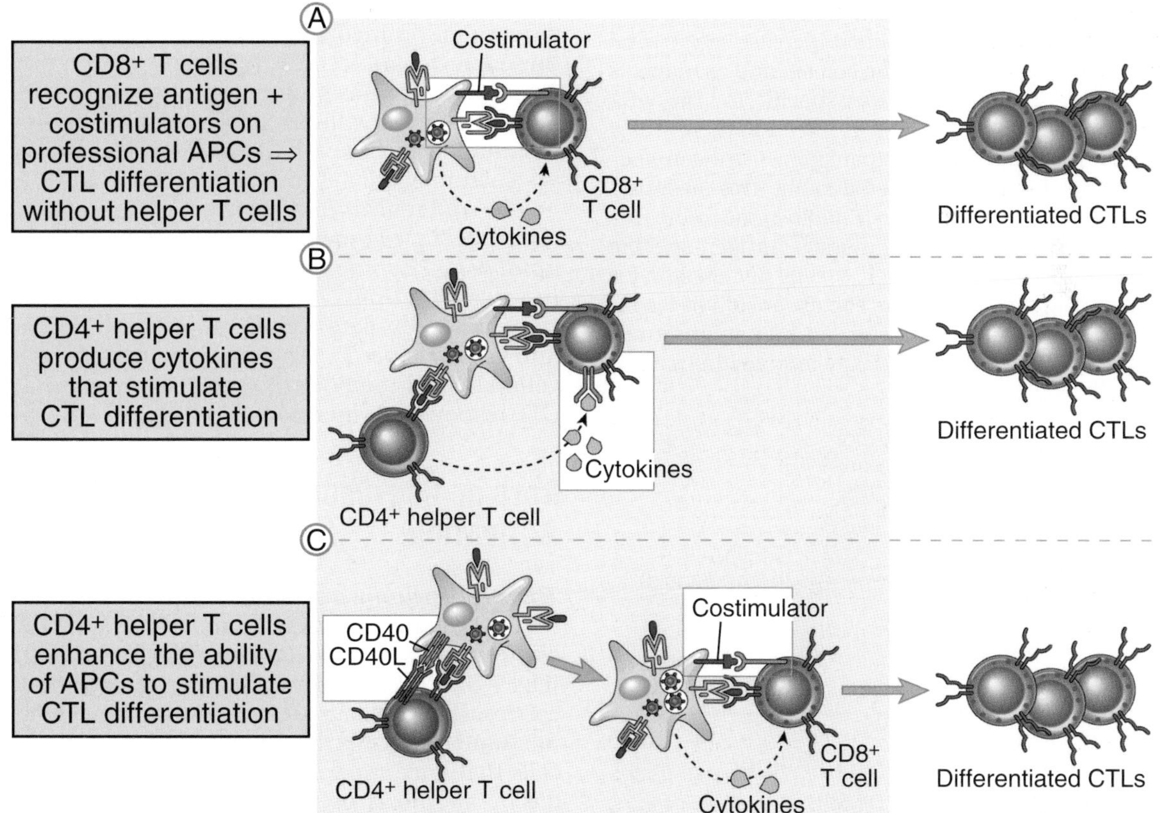

FIGURE 9–4 Role of costimulation and helper T cells in the differentiation of CD8⁺ T lymphocytes. Differentiation of naive $CD8^+$ T cells into effector cytotoxic T lymphocytes (CTLs) requires antigen recognition (signal 1) and additional stimuli such as costimulators or cytokines expressed by professional antigen-presenting cells (APCs) (A) or by cytokines produced by $CD4^+$ helper T cells (B). $CD4^+$ helper T cells may also activate APCs and make them able to stimulate CTL development, for example, by stimulating expression of costimulators or cytokines (C).

CD8⁺ T cells. Antigen-stimulated helper T cells express the trimeric tumor necrosis factor (TNF) family member called CD40 ligand (CD40L), which binds to CD40 on APCs and activates these APCs to make them more efficient at stimulating the differentiation of $CD8^+$ T cells. The effects of helper T cells appear to be mostly on the differentiation of $CD8^+$ cells into fully functional memory cells, and less on the initial clonal expansion and early CTL development.

Clonal Expansion of $CD8^+$ T Cells

Before antigen exposure, the frequency of naive $CD8^+$ T cells specific for any antigen is 1 in 10^5 to 10^6 lymphocytes. Following antigen exposure, the number of $CD8^+$ T cells specific for that antigen may increase to as high as 1 in 10 (Fig. 9–5).

Studies in mice have revealed an unexpectedly large expansion of $CD8^+$ T cells during the acute phase of infections with intracellular microbes. In one such study, T cells specific for a dominant epitope of the lymphocytic choriomeningitis virus (LCMV) were identified by staining cell populations with a fluorescent tetramer of an appropriate MHC molecule loaded with the viral peptide. It was estimated that the frequency of LCMV-specific T cells in uninfected mice is about 1 in 10^5 $CD8^+$ cells. Following infection with the virus, at the peak of the immune response there was a twofold to threefold increase in the total number of $CD8^+$ T cells in the spleen, and as many as one in five of these cells was specific for the viral peptide. In other words, in this infection there was a greater than 50,000-fold expansion of antigen-specific $CD8^+$ T cells, and, remarkably, this occurred within 1 week after infection. Equally remarkable was the finding that during this massive antigen-specific clonal expansion, "bystander" T cells not specific for the virus did not proliferate. The expansion of T cells specific for Epstein-Barr virus and human immunodeficiency virus (HIV) in acutely infected humans is also on this order of magnitude. Although it has been more difficult to quantitate the antigen-stimulated expansion of $CD4^+$ cells, it appears to be much less than the clonal expansion of $CD8^+$ cells. This may be expected, because $CD8^+$ CTLs perform their effector functions by directly attacking infected cells, whereas a single $CD4^+$ helper cell may secrete cytokines that activate many effector cells such as macrophages, and therefore a greater number of CTLs may be needed for protective immunity.

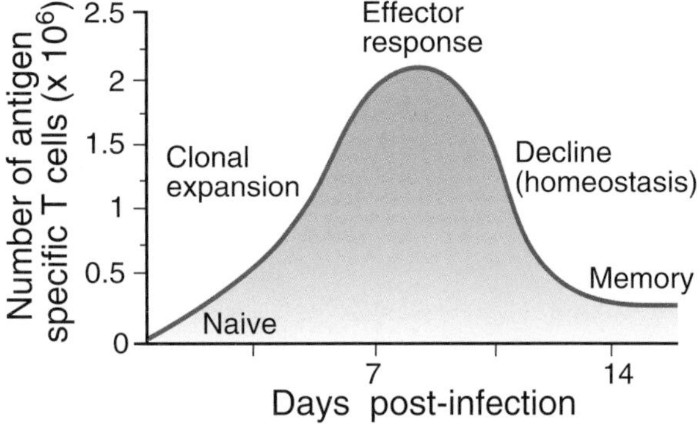

FIGURE 9–5 Clonal expansion of T cells. T cells expand in response to infection, some of the progeny differentiate into effector cells, the majority die, and memory cells persist. The kinetics and numbers of cells are typical of the response of $CD8^+$ T cells in the spleen of a mouse infected with a virus, such as lymphocytic choriomengitis virus; other intracellular microbes elicit qualitatively similar responses.

Several cytokines may function as growth factors to drive the clonal expansion of $CD8^+$ T cells; these include IL-12, IL-15, and IL-7 (see Chapter 12). A role for IL-2, the first identified T cell growth factor, in $CD8^+$ T cell clonal expansion is not at all clear.

Differentiation of $CD8^+$ T Cells into CTLs

Differentiation of $CD8^+$ T cells into effector CTLs involves acquisition of the machinery to perform target cell killing. The most specific feature of CTL differentiation is the development of membrane-bound cytoplasmic granules that contain proteins, including perforin and granzymes, whose function is to kill other cells (described later). In addition, differentiated CTLs are capable of secreting cytokines, mostly IFN-γ, lymphotoxin, and TNF, which function to activate phagocytes and induce inflammation. The molecular events in CTL differentiation involve transcription of genes encoding these effector molecules. Two transcription factors that are required for this program of new gene expression are T-bet (which we will discuss in relationship to T_H1 differentiation in Chapter 13), and eomesodermin, which is structurally related to T-bet.

The differentiation of naive $CD8^+$ T cells into functional CTLs requires antigen recognition, cytokines, notably IL-12, and the participation of $CD4^+$ helper cells in some situations. Antigens initiate the response and cytokines stimulate proliferation and differentiation into CTLs. Helper T cells may be more important for the generation of memory $CD8^+$ T cells than for a primary CTL response, as mentioned before.

Role of Costimulators in T Cell Activation

The proliferation and differentiation of naive T cells require signals provided by molecules on APCs, called costimulators, in addition to antigen-induced signals (Fig. 9–6). The second signal for T cell activation is called costimulation because it functions together with antigen to stimulate T cells. In the absence of costimulation, T cells that encounter antigens either fail to respond and die by apoptosis or enter a state of unresponsiveness called anergy (see Chapter 11).

The best characterized costimulatory pathway in T cell activation involves the T cell surface molecule CD28, which binds the costimulatory molecules B7-1 (CD80) and B7-2 (CD86) expressed on activated APCs (Box 9–1).

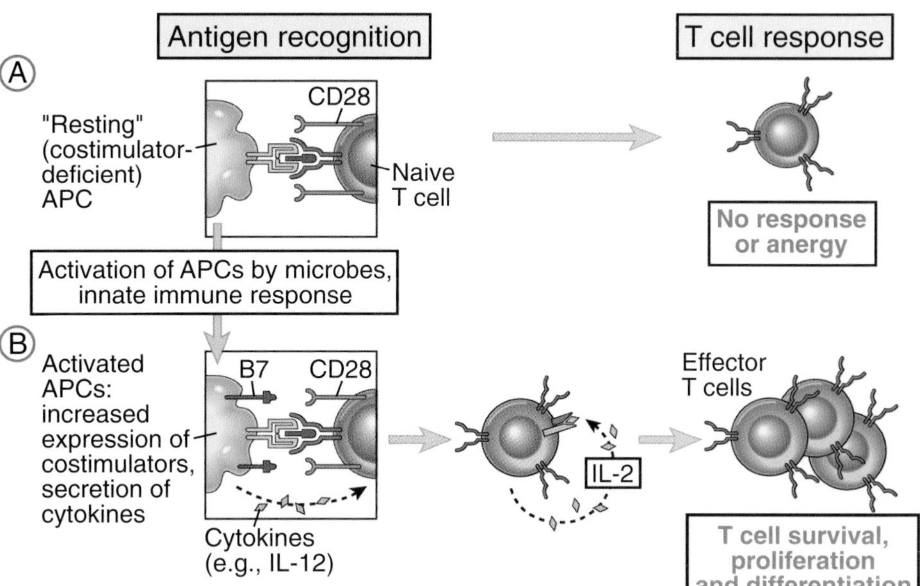

FIGURE 9–6 Functions of costimulators in T cell activation. The resting antigen-presenting cell (APC) expresses few or no costimulators and fails to activate naive T cells (A). (Sometimes antigen recognition without costimulation may make the T cells anergic; this phenomenon will be discussed in Chapter 11.) Microbes and cytokines produced during innate immune responses activate the APCs to express costimulators, such as B7 molecules (B). The APCs then become capable of activating naive T cells. Activated APCs also produce cytokines such as IL-12, which stimulate the differentiation of naive T cells into effector cells.

CD28 delivers signals that enhance many T cell responses to antigen, including cell survival, production of cytokines such as IL-2, and differentiation of naive T cells into effector and memory cells. The structure of CD28 was briefly described in Chapter 7. B7-1 and B7-2 are structurally similar integral membrane single-chain glycoproteins, each with two extracellular immunoglobulin (Ig)-like domains, although on the cell surface B7-1 exists as a dimer and B7-2 as a monomer. The B7 molecules are expressed mainly on APCs, including dendritic cells, macrophages, and B lymphocytes. They are absent or expressed at low levels on resting APCs and are induced by various stimuli (discussed later).

The essential role of the B7 costimulators in T cell activation has been established by several types of experiments.

- In vitro, purified populations of $CD4^+$ T cells respond to antigen by cytokine secretion and proliferation when the antigen is presented by APCs that express B7 molecules but not when the antigen is presented by APCs that lack B7 expression. An activating antibody that binds to CD28 can provide an artificial costimulatory signal and induce T cell responses even if the APCs lack B7 molecules.
- If a pure population of $CD4^+$ T cells is cultured with agents that cross-link the TCR, such as anti-CD3 antibodies, the T cells produce very little cytokine and do not proliferate. Again, if an additional costimulatory signal is provided by antibodies that bind to CD28, the T cells are able to respond. The costimulatory signal provided by anti-CD28 antibody in the absence of the TCR signal does not by itself induce T cell responses.
- Knockout mice lacking B7-1 and B7-2 are deficient in T cell–dependent responses to immunization with protein antigens.

The expression of costimulators is regulated and ensures that T lymphocyte responses are initiated at the correct time and place. The expression of B7 costimulators is increased by microbial products that bind Toll-like receptors, and by cytokines such as interferon (IFN)-γ produced during innate immune reactions to microbes. The induction of costimulators by microbes and by the cytokines of innate immunity promotes T cell responses to microbial antigens (see Chapter 13). In addition, activated T cells express CD40L on their surface, which binds to CD40 expressed on APCs and delivers signals that enhance the expression of B7 costimulators on the APCs. Of all potential APCs, mature dendritic cells express the highest levels of costimulators and, as a result, are the most potent stimulators of naive T cells (which are completely dependent on costimulation for activation). In Chapter 6, we mentioned the essential role of adjuvants in inducing primary T cell responses to protein antigens such as vaccines. Many adjuvants are products of microbes, or mimic microbes, and one of their major functions in T cell activation is to stimulate the expression of costimulators on APCs. The absence of costimulators on unactivated, or "resting," APCs in normal tissues contributes to the maintenance of tolerance to self antigens. Because such tissue APCs are capable of presenting self antigens to T cells, the lack of costimulator expression ensures that potentially self-reactive T cells are not activated and may be rendered anergic (see Chapter 11).

Previously activated effector and memory T cells are less dependent on costimulation by the B7:CD28 pathway than are naive cells. This property of effector and memory cells enables them to respond to antigens presented by various APCs that may reside in nonlymphoid tissues and may express no or low levels of B7. For instance, the differentiation of $CD8^+$ T cells into effector CTLs requires costimulation, but effector CTLs can

Box 9–1 ■ IN DEPTH: THE B7–CD28 FAMILIES OF COSTIMULATORS AND INHIBITORY RECEPTORS

The best defined costimulators for T lymphocytes are the B7 family of molecules on APCs that bind to members of the CD28 family of receptors on T cells. The first proteins to be discovered in these families were CD28 and B7-1. The existence and functions of B7-1 and CD28 were originally surmised from experiments with monoclonal antibodies specific for these molecules. The cloning of the genes encoding B7-1 and CD28 opened the way for a variety of experiments in mice that have clarified the role of these molecules and led to the identification of additional homologous proteins involved in T cell costimulation. For example, residual costimulatory activity of APCs from B7-1 knockout mice suggested the existence of additional costimulatory molecules, and homology-based cloning strategies led to the identification of the B7-2 molecule. B7-1 and B7-2 both bind to CD28 and together account for the majority of costimulatory activity provided by APCs for the activation of naive T cells. This is evident from the phenotype of B7-1/B7-2 double knockout mice, which have profound defects in adaptive immune responses to protein antigens.

Although costimulatory pathways were discovered as mediators of T cell activation, it is now clear that homologous molecules are involved in inhibiting T cell responses. The first and best defined example of an inhibitory receptor on T cells is CTLA-4, a member of the CD28 family, which was discovered and characterized by the use of monoclonal antibodies. The name CTLA-4 is based on the fact that this molecule was the fourth receptor identified in a search for molecules expressed in CTLs, but its expression and function are not restricted to CTLs. CTLA-4 is structurally homologous to CD28 and is a receptor for both B7-1 and B7-2. Unlike CD28, CTLA-4 serves as a negative regulator of T cell activation. CTLA-4 knockout mice show excessive T cell activation, proliferation, and systemic autoimmunity.

Several other proteins structurally related to B7-1 and B7-2 or to CD28 and CTLA-4 have recently been identified by homology-based cloning strategies, and their functions are now being studied. These proteins can be considered members of the B7 and CD28 families, respectively. Two other members of the CD28 family are called ICOS (inducible costimulator) and PD-1 (programmed death-1, because this molecule was thought to regulate programmed death of T cells). The available data indicate that CD28 is important for activating naive T cells, and ICOS plays a greater role in effector responses, particularly IL-10 and IL-4 production. CTLA-4 and PD-1 are inhibitory receptors. How diverse signals from this receptor family are integrated during immune responses is a major question in the field.

Members of the B7 family include B7-1, B7-2, ICOS-ligand, B7-H1 (PD-L1), B7-DC (PD-L2), B7-H3, and B7-H4 (see Figure). All these proteins are transmembrane proteins consisting of two extracellular Ig-like domains, including an N-terminal V-like domain and a membrane proximal C-like domain. B7-H3 may be expressed in alternative forms, with either one pair of V and C domains like the other B7 family members or two tandem pairs of V and C domains. The main function of these molecules is to bind to CD28 family receptors on T cells, thereby stimulating signal transduction pathways in the T cells. There is no compelling evidence that the cytoplasmic tails of the B7 family members transduce activating signals in the cells on which they are expressed. B7-1 and B7-2 are mainly expressed on APCs, including dendritic cells, macrophages, and B cells. Although there is some constitutive expression on dendritic cells, expression of both molecules is strongly induced by various signals, including endotoxin, inflammatory cytokines (e.g., IL-12, IFN-γ), and CD40-CD40 ligand interactions. The temporal patterns of expression of B7-1 and B7-2 differ; B7-2 is expressed constitutively at low levels and induced early after activation of APCs, whereas B7-1 is not expressed constitutively and is induced hours or days later. The other members of the B7 family, ICOS ligand, PD-L1 and PD-L2, are also expressed on APCs, but in addition, there is significant expression on a variety of non-immune cells, such as endothelial cells. The nonlymphoid expression of these molecules suggests they play a role in regulating T cell activation in peripheral tissues and perhaps in the maintenance of self-tolerance.

The CD28 family of receptors are all expressed on T cells, but PD-1 is also expressed on B cells and myeloid cells. These receptors are transmembrane proteins, all of which include a single Ig V-like domain and a cytoplasmic tail with tyrosine residues. CD28, CTLA-4, and ICOS exist as disulfide-linked homodimers; PD-1 is expressed as a monomer. Both CD28 and CTLA-4 bind both B7-1 and B7-2, with different affinities, and share a sequence motif, MYPPPY, in the V domain, which is essential for B7 binding. ICOS has an FDPPPF motif in the corresponding position, which mediates binding to ICOS-ligand but not to B7-1 or B7-2. PD-1 has neither motif and binds to PD-L1 or PD-L2 but not to B7-1, B7-2, or ICOS-ligand. The cytoplasmic tails of the CD28 family molecules contain structural motifs that mediate interaction with signaling molecules, although the signal transduction pathways that are engaged are incompetently understood. Tyrosine residues in the tails of CD28 become phosphorylated on B7-1 or B7-2 binding, and they serve as docking sites for PI-3 kinase and Grb-2. PI-3 kinase activation is linked to the activation of the serine/threonine kinase Akt. PI-3 kinase can also be activated by recruitment to the cytoplasmic tail of CTLA-4, and perhaps of ICOS as well. Consistent with their roles in negative regulation of cellular activation, both CTLA-4 and PD-1 have variations of the ITIMs in their cytoplasmic tails (see Box 9–3) and recruit the tyrosine phosphatase SHP-2. CD28 is constitutively expressed on CD4$^+$ and CD8$^+$ T cells. ICOS is expressed on CD4$^+$ and CD8$^+$ T cells only after TCR binding to antigen, and its induction is enhanced by CD28 signals.

X-ray crystallographic analyses of B7-1 and B7-2 interactions with CTLA-4 suggest that these molecules form a repeating lattice structure in the immunological

Continued on following page

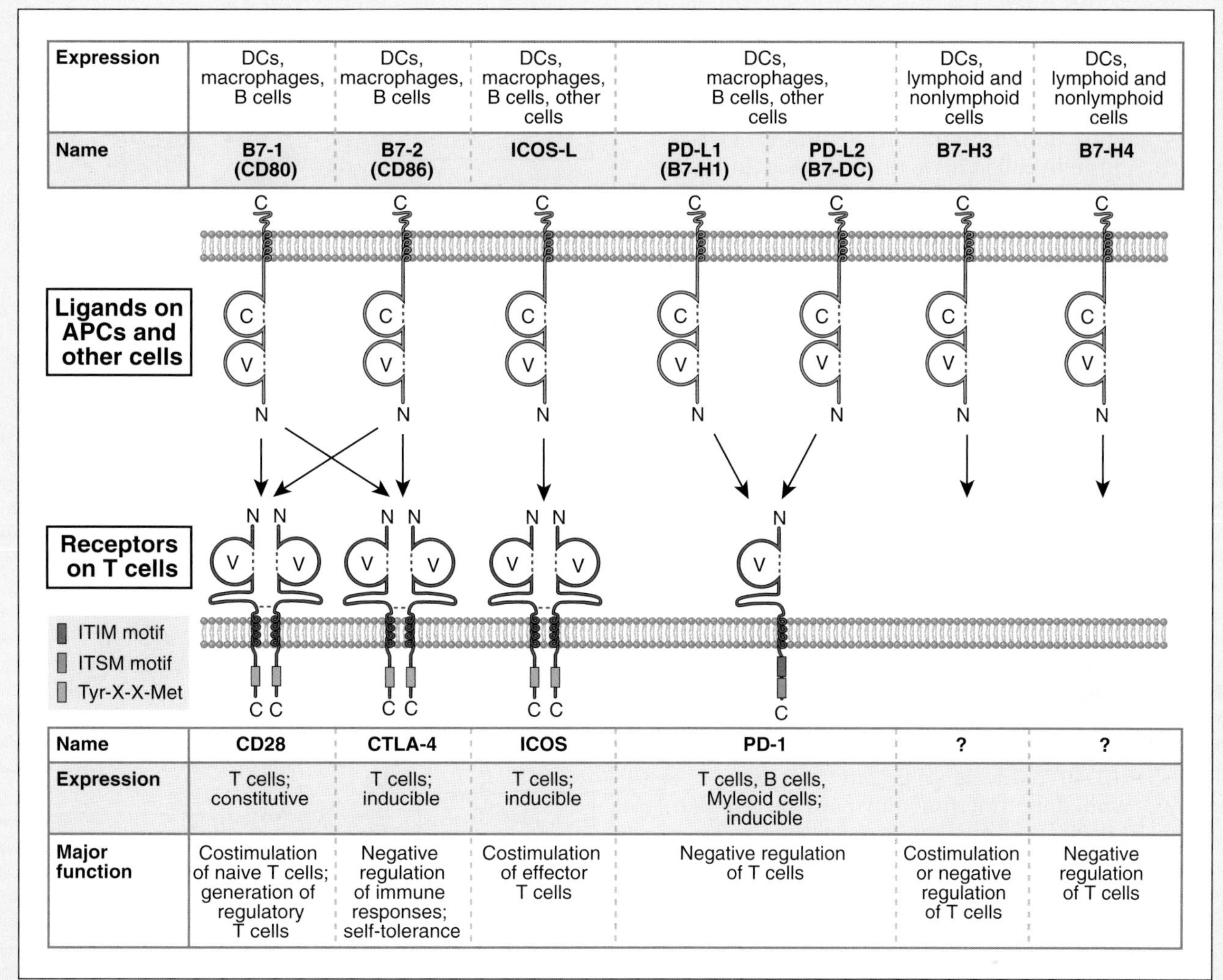

synapse. B7-1 or B7-2 may dimerize in the APC membrane, and each monomeric subunit could bind to one chain of a different CTLA-4 dimer. Such an arrangement could enhance the local concentration of the ligands and receptors and presumably enhance signaling. It is not known if such an arrangement also applies to other B7:CD28 family ligand-receptor interactions.

Expression
DCs, macrophages, B cells
DCs, macrophages, B cells
DCs, macrophages, B cells, other cells
DCs, macrophages, B cells, other cells
DCs, lymphoid and nonlymphoid cells
DCs, lymphoid and nonlymphoid cells
Name
B7-1 (CD80)
B7-2 (CD86)
ICOS-L
PD-L1 (B7-H1)
PD-L2 (B7-DC)
B7-H3
B7-H4
Ligands on APCs and other cells
Receptors on T cells
ITIM motif
ITSM motif
Tyr-X-X-Met
Name
CD28
CTLA-4
ICOS
PD-1
?
?
Expression
T cells; constitutive
T cells; inducible
T cells; inducible
T cells, B cells, Myleoid cells; inducible
Major function
Costimulation of naive T cells; generation of regulatory T cells
Negative regulation of immune responses; self-tolerance
Costimulation of effector T cells
Negative regulation of T cells
Costimulation or negative regulation of T cells
Negative regulation of T cells

The functional consequences of signaling by CD28 family members differ for each molecule. As discussed in the text, CD28 is essential for initiating responses of $CD4^+$ T cells, whereas ICOS may be more important for activation of effector T cells. CTLA-4 and PD-1 are inhibitory receptors that may play different roles in terminating immune responses. It has been proposed that CTLA-4 inhibits acute responses in lymphoid organs, and PD-1 inhibits chronically activated cells and responses in peripheral, non-lymphoid tissues. The physiologic functions of the other recently described B7 family members are not yet defined.

kill other cells that do not express costimulators (see Chapter 13).

A major essential function of the B7:CD28 pathway is in the generation of regulatory T cells. Regulatory T cells are $CD4^+CD25^+$ T cells that can suppress the function of effector T cells (see Chapter 11). A large proportion of these cells develop in the thymus, and are known as natural regulatory T cells. The development of natural regulatory T cells requires both B7 and CD28, as shown by the failure of these cells to emerge in knockout mice lacking CD28 or B7 proteins. The mechanisms underlying this role of CD28 are not fully defined.

The biochemical mechanism by which CD28:B7 interactions promote T cell activation is incompletely understood. CD28-mediated signals increase the production of cytokines, especially the T cell autocrine growth factor IL-2. This may occur by a combination of enhanced transcription and stabilization of IL-2 messenger RNA. In addition, CD28 signals promote the survival of T cells, in part by increasing expression of the anti-apoptotic protein Bcl-x (see Chapter 11, Box 11–2).

We will describe signaling responses to costimulators later in the chapter, after we discuss the biochemistry of T cell activation.

The CD28:B7 pathway of costimulation is the prototype of a much larger family of receptors and ligands that function to stimulate and inhibit T cells (see Box 9–1). A protein called ICOS (inducible costimulator) is homologous to CD28 and is so named because it is induced on T cells after activation. The ligand for ICOS is homologous to B7-1 and B7-2. ICOS appears to be particularly important for stimulating the production of certain cytokines, notably IL-10, and for the activation of previously differentiated effector T cells. A protein called CTLA-4 (CD152) is also homologous to CD28, binds to B7-1 and B7-2, and is expressed on activated T cells. Unlike CD28, CTLA-4 functions to terminate T cell responses and plays a role in self-tolerance (Chapter 11). We will briefly discuss CTLA-4 and another inhibitory receptor, PD-1, later in this chapter.

The interaction of CD40L on T cells with CD40 on APCs enhances T cell activation. The likely mechanism of this effect is that the engagement of CD40 on the APCs activates the APCs to make them more potent, perhaps by enhancing their expression of B7 molecules and secretion of cytokines such as IL-12 that promote T cell differentiation. This phenomenon is sometimes called "licensing," since activated T cells license additional APCs to participate in an immune response (Fig. 9–7). Thus, the CD40 pathway indirectly amplifies T cell responses and does not function as a costimulatory pathway by itself.

Many new therapeutics are being developed based on the understanding of costimulatory pathways. CTLA-4Ig, a fusion protein consisting of the extracellular domain of CTLA-4 and the Fc portion of human IgG, binds to B7-1 and B7-2 and blocks the B7:CD28 interaction when administered to patients. It is an approved therapy for rheumatoid arthritis, and clinical trials are currently assessing its efficacy in the treatment of psoriasis, Crohn's disease and transplant rejection. Inhibitors of the CD40L:CD40 pathway are also being currently assessed in clinical trials for use in transplant rejection and in chronic inflammatory diseases of presumed autoimmune origin. Antibodies that block the inhibitory receptor CTLA-4 attenuate inhibitory signals and thus enhance immune responses. These agents are in clinical trials for the immunotherapy of tumors.

Many other T cell surface molecules, including CD2 and integrins, have been shown to deliver costimulatory signals in vitro, but their physiologic role in mice and humans is less clear. We have discussed the functions of CD2 family proteins in Chapter 7, and of integrins in Chapter 2.

Having described the main steps in the functional responses of T cells, we can proceed to a consideration of the biochemistry of T cell activation.

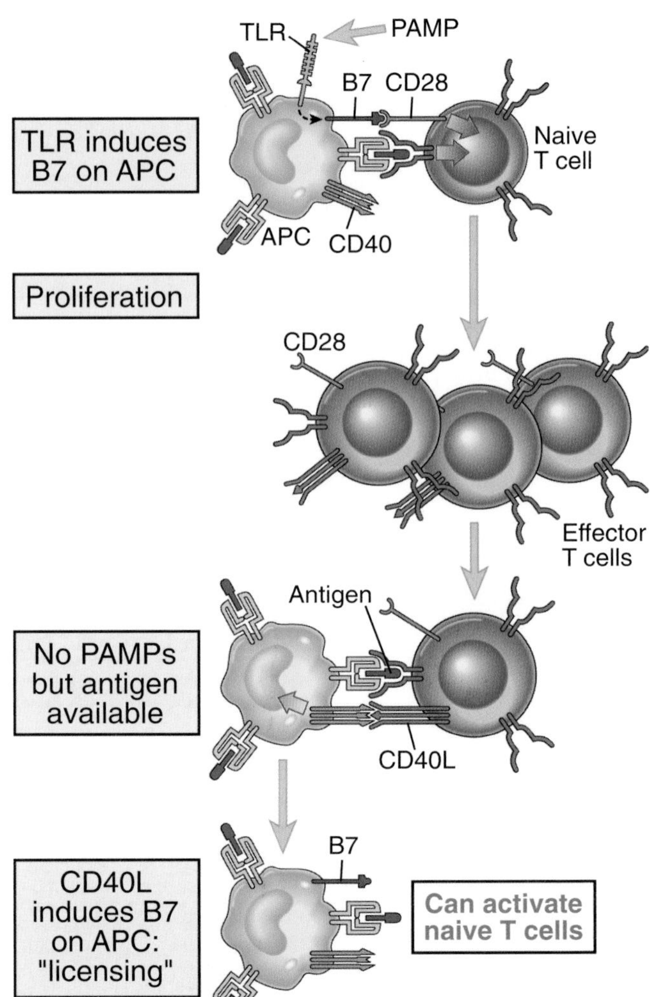

FIGURE 9–7 Role of CD40 in T cell activation. Naive T cells are activated by peptide-MHC complexes on antigen-presenting cells (APCs) previously activated by the binding of pathogen-associated molecular patterns (PAMP) to Toll-like receptors (TLRs). Antigen recognition by T cells in conjunction with CD28 activation induces the expression of CD40 ligand (CD40L) on activated T cells. CD40L engages CD40 on the APC and may stimulate the expression of B7 molecules and the secretion of cytokines that activate T cells. Thus, CD40L on the T cells makes the APCs "better" APCs, and the B7 and CD40 pathways stimulate each other.

SIGNAL TRANSDUCTION BY THE TCR COMPLEX

T cell signaling pathways coordinately activate the transcription of genes that are silent in naive cells and whose products mediate the responses and functions of activated T cells. The recognition of antigen by the TCR initiates a sequence of biochemical signals in T cells that result in transcriptional activation of particular genes and the entry of the cells into the cell cycle. The genes that are expressed in T cells after antigen recognition encode many of the proteins that mediate the biologic responses of these cells (Fig. 9–8). The signaling cascades triggered by the TCR have been defined largely by *in vitro* analyses of various T cell populations that can be activated by the engagement of their antigen receptors. From such studies, several important general features of T cell signal transduction are now well established.

- ***Activation of T cells involves the integration of signals from multiple receptors.*** The TCR provides specificity,

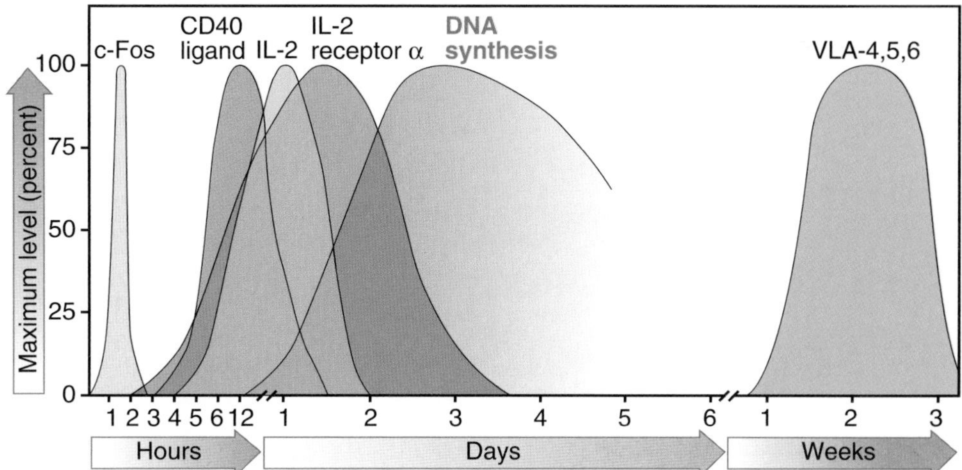

FIGURE 9–8 Kinetics of gene expression in antigen-stimulated T lymphocytes. T lymphocytes activated by antigens and costimulators express new genes. The approximate time course of the expression of selected genes is shown; the actual kinetics may vary in different T cell populations exposed to different stimuli.

and costimulatory and cytokine receptors play key rates in clonal expansion and differentiation.

- ***The early biochemical response to antigen recognition consists of clustering of coreceptors with the antigen receptor, and tyrosine phosphorylation of immunoreceptor tyrosine-based activation motif (ITAM) tyrosine residues*** (Fig. 9–9). The TCR does not have intrinsic enzymatic activity, but it is associated with the CD3 complex and ζ proteins that bind enzymes and contain ITAMs, as discussed below. Phosphorylation of ITAM tyrosines initiates signal transduction and the activation of downstream tyrosine kinases, which in turn phosphorylate tyrosine residues on other adapter proteins. The subsequent events in signal transduction are generated by the specific recruitment of key enzymes that each initiate distinct downstream signaling pathways.
- ***Signals from the antigen receptor coordinately activate a number of important biochemical pathways, some of the major ones being the Ras-MAP kinase pathway, the protein kinase C (PKC) pathway, and the calcium-calcineurin pathway*** (see Fig. 9–9). Activation of these enzymes occurs within minutes after antigen recognition. The enzymes activated by each of these pathways induce transcription factors that stimulate the expression of various genes in the T cells, a process that takes several hours.

In the following sections, we describe the major steps in signaling by the TCR complex, starting with the earliest responses at the plasma membrane and culminating in the transcriptional activation of many T cell–specific genes.

Early Membrane Events: Activation of Protein Tyrosine Kinases, Recruitment of Adapter Proteins, and Formation of the Immunological Synapse

Antigen recognition by the TCR induces the activation of T cell signaling initially by the activation of Src family kinases, and this is followed by the activation of downstream signaling pathways following the recruitment and phosphorylation of specific adapters. Eventually a relatively stable interface is formed between the T cell and the APC, and this interface is known as the immunological synapse.

Activation of Tyrosine Kinases

The earliest biochemical events within the T cell that follow clustering of the TCR complex and coreceptor are the activation of protein tyrosine kinases associated with the cytoplasmic domains of the clustered CD3 and coreceptor proteins and phosphorylation of tyrosines in CD3 and ζ chains (Fig. 9–10). Protein tyrosine kinases are enzymes that catalyze the phosphorylation of tyrosine residues in various protein substrates (Box 9–2). In T cells, several components of the TCR complex, as well as downstream intermediates, are targets of protein tyrosine kinases. The cytoplasmic portions of the CD3 chains and the ζ chains contain a total of ten conserved tyrosine-containing peptide sequences called ITAMs (see Chapter 7). When TCRs bind to peptide-MHC complexes, CD4 or CD8 binds at the same time to nonpolymorphic regions of the class II or class I MHC molecule on the APC (see Fig. 9–10). Lck, a Src family tyrosine kinase that is associated with the cytoplasmic tails of CD4 and CD8, is thus brought close to the ITAMs in the CD3 and ζ chains. The clustering of the TCR complex and coreceptor leads to activation of Lck, by mechanisms that are not clear. The active Lck then phosphorylates the tyrosines in the ITAMs of the CD3 and ζ chains. Thus, within seconds of TCR clustering, many of the tyrosine residues within the ITAMs of the CD3 and ζ chains become phosphorylated. Another cytoplasmic tyrosine kinase that is found in physical association with the TCR complex is CD3-associated Fyn, and it may play a role similar to that of Lck. It is believed that Fyn may be activated by a conformational alteration of TCR and CD3 molecules following TCR binding to MHC-peptide complexes. Mice lacking Lck show some defects in T cell development, and double knockout mice lacking both Lck and Fyn show even more severe defects.

The tyrosine phosphorylated ITAMs in the ζ chain become "docking sites" for the tyrosine kinase called

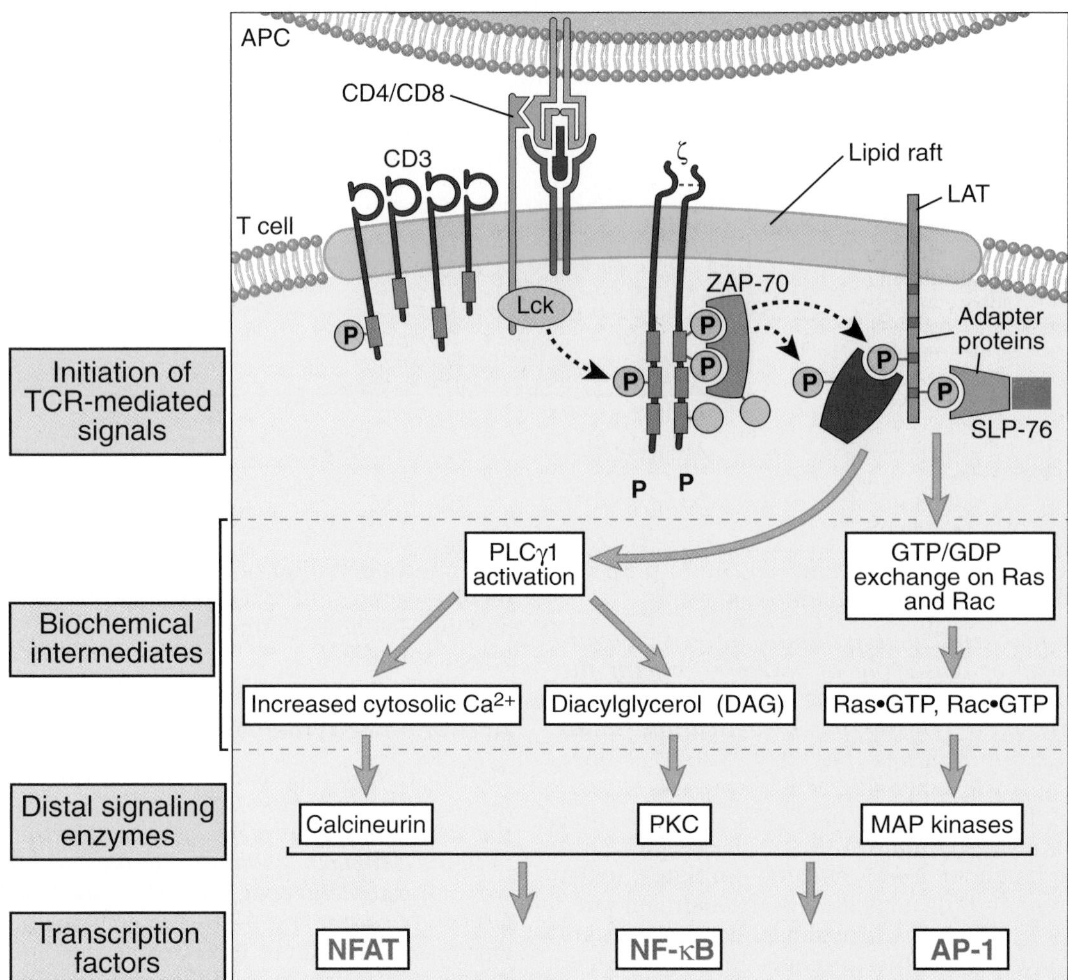

FIGURE 9–9 Intracellular signaling events during T cell activation. Binding of the TCR and coreceptors to peptide-MHC complexes on the antigen-presenting cell (APC) initiates proximal signaling events, which result in phosphorylation of the ζ chain, binding and activation of ZAP-70, phosphorylation of adapter proteins, and activation of various cellular enzymes. These enzymes then activate transcription factors that stimulate the expression of various genes involved in T cell responses.

ZAP-70 (ζ-associated protein of 70 kD). ZAP-70 is a member of a family of tyrosine kinases distinct from the Src family. (Another member of this family is Syk, which plays an important role in signal transduction in B cells and in some populations of T cells, such as γδ T cells from the intestine.) ZAP-70 contains two conserved domains called Src homology 2 (SH2) domains that can bind to phosphotyrosines (see Box 9–2). Each ITAM has two tyrosine residues, and both of these must become phosphorylated to form a docking site for one ZAP-70 molecule. The bound ZAP-70 becomes a substrate for the adjacent Lck, which phosphorylates specific tyrosine residues of ZAP-70. As a result, ZAP-70 acquires its own tyrosine kinase activity and is then able to phosphorylate a number of other cytoplasmic signaling molecules. A critical threshold of ZAP-70 activity may be needed before downstream signaling events will proceed, and this threshold is achieved by the recruitment of multiple ZAP-70 molecules to the phosphorylated ITAMs on the ζ chains and on CD3 tails.

Another kinase pathway in T cells involves the activation of PI-3 (phosphatidylinositol-3) kinase, which phosphorylates a specific membrane-associated inositol lipid. This enzyme is recruited to the TCR complex and associated adapter proteins and generates phosphatidylinositol trisphosphate (PIP_3) from membrane phosphatidylinositol bisphosphate (PIP_2). PIP_3 provides a binding site on the inside of the plasma membrane for signaling intermediates that contain pleckstrin homology domains, including phospholipase Cγ and kinases such as Itk (and Btk in B cells). Another important PIP_3-dependent kinase is PDK1, which is required for the activation of an important downstream kinase called Akt. Akt is a crucial regulator of cell survival. PI-3 kinase is most efficiently activated downstream of the CD28 costimulatory receptor, as we will discuss later in this chapter.

The activity of kinases in T cell signaling pathways may be regulated by protein tyrosine phosphatases. These phosphatases can remove phosphates from tyrosine residues of the kinases as well as from adapter

Box 9–2 ▪ IN DEPTH: PROTEIN TYROSINE KINASES AND PHOSPHATASES

Protein-protein interactions and the activities of cellular enzymes are often regulated by phosphorylation of tyrosine residues. Inducible phosphorylation of tyrosines is much less common than phosphorylation of serine or threonine residues and is usually reserved for critical regulatory steps. It is not surprising, therefore, that the kinases that catalyze tyrosine phosphorylation are essential components of many intracellular signaling cascades in lymphocytes and other cell types. These protein tyrosine kinases (PTKs) mediate the transfer of the terminal phosphate of ATP to the hydroxyl group of a tyrosine residue in a substrate protein. A particular PTK will phosphorylate only a limited set of substrates, and this specificity is determined by the amino acid sequences flanking the tyrosine as well as by the tertiary structural characteristics of the substrate protein.

Some tyrosine kinases are intrinsic components of the cytoplasmic tails of cell surface receptors, such as the receptors for platelet-derived growth factor (PDGF) and epidermal growth factor (EGF). Examples of receptor tyrosine kinases that are involved in hematopoiesis include c-Kit, a receptor for stem cell factor, and the receptor for monocyte colony-stimulating factor (M-CSF). Many PTKs of importance in the immune system, however, are cytoplasmic proteins that are noncovalently associated with the cytoplasmic tails of cell surface receptors or with adapter proteins. Sometimes this association is only transiently induced in the early stages of signaling cascades. Three families of cytoplasmic PTKs that are prominent in B and T cell antigen receptor signaling, as well as Fc receptor signaling, are the Src, Syk/ZAP-70, and Tec families (see Figure). The Janus kinases are another group of nonreceptor PTKs involved in many cytokine-induced signaling cascades and are discussed in Chapter 12.

Src family kinases are homologous to, and named after, the transforming gene of Rous sarcoma virus, the first animal tumor virus identified. Members of this family include Src, Yes, Fgr, Fyn, Lck, Lyn, Hck, and Blk. All Src family members share tertiary structural characteristics that are distributed among four distinct domains and are critical for their function and regulation of enzymatic activity. The amino-terminal end of most Src family kinases contains a consensus site for addition of a myristic acid group; this type of lipid modification serves to anchor cytoplasmic proteins to the inner side of the plasma membrane. Otherwise, the amino-terminal domains of Src family PTKs are highly variable among different family members, and this region determines the ability of each member to interact specifically with different proteins. For example, the amino-terminal region of the Lck protein is the contact site for interaction with the cytoplasmic tails of CD4 and CD8. The Src family PTKs have two internal domains called **Src homology 2 (SH2)** and **Src homology 3 (SH3) domains,** each of which has a distinct three-dimensional structure that permits specific noncovalent interactions with other proteins. SH2 domains are about 100 amino acids long and bind to phosphotyrosines on other proteins or on themselves. Each SH2 domain has a unique binding specificity, which is

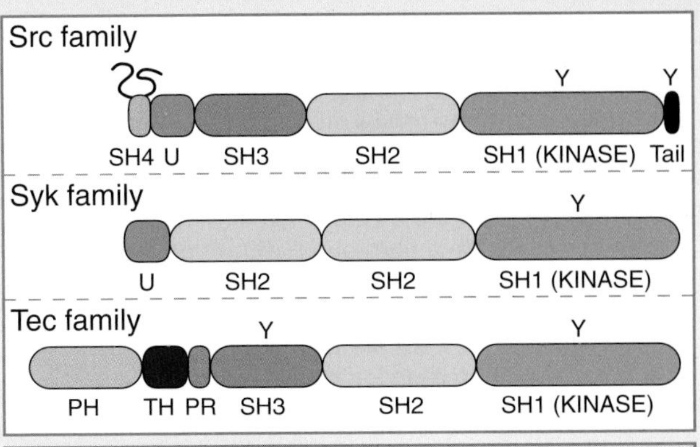

SH1: Src homology 1 domain
SH2: Src homology 2 domain
SH3: Src homology 3 domain
SH4: Src homology 4 domain (lipid attachment motif)
U: Unique region
PH: Pleckstrin homology domain
TH: Tec homology domain
PR: Proline rich region
Y: Regulatory tyrosine
T: Tail

determined by the three residues that follow the phosphotyrosine on the target protein. SH2 domains are also found on many signaling molecules outside the Src family. SH3 domains are approximately 60 amino acids long and also mediate protein-protein binding. SH3 domains bind to proline residues and may function cooperatively with the SH2 domains of the same protein. The critical role of SH3 domains in PTK function is illustrated by mutations in the SH3 domain of Bruton's tyrosine kinase; these mutations do not alter the protein's stability or kinase activity but result in defective B cell receptor signaling and agammaglobulinemia. The carboxy-terminal SH1 domain in Src PTKs is the tyrosine kinase enzymatic domain. It contains binding sites for the substrate and for the ATP phosphate donor and an autophosphorylation site (a tyrosine residue) whose phosphorylation is needed for kinase activity. A tyrosine residue at the C-terminal end of the Src family kinase serves as a regulatory switch for the PTK. When it is phosphorylated, the PTK is inactive, and when the phosphate is removed by tyrosine phosphatases, the enzyme activity is turned on. The PTKs that phosphorylate Src family PTKs at this inhibitory site form yet another subfamily of PTKs, the best described member being c-Src kinase-1 (Csk-1).

The Syk/ZAP-70 family of PTKs includes only two identified members so far. Syk is abundantly expressed in B lymphocytes but is also found in lower amounts in other hematopoietic cells, including some T cells. ZAP-70 is expressed in only T lymphocytes and natural killer cells. Syk and ZAP-70 play similar roles in BCR and TCR signaling cascades, respectively. There are two SH2 domains in the Syk/ZAP-70 PTKs, but no SH3 domain and

Continued on following page

Box 9–2 ▪ IN DEPTH: PROTEIN TYROSINE KINASES AND PHOSPHATASES (Continued)

no inhibitory tyrosine. Syk and ZAP-70 are inactive until they bind, through their two SH2 domains, to paired phosphotyrosines within ITAMs of antigen-receptor complex proteins (see text). Furthermore, activation of ZAP-70 probably requires Src family PTK (e.g., Lck)-mediated phosphorylation of one or more tyrosine residues.

The Tec PTKs are a third group of nonreceptor kinases that are activated by antigen receptors in B and T cells as well as by many other signals in other cell types. This family includes Btk, Tec, Itk, DSrc29, Etk, and Rlk. Btk is expressed in all hematopoietic cells, but mutations of the Btk gene primarily affect B cell development in humans, causing X-linked agammaglobulinemia. The major Tec kinases expressed by T cells are Itk, Rlk, and Tec. All the Tec family members contain a Tec homology (TH) domain, which includes sequences unique to this family (Btk homology domain) and sequences homologous with GTPase-activating protein domains. The TH domain mediates interactions with other signaling molecules. In addition, Tec kinases share structural similarities with the Src family kinases, including SH3 and SH2 domains that mediate interactions with other signaling molecules and a catalytic SH1 domain. Unlike the Src kinases, the Tec kinases do not have N-terminal myristoylation sites. In contrast, most Tec family kinases contain a pleckstrin homology (PH) domain, which promotes membrane localization by binding to PIP_3 generated by PI-3 kinase. The Tec kinases also do not contain a C-terminal regulatory tyrosine. Activation of a Tec kinase requires membrane localization, phosphorylation by a Src kinase, and autophosphorylation of the SH3 domain. The SH2 domains of Btk and Itk bind the phosphorylated adapter proteins BLNK/SLP-65 and SLP-76, in B and T cells, respectively, shortly after antigen recognition. Once bound to these adapter proteins, Btk and Itk can phosphorylate and activate phospholipase C.

Protein tyrosine phosphatases (PTPs) are enzymes that remove phosphate moieties from tyrosine residues, countering the actions of PTKs. PTPs may be membrane receptors or cytoplasmic proteins. One important receptor PTP, which has a role in lymphocyte activation, is CD45, a membrane-bound protein that removes autoinhibitory C-terminal phosphates from Src family kinases, such as Lck and Fyn, and is essential for T and B cell activation. The phosphatase activity of CD45 appears to require dimerization for activation, and mutations that prevent dimerization result in defective CD45 function and uncontrolled activation of lymphocytes. Cytoplasmic PTPs are loosely associated with receptors or are recruited to tyrosine phosphorylated receptors through SH2 domains. These enzymes include two PTPs commonly called SHP-1 and SHP-2. SHP-1 is particularly abundant in hematopoietic cells. SHP-1 is a negative regulator of lymphocytes and contributes to the inhibitory signals mediated by inhibitory receptors of the immune system, such as killer inhibitory receptors of NK cells (see Chapter 2). These inhibitory receptors bind SHP-1 through special motifs called ITIMs by analogy to the ITAMs of the TCR and other activating receptors. The central role of SHP-1 in regulating lymphocyte function is illustrated by the "moth-eaten" mouse strain, which carries a mutation in the SHP-1 gene and is characterized by autoimmunity and defects in homeostasis. SHP-2 plays a positive role in signaling by certain receptors, such as the EGF receptor, but may also be involved in negative regulation in CTLA-4 signaling.

Other phosphatases act on phosphorylated inositol lipids and inhibit cellular responses; an example is SHIP-1, an SH2 domain-containing inositol phosphatase that is associated with an Fc receptor of B cells and serves to terminate B cell responses (see Chapter 10, Fig. 10–19).

proteins. In the case of tyrosine phosphatases that dephosphorylate tyrosine kinases, depending on which tyrosine residue is involved the effect may be to activate or to inhibit the enzymatic function of the kinases. Two phosphatases that are recruited to the TCR complex are SHP-1 and SHP-2 (for SH2 domain-containing phosphatases). These phosphatases serve to inhibit signal transduction by removing phosphates from tyrosine residues in key signaling molecules. Another inhibitory phosphatase is specific for inositol phospholipids and is called SHIP (SH2 domain containing inositol phosphatase). The CD45 protein is an integral membrane protein whose cytoplasmic tail contains tandem protein tyrosine phosphatase domains. CD45 dephosphorylates inhibitory tyrosine residues in Src family kinases such as Lck and may thus contribute to the generation of potentially active Lck and Fyn, perhaps even before antigen recognition occurs. CD45 has complex activating and inhibitory roles in lymphocytes, and how its activity is regulated during T cell signaling is still not clearly understood.

Formation of the Immunological Synapse

When the TCR complex recognizes MHC-associated peptides on an APC, several T cell surface proteins and intracellular signaling molecules are rapidly mobilized to the site of T cell–APC contact (Fig. 9–11). This region of physical contact between the T cell and the APC forms a bull's-eye-like structure that is called an **immunological synapse**, or a supramolecular activation cluster (SMAC). The T cell molecules that are rapidly mobilized to the center of the synapse include the TCR complex (the TCR, CD3, and ζ chains), CD4 or CD8 coreceptors, receptors for costimulators (such as CD28), enzymes such as PKC-θ, and adapter proteins that associate with the cytoplasmic tails of the transmembrane receptors. At this portion of the synapse, called the c-SMAC (for central supramolecular activation cluster), the distance between the T cell plasma membrane and that of the APC is about 15 nm. Integrins remain at the periphery of the synapse, where they function to stabilize the binding

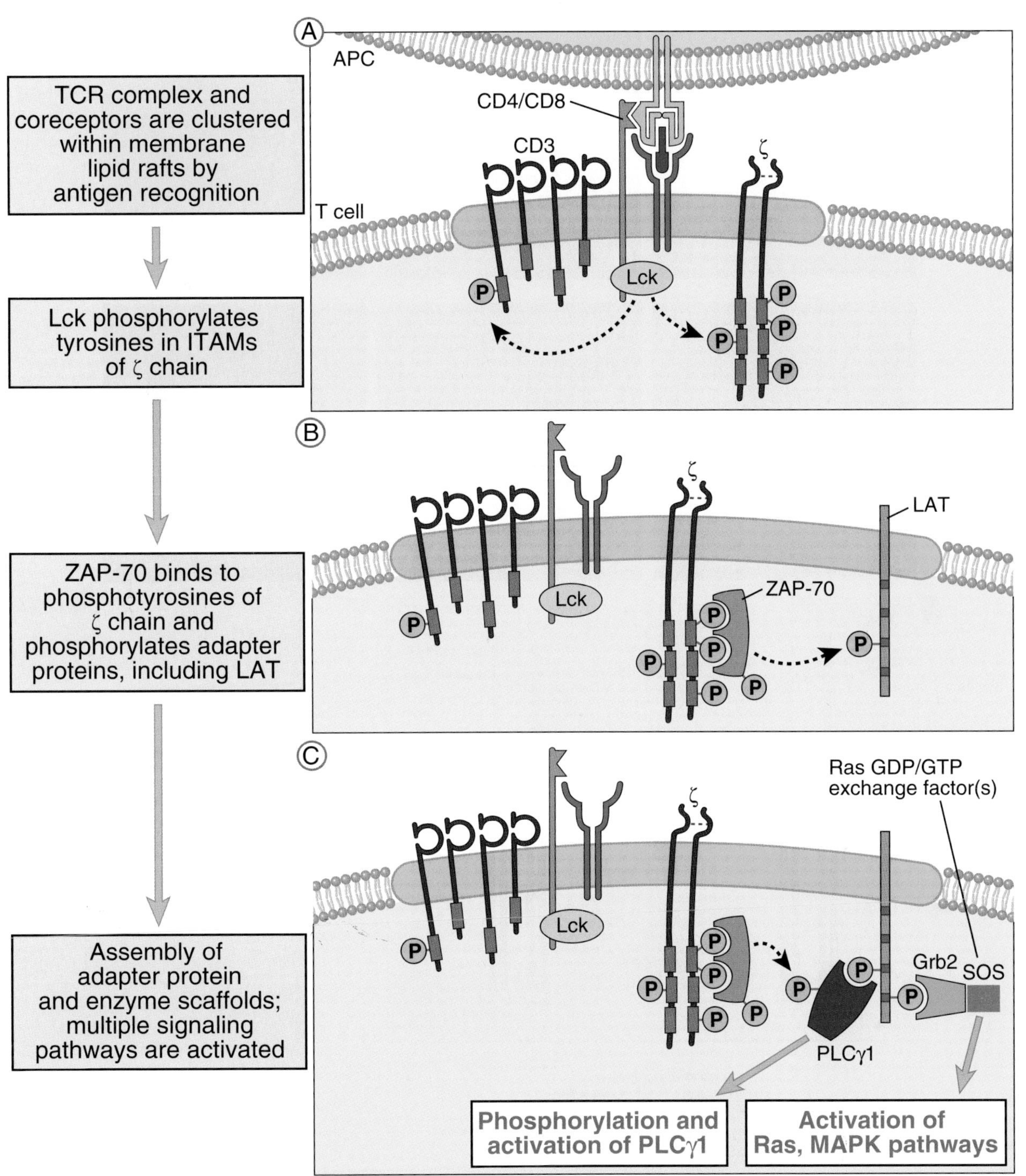
TCR complex and coreceptors are clustered within membrane lipid rafts by antigen recognition
Lck phosphorylates tyrosines in ITAMs of ζ chain
ZAP-70 binds to phosphotyrosines of ζ chain and phosphorylates adapter proteins, including LAT
Assembly of adapter protein and enzyme scaffolds; multiple signaling pathways are activated
A
APC
CD4/CD8
CD3
ζ
T cell
Lck
P
B
LAT
ZAP-70
C
Ras GDP/GTP exchange factor(s)
Grb2
SOS
PLCγ1
Phosphorylation and activation of PLCγ1
Activation of Ras, MAPK pathways

FIGURE 9–10 Early tyrosine phosphorylation events in T cell activation. On antigen recognition, there is clustering of TCR complexes with coreceptors (CD4, in this case). CD4-associated Lck becomes active and phosphorylates tyrosines in the ITAMs of CD3 and ζ chains (A). ZAP-70 binds to the phosphotyrosines of the ζ chains and is itself phosphorylated and activated. (The illustration shows one ZAP-70 molecule binding to two phosphotyrosines of one ITAM in the ζ chain, but it is likely that initiation of a T cell response requires the assembly of multiple ZAP-70 molecules on each ζ chain.) Active ZAP-70 then phosphorylates tyrosines on various adapter molecules, such as LAT (B). The adapters become docking sites for cellular enzymes such as PLCγ1 and exchange factors that activate Ras and other small G proteins upstream of MAP kinases (C), and these enzymes activate various cellular responses.

of the T cell to the APC, forming the peripheral portion of the SMAC called the p-SMAC. In this part of the synapse the two membranes are about 40 nm apart. Many signaling molecules found in synapses are localized to regions of the plasma membrane that have a lipid content different from the rest of the cell membrane and are called **lipid rafts** or glycolipid-enriched microdomains.

TCR and costimulatory receptor signaling is initiated in these rafts and induces cytoskeletal rearrangements that allow rafts to coalesce and form the immunological synapse. Immunological synapses

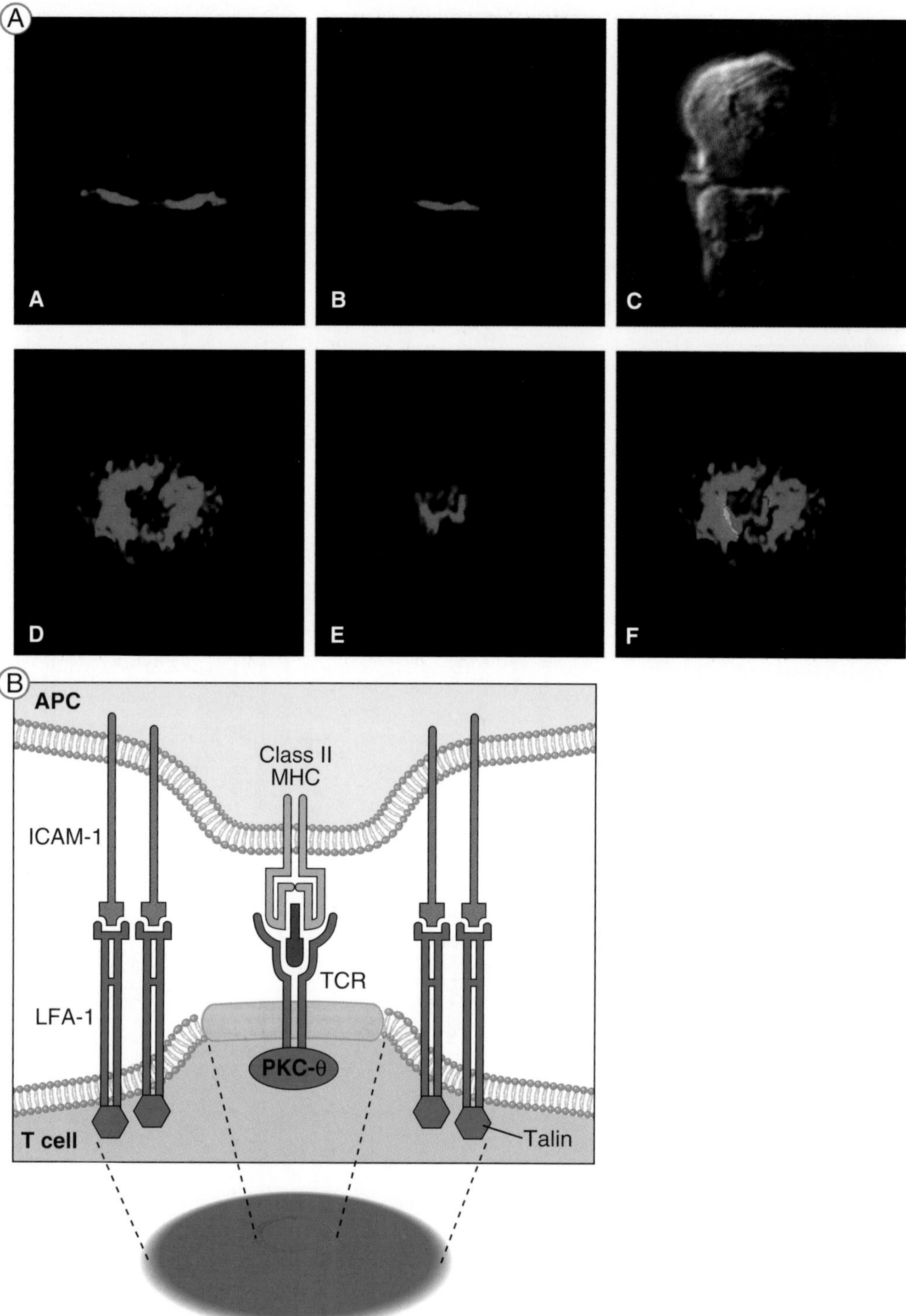

FIGURE 9-11 The immunological synapse. A, This figure shows two views of the immunological synapse in a T cell-APC conjugate (shown as a Nomarski image in panel C). Talin, a protein that associates with the cytoplasmic tail of the LFA-1 integrin was revealed by an antibody labeled with a green fluorescent dye, and PKC-θ, which associates with the TCR complex, was visualized by antibodies conjugated to a red fluorescent dye. In panels A and B, a two-dimensional optical section of the cell contact site along the *x-y* axis is shown, revealing the central location of PKC-θ, and the peripheral location of talin, both in the T cell. In panels D–F, a three-dimesional view of the entire region of cell-cell contact along the x-z axis is provided. Note, again, the central location of PKC-θ and the peripheral accumulation of talin. (Reprinted with permission from Macmillan Publishers Ltd. Monks, CRF, BA Freiburg, H Kupfer, N Sciaky, and A Kupfer. Three dimensional segregation of supramolecular activation clusters in T cells. Nature, 395:82–86, copyright 1998.) B, A schematic view of the synapse, showing talin and LFA-1 in the p-SMAC (green) and PKC-θ and the TCR in the c-SMAC (red).

may serve a number of functions during and after T cell activation:

- Although TCR signal transduction is clearly initiated before the formation of the synapse and is required for synapse formation, the immunological synapse itself may provide a unique interface for TCR triggering. T cell activation needs to overcome the problems of a generally low affinity of TCRs for peptide-MHC ligands, and the presence of few MHC molecules displaying any one peptide on an APC. The formation of the synapse overcomes these problems. The synapse represents a site at which repeated engagement of TCRs may be sustained by this small number of peptide-MHC complexes on the APC, thus facilitating prolonged and effective T cell signaling.
- The synapse may ensure the specific delivery of secretory granules and signals to appropriate APCs or targets. Vectorial delivery of secretory granules containing perforin and granzymes by CTLs to target cells has been shown to occur at the synapse. Similarly, CD40L-CD40 interactions are facilitated by the accumulation of these molecules on the T cell and APC interfaces of the immunological synapse. Some cytokines are also secreted in a directed manner into the synaptic cleft.
- The synapse may be an important site for the turnover of signaling molecules, primarily by ubiquitination and delivery to late endosomes and lysosomes. This degradation of signaling proteins may contribute to the termination of T cell activation.

Recruitment and Activation of Adapter Proteins

Activated ZAP-70 phosphorylates several adapter proteins that are able to bind signaling molecules (see Fig. 9–10). Adapter proteins serve to bring many signaling molecules into specific cellular compartments and thereby promote the activation of signal transduction pathways. Adapter proteins contain structural motifs, or domains, that bind other proteins. These domains include motifs that bind SH2 and SH3 domains, and phosphotyrosine-binding (PTB) domains, among others. Both transmembrane and cytoplasmic adapter proteins contribute to the rapid assembly of scaffolds of signaling molecules after T cells recognize antigen on APCs. A key early event in T cell activation is the ZAP-70–mediated tyrosine phosphorylation of the membrane-anchored adapter protein LAT (linker for the activation of T cells). The phosphorylated tyrosines of LAT serve as docking sites for SH2 domains of other adapter proteins and enzymes involved in several signaling cascades. LAT also contains proline-rich regions that bind SH3 domains of other proteins. Phosphorylated LAT directly binds phospholipase Cγ1, a key enzyme in T cell activation (discussed later), and coordinates the recruitment of several other adapter proteins, including SLP-76 (SH2-binding leukocyte phosphoprotein of 76 kD) and Grb-2, to the cluster of TCR and TCR-associated proteins often referred to as the signalosome. Thus, LAT serves to bring a variety of downstream components of TCR signaling pathways close to their upstream activators. Because the function of many of these adapters depends on their tyrosine phosphorylation by active ZAP-70, only antigen recognition (the physiologic stimulus for ZAP-70 activation) triggers the signal transduction pathways that lead to functional T cell responses.

MAP Kinase Signaling Pathways in T Lymphocytes

The Ras pathway is activated in T cells following TCR ligation, leading to the activation of the extracellular receptor–activated kinase (ERK), a prominent member of the mitogen-activated protein (MAP) kinase family, and eventually to the activation of downstream transcription factors. Ras is a member of a family of guanine nucleotide-binding proteins (small G proteins) that are involved in diverse activation responses in different cell types. Ras is loosely attached to the plasma membrane through covalently attached lipids. In its inactive form, the guanine nucleotide-binding site of Ras is occupied by guanosine diphosphate (GDP). When the bound GDP is replaced by guanosine triphosphate (GTP), Ras undergoes a conformational change and can then recruit or activate various cellular enzymes. Activation of Ras by GDP/GTP exchange is seen in response to the engagement of many types of receptors in many cell populations, including the TCR complex in T cells. Mutated Ras proteins that are constitutively active (i.e., they assume the GTP-bound conformation) are associated with neoplastic transformation of many cell types.

The mechanism of Ras activation in T cells involves the adapter proteins LAT and Grb-2 (Fig. 9–12). When LAT is phosphorylated by ZAP-70 at the site of TCR clustering, it serves as the docking site for the SH2 domain of Grb-2. Once attached to LAT, Grb-2 recruits to the membrane the Ras GTP/GDP exchange factor called Sos (so named because it is the mammalian homologue of a *Drosophila* protein called son of sevenless). Sos catalyzes GTP for GDP exchange on Ras. This generates the GTP-bound form of Ras (written as Ras·GTP), which then activates one member of a family of enzymes called **MAP kinases**. There are three main MAP kinases in T cells, the prototype being the enzyme called ERK. ERK activation results from Ras·GTP-induced sequential activation of two different kinases, each of which phosphorylates (and thus activates) the next enzyme in the cascade. The final enzyme prior to ERK is a dual specificity kinase that phosphorylates this MAP kinase on closely spaced threonine and tyrosine residues. The activated ERK translocates to the nucleus and phosphorylates a protein called Elk, and phosphorylated Elk stimulates transcription of Fos, a component of the activation protein-1 (AP-1) transcription factor.

In parallel with the activation of Ras through recruitment of Grb-2 and Sos, the adapters phosphorylated by TCR-associated kinases also recruit and activate a GTP/GDP exchange protein called Vav that acts on another small guanine nucleotide-binding protein called Rac. The Rac·GTP that is generated initiates a par-

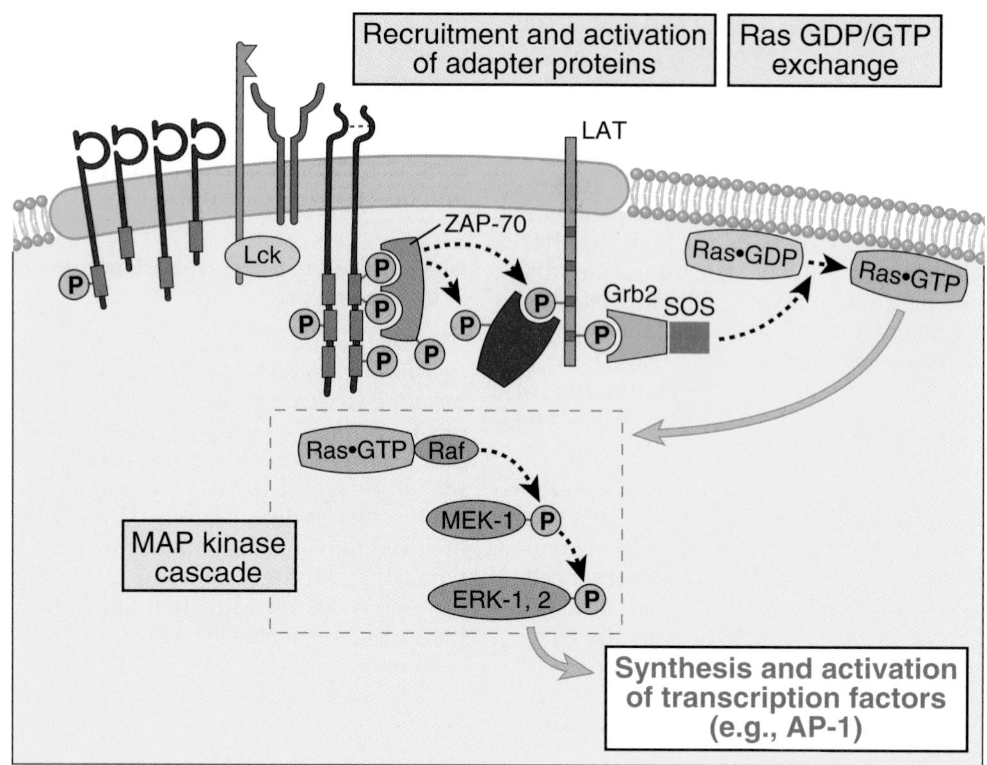

FIGURE 9–12 The Ras-MAP kinase pathway in T cell activation. ZAP-70 that is activated by antigen recognition (see Fig. 9–7) phosphorylates membrane-associated adapter proteins (such as LAT), which then bind another adapter, Grb-2, which provides a docking site for the GTP/GDP exchange factor Sos. Sos converts Ras·GDP to Ras·GTP. Ras·GTP activates a cascade of enzymes, which culminates in the activation of the MAP kinase ERK. A parallel Rac-dependent pathway generates another active MAP kinase, JNK (not shown).

allel enzyme cascade, resulting in the activation of a distinct MAP kinase called c-Jun N-terminal kinase (JNK). JNK is sometimes called stress-activated protein (SAP) kinase because in many cells it is activated by various forms of noxious stimuli such as ultraviolet light, osmotic stress, or proinflammatory cytokines such as TNF and IL-1. Activated JNK then phosphorylates c-Jun, the second component of the AP-1 transcription factor. A third member of the MAP kinase family, in addition to ERK and JNK, is p38, and it too is activated by Rac·GTP and in turn activates various transcription factors. Rac·GTP also induces cytoskeletal reorganization and may play a role in the clustering of TCR complexes, coreceptors, and other signaling molecules into the synapse. ***Thus, active G proteins induced by antigen recognition stimulate at least three different MAP kinases, which in turn activate transcription factors.***

The activities of ERK and JNK are eventually shut off by the action of dual-specificity protein tyrosine/threonine phosphatases. These phosphatases are induced or activated by ERK and JNK themselves, providing a negative feedback mechanism to terminate T cell activation.

Calcium- and PKC–Mediated Signaling Pathways in T Lymphocytes

TCR signaling leads to the activation of the γ1 isoform of the enzyme phospholipase C (PLCγ1), and the products of PLCγ1-mediated hydrolysis of membrane lipids activate enzymes that induce specific transcription factors in T cells (Fig. 9–13). PLCγ1 is a cytosolic enzyme specific for inositol phospholipids that is recruited to the plasma membrane by tyrosine phosphorylated LAT within minutes of ligand binding to the TCR. Here the enzyme is phosphorylated by ZAP-70 and by other kinases, such as the Tec family kinase called Itk (see Box 9–2). Phosphorylated PLCγ1 catalyzes the hydrolysis of a plasma membrane phospholipid called PIP_2, generating two breakdown products, inositol 1,4,5-trisphosphate (IP_3) and diacylglycerol (DAG). IP_3 and DAG then activate two distinct downstream signaling pathways in T cells.

IP_3 produces a rapid increase in cytosolic free calcium within minutes after T cell activation. IP_3 diffuses through the cytosol to the endoplasmic reticulum, where it binds to its receptor and stimulates release of membrane-sequestered calcium stores. The released calcium causes a rapid rise (during a few minutes) in the cytosolic free calcium ion concentration, from a resting level of about 100 nM to a peak of 600 to 1000 nM. The depletion of ER calcium activates a "store-operated" plasma membrane ion channel called CRAC (Calcium Release Activated Calcium) channel, which facilitates the influx of extracellular calcium. (A key component of the CRAC channel is a protein called Orai, which was discovered as a gene that is defective in a rare human immunodeficiency disease.) This CRAC channel-mediated influx of extracellular calcium allows the T cell to sustain an increase in cytosolic free calcium for more than an hour. Cytosolic free calcium acts

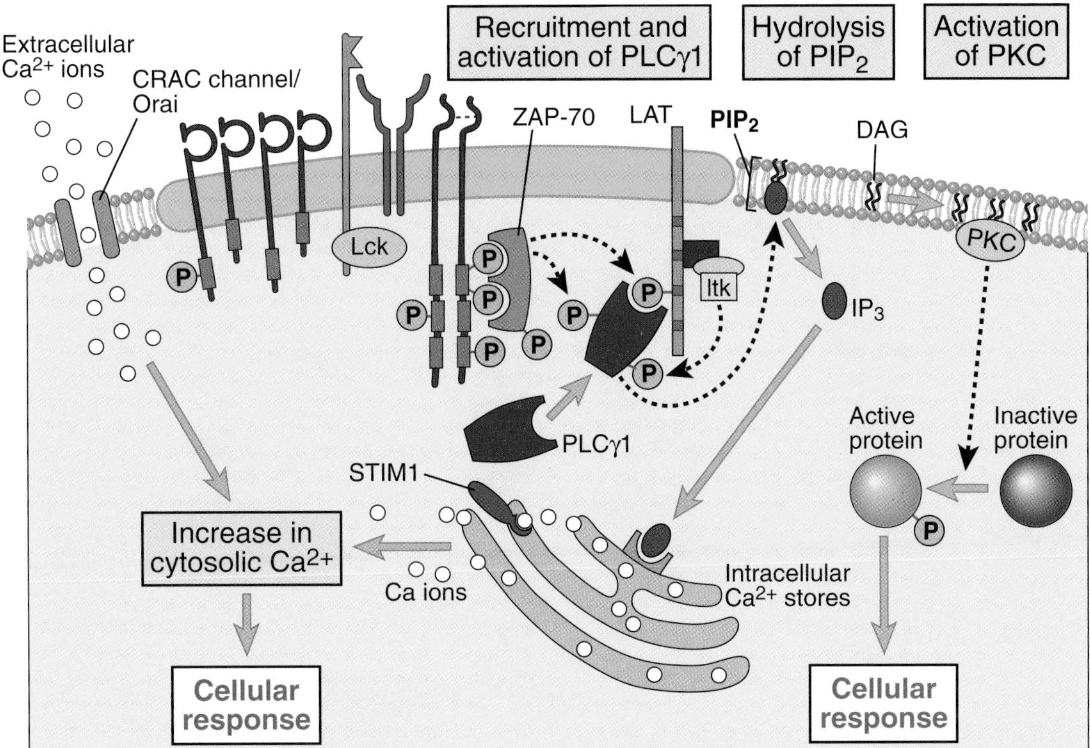

FIGURE 9–13 T cell signaling downstream of PLCγ1. The LAT adapter protein that is phosphorylated on T cell activation binds the cytosolic enzyme PLCγ1, which is phosphorylated by ZAP-70 and other kinases, such as Itk, and activated. Active PLCγ1 hydrolyzes membrane PIP_2 to generate IP_3, which stimulates an increase in cytosolic calcium, and DAG, which activates the enzyme PKC. Depletion of ER calcium is sensed by STIM1, which induces the opening of the CRAC channel that facilitates entry of extracellular calcium into the cytosol. Orai is a component of the CRAC channel. Increased cytosolic calcium and PKC then activate various transcription factors, leading to cellular responses.

as a signaling molecule by binding to a ubiquitous calcium-dependent regulatory protein called calmodulin. Calcium-calmodulin complexes activate several enzymes, including a protein serine/threonine phosphatase called **calcineurin** that is important for transcription factor activation, as discussed later.

DAG, the second breakdown product of PIP_2, activates the enzyme PKC, which has several isoforms and also participates in the generation of active transcription factors (see Fig. 9–13). DAG is hydrophobic, and it remains in the membrane where it is formed. The combination of elevated free cytosolic calcium and DAG activates certain isoforms of membrane-associated PKC by inducing a conformational change that makes the catalytic site of the kinase accessible to substrate. The PKCθ isoform localizes to the immunological synapse and is involved in the activation and nuclear translocation of the nuclear factor κB (NF-κB) transcription factor, via a trimeric protein complex made up of two proteins (called MALT1 and Bcl-10) that were identified in lymphoid tumors and a third (called CARMA1). This complex has ubiquitin ligase activity and is required for the activation of NF-κB following TCR ligation.

So far, we have described several signal transduction pathways initiated by ligand binding to the TCR that result in the activation of different types of enzymes: small G protein–MAP kinase pathways leading to activation of kinases such as ERK and JNK, a PLCγ1-calcium-dependent pathway leading to activation of the phosphatase calcineurin, and a PLCγ1–DAG-dependent pathway leading to activation of PKC (see Fig. 9–9). Each of these pathways contributes to the expression of genes encoding proteins needed for T cell clonal expansion, differentiation, and effector functions. In the following section, we describe the mechanisms by which these different signaling pathways stimulate the transcription of various genes in T cells.

Activation of Transcription Factors That Regulate T Cell Gene Expression

The enzymes generated by TCR signaling activate transcription factors that bind to regulatory regions of numerous genes in T cells and thereby enhance transcription of these genes (Fig. 9–14). Much of our understanding of the transcriptional regulation of genes in T cells is based on analyses of cytokine gene expression. The transcriptional regulation of most cytokine genes in T cells is controlled by the binding of transcription factors to nucleotide sequences in the promoter and enhancer regions of these genes. For instance, the IL-2 promoter, located 5′ of the gene, contains a segment of

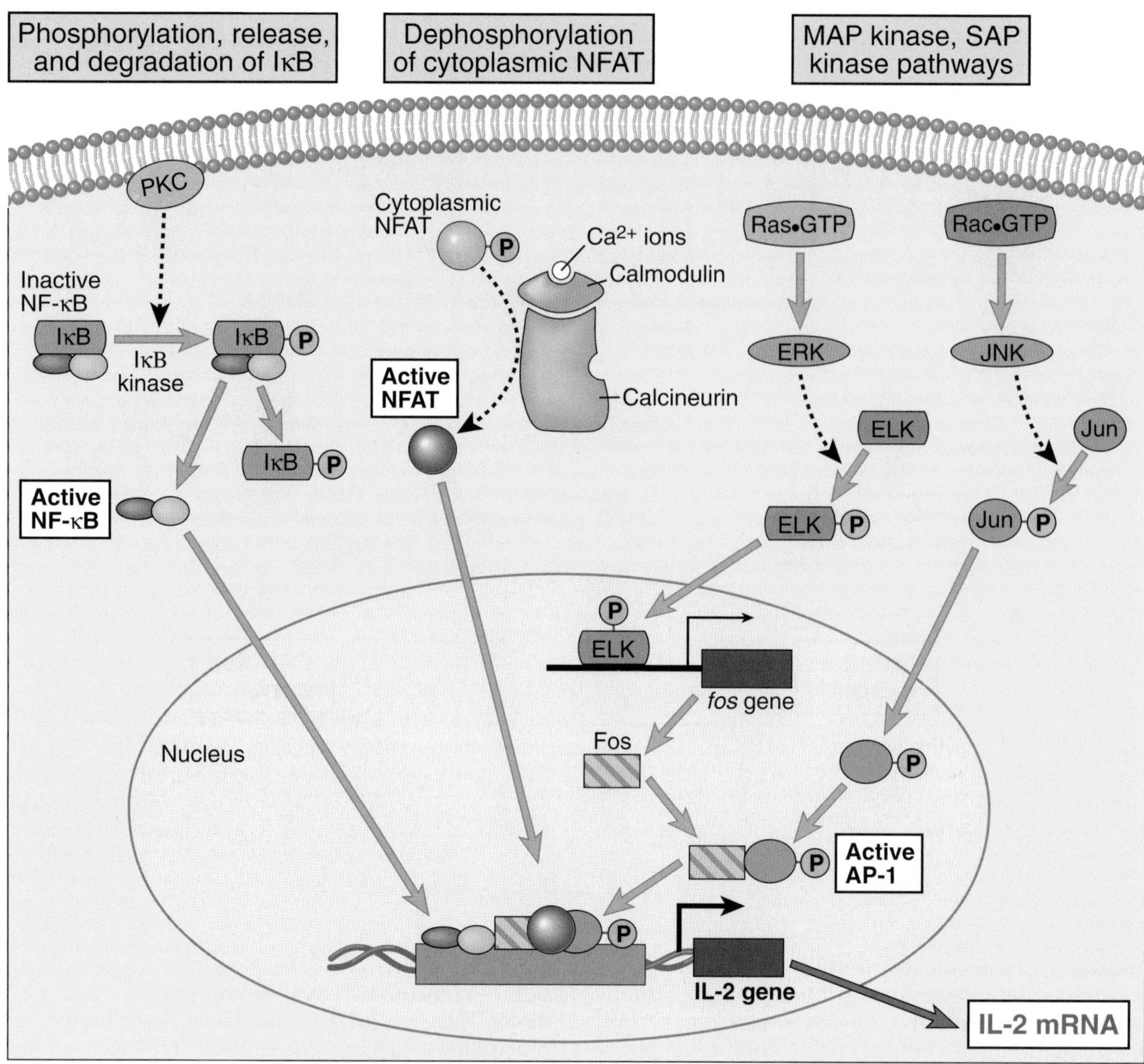

FIGURE 9–14 Activation of transcription factors in T cells. Multiple signaling pathways converge in antigen-stimulated T cells to generate transcription factors that stimulate expression of various genes (in this case, the IL-2 gene). The calcium-calmodulin pathway activates NFAT, and the Ras and Rac pathways generate the two components of AP-1. Less is known about the link between TCR signals and NF-κB activation. (NF-κB is shown as a complex of two subunits, which in T cells are typically the p50 and p65 proteins, named for their molecular sizes in kilodaltons.) PKC is important in T cell activation, and the PKCθ isoform is particularly important in activating NF-κB. These transcription factors function coordinately to regulate gene expression. Note also that the various signaling pathways are shown as activating unique transcription factors, but there may be considerable overlap, and each pathway may play a role in the activation of multiple transcription factors.

approximately 300 base pairs in which are located binding sites for several different transcription factors. All these sites must be occupied by transcription factors for maximal transcription of the IL-2 gene. Different transcription factors are activated by different cytoplasmic signal transduction pathways, and the requirement for multiple transcription factors accounts for the need to activate many signaling pathways following antigen recognition. It is likely that the same principles are true for many genes in T cells, including genes encoding cytokine receptors and effector molecules, although different genes may be responsive to different combinations of transcription factors.

Three transcription factors that are activated in T cells by antigen recognition and appear to be critical for most T cell responses are nuclear factor of activated T cells (NFAT), AP-1, and NF-κB.

NFAT is a transcription factor required for the expression of IL-2, IL-4, TNF, and other cytokine genes. There are four different NFATs, each encoded by separate genes; NFAT1 and NFAT2 are the types found in T cells. NFAT is present in an inactive, serine phosphorylated form in the cytoplasm of resting T lymphocytes. It is activated by the calcium-calmodulin–dependent phosphatase calcineurin. Calcineurin dephosphorylates cytoplasmic NFAT, thereby uncovering a nuclear localization signal that permits NFAT to translocate into the nucleus. Once in the nucleus, NFAT binds to the regulatory regions of IL-2, IL-4, and other cytokine genes, usually in association with other transcription factors, such as AP-1.

The mechanism of activation of NFAT was discovered indirectly by studies of the mechanism of action of the immunosuppressive drugs cyclosporin A and FK-506 (see Chapter 16). These drugs, which are natural products of fungi, are the main therapeutic agents used to prevent allograft rejection, and they function largely by blocking T cell cytokine gene transcription. Cyclosporin A binds to a cytosolic protein called cyclophilin, and FK-506 binds to a structurally homologous protein called FK-506-binding protein (FKBP). Cyclophilin and FKBP are also called immunophilins. Cyclosporin A-cyclophilin complexes and FK-506–FKBP complexes bind to and inhibit calcineurin, and thereby block translocation of NFAT into the nucleus.

AP-1 is a transcription factor found in many cell types; it is specifically activated in T lymphocytes by TCR-mediated signals. AP-1 is actually the name for a family of DNA-binding factors composed of dimers of two proteins that bind to one another through a shared structural motif called a leucine zipper. The best characterized AP-1 factor is composed of the proteins Fos and Jun. TCR-induced signals lead to the appearance of active AP-1 in the nucleus of T cells. Activation of AP-1 typically involves synthesis of the Fos protein and phosphorylation of preexisting Jun protein. Transcription and synthesis of Fos can be enhanced by the ERK pathway, as described before, and also by PKC. JNK phosphorylates c-Jun, and AP-1 complexes containing the phosphorylated form of Jun have increased transcription enhancing activity. AP-1 appears to physically associate with other transcription factors in the nucleus, including NFAT, and works best in combination with NFAT. Thus, AP-1 activation represents a convergence point of several TCR-initiated signaling pathways.

NF-κB is a transcription factor that is activated in response to TCR signals and is essential for cytokine synthesis. NF-κB proteins are homodimers or heterodimers of proteins that are homologous to the product of a cellular proto-oncogene called c-*rel* and are important in the transcription of many genes in diverse cell types, particularly in cells of innate immunity (see Chapter 2). In resting T cells, NF-κB is present in the cytoplasm in a complex with other proteins called inhibitors of κB (IκBs), which block the entry of NF-κB into the nucleus. TCR signals lead to serine phosphorylation of IκB, and then its ubiquitination and proteasomal degradation. The enzymes responsible for phosphorylation of IκB are called IκB kinases.

The links between different signaling proteins, activation of transcription factors, and functional responses of T cells are often difficult to establish because there are complex and incompletely understood interactions between signaling pathways. Also, we have focused on selected pathways to illustrate how antigen recognition may lead to biochemical alterations, but it is clear that many other signaling molecules are also involved in antigen-induced lymphocyte activation.

Biochemistry of Costimulation

Costimulatory signals delivered by receptors, such as CD28 cooperate with TCR signals to augment the activation of transcription factors. CD28 engagement leads to the activation of a myriad of signaling pathways. The cytoplasmic tail of CD28 includes a tyrosine-containing motif that, following tyrosine phosphorylation, can recruit the regulatory subunit of PI-3 kinase. It also contains two proline-rich motifs, one of which can bind the Tec kinase Itk (functionally similar to Btk in the B lineage), and the other binds to the Src family kinase, Lck. Mutation of the Lck binding motif abrogates the ability of CD28 to induce IL-2 gene expression.

CD28 clustering induced by antibodies or by binding to B7 costimulators can activate PI-3 kinase and facilitate the activation of the Ras/ERK MAP kinase pathway as well as activation of the Akt kinase. PI-3 kinase, as discussed earlier, creates PIP_3 moieties on the inner leaflet of the plasma membrane that can contribute to the recruitment and activation of the Itk tyrosine kinase, the phospholipase PLCγ, and another pleckstrin homology domain containing kinase called PDK1. PDK1 can phosphorylate and activate Akt. Akt in turn phosphorylates a number of targets, inactivating pro-apoptotic proteins and activating anti-apoptotic factors, thus contributing to cell survival. CD28 also provides an independent pathway for the activation of the Vav exchange factor and the subsequent activation of the Rac/JNK pathway. In some cultured T cell lines, CD28 signals have been shown to induce NF-κB binding to a site in the IL-2 gene promoter, called the CD28 response element, that is not activated by TCR-mediated signals. All these pathways promote T cell survival, cytokine production, and proliferation. CD28 may also block inhibitory signals in T cells (discussed below).

T Cell Signal Attenuation: Roles of Inhibitory Receptors and Ubiquitin Ligases

Inhibitory signaling in T cells is mediated by a number of mechanisms including the recruitment of tyrosine phosphatases such as SHP-1 (see Box 9–3), the activation of inhibitory receptors of the CD28 family, and the recruitment of proteins known as E3 ubiquitin ligases that mark certain signaling molecules for degradation. The functional responses of all cells are regulated by a balance being stimulatory and inhibitory signals, and T cells are no exception. Below we discuss the main features of selected inhibitory receptors and ubiquitination pathways in T cells.

Inhibitory receptors of the CD28 family

We have mentioned the prototypical inhibitory receptor of the CD28 family, **CTLA-4** (also called CD152) previously, in the discussion of costimulation. The ability of CTLA-4 to inhibit T cell responses was discovered by studies looking at the effects of anti-CTLA-4 antibodies on in vitro responses. Several types of results have clearly established the role of this receptor in controlling T cell responses to self and foreign antigens.

- Mice in which the CTLA-4 gene is knocked out develop severe systemic inflammatory reactions against multiple tissues with massive accumulation of activated lymphocytes in lymphoid organs. This result was the first to clearly show that CTLA-4 is involved in the maintenance of unresponsiveness (tolerance) to self antigens (see Chapter 11).

- A polymorphism in the *CTLA4* gene that interferes with the production of a splice variant is associated with some human autoimmune diseases, suggesting that this receptor functions to inhibit T cell responses to self antigens in humans, as well.
- Antibodies that block CTLA-4 enhance T cell responses to tumors, indicating that this pathway limits anti-tumor immunity. This finding has been exploited to develop anti-CTLA-4 antibody as a mode of tumor immunotherapy; clinical trials of the antibody combined with tumor vaccines are ongoing.

Very little is known about the biochemical mechanisms by which CTLA-4 inhibits T cell activation. The majority of cell-associated CTLA-4 is normally in intracellular vesicles, and it is rapidly recruited to the immune synapse at the time of T cell activation. Here, CTLA-4 may either competitively inhibit the ability of CD28 to bind to B7 molecules, or CTLA-4 may recruit a phosphatase (SHP-2) to the synapse and thus block the normal phosphorylation of TCR-associated ζ chains (Fig. 9–15). Whether a T cell uses CD28 or CTLA-4 to bind to B7 molecules on APCs is a key determinant of the outcome of antigen recognition, but how this choice is made is not known. One possibility is that because CTLA-4 binds to B7-1 and B7-2 with ~50-fold higher affinity than does CD28, APCs with low expression of B7 may preferentially engage CTLA-4. Thus, normal resting APCs, which may be displaying self antigens but express little B7, engage CTLA-4 and induce tolerance in self-reactive T cells. Infections up-regulate B7 expression, leading to engagement of CD28 and T cell activation. It is also known that naive T cells express CD28, but CTLA-4 expression requires T cell activation. Therefore, naive T cells may use CD28 to initiate responses, but at later times, more CTLA-4 may be expressed, and its binding to B7 molecules may function to terminate the responses.

The other inhibitory receptor of the CD28 family that is of growing interest in T cells is **PD-1**. It is induced on T cells, B cells, and monocytes upon activation of the cells. PD-1 has two ligands PD-L1 and PD-L2, which are homologous to B7-1 and B7-2, and are induced on activated dendritic cells, monocytes, and many other cell types. The importance of PD-1 has also been established by several types of evidence.

- Mice in which the PD-1 gene is knocked out develop either autoimmune cardiomyopathy or a lupus-like syndrome, depending on the mouse strain, establishing the role of PD-1 in self-tolerance.
- In one form of a chronic viral infection in mice, virus-specific T cells become functionally paralyzed and they can be rescued by blocking PD-1. This result suggests that the virus has "learned" to use a normal regulatory pathway to evade host immunity. In humans, part of the immune deficiency associated with HIV infection may also be because of PD-1-mediated inhibition of T cell activation.

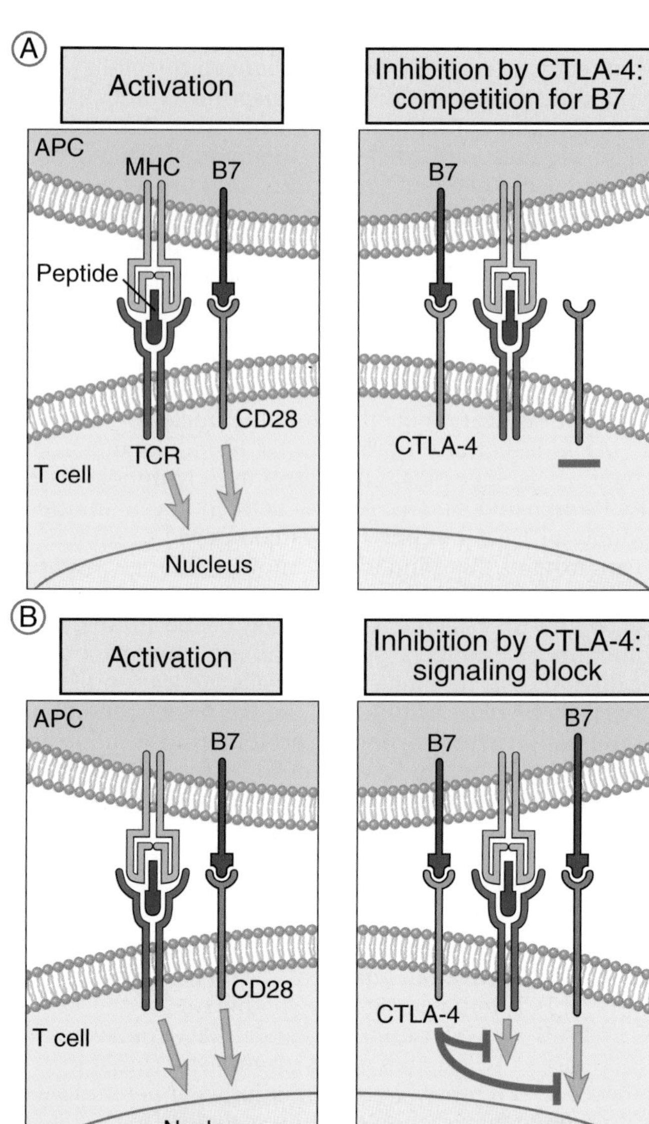

FIGURE 9–15 Mechanisms of action of the inhibitory receptor CTLA-4. CTLA-4 may inhibit T cell responses by competitively preventing CD28 binding to B7 costimulators (A), or by generating inhibitory signals (e.g. by associated phosphatases) that attenuate activation via the TCR and CD28 (B).

The cytoplasmic tail of PD-1 contains inhibitory tyrosine based motifs, including an ITIM (immunoreceptor tyrosine based inhibitory motif) and an ITSM (immunoreceptor tyrosine based switch motif) that may both contribute to the recruitment of tyrosine phosphatases such as SHP-1 and SHP-2 that can attenuate T cell signaling.

Ubiquitin-dependent degradation of signaling proteins

Ubiquitin moieties attached to proteins mark them for degradation, but in some cases this modification can also enhance signaling without targeting proteins for degradation (Box 9–3). Ubiquitin E3 ligases are

Box 9–3 ▪ IN DEPTH: UBIQUITINATION IN PROTEIN DEGRADATION AND SIGNALING

Approximately 10% of all the proteins in a cell are involved in the identification of other proteins, marking proteins for poteolytic destruction. One of the major ways of degrading cytosolic and nuclear proteins involves the covalent attachment of ubiquitin residues to these proteins. Although ubiquitination of proteins is frequently linked to the degradation of these proteins in proteasomes, proteins can be ubiquitinated in a number of ways, each form of ubiquitination serving a very different function.

Ubiquitination was briefly discussed in Chapter 6 in the context of Class I MHC based antigen processing and presentation. Ubiquitin is a 76 amino acid protein that is activated in an ATP dependent fashion by an E1 enzyme, is then "carried" by an E2 enzyme and transferred to lysine residues on specific substrates recognized by specific E3 ubiquitin ligases (see Figure). E3 ligases are enzymes that simultaneously recognize an E2 enzyme poised to conjugate ubiquitin and a specific protein substrate that can then be ubiquitinated by the E2 now brought in close proximity to its target. In most cases a poly-ubiquitin chain is added, but for some functions only a single ubiquitin moiety need be attached to a protein target.

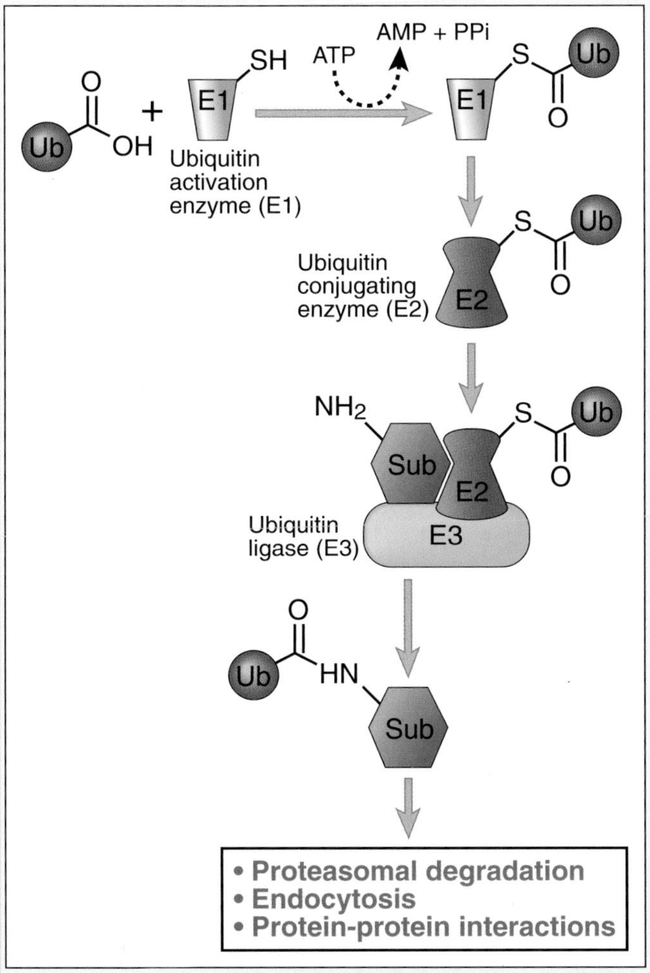

E3 ubiquitin ligases attenuate T cell signaling. The C terminus of ubiquitin is activated by a ubiquitin-activating enzyme (E1) which forms a thioester linkage to ubiquitin in an ATP-dependent manner. The activating ubiquitin is transferred to a ubiquitin-conjugating enzyme (E2), to which it is also attached by a thioester linkage. The E2 is assisted by an E3 ubiquitin ligase in identifying specific target proteins (substrates). Ubiquitin is covalently attached to a lysine residue on the substrate (sub).

PATHWAYS OF UBIQUITINATION. Although the process of ubiquitination was discovered as a mechanism for degrading cellular proteins, it is now clear that it serves different functions. In fact, attachment of ubiquitin moieties to different residues on an attached ubiquitin induces quite distinct functional outcomes.

Proteasomal Degradation and K48 Polyubiquitination. After the C-terminus of a ubiquitin moiety is covalently linked to a lysine residue on a target protein, the C-terminal ends of subsequent ubiquitin moieties may be covalently attached to lysine residues on the preceding ubiquitin in order to generate a poly-ubiquitin chain. There are two major types of poly-ubiquitin chains, which mediate very different cellular functions. In one type of poly-ubiquitination, the second and subsequent ubiquitins in the chain are each covalently linked to lysine 48 (K48) on the preceding ubiquitin in the chain. Once at least four ubiquitins, attached to one another via K48 ubiquitination, are serially linked to a protein, this marked protein may be recognized by the 19S cap of the proteasome and is degraded in the proteasome. The substrate is cleaved into peptides and the ubiquitin is recycled. A second type of poly-ubiqitination that has a distinct function is discussed below.

Cell Signaling and K63 Ubiquitination. A distinct type of poly-ubiquitin chain is attached by certain E2 enzymes and their partner E3 ligases. In this type of chain the C-terminus of the second and subsequent ubiquitin moieties are attached to preceding ubiquitins in the chain via lysine 63 (K63) of ubiquitin. Such a ubiquitin chain modifies the target protein and thus alters its ability to associate with other proteins without marking the target protein for destruction. The NEMO or IKKγ subunit of the IκB kinase, for instance, must be poly-ubiquitinated in a K63 manner in order for the IκB kinase to be able to phosphorylate its target protein, IκBα (inhibitor of NFκB). Certain TRAF proteins, such as those downstream of Toll Like Receptors, are ubiquitin E3 ligases that facilitate K63 poly-ubiquitination of NEMO/IKKγ and thus facilitate NFκB activation. It should be noted that while the IκB kinase complex needs to have K63 ubiquitin chains attached to NEMO in order for the complex to be active and phosphorylate IκBα, in contrast, in order to permit NFκB to enter the nucleus, IκBα itself must undergo K48 poly-ubiquitination so that it may be degraded in the proteasome.

Continued on following page

Box 9–3 ■ IN DEPTH: UBIQUITINATION IN PROTEIN DEGRADATION AND SIGNALING (Continued)

Mono-ubiquitination for Endocytosis and Lysosomal Degradation. Mono-ubiquitination of intracellular domains of receptors can contribute to endocytosis and lysosomal degradation. An E3 ligase called Cbl-b (discussed in the text) facilitates the mono-ubiqitination of ZAP70 and of the cytosolic domains of CD3 proteins, thus targeting the activated TCR-CD3 complex and associated ZAP-70 for lysosomal degradation.

UBIQUITIN E3 LIGASES AND THE ATTENUATION OF T CELL SIGNALING. E3 proteins are very important components of the cellular machinery that attenuates T cell signaling. Two important types of E3 ligases are found in T cells defined by the presence of either a RING finger or of a HECT domain. RING finger containing E3 ligases such as Cbl-b, c-Cbl, and GRAIL, and HECT-family ubiquitin ligases, such as Itch and Nedd4, may all contribute to the attenuation of T cell signaling. In addition specific E3 ligases contribute to a number of signaling events during lymphocyte development, lymphocyte activation, and the induction of tolerance.

As discussed in the text Cbl-b and c-Cbl can contribute to the monoubiquitination, endocytosis, and lysosomal degradation of the T cell receptor complex, and this may be a major mechanism for the attenuation of TCR signaling and the induction of T cell anergy (see Chapter 11). The HECT family E3 ligases, Nedd4 and Itch, may ubiquitinate signaling molecules downstream of the TCR such as activated PLC-γ and PCK-θ, and target these proteins for lysosomal degradation as well. These HECT family proteins therefore collaborate with RING finger proteins such as Cbl-b and c-Cbl to degrade signaling components and maintain the anergic state.

enzymes that attach ubiquitin moieties to specific target proteins. In T cells, several E3 ligases are believed to mediate the targeted degradation of specific signaling molecules, and these E3 proteins are therefore important components of the cellular machinery that attenuates T cell signaling (Fig. 9–16). The prototype of these ligases is Cbl-b, but several others are involved in terminating T cell responses. Proteins are often marked for ubiquitination and degradation by specific phosphorylation events. When the LAT and the SLP-76

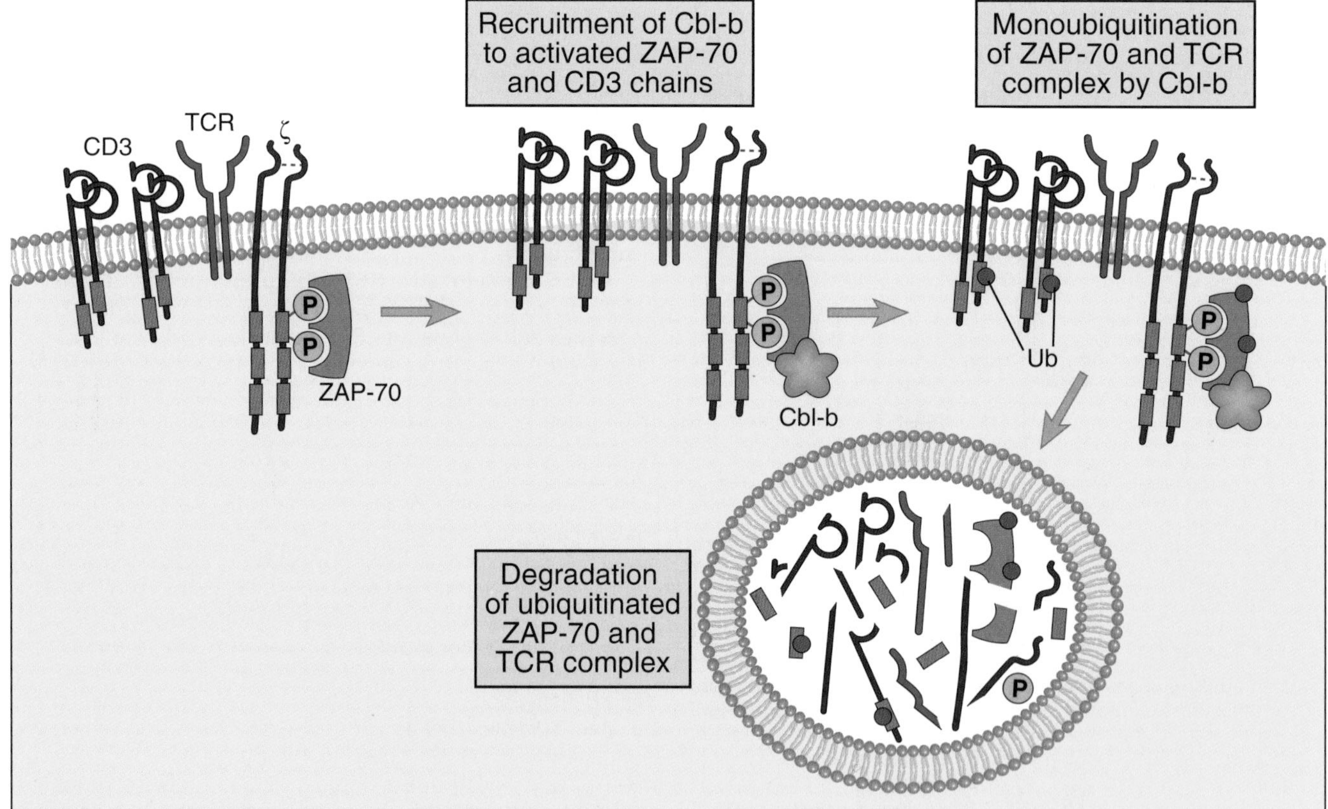

FIGURE 9–16 Role of the ubiquitin ligase Cbl-b in terminating T cell responses. Cbl-b is recruited to the TCR complex, where it facilitates the monoubiquitination of CD3, ZAP-70, and other proteins of the TCR complex. These proteins are targeted for proteolytic degradation in lysosomes and other organelles (not shown).

adapters are tyrosine phosphorylated and recruited to the T cell receptor signalosome, the Cbl-b E3 ligase may be recruited to the complex as well. Recruitment of Cbl-b leads to the monoubiquitination, endocytosis, and lysosomal degradation of the T cell receptor complex, and this may be a major mechanism for the attenuation of TCR signaling. CD28 signals, through activation of Vav and the Rac pathway, block the inhibitory activity of Cbl-b and thus augment TCR signals. In knockout mice lacking Cbl-b, the T cells respond to antigen even without CD28-mediated costimulation and produce abnormally high amounts of IL-2. These mice develop autoimmunity as a result of hyperactivation of their T cells.

SUMMARY

- T cell responses are initiated by signals that are generated by the association of TCR complexes with specific peptide-MHC protein complexes on the surface of an APC and through signals provided by costimulators expressed on APCs.

- T cell responses to antigen and costimulators include synthesis of cytokines and effector molecules, cellular proliferation, differentiation into effector and memory cells, and performance of effector functions.

- Naive T cells of the CD4+ subset proliferate and differentiate into effector cells that mediate cell-mediated immune responses and can also facilitate B cell activation in response to protein antigens.

- Naive T cells of the CD8+ subset proliferate and differentiate into effector cells that can kill infected targets and these effectors are known as cytotoxic T lymphocytes (CTLs).

- The best defined costimulators for T cells are the B7 proteins, which are recognized by CD28 on T cells. B7 molecules are expressed on professional APCs, and their expression is enhanced by microbes and by cytokines produced during innate immune reactions to microbes. The requirement for costimulation, especially for activation of naive T cells, ensures that T cell responses are induced in lymphoid organs, where professional APCs are concentrated, and against microbes and microbial products, which stimulate expression of costimulators on the APCs.

- Signaling molecules in T cell plasma membranes accumulate in specialized membrane microdomains known as lipid rafts. T cell activation via the TCR-coreceptor complex and through costimulatory receptors initially occurs in lipid rafts. During T cell activation, cytoskeletal reorganization results in a polarized cell, and the rafts coalesce to form tight interfaces with APCs. Each of these junctions is known as an immunological synapse. The synapses represent sites of ongoing signals and provide interfaces that ensure the specificity of T cell-APC communication.

- Ligation of TCRs by peptide-MHC complexes triggers intracellular signaling pathways that result in the production of transcription factors, which activate a variety of genes in T cells. Intracellular signaling may be divided into membrane events, cytoplasmic signaling pathways, and nuclear transcription of genes. Membrane events include the recruitment and activation of Src family protein tyrosine kinases closely associated with the TCR, the phosphorylation of TCR complex constituents (e.g., the ζ chains), and the recruitment of protein tyrosine kinases, especially ZAP-70, and adapter proteins. Cytoplasmic signaling pathways lead to the activation of effector enzymes, such as the kinases ERK, JNK, and PKC, and the phosphatase calcineurin. These enzymes contribute to the activation of transcription factors such as NFAT, AP-1, and NF-κB, which function to enhance gene expression in antigen-stimulated T cells.

- Signaling in T cells may be attenuated by a number of phosphatases, inhibitory receptors, and E3 ubiquitin ligases.

Selected Readings

Acuto O, VD Bartolo, and F Michel. Tailoring T-cell receptor signals by proximal negative feedback mechanisms. Nature Reviews Immunology 8:699–712, 2008.

Burkhardt JK, E Carrizosa, and MH Shaffer. The actin cytoskeleton in T cell activation. Annual Review of Immunology 26:233–259, 2008.

Call ME, and KW Wucherpfennig. The T cell receptor: critical role of the membrane environment in receptor assembly and function. Annual Review of Immunology 23:101–125, 2005.

Chen L. Co-inhibitory molecules of the B7-CD28 family in the control of T-cell immunity. Nature Reviews Immunology 4:336–347, 2004.

Croft M. Co-stimulatory members of the TNFR family: keys to effective T cell immunity? Nature Reviews Immunology 3:609–620, 2003.

Davis DM, and ML Dustin. What is the importance of the immunological synapse? Trends in Immunology 25:323–327, 2004.

Davis SJ, and PA van der Merwe. The kinetic-segregation model: TCR triggering and beyond. Nature Immunology 7:803–809, 2006.

Dustin ML. A dynamic view of the immunological synapse. Seminars in Immunology 17:400–410, 2005.

Gallo EM, K Cante-Barrett, and GR Crabtree. Lymphocyte calcium signaling from membrane to nucleus. Nature Immunology 7:25–32, 2006.

Greenwald RJ, GJ Freeman, and AH Sharpe. The B7 family revisited. Annual Review of Immunology 23:515–548, 2005.

Huse M, EJ Quann, and MM Davis. Shouts, whispers and the kiss of death: directional secretion in T cells. Nature Immunology 9:1105–1111, 2008.

Kuhns MS, MM Davis, and KC Garcia. Deconstructing the form and function of the TCR/CD3 complex. Immunity 24:133–139, 2006.

Oh-hora M, and A Rao. Calcium signaling in lymphocytes. Current Opinion in Immunology 20:250–258, 2008.

Pao LI, K Badour, KA Siminovitch, and BG Neel. Nonreceptor protein-tyrosine phosphatases in immune cell signaling. Annual Review of Immunology 25:473–523, 2007.

Rudolph MG, RL Stanfield, and IA Wilson. How TCRs bind MHCs, petides, and coreceptors. Annual Review of Immunology 24:419–466, 2006.

Samelson LE. Signal transduction mediated by the T cell antigen receptor: the role of adapter proteins. Annual Reviews of Immunology 20:371–394, 2002.

Sun SC. Deubiquitylation and regulation of the immune response. Nature Reviews Immunology 8:501–511, 2008.

Watts TH. TNF/TNFR family members in costimulation of T cell responses. Annual Review of Immunology 23:23–68, 2005.

Weil R and A Israel. Deciphering the pathway from the TCR to NF-Kappa B. Cell Death and Differentiation 13:826–833, 2006.

Chapter 10

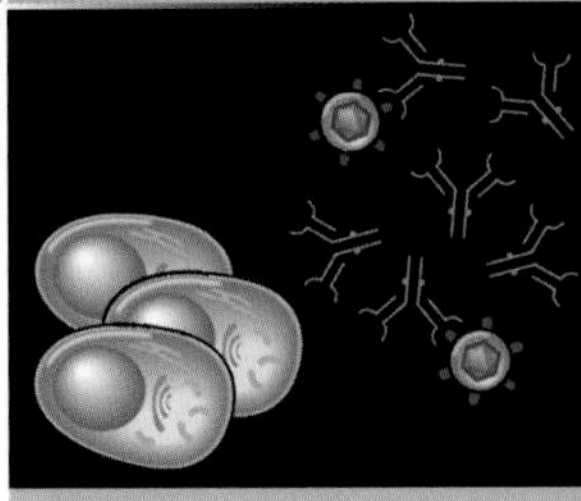

B CELL ACTIVATION AND ANTIBODY PRODUCTION

Humoral immunity is mediated by secreted antibodies, which are produced by cells of the B lymphocyte lineage. Antibodies bind to the antigens of extracellular microbes and function to neutralize and eliminate these microbes. The elimination of different types of microbes requires several effector mechanisms, which are mediated by distinct classes, or isotypes, of antibodies. This chapter describes the molecular and cellular events of the humoral immune response, in particular the stimuli that induce B cell proliferation and differentiation and how these stimuli influence the type of antibody that is produced.

General Features of Humoral Immune Responses

The earliest studies of adaptive immunity were devoted to analyses of serum antibodies produced in response to microbes, toxins, and model antigens. Much of our current understanding of adaptive immune responses and the cellular interactions that take place during such responses has evolved from studies of antibody production. The type and amount of antibodies produced vary according to the type of antigen, involvement of T cells, prior history of antigen exposure, and anatomic site.

- ***The process of activation of B cells and generation of antibody-producing cells consists of sequential phases*** (Fig. 10–1). As we discussed in Chapter 8, mature antigen-responsive B lymphocytes develop from bone marrow precursors before antigenic stimulation and populate peripheral lymphoid tissues, which are the sites of interaction with foreign antigens. Humoral immune responses are initiated by the recognition of antigens by B lymphocytes specific for each antigen. Antigen binds to membrane immunoglobulin M (IgM) and IgD antigen receptors on naive B cells and activates these cells. B cell activation may occur in a T cell-dependent or T cell-

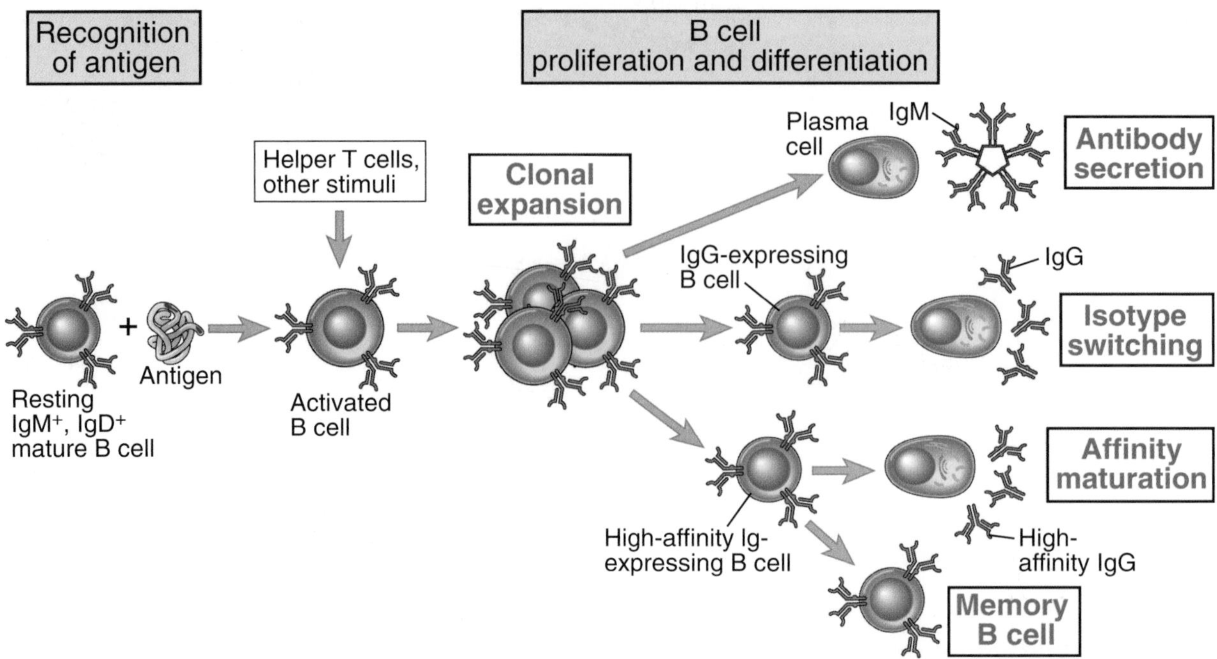

FIGURE 10–1 Phases of the humoral immune response. The activation of B cells is initiated by specific recognition of antigens by the surface Ig receptors of the cells. Antigen and other stimuli, including helper T cells, stimulate the proliferation and differentiation of the specific B cell clone. Progeny of the clone may produce IgM or other Ig isotypes (e.g., IgG), may undergo affinity maturation, or may persist as memory cells.

independent manner, as discussed below. Activation can lead to **proliferation,** resulting in expansion of the clone of antigen-specific cells, and **differentiation,** resulting in the generation of plasma cells that actively secrete antibodies and also of memory B cells. Some activated B cells begin to produce antibodies other than IgM and IgD; this process is called heavy chain isotype (class) switching. Activated B cells that produce antibodies that bind to antigens with much higher affinity are selected and preferentially expanded; this process is called affinity maturation. A single B cell may, within a week, give rise to approximately 4000 antibody-secreting cells, which produce greater than 10^{12} antibody molecules per day. This prodigious expansion is needed to keep pace with rapidly dividing microbes.

- ***Antibody responses to protein antigens require CD4⁺ helper T lymphocytes that recognize the antigen and play an essential role in activating B lymphocytes.*** For this reason, proteins are classified as thymus-dependent or T-dependent antigens. The term *helper* T lymphocyte arose from the realization that these cells stimulate, or help, B lymphocytes to produce antibodies.
- ***Antibody responses to multivalent antigens with repeating determinants, such as polysaccharides and lipids, do not require antigen-specific helper T lymphocytes.*** Therefore, polysaccharide and lipid antigens are called thymus-independent or T-independent (TI) antigens.
- ***Activated B cells differentiate into antibody-secreting plasma cells, some of which continue to produce antibodies for long periods, and into long-lived memory cells.*** Humoral immune responses are initiated in peripheral lymphoid organs, such as the spleen for blood-borne antigens, draining lymph nodes for antigens entering through the skin and other epithelia, and mucosal lymphoid tissues for some inhaled and ingested antigens. Antibodies enter the circulation or are transported into the lumens of mucosal organs and mediate their protective effects wherever antigens are present. Some plasma cells migrate from the peripheral lymphoid organs to the bone marrow, where they live for many years and produce low levels of antibodies that provide immediate protection whenever a microbe recognized by those antibodies infects the individual. Some progeny of activated B cells may differentiate into memory cells, which mount rapid responses to subsequent encounters with the antigen.
- ***Heavy chain isotype switching and affinity maturation are typically seen in helper T cell–dependent humoral immune responses to protein antigens.*** As we shall discuss later, isotype switching is stimulated by helper T cell signals, including the membrane molecule CD40 ligand and cytokines, and affinity maturation is also dependent on the activation of B cells by T cells. Affinity maturation involves the generation of somatic mutation at a high frequency in rearranged Ig V genes and the subsequent selection of B cells with a high affinity for the original antigen. The nature of the humoral immune response also varies at distinct anatomic sites. For instance, mucosal lymphoid tissues are uniquely adapted to produce high levels of

IgA in response to the same antigens that stimulate other antibody isotypes in nonmucosal lymphoid tissues.

- ***Primary and secondary antibody responses to protein antigens differ qualitatively and quantitatively*** (Fig. 10–2). Primary responses result from the activation of previously unstimulated naive B cells, whereas secondary responses are due to stimulation of expanded clones of memory B cells. Therefore, the secondary response develops more rapidly than does the primary response, and larger amounts of antibodies are produced in the secondary response (see Fig. 10–2). Heavy chain isotype switching and affinity

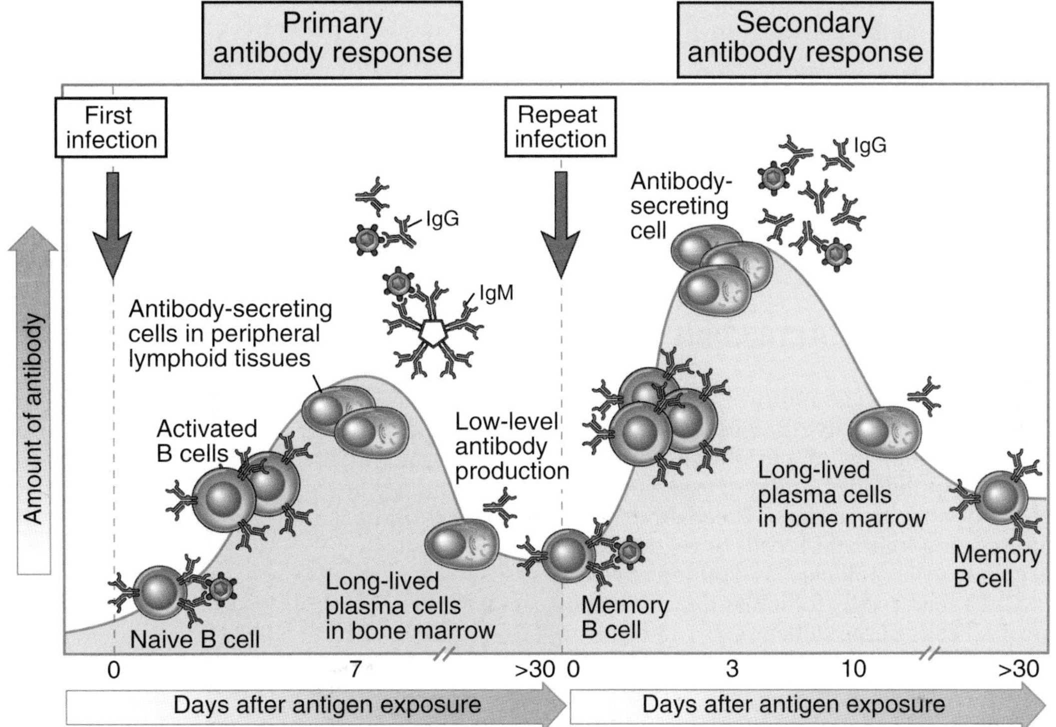

Feature	Primary response	Secondary response
Time lag after immunization	Usually 5–10 days	Usually 1–3 days
Peak response	Smaller	Larger
Antibody isotype	Usually IgM > IgG	Relative increase in IgG and, under certain situations, in IgA or IgE
Antibody affinity	Lower average affinity, more variable	Higher average affinity (affinity maturation)
Induced by	All immunogens	Only protein antigens
Required immunization	Relatively high doses of antigens, optimally with adjuvants (for protein antigens)	Low doses of antigens; adjuvants may not be necessary

FIGURE 10–2 Primary and secondary humoral immune responses. In a primary immune response, naive B cells are stimulated by antigen, become activated, and differentiate into antibody-secreting cells that produce antibodies specific for the eliciting antigen. Some of the antibody-secreting plasma cells survive in the bone marrow and continue to produce antibodies for long periods. Long-lived memory B cells are also generated during the primary response. A secondary immune response is elicited when the same antigen stimulates these memory B cells, leading to more rapid proliferation and differentiation and production of greater quantities of specific antibody than are produced in the primary response. The principal characteristics of primary and secondary antibody responses are summarized in the Table. These features are typical of T cell-dependent antibody responses to protein antigens.

maturation also increase with repeated exposures to protein antigens.

- *Distinct subsets of B cells respond preferentially to different types of antigens.* Follicular B cells in peripheral lymphoid organs make antibody responses to protein antigens, which require collaboration with helper T cells. Marginal zone B cells in the spleen and other lymphoid tissues recognize multivalent atigens, such as blood-borne polysaccharides, and mount T cell-independent antibody responses. B-1 B cells also primarily mediate T cell-independent responses, but in mucosal tissues and the peritoneum.

In the following sections, we first describe how antigens initiate the process of B cell activation. We then discuss the role of helper T cells in B cell responses to protein antigens and the mechanisms of isotype switching and affinity maturation. We will describe TI antibody responses at the end of the chapter.

Antigen Recognition and Antigen-Induced B Cell Activation

The activation of B lymphocytes requires antigen recognition in lymphoid tissues. Naive B cells reside in and circulate through the follicles of peripheral lymphoid organs (the spleen, lymph nodes, and mucosal lymphoid tissues) in search of cognate antigen. B cells that enter follicles are often called follicular B cells or recirculating B cells. Entry into the follicles is guided by the chemokine CXCL13 secreted by follicular dendritic cells (FDCs) and stromal cells in the follicle. CXCL13 binds to the CXCR5 chemokine receptor on recirculating B cells, and attracts these cells into the follicles. The same chemokine–receptor pair is also important during immune responses since it can attract activated T cells to the follicle. Naive follicular B cells survive for limited periods until they encounter antigen (see Chapter 3). Follicular B cell survival may depend on signals derived from the B cell receptor (BCR) as well as on inputs received from a tumor necrosis factor (TNF) family cytokine called BAFF (B cell activating factor of the TNF family; also known as BLyS, for B lymphocyte stimulator), which provides maturation and survival signals via the BAFF receptor. BAFF, and a related ligand, APRIL, can also activate two other receptors, TACI and BCMA, which participate in later stages of B cell activation and differentiation (and will be discussed later in this chapter). These cytokines are produced mainly by myeloid cells in the follicle and the bone marrow.

Antigens enter secondary lymphoid organs through the blood or lymph, often following capture by dendritic cells (DCs), and bind to the antigen receptors on specific B cells. DCs can internalize antigen for presentation to T cells, but can also separately recycle antigen to the cell surface in an intact form where it can be made available to antigen-specific B cells. Soluble antigen may also enter follicles and be recognized by B cells.

The activation of antigen-specific B lymphocytes is initiated by the binding of antigen to membrane Ig molecules, which, in conjunction with the associated Igα and Igβ chains, make up the antigen receptor complex of mature B cells. The B lymphocyte antigen receptor serves two key roles in B cell activation. First, antigen-induced clustering of receptors delivers biochemical signals to the B cells that initiate the process of activation. Second, the receptor binds antigen and internalizes it into endosomal vesicles, and if the antigen is a protein, it is processed into peptides that are presented on the B cell surface for recognition by helper T cells. This antigen-presenting function of B cells will be discussed later.

Signal Transduction by the B Lymphocyte Antigen Receptor Complex

The B cell antigen receptor delivers activating signals to a B cell when two or more receptor molecules are brought together, or cross-linked, by multivalent antigens. Membrane IgM and IgD, the antigen receptors of naive B cells, have short cytoplasmic tails consisting of only three amino acids (lysine, valine, and lysine). These tails are too small to transduce signals generated by the clustering of Ig. Ig-mediated signals are transduced by two other molecules, called Igα and Igβ, that are disulfide linked to one another and are expressed in B cells noncovalently associated with membrane Ig (Fig. 10–3). Igα and Igβ are also required for the surface expression of membrane Ig molecules and together with membrane

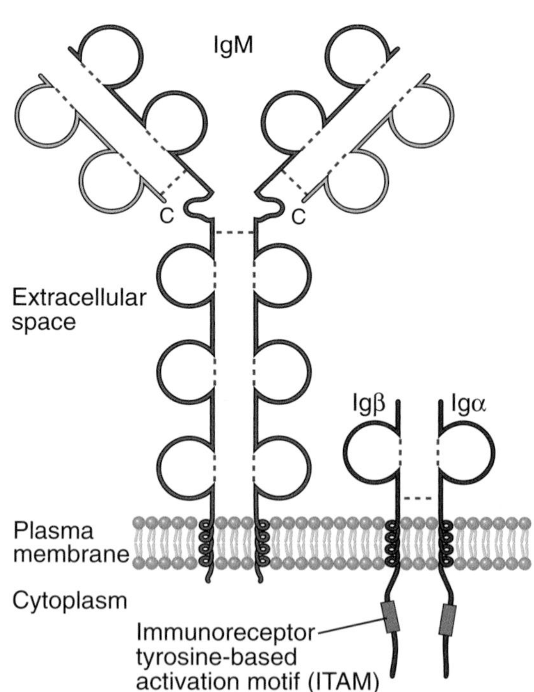

FIGURE 10–3 B cell antigen receptor complex. Membrane IgM (and IgD) on the surface of mature B cells is associated with the invariant Igα and Igβ molecules, which contain ITAMs in their cytoplasmic tails that mediate signaling functions. Note the similarity to the TCR complex (see Chapter 7, Fig. 7–2).

Ig form the **B cell receptor (BCR) complex.** Thus, Igα and Igβ serve the same functions in B cells as the CD3 and ζ proteins do in T lymphocytes (see Chapter 7). The cytoplasmic domains of Igα and Igβ contain tyrosine motifs (immunoreceptor tyrosine-based activation motifs, or ITAMs) that are also found in CD3 and ζ proteins and are required for signal transduction. Igα and Igβ are also loosely associated with Src-family tyrosine kinases.

The early signaling events initiated by the BCR complex are similar to the events described in TCR complex signaling (see Chapter 9).

- ***Antigen-mediated cross-linking of membrane Ig induces phosphorylation of the tyrosines in the ITAMs of Igα and Igβ.*** Cross-linking of membrane Ig brings Src family kinases together and, by promoting their physical interaction, activates these enzymes, instigating them to then phosphorylate the tyrosine residues on ITAMs. This phosphorylation of ITAM tyrosine residues triggers all subsequent signaling events (Fig. 10–4). Cross-linked Ig receptors enter specialized membrane domains, or lipid rafts, where many adapter proteins and signaling molecules may be concentrated, as in T cells. Igα and Igβ are loosely connected to Src-family tyrosine kinases such as Lyn, Fyn, or Blk, and these enzymes are also linked by lipid anchors to the inside of the plasma membrane. The phosphorylation of the tyrosine residues in the ITAMs of Igα and Igβ provides a docking site for the tandem Src homology 2 (SH2) domains of the tyrosine kinase Syk. Syk is the B cell equivalent of ZAP-70 in T lymphocytes. Syk is activated when it associates with phosphorylated tyrosines of ITAMs and may itself be phosphorylated on specific tyrosine residues by BCR-associated Src-family kinases, leading to further activation.
- ***Syk, and other tyrosine kinases, activate numerous downstream signaling pathways that are regulated by adapter proteins.*** In B cells, phosphorylation by activated Syk of critical tyrosine residues on adapter proteins such as SLP-65 (for SH2-binding leukocyte

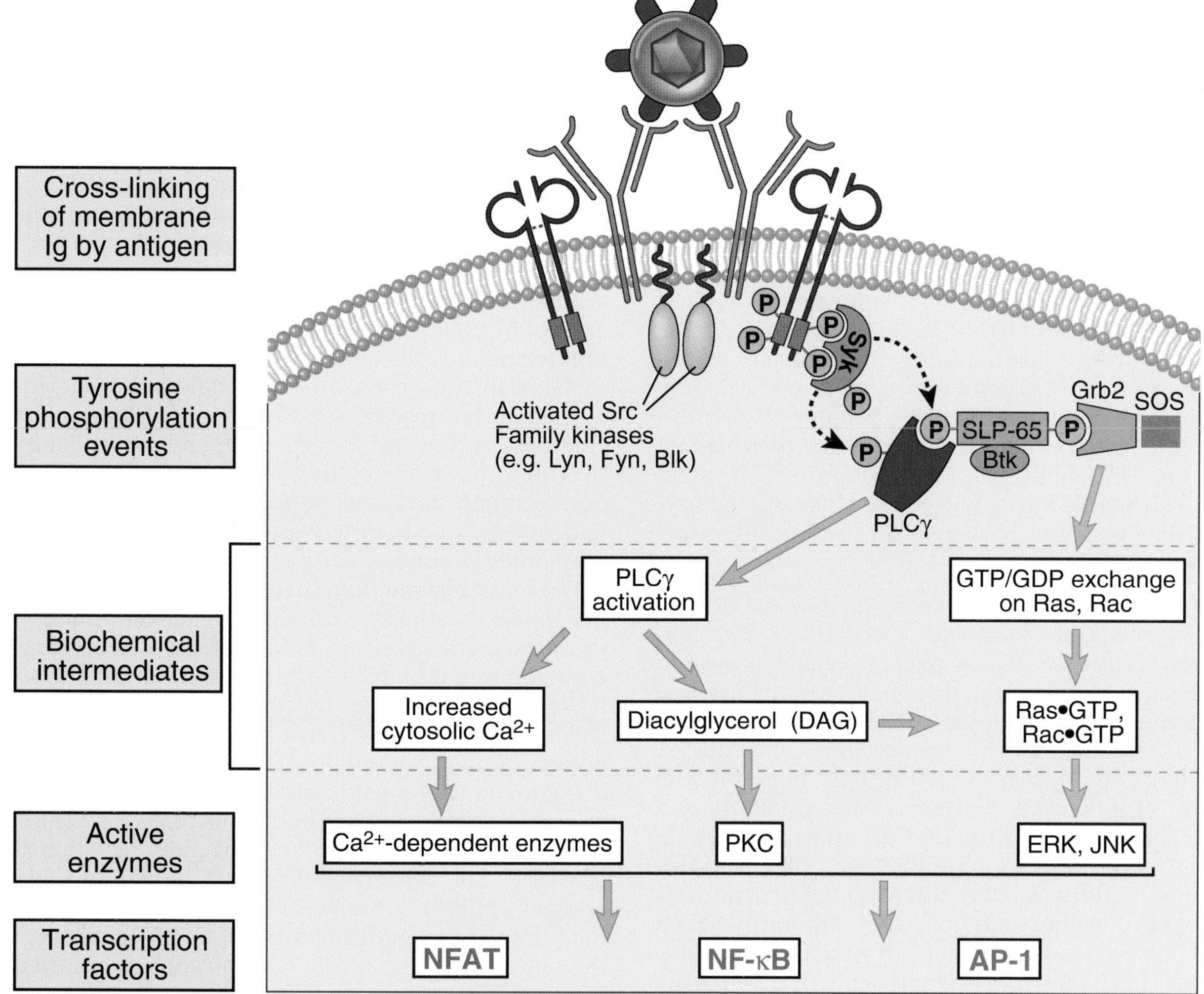

FIGURE 10–4 Signal transduction by the BCR complex. Antigen-induced cross-linking of membrane Ig on B cells leads to clustering and activation of Src-family tyrosine kinases and tyrosine phosphorylation of the ITAMs in the cytoplasmic tails of the Igα and Igβ molecules. This leads to docking of Syk and subsequent tyrosine phosphorylation events as depicted. Several signaling cascades follow these events, as shown, leading to the activation of several transcription factors. These signal transduction pathways are similar to those described in T cells (Chapter 9).

phosphoprotein of 65 kD, also called BLNK, for B cell linker protein) facilitates the recruitment to these adapter proteins of other SH2 domain and phosphotyrosine-binding (PTB) domain–containing enzymes. These include guanine nucleotide exchange proteins that can separately activate Ras and Rac, phospholipase Cγ and the Btk tyrosine kinase, among others. Recruitment facilitates the activation of these downstream effectors, each generally contributing to the activation of a distinct signaling pathway.

- ***The Ras-MAP kinase (mitogen-activated protein kinase) pathway is activated in antigen-stimulated B cells.*** The guanosine triphosphate/ guanosine diphosphate (GTP/GDP) exchange factor Sos is recruited to the SLP-65 complex, probably through the binding of the Grb-2 adapter protein; the subsequent activation of Ras proceeds in the same manner as in T cells, Ras being converted from an inactive GDP bound form to an active GTP bound form (see Chapter 9, Fig. 9–9). In a parallel fashion, the activation of the Rac small GTP proteins may contribute to the activation of the JNK MAP kinase pathway.
- ***A specific phosphatidylinositol-specific phospholipase C (PLC) is activated in response to BCR signaling, and this in turn facilitates the activation of downstream signaling pathways.*** (In B cells, the dominant isoform of PLC is the γ2 isoform, whereas T cells express the related γ1 isoform of the enzyme.) PLCγ2 becomes active when it binds to SLP-65 and is phosphorylated by Syk and Btk. Active PLC breaks down membrane phosphatidylinositol bisphosphate (PIP_2) to yield soluble inositol trisphosphate (IP_3) and leaves diacylglycerol (DAG) in the plasma membrane. IP_3 mobilizes calcium from intracellular stores, leading to a rapid elevation of cytoplasmic calcium, which may be augmented by an influx of calcium from the extracellular milieu. In the presence of calcium, DAG activates some isoforms of protein kinase C (mainly PKC-β in B cells), which phosphorylate downstream proteins on serine/threonine residues.
- ***PKC-β activation contributes in turn to the activation of nuclear factor-κB (NF-κB) in antigen-stimulated B cells.*** PKC-β phosphorylates a protein called CARMA1 that contains an N-terminal caspase recruitment domain (CARD) that mediates protein-protein interactions. Phosphorylation of CARMA1 contributes to its recruitment to lipid rafts, the formation of a complex between CARMA1, Bcl10, and MALT1 (described in Chapter 9), and the resulting activation of the IκB kinase (IKK) complex. The IKK complex is critical for NF-κB activation by virtue of its ability to phosphorylate IκBα, an inhibitor of NF-κB (see Chapter 2) and target it for proteasomal degradation. This releases NF-κB and allows it to enter the nucleus.
- ***These signaling cascades ultimately lead to the activation of transcription factors that induce the expression of genes whose products are required for functional responses of B cells.*** Some of the transcription factors that are known to be activated by antigen receptor-mediated signal transduction in B cells are Fos (downstream of Ras and ERK activation), JunB (downstream of Rac and JNK activation), and NF-κB (downstream of Btk, PLCγ2, and PKC-β activation). A variety of transcription factors, many not mentioned here, are involved in stimulating proliferation and differentiation of B cells.

As in T cells, our knowledge of the antigen-induced signaling pathways in B cells and their links with subsequent functional responses is incomplete. We have described some of these pathways to illustrate the main features, but others may play important roles in B cell activation. The same signaling pathways are used by membrane IgM and IgD on naive B cells and by IgG, IgA, and IgE on B cells that have undergone isotype switching, because all these membrane isotypes associate with Igα and Igβ. Also, other surface molecules, including receptors for complement proteins and Fc receptors, augment or inhibit signals transduced by the antigen receptors, as we will discuss shortly.

Role of the CR2/CD21 Complement Receptor as a Coreceptor for B Cells

The activation of B cells is enhanced by signals that are provided by complement proteins and the CD21 coreceptor complex, which link innate immunity to the adaptive humoral immune response. The complement system consists of a collection of plasma proteins that are activated either by binding to antigen-complexed antibody molecules (the classical pathway) or by binding directly to some polysaccharides and microbial surfaces in the absence of antibodies (the alternative and lectin pathways) (see Chapter 14). Thus, polysaccharides and other T cell-independent antigens of microbes may activate the complement system directly, during innate immune responses. Protein (and other) antigens may be bound by preexisting antibodies or by antibodies produced early in the response, and these antigen-antibody complexes activate complement by the classical pathway. Complement activation results in the proteolytic cleavage of complement proteins. The key component of the system is a protein called C3, and its cleavage results in the production of a molecule called C3b that binds covalently to the microbe or antigen-antibody complex. C3b is further degraded into a fragment called C3d, which remains bound to the microbial surface. B lymphocytes express a receptor for C3d that is called the type 2 complement receptor (CR2, or CD21). The complex of C3d and antigen or C3d and antigen-antibody complex binds to B cells, with the membrane Ig recognizing antigen and CR2 recognizing the bound C3d (Fig. 10–5). CR2 is expressed on mature B cells as a complex with two other membrane proteins, CD19 and CD81 (also called TAPA-1). The CR2-CD19-CD81 complex is often called the B cell coreceptor complex because CR2 binds to antigens through attached C3d at the same time that membrane Ig binds

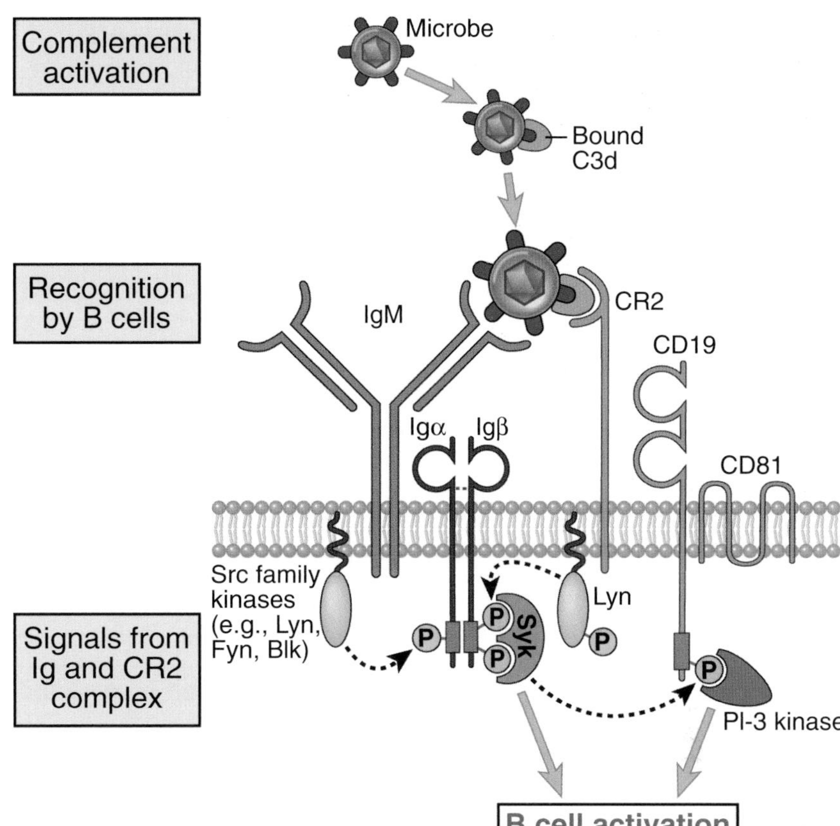

FIGURE 10–5 Role of complement in B cell activation. B cells express a complex of the CR2 complement receptor, CD19, and CD81. Microbial antigens that have bound the complement fragment C3d can simultaneously engage both the CR2 molecule and the membrane Ig on the surface of a B cell. This leads to the initiation of signaling cascades from both the BCR complex and the CR2 complex, because of which the response to C3d-antigen complexes is greatly enhanced compared with the response to antigen alone.

directly to the antigen. Binding of C3d to the B cell complement receptor brings CD19 in proximity to BCR-associated kinases, and the cytoplasmic tail of CD19 rapidly becomes tyrosine phosphorylated. Phosphorylation of the tail of CD19 results in the efficient recruitment of Lyn, a Src family kinase, that can amplify BCR signaling by greatly enhancing the phosphorylation of ITAM tyrosines in Igα and Igβ. Phosphorylated CD19 also activates other signaling pathways, notably one dependent on the enzyme PI-3 kinase, which in turn further augment the signaling pathways initiated by antigen binding to membrane Ig. PI-3 kinase enhances the activation of Btk and PLCγ2 by facilitating their recruitment to PIP_3 on the inner leaflet of the plasma membrane. The net result of coreceptor activation is that the response of the antigen-stimulated B cell is greatly enhanced.

The importance of the complement system in humoral immune responses has been established by several experiments.

- If C3d is covalently attached to a protein antigen, the modified antigen is about 1000-fold more immunogenic than the native antigen.
- Knockouts of the C3, CR2, or CD19 genes in mice result in defects in antibody production.

While C3d bound to antigen binds to CD21 and augments BCR signaling similar to the way that CD4 and CD8 coreceptors enhance TCR signaling, C3d has sometimes been regarded as a "second signal" for B cell activation because it ensures that B cell responses will most likely occur when microbes and antigens that activate complement are encountered. However, it is more useful to consider CD21 as part of "signal one" since it contributes mainly to antigen receptor signal strength. "Second signals" for B cell activation that reflect antigen-receptor independent costimulation, induced directly or indirectly by the presence of pathogens, are provided by CD40 and Toll-like receptors (TLRs), as will be discussed below. The participation of complement in B cell activation provides an amplification mechanism for humoral immune responses because antibodies are able to activate complement and thus contribute to more B cell stimulation. As we will see later, the complement system enhances antibody production not only by CR2-mediated B cell activation but also by promoting the display of antigens in germinal centers.

Functional Responses of B Cells to Antigen

The early cellular events that are induced by antigen-mediated cross-linking of the BCR complex initiate B cell proliferation and differentiation and prepare the cells for subsequent interactions with helper T cells (Fig. 10–6). Antigen recognition stimulates the entry of previously resting cells into the G1 stage of the cell cycle, accompanied by increases in cell size, cytoplasmic RNA, and biosynthetic organelles such as ribosomes. The sur-

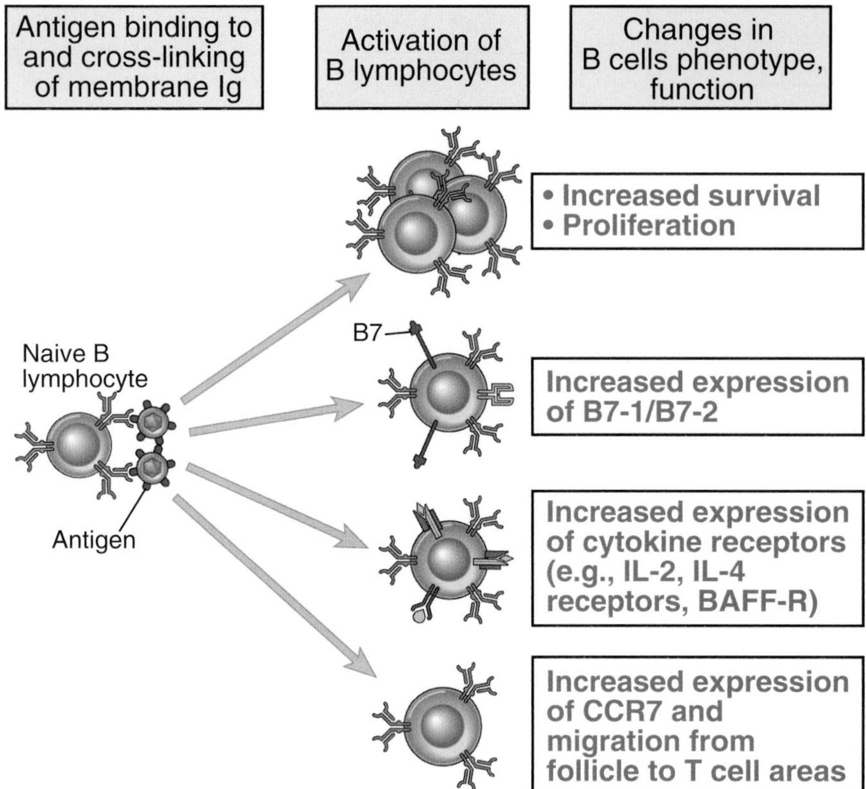

FIGURE 10–6 Functional responses induced by antigen-mediated cross-linking of the BCR complex. Antigen-mediated cross-linking of the B cell antigen receptor induces several cellular responses, including mitosis, expression of new surface molecules, including costimulators and cytokine receptors, and altered migration of the cells as a result of the expression of CCR7.

vival of the B cells is enhanced as a result of the induction of various anti-apoptotic genes. The activated B cells also show low levels of proliferation and antibody secretion. As we will discuss later, although proliferation and Ig secretion can be induced in the absence of T cell help, they are enhanced by signals from helper T cells. Activated B cells show increased expression of class II major histocompatibility complex (MHC) molecules and costimulators, first B7-2 (CD86) and later B7-1 (CD80), because of which antigen-stimulated B cells are more efficient activators of helper T lymphocytes than are naive B cells. The expression of receptors for several T cell–derived cytokines is also increased, which enables antigen-specific B lymphocytes to respond to T cell help. At the same time, the B cells change their expression of chemokine receptors, which enables them to migrate toward and interact with helper T cells (discussed in more detail below).

The importance of signaling by the BCR complex for the subsequent responses of the cells may vary with the nature of the antigen. Most TI antigens, such as polysaccharides and membrane-associated glycolipids or proteins, display multiple identical epitopes in a polyvalent array on each molecule or on a cell surface. Therefore, such antigens effectively cross-link B cell antigen receptors and initiate responses even though they are not recognized by helper T lymphocytes. In contrast, many naturally occurring globular protein antigens possess only one copy of each epitope per molecule. Therefore, such protein antigens cannot simultaneously bind to and cross-link two Ig molecules, and their ability to activate the BCR might be limited. However, some protein antigens may be displayed as multivalent arrays on cell surfaces, or if they are aggregated by antibody. Irrespective of how strongly they trigger the BCR, protein antigens are internalized by the BCR and recruit T cell help, and helper T cells and their products are potent stimulators of B lymphocyte proliferation and differentiation. Therefore, protein antigens may need to initiate minimal signals by the BCR complex to induce humoral immune responses. In such responses, a major function of membrane Ig may be to bind and internalize the antigen for subsequent presentation to helper T cells, as discussed below.

HELPER T CELL–DEPENDENT ANTIBODY RESPONSES TO PROTEIN ANTIGENS

Antibody responses to protein antigens require recognition of the antigen by helper T cells and cooperation between the antigen-specific B and T lymphocytes. The helper function of T lymphocytes was discovered by experiments done in the late 1960s, even before the classification of lymphocytes into T and B cell subsets was established. Subsequent studies established that most helper T cells are $CD4^+CD8^-$ and recognize peptide antigens presented by class II MHC molecules.

- If irradiated mice were given bone marrow cells (which contain mature B lymphocytes but no mature T cells) and immunized, specific antibody was not produced, but the transfer of both B cells and thymocytes (a source of mature T cells) resulted in antibody production after immunization.

- Purified B cells proliferate and differentiate in vitro in response to protein antigens only if helper T lymphocytes are also present.
- Humans or knockout mice with reduced numbers of $CD4^+$ T cells, or mice treated with a depleting anti-CD4 antibody, show defective antibody responses to protein antigens.

Helper T lymphocytes stimulate B cell clonal expansion, isotype switching, affinity maturation, and differentiation into memory B cells (see Fig. 10–1). Different phases of T cell–dependent B cell activation occur in different anatomic regions within peripheral lymphoid organs (Fig. 10–7). The early phase occurs at the border of T cell–rich zones and primary follicles and results in B cell proliferation, initial antibody secretion, and some isotype (class) switching. The late phase of T cell–dependent humoral immune responses takes place in the specialized microenvironment of the germinal centers within lymphoid follicles and results in affinity maturation, memory B cell generation, and much more isotype switching. The molecular and anatomic details of each of the early and late events in T cell–dependent B cell responses are described next.

Sequence of Events in T Cell–Dependent Antibody Responses

Protein antigens are recognized by specific B and T lymphocytes in peripheral lymphoid organs, and the activated cell populations come together in these organs to initiate humoral immune responses. The interaction between helper T cells and B lymphocytes is initiated by the recognition of protein antigens. The sequence of events that lead to the interaction of helper T cells with B cells, and the subsequent events that drive further B cell differentiation, are listed below:

1. Antigen is taken up by dendritic cells (DCs) and presented to helper T cells.
2. Helper T cells are activated and induced to express membrane proteins (CD40L) and cytokines.
3. Activated helper T cells are instructed to migrate toward the follicle following a chemokine gradient.
4. B cells are activated by antigen that may be in soluble form or displayed by DCs.
5. B cells process and present antigen, alter their cell surface chemokine receptor profile, and migrate toward the T cell zone.
6. T and B cells interact at the T-B interface, and B cells are activated by CD40L and cytokines.
7. Small extrafollicular B cell foci form in T cell zones, and some isotype switching and Ig secretion occur.
8. Activated B cells migrate back into the follicle. Germinal centers form within the follicles and

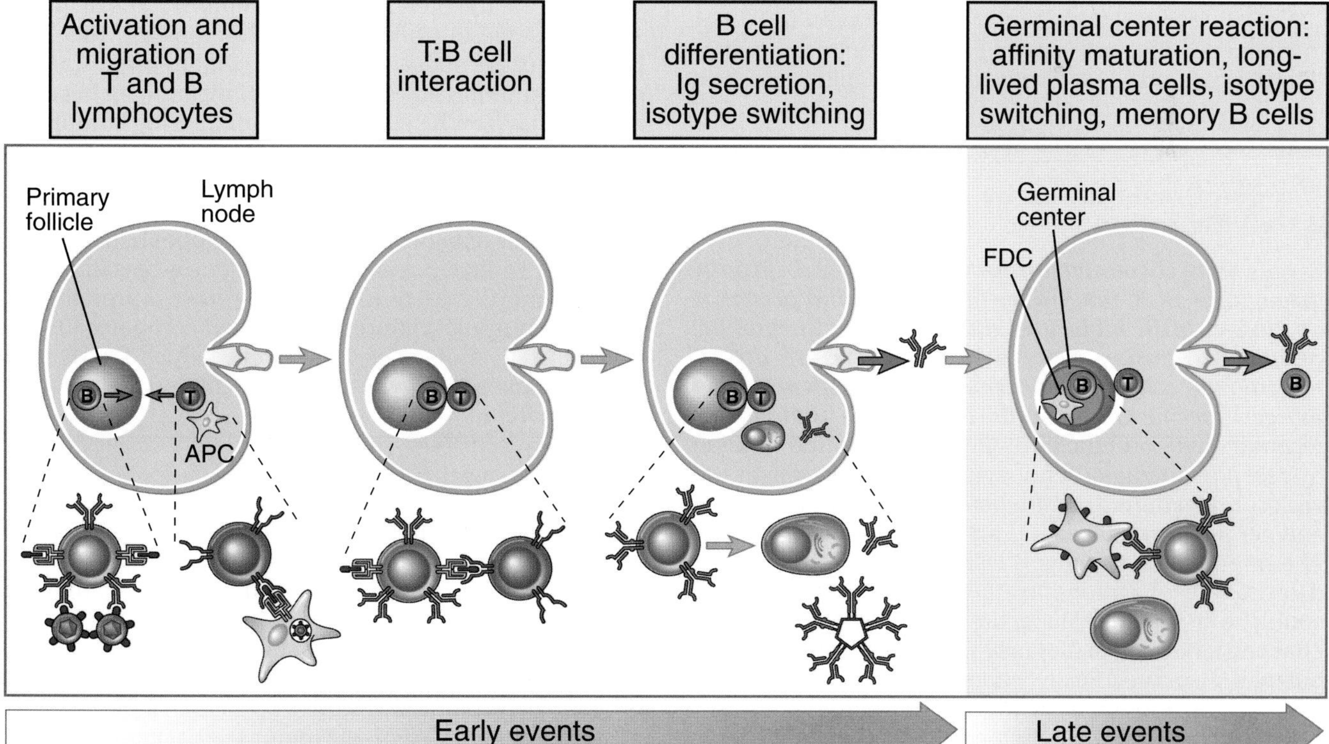

FIGURE 10–7 Early and late events in humoral immune responses to T cell–dependent protein antigens. Immune responses are initiated by the recognition of antigens by B cells and helper T cells. The activated lymphocytes migrate toward one another and interact, resulting in B cell proliferation, differentiation into antibody-secreting cells, and early isotype switching. The late events occur in germinal centers and include affinity maturation of the response and additional isotype switching, and memory B cell generation.

are the sites of extensive isotype switching, somatic mutation, the selection events that lead to affinity maturation, and memory B cell generation.

9. Long-lived plasma cells are generated from cells activated in the germinal center reaction, and some of these terminally differentiated plasma cells migrate to the bone marrow.

In the following sections we describe each of these steps in some detail.

Helper T Cell Activation

Even after specific B and T cells respond to antigen, they are relatively rare in lymphoid organs and need to be brought into proximity to enhance the possibility that antigen-specific B and T cells will physically interact (Fig. 10–8). The frequency of naive B cells or T cells specific for a given epitope on an antigen is as low as 1 in 10^5 to 10^6. The cells that initially and most readily access protein antigens are DCs. These cells present peptides derived from protein antigens and displayed on class II MHC molecules to naive $CD4^+$ T cells. The DCs are also induced by TLR ligands to express B7-1 and B7-2, and thus provide second signals for helper T cell activation. T cells that have been activated by DCs are induced to proliferate, express CD40L, and secrete cytokines. They also alter their chemokine receptor profile, downregulating the CCR7 chemokine receptor, and increasing the expression of CXCR5, and as a result leave the T cell zone and migrate toward the follicle. CXCL13, the ligand for CXCR5, is secreted by follicular dendritic cells and other follicular stromal cells and it contributes to the migration of activated $CD4^+$ T cells toward the follicle.

Antigen Presentation by B Cells and B Cell Migration

B cells that encounter antigen are activated initially through the BCR, internalize the antigen and present it on class II MHC molecules, and alter their chemokine receptor expression pattern so that they are drawn toward the T cell zone in order to interact with activated antigen-specific helper T cells. The BCR is a high-affinity receptor that can efficiently internalize bound antigen by receptor-mediated endocytosis and deliver it to the endosomal compartment where proteins are processed and peptides bind to class II MHC molecules (Fig. 10–9). The rare antigen-specific B cells that recognize a B cell determinant or epitope on the protein antigen (which could be a specific shape on the protein or even an attached small molecule) may receive some BCR signals but will also specifically endocytose the antigen and process and present it in an MHC class II–dependent manner to activated T helper cells.

Several "second signals" enable a B cell responding to a protein antigen to discriminate between a potentially innocuous and a dangerous antigen. First, T cell help will be provided only by T cells that have responded to activated DCs expressing B7, which in turn is typically induced by the engagement of TLRs by microbial products (see Chapter 2). Second, B cells also directly sense the presence of pathogens by being triggered by ligands for one or more TLRs such as TLR4, TLR5, or TLR9, all of which are expressed by B cells. Antigen-activated B cells down-regulate CXCR5, the chemokine receptor that retains them in follicles, and are induced to express CCR7. As a result, they are drawn toward the T-B interface and the T cell zone. This, of course, is the mirror image of the change in migration exhibited by activated $CD4^+$ T cells.

In any humoral immune response, B cells specific for the antigen that initiates the response are preferentially activated, compared with cells that are not specific for the antigen. There are several reasons for this. First, only B cells expressing membrane Ig molecules that specifically bind the antigen receive the signals that initiate B cell activation. Second, B cells are able to present the antigen they recognize at 10^4- to 10^6-fold lower concentrations than antigens for which they do not express specific receptors (in which case the antigen is internalized far less efficiently by fluid-phase pinocytosis), because receptor mediated endocytosis via the BCR is extremely efficient. Third, the B cells in T cell–B cell conjugates are exposed to signals delivered by CD40L and other T cell surface molecules and to very high local concentrations of T cell–derived cytokines, in part because of the formation of immunological synapses between specific T and B cells and the vectorial delivery of T cell cytokines into the synaptic cleft. Therefore, antigen-specific B lymphocytes are the preferential recipients of T cell help and are stimulated to proliferate and differentiate. The antibodies that are subsequently secreted are often specific for conformational determinants of the antigen because membrane Ig on B cells is capable of binding conformational epitopes of native antigens. This feature of B cell antigen recognition determines the fine specificity of the antibody response and is independent of the fact that helper T cells recognize only linear epitopes of processed peptides. In fact, a single B lymphocyte specific for a native epitope may bind and endocytose a protein and present multiple different peptides complexed with class II MHC molecules to different helper T cells, but the resultant antibody response remains specific for the native protein.

The Hapten-Carrier Effect

The principles outlined here for T-B cell collaboration provide the basis for understanding a phenomenon that is known as the **hapten-carrier effect**. Analysis of antibody responses to hapten-carrier conjugates was among the earliest approaches that demonstrated how antigen presentation by B lymphocytes contributes to the development of humoral immune responses. Haptens, such as dinitrophenol, are small chemicals that can be bound by specific antibodies but are not immunogenic by themselves. If, however, haptens are coupled to proteins, which serve as carriers, the conjugates are able to induce

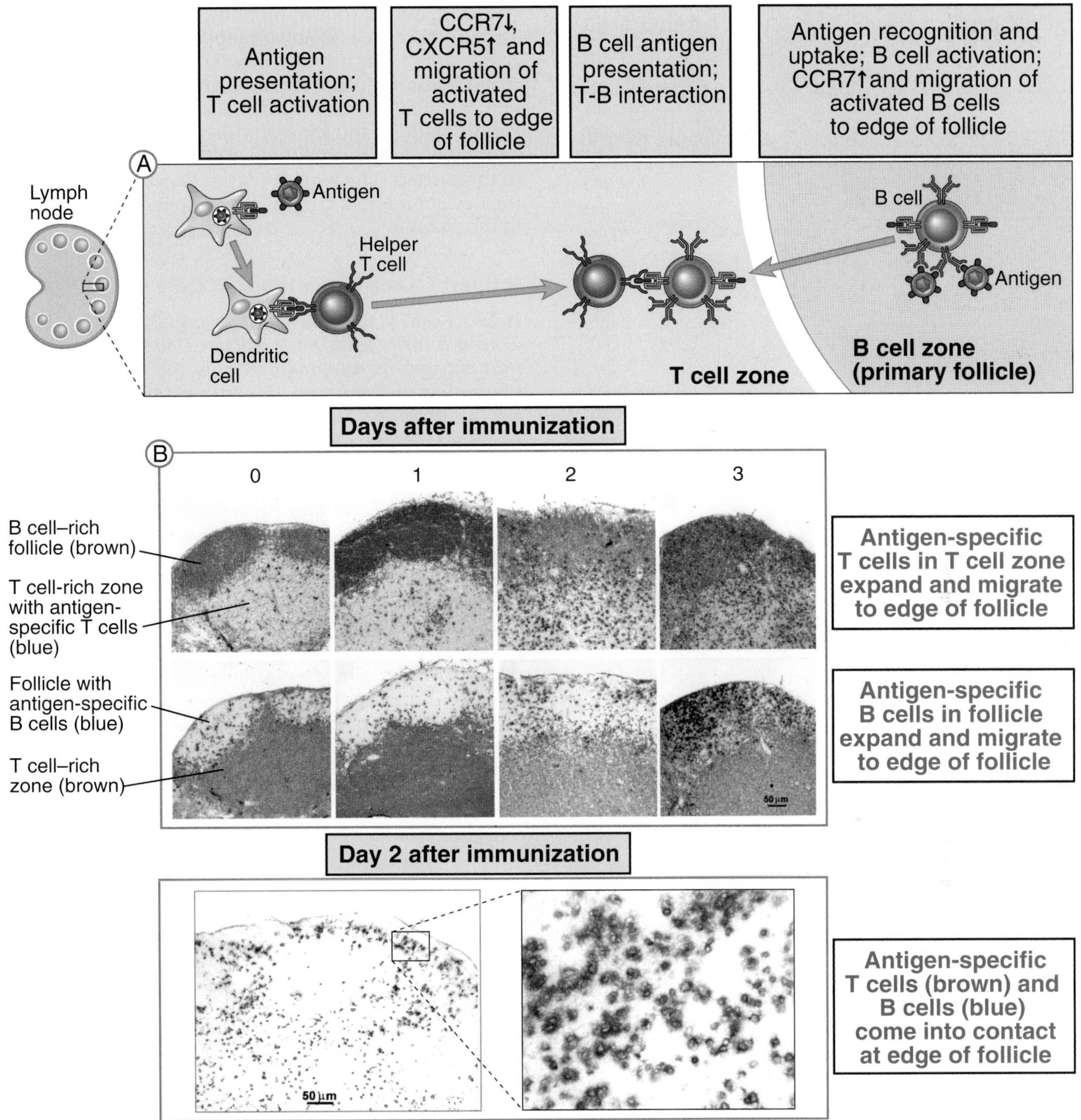

FIGURE 10–8 Migration and interactions of B cells and helper T cells. A. The initiation of humoral immune responses to protein antigens in lymph nodes is shown schematically. Antigen-activated helper T cells and B cells move toward one another and make contact adjacent to the edge of primary follicles. In this location, the B cell presents antigen to the T cell, and the B cell receives activating signals from the T cell. B. An immunohistochemical analysis of antigen-dependent T cell–B cell interactions in a lymph node is shown. In this experiment, T cells expressing a TCR specific for the protein antigen ovalbumin and B cells specific for the protein hen egg lysozyme were adoptively transferred into normal mice, and the mice were immunized with a conjugate of ovalbumin–hen egg lysozyme. (The T cells and B cells were obtained from TCR- and Ig-transgenic mice, respectively. See Appendix III for a description of antigen receptor transgenic mice.) The locations of the antigen-specific T cells and B cells in draining lymph nodes were followed after immunization with use of antibodies specific for the cell populations and two-color immunohistochemistry. (Adapted with permission from Garside P, E Ingulli, RR Merica, JG Johnson, RJ Noell, and MK Jenkins. Visualization of specific B and T lymphocyte interactions in the lymph node. Science 281:96–99, 1998. Copyright 1998, AAAS.)

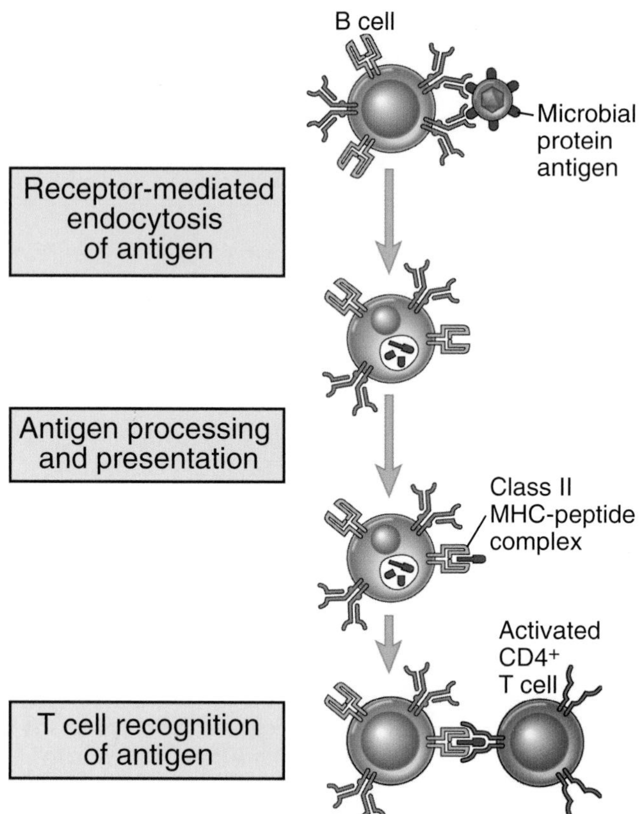

FIGURE 10–9 B cell antigen presentation to activated helper T cells. Protein antigens bound to membrane Ig are endocytosed and processed, and peptide fragments are presented in association with class II MHC molecules. Activated helper T cells recognize the MHC-peptide complexes and then stimulate B cell responses. Activated B cells also express costimulators (not shown) that enhance helper T cell responses.

antibody responses against the haptens. There are three important characteristics of antihapten antibody responses to hapten-protein conjugates. First, such responses require both hapten-specific B cells and protein (carrier)-specific helper T cells. Second, to stimulate a response, the hapten and carrier portions have to be physically linked and cannot be administered separately. Third, the interaction is class II MHC restricted (i.e., the helper T cells cooperate only with B lymphocytes that express class II MHC molecules recognized as self by the T cells). All these features of antibody responses to hapten-protein conjugates can be explained by the antigen-presenting functions of B lymphocytes. Hapten-specific B cells bind the antigen through the hapten determinant, endocytose the hapten-carrier conjugate, and present peptides derived from the carrier protein to carrier-specific helper T lymphocytes (Fig. 10–10). Thus, the two cooperating lymphocytes recognize different epitopes of the same complex antigen. The hapten is responsible for efficient carrier uptake, which explains why hapten and carrier must be physically linked. The requirement for MHC-associated antigen presentation for T cell activation accounts for the MHC restriction of T cell–B cell interactions.

The characteristics of humoral responses elucidated for hapten-carrier conjugates apply to all protein antigens in which one intrinsic determinant, usually a native conformational determinant, is recognized by B cells (and is, therefore, analogous to the hapten) and another determinant, in the form of a class II–associated linear peptide, is recognized by helper T cells (and is analogous to the carrier). The hapten-carrier effect is the basis for the devleopment of **conjugate vaccines**, discussed later in the chapter.

Helper T Cell–Dependent B Cell Activation

Helper T cells activated by antigen and B7 costimulation express a surface molecule called CD40 ligand (CD40L) that engages its receptor, CD40, on the B cells that are presenting antigen, and this interaction stimulates B cell proliferation and both early differentiation and germinal center formation (Fig. 10–11). **CD40** is a member of the TNF receptor family. **CD40L** (CD154) is a trimeric T cell membrane protein that is structurally homologous to TNF and Fas ligand. CD40 is constitutively expressed on B cells, and CD40L is expressed on the surface of helper T cells after activation by antigen and costimulators. When these activated helper T cells bind to antigen-presenting B cells, CD40L interacts with CD40 on the B cell surface. CD40L binding to CD40 results in the conformational alteration of preformed CD40 trimers, and this induces the association of cytosolic proteins called TRAFs (TNF receptor–associated factors) with the cytoplasmic domain of CD40. The TRAFs recruited to CD40 initiate enzyme cascades that lead to the activation and nuclear transloca-

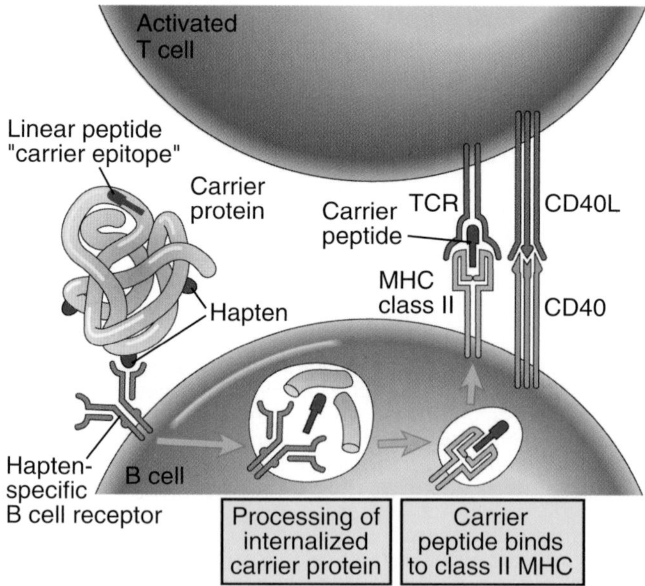

FIGURE 10–10 T-B collaboration and the hapten-carrier effect. A monovalent protein conjugated to a hapten is internalized by a hapten-specific B cell that processes the antigen and presents the linear peptide or "carrier determinant" on class II MHC molecules to an activated helper T cell, which then triggers the B cell via a CD40L-CD40 interaction.

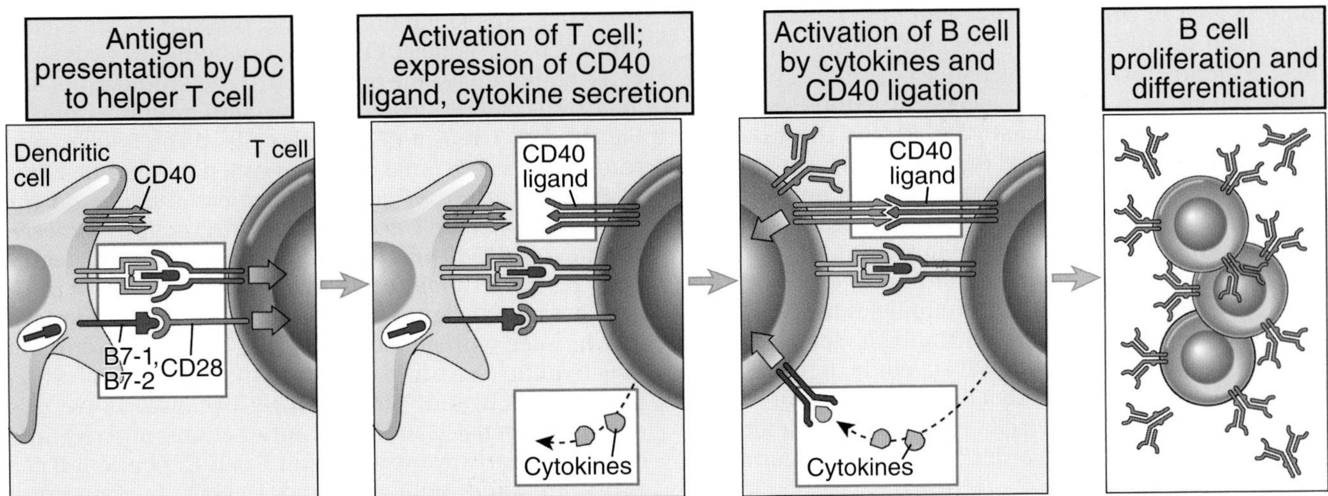

FIGURE 10–11 Mechanisms of helper T cell–mediated B cell activation. Dendritic cells initially display processed peptides derived from endocytosed protein antigens and express the costimulators B7-1 and B7-2. Helper T cells recognize the antigen (in the form of peptide-MHC complexes) and the costimulators and are stimulated to express CD40 ligand and to secrete cytokines. CD40 ligand on activated helper T cells then binds to CD40 on B cells and initiates B cell proliferation and differentiation. Cytokines bind to cytokine receptors on the B cells and also stimulate B cell responses.

tion of transcription factors, including NF-κB and AP-1. Similar signaling pathways are activated by TNF receptors (see Chapter 2). CD40-induced transcription factor induction is crucial for subsequent germinal center formation and also contributes to the expression of the gene encoding activation-induced deaminase (AID), an enzyme that is critical for somatic mutation and isotype switching, as will be discussed below. T cell–mediated DC and macrophage activation also involves the interaction of CD40L on T cells with CD40 on DCs and macrophages (see Chapter 13). Thus, this pathway of contact-mediated cellular responses is a general mechanism for the activation of target cells by helper T lymphocytes and is not unique to antibody production.

The importance of the CD40L-CD40 pathway is demonstrated in CD40 or CD40L gene knockout mice. The mice exhibit profound defects in antibody production, isotype switching, affinity maturation, and memory B cell generation in response to protein antigens. Similar abnormalities are found in humans with mutations in the CD40L gene, which results in a disease called the X-linked hyper-IgM syndrome (see Chapter 20).

Interestingly, a DNA virus called the Epstein-Barr virus (EBV) infects human B cells and induces their proliferation. This may lead to immortalization of the cells and the development of lymphomas (see Chapter 17, Box 17–2). The cytoplasmic tail of a transforming protein of EBV called LMP1 (latent membrane protein 1) associates with the same TRAF molecules as does the cytoplasmic domain of CD40, and this apparently triggers B cell proliferation. Thus, EBV LMP1 is functionally homologous to a physiologic B cell signaling molecule, and EBV has apparently co-opted a normal pathway of B lymphocyte activation for its own purposes, which are to promote survival and proliferation of cells that the virus has infected.

Activated helper T lymphocytes secrete cytokines that act in concert with CD40L to stimulate B cell proliferation and production of antibodies of different isotypes. We have mentioned cytokines previously as important secreted products of T lymphocytes and other cells of the immune system, and they will be discussed in more detail in Chapter 12. The roles of these proteins in humoral immunity have been most clearly established by showing that various aspects of antibody responses can be inhibited by cytokine antagonists or are deficient in mice in which particular cytokine genes are knocked out.

Cytokines serve two principal functions in antibody responses: they increase B cell proliferation and differentiation (which were initiated by CD40 signals), and they promote switching to different heavy chain isotypes. Different cytokines play distinct but often overlapping roles in antibody production, and their actions may be synergistic or antagonistic. Antigen recognition by B cells enhances the expression of receptors for cytokines, and, as we have described earlier, B cells in direct contact with helper T lymphocytes are exposed to high concentrations of these secreted proteins. As a result, antigen-specific B cells respond to cytokines more than do bystander B cells that are not specific for the initiating antigen but happen to be close to the antigen-stimulated lymphocytes. Helper T cell–derived cytokines, most notably interleukin-2 (IL-2), IL-4, and IL-21, can enhance B cell proliferation and differentiation, as do the TNF family cytokines BAFF and APRIL. IL-6, which is produced by macrophages, T cells, and many other cell types, is a growth factor for already differentiated, antibody-secreting B cells. The effects of specific cytokines on isotype switching are described later.

The activation of B cells by T cells via CD40L and cytokines contributes to the initial formation of extrafollicular foci of activated B cells that may undergo

some degree of differentiation and isotype switching. Each such focus may contain about 100 to 200 short-lived antibody secreting plasmablasts and plasma cells. In the spleen, extrafollicular foci occur in the T cell–rich periarteriolar lymphoid sheath (PALS), and these collections of cells are often called PALS foci. This generation of PALS foci has been shown to be T cell dependent. The small amount of low-affinity antibody generated in these foci may contribute to the formation of immune complexes (containing antigen, antibody, and complement) that are trapped by FDCs in follicles in secondary lymphoid organs. It is believed that this deposition of immune complexes is a necessary prelude to the release of chemokines from FDCs that draw in a few (often only one or two) activated B cells from the extrafollicular focus into the follicle, in order to initiate the germinal center reaction.

The Germinal Center Reaction

A number of events that are characteristic of helper T cell–dependent antibody responses, including affinity maturation, isotype switching, and the generation of memory B cells, occur primarily in the germinal centers of lymphoid follicles. As we discussed earlier, the initial B cell response to protein antigens occurs at the boundaries between lymphoid follicles and T cell zones (see Fig. 10–8). Within 4 to 7 days after antigen exposure, some of the activated B cells migrate deep into the follicle and begin to proliferate rapidly, forming the lightly staining central region of the follicle, called the germinal center (Fig. 10–12). Within the germinal center is a "dark zone" that contains rapidly proliferating B cells. The doubling time of these proliferating germinal center B cells, also called centroblasts, is estimated to be 6 to 12 hours, so that within 5 days, a single lymphocyte may give rise to almost 5000 progeny. Each fully formed germinal center contains cells derived from only one or a few antigen-specific B cell clones. The progeny of the proliferating B cells in the germinal center are smaller cells, sometimes called centrocytes, that undergo differentiation and selection processes in the "light zone," as described below.

The architecture of lymphoid follicles and the germinal center reactions within follicles depend on the presence of **follicular dendritic cells (FDCs)**. FDCs are found only in lymphoid follicles and express complement receptors (CR1, CR2, and CR3) and Fc receptors. All of these molecules are involved in the selection of germinal center B cells, as described below. FDCs do not express class II MHC molecules. The origin of FDCs is unclear. They are not derived from the bone marrow, and they are clearly different from the class II MHC-expressing DCs that capture antigens in tissues and transport them to secondary lymphoid organs where they present peptide antigens to T lymphocytes, and may make antigen available to naive B cells as well. The long cytoplasmic processes of FDCs form a meshwork around which germinal centers are formed. Proliferating B cells accumulate in the histologically identifiable dark zone of the germinal center, which has few FDCs. The small nondividing progeny of the B cells migrate to the adjacent light zone, where they come into close contact with the processes of the abundant FDCs, and this is where subsequent selection events occur (see Fig. 10–12). The rim of naive B cells in the follicle, surrounding the germinal center, is called the mantle zone.

The formation of germinal centers depends on the presence of helper T cells and the interactions between CD40L and CD40 and is therefore observed only in antibody responses to helper T cell–dependent protein antigens. Germinal center formation is impaired in humans and in mice with genetic defects in T cell development or activation (see Chapter 20) or with mutations of either CD40 or its ligand. This is partly because, as we discussed earlier, CD40:CD40L interactions are required during the early events of helper T cell–dependent B cell activation, and only activated B cells migrate from extrafollicular foci back into follicles to form germinal centers. In addition, germinal centers contain small numbers of helper T cells, which express CD40L and may stimulate the proliferation and selection of germinal center B cells by CD40 engagement.

Heavy Chain Isotype (Class) Switching

In response to CD40 engagement and cytokines, some of the progeny of activated IgM- and IgD-expressing B cells undergo the process of heavy chain isotype (class) switching, leading to the production of antibodies with heavy chains of different classes, such as γ, α, and ε (Fig. 10–13). Isotype switching occurs in peripheral lymphoid tissues, in B cells that are activated at the edges of the follicles, and in germinal centers. The requirement for CD40 signaling to promote isotype switching in B cells is well documented by analysis of mice and humans lacking CD40 or its ligand. In all these cases, the antibody response to protein antigens is dominated by IgM antibodies, and there is limited switching to other isotypes.

Cytokines play essential roles in regulating switching to particular heavy chain isotypes. For instance, IL-4, which is produced mainly by $CD4^+$ T cells, is the principal switch factor for IgE in all species examined, and the production of IgG2a in mice is dependent on interferon-γ (IFN-γ), which is secreted by T cells and by natural killer (NK) cells.

- Addition of IL-4 or IFN-γ induces specific isotype switching in cultures of mature IgM- and IgD-expressing B cells stimulated with antigens or polyclonal activators (Table 10–1).
- IgE responses to antigen-specific or polyclonal stimulation are inhibited by antibodies that neutralize IL-4, and IgG2a responses are blocked by antibodies that neutralize IFN-γ.
- IL-4-deficient mice created by gene knockout have no serum IgE, and IFN-γ knockout mice have greatly reduced serum IgG2a.
- Some individuals with a selective deficiency of IgA production (as well as patients with Combined Variable Immunodeficiency) inherit mutant versions of the *TACI gene* (see Chapter 20). This gene encodes

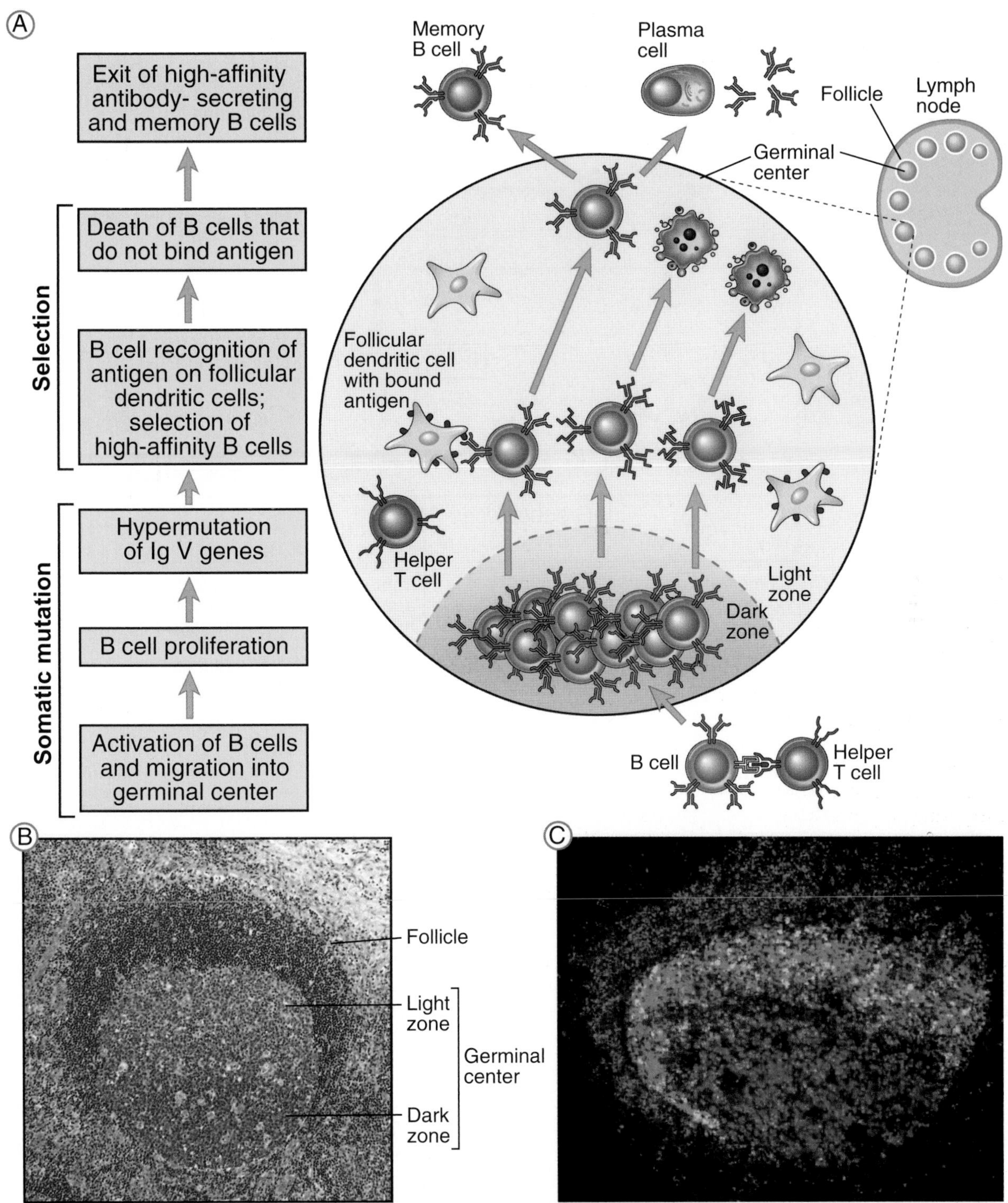

FIGURE 10–12 Germinal center reactions in T cell–dependent antibody responses. A. Schematic diagram of germinal center reactions in a lymph node. B cells that have been activated by helper T cells at the edge of a primary follicle migrate into the follicle and proliferate, forming the dark zone. Somatic mutations of Ig V genes occur in these B cells, and they migrate into the light zone where they encounter follicular dendritic cells displaying antigen. B cells with the highest affinity Ig receptors are selected to survive, and they differentiate into antibody-secreting or memory B cells. B. Histology of a secondary follicle with a germinal center in a lymph node. The germinal center is contained within the follicle and includes a basal dark zone and an adjacent light zone. The mantle zone is the parent follicle within which the germinal center has formed. (Courtesy of Dr. James Gulizia, Department of Pathology, Brigham and Women's Hospital, Boston.) C. Cellular components of the germinal center. A secondary follicle has been stained with an anti-CD23 antibody (green), which brightly stains follicular dendritic cells in the light zone and dimly stains naive B cells in the mantle zone. Anti-Ki67 (red), which detects cycling cells, stains mitotically active B cell blasts in the dark zone. (Adapted from Liu YJ, GD Johnson, J Gordon, and IC MacLennan. Germinal centres in T-cell-dependent antibody responses. Immunology Today 13:17–21, Copyright 1992, with permission from Elsevier.)

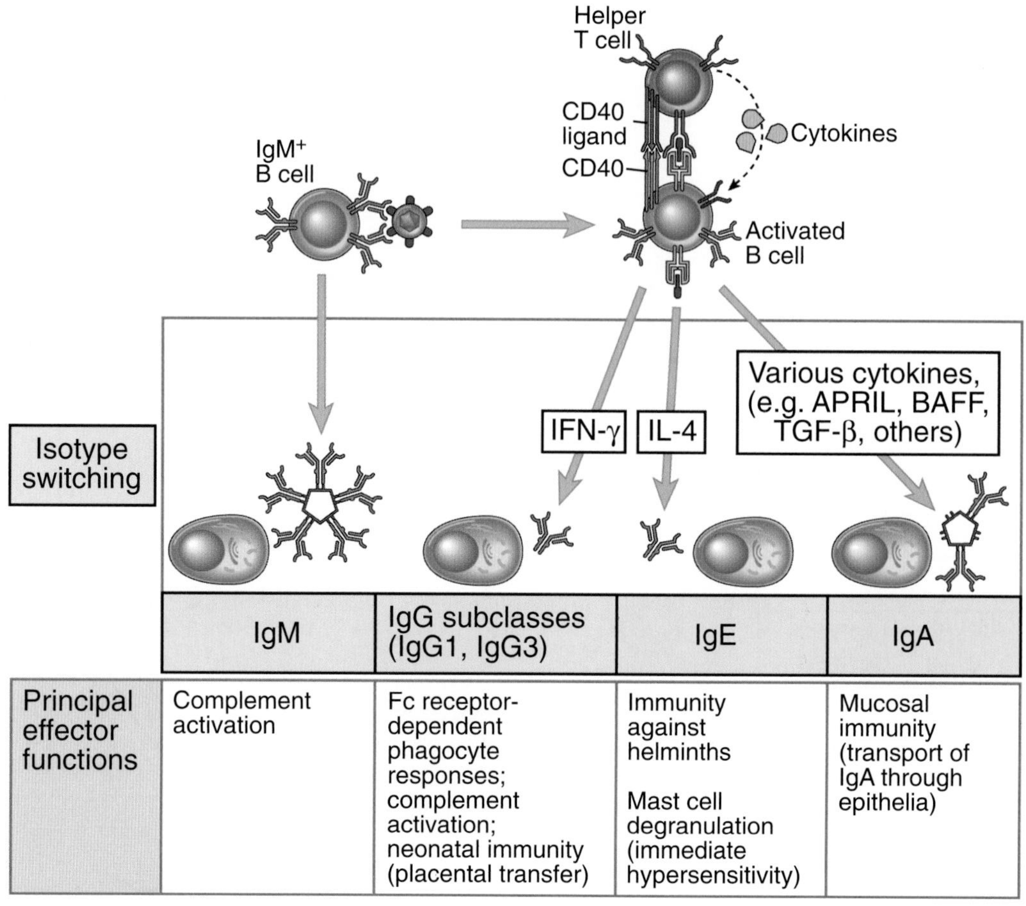

FIGURE 10–13 Ig heavy chain isotype switching. B cells activated by helper T cell signals (CD40L, cytokines) undergo switching to different Ig isotypes, which mediate distinct effector functions. Selected examples of switched isotypes in humans are shown.

a protein of the TNF receptor family that is present on B cells and is a receptor for the TNF family cytokines BAFF and APRIL.

The major mechanism by which CD40 signals induce isotype switching is the induction of the AID gene downstream of CD40. AID, as we shall see, is an activation-induced deaminase that is crucial for both isotype switching and somatic mutation. While CD40 is the major signaling receptor that contributes to the induction of AID, cytokines induce transcription factors that identify which Ig heavy chain loci will be the target of isotype switching mediated by AID in a given activated B cell. Cytokines may initiate transcription and create

Table 10–1. Heavy Chain Isotype Switching Induced by Cytokines

B cells cultured with		**Ig isotype secreted (percent of total Ig produced)**				
Polyclonal Activator	Cytokine	IgM	IgG1	IgG2a	IgE	IgA
LPS	None	85	2	<1	<1	<1
LPS	IL-4	70	**20**	<1	**5**	<1
LPS	IFN-γ	80	2	**10**	<1	<1
LPS	TGF-β + IL-5	75	2	<1	<1	**15**

Addition of various cytokines to purified IgM^+IgD^+ mouse B cells cultured with the polyclonal activator lipopolysaccharide (LPS) induces switching to different heavy chain isotypes (bold). The values of the isotypes shown are approximations and do not add up to 100% because not all were measured. (Courtesy of Dr. Robert Coffman, Dynavax Technologies Corp., California) single-stranded DNA segments in specific Ig loci that can be targets of AID-induced DNA deamination for class switching (discussed below).

The capacity of B cells to produce different antibody isotypes provides a remarkable plasticity in humoral immune responses by generating antibodies that perform distinct effector functions and are involved in defense against different types of infectious agents (see Fig. 10–13). Isotype switching in response to different types of microbes is regulated by the types of helper T cells that are activated by these microbes. For instance, the major protective humoral immune response to bacteria with polysaccharide-rich capsules consists of IgM antibodies, which bind to the bacteria, activate the complement system, and induce phagocytosis of the opsonized bacteria. Polysaccharide antigens, which do not elicit T cell help, stimulate mainly IgM antibodies, with little, if any, isotype switching to some IgG subclasses. The response to many viruses and bacteria consists of production of IgG antibodies, which block entry of the microbes into host cells and also promote phagocytosis by macrophages. Viruses and many bacteria activate helper T cells of the T_H1 subset, which produce the cytokine IFN-γ, the main inducer of B cell switching to opsonizing and complement-fixing IgG subclasses. The immune response to many helminthic parasites is mainly production of IgE, which participates in eosinophil-mediated killing of the helminths (see Chapter 15); IgE antibodies also mediate immediate hypersensitivity (allergic) reactions (see Chapter 19). Helminths activate the T_H2 subset of helper T cells, which produces IL-4, the cytokine that induces switching to IgE. (We will discuss the development and functions of helper T cell subsets in more detail in Chapter 13.) In addition, B cells in different anatomic sites switch to different isotypes. Specifically, B cells in mucosal tissues switch to IgA, which is the antibody class that is most efficiently transported through epithelia into mucosal secretions, where it defends against microbes that try to enter through the epithelia. Switching to IgA is stimulated by transforming growth factor-β (TGF-β), which is produced by many cell types in mucosal and other tissues. The TNF family cytokine receptor TACI (which can be recognized by both APRIL and BAFF) is also a critical player in IgA class switching but may contribute mainly to AID induction for T cell-independent activation of IgA responses (discussed later in this chapter). These examples of isotype switching illustrate how helper T cells function as controllers of immune responses—these T cells secrete different cytokines in response to distinct microbes, and the cytokines stimulate antibody responses that are best at combating those microbes.

The principal molecular mechanism of isotype switching is a process called **switch recombination,** in which the rearranged VDJ (variable-diversity-joining) gene segment in a B cell recombines with a downstream C region gene and the intervening DNA is deleted. These DNA recombination events involve nucleotide sequences called switch regions, which are located in the J-C introns at the 5′ ends of each C_H locus. Switch regions are 1 to 10 kilobases long, contain numerous tandem repeats of GC–rich DNA sequences, and are found upstream of every heavy chain gene other than the δ gene. Upstream of each switch region is a small exon called the I exon (for initiator of transcription) preceded by an I region promoter. CD40 and cytokines trigger isotype switching by increasing the accessibility of the DNA at a specific C region and then inducing transcription through the I exon, switch region, and C_H exons. These transcripts, known as germline transcripts since they do not encode specific proteins, participate in switching in a major way.

Germline transcription is accompanied by accessibility of a particular C gene to DNA breaks and repair, as explained below. As a result, the rearranged VDJ exon just upstream of the μ switch region in the B cell recombines with the transcriptionally active downstream C region. For instance, IL-4 induces germline transcription through the I_ε-S_ε-C_ε locus, and IFN–γ induces germline transcription in mice through the $I_\gamma2a$-$S_\gamma2a$-$C_\gamma2a$ locus (see Fig. 10–14). This leads first to the production of germline ε or γ2a transcripts in an IgM-expressing B cell (depending on which cytokine is present, IL-4 or IFN-γ) and then to switch recombination and the production of IgE or IgG2a, respectively, with the same VDJ exon as that of the original IgM produced by that B cell. Knockout of the I exon or switch region for any heavy chain isotype leads to an inability to switch to that isotype.

The key enzyme known to be required for isotype switching and affinity maturation is **activation-induced deaminase (AID).** Humans with a deficiency of this enzyme develop a disease similar to the hyper-IgM syndrome caused by mutations in CD40L, and knockout mice lacking this enzyme have profound defects in isotype switching and affinity maturation. AID is a DNA deaminase that deaminates cytosines in single-stranded DNA templates converting C residues to uracil (U) residues (Fig. 10–15). The requirement for transcription at Ig loci for subsequent switching is linked to the generation of single-stranded DNA templates for AID. Transcription always results in a small single-stranded DNA bubble as the RNA polymerase complex slides down the coding strand. Since the DNA in the bubble is single stranded, AID can convert Cs to Us in the bubble region. More importantly switch transcripts tend to form very stable DNA-RNA hybrids involving the coding (top) strand of DNA, thus freeing up the bottom or nontemplate strand, which forms an open single-stranded DNA loop called an R loop. The R loop is where a large number of C residues in the switch DNA sequence are converted to U residues by AID. An enzyme called **uracil N-glycosylase** removes the U residues, leaving abasic sites. The **Ape1 endonuclease** cleaves these abasic sites, generating a nick at each position. Nicks on both strands contribute to double-strand breaks both at the Sμ region as well as at the downstream switch locus that is involved in a particular isotype switch event. The existence of double-strand breaks in two switch regions results in the deletion of the intervening DNA and joining together of the two broken switch junctions using the machinery involved in double-strand break repair/nonhomologous end joining. This latter machin-

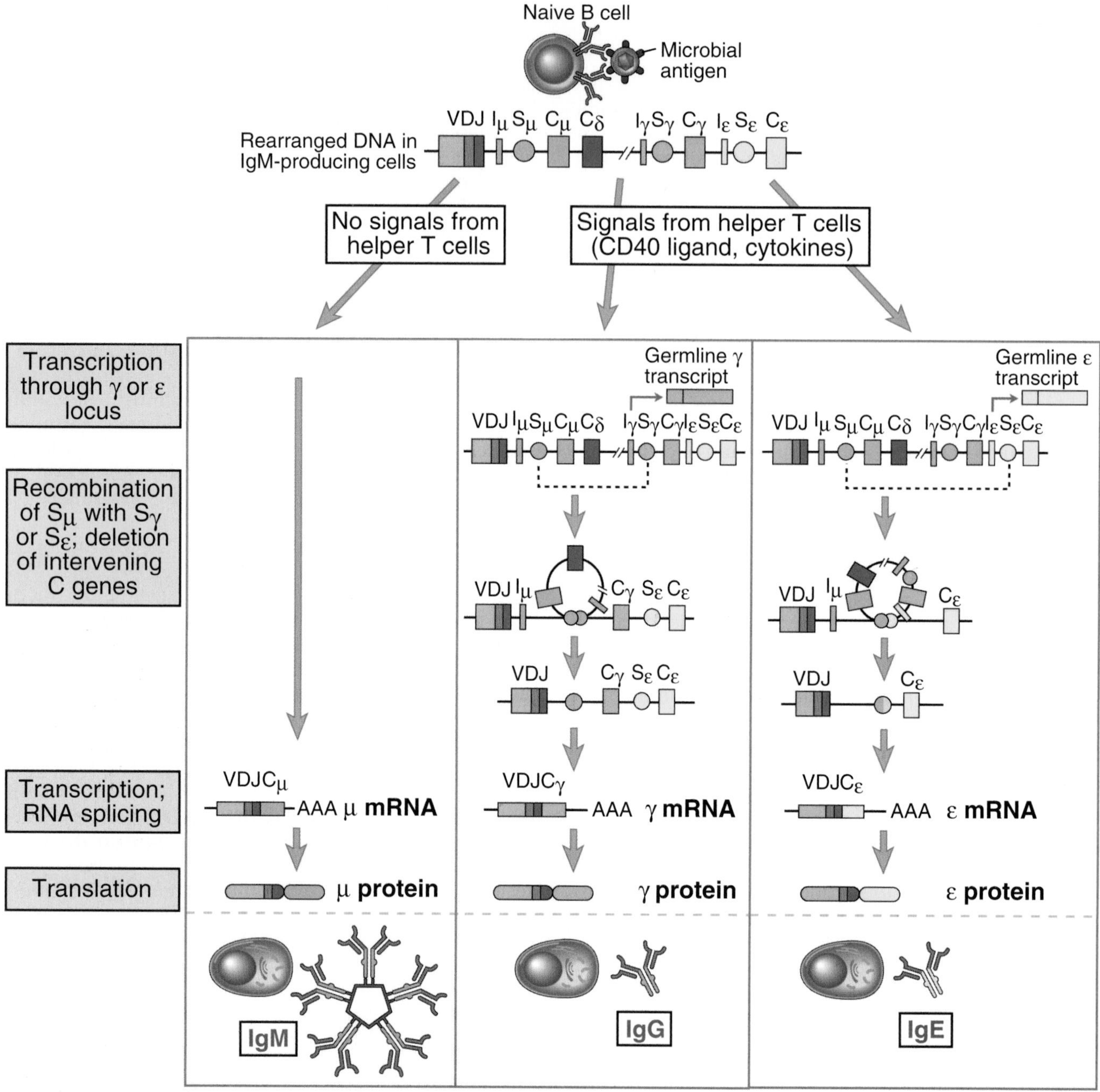

FIGURE 10–14 Molecular mechanisms of heavy chain isotype switching. In the absence of helper T cell signals, B cells produce IgM. When antigen-activated B cells encounter helper T cell signals (CD40L and, in this example, IL-4), the B cells undergo switching to other Ig isotypes (in this example, IgE). These stimuli initiate germline transcription through the $I_ε$-$S_ε$-$C_ε$ locus. The proximal C_H genes are deleted in a circle of DNA, leading to recombination of the VDJ complex with the $C_ε$ gene. Switch regions are indicated by circles labeled $S_μ$ or $S_γ$. $I_γ$ represents an initiation site for germline transcription. (Note that there are multiple $C_γ$ genes located between $C_δ$ and $C_ε$, but these are not shown.)

ery is also used to repair double-strand breaks during VDJ recombination.

Affinity Maturation: Somatic Mutations in Ig Genes and Selection of High-Affinity B Cells

Affinity maturation is the process that leads to increased affinity of antibodies for a particular antigen as a T-dependent humoral response progresses, and is the result of somatic mutation of Ig genes followed by selective survival of the B cells producing the antibodies with the highest affinities (Figs. 10–16 and 10–17). The process of affinity maturation generates antibodies with increasing capacity to bind antigens and thus to more efficiently bind to, neutralize, and eliminate microbes. Helper T cells and CD40:CD40L interactions are required for affinity maturation to proceed, and therefore affinity maturation occurs only in antibody responses to helper T cell–dependent protein antigens. As discussed earlier,

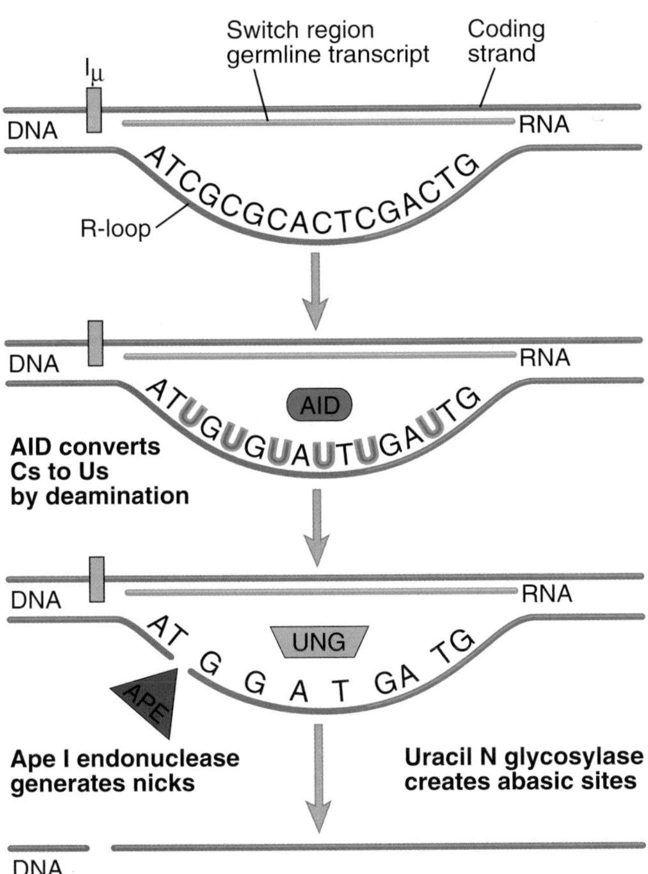

FIGURE 10–15 Mechanism by which AID and germline transcription collaborate to generate double-strand breaks at switch regions. Germline transcripts form DNA RNA hybrids in the switch region freeing up the nontemplate strand as an R-loop of single-stranded DNA. This is a particularly good template for AID, which deaminates C residues to generate U residues in single-stranded DNA. Uracil N-glycosylase (UNG) removes U residues to generate abasic sites that can be sites of nick generation following the action of the Ape I endonuclease. Two nicks roughly opposite each other contribute to a double-strand break. The mechanism of generation of the nick in the template strand is less well understood.

the need for CD40 reflects the ability of this receptor to induce AID in B cells when triggered.

In proliferating dark zone germinal center B cells, the Ig V genes undergo point mutations at an extremely high rate. This rate is estimated to be 1 in 10^3 V gene base pairs per cell division, which is 10^3 to 10^4 times higher than the spontaneous rate of mutation in other mammalian genes. (For this reason, mutation in Ig V genes is also called hypermutation.) The V genes of expressed heavy and light chains in each B cell contain a total of about 700 nucleotides; this implies that mutations will accumulate in expressed V regions at an average rate of almost one per cell division. Ig V gene mutations continue to occur in the progeny of individual B cells. As a result, any B cell clone can accumulate more and more mutations during its life in the germinal center. It is estimated that as a result of somatic mutations, the nucleotide sequences of IgG antibodies derived from one clone of B cells can diverge as much as 5% from the original germline sequence. This usually translates to up to 10 amino acid substitutions. The importance of somatic hypermutation in the process of affinity maturation is well established.

- Analysis of the Ig genes of B cell clones isolated at different stages of antibody responses to proteins or hapten-protein conjugates first showed the accumulation of point mutations in the V regions of the antibodies (Fig. 10–16). Several features of these mutations are noteworthy. First, the mutations are clustered in the V regions, mostly in the antigen-binding complementarity-determining regions. Second, there are more mutations in IgG than in IgM antibodies. Third, the presence of mutations correlates with the increasing affinities of the antibodies for the antigen that induced the response.
- Mutations in Ig genes were also found in clones of B cells isolated from germinal centers microdissected from the spleens of mice that had been immunized with an antigen. Analyses of these Ig genes showed that the progeny of a single antigen-specific B cell clone progressively accumulate mutations with time after immunization.

The mechanisms underlying somatic mutation in Ig genes are poorly understood. It is clear that the rearranged Ig VDJ DNA becomes highly susceptible to mutation, suggesting enhanced susceptibility of this region to DNA-binding factors that promote mutation. It is not known whether germinal center T cells provide specific contact-mediated signals or cytokines that stimulate somatic hypermutation in B cells. The enzyme AID, discussed above, plays an essential role in affinity maturation. It is a DNA deaminase that converts C residues to U residues at hotspots for mutation. The Us may be changed to Ts when DNA replication occurs, thus generating a common type of C $\rightarrow$ T mutation, or the U may be excised by uracil N-glycosylase, and the abasic site repaired by an error-prone repair process, thus generating all types of substitutions at each site of AID-induced cytidine deamination.

On the basis of the studies described, it is believed that repeated stimulation by T cell–dependent protein antigens leads to increasing numbers of mutations in the Ig genes of antigen-specific germinal center B cells. Some of these mutations are likely to be useful because they will generate high-affinity antibodies. However, many of the mutations may result in a decline or even in a loss of antigen binding. Therefore, the next and crucial step in the process of affinity maturation is the selection of the useful, high-affinity B cells.

FDCs in the germinal centers display antigens, and the B cells that bind these antigens with high affinity are selected to survive (see Fig. 10–17). The early response to antigen results in the production of antibodies, some of which form complexes with residual antigen and may activate complement. FDCs express receptors for the Fc portions of antibodies and for products of complement activation, including C3b and C3d. These receptors bind and display antigens that are complexed with antibodies or complement products. Antigen may also be dis-

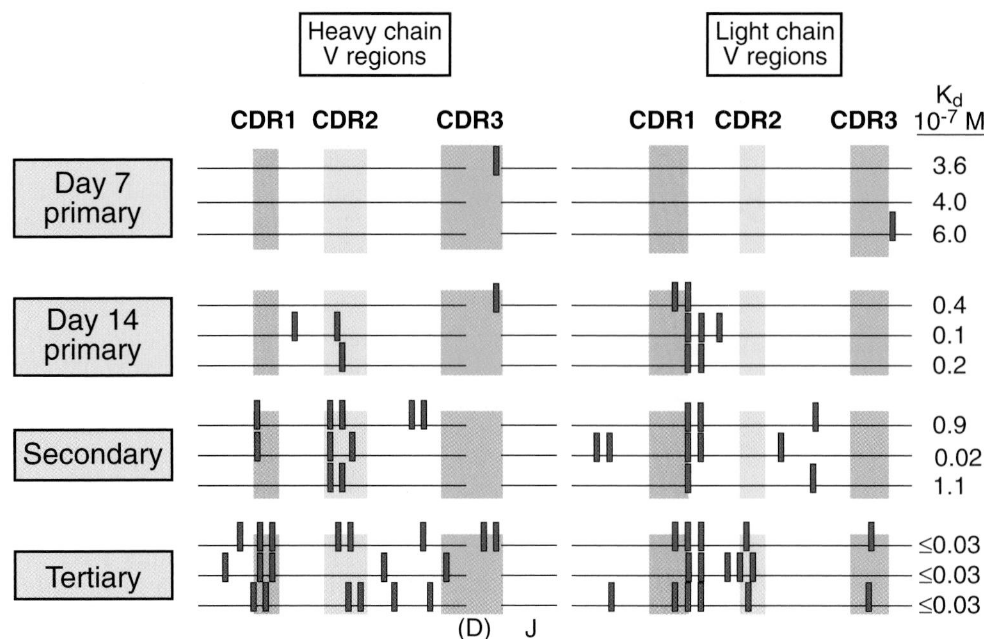

FIGURE 10–16 Somatic mutations in Ig V genes. Hybridomas were produced from spleen cells of mice immunized 7 or 14 days previously with a hapten, oxazolone, coupled to a protein, and from spleen cells obtained after secondary and tertiary immunizations with the same antigen. Hybridomas producing oxazolone-specific monoclonal antibodies were isolated, and the nucleotide sequences of the V genes encoding the Ig heavy and light chains were determined. Mutations in V genes increase with time after immunization and with repeated immunizations and are clustered in the complementarity-determining regions (CDRs). The location of CDR3 in the heavy chains is approximate. The affinities of the antibodies produced also tend to increase with more mutations, as indicated by the lower dissociation constants (K_d) for hapten binding. (Adapted from Berek C, and C Milstein. Mutation drift and repertoire shift in maturation of the immune response. Immunological Reviews 96:23–41, 1987, Blackwell Publishing.)

played in free form in the germinal center. Meanwhile, germinal center B cells that have undergone somatic hypermutation migrate into the FDC-rich light zone of the germinal center. These B cells die by apoptosis unless they are rescued by recognition of antigen. Therefore, the B cells that specifically recognize the antigen displayed by FDCs are selected to live. Helper T cells in the germinal center may also play a role in the selection of B cells. High-affinity B cells will be better able to bind antigens and present peptides to T cells, and will thus be the preferential recipients of T cell help. As more antibody is produced, more of the antigen is eliminated and less is available in the germinal centers. Therefore, the B cells that will be able to specifically bind this antigen and to be rescued from death need to express antigen receptors with higher and higher affinity for the antigen. As a result, as the antibody response to an antigen progresses, the B cells that are selected in germinal centers produce Ig of increasing affinity for the antigen. This selection process results in affinity maturation of the antibody response. Because somatic mutations also generate many B cells that do not express high-affinity receptors for antigen and cannot, therefore, be selected to survive, the germinal centers are sites of tremendous apoptosis.

Somatic mutation occurs in the basal dark zone of germinal centers in centroblasts that contain nuclear AID, and then mutated cells migrate from the basal dark zone to the apical light zone, where they differentiate into centrocytes, may be selected on FDCs, and may undergo additional isotype switching. The cells then exit the germinal center and either develop into memory B cells or differentiate into high-affinity antibody-secreting plasma cells outside the germinal centers.

B Cell Differentiation into Antibody-Secreting Plasma Cells

Some of the progeny of the B cells that have proliferated in response to antigen and T cell help differentiate into antibody-secreting plasma cells. Antibody synthesis and secretion in response to protein antigens, like B cell proliferation, are stimulated by CD40-mediated signals and cytokines. Both stimuli activate transcription factors that enhance the transcription of Ig genes and therefore Ig synthesis. Cytokines may also affect RNA processing to increase the amount of transcripts encoding the secretory form of Ig. Multiple cytokines, including IL-2, IL-4, and IL-6, have been shown to stimulate antibody synthesis and secretion by activated B lymphocytes.

Within lymphoid organs, antibody-secreting **plasma cells** are found mainly in extrafollicular sites, such as the red pulp of the spleen and the medulla of the lymph nodes. Plasma cells are morphologically distinct, terminally differentiated B cells committed to abundant antibody production (see Chapter 3). They are generated following the activation of B cells via the BCR, CD40, TLRs, and other receptors including cytokine receptors. Development of plasma cells depends on the induction of a key transcription factor called BLIMP-1 that orchestrates the process of differentiation. There are two types of plasma cells. Short-lived plasma cells are generated

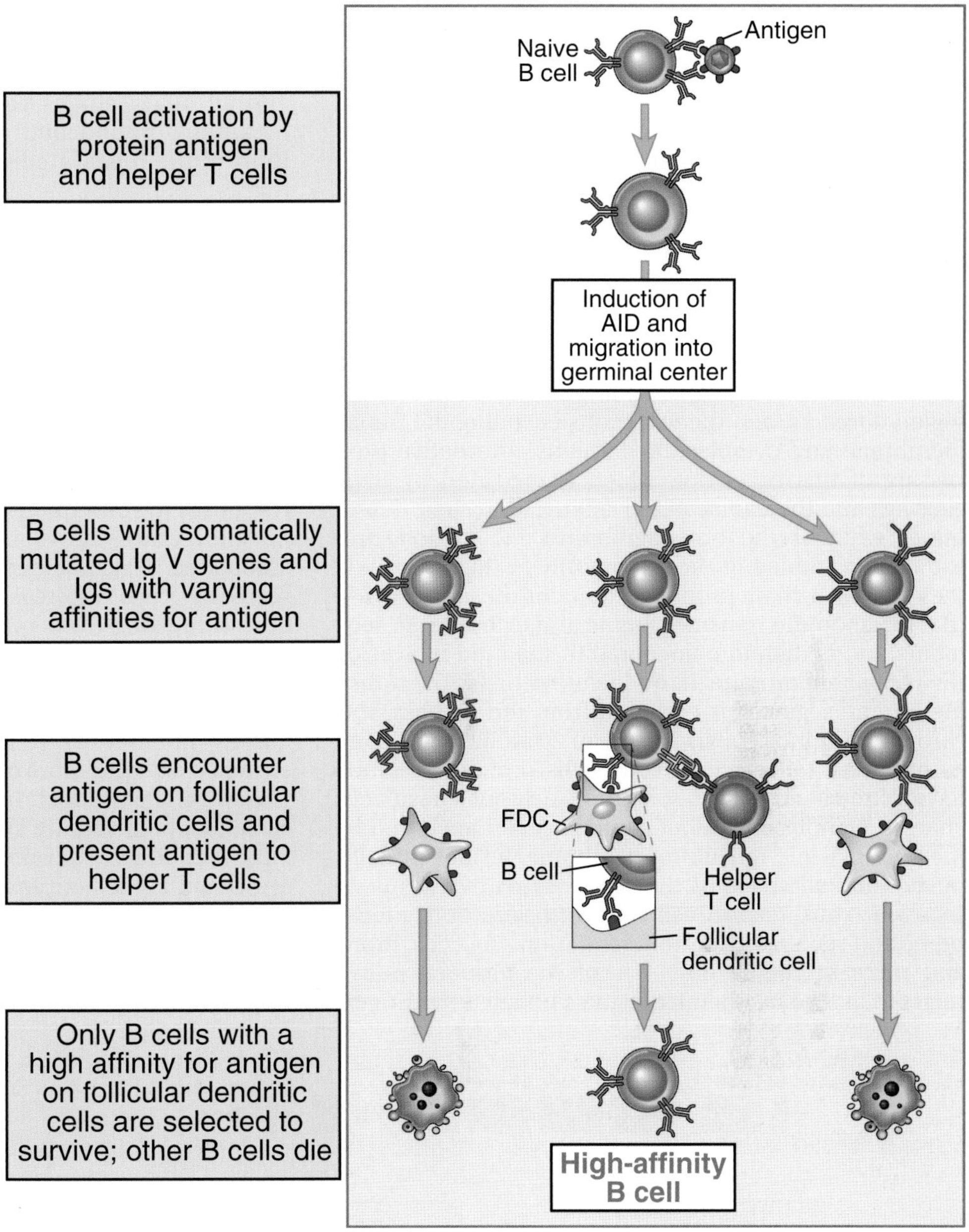

FIGURE 10–17 B cell selection in germinal centers. Somatic mutation of V region genes in germinal center B cells generates antibodies with different affinities for antigen. Subsequently, binding of the B cells to antigen displayed on follicular dendritic cells is necessary to rescue the B cells from programmed cell death. B cells may also present antigen to germinal center helper T cells, which may promote B cell survival (not shown). The B cells with the highest affinity for antigen will have a selective advantage for survival as the amount of available antigen decreases during an immune response. This leads to an average increase in the affinity of antibodies for antigen as the humoral immune response progresses.

during TI responses early during a T cell–dependent response in B cell foci such as the PALS foci described earlier. These cells are generally found in secondary lymphoid organs and in peripheral non-lymphoid tissues. Following the germinal center reaction, plasma cells acquire the ability to home to the bone marrow, where they are maintained via a receptor of the BAFF family called BCMA, and these plasma cells are called long-lived plasma cells. Typically 2 to 3 weeks after immunization with a T cell–dependent antigen, the bone marrow becomes a major site of antibody production. Plasma cells in the bone marrow may continue to secrete antibodies for months or even years after the antigen is no longer present. These antibodies can provide immediate protection if the antigen, such as a microbe, is encountered later. It is estimated that almost half the antibody in the blood of a healthy adult is produced by long-lived plasma cells and is specific for antigens that were encountered in the past. Secreted antibodies enter the circulation and mucosal secretions, but antibody-producing cells do not circulate.

The differentiation of B cells from antigen-recognizing cells that express membrane Ig receptors for antigens into effector cells that actively secrete antibodies involves major morphologic alterations, especially of components of the endoplasmic reticulum and secretory

pathway, and also involves a change in Ig heavy chain gene expression from the membrane to the secreted form. Membrane and secreted Ig molecules differ in their carboxyl termini (see Chapter 4, Fig. 4–6). For instance, in secreted IgM, the $C_\mu4$ domain is followed by a tail piece containing polar amino acids. In membrane μ, on the other hand, $C_\mu4$ is followed by a short spacer, 26 hydrophobic transmembrane residues, and a cytoplasmic tail of three amino acids (lysine, valine, and lysine). The transition from membrane to secreted Ig reflects a change in the processing of the heavy chain messenger RNA (mRNA). The primary RNA transcript in all IgM-producing B cells contains the rearranged VDJ cassette, the four C_μ exons coding for the constant (C) region domains, and the two exons encoding the transmembrane and cytoplasmic domains. Alternative processing of this transcript, which is regulated by RNA cleavage and the choice of polyadenylation sites, determines whether the transmembrane and cytoplasmic exons are included in the mature mRNA (Fig. 10–18). If they are, the μ chain produced contains the amino acids that make up the transmembrane and cytoplasmic segments and is therefore anchored in the lipid bilayer of the plasma membrane. If, on the other hand, the transmembrane segment is excluded from the μ chain, the carboxyl terminus consists of about 20 amino acids constituting the tail piece. Because this protein does not have a stretch of hydrophobic amino acids or a positively charged cytoplasmic tail, it cannot remain anchored in the endoplasmic reticulum membrane, resides initially in the luminal space of the secretory pathway, and is secreted. Thus, each B cell can synthesize both membrane and secreted Ig. As differentiation proceeds, more and more of the Ig mRNA is of the form encoding secreted Ig. The biochemical signals initiated by antigen binding to membrane Ig and by helper T cells that regulate this process of alternative RNA splicing are not known. All C_H genes contain similar membrane exons, and all heavy chains can apparently be expressed in membrane-bound and secreted forms. The secretory form of the δ heavy chain is rarely made, however, so that IgD is usually present only as a membrane-bound protein.

Generation of Memory B Cells and Secondary Humoral Immune Responses

Some of the antigen-activated B cells emerging from germinal centers acquire the ability to survive for long periods, apparently without antigenic stimulation. These are **memory cells,** capable of mounting rapid responses to subsequent introduction of antigen. We do not know exactly how some of the progeny of an antigen-stimulated B cell clone differentiate into antibody-secreting cells whereas others become functionally quiescent, long-lived memory cells. Some memory B cells may remain in the lymphoid organ whereas others exit germinal centers and recirculate between the spleen and lymph nodes. Memory cells typically bear high-affinity (mutated) antigen receptors and Ig molecules of switched isotypes more commonly than do naive B lymphocytes. The production of large quantities of isotype-switched, high-affinity antibodies is greatly accelerated after secondary exposure to antigens, and this can be attributed to the activation of memory cells in germinal centers and the rapid formation of immune complexes that can be concentrated by FDCs.

Many of the features of secondary antibody responses to protein antigens, and their differences from primary

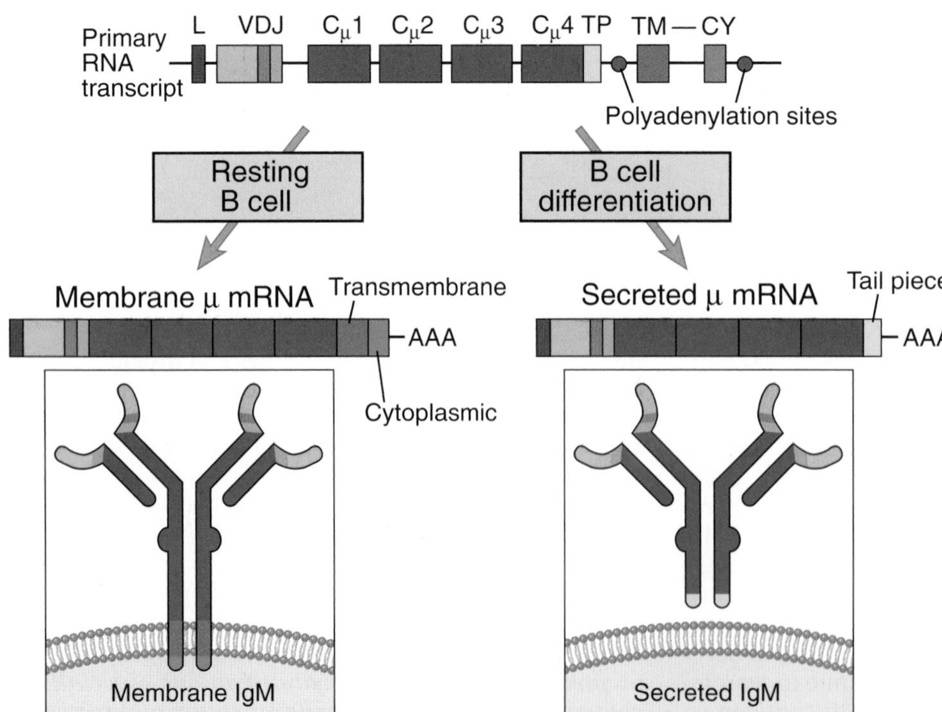

FIGURE 10–18 Production of membrane and secreted μ chains in B lymphocytes. Alternative processing of a primary RNA transcript results in the formation of mRNA for the membrane or secreted form of the μ heavy chain. B cell differentiation results in an increasing fraction of the μ protein produced as the secreted form. TP, TM, and CY refer to tail piece, transmembrane, and cytoplasmic segments, respectively. $C_\mu1$, $C_\mu2$, $C_\mu3$, and $C_\mu4$ are four exons of the C_μ gene.

responses (see Fig. 10–2), reflect the prior activation of B cells by $CD4^+$ helper T cells. Thus, heavy chain class switching, which is typical of secondary responses, is induced by helper T cells and their cytokines. Affinity maturation, which increases with repeated antigenic stimulation, is also secondary to helper T cell–induced B cell activation and somatic mutation. These features are usually seen in responses to protein antigens because only protein antigens stimulate specific helper T cells. High-affinity antibodies are required to neutralize the infectivity of many microbes and the pathogenicity of microbial toxins. Therefore, effective vaccines against these microorganisms must induce affinity maturation and memory B cell formation, and both these events will occur only if the vaccines are able to activate helper T cells. This concept has been applied to the design of vaccines for some bacterial infections in which the target antigen is a capsular polysaccharide, which is incapable of stimulating T cells. In these cases, the polysaccharide is covalently linked to a foreign protein to form the equivalent of a hapten-carrier conjugate, which does activate helper T cells. Such vaccines, which are called **conjugate vaccines,** more readily induce high-affinity antibodies and memory than do polysaccharide vaccines without linked proteins.

ANTIBODY RESPONSES TO T CELL–INDEPENDENT ANTIGENS

Many nonprotein antigens, such as polysaccharides and lipids, stimulate antibody production in the absence of helper T cells, and these antigens and the responses they elicit are termed thymus-independent or T-independent. These antibody responses differ in several respects from responses to T cell–dependent protein antigens (Table 10–2). As we have discussed in the previous sections, antibody responses to protein antigens require the participation of helper T cells, and helper T cells stimulate isotype switching, affinity maturation, and long-lived memory. In contrast, the antibodies that are produced in the absence of T cell help are generally of low affinity and consist mainly of IgM with limited isotype switching to some IgG subtypes.

The most important TI antigens are polysaccharides, membrane glycolipids, and nucleic acids, all of which induce specific antibody production in T cell–deficient

Table 10–2. Properties of Thymus-Dependent and Thymus-Independent Antigens

	Thymus-dependent antigen	Thymus-independent antigen
Chemical nature	Proteins	Polymeric antigens, especially polysaccharides; also glycolipids, nucleic acids
Features of anitbody response		
Isotype switching	Yes (IgM → IgG, IgE, IgA)	Little or no: may be some IgG (IgM, IgG)
Affinity maturation	Yes	No
Secondary response (memory B cells)	Yes	Only seen with some antigens (e.g., polysaccharides)

animals. These antigens cannot be processed and presented in association with MHC molecules, and therefore they cannot be recognized by helper T cells. Most TI antigens are polyvalent, being composed of multiple identical antigenic epitopes. Such polyvalent antigens may induce maximal cross-linking of the BCR complex on specific B cells, leading to activation without a requirement for cognate T cell help. In addition, many polysaccharides activate the complement system by the alternative pathway, generating C3d, which binds to the antigen and augments B cell activation (see Fig. 10–5). B cell responses to TI antigens also depend on additional signals from BAFF family receptors that respond to growth factors produced by DCs and macrophages, and from TLRs.

Antibody responses to TI antigens occur at particular anatomic sites in lymphoid tissues. TI responses may be initiated in the spleen, bone marrow, peritoneal cavity, and mucosal sites. Macrophages located in the marginal zones surrounding lymphoid follicles in the spleen are particularly efficient at trapping polysaccharides when these antigens are injected intravenously. **Marginal zone B cells** are a distinct subset of B cells that mainly respond to polysaccharides and produce IgM following activation and differentiation into short-lived plasma cells. TI antigens may persist for prolonged periods on the surfaces of marginal zone macrophages, where they are recognized by specific B cells. Another lineage of B cells that responds readily to TI antigens is the **B-1 B cell** lineage. Most B-1 B cells are derived from fetal liver stem cells and are exposed to antigen mainly in the peritoneum and in mucosal sites.

The practical significance of TI antigens is that many bacterial cell wall polysaccharides belong to this category, and humoral immunity is the major mechanism of host defense against infections by such encapsulated bacteria. For this reason, individuals with congenital or acquired deficiencies of humoral immunity are especially susceptible to life-threatening infections with encapsulated bacteria, such as *Pneumococcus, Meningococcus,* and *Haemophilus.* In addition, TI antigens contribute to the generation of **natural antibodies,** which are present in the circulation of normal individuals and are apparently produced without overt exposure to pathogens. Most natural antibodies are low-affinity anti-carbohydrate antibodies, postulated to be produced by B-1 peritoneal B cells stimulated by bacteria that colonize the gastrointestinal tract and by marginal zone B cells in the spleen. Antibodies to the A and B glycolipid blood group antigens are examples of these natural antibodies.

Some T cell-independent nonprotein antigens do induce Ig isotypes other than IgM. In humans, the dominant antibody class induced by pneumococcal capsular polysaccharide is IgG2. In mice engineered to lack CD40, IgE and many IgG isotypes are barely detectable in the serum, but IgG3 (which resembles human IgG2) and IgA levels in serum are only reduced to about half their normal levels. In the absence of T cells, BAFF and APRIL on cells of myeloid origin, such as DCs and macrophages, can induce the synthesis of AID in antigen-activated B cells. This may be further facilitated by the activation of TLRs on these B cells. In addition, cytokines such as TGF-β that help mediate the IgA switch are secreted by many nonlymphoid cells at mucosal sites and may contribute to the generation of IgA antibodies directed against non-protein antigens.

Despite their inability to specifically activate helper T cells, many polysaccharide vaccines, such as the pneumococcal vaccine, induce long-lived protective immunity. Rapid and large secondary responses typical of memory (but without much isotype switching or affinity maturation) do occur on secondary exposure to these carbohydrate antigens. The phenomenon of IgM memory has been clearly demonstrated in the mouse, and in both mice and humans TI memory B cells can be phenotypically defined by specific cell surface markers. In humans these memory cells express high levels of CD27 and IgM or IgD, whereas in mice peritoneal IgM memory cells, also known as B-1b B cells, express high levels of IgM and the Mac-1 integrin.

Antibody Feedback: Regulation of Humoral Immune Responses by Fc Receptors

Secreted antibodies inhibit continuing B cell activation by forming antigen-antibody complexes that simultaneously bind to antigen receptors and Fcγ receptors on antigen-specific B cells (Fig. 10–19). This is the explanation for a phenomenon called **antibody feedback**, which refers to the down-regulation of antibody production by secreted IgG antibodies. IgG antibodies inhibit B cell activation by forming complexes with the antigen, and these complexes bind to a B cell receptor for the Fc portions of the IgG, called the Fcγ receptor II (FcγRIIB, or CD32). (The biology of Fc receptors is discussed in Chapter 14.) The cytoplasmic domain of FcγRIIB contains a six–amino acid (isoleucine-x-tyrosine-x-x-leucine) motif shared by other receptors in the immune system that mediate negative signals, including inhibitory receptors on NK cells (see Chapter 2). By analogy to ITAMs, this inhibitory motif is called the immunoreceptor tyrosine-based inhibition motif (ITIM). When the Fcγ receptor of B cells is engaged, the ITIM of the receptor is phosphorylated on tyrosine residues, and it forms a docking site for the inositol 5-phosphatase SHIP (SH2 domain-containing inositol phosphatase). The recruited SHIP hydrolyses a phosphate on the signaling lipid intermediate PIP_3. By this mechanism, engagement of FcγRII terminates the B cell response to antigen. The antigen-antibody complexes simultaneously interact with the antigen receptor (through the antigen) and the FcγRIIB (through the antibody), and this brings the inhibitory phosphatases close to the antigen receptors whose signaling is blocked.

Fc receptor–mediated antibody feedback is a physiologic control mechanism in humoral immune responses because it is triggered by secreted antibody and blocks further antibody production. We have stated earlier in

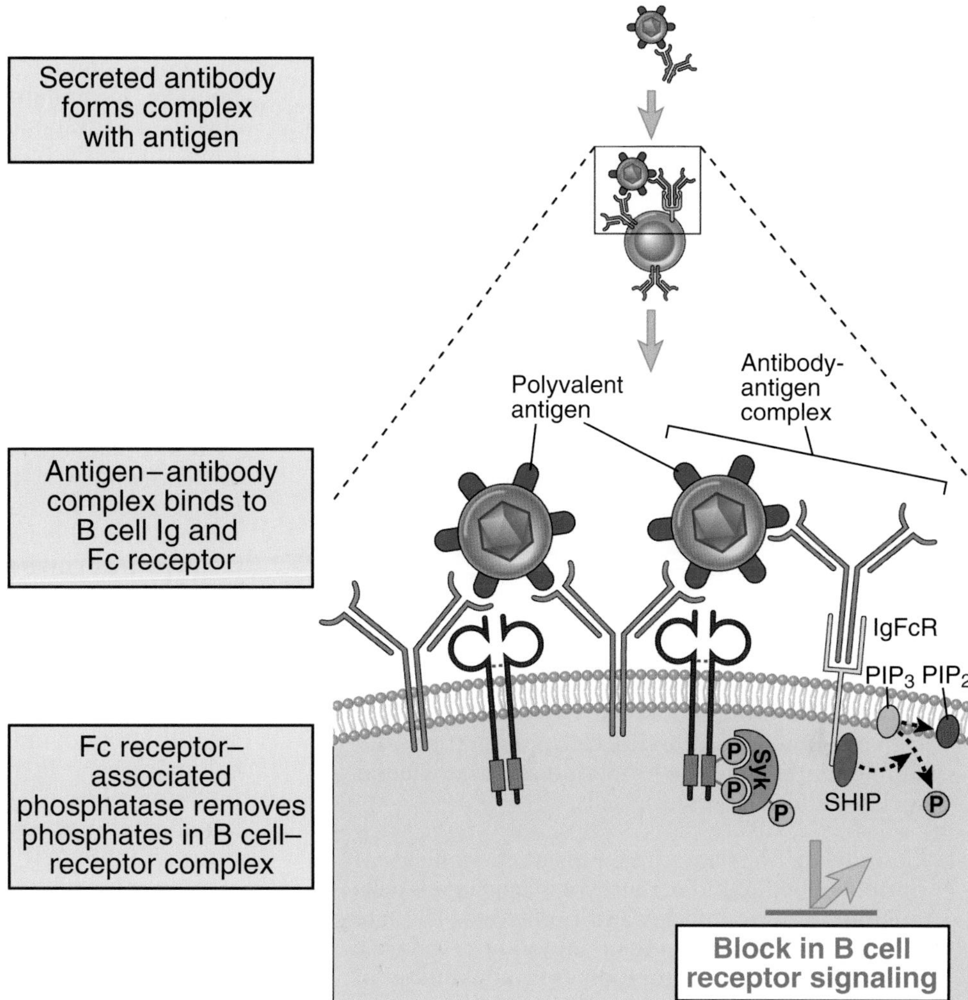

Secreted antibody forms complex with antigen
Antigen–antibody complex binds to B cell Ig and Fc receptor
Fc receptor–associated phosphatase removes phosphates in B cell–receptor complex
Polyvalent antigen
Antibody-antigen complex
IgFcR
PIP3 PIP2
Syk
P
SHIP
Block in B cell receptor signaling

FIGURE 10–19 Regulation of B cell activation by Ig Fc receptors. Antigen-antibody complexes can simultaneously bind to membrane Ig (through antigen) and the FcγRIIB receptor through the Fc portion of the antibody. As a consequence of this simultaneous ligation of receptors, phosphatases associated with the cytoplasmic tail of the FcγRIIB inhibit signaling by the BCR complex and block B cell activation.

the chapter that antibodies can also amplify antibody production by activating complement and generating C3d. It is not clear under which circumstances secreted antibodies provide complement-mediated amplification or Fc receptor–mediated inhibition. A likely scenario is that early in humoral immune responses, IgM antibodies (which activate complement but do not bind to the Fcγ receptor) are involved in amplification, whereas increasing production of IgG leads to feedback inhibition.

The importance of FcγRIIB mediated inhibition is demonstrated by the uncontrolled antibody production seen in mice in which the gene encoding this receptor has been knocked out. A polymorphism in the *FcγRIIB* gene has been linked to susceptibility to systemic lupus erythematosus (SLE) in humans. Also, intraveous immunoglobulin (IVIG) is a treatment for various inflammatory diseases that was devleoped empirically. It is postulated now that at high concentrations, the administered antibodies, which contain substantial amounts of aggregated IgG, engage FcγRIIB on B cells sufficiently to deliver inhibitory signals.

B cells express another inhibitory receptor called CD22. CD22 is an α2,6 sialic acid-binding lectin; its natural ligand is not known, and we do not know how it is engaged during physiologic B cell responses. However, knockout mice lacking CD22 show greatly enhanced B cell activation, as do mice in which CD22 has been mutated so that it can no longer bind α2,6 sialic acid–containing ligands. The cytoplasmic tail of this molecule contains an ITIM, which, when phosphorylated, binds the SH2 domain of the SHP-1 tyrosine phosphatase. SHP-1 removes phosphates from the tyrosine residues of the Igα and Igβ ITAMs and thus abrogates BCR signaling. A mouse strain called *motheaten,* which develops severe autoimmunity with uncontrolled B cell activation and autoantibody production, has a naturally occurring mutation in SHP-1.

SUMMARY

- In humoral immune responses, B lymphocytes are activated by antigen and secrete antibodies that act to eliminate the antigen. Both protein and nonprotein antigens can stimulate antibody responses. B cell responses to protein antigens require the contribution of $CD4^+$ helper T cells specific for the antigen.

- B cell activation is initiated by the clustering of antigen receptors (membrane IgM and IgD on naive B cells) by the binding of multivalent antigen. Membrane Ig-associated signaling molecules Igα and Igβ transduce signals on antigen binding to the Ig, and these signals lead to activation of transcription factors and expression of various genes.

- Helper T cell–dependent B cell responses to protein antigens require initial activation of naive T cells in the T cell zones and of B cells in lymphoid follicles in lymphoid organs. The activated lymphocytes migrate toward one another and interact at the edges of follicles, where the B cells present the antigen to helper T cells.

- Activated helper T cells express CD40L, which engages CD40 on the B cells, and the T cells secrete cytokines that bind to cytokine receptors on the B cells. The combination of CD40 and cytokine signals stimulates initial B cell proliferation and differentiation and the formation of extrafollicular foci of antibody-secreting cells.

- Germinal centers are formed inside the follicles of peripheral lymphoid organs when activated B cells migrate into the follicles and proliferate. The late events in T cell–dependent antibody responses, including affinity maturation and generation of memory B cells, as well as extensive isotype switching, take place within germinal centers.

- Helper T cell–derived signals, including CD40L and cytokines, induce isotype switching in B cells by a process of switch recombination, leading to the production of various Ig isotypes. Isotype switching requires the induction of AID, a cytidine deaminase that converts cytosine to uracil in single-stranded DNA, and different cytokines allow AID to access distinct downstream heavy chain loci. Different isotypes mediate different effector functions.

- Affinity maturation leads to increased affinity of antibodies during the course of a T cell–dependent humoral response. Affinity maturation is a result of somatic hypermutation of Ig heavy and light chain genes followed by selective survival of the B cells that produce the high-affinity antibodies and bind to antigen displayed by FDCs in the germinal centers.

- Some of the progeny of germinal center B cells differentiate into antibody-secreting plasma cells that migrate to extrafollicular regions of secondary lymphoid organs and to the bone marrow. Other progeny become memory B cells that live for long periods, recirculate between lymph nodes and spleen, and respond rapidly to subsequent exposures to antigen by differentiating into high-affinity antibody secretors.

- TI antigens are nonprotein antigens that induce humoral immune responses without the involvement of helper T cells. Many TI antigens, including polysaccharides, membrane glycolipids, and nucleic acids, are polyvalent, can cross-link multiple membrane Ig molecules on a B cell, and activate complement, thereby activating the B cells without T cell help. TI antigens stimulate antibody responses in which there is limited or no heavy chain class switching, affinity maturation, or memory B cell generation because these features are dependent on helper T cells, which are not activated by nonprotein antigens.

- Antibody feedback is a mechanism by which humoral immune responses are down-regulated when enough antibody has been produced and soluble antibody-antigen complexes are present. B cell membrane Ig and the receptor on B cells for the Fc portions of IgG, called FcγRIIB, are clustered together by antibody-antigen complexes. This activates an inhibitory signaling cascade through the cytoplasmic tail of FcγRIIB that terminates the activation of the B cell.

Selected Readings

Batista FD and NE Harwood. The who, how and where of antigen presentation to B cells. Nature Reviews Immunology 9:15–27, 2009.

Calame KL, K-I Lin, and C Tunyaplin. Regulatory mechanisms that determine the development and function of plasma cells. Annual Review of Immunology 21:205–230, 2003.

Carroll MC. The complement system in B cell regulation. Molecular Immunology 41:141–146, 2004.

Cerutti A. The regulation of IgA class switching. Nature Reviews Immunology 8:421–434, 2008.

Chaudhuri J, and FW Alt. Class-switch recombination: interplay of transcription, DNA deamination and DNA repair. Nature Reviews Immunology 4:541–552, 2004.

DeFranco AL. B-cell activation 2000. Immunological Reviews 176:5–9, 2000.

De Villartay JP, A Fischer, and A Durandy. The mechanisms of immune diversification and their disorders. Nature Reviews Immunology 3:962–972, 2003.

Hardy RR. B-1 B cell development. Journal of Immunology 176:2749–2754, 2006.

Harwood NE, and FD Batista. New insights into the early molecular events underlying B cell activation. Immunity 28:609–619, 2008.

Honjo T, H Nagaoka, R Shinkura, and M Muramatsu. AID to overcome the limitations of genomic information. Nature Immunology 6:655–661, 2005.

Kurosaki T. Regulation of B cell signal transduction by adapter proteins. Nature Reviews Immunology 2:354–363, 2002.

Manz RA, AE Hauser, F Hiepe, and A Radbruch. Maintenance of serum antibody levels. Annual Review of Immunology 23:367–386, 2005.

Martin F, and AC Chan. B cell immunobiology in disease: evolving concept from the clinic. Annual Review of Immunology 24:467–496, 2006.

McHeyzer-Williams LJ, and MG McHeyzer-Williams. Antigen-specific memory B cell development. Annual Review of Immunology 23:487–513, 2005.

Mills DM, and JC Cambier. B lymphocyte interactions during cognate interactions with $CD4^+$ T lymphocytes: molecular dynamics and immunological consequences. Seminars in Immunology 15:325–329, 2003.

Neuberger MS, RS Harris, J Di Noia, and SK Petersen-Mahrt. Immunity through DNA deamination. Trends in Biochemical Sciences 28:305–312, 2003.

Peled JU, FL Kuang, MD Iglesias-Ussel, S Roa, SL Kalis, MF Goodman, and MD Scharff. The biochemistry of somatic hypermutation. Annual Review of Immunology 26:481–511, 2008.

Pierce SK. Lipid rafts and B cell activation. Nature Reviews Immunology 2:96–105, 2002.

Radbruch A et al. Competence and competition: the challenge of becoming a long-lived plasma cell. Nature Reviews Immunology 6:741–750, 2006.

Ravetch JV, and LL Lanier. Immune inhibitory receptors. Science 290:84–89, 2000.

Stavnezer J, JE Guikema, and CE Schrader. Mechanism and regulation of class switch recombination. Annual Review of Immunology 26:261–292, 2008.

Chapter 11

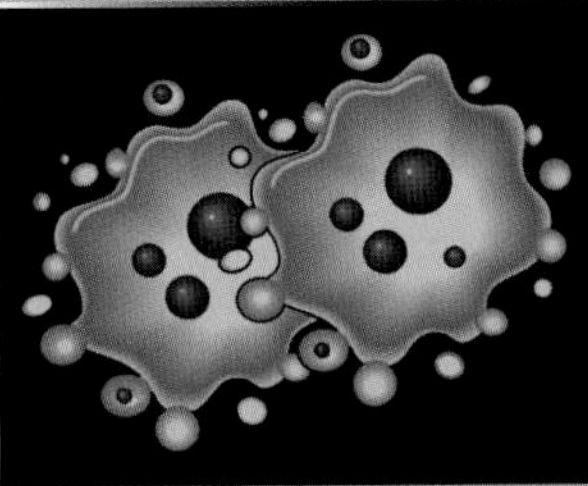

IMMUNOLOGICAL TOLERANCE

Immunological tolerance is defined as unresponsiveness to an antigen that is induced by previous exposure to that antigen. When specific lymphocytes encounter antigens, the lymphocytes may be activated, leading to immune responses, or the cells may be inactivated or eliminated, leading to tolerance. Different forms of the same antigen may induce an immune response or tolerance. Antigens that induce tolerance are called **tolerogens,** or tolerogenic antigens, to distinguish them from immunogens, which generate immunity. A single antigen may be an immunogen or a tolerogen depending on how it is recognized by specific lymphocytes. Tolerance to self antigens, also called **self-tolerance,** is a fundamental property of the normal immune system. In this chapter, we discuss immunological tolerance mainly in the context of self-tolerance and summarize how self-tolerance may fail. We also mention the relevance of this phenomenon to unresponsiveness to foreign antigens. We conclude with a discussion of the mechanisms by which normal immune responses are terminated.

Immunological tolerance is important for several reasons:

- ***Normal individuals are tolerant of their own (self) antigens because the lymphocytes that recognize self antigens are killed or inactivated, or change their specificity*** (Fig. 11–1). All individuals inherit essentially the same antigen receptor genes, and these genes recombine and are expressed in lymphocytes as the lymphocytes arise from stem cells. The molecular mechanisms that produce functional antigen receptor genes from germline sequences are random and are not influenced by what is foreign or self for each individual. It is not surprising that during this process of generating a diverse repertoire, some developing T and B cells in every individual may express receptors capable of recognizing normal molecules in that individual, i.e., self antigens. Therefore, there is a risk for lymphocytes reacting against that individual's cells and tissues, and causing damage. The mechanisms of immunologic tolerance are designed to prevent such reactions.

The importance of self-tolerance for the health of individuals was appreciated from the early days of immunology. In Chapter 1, we introduced the concept of self-nonself discrimination, which is the ability of the immune system to recognize and respond to foreign antigens but not to self antigens. Burnet added to his clonal selection hypothesis the corollary that lymphocytes specific for self antigens are eliminated to prevent immune reactions against one's own antigens. As we shall see later in this chapter, self-tolerance is maintained by several different mechanisms that prevent the maturation and activation of potentially harmful self-reactive lymphocytes. Failure of self-tolerance results in immune reactions against self (autologous) antigens. Such reactions are called autoimmunity, and the diseases they cause are called autoimmune diseases. The pathogenesis and clinicopathologic features of autoimmune diseases will be discussed in Chapter 18.

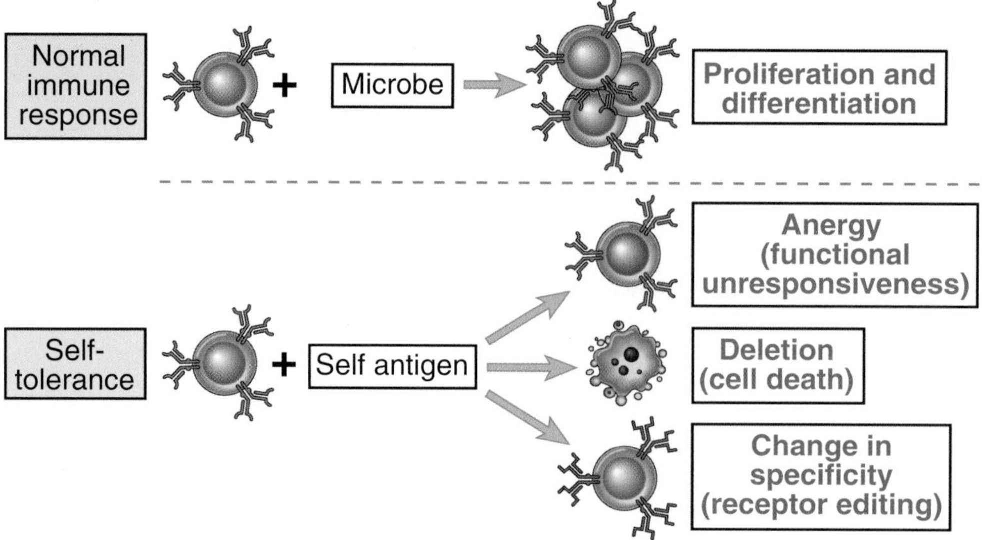

FIGURE 11–1 Fates of lymphocytes after encounter with antigens. In a normal immune response, microbes stimulate the proliferation and differentiation of antigen-specific lymphocytes. (Microbial antigens are typically recognized by lymphocytes in the presence of costimulators and innate immune responses, which are not shown.) Self antigens may induce functional unresponsiveness or death of antigen-specific lymphocytes or a change in the specificity of the receptors, making these cells incapable of responding to the antigen (self-tolerance). Some antigens elicit no response (ignorance), but the lymphocytes are able to respond to subsequent antigen challenge (not shown). This illustration depicts B lymphocytes; the same general principles apply to T lymphocytes.

Defining the mechanisms of self-tolerance is the key to understanding the mechanisms of autoimmunity.

- ***Foreign antigens may be administered in ways that inhibit immune responses by inducing tolerance in specific lymphocytes.*** Some microbes and tumors may evade immune attack by inducing unresponsiveness in specific lymphocytes. Many of the mechanisms of tolerance to foreign antigens are similar to those of self-tolerance in mature lymphocytes. Effective immunization methods are designed to enhance the immunogenicity of antigens by administering them in ways that promote lymphocyte activation and prevent tolerance induction.

- ***The induction of immunological tolerance may be exploited as a therapeutic approach for preventing harmful immune responses.*** A great deal of effort is being devoted to the development of strategies for inducing tolerance to treat autoimmune and allergic diseases and to prevent the rejection of organ transplants. Tolerance induction may also be useful for preventing immune reactions to the products of newly expressed genes in gene therapy protocols and preventing reactions to injected proteins in patients with deficiencies of these proteins (e.g., hemophiliacs treated with factor VIII).

General Features and Mechanisms of Immunological Tolerance

There are several characteristics of self-tolerance in T and B lymphocyte populations, and many of these are also features of tolerance to foreign antigens.

- ***Tolerance results from the recognition of antigens by specific lymphocytes.*** The key advances that allowed immunologists to study tolerance were the ability to induce this phenomenon in animals by exposure to defined antigens under various conditions, and later to analyze the functions of the lymphocytes that had encountered tolerogenic antigens. The earliest studies of tolerance showed that it could be induced by recognition of antigens during fetal or neonatal life. These initial studies also demonstrated that the phenomenon of tolerance exhibited one of the main characteristics of lymphocytes, namely specificity for antigens.

  - The results that definitively established tolerance as an immunologically specific phenomenon that could be induced experimentally came from studies of graft rejection in inbred mice done by Peter Medawar and colleagues in the 1950s. An adult mouse of strain A will reject a skin graft from an allogeneic mouse of strain B that differs from strain A at the major histocompatibility complex (MHC). If the strain A mouse is injected with blood cells of strain B during neonatal life (the blood cells serving as a source of strain B antigens), the injected cells will not be rejected (because the neonate is immunodeficient), and small numbers will survive indefinitely in the recipient, which now becomes a chimera. This strain A recipient will accept a graft from strain B even after it becomes an adult. However, the strain A recipient will reject skin grafts from all mouse strains whose MHC is different from that of strain B. Thus, tolerance to the graft is immunologically specific. Such experiments led to the concept that exposure of developing lymphocytes to foreign antigens induces tolerance to these antigens. The persistence of allogeneic lymphoid cells in a host is called hematopoietic microchimerism, and it is being studied as a possible approach for preventing graft rejection in humans. The mechanism of this form of tolerance remains poorly defined.

- ***Self-tolerance may be induced in immature self-reactive lymphocytes in generative lymphoid organs (central tolerance), or in mature lymphocytes in peripheral sites (peripheral tolerance)*** (Fig. 11–2). Central tolerance ensures that the repertoire of mature lymphocytes cannot recognize self antigens that are present in the generative lymphoid organs (the thymus for T cells and the bone marrow for B lymphocytes, also called "central" lymphoid organs). Such antigens include ubiquitous, or widely disseminated, self antigens as well as some peripheral tissue antigens that are expressed in generative lymphoid organs, specifically the thymus. However, central tolerance cannot account for unresponsiveness to antigens that are expressed only in peripheral tissues. Tolerance to such tissue-specific self antigens is maintained by peripheral mechanisms.

- ***Central tolerance occurs because during their maturation in the generative lymphoid organs, all lymphocytes pass through a stage in which encounter with antigen leads to cell death or the expression of new antigen receptors or a change in functional capabilities.*** The only antigens normally present in the thymus and bone marrow are self antigens because foreign antigens that enter from the external environment are not transported to the thymus but rather are captured and transported to peripheral lymphoid organs, such as the lymph nodes, spleen, and mucosal lymphoid tissues. Therefore, in the generative lymphoid organs, developing lymphocytes normally encounter only self antigens at high concentrations. This interaction of immature lymphocytes with self antigens has several possible outcomes—the cells may die by apoptosis (called

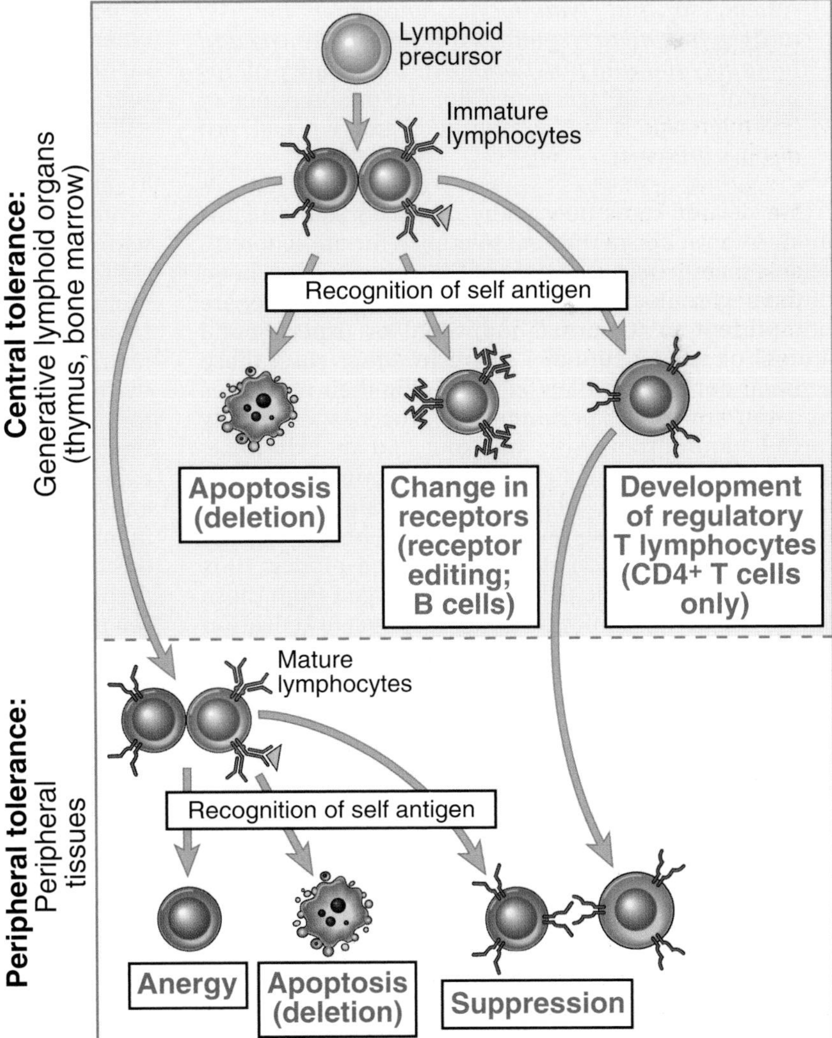

FIGURE 11–2 Central and peripheral tolerance to self antigens. Immature lymphocytes specific for self antigens may encounter these antigens in the generative lymphoid organs and are deleted, change their specificity (B cells only), or (in the case of $CD4^+$ T cells) develop into regulatory lymphocytes (central tolerance). Some self-reactive lymphocytes may mature and enter peripheral tissues and may be inactivated or deleted by encounter with self antigens in these tissues, or are suppressed by the regulatory T cells (peripheral tolerance). (Note that T cells recognize antigens presented by antigen-presenting cells, which are not shown.)

clonal deletion, see Chapter 8); many immature B cells do not die but change their receptors and stop recognizing the self antigen (called **receptor editing**); and some CD4⁺ T cells differentiate into **regulatory T cells,** which migrate to the periphery and prevent responses to the self antigens (see Fig. 11–2). Both clonal deletion and receptor editing represent mechanisms of negative selection during lymphocyte development.

- ***Peripheral tolerance occurs when mature lymphocytes that recognize self antigens become incapable of responding to that antigen, or lose their viability and become short-lived cells, or are induced to die by apoptosis.*** Peripheral tolerance is most important for maintaining unresponsiveness to self antigens that are expressed in peripheral tissues and not in the generative lymphoid organs, and for tolerance to self antigens that are expressed in adult life, after mature lymphocytes have been generated. The mature lymphocyte repertoire contains cells capable of recognizing such self antigens, and the responses of the mature lymphocytes to these antigens are tightly regulated to maintain self-tolerance.
- ***Some self antigens may be ignored by the immune system, so that lymphocytes encounter the self antigen but fail to respond in any detectable way and remain viable and functional.*** The importance of this phenomenon of "ignorance" for the maintenance of self-tolerance is not established, and we will not discuss it further.

We do not know how many or which self antigens induce central or peripheral tolerance (or are ignored). This is mainly because study of self-tolerance has been difficult; lymphocytes specific for self antigens either are not present in a normal individual or experimental animal or are functionally silent. In either case, these cells cannot be identified by examining their responses to a self antigen. Experimental approaches, especially the creation of transgenic knockout and knockin mice, and the identification of genes that are mutated in some autoimmune diseases, have provided valuable models for analyzing self-tolerance, and many of our current concepts are based on studies with such models (Box 11–1). A general principle that has emerged from these studies is that the choice between lymphocyte activation and tolerance is determined by the properties of the antigens, by the state of maturation of the antigen-specific lymphocytes, and by the types of stimuli received when these lymphocytes encounter self antigens. In the sections that follow, we will discuss central and peripheral tolerance first in T cells and then in B lymphocytes, but many aspects of the processes are common to both lineages.

T Lymphocyte Tolerance

Tolerance in CD4⁺ helper T lymphocytes is an effective way of preventing immune responses to protein antigens because helper T cells are necessary inducers of both cell-mediated and humoral immune responses to proteins. This realization has been the impetus for a large amount of work on the mechanisms of tolerance in CD4⁺ T cells. Immunologists have also developed experimental models for studying tolerance in CD4⁺ T cells that have proved to be quite informative. Also, many of the therapeutic strategies that are being developed to induce tolerance to transplants and autoantigens are targeted to these T cells. Much less is known about tolerance in CD8⁺ T cells.

Central Tolerance in T Cells

During their maturation in the thymus, many immature T cells that recognize antigens with high avidity are deleted (Fig. 11–3). This process of deletion, or negative selection, of T lymphocytes was described in Chapter 8, when the maturation of T cells in the thymus was discussed. The two main factors that determine if a particular self antigen will induce negative selection of self-reactive thymocytes are the concentration of that antigen in the thymus and the affinity of the thymocyte T cell receptors (TCRs) that recognize the antigen. Self proteins are processed and presented in association with MHC molecules on thymic antigen-presenting cells (APCs). The self antigens that are present in the thymus include many circulating and cell-associated proteins. In addition, some proteins that were thought to be restricted to peripheral tissues are also expressed in thymic epithelial cells under the control of the autoimmune regulator *(AIRE)* gene (see later). The AIRE protein may function as a transcription factor to promote the expression of selected tissue antigens in the thymus and/or to stimulate production of proteins that are involved in the presentation of these antigens. Among the immature T cells that arise from precursors in the thymus are some whose receptors specifically recognize self peptide–MHC complexes with high affinity. If immature thymocytes with such high-affinity receptors encounter self antigens in the thymus, one result is apoptotic death of the cells. Deletion may occur in double-positive T cells in the thymic cortex or newly generated single-positive cells in the medulla. The death sensitivity of immature lymphocytes suggests that

Box 11–1 ▪ IN DEPTH: TRANSGENIC AND KNOCKOUT MOUSE MODELS FOR THE ANALYSIS OF SELF-TOLERANCE AND AUTOIMMUNITY

The experimental analysis of self-tolerance is confounded by two important technical problems. First, it is not possible to identify self-reactive lymphocytes by functional assays because these cells are normally deleted or functionally inactive (anergic). Second, in normal animals or humans, it has been difficult or impossible to define the self antigens that actually induce and maintain tolerance in T and B lymphocytes. For these reasons, much of our early understanding of tolerance was based on administering tolerogenic forms of foreign antigens to animals and studying subsequent immune responses to immunogenic forms of the same antigens. Conclusions about self-tolerance were largely extrapolations from these studies with foreign antigens. Transgenic technology has provided a valuable tool for studying self-tolerance in mice. Rearranged antigen receptor genes can be expressed as transgenes in T or B lymphocytes. Because these antigen receptor genes inhibit recombination at other, endogenous, antigen receptor gene loci (the phenomenon of allelic exclusion), a large fraction of the T or B lymphocytes in these mice express the introduced, transgene-encoded antigen receptor. Therefore, lymphocytes with a known specificity may be detected and followed quantitatively for the life of a mouse. The second application of transgenic technology is to express known proteins in different tissues. These transgene-encoded antigens are present throughout the development of the animal, and therefore they are effectively self antigens for the mouse. Transgenic technology is often combined with spontaneous or induced single-gene mutations or deletions (knockouts) that give rise to autoimmunity. Although autoimmunity caused by abnormalities in single genes is rare, these models have been very informative for elucidating the mechanisms of self-tolerance.

Transgenic approaches may be used to study self-tolerance in many ways.

- It is possible to express transgenic antigen receptors specific for self antigens that are targets of autoimmune diseases. Examples include mice expressing a TCR specific for a protein in pancreatic islet β cells (a target for autoreactive T cells in type 1 diabetes), a TCR specific for myelin basic protein (which is a central nervous system autoantigen), and Ig specific for self DNA (involved in the autoimmune disease lupus).
- Both the antigen receptors of T or B lymphocytes and the antigen that is recognized by these receptors may be coexpressed. Two examples we mention in the text are T cells specific for a viral glycoprotein expressed in islet β cells and B cells specific for HEL expressed in different tissues. By changing the promoters used to drive transgene expression, it is possible to vary the site of expression of the antigen. The use of inducible promoters allows investigators to turn the expression of the antigen on and off during the life of the mouse. It is also possible to express the same antigen in different forms (secreted, membrane bound, and cytoplasmic) and thus to analyze tolerance to different types of self antigens.
- Genes encoding particular immunoregulatory molecules, such as costimulators and cytokines, may be coexpressed with antigens, thus modeling the consequences of local alterations in the tissues where particular self antigens are present. In addition, by breeding antigen receptor transgenics with appropriate knockout mice, investigators have generated mice in which lymphocytes of known specificities lack genes encoding lymphocyte regulatory molecules, such as CTLA-4 and FasL. The same types of studies have been done in mice with mutated or deleted *AIRE* and *FOXP3* genes. All of these mutations result in selective defects in lymphocyte selection or regulation (see text).

Experimental systems using transgenic and knockout mice have allowed investigators to analyze the types of antigens that induce central and peripheral tolerance in T and B cells, the mechanisms of these pathways of tolerance, and the genetic control of self-tolerance. Experimental protocols have been developed to compare the consequences of self antigen recognition by immature or mature lymphocytes. For instance, as described in the text, by mating one mouse expressing a transgenic antigen receptor with another mouse expressing the antigen, in the offspring the immature lymphocytes are exposed to the antigen throughout development. Alternatively, mature lymphocytes expressing the antigen receptor may be transferred into mice expressing the antigen as a self protein, and the consequences of this encounter may be analyzed.

Despite the value of transgenic technology, several important caveats should be mentioned. Expression of a single antigen receptor markedly limits the normal lymphocyte repertoire. Transgene-encoded protein antigens may be expressed at higher concentrations than are normal self proteins. Transgene-encoded immunoregulatory molecules may be expressed at high levels and constitutively and constantly, which is rarely the case with normal immunoregulatory molecules. Therefore, many of the normal controls on lymphocyte activation and regulation may be lost in transgenic mice.

Finally, the type of transgene may influence the result. For instance, in conventional immunoglobulin (Ig) transgenic mice, the rearranged Ig genes are integrated randomly in the genome. When B cells in these mice encounter a self antigen (also transgenically expressed), the integrated Ig light chain is not deleted, so it appears that the specificity does not change. However, when Ig "knock-in" mice are made, the rearranged Ig gene is integrated into its own locus. When immature B cells encounter their cognate antigen, the integrated Ig light chain is deleted and a new light chain is expressed. In fact, "knock-in" mice have revealed that this process of receptor editing, and not deletion, is the major mechanism of central tolerance in B cells.

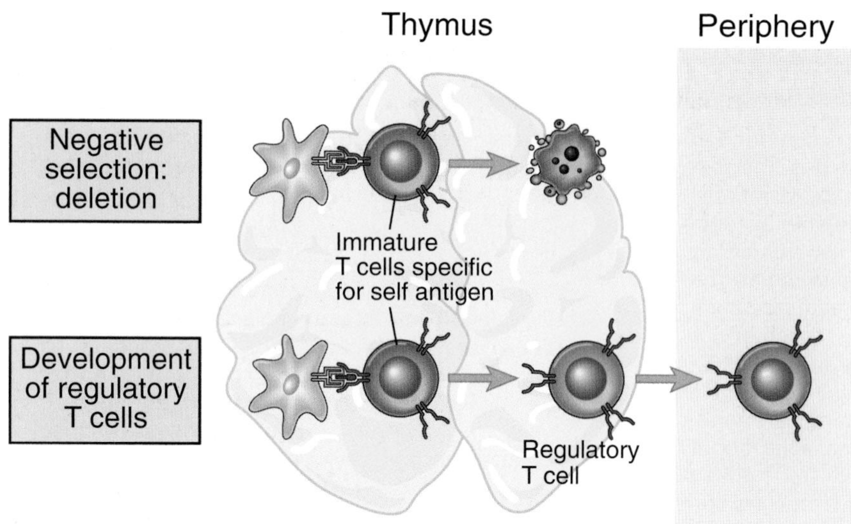

FIGURE 11–3 Central T cell tolerance. Recognition of self antigens by immature T cells in the thymus may lead to death of the cells (negative selection, or deletion) or the development of regulatory T cells that enter peripheral tissues.

immature and mature T cells interpret antigen receptor signals differently. However, we do not know what these signaling differences might be or how they determine the outcome of antigen recognition. This process affects both class I and class II MHC-restricted T cells and is therefore important for tolerance in both $CD8^+$ and $CD4^+$ lymphocyte populations. Negative selection of thymocytes is responsible for the fact that the repertoire of mature T cells that leave the thymus and populate peripheral lymphoid tissues is unresponsive to the self antigens that are present at high concentrations in the thymus. The importance of negative selection in self-tolerance is illustrated by the autoimmune disorders that develop when this process fails.

- The best-defined example of autoimmunity resulting from a defect in negative selection in the thymus is the **autoimmune polyendocrine syndrome (APS).** This group of diseases is caused by mutations in the *AIRE* gene, and is characterized by antibody- and lymphocyte-mediated injury to multiple endocrine organs, including the parathyroids, adrenals, and pancreatic islets. A mouse model of APS has been developed by knockout of the *AIRE* gene. These mice develop T cell infiltrates in and autoantibodies against multiple endocrine organs. In normal mice, protein antigens thought to be restricted to these organs are expressed in thymic epithelial cells, and immature T cells specific for these antigens are deleted in the thymus. In the *AIRE*-knockout mice, these antigens are not displayed in the thymus, and T cells specific for the antigens escape deletion, mature, and enter the periphery, where they attack the target tissues.
- A strain of mice with a mutation in the TCR-associated kinase, ZAP-70, develops arthritis and other manifestations of autoimmunity. The reason for this is that the mutation decreases TCR-induced signaling in the thymus enough to interfere with negative selection (but not with positive selection, which requires weaker signals; see Chapter 8). Thus, self-reactive T cells escape deletion and cause autoimmunity.
- In the non-obese diabetic (NOD) mouse strain, there is autoimmune attack against multiple organs. These mice appear to have a defect in negative selection (in addition to many other defects in self-tolerance), but the underlying mechanisms and the genetic basis of this defect are not yet known.

Some self-reactive $CD4^+$ T cells that see self antigens in the thymus are not deleted but instead differentiate into regulatory T cells (see Fig. 11–3) that leave the thymus and inhibit responses against self tissues in the periphery (discussed later). Interestingly, deficiency of the AIRE protein, which interferes with deletion of T cells reactive with some antigens in the thymus, does not appear to prevent the development of regulatory T cells specific for the same self antigens. This observation suggests that the requirements for T cell deletion and regulatory T cell development in the thymus are different, but what determines the choice between cell death and development of regulatory T cells is not known.

Peripheral T Cell Tolerance

Peripheral tolerance is the mechanism by which mature T cells that recognize self antigens in peripheral tissues become incapable of subsequently responding to these antigens. Peripheral tolerance mechanisms are responsible for T cell tolerance to tissue-specific self antigens that are not abundant in the thymus. The same mechanisms may induce unresponsiveness to tolerogenic forms of foreign antigens. Peripheral tolerance is due to anergy, deletion, or suppression of T cells (see Fig. 11–2), and each of these mechanisms has been defined in several experimental models. We do not know if tolerance to different self antigens is maintained by one or another mechanism or if all these mechanisms function cooperatively to prevent dangerous autoimmunity.

Anergy (Functional Unresponsiveness) Induced by Recognition of Self Antigen

Exposure of CD4⁺ T cells to an antigen in the absence of costimulation or innate immunity may make the cells incapable of responding to that antigen. We previously introduced the concept that full activation of T cells requires the recognition of antigen by the TCR (signal 1) and recognition of costimulators, mainly B7-1 and B7-2, by CD28 (signal 2) (see Chapter 9). Prolonged signal 1 (i.e., antigen recognition) alone may lead to anergy. It is likely that self antigens are displayed to specific T cells in the absence of innate immunity and strong costimulation. Antigen-induced anergy has been demonstrated in a variety of experimental models.

- The first experimental demonstration of T cell anergy came from in vitro studies with cloned lines of mouse $CD4^+$ T cells. If these cells are exposed to peptide-MHC complexes presented on synthetic lipid membranes, on APCs that lack costimulators like B7 molecules, or on APCs that are treated with chemicals that destroy costimulators, the T cells remain viable but are incapable of responding to the antigen even if it is subsequently presented by competent APCs. Similarly, normal T cells exposed to anti-TCR antibodies in the absence of APCs or costimulation become refractory to subsequent activating stimuli. Anergy can be prevented if activated APCs are added to the cultures or if costimulatory receptors on the T cells, such as CD28, are stimulated with antibodies. The physiologic importance of this type of T cell anergy is uncertain because the phenomenon has mostly been demonstrated in vitro.

- T cell anergy can be induced by administering foreign antigens in ways that result in antigen recognition without costimulation or inflammation. In one experimental model, small numbers of T cells from transgenic mice expressing a TCR specific for a known antigen are transferred into normal mice, and the recipients are exposed to the antigen in different forms. If the antigen is administered subcutaneously with adjuvants (the immunogenic form), antigen-specific T cells proliferate in the draining lymph nodes, differentiate into effector cells, and migrate toward lymphoid follicles, where T cell–B cell interactions occur. In contrast, if a large dose of the antigen is administered in aqueous form, without adjuvants (the tolerogenic form), the antigen-specific T cells remain viable but with a greatly reduced ability to proliferate, differentiate, or migrate toward follicles (Fig. 11–4). It is believed that in this model, the aqueous antigen induces anergy in the antigen-specific T cells, resulting in an inability of these cells to proliferate and differentiate in response to the antigen. These experiments also illustrate an important principle mentioned earlier in the chapter—that the same antigen may be immunogenic or tolerogenic, depending on how it is administered.

- An antigen, such as a viral glycoprotein, may be expressed in the tissues of a mouse as a transgene. This may be done by expressing the antigen under the control of the insulin promoter, in which case it is produced mainly by pancreatic islet β cells. In effect, this viral protein becomes a tissue-specific self antigen for the mouse. If the antigen-expressing transgenic mouse is bred with another mouse that expresses the antigen-specific TCR as a transgene, large numbers of the specific T cells encounter the self antigen. These T cells may become anergic and lose their ability to respond to the viral antigen (Fig. 11–5). Presumably, the transgene-encoded viral protein is presented by the β cells or by APCs in the pancreatic islets or draining lymph nodes that do not express adequate levels of costimulators needed to elicit T cell responses, and recognition of the antigen leads to T cell anergy. In the same experimental model, coexpression of the viral antigen and B7 costimulators in islet cells results in the breakdown of anergy and immune responses against the islets. This result illustrates how aberrant expression of costimulators may trigger autoimmune reactions, a concept we will return to in Chapter 18.

- A protein antigen can also be expressed as a systemic, cell-associated or secreted, self antigen in a transgenic mouse. If T cells specific for this protein encounter the antigen, the T cells lose their ability to respond to that antigen. In some of these models, unresponsiveness requires continuous exposure to the self antigen, and the cells recover if they no longer see that antigen.

Anergy results from biochemical or genetic alterations that reduce the ability of lymphocytes to respond to self antigens (Fig. 11–6). The process of anergy is one in which the responsiveness of self-reactive lymphocytes is "tuned" to prevent harmful self-reactivity. Several biochemical alterations are believed to cooperate to maintain this unresponsive state.

- Anergic cells show a block in TCR-induced signal transduction. The mechanisms of this signaling block are not fully known. In different experimental models, it is attributable to decreased TCR expression (perhaps because of increased degradation; see below) and recruitment to the TCR complex of inhibitory molecules such as tyrosine phophatases.

- Self antigen recognition may activate cellular ubiquitin ligases, which may ubiquitinate TCR-associated proteins and target them for proteolytic degradation in proteasomes or lysosomes. The net result is loss of these signaling molecules and defective T cell activation.
  - One ubiquitin ligase that is important in T cells is called Cbl-b. Mice in which Cbl-b is knocked out show "spontaneous" T cell proliferation and manifestations of autoimmunity, suggesting that this enzyme is involved in maintaining T cell unresponsiveness to self antigens.

- When T cells recognize self antigens, they may engage inhibitory receptors of the CD28 family, whose func-

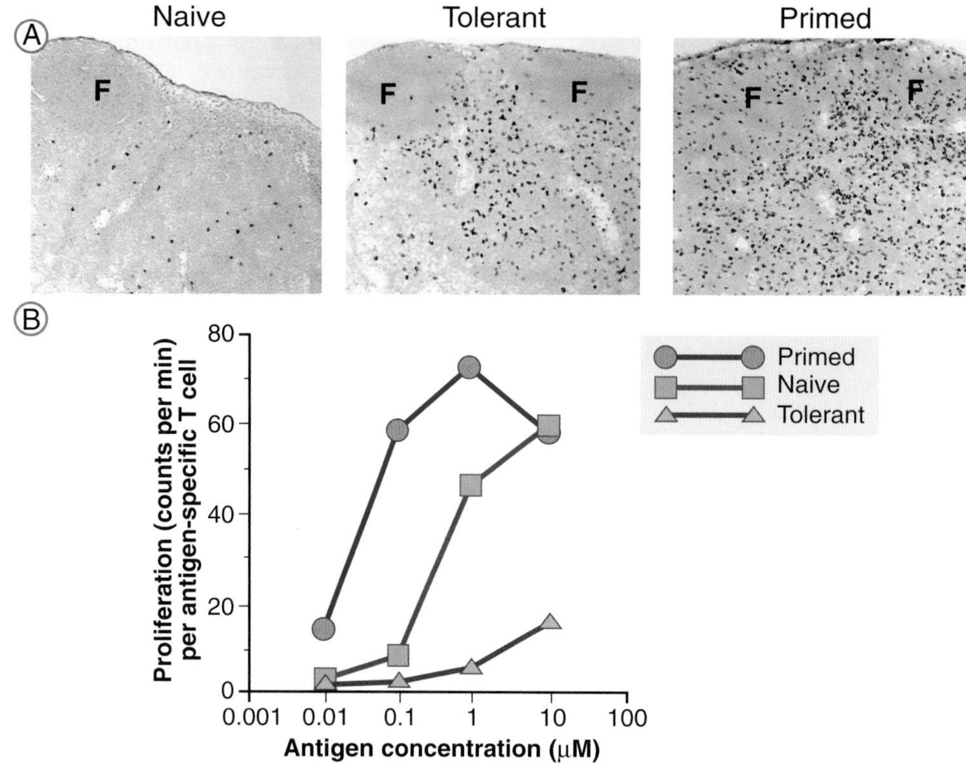

FIGURE 11–4 Induction of T cell tolerance by an aqueous antigen. T cells from transgenic mice expressing an antigen receptor specific for a peptide of ovalbumin are transferred into normal recipient mice, and the recipients are left untreated or are exposed to the peptide in immunogenic form (with adjuvant) or in tolerogenic form (large dose of aqueous peptide without adjuvant). A. Lymph nodes of the recipient mice are stained with an antibody that recognizes the ovalbumin-specific T cells. Untreated (naive) mice contain few of these T cells. In mice given tolerogenic antigen (tolerant), there is some expansion in the number of T cells, but the cells fail to enter the B cell–rich lymphoid follicles (F). In mice given immunogenic antigen (primed), there is greater expansion of T cells, and these cells do enter the follicles. (From Pape KA, ER Kearney, A Khoruts, A Mondino, R Mevica, ZM Chen, E Ingulli, J White, JG Johnson, and MK Jenkins. Use of adoptive transfer of T-cell antigen-receptor-transgenic T cells for the study of T-cell activation *in vivo*. Immunological Reviews 156:67–78, 1997. Copyright 1997 by Blackwell Publishing.) B. The T cells are recovered from the transfer recipients and stimulated with ovalbumin peptide in culture, and their proliferative responses are measured by the incorporation of ^{3}H-thymidine into DNA (expressed as counts per minute per T cell). Naive T cells respond to antigen, cells from primed mice show an increased response, and cells from tolerant mice fail to respond, an indication of anergy. (From Kearney ER, KA Pape, DY Loh, and MK Jenkins. Visualization of peptide-specific T cell immunity and peripheral tolerance induction *in vivo*. Immunity 1:327–339, 1994. Copyright 1994, with permission from Elsevier Science.)

tion is to terminate T cell responses. Although many such inhibitory receptors have been described, the two whose physiologic role in self-tolerance is best established are CTLA-4 and PD-1 (see Chapter 9). **CTLA-4** competes with CD28 for B7 costimulators, and thus excludes CD28 from the site of T cell recognition (the "immune synapse"); in addition, CTLA-4 delivers inhibitory signals that negate the signals triggered by the TCR.

- The importance of CTLA-4 in tolerance induction is illustrated by the finding that knockout mice lacking CTLA-4 develop uncontrolled lymphocyte activation with massively enlarged lymph nodes and spleen and fatal multiorgan lymphocytic infiltrates suggestive of systemic autoimmunity. In other words, eliminating this one control mechanism results in a severe T cell-mediated disease.
- Blocking CTLA-4 with antibodies also enhances autoimmune diseases in animal models, such as encephalomyelitis induced by immunization with myelin antigens and diabetes induced by injection of T cells reactive with antigens in the β cells of pancreatic islets.
- In the antigen-induced model of anergy described earlier (see Fig. 11–4), T cells lacking CTLA-4 do not become unresponsive after exposure to aqueous protein antigen.

These findings indicate that in normal animals, CTLA-4 functions continuously to keep T cells in check. We do not know the factors that determine why, under some conditions, T cells use the activating receptor CD28 to recognize B7 molecules and induce immune responses and, at other times, recognize the same B7 molecules with the inhibitory receptor CTLA-4 to induce tolerance. It is possible that APCs that express low levels of B7 normally engage CTLA-4 preferentially because CTLA-4 binds to B7 molecules with higher affinity than does CD28.

Another inhibitory receptor of the CD28 family is **PD-1** (so called because it was originally thought to be involved in programmed cell death, but now known to not have a role in T cell deletion). PD-1 recognizes

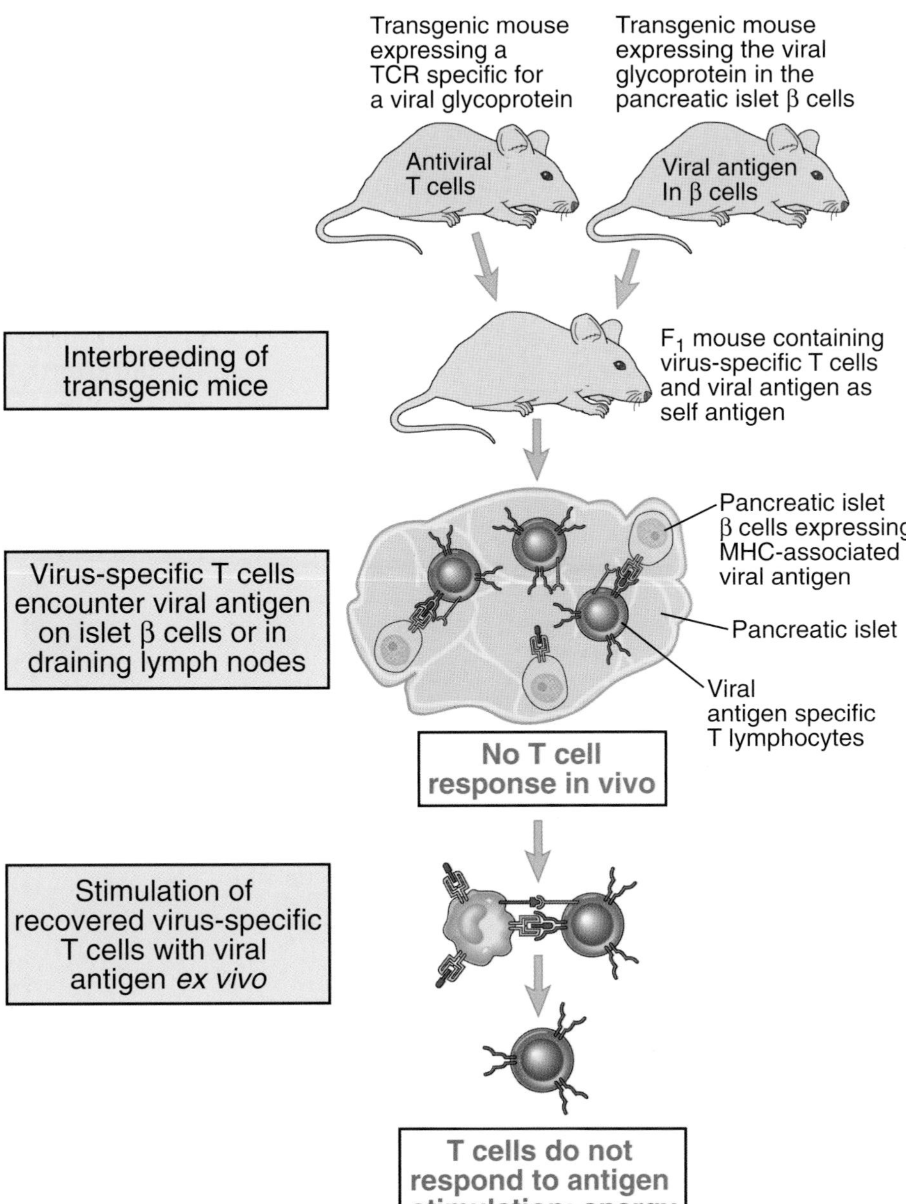

FIGURE 11–5 T cell tolerance induced by a self antigen in a transgenic mouse model. Two sets of transgenic mice are created, one that expresses a TCR specific for a viral glycoprotein antigen and another that expresses the antigen in the β cells of pancreatic islets. When these two mice are interbred, in the F_1 offspring the T cells encounter this islet self antigen but do not attack the antigen-expressing islet cells. If the T cells are recovered and challenged with the viral antigen, the cells fail to respond, indicating that the cells became anergic in vivo. In some similar experiments, the T cells fail to respond in vivo but remain functionally responsive, indicating that they have ignored the presence of the self antigen. Although the T cells are shown recognizing the antigen directly on islet β cells, it is possible that the antigen is recognized on dendritic cells in the islets or in draining lymph nodes.

two ligands that are expressed on APCs and many other cells, and this recognition leads to inactivation of the T cells.

- Mice in which PD-1 is knocked out develop autoimmune diseases, including lupus-like kidney disease, arthritis, and autoimmune cardiomyopathy in different strains of mice.

Dendritic cells that are resident in lymphoid organs and nonlymphoid tissues may present self antigens to T lymphocytes and maintain tolerance. Tissue dendritic cells are normally in a resting (immature) state and express few or no costimulators. Such APCs may be constantly presenting self antigens without activating signals, and T cells that recognize these antigens become anergic. Thus, dendritic cells that are activated by microbes are the principal APCs for initiating T cell responses (Chapter 6), whereas resting dendritic cells may be tolerogenic. As we shall discuss in Chapter 18, local infections and inflammation may activate resident APCs, leading to increased expression of costimulators, breakdown of tolerance, and autoimmune reactions against the tissue antigens.

- In one experimental model, a protein antigen is targeted to resting dendritic cells by coupling the antigen to a dendritic cell–specific antibody. The antigen is captured and presented by resting dendritic cells, and T cells that recognize the antigen become anergic. If, however, the dendritic cells are activated (e.g., by engaging Toll-like receptors or by ligating CD40), T cells that recognize the presented antigen respond as they would in a normal immune response to a microbe.

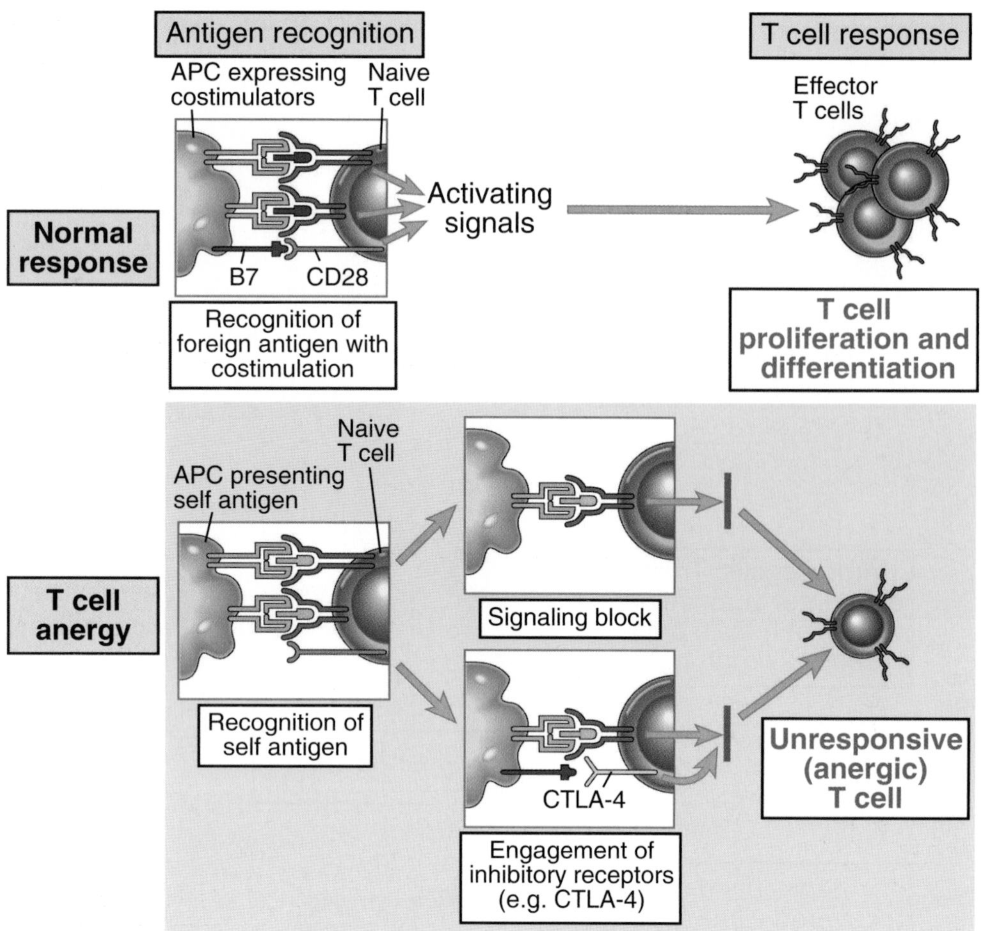

FIGURE 11–6 Mechanisms of T cell anergy. T cell responses are induced when the cells recognize an antigen presented by a professional antigen-presenting cell (APC) and activating receptors on the T cells (such as CD28) recognize costimulators on the APCs (such as B7). If the T cell recognizes a self antigen without costimulation, the T cell becomes unresponsive to the antigen because of a block in signaling from the TCR complex, or engagement of inhibitory receptors (such as CTLA-4). The signaling block may be the result of recruitment of phosphatases to the TCR complex, or the activation of ubiquitin ligases that degrade signaling proteins. Regardless of the mechanism, the T cell remains viable but is unable to respond to the self antigen.

The characteristics of dendritic cells that make them tolerogenic are not defined. There is great interest in manipulating the properties of dendritic cells as a way of enhancing or inhibiting immune responses for therapeutic purposes.

Suppression of Self-Reactive Lymphocytes by Regulatory T Cells

Regulatory T lymphocytes are a subset of CD4⁺ T cells whose function is to suppress immune responses and maintain self-tolerance (Fig. 11–7). The majority of these $CD4^+$ regulatory T lymphocytes express high levels of the interleukin-2 (IL-2) receptor α chain (CD25) but not other markers of activation. Regulatory T cells are generated mainly by self antigen recognition in the thymus, but they also develop in peripheral lymphoid organs. The generation and survival of regulatory T cells are dependent on the cytokines TGF-β and IL-2, and costimulation by the B7: CD28 pathway. Exactly what these signals do in the development of regulatory T cells is unclear. It is also not known what stimuli determine if a T cell will become an effector or memory cell or a regulatory cell. A transcription factor called FoxP3, a member of the forkhead family of transcription factors, is critical for the development and function of the majority of regulatory T cells. The importance of regulatory cells in maintaining self-tolerance is illustrated by many observations in experimental animals and in humans.

- If $CD4^+$ T cells from a normal mouse are depleted of $CD25^+$ cells and transferred into a lymphocyte-deficient syngeneic mouse, the recipient develops multiorgan autoimmune disease involving the thyroid, colon, stomach, and other organs. If $CD4^+$ $CD25^+$ T cells from the normal mouse are transferred together with the $CD25^-$ cells, the induction of the disease is prevented. The interpretation of this experiment is that in the normal mouse, there are T cells capable of reacting to self antigens, and they are kept in check by regulatory cells that have developed in response to recognition of the same self antigens. When the $CD25^-$ T cells are transferred into a recipient that has no other lymphocytes, they cannot be controlled, and this leads to autoimmunity. Cotransfer of $CD25^+$ regulatory T cells prevents autoimmunity.
- Mice with mutations in the *foxp3* gene, or mice in which this gene is knocked out, develop a multisystem autoimmune disease associated with an absence of $CD25^+$ regulatory T cells. A rare autoimmune disease in humans called IPEX (immune dysregula-

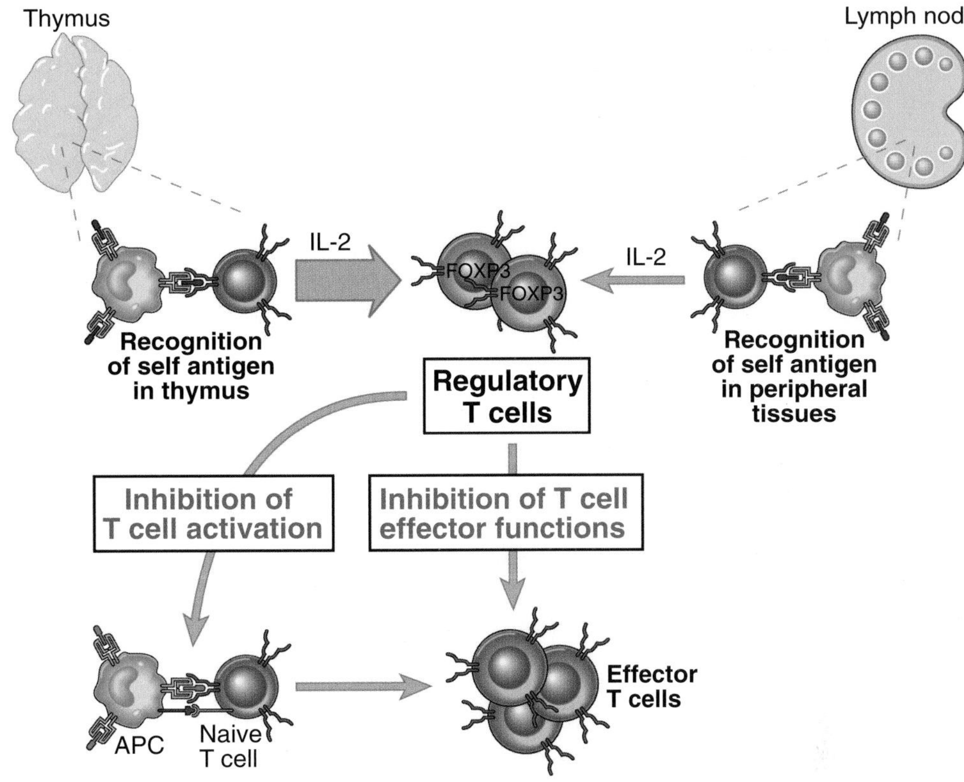

FIGURE 11–7 T cell–mediated suppression. Regulatory T cells are generated by self antigen recognition in the thymus (sometimes called "natural" regulatory cells), and (probably to a lesser extent) by antigen recognition in peripheral lymphoid organs (called "adaptive" regulatory cells). The development and survival of these regulatory T cells require IL-2 and the transcription factor FoxP3. In peripheral tissues, regulatory T cells suppress the activation and effector functions of other, self-reactive and potentially pathogenic lymphocytes.

tion, polyendocrinopathy, enteropathy, X-linked syndrome) is also associated with deficiency of regulatory T cells and is now known to be caused by mutations in the *FOXP3* gene.

- Mice in which the gene for IL-2 or for the α or β chains of the IL-2 receptor are knocked out develop autoimmunity, manifested by inflammatory bowel disease, autoimmune hemolytic anemia, and multiple autoantibodies (including anti-erythrocyte and anti-DNA). These mice lack CD25$^+$ regulatory T cells, and their disease can be corrected by injecting into the IL-2R knockouts normal CD25$^+$CD4$^+$ T lymphocytes.

Regulatory T cells recognize self antigens, and are generated by recognition of self antigens, but the range of their receptor specificity and diversity in normal individuals is not defined. One mechanism by which these cells control immune responses is by secreting immunosuppressive cytokines such as IL-10, which inhibits the function of macrophages and dendritic cells. In many experimental models, the function of regulatory T cells also appears to depend on the cytokine transforming growth factor-β (TGF-β), which inhibits the responses of lymphocytes and macrophages. Therefore, T cells that secrete these inhibitory cytokines may block the activation and effector functions of other T cells. Other mechanisms of inhibition have been suggested; some experiments indicate that regulatory T cells work by directly contacting APCs or responding T lymphocytes, but how they suppress is unclear. Although we have emphasized CD4$^+$ CD25$^+$ FoxP3-expressing regulatory T cells, many other populations have been described that are able to suppress immune responses, but the significance of these populations is not as well established. Attempts are being made to identify defects in the development or function of regulatory T cells in autoimmune diseases, such as type 1 diabetes and multiple sclerosis, in humans. It is also possible that in such disorders, the pathogenic self-reactive lymphocytes are resistant to suppression by regulatory T cells. There is enormous potential for generating regulatory cells and using them to control abnormal immune responses, and many attempts are ongoing to develop such therapeutic strategies.

Deletion of T Cells by Apoptotic Cell Death

T lymphocytes that recognize self antigens without inflammation or that are repeatedly stimulated by antigens die by apoptosis (Fig. 11–8). Cell death that occurs as a consequence of antigen recognition has been called activation-induced cell death. Apoptotic death may be induced by two biochemical pathways (Box 11–2).

- ***T cells that recognize self antigens without costimulation or an accompanying innate immune response may activate a pro-apoptotic protein called Bim, resulting in apoptosis by the mitochondrial pathway.*** In normal lymphocyte responses, signals from the TCR, costimulators, and growth factors stimulate the expression of anti-apoptotic proteins of the Bcl-2 family (Bcl-2, Bcl-x), and these proteins promote cell survival and subsequent proliferation. Bim is a pro-apoptotic member of the Bcl-2 family (see Box 11–2). Bim may be activated by self antigen recognition in the absence of costimulation and growth factors, and it in turn activates effector proteins that trigger death by the mitochondrial pathway. In the absence of strong T cell activation, growth factors such as IL-2 are not produced, and the effects of activated Bim are not counteracted by the anti-apoptotic members of the family (such as Bcl-2 or Bcl-x). The Bim-dependent mitochondrial pathway of apoptosis has been implicated in many situations, not just the elimination of self-reactive lymphocytes. Its role in self-tolerance has been demonstrated experimentally.

- If T cells specific for a protein are injected into mice expressing this protein in islet β cells or in the circulation, the T cells recognize the "self" antigen and die. Bim-deficient T cells do not die under the same conditions.

- ***Repeated stimulation of T cells results in the co-expression of death receptors and their ligands, and engagement of the death receptors triggers apoptotic death.*** In $CD4^+$ T cells, the relevant death receptor is called Fas (CD95) and its ligand is Fas ligand (FasL). Fas is a member of the tumor necrosis factor (TNF) receptor family, and FasL is homologous to the cytokine TNF. When T cells are repeatedly activated, FasL is expressed on the cell surface, and it binds to surface Fas on the same or adjacent T cells. This activates a cascade of intracellular cysteine proteases, called caspases, which ultimately cause the apoptotic death of the cells. Much of the evidence for the role of the Fas pathway in activation-induced cell death has come from in vitro studies and experiments with transgenic mice.

  - If $CD4^+$ T cells that have been recently activated in vitro with antigen or polyclonal activators are restimulated with the same activators, the T cells undergo apoptosis. Fas- or FasL-deficient T cells are resistant to death under these conditions.

  - If mice expressing a transgenic TCR on most of their T cells are injected with high doses of the antigen that is recognized by that TCR, again the T cells are first activated and then undergo apoptosis, and death is dependent on the presence of Fas.

Mice with defects in the expression of Fas or mutations in FasL, and children with Fas mutations, develop autoimmune diseases with some similarity to systemic lupus erythematosus (see Chapter 18). The same pathway of apoptosis is involved in the elimination of self-reactive B lymphocytes (discussed later). It is not established if the autoimmune disease associated with defects in the Fas pathway is due to defective elimination of self-reactive helper T cells or B cells or both.

Peripheral Tolerance in $CD8^+$ T Lymphocytes

Most of our knowledge of peripheral T cell tolerance is limited to $CD4^+$ T cells, and much less is known about the mechanisms of tolerance in mature $CD8^+$ T cells. It

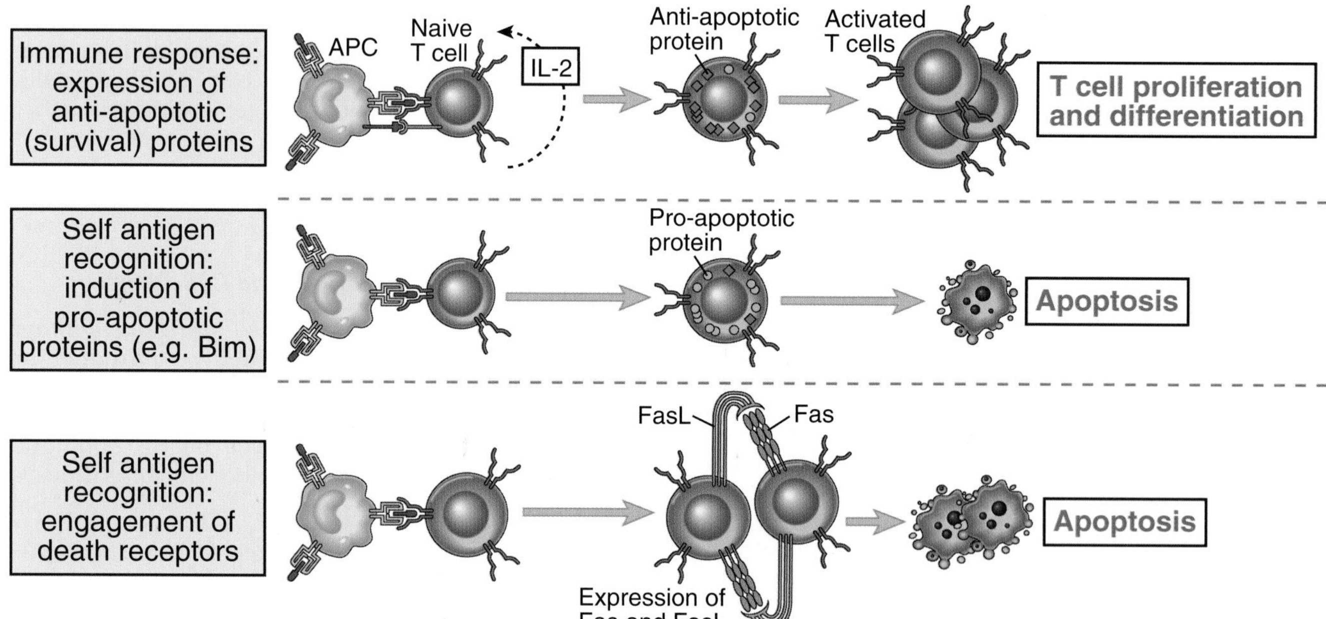

FIGURE 11–8 Self antigen–induced death of peripheral T lymphocytes. In response to immunogenic antigens and growth factors, lymphocytes express anti-apoptotic proteins that promote their survival and allow immune responses to develop *(top panel).* Self antigens may kill T cells by inducing an excess of pro-apoptotic proteins *(middle panel),* or by coexpression of Fas and FasL and engagement of Fas *(lower panel).*

Box 11–2 ▪ IN DEPTH: APOPTOSIS IN LYMPHOCYTES

Apoptosis is a form of death in which a cell initiates a suicide program and characteristic morphologic alterations are observed in dying and dead cells. These changes include chromatin condensation, nucleolar disruption, cytoplasmic contraction, and membrane blebbing. This type of cell death is typically accompanied by the cleavage of DNA into a "ladder" of oligonucleosome length fragments. Apoptotic cells are systematically dismantled into "bite-size" packages, called apoptotic bodies, that are recognized and disposed of by tissue macrophages without the concomitant activation of the innate immune system. This form of death is not associated with inflammation, and is also referred to as "programmed cell death" or "physiologic cell death."

Apoptosis may be initiated in a variety of circumstances, including, but not limited to, the induction of DNA damage by radiation or chemical toxins, the activation of a stress response, the withdrawal of growth factors, and the triggering of specific signaling receptors. This type of cell death is of critical importance in the development of every multicellular organism. In the immune system, as will be discussed below, apoptosis is an essential process during the development of lymphocytes, in the shaping of the immune repertoire, in the regulation of immune responses, and in the elimination of infected cells.

There are two major pathways that lead to apoptosis, both of which culminate in a common death program (see Figure). The "mitochondrial" or "intrinsic" pathway involves the induction of specialized proteins that induce mitochondrial leakiness, leading to the release of death-inducing proteins that are normally sequestered within mitochondria. In the "death receptor" or "extrinsic"

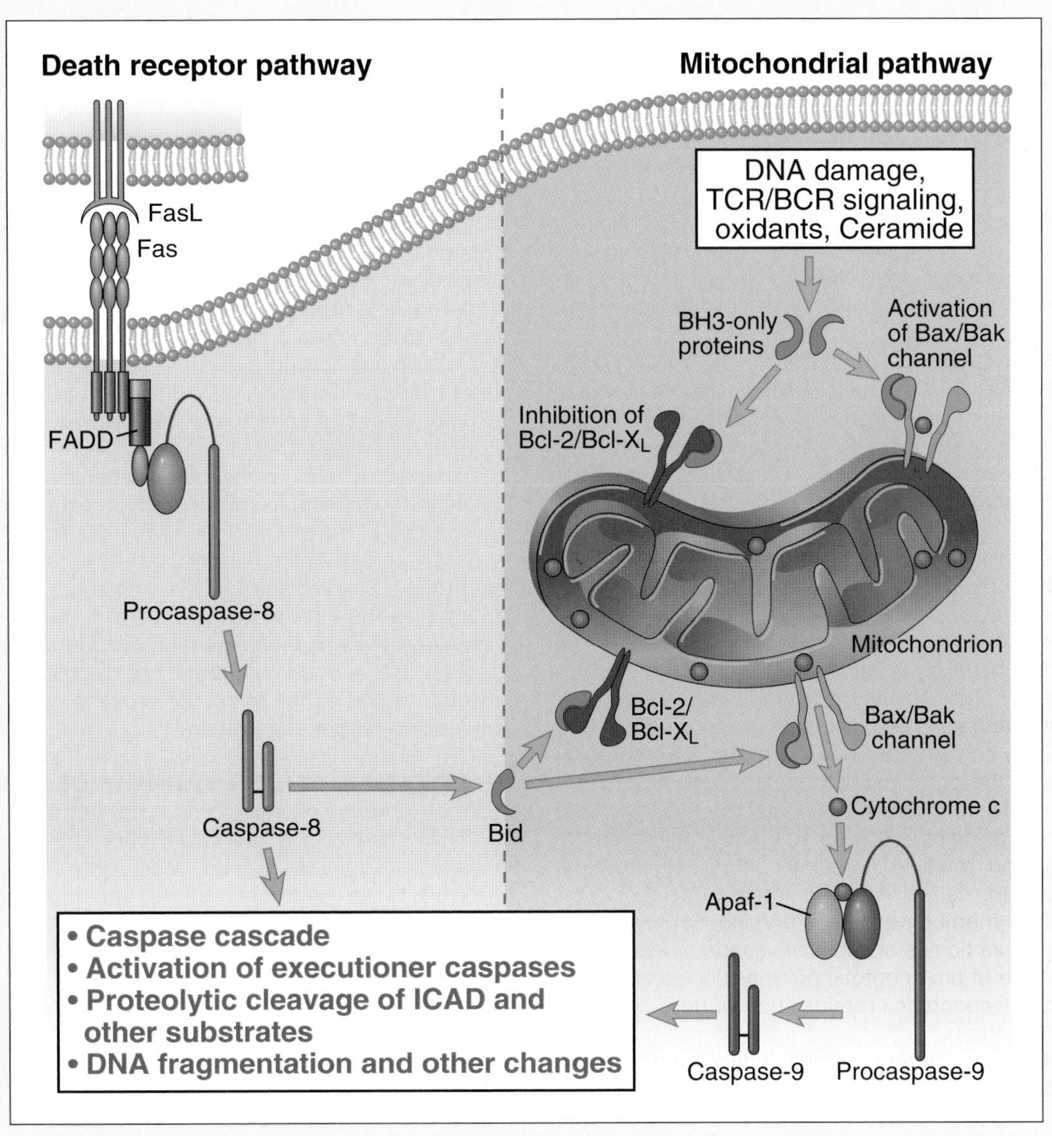

Continued on following page

pathway, the triggering of cell surface receptors of the TNF-receptor family results in activation of the common death pathway.

THE INDUCTION OF APOPTOSIS DEPENDS ON THE ACTIVATION OF CASPASES. The induction of death is generally linked to the activation of a set of proteolytic enzymes that are called caspases (**c**ysteine proteases that cleave proteins immediately after **asp**artic acid residues). The first such enzyme to be identified was the *Caenorhabditis elegans* cell death protein, Ced-3. Caspases exist as latent pro-enzymes that are activated in a cascade-like fashion following cleavage of a pro-piece that ends in an aspartyl residue. All caspases contain a QACRG motif in which the cysteine residue is a part of the active site. Signals from the mitochondrial pathway and the death receptor pathway activate "initiator" caspases, which cleave and activate "executioner" caspases of the common death pathway. Executioner caspases in turn cleave specific substrates and thus contribute to the dismantling and packaging of the dying cell. The caspase that has been best characterized in the context of the common death pathway is caspase-3.

A number of substrates of caspase-3 have been identified. A particularly interesting substrate is the caspase-activated DNase (CAD). CAD is a latent nuclease that can cleave chromosomal DNA into nucleosome-sized fragments but is held in check by an inhibitor called ICAD (for inhibitor of CAD). The nuclease activity of CAD is released by caspase-3-mediated cleavage of two specific aspartyl residues in ICAD. Activated CAD is responsible in part for the fragmentation of DNA that is characteristic of apoptosis.

THE MITOCHONDRIAL PATHWAY OF APOPTOSIS AND PROTEINS OF THE Bcl-2 FAMILY. The major mechanism of apoptosis in all metazoan cells involves the regulation of mitochondrial integrity by members of the Bcl-2 family of proteins. Bcl-2 was initially identified during the molecular characterization of a chromosomal translocation in follicular lymphoma that brings the Ig heavy chain locus on chromosome 14 in apposition with the Bcl-2 gene on chromosome 18. Bcl-2 represents the vertebrate homologue of *Ced-9,* a *C. elegans* gene that inhibits apoptosis in nematodes. Like Ced-9, Bcl-2 is an inhibitor of the mitochondrial pathway of apoptosis.

Bcl-2 family proteins can be divided into three groups. Multidomain anti-apoptotic proteins such as Bcl-2 and Bcl-X_L typically contain four Bcl-2 homology (BH) domains and reside in the outer mitochondrial membrane where they contribute to mitochondrial stability. Multidomain pro-apoptotic proteins, such as Bax and Bak, resemble Bcl-2 in having multiple domains, but these proteins, when activated, can disrupt the integrity of the outer mitochondrial membrane. Single-domain BH3-only proteins, which function as sensors of various stresses, can bind to a range of pro-apoptotic proteins such as Bak and Bax and to anti-apoptotic proteins such as Bcl-2, and regulate their functions.

A number of different stimuli induce and activate distinct BH3-only proteins by transcriptional and posttranscriptional means. DNA damage contributes to the p53-mediated transcriptional induction of genes encoding BH3-only proteins called Puma and Noxa. B cell receptor and TCR signals in developing B and T cells activate a BH3-only protein called Bim by several mechanisms, including increased synthesis and posttranslational modification by phosphorylation. Depriving T and B cells of necessary growth and survival factors also activates Bim. Activation of caspase-8 by death receptors, as discussed below, can induce the activation of a latent BH3-only protein called Bid by proteolytic processing.

Generation of the active forms of BH3-only proteins may set in train a series of events that leads to mitochondrial leakiness, resulting in the release from this organelle of apoptosis-inducing proteins that inexorably drive a cell down the common death pathway. The BH3-only proteins contribute to the disruption of mitochondrial integrity in two major ways. They may bind to the pro-apoptotic Bak and Bax proteins in the cytoplasm, cause them to change conformation, oligomerize, translocate to the outer mitochondrial membrane, and generate an increase in mitochondrial permeability. They may also bind to and inhibit anti-apoptotic proteins such as Bcl-2 or Bcl-X_L in the mitochondrial outer membrane, preventing the latter from interacting with and antagonizing Bak or Bax.

The loss of mitochondrial membrane integrity results in the release of key mitochondrial inducers of apoptosis, including cytochrome c, Smac/Diablo, and Omi/HtrA2 (discussed below). Cytochrome c released from mitochondria binds to a protein called apoptosis-activating factor-1 (Apaf-1), which is the vertebrate homologue of Ced-4, a key regulator of apoptosis in *C. elegans.* The Apaf-1–cytochrome c complex, also known as the apoptosome, binds to and activates procaspase-9, a key initiator caspase in the mitochondrial pathway. Caspase-9 in turn activates the common death pathway.

Other released mitochondrial proteins contribute to caspase activation in a less direct manner. Activated caspases in the cytosol associate with and are held in check by a family of inhibitors, known as IAPs (for inhibitors of apoptosis). Two mitochondrial proteins released during apoptosis, Smac/Diablo and Omi/HtrA2, bind to and antagonize the activity of the IAPs and thereby promote caspase activity and the induction of apoptosis. A number of other mitochondrial proteins, not discussed here, may also contribute to the apoptotic process without directly influencing caspase activation.

THE DEATH RECEPTOR PATHWAY OF APOPTOSIS. Several trimeric cell surface receptors of the TNF receptor family can induce apoptosis when they bind to their physiologic ligands. These receptors are generically referred to as death receptors. The prototypic death receptor is Fas. FasL induced in activated $CD4^+$ T cells may interact with Fas on the same or neighboring cells and contribute to the contraction of some helper T cell responses and the maintenance of self-tolerance. FasL on activated helper T cells also interacts with Fas on B cells to mediate the elimination of anergic self-reactive B cells.

Continued on following page

Box 11–2 ▪ IN DEPTH: APOPTOSIS IN LYMPHOCYTES (Continued)

The intracellular portion of Fas contains a protein-protein interaction domain known as a death domain. A death domain–containing adapter protein called FADD (Fas-associated death domain) links Fas to another initiator caspase, procaspase-8, on the inner face of the plasma membrane. Ligation of Fas by FasL leads to the activation of caspase-8 and consequently the induction of apoptosis.

Although death receptor pathways can induce apoptosis without requiring mitochondrial changes, death receptor signaling is amplified in some cell types by a positive feedback mechanism involving mitochondria. In these cells, caspase-8 cleaves and activates a pro-apoptotic BH3-only protein called Bid, which contributes to the mitochondrial pathway via Bak and Bax, as discussed above.

THE ROLE OF APOPTOSIS IN THE IMMUNE SYSTEM. Apoptotic death is initiated at many steps during lymphoid development and immune activation. Both pro-apoptotic and anti-apoptotic mechanisms are crucial during the development and activation of immune cells, and many of the molecules that regulate these processes are exquisitely regulated.

Early in T cell development, the IL-7 receptor provides survival signals by transiently increasing the levels of Bcl-2. Apoptosis is the fate of pro-B and pro-T cells that fail to express functional antigen receptors, in part because Bcl-2 levels drop just before these pre-B receptor and pre-T receptor checkpoints. Deletion of immature lymphocytes by high-avidity self antigen recognition in both the thymus and the bone marrow results at least in part from the induction of Bim, a pro-apoptotic BH3-only protein. Positive selection by lower-avidity self antigens in the thymus depends on TCR-induced survival signals, and lymphocytes that fail to be positively selected are eliminated by apoptosis. The molecular mechanisms that contribute to survival during the positive selection of T cells are unclear, but antigen receptor signaling can activate many pathways and molecules that protect cells from apoptosis, including nuclear factor κB, which stimulates expression of several anti-apoptotic proteins.

Following immune activation, the contraction phase of immune responses involves the apoptotic loss of numerous activated lymphocytes. Much of this loss is attributed to decreased expression of Bcl-2 and Bcl-x, and possibly activation of Bim, because of deprivation of growth factor–induced survival signals. It is unclear if Fas-mediated activation-induced cell death contributes to the contraction of immune responses. The majority of activated B cells in germinal centers are also eliminated by apoptosis, primarily because these cells fail to be positively selected by antigen.

Cytotoxic $CD8^+$ T lymphocytes and natural killer cells synthesize perforin and granzymes, molecules that are designed to assist in the execution of target cells by apoptosis. Granzyme B is a serine protease that, like caspases, cleaves proteins after aspartyl residues, and can directly activate the caspase cascade.

Finally, survival signals contribute to the generation of memory lymphocytes, the hallmark of which is the prolonged survival of previously activated cells without continuing stimulation. The induction of anti-apoptotic Bcl-2 family proteins, the induced degradation of pro-apoptotic Bcl-2 family proteins, and the expression of caspase inhibitors such as the IAP proteins are some of the mechanisms by which apoptosis may be held at bay in cells that acquire a memory phenotype.

is possible that if $CD8^+$ T cells recognize class I MHC-associated peptides without costimulation, innate immunity, or T cell help, the $CD8^+$ cells become anergic. In this situation, the $CD8^+$ T cells would encounter signal 1 (antigen) without second signals, and the mechanism of anergy would be essentially the same as for helper T lymphocytes. The role of CTLA-4 and other inhibitory receptors in inducing anergy in $CD8^+$ T cells is not established. $CD25^+$ regulatory T cells can directly inhibit the activation of $CD8^+$ T cells. $CD8^+$ T cells that are exposed to high concentrations of self antigens may also undergo apoptotic cell death; this process may result from Bim activation (as mentioned above) and does not appear to involve the Fas death receptor.

Factors That Determine the Tolerogenicity of Self Antigens

Studies with a variety of experimental models have shown that many features of protein antigens determine whether these antigens will induce T cell activation or tolerance (Table 11–1). Self antigens have special properties that make them tolerogenic. Some self antigens are present at high concentrations in the generative lymphoid organs, and these antigens may induce negative selection or the development of regulatory T cells. In the periphery, self antigens are normally displayed to the immune system without inflammation or innate immunity. Under these conditions, APCs express few or no costimulators, and antigen recognition may either elicit no response (ignorance) or induce anergy or cell death. Because self antigens cannot be eliminated, they are capable of chronically engaging the antigen receptors of specific T lymphocytes, and chronic stimulation without activating signals may induce anergy or activation-induced cell death, or promote the development of regulatory T cells. These concepts are based largely on experimental models in which antigens are administered to mice or are expressed as transgenes in mice. One of the continuing challenges in this field is to

Table 11–1. Factors That Determine the Immunogenicity and Tolerogenicity of Protein Antigens

Factor	Factors that favor stimulation of immune responses	Factors that favor tolerance
Amount	Optimal doses vary for different antigens	High doses
Persistence	Short lived (eliminated by immune response)	Prolonged
Portal of entry; location	Subcutaneous, intradermal; absence from generative organs	Intravenous, oral; presence in generative organs
Presence of adjuvants	Antigens with adjuvants: stimulate helper T cells	Antigens without adjuvants: nonimmunogenic or tolerogenic
Properties of antigen-presenting cells	High levels of costimulators	Low levels of costimulators and cytokines

define the mechanisms by which various normally expressed self antigens induce tolerance, especially in humans.

B Lymphocyte Tolerance

Tolerance in B lymphocytes is necessary for maintaining unresponsiveness to thymus-independent self antigens, such as polysaccharides and lipids. B cell tolerance also plays a role in preventing antibody responses to protein antigens. Experimental studies have led to the concept that during B cell maturation and activation, there are multiple mechanisms by which encounter with self antigens may abort these processes (Fig. 11–9).

Central Tolerance in B Cells

Immature B lymphocytes that recognize self antigens in the bone marrow with high affinity either change their specificity or are deleted. If immature B cells recognize self antigens that are present at high concentration in the bone marrow and especially if the antigen is displayed in multivalent form (e.g., on cell surfaces), the B cells reactivate their *RAG1* and *RAG2* genes and express a new immunoglobulin (Ig) light chain, thus acquiring a new specificity. This process is called **receptor editing** (see Chapter 8) and is an important mechanism for eliminating self-reactivity from the mature B cell repertoire. If editing fails to eliminate autoreactivity, the immature B cells may be deleted (i.e., they die by apoptosis). Weaker recognition of self antigens may lead to functional inactivation (anergy) rather than cell death.

- The mechanisms of self-tolerance in B lymphocytes have been examined mainly in experimental models using transgenic mice. In one such model (Fig. 11–10), one set of mice is created in which an Ig receptor specific for a model protein antigen, hen egg lysozyme (HEL), is expressed as a transgene. Most of the B cells in these transgenic mice are HEL specific and can be stimulated to produce anti-HEL antibody. The antigen HEL is expressed in another set of transgenic mice; because this protein is present throughout development, in effect it is a self antigen (like the viral protein expressed in pancreatic islets, referred to earlier). The antigen can be expressed as a multivalent membrane protein, in which case it is recognized with high avidity, or as a secreted protein, in which case it is present at low valency and is recognized with low avidity. If the Ig transgenic mice and the HEL transgenic mice are mated, in the F_1 offspring, immature B cells specific for HEL are exposed to HEL. Immature B cells that encounter the multivalent form of this self antigen are killed and do not attain maturity. B cells that recognize the soluble antigen with lower avidity do mature and exit the bone marrow, but they decrease their expression of antigen receptors and are unable to respond to the self antigen. In these Ig transgenics, it is difficult to assess receptor editing because the transgenic Ig is randomly integrated in the genome and is not eliminated. However, if the transgenic Ig is "knocked-in" to the normal Ig locus, antigen recognition leads to deletion of the Ig light chain and expression of a new light chain. In fact, such knock-in mice have revealed that receptor editing is the major mechanism of tolerance in developing B cells.

- In another transgenic system, if the genes encoding an Ig specific for a class I MHC allele are introduced into mice expressing that allele, B cells expressing the transgenic Ig fail to mature and exit the marrow. Many of the immature B cells die, but as many as 25% undergo receptor editing and express a new Ig light chain, and lose their reactivity with the MHC antigen. The class I MHC molecule is an example of a membrane-bound self antigen that is displayed on cell surfaces in a multivalent form able to cross-link B cell Ig molecules.

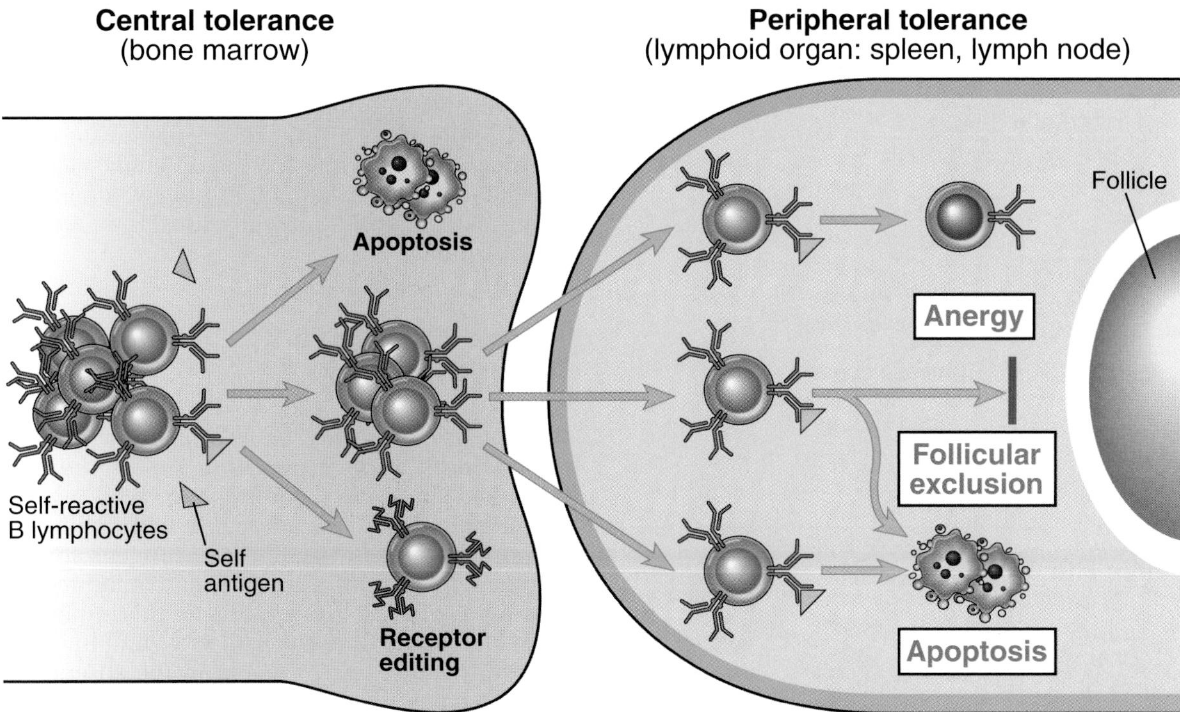

FIGURE 11–9 Central and peripheral tolerance in B cells. Immature B cells that encounter self antigens in the bone marrow die by apoptosis or change the specificity of their antigen receptors (receptor editing). B cells that encounter self antigens in peripheral tissues become anergic, are excluded from lymphoid follicles, or die by apoptosis.

Peripheral B Cell Tolerance

Mature B lymphocytes that recognize self antigens in peripheral tissues in the absence of specific helper T cells may be rendered functionally unresponsive or die by apoptosis (see Fig. 11–9). The biochemical mechanisms of B cell anergy are probably similar to the process of "tuning" that we mentioned earlier in our discussion of T cell anergy. Encounter with self antigens reduces B cell survival and promotes death by the mitochondrial pathway. B cells that encounter self antigens in the periphery are less able to migrate into lymphoid follicles than are normal, naive B cells. A likely mechanism of follicular exclusion is that chronic antigen recognition leads to reduced expression of the chemokine receptor (CXCR5) that normally brings naive B lymphocytes into the follicles. Cells that are excluded from follicles do not receive necessary survival signals and die. If anergic B cells do encounter any antigen-specific helper T cells, the B cells may be killed by FasL on the T cells engaging Fas on the B cells. This mechanism of elimination of self-reactive B lymphocytes fails in mice and humans with mutations in Fas or FasL, and such a failure may contribute to autoantibody production.

- Many of these mechanisms of peripheral B cell tolerance have been analyzed in the HEL transgenic system mentioned before. In such experimental systems, HEL-specific B cells can be transferred into mice expressing the soluble form of HEL in the periphery in the absence of T cell help. The principal fate of these self-recognizing B cells is functional anergy, resulting in an inability to respond to antigen. The anergic B cells appear incapable of activating receptor-associated tyrosine kinases or maintaining sustained increases in intracellular calcium on exposure to the antigen. The B cells also show increased levels of the pro-apoptotic protein Bim and increased dependence on survival factors such as BAFF (see Chapter 10). As a result, the B cells that have encountered self antigen cannot compete effectively with other lymphocytes and die since they do not get adequate survival signals.

Many other mechanisms of B cell tolerance have been demonstrated in experimental models. The inhibitory Fcγ receptor, FcγRII, the phosphatase-associated ITIM-containing protein CD22, and some tyrosine kinases (e.g. Lyn) all play a role in B cell self-tolerance. This is deduced from the observation that knockout of genes encoding any of these proteins results in autoantibody production. How these pathways are engaged by encounter with self antigens is not known.

It is suspected that many diseases caused by autoantibodies are due to a failure of B cell tolerance, but little is known about which pathway of tolerance fails or why in any of these disorders. Normal individuals do not produce pathogenic, high-affinity autoantibodies against self protein antigens, and this may be due to deletion or tolerance of helper T lymphocytes even if functional B cells are present. In these cases, defects in the maintenance of T cell tolerance may result in autoantibody production.

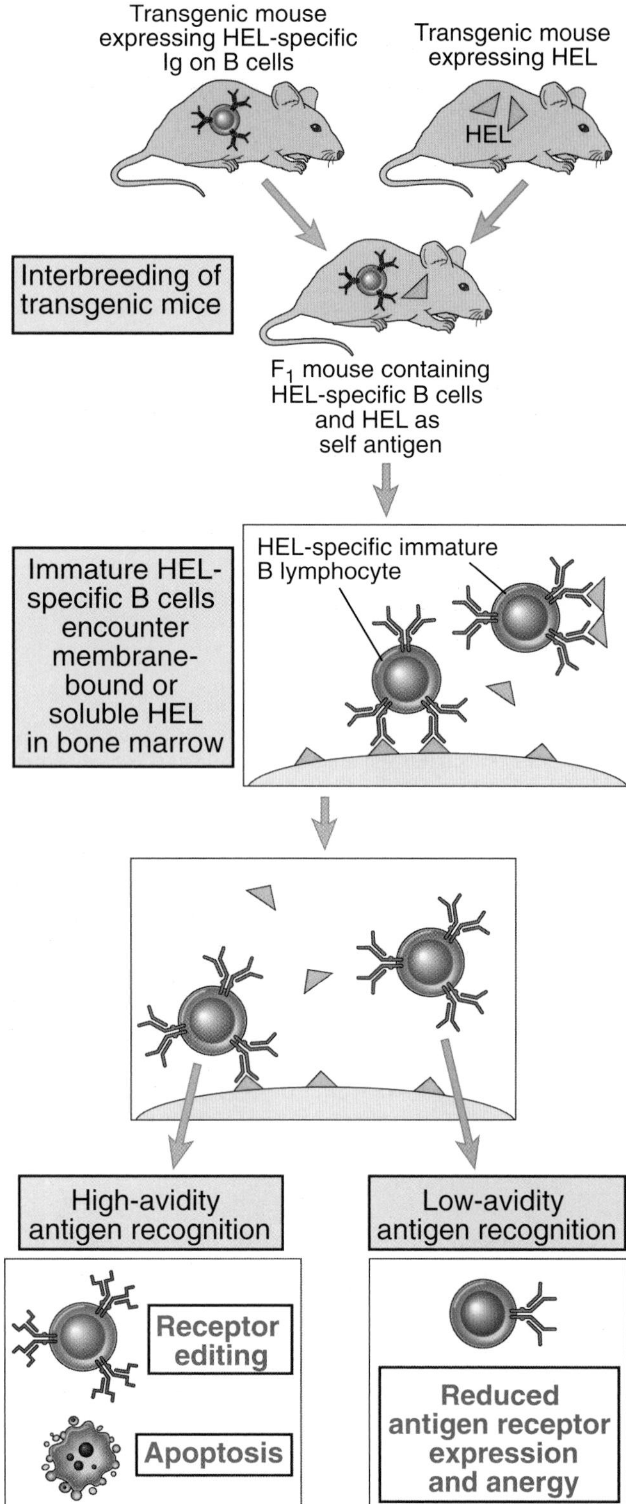

FIGURE 11–10 B cell tolerance in a transgenic mouse model. A transgenic mouse expressing an Ig specific for the antigen HEL is bred with another transgenic mouse that produces HEL as a self antigen. In the "double-transgenic" F_1 mouse, most B cells express HEL-specific receptors that recognize the self HEL. When immature B cells recognize the antigen in the bone marrow, the B cells may change their receptors, be deleted by apoptosis, or leave the bone marrow with greatly reduced levels of receptor expression. Receptor editing is seen only if the Ig transgene is expressed in the normal Ig locus in the genome.

The mechanisms of tolerance in T and B lymphocytes are similar in many respects, but there are also important differences (Table 11–2). Much has been learned from the use of animal models, especially transgenic mice. Application of this knowledge to understanding the mechanisms of tolerance to different self antigens in normal individuals, and to defining why tolerance fails, giving rise to autoimmune diseases, is an area of active investigation.

TOLERANCE INDUCED BY FOREIGN PROTEIN ANTIGENS

Foreign antigens may be administered in ways that preferentially induce tolerance rather than immune responses. In general, protein antigens administered subcutaneously or intradermally with adjuvants favor immunity, whereas high doses of antigens administered systemically without adjuvants tend to induce tolerance (see Fig. 11–4). The likely reason for this is that adjuvants stimulate innate immune responses and the expression of costimulators on APCs, and in the absence of these second signals, T cells that recognize the antigen may become anergic or die. Tolerogenic antigens may also activate regulatory T cells, but the signals that lead to the development of regulatory T lymphocytes in response to such antigens are not yet defined. Many other features of antigens, and how they are administered, may influence the balance between immunity and tolerance (see Table 11–1).

The oral administration of a protein antigen often leads to suppression of systemic humoral and cell-mediated immune responses to immunization with the same antigen. This phenomenon is called **oral tolerance.** It has been postulated that the physiologic importance of oral tolerance may be as a mechanism for preventing immune responses to food antigens and to bacteria that normally reside as commensals in the intestinal lumen and are needed for digestion and absorption. Different doses of orally administered antigens may induce anergy in antigen-specific T cells or may induce suppressor cells that produce cytokines, such as TGF-β, that inhibit immune responses. It is unclear why oral administration of some antigens, such as soluble proteins in large doses, induces systemic T cell tolerance, whereas oral immunization with other antigens, such as attenuated polio virus vaccines, induces protective T cell–dependent antibody responses and long-lived memory.

HOMEOSTASIS IN THE IMMUNE SYSTEM: TERMINATION OF NORMAL IMMUNE RESPONSES

So far in this chapter, we have mainly discussed how the immune system becomes unresponsive to self antigens. Lymphocyte death and inactivation are also important for maintaining a steady number of these cells throughout the life of an individual, despite the constant

Table 11–2. Self-Tolerance in T and B Lymphocytes

Feature	T lymphocytes	B lymphocytes
Principal sites of tolerance induction	Thymus (cortex); periphery	Bone marrow; periphery
Tolerance-sensitive stage of maturation	$CD4^+CD8^+$ (double positive) thymocyte	Immature (IgM^+IgD^-) B lymphocyte
Stimuli for tolerance induction	Central: high-avidity recognition of antigen in thymus	Central: recognition of multivalent antigen in bone marrow
	Peripheral: antigen presentation by APCs lacking costimulators; repeated stimulation by self antigen	Peripheral: antigen recognition without T cell help or second signals
Principal mechanisms of tolerance	Central tolerance: deletion (apoptosis); development of regulatory T cells	Central tolerance: deletion (apoptosis); receptor editing
	Peripheral tolerance: anergy, apoptosis, suppression	Peripheral tolerance: block in signal transduction (anergy); failure to enter lymphoid follicles; apoptosis

Abbreviations: APCs, antigen-presenting cells.

production of new lymphocytes in the generative lymphoid organs and the tremendous clonal expansion that may occur during responses to potent immunogenic antigens. The maintenance of constant numbers of cells is called **homeostasis.** In the following section, we discuss the known mechanisms that function to maintain homeostasis after lymphocyte activation.

Immune responses to foreign antigens are self-limited and wane as the antigens are eliminated, returning the immune system to its basal resting state. In previous chapters, we discussed the expansion of T and B lymphocytes after stimulation with antigens and other signals and the differentiation of these lymphocytes into effector and memory cells. Following elimination of the antigen, there is a phase of contraction, in which most of the cells that have responded to the antigen are lost. This contraction phase is largely because of apoptotic death of previously activated lymphocytes. Antigens, costimulators, and cytokines (growth factors) produced during immune responses prevent lymphocytes from dying and allow clonal expansion and differentiation of the lymphocytes into effector cells. Survival stimuli for lymphocytes function mainly by inducing the expression of anti-apoptotic proteins, the most important of which are members of the Bcl-2 family. The effector cells that develop during adaptive immune responses function to eliminate the antigen, as a result of which the innate immune response also subsides. Therefore, the clones of lymphocytes that were activated by the antigen are deprived of essential survival stimuli, and they die by apoptosis (Fig. 11–11). Apoptosis is mainly the result of activation of death sensors such as Bim and reduced levels of survival proteins such as Bcl-2 and Bcl-x (see Box 11–2). Thus, homeostasis is restored after the antigen is eliminated, and the only sign of the earlier immune response is the persistence of long-lived but functionally quiescent memory lymphocytes.

In addition to this contraction of immune responses because of cell death, antigens may trigger active regulatory mechanisms that also serve to terminate immune responses. Two of these mechanisms have been mentioned before as mechanisms of peripheral T cell tolerance. Activated T cells begin to express CTLA-4, which interacts with B7 molecules and inhibits continued lymphocyte proliferation. CTLA-4 appears after 3 or 4 days of T cell activation, and this may herald the decline of the T cell response. Thus, CTLA-4 may be a physiologic terminator of T cell activation. Other inhibitory receptors such as PD-1 may serve a similar function. Activated T cells may also express death receptors such as Fas and ligands for these receptors, and the interaction of these molecules results in apoptosis (see Box 11–2). Because coexpression of Fas and FasL and Fas-mediated apoptosis are induced by repeated antigen stimulation, they are most likely to be triggered in situations of persistent antigen exposure (e.g., with self antigens, or during chronic infections). However, inhibitory receptors such as CTLA-4 and death receptors appear to be more important for tolerance to self antigens than for terminating normal immune responses to foreign antigens, such as microbial proteins. Similarly, we do not know whether regulatory T cells play a role in limiting responses to most immunogens.

The responses of B lymphocytes are also actively controlled because IgG antibodies produced by the B cells form complexes with the antigen, and the complexes bind to Fcγ receptors on the B cells and inhibit these cells. This process of **antibody feedback** was described in Chapter 10.

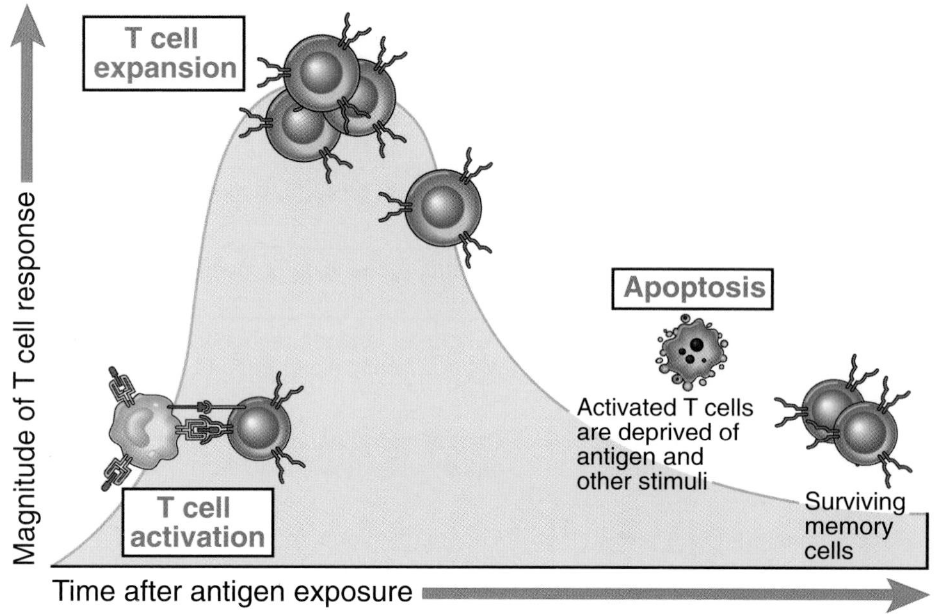

FIGURE 11–11 Mechanisms of the decline of normal immune responses (homeostasis). T lymphocytes proliferate and differentiate in response to antigen. As the antigen is eliminated, many of the activated T cells die by apoptosis. At the end of the immune response, memory cells are the only surviving cells. Although many active regulatory mechanisms have been suggested as mechanisms for termination of normal immune responses, apoptosis is probably the principal mechanism for the decline of both T cell and B cell responses (only T cells are shown).

Another mechanism for regulating adaptive immune responses was proposed by Niels Jerne in the 1970s as the **network hypothesis.** This idea is based on the fact that lymphocyte antigen receptors are extremely diverse and that receptors of any one specificity have amino acid sequences different from the receptors of all other specificities. These unique sequences form determinants, called **idiotypes,** that may be recognized by other lymphocytes with complementary, or anti-idiotypic, specificities (see Chapter 4, Box 4–3). Thus, lymphocytes may respond to the unique antigen receptors of other lymphocytes; such responses are said to be anti-idiotypic. The basic tenet of the network hypothesis is that complementary interactions involving idiotypes and anti-idiotypes reach a steady state at which the immune system is at homeostasis. When a foreign antigen enters the system, one or a few clones of lymphocytes respond, their idiotypes are expanded, and anti-idiotype responses are triggered that function to shut off the antigen-specific (idiotype-expressing) lymphocytes. Although this concept remains an intriguing idea, it has not been proved experimentally that idiotypic networks are actually involved in regulating physiologic immune responses.

SUMMARY

- Immunological tolerance is unresponsiveness to an antigen induced by the exposure of specific lymphocytes to that antigen. Tolerance to self antigens is a fundamental property of the normal immune system, and the failure of self-tolerance leads to autoimmune diseases. Antigens may be administered in ways that induce tolerance rather than immunity, and this may be exploited for the prevention and treatment of transplant rejection and autoimmune and allergic diseases.

- Central tolerance is induced in the generative lymphoid organs (thymus and bone marrow) when immature lymphocytes encounter self antigens present in these organs. Peripheral tolerance occurs when mature lymphocytes recognize self antigens in peripheral tissues under particular conditions.

- In T lymphocytes, central tolerance (negative selection) occurs when immature thymocytes with high-affinity receptors for self antigens recognize these antigens in the thymus. Some immature T cells that encounter self antigens in the thymus die and others develop into $CD4^{+}CD25^{+}$ regulatory T lymphocytes, which function to control responses to self antigens in peripheral tissues.

- Several mechanisms account for peripheral tolerance in mature T cells. In $CD4^{+}$ T cells, anergy is induced by antigen recognition without adequate costimulation or with engagement of inhibitory receptors like CTLA-4 and PD-1. Regulatory T cells inhibit immune responses in part by producing immunosuppressive cytokines. T cells that encounter self antigens without other stimuli or that are repeatedly stimulated die by apoptosis.

- In B lymphocytes, central tolerance is induced when immature B cells recognize multivalent self antigens in the bone marrow. The usual result is apoptotic death of the B cells or the acquisition of a new specificity, called receptor editing. Mature B cells that recognize self antigens in the periphery in the absence of T cell help may be rendered anergic or are excluded from lymphoid follicles, cannot be activated by antigen, and ultimately die by apoptosis.

- Immune responses to foreign antigens decline with time after immunization. This is mainly because of apoptotic death of activated lymphocytes that are deprived of survival stimuli as the antigen is eliminated and innate immunity wanes. Various active mechanisms of lymphocyte inhibition may also function to terminate immune responses.

Selected Readings

Baxter AG, and PD Hodgkin. Activation rules: the two-signal theories of immune activation. Nature Reviews Immunology 2:439–446, 2002.

Fontenot JD, and AY Rudensky. A well adapted regulatory contrivance: regulatory T cell development and the forkhead family transcription factor FoxP3. Nature Immunology 6:331–337, 2005.

Goodnow CC, J Sprent, B Fazekas de St Groth, and CG Vinuesa. Cellular and genetic mechanisms of self tolerance and autoimmunity. Nature 435:590–597, 2005.

Greenwald RJ, GJ Freeman, and AH Sharpe. The B7 family revisited. Annual Review of Immunology 23:515–548, 2005.

Hogquist KA, TA Baldwin, and SC Jameson. Central tolerance: learning self-control in the thymus. Nature Reviews Immunology 5:772–782, 2005.

Jun JE, and CC Goodnow. Scaffolding of antigen receptors for immunogenic versus tolerogenic signaling. Nature Immunology 4:1057–1064, 2003.

Keir ME, MJ Butte, GJ Freeman, and AH Sharpe. PD-1 and its ligands in tolerance and immunity. Annual Review of Immunology 26:677–704, 2008.

Kronenberg M, and A Rudensky. Regulation of immunity by self-reactive T cells. Nature 435:598–604, 2005.

Kyewski B, and L Klein. A central role for central tolerance. Annual Review of Immunology 24:571–606, 2006.

Malek TR. The biology of interleukin-2. Annual Review of Immunology 26:453–479, 2008.

Marsden VS, and A Strasser. Control of apoptosis in the immune system: Bcl-2, BH3-only proteins, and more. Annual Review of Immunology 21:71–105, 2003.

Mathis D, and C Benoist. Back to central tolerance. Immunity 20:509–516, 2004.

Matzinger P. The danger model: a renewed sense of self. Science 296:301–305, 2002.

Mueller DL. E3 ubiquitin ligases as T cell anergy factors. Nature Immunology 5:883–890, 2004.

Nemazee D. Receptor editing in lymphocyte development and central tolerance. Nature Reviews Immunology 6:728–740, 2006.

Parish IA, and WR Heath. Too dangerous to ignore: self-tolerance and the control of ignorant autoreactive T cells. Immunology Cell Biology 86:146–152, 2008.

Redmond WL, and LA Sherman. Peripheral tolerance of CD8 T lymphocytes. Immunity 22:275–284, 2005.

Sakaguchi S, T Yamaguchi, T Nomura, and M Ono. Regulatory T cells and immune tolerance. Cell 133:775–787, 2008.

Schwartz RH. T cell anergy. Annual Review of Immunology 21:305–334, 2003.

Shevach EM. $CD4^+$ $CD25^+$ suppressor T cells: more questions than answers. Nature Reviews Immunology 2:389–400, 2002.

Siegel RM, FK-M Chan, and MJ Lenardo. The multifaceted role of Fas signaling in immune cell homeostasis and autoimmunity. Nature Immunology 1:469–474, 2000.

Singh NJ, and RH Schwartz. Primer: mechanisms of immunologic tolerance. Nature Clinical Practice Rheumatology 2:44–51, 2006.

Steinman RM, D Hawiger, and MC Nussenzweig. Tolerogenic dendritic cells. Annual Review of Immunology 21:685–711, 2003.

Tang Q, and JA Bluestone. The Foxp3+ regulatory T cell: a jack of all trades, master of regulation. Nature Immunology 9:239–244, 2008.

Walker LS, and AK Abbas. The enemy within: keeping self-reactive T cells at bay in the periphery. Nature Reviews Immunology 2:11–19, 2002.

Zheng Y, Y Zha, and TF Gajewski. Molecular regulation of T-cell anergy. EMBO Reports 9:50–55, 2008.

Ziegler SF. FoxP3: of mice and men. Annual Review of Immunology 6:209–226, 2006.

Section IV

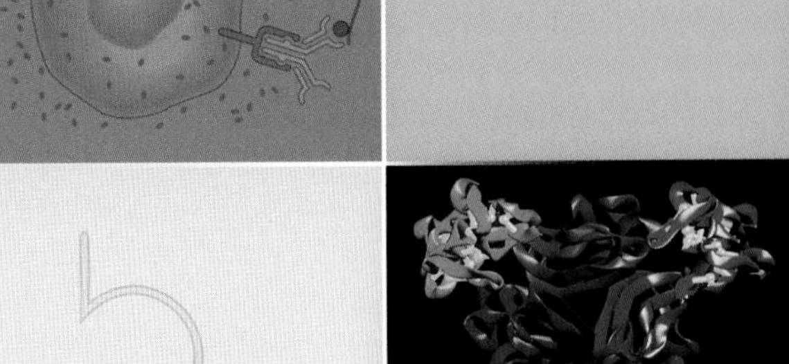

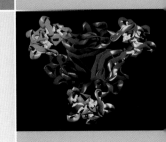

Effector Mechanisms of Immune Responses

The physiologic function of all immune responses is to eliminate microbes and other foreign antigens. The mechanisms by which specific lymphocytes recognize and respond to foreign antigens (i.e., the recognition and activation phases of adaptive immune responses) were discussed in Sections II and III. Section IV is devoted to the effector mechanisms that are activated during immune responses and to how these mechanisms function in host defense.

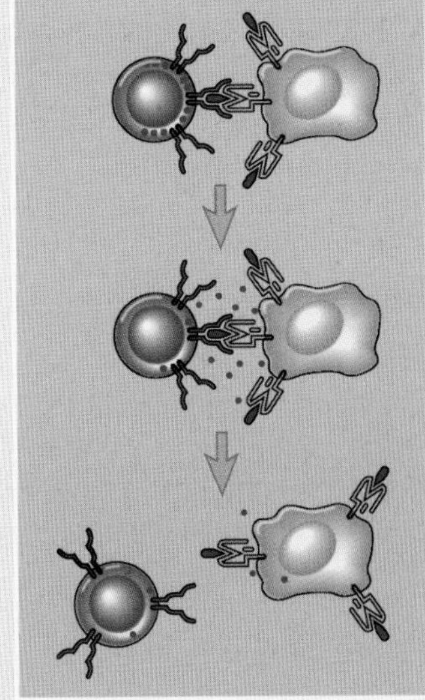

In Chapter 12 we describe cytokines, the soluble mediators of innate and adaptive immunity and the mechanisms by which leukocytes communicate with one another and with other cells. In Chapter 13 we describe the effector cells of cell-mediated immunity, namely T lymphocytes and macrophages, which function as defense mechanisms against intracellular microbes. Chapter 14 is devoted to the effector mechanisms of antibody-mediated humoral immunity, including the complement system, which are involved in host defense against extracellular microbes.

Chapter 12

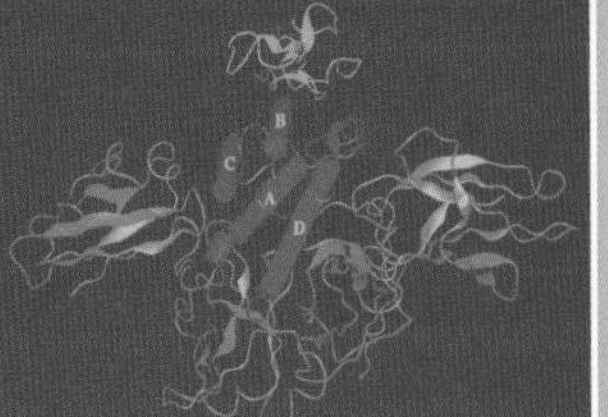

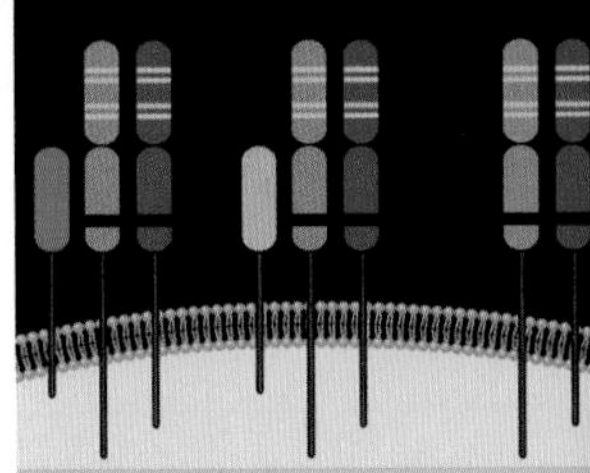

CYTOKINES

Cytokines are proteins secreted by the cells of innate and adaptive immunity that mediate many of the functions of these cells. Cytokines are produced in response to microbes and other antigens, and different cytokines stimulate diverse responses of cells involved in immunity and inflammation. In the activation phase of adaptive immune responses, cytokines stimulate the growth and differentiation of lymphocytes, and in the effector phases of innate and adaptive immunity, they activate different effector cells to eliminate microbes and other antigens. Cytokines also stimulate the development of hematopoietic cells. In clinical medicine, cytokines are important as therapeutic agents and as targets for specific antagonists in numerous immune and inflammatory diseases.

The nomenclature of cytokines is often based on their cellular sources. Cytokines that are produced by mononuclear phagocytes were originally called **monokines,** and those produced by lymphocytes were called **lymphokines.** With the development of anticytokine antibodies and molecular probes, it became clear that the same protein may be synthesized by lymphocytes, monocytes, and a variety of tissue cells, including endothelial cells and some epithelial cells. Therefore, the generic term **cytokines** is the preferred name for this class of mediators. Because many cytokines are made by leukocytes (e.g., macrophages or T cells) and act on other leukocytes, they are also called **interleukins.** This term is imperfect because many cytokines that are synthesized only by leukocytes and that act only on leukocytes are not called interleukins, for historical reasons, whereas many cytokines called interleukins are made by or act on cells other than leukocytes. Nevertheless, the term has been useful because as new cytokines are molecularly characterized, they are assigned an interleukin (IL) number (e.g., IL-1, IL-2, and so on) to maintain a standard nomenclature. Cytokines are also increasingly used in clinical situations and in animal studies to stimulate or inhibit inflammation, immunity, and hematopoiesis. In this setting, cytokines are often referred to as biologic response modifiers. Throughout this book, we use the term *cytokine,* which does not imply restricted cellular sources or biologic activities. We have discussed many different cytokines in previous chapters, which are important in innate immunity, and in the development, activation, trafficking, and effector functions of lymphocytes. In this chapter, we will present a comprehensive overview of cytokine biology, including the structure, production, and biologic actions of cytokines. Before describing the individual molecules, we begin with a summary of the general properties of cytokines.

General Properties of Cytokines

Cytokines are polypeptides produced in response to microbes and other antigens that mediate and regulate immune and inflammatory reactions (Fig. 12–1). Although cytokines are structurally diverse, they share several properties.

- ***Cytokine secretion is a brief, self-limited event.*** Cytokines are not usually stored as preformed molecules, and their synthesis is initiated by new gene transcription as a result of cellular activation. Such transcriptional activation is transient, and the messenger RNAs encoding most cytokines are unstable, so cytokine synthesis is also transient. The production of some cytokines may additionally be controlled by RNA processing and by posttranslational mechanisms, such as proteolytic release of an active product from an inactive precursor. Proteolytic processing is important, for example, in production of active tumor necrosis factor (TNF), IL-1, and transforming growth factor-β (TGF-β). Once synthesized, cytokines are rapidly secreted, resulting in a burst of release when needed.
- ***The actions of cytokines are often pleiotropic and redundant*** (Fig. 12–2). Pleiotropism refers to the ability of one cytokine to act on different cell types. This property allows a cytokine to mediate diverse biologic effects, but it greatly limits the therapeutic use of cytokines because administration of a cytokine for a desired clinical effect may result in numerous unwanted side effects. Redundancy refers to the property of multiple cytokines having the same functional effects. Because of this redundancy, antagonists against a single cytokine or mutation of one cytokine gene may not have functional consequences, as other cytokines may compensate.

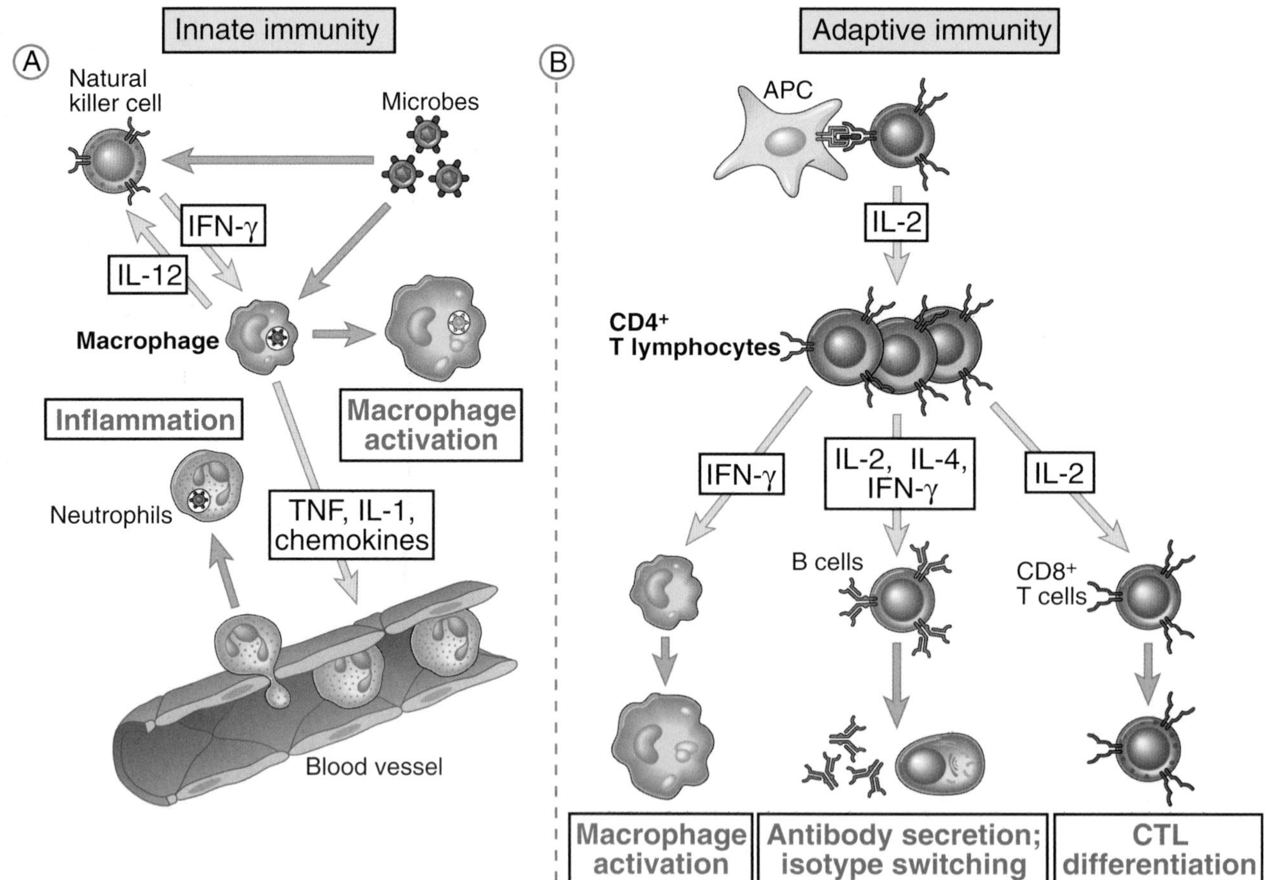

FIGURE 12–1 Functions of selected cytokines in host defense. In innate immunity, cytokines produced by macrophages and NK cells mediate the early inflammatory reactions to microbes and promote the elimination of microbes. In adaptive immunity, cytokines stimulate proliferation and differentiation of antigen-stimulated lymphocytes and activate specialized effector cells, such as macrophages. The properties of the cytokines shown in this figure are discussed later in this chapter. APC, antigen-presenting cell.

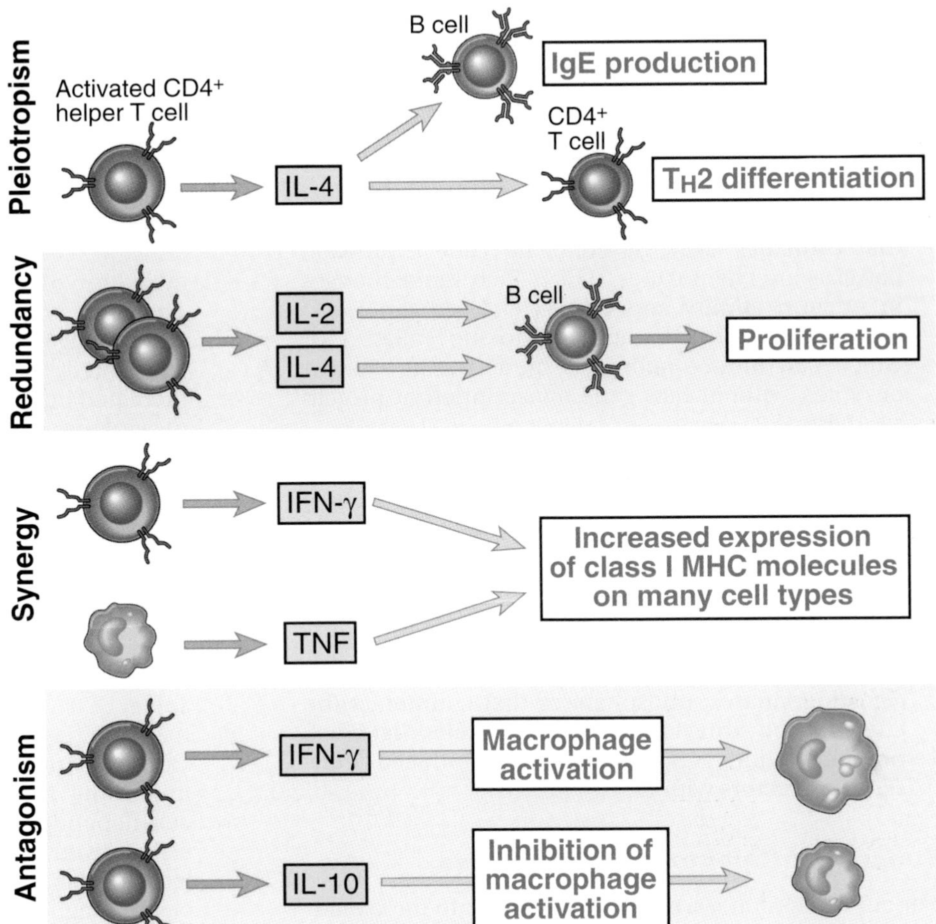

FIGURE 12–2 Properties of cytokines. Selected examples are shown to illustrate the following properties of cytokines: pleiotropism, one cytokine having multiple effects on diverse cell types; redundancy, multiple cytokines having the same or overlapping actions; synergy, two or more cytokines having greater than additive effects; and antagonism, one cytokine inhibiting the action of another.

- ***Cytokines often influence the synthesis and actions of other cytokines.*** The ability of one cytokine to stimulate production of others leads to cascades in which a second or third cytokine may mediate the biologic effects of the first. Two cytokines may antagonize each other's action, produce additive effects, or, in some cases, produce greater than anticipated, or synergistic, effects (see Fig. 12–2).
- ***Cytokine actions may be local and systemic.*** Most cytokines act close to where they are produced, either on the same cell that secretes the cytokine **(autocrine action)** or on a nearby cell **(paracrine action).** T cells often secrete cytokines at the site of contact with antigen-presenting cells (APCs), the so-called immune synapse (see Chapter 9). This may be one reason why cytokines often act on cells that are in contact with the cytokine producers. When produced in large amounts, cytokines may enter the circulation and act at a distance from the site of production **(endocrine action).** TNF is an example of a cytokine that has important local and systemic effects.
- ***Cytokines initiate their actions by binding to specific membrane receptors on target cells.*** Receptors for cytokines often bind their ligands with high affinities, with dissociation constants (K_d values) in the range of 10^{-10} to 10^{-12} M. (For comparison, recall that antibodies typically bind antigens with a K_d of 10^{-7} to 10^{-11} M and that T cell antigen receptors bind MHC-associated peptides with a K_d of 10^{-5} to 10^{-7} M.) Therefore, only small quantities of a cytokine are needed to occupy receptors and elicit biologic effects. Most cells express low levels of cytokine receptors (on the order of 100 to 1000 receptors per cell), but this is adequate for inducing responses.
- ***External signals regulate the expression of cytokine receptors and thus the responsiveness of cells to cytokines.*** For instance, stimulation of T or B lymphocytes by antigens leads to increased expression of cytokine receptors. For this reason, during an immune response, the antigen-specific lymphocytes are the preferential responders to secreted cytokines. This is one mechanism for maintaining the specificity of immune responses, even though cytokines themselves are not antigen specific. Receptor expression is also regulated by cytokines themselves, including the same cytokine that binds to the receptor, permitting positive amplification or negative feedback.
- ***The cellular responses to most cytokines consist of changes in gene expression in target cells, resulting in the expression of new functions and sometimes in the***

proliferation of the target cells. Many of the changes in gene expression induced by cytokines result in differentiation of T and B lymphocytes and activation of effector cells such as macrophages. For instance, cytokines stimulate switching of antibody isotypes in B cells, differentiation of helper T cells into T_H1 and T_H2 subsets, and activation of microbicidal mechanisms in phagocytes. Exceptions to the rule that cytokines work by changing gene expression patterns are chemokines, which elicit rapid changes in integrin affinity and cytoskeletal reorganization that favor migration, and a cytokine called TNF, which can induce apoptosis by activating cellular enzymes, without new gene transcription or protein synthesis.

- ***Cellular responses to cytokines are tightly regulated, and feedback inhibitory mechanisms exist to turn down these responses.*** These mechanisms include cytokine induction of genes encoding inhibitors of the cytokine receptors or the downstream signaling pathways activated by the receptors. The inhibitors include decoy cytokine receptors expressed on the cell surface, molecules that block interactions of signaling kinases, phosphatases that counteract the effects of activating kinases, and molecules that block productive interactions of cytokine-induced transcription factors with DNA.

Functional Categories of Cytokines

For our discussion, we classify cytokines into three main functional categories based on their principal biologic actions:

1. ***Mediators and regulators of innate immunity*** are produced mainly by mononuclear phagocytes in response to infectious agents (Table 12–1). Pathogen-associated molecular patterns, such as bacterial lipopolysaccharide (LPS) and viral double-stranded RNA (dsRNA), bind to Toll-like receptors (TLRs) on the cell surface or in endosomes of macrophages and stimulate the synthesis and secretion of some of the important cytokines of innate immunity (see Chapter 2). The same cytokines may also be secreted by macrophages that are activated by antigen-stimulated T cells (i.e., as part of adaptive cell-mediated immunity). Most members of this group of cytokines act on endothelial cells and leukocytes to stimulate the early inflammatory reactions to microbes, and some function to control these responses. Natural killer (NK) cells and NK-T cells also produce cytokines during innate immune reactions.
2. ***Mediators and regulators of adaptive immunity*** are produced mainly by T lymphocytes in response to specific recognition of foreign antigens (see Table 12–1). Some T cell cytokines function primarily to regulate the growth and differentiation of various lymphocyte populations and thus play important roles in the activation phase of T cell–dependent immune responses. Other T cell–derived cytokines recruit, activate, and regulate specialized effector cells, such as mononuclear phagocytes, neutrophils, and eosinophils, to eliminate antigens in the effector phase of adaptive immune responses.

Table 12–1. Comparative Features of the Cytokines of Innate and Adaptive Immunity

Features	Innate immunity	Adaptive immunity
Examples	TNF, IL-1, IL-12, IFN-γ *	IL-2, IL-4, IL-5, IFN-γ *
Major cell source	Macrophages, NK cells	T lymphocytes
Principal physiologic functions	Mediators of inflammation (local and systemic)	Regulation of lymphocyte growth and differentiation; activation of effector cells (macrophages, eosinophils, mast cells)
Stimuli	LPS (endotoxin), bacterial peptidoglycans, viral RNA, T cell-derived cytokines (IFN-γ)	Protein antigens
Amounts produced	May be high; detectable in serum	Generally low; usually undetectable in serum
Local or systemic effects	Both	Usually local only
Roles in disease	Systemic diseases (e.g., septic shock)	Local tissue injury (e.g., granulomatous inflammation)
Inhibitors	Corticosteroids	Cyclosporine, FK-506

*IFN-γ plays important roles in innate and adaptive immunity.
Abbreviations: IFN, interferon; IL, interleukin; LPS, lipopolysaccharide; NK, natural killer; TNF, tumor necrosis factor

3. ***Stimulators of hematopoiesis*** are produced by bone marrow stromal cells, leukocytes, and other cells, and stimulate the growth and differentiation of immature leukocytes.

In general, the cytokines of innate and adaptive immunity are produced by different cell populations and act on different target cells (see Table 12–1). However, these distinctions are not absolute because the same cytokine may be produced during innate and adaptive immune reactions, and different cytokines produced during such reactions may have overlapping actions.

Cytokine Receptors and Signaling

Before we describe the functions of individual cytokines, it is useful to summarize the characteristics of cytokine receptors and how they transduce signals as a consequence of the binding of the cytokines. All cytokine receptors consist of one or more transmembrane proteins whose extracellular portions are responsible for cytokine binding and whose cytoplasmic portions are responsible for initiating intracellular signaling pathways. These signaling pathways are typically activated by ligand-induced receptor clustering, bringing together the cytoplasmic portions of two or more receptor molecules in a process analogous to signaling by T and B cell receptors for antigens (see Chapters 9 and 10).

There are several criteria by which cytokine receptors are classified. The most widely used classification is based on structural homologies of the extracellular cytokine-binding domains and shared intracellular signaling mechanisms. According to this classification, cytokine receptors can be divided into several families (Fig. 12–3 and Table 12–2).

- ***Type I cytokine receptors,*** also called hemopoietin receptors, contain one or more copies of a domain with two conserved pairs of cysteine residues and a membrane proximal sequence of tryptophan-serine-X-tryptophan-serine (WSXWS), where X is any amino acid. These receptors typically bind cytokines that fold into four α-helical strands, called type I cytokines. The conserved features of the receptors form structures that bind four α-helical cytokines, but the specificity for individual cytokines is determined by amino acid residues that vary from one receptor to another. These receptors consist of unique ligand-binding chains and one or more signal-transducing chains, which are often shared by receptors for different cytokines (Fig. 12–3B). All the type I cytokine receptors engage Jak-STAT signaling pathways, described later in this chapter, that induce new gene transcription.
- ***Type II cytokine receptors*** are similar to type I receptors by virtue of two extracellular domains with conserved cysteines, but type II receptors do not contain the WSXWS motif. These receptors consist of one ligand-binding polypeptide chain and one signal-transducing chain. All the type II cytokine receptors engage Jak-STAT signaling pathways.
- ***IL-1 family receptors*** share a conserved cytosolic sequence, called the Toll-like/IL-1 receptor (TIR) domain, and engage similar signal transduction pathways that induce new gene transcription.

Table 12–2. Signal Transduction Mechanisms of Cytokine Receptors

Signal transduction pathway	Cytokine receptors using this pathway	Signaling mechanism
Jak-STAT pathway	Type I and type II cytokine recptors	Jak-mediated phosphorylation and activation of STAT transcription factors (See Box 12-2)
TNF receptor signaling by TRAFs	TNF receptor family: TNR-RII, CD40	Binding of TRAF family adapter proteins, activation of transcription factors (see Box 12-1)
TNF receptor signaling by death domains	TNF receptor family: TNF-RI, Fas	Binding of death domain family adapter proteins, caspase activation (see Box 12-1)
TIR-domain/IRAK pathway	IL-1 and IL-18 receptors	Binding of IRAK family kinases to TIR domains, activation of transcription factors
Receptor-associated kinases	TGF-β receptor, M-CSF receptor, stem cell factor receptor	Intrinsic kinase activity in receptor, activation of transcription factors
G protein signaling	Chemokine receptors	GTP exchange and dissociation of Gα · GTP from Gβγ, Gα · GTP activates various cellular enzymes

Abbreviations: GTP, guanosine triphosphate; IRAK, IL-1 receptor-associated kinase; Jak, Janus kinase; M-CSF, monocyte colony-stimulating factor; STAT, signal transducer and activator of transcription; TNF, tumor necrosis factor; TNF-RI, type I TNF receptor; TNF-RII, type II TNF receptor; TIR, Toll-IL-1 receptor; TRAF, TNF receptor–associated factor

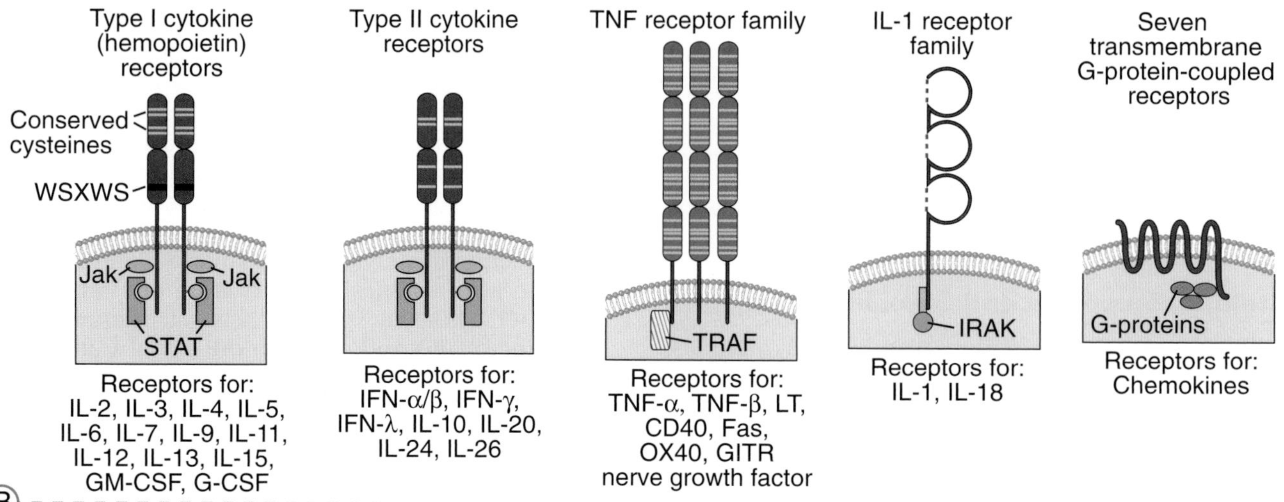

B

Subunit composition of cytokine receptors

Common γ chain family

γc γc γc

α α α

β β

IL-2 IL-15 IL-4

(also: IL-7, IL-9, IL-21)

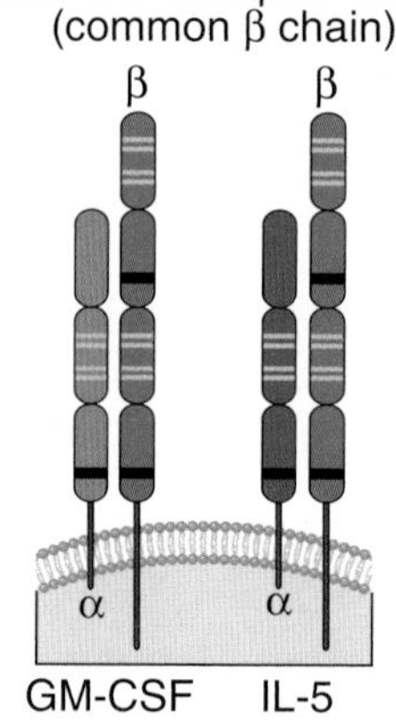

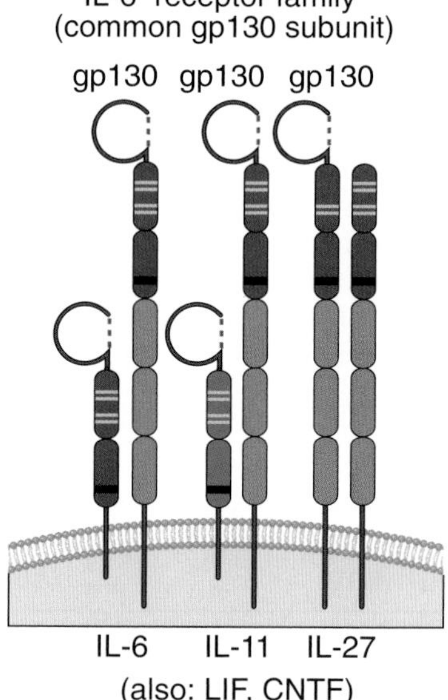

FIGURE 12–3 Structure of cytokine receptors. A. Receptors for different cytokines are classified into families on the basis of conserved extracellular domain structures and signaling mechanisms. The cytokines or other ligands that bind to each receptor family are listed below the schematic drawings. WSXWS, tryptophan-serine-X-tryptophan-serine. B. Groups of cytokine receptors share identical or highly homologous subunit chains. Selected examples of cytokine receptors in each group are shown.

- ***TNF receptors*** are part of a large family of proteins (some of which are not cytokine receptors) with conserved trimeric, cysteine-rich extracellular domains, and shared intracellular signaling mechanisms that induce apoptosis and/or stimulate gene expression.

- ***Seven-transmembrane α-helical receptors*** are also called serpentine receptors, because their transmembrane domains appear to "snake" back and forth through the membrane, and **G protein–coupled receptors**, because their signaling pathways involve guanosine triphosphate (GTP)-binding proteins (G proteins). The mammalian genome encodes many such receptors involved in many types of cellular responses. In the immune system, members of this receptor class mediate rapid and transient responses to chemokines and several different inflammatory mediators.

Members of a family defined by extracellular domains usually engage similar signal transduction pathways, although there are exceptions. We describe the principal features of the different signaling pathways that cytokine receptors utilize when we consider the individual cytokines.

With this introduction to the shared properties of cytokines, we proceed to discussions of individual cytokines. We conclude each section with an overview of the roles of the cytokines in the relevant host response.

Cytokines That Mediate and Regulate Innate Immunity

An important component of the early innate immune response to viruses and bacteria is the secretion of cytokines, which mediate many of the effector functions of innate immunity (see Chapter 2). In this section, we first describe the individual cytokines of innate immunity (Table 12–3), and then we summarize how these cytokines function in host defense and inflammation. One cytokine, IFN-γ, plays important roles in both innate and adaptive immunity; it is discussed later in this chapter.

Tumor Necrosis Factor

TNF is the principal mediator of the acute inflammatory response to gram-negative bacteria and other infectious microbes and is responsible for many of the systemic complications of severe infections. The name of this cytokine derives from its original identification as a serum factor that caused necrosis of tumors. TNF is also called TNF-α to distinguish it from the closely related TNF-β, also called lymphotoxin (LT).

Production, Structure, and Receptors

The major cellular source of TNF is activated mononuclear phagocytes, although antigen-stimulated T cells, NK cells, and mast cells can also secrete this protein. The most potent stimulus for eliciting TNF production by macrophages is TLR engagement with LPS and other microbial products, and large amounts of this cytokine may be produced during infections by gram-negative bacteria, which release LPS. IFN-γ, produced by T cells and NK cells, augments TNF synthesis by LPS-stimulated macrophages.

In mononuclear phagocytes, TNF is synthesized as a nonglycosylated type II membrane protein with an intracellular amino terminus and a large extracellular carboxyl terminus. Membrane TNF is expressed as a homotrimer and is able to bind to type II TNF receptor (TNF-RII), described below. The membrane form of TNF is cleaved by a membrane-associated metalloproteinase, releasing a 17-kD polypeptide. Three of these polypeptide chains polymerize to form the 51-kD circulating TNF protein. Secreted TNF assumes a triangular pyramid shape, each side of the pyramid being formed by one subunit (Fig. 12–4). The receptor-binding sites are at the base of the pyramid, allowing simultaneous binding of the cytokine to three receptor molecules.

There are two distinct TNF receptors of molecular sizes 55 kD (type I TNF receptor [TNF-RI]) and 75 kD (TNF-RII). The affinities of TNF for its receptors are unusually low for a cytokine, the K_d being only ~1×10^{-9} M for binding to TNF-RI and approximately 5×10^{-10} M for binding to TNF-RII. Both TNF receptors are present on most cell types. The TNF receptors are members of a large family of proteins, many of which are involved in immune and inflammatory responses. These receptors exist as trimers in the plasma membrane, even before binding of TNF (Box 12–1). Cytokine binding to some TNF receptor family members, such as TNF-RI, TNF-RII, and CD40 leads to the recruitment of proteins, called TNF receptor-associated factors (TRAFs), to the cytoplasmic domains of the receptors. The TRAFs activate transcription factors, notably nuclear factor κB (NF-κB) and activation protein-1 (AP-1). Cytokine binding to other family members, such as TNF-RI, leads to recruitment of an adapter protein that activates caspases and triggers apoptosis. Thus, different members of the TNF receptor family can induce gene expression and cell death, and some can do both. TNF-RI knockout mice show more impaired host defense than do TNF-RII knockout mice, suggesting that TNF-RI is more important for the function of the cytokine.

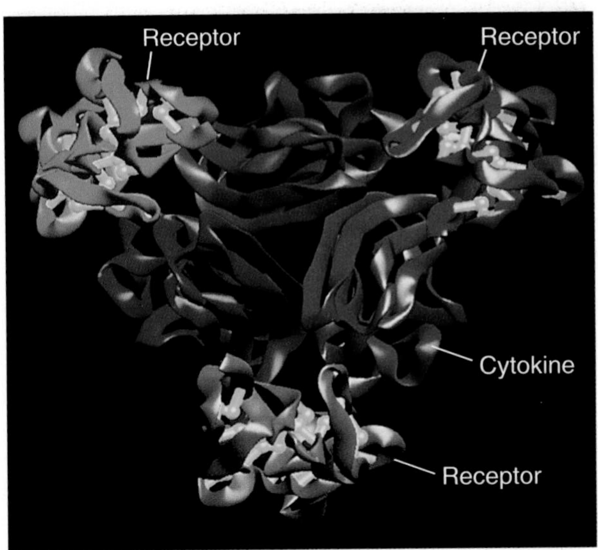

FIGURE 12–4 Structure of the TNF receptor with bound LT. The ribbon structure depicts a top view of a complex of three TNF receptors (TNF-RI) and one molecule of the bound cytokine, revealed by x-ray crystallography. LT is a homotrimer in which the three subunits are colored dark blue. The LT homotrimer forms an inverted three-sided pyramid with its base at the top and its apex at the bottom. Three TNF-RI molecules, colored magenta, cyan, and red, bind one homotrimer of LT, with each receptor molecule interacting with two different LT monomers in the homotrimer complex. Disulfide bonds in the receptor are colored yellow. TNF is homologous to LT and presumably binds to its receptors in the same way. (From Banner DW, A D'Arcy, W Jones, R Gentz, HJ Schoenfeld, C Broger, H Loetscher, and W Lesslauer. Crystal structure of the soluble human 55kd TNF receptor-human TNFbeta complex; implications for TNF receptor activation. Cell 73:431–445, 1993. Copyright 1993, with permission from Elsevier Science.)

Biologic Actions

The principal physiologic function of TNF is to stimulate the recruitment of neutrophils and monocytes to sites of infection and to activate these cells to eradicate

Table 12–3. Cytokines of Innate Immunity

Cytokine	Size (kD)	Principal cell source	Principal cellular targets and biologic effects
Tumor necrosis factor (TNF)	17 kD; 51 kD homotrimer	Macrophages, T cells	Endothelial cells: activation (inflammation, coagulation) Neutrophils: activation Hypothalamus: fever Liver: synthesis of acute phase proteins Muscle, fat: catabolism (cachexia) Many cell types: apoptosis
Interleukin-1 (IL-1)	17 kD mature form; 33 kD precursors	Macrophages, endothelial cells, some epithelial cells	Endothelial cells: activation (inflammation, coagulation) Hypothalamus: fever Liver: synthesis of acute phase proteins
Chemokines (see Table 12-4)	8–12 kD	Macrophages, endothelial cells, T cells, fibroblasts, platelets	Leukocytes: chemotaxis, activation; migration into tissues
Interleukin-12 (IL-12)	Heterodimer of 35 kD + 40 kD subunits	Macrophages, dendritic cells	T cells: T_H1 differentiation NK cells and T cells: IFN-γ synthesis, increased cytotoxic activity
Type I IFNs (IFN-α, IFN-β)	IFN-α: 15–21 kD IFN-β: 20–25 kD	IFN-α: macrophages IFN-β: fibroblasts	All cells: antiviral state, increased class I MHC expression NK cells: activation
Interleukin-10 (IL-10)	Homodimer of 34–40 kD; 18 kD subunits	Macrophages, T cells (mainly regulatory T cells)	Macrophages, dendritic cells: inhibition of IL-12 production and expression of costimulators and class II MHC molecules
Interleukin-6 (IL-6)	19–26 kD	Macrophages, endothelial cells, T cells	Liver: synthesis of acute phase proteins B cells: proliferation of antibody-producing cells
Interleukin-15 (IL-15)	13 kD	Macrophages, others	NK cells: proliferation T cells: proliferation (memory $CD8^+$ cells)
Interleukin-18 (IL-18)	17 kD	Macrophages	NK cells and T cells: IFN-γ synthesis
Interleukin-23 (IL-23)	Heterodimer of unique 19 kD subunit and 40 kD subunit of IL-12	Macrophages and dendritic cells	T cells: maintenance of IL-17 producing T cells
Interleukin-27 (IL-27)	Heterodimer of 28 kD and 13 kD subunits	Macrophages and dendritic cells	T cells: inhibition of T_H1 cells; role in T_H1 differentiation? NK cells: IFN-γ synthesis

Abbreviations: IFN, interferon; kD, kilodalton; MHC, major histocompatibility complex; NK, natural killer.

microbes (Fig. 12–5). TNF mediates these effects by several actions on vascular endothelial cells and leukocytes.

- TNF induces vascular endothelial cells to express adhesion molecules that make the endothelial surface adhesive for leukocytes, initially for neutrophils and subsequently for monocytes and lymphocytes. The most important of these adhesion molecules are selectins and ligands for leukocyte integrins (see Chapter 2, Boxes 2–2 and 2–3). The sequence of events in the recruitment of leukocytes to sites of infection was described in Chapter 2.
- TNF stimulates endothelial cells and macrophages to secrete chemokines (discussed later) that enhance the affinity of leukocyte integrins for their ligands and induce leukocyte chemotaxis and recruitment. TNF also acts on mononuclear phagocytes to stimulate secretion of IL-1, which functions much like TNF itself (see later). This is an example of a cascade of cytokines that have similar or complementary biologic activities.

Box 12–1 ▪ IN DEPTH: SIGNALING BY THE TNF-R FAMILY

The TNF family of proteins includes secreted cytokines and membrane proteins that share sequence homologies and fold into homotrimeric triangular pyramidal complexes, which bind to structurally similar cell surface receptors. Members of this family include TNF, LT (TNF-β), CD40 ligand, Fas ligand, GITR ligand, OX40 ligand, RANK ligand, TNF-related apoptosis-inducing ligand (TRAIL), and several other proteins. The cell surface receptors for the TNF family of proteins are type I membrane proteins that can also be grouped into a family, called the TNF-R family, on the basis of sequence homology in their cysteine-rich extracellular ligand-binding domains. Members of the TNF-R family include TNF-RI, TNF-RII, lymphotoxin-β receptor (LT-βR), Fas, CD40, OX40, RANK, and

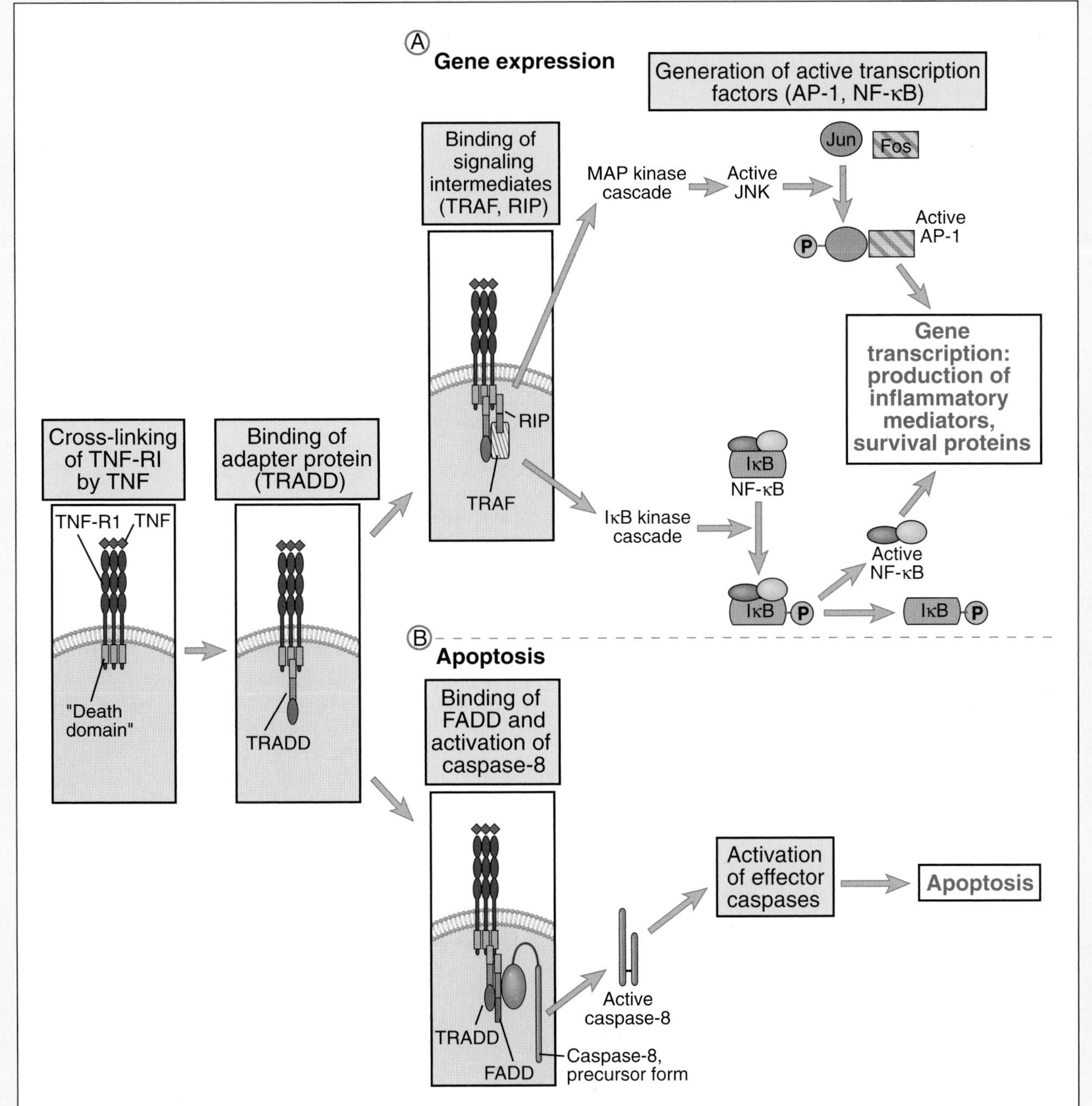

Signal transduction by TNF receptors. TNF-RI may stimulate gene expression (A) or induce apoptosis (B). These distinct effects are both initiated by the binding of the adapter protein TRADD followed by either TRAF and RIP, leading to new gene expression, or binding of the adapter protein FADD, leading to apoptosis. The cytoplasmic tails of other members of the TNF-R family may directly bind FADD (e.g., Fas), leading to apoptosis, or directly bind TRAFs (e.g., TNF-RII or CD40), leading to gene expression. The genes induced by TNF-R family members encode mainly mediators of inflammation and anti-apoptotic proteins.

Continued on following page

Box 12–1 ▪ IN DEPTH: SIGNALING BY THE TNF-R FAMILY (Continued)

others. The binding of TNF family members to their respective receptors initiates a wide variety of responses. Many of these responses are proinflammatory and depend on activation of the NF-κB and AP-1 transcription factors leading to new gene transcription. In contrast, some TNF-R family members (TNF-RI and Fas) deliver signals that cause apoptotic cell death. The specific responses to the cytokines depend on the particular receptor and cell type. Many of the molecular details of the signaling pathways engaged by TNF-R family molecules are now known. Although the members of this receptor family share structural features in their extracellular ligand-binding regions, they have widely divergent cytoplasmic domain structures. Nonetheless, there are shared features in the signaling pathways associated with these receptors. We discuss signaling by the TNF-R family, with an emphasis on how a protypical member of the family, TNF-RI, can induce anti-apoptotic and inflammatory responses in some circumstances or apoptosis in others (see Figure).

As is the case with many membrane receptors in the immune system, the cytoplasmic tails of the TNF-R family members do not contain intrinsic enzymatic activities, but they do contain structural motifs that bind to cytoplasmic signaling molecules and promote the assembly of signaling complexes. One of these structural motifs is called the **death domain,** and it binds, by homotypic interactions, to death domains in a variety of cytoplasmic signaling/adapter molecules. The cytoplasmic tails of both TNF-RI and Fas contain death domains, and mutation or deletion of this region prevents TNF-RI or Fas molecules from delivering apoptosis-inducing signals. However, death domain interactions are also essential for the anti-apoptotic, proinflammatory signaling pathways. The cytoplasmic signaling molecules that contain death domains and that are involved in TNF-R signaling include TRADD (TNF receptor-associated death domain), FADD (Fas-associated death domain), and RIP (receptor interacting protein).

The second type of motif that plays a key role in signaling by several TNF-R family members binds to one of a family of molecules called **TNF receptor-associated factors** (TRAFs). TNF-RII, LT-βR, and CD40 all bind TRAF proteins. To date, seven TRAFs have been identified, and they are called TRAF-1 to TRAF-7. All TRAFs share a C-terminal region of homology called a TRAF domain, which mediates binding to the cytoplasmic domains of TNF-R family members, and TRAFs 2 to 6 have RING and zinc finger motifs that are involved in signaling.

Multiple different interactions of death domain proteins and TRAFs are known to occur in the signaling pathways associated with the different TNF-R family members. In the case of TNF-RI, TNF may lead to either apoptosis or inflammatory responses (see Figure). The death domain protein TRADD binds directly to the TNF-RI death domain and acts as a pivotal adapter molecule leading to one of two different signaling cascades. In one of these pathways, the death domain protein FADD binds to TRADD, and the aspartyl-directed cysteine protease caspase-8 binds to FADD. Caspase-8 binding initiates the activation of a cascade of caspases that eventually causes apoptosis. In response to Fas ligand binding, Fas mediates apoptosis by a similar pathway, but in this case, FADD binds directly to the cytoplasmic tail of Fas (see Chapter 11, Box 11–2). The alternative proinflammatory and anti-apoptotic pathway involves the binding of TRAF-2 and RIP-1 to TRADD and results in NF-κB- and AP-1–dependent gene transcription. Both TRAF-2 and RIP-1 are involved in the activation of IκB kinases, which mediate the initial steps in NF-κB activation. TRAF-2 also activates the mitogen-activated protein kinase (MAP kinase) cascade that leads to JNK activation, phosphorylation of c-Jun, and formation of the AP-1 transcription factor. The combination of NF-κB and AP-1 activation promotes the transcription of a variety of genes involved in inflammation, including endothelial adhesion molecules, cytokines, and chemokines. Furthermore, NF-κB also enhances expression of a family of cellular inhibitors of apoptosis (cIAPs), which block the function of caspases. Therefore, when the proinflammatory pathway is engaged, there is active inhibition of the apoptotic pathway. It is still unclear what determines whether TNF binding to TNF-RI will activate the inflammatory or apoptotic signaling pathways.

Other members of the TNF-R family use TRAF-dependent signaling pathways that lead to NF-κB and AP-1 activation similar to the TNF-RI pathway, but in contrast to TNF-RI, these other receptors directly bind TRAFs to their cytoplasmic tails. TRAF-1 and TRAF-2 interact with TNF-RII, TRAF-2 and TRAF-3 interact with CD40, and TRAF-4 interacts with LT-βR. CD40 delivers activating signals to B cells and macrophages through TRAF binding (see Chapters 10 and 13). Interestingly, one of the transforming gene products of the Epstein-Barr virus encodes a self-aggregating TRAF domain-containing protein that binds TRAF molecules, and therefore infection by the virus mimics TNF- or CD40-induced signals.

- TNF stimulates the microbicidal activities of neutrophils and macrophages.

The actions of TNF on endothelium and leukocytes are critical for local inflammatory responses to microbes. If inadequate quantities of TNF are present (e.g., in animals treated with neutralizing anti-TNF antibodies or in TNF gene knockout mice), a consequence may be failure to contain infections. TNF also contributes to local inflammatory reactions that are injurious to the host (e.g., in autoimmune diseases) (see Chapter 18). Neutralizing antibodies to TNF and soluble TNF receptors are in clinical use to reduce inflammation in patients with rheumatoid arthritis and inflammatory bowel disease.

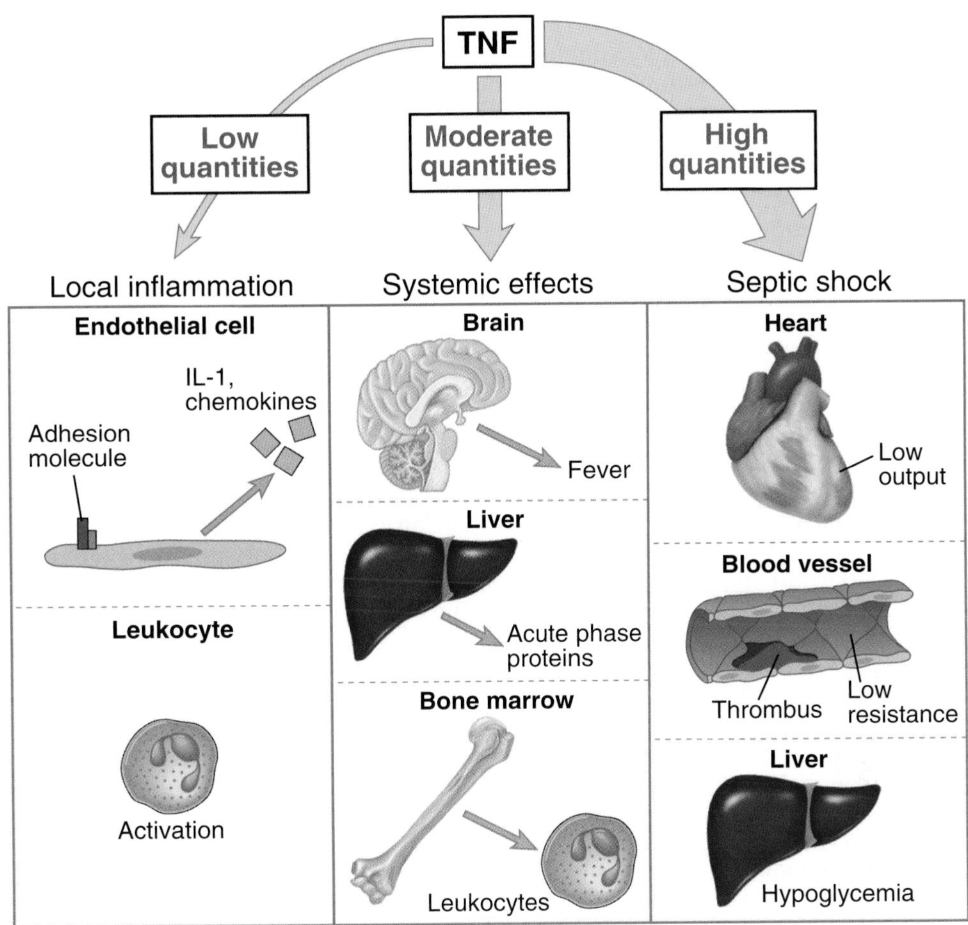

FIGURE 12–5 Biologic actions of TNF. At low concentrations, TNF acts on leukocytes and endothelium to induce acute inflammation. At moderate concentrations, TNF mediates the systemic effects of inflammation in part via the induction of IL-1 and IL-6. At high concentrations, TNF causes the pathologic abnormalities of septic shock.

TNF also induces apoptosis of some cell types in vitro; the physiologic role of this activity is not known.

In severe infections, TNF is produced in large amounts and causes systemic clinical and pathologic abnormalities. If the stimulus for TNF production is sufficiently strong, the quantity of the cytokine produced is so large that it enters the blood stream and acts at distant sites as an endocrine hormone (see Fig. 12–5). The principal systemic actions of TNF are the following:

- TNF acts on the hypothalamus to induce fever and is therefore called an endogenous (i.e., host-derived) pyrogen (to distinguish it from LPS, which functions as an exogenous, microbe-derived, pyrogen). Fever production in response to TNF (and IL-1) is mediated by increased synthesis of prostaglandins by cytokine-stimulated hypothalamic cells. Prostaglandin synthesis inhibitors, such as aspirin, reduce fever by blocking this action of TNF and IL-1.

- TNF acts on hepatocytes to increase synthesis of certain serum proteins, such as serum amyloid A protein and fibrinogen. The increase in hepatocyte-derived plasma proteins induced by TNF and by IL-1 and IL-6, two other cytokines of innate immunity, constitutes the acute-phase response to inflammatory stimuli (see Chapter 15, Box 15–1).

- Prolonged production of TNF causes wasting of muscle and fat cells, called cachexia. This wasting results from TNF-induced appetite suppression and reduced synthesis of lipoprotein lipase, an enzyme needed to release fatty acids from circulating lipoproteins so that they can be used by the tissues.

- When large amounts of TNF are produced, with serum concentrations reaching 10^{-7}M or more, myocardial contractility and vascular smooth muscle tone are inhibited, resulting in a marked fall in blood pressure, or shock.

- TNF causes intravascular thrombosis, mainly as a result of loss of the normal anticoagulant properties of the endothelium. TNF stimulates endothelial cell expression of tissue factor, a potent activator of coagulation, and inhibits expression of thrombomodulin, an inhibitor of coagulation. The endothelial alterations are exacerbated by activation of neutrophils, leading to vascular plugging by these cells. The ability of this cytokine to cause necrosis of tumors, which is the basis of its name, is mainly a result of thrombosis of tumor blood vessels.

- High circulating levels of TNF cause severe metabolic disturbances, such as a fall in blood glucose concentrations to levels incompatible with life. This is due to overuse of glucose by muscle and failure of the liver to replace the glucose.

A complication of severe gram-negative bacterial sepsis is a syndrome called **septic shock** (or endotoxin shock), which is characterized by vascular collapse, disseminated intravascular coagulation, and metabolic disturbances. This syndrome is due to LPS-induced production of TNF and other cytokines, including IL-12, IFN-γ, and IL-1. The concentration of serum TNF may be predictive of the outcome of severe gram-negative infections. This is one of the few examples of a disorder in which measuring levels of a circulating cytokine is informative. Septic shock can be reproduced in experimental animals by administration of LPS or TNF (see Chapter 15, Box 15–1). Antagonists of TNF can prevent mortality in the experimental models, but clinical trials with anti-TNF antibodies or with soluble TNF receptors have not shown benefit in patients with sepsis. The cause of this therapeutic failure is not known, but it may be because other cytokines elicit the same responses as TNF, an example of redundancy.

There are many cytokines and membrane proteins belonging to the TNF–TNF receptor families, and they serve important functions in innate and adaptive immune responses. Two TNF family membrane proteins expressed on activated T lymphocytes are CD40 ligand and Fas ligand. CD40 ligand mediates activation of macrophages and B cells (see Chapters 10 and 13), and Fas ligand is involved in killing of some cell types (see Chapter 11). BAFF and APRIL are TNF family members that play critical roles in B cell survival and differentiation (see Chapter 10). Glucocorticoid-induced TNF-related (GITR) ligand and OX40 ligand are TNF family molecules that may be involved in regulation of T cell responses. Receptor activator of NF-κB (RANK) is a TNF-R family member that is expressed on osteoclasts and some macrophages and dendritic cells. RANK is the receptor for the cytokine RANK-ligand, which is made by activated T cells. RANK-ligand activates osteoclasts and thus plays an important role in bone resorption in many disease states, notably rheumatoid arthritis.

Interleukin-1

The principal function of IL-1, similar to that of TNF, is as a mediator of the host inflammatory response to infections and other stimuli. IL-1 works together with TNF in innate immunity and inflammation.

Production, Structure, and Receptors

The major cellular source of IL-1, like that of TNF, is activated mononuclear phagocytes. IL-1 production by mononuclear phagocytes is induced by bacterial products such as LPS and by other cytokines such as TNF. Unlike TNF, IL-1 is also produced by many cell types other than macrophages, such as neutrophils, epithelial cells (e.g., keratinocytes), and endothelial cells.

There are two forms of IL-1, called IL-1α and IL-1β, that are less than 30% homologous to each other, but they bind to the same cell surface receptors and have the same biologic activities. Both IL-1 polypeptides are synthesized as 33-kD precursors and are secreted as 17-kD mature proteins. The active form of IL-1β is the cleaved product, but IL-1α is active either as the 33-kD precursor or as the smaller cleaved product. IL-1β is proteolytically cleaved by the cysteine protease caspase-1 (also called IL-1β-converting enzyme) to generate the biologically active secreted protein. Caspase-1 was the first described mammalian member of the caspase family, many other members of which are involved in apoptotic death in a variety of cells (see Chapter 11, Box 11–2). Activation of caspase-1 requires the assembly of a complex of proteins termed the **inflammasome**. NALP family proteins, which are cytoplasmic innate immune sensors (see Chapter 2), are critical components of the inflammasome. Gain-of-function mutations affecting NALP proteins lead to uncontrolled IL-1 production and "auto-inflammatory syndromes".

IL-1 mediates its biologic effects through a membrane receptor called the type I IL-1 receptor, which engages signal transduction pathways that activate NF-κB and AP-1 transcription factors. The type I IL-1 receptor is a member of a family of integral membrane proteins that contain an extracellular ligand-binding Ig domain and a TIR signaling domain in the cytoplasmic region. The TIR domain was described in reference to TLRs in Chapter 2. Another member of this family is the IL-18 receptor (IL-18 is discussed later in this chapter). The signaling events that occur when IL-1 binds to the type I IL-1 receptor are similar to those associated with TLRs. Upon IL-1 binding, the adapter protein MyD88 is recruited to the TIR domain, followed by two protein kinases, IL-1 receptor-associated kinase-4 (IRAK4) and IRAK-1, and another adapter protein, TRAF-6. Downstream signaling involves several phosphorylation events and formation of new complexes with other kinases and adapter proteins, eventually leading to the activation of NF-κB.

Biologic Actions

The biologic effects of IL-1 are similar to those of TNF and depend on the quantity of cytokine produced.

- When secreted at low concentrations, IL-1 functions as a mediator of local inflammation. It acts on endothelial cells to increase expression of surface molecules that mediate leukocyte adhesion, such as ligands for integrins.
- When secreted in larger quantities, IL-1 enters the blood stream and exerts endocrine effects. Systemic IL-1 induces fever, synthesis of acute-phase plasma proteins by the liver, directly and indirectly through stimulation of IL-6 production, and neutrophil and platelet production by the bone marrow.

The similarities between IL-1 actions and those of TNF appear surprising at face value because the cytokines and their receptors are structurally different. The likely explanation for the similar biologic effects is that receptors for both cytokines signal by homologous proteins and activate the same transcription factors (see Box 12–1). However, there are several differences between IL-1 and TNF. For instance, IL-1 does not induce the apoptotic death of cells, and even at high systemic concentrations, by itself it does not cause the pathophysiologic changes of septic shock.

Mononuclear phagocytes produce a natural antagonist of IL-1 that is structurally homologous to the cytokine and binds to the same receptors but is biologically inactive, so that it functions as a competitive inhibitor of IL-1. It is therefore called IL-1 receptor antagonist (IL-1ra). IL-1ra may be an endogenous regulator of IL-1 action. IL-1ra is used to treat systemic juvenile rheumatoid arthritis. Regulation of IL-1-mediated inflammation may also occur by expression of the type II receptor, which binds IL-1, but does not transduce activating signal. The major function of this receptor may be to act as a "decoy" that competitively inhibits IL-1 binding to the type I signaling receptor.

Chemokines

Chemokines are a large family of structurally homologous cytokines that stimulate leukocyte movement and regulate the migration of leukocytes from the blood to tissues. The name *chemokine* is a contraction of "chemotactic cytokine." Some chemokines may be produced by various cells in response to inflammatory stimuli and recruit leukocytes to sites of inflammation; other chemokines are produced constitutively in various tissues and recruit leukocytes (mainly lymphocytes) to these tissues in the absence of inflammation.

Structure, Production, and Receptors

There are about 50 human chemokines, all of which are 8- to 12-kD polypeptides that contain two internal disulfide loops. The chemokines are classified into four families on the basis of the number and location of N-terminal cysteine residues. The two major families are the CC chemokines, in which the cysteine residues are adjacent, and the CXC family, in which these residues are separated by one amino acid. These differences correlate with organization of the subfamilies into separate gene clusters. A small number of chemokines have a single cysteine (C family) or two cysteines separated by three amino acids (CX_3C). Chemokines were originally named on the basis of how they were identified and what responses they triggered. More recently, a standard nomenclature is being used based in part on which receptors the chemokines bind to (Table 12–4).

The chemokines of the CC and CXC subfamilies are produced by leukocytes and by several types of tissue cells, such as endothelial cells, epithelial cells, and fibroblasts. In many of these cells, secretion of chemokines is induced by microbes, via TLR signaling, and by inflammatory cytokines, mainly TNF and IL-1. Several CC chemokines are also produced by antigen-stimulated T cells, providing a link between adaptive immunity and recruitment of inflammatory leukocytes. Chemokines that are produced constitutively (i.e., without any inflammatory stimulus) in lymphoid organs are involved in the physiologic traffic of lymphocytes through the organs. Chemokines bind to heparan sulfate proteoglycans on endothelial cells and are displayed in this way to circulating leukocytes that have bound to the endothelial surfaces via selectin-dependent interactions (see Chapter 2). The endothelial display provides a high local concentration of chemokines, which causes activation of leukocyte integrins, thereby strengthening adhesion, and stimulation of leukocyte motility and transmigration through the blood vessel wall.

The receptors for chemokines are G protein–coupled receptors with seven-transmembrane α-helical domains. When occupied by ligand, these receptors act as GTP exchange proteins, catalyzing the replacement of bound guanosine diphosphate (GDP) by GTP. The GTP-associated form of these G proteins can activate a variety of cellular enzymes that modulate cytoskeletal protein configuration and integrin affinity. Chemokine receptors may be rapidly down-regulated by exposure to the chemokine, and this is a likely mechanism for terminating responses. At least 10 distinct receptors for CC chemokines (called CCR1 through CCR10) and six for CXC chemokines (called CXCR1 through CXCR6) have already been identified, and this list may be incomplete (see Table 12–4). Chemokine receptors are expressed on leukocytes, with the greatest number and diversity seen on T cells. The receptors exhibit overlapping specificity for chemokines within each family, and the pattern of cellular expression of the receptors determines which cell types respond to which chemokines. Certain chemokine receptors, notably CCR5 and CXCR4, act as coreceptors for the human immunodeficiency virus (HIV) (see Chapter 20). Some activated T lymphocytes secrete chemokines that bind to CCR5 and block infection with HIV by competing with the virus.

Biologic Actions

Chemokines involved in inflammatory reactions are produced by leukocytes in response to external stimuli, and chemokines that regulate cell traffic through tissues are produced constitutively by various cells in these tissues. Chemokines were discovered on the basis of their activities as leukocyte chemoattractants, but we now know that they serve many important functions in the immune system and in other systems.

- ***Chemokines recruit the cells of host defense to sites of infection.*** Leukocyte recruitment is regulated by several sequential actions of chemokines on these cells. Chemokines bound to heparan sulfate proteoglycans on endothelial cells act on leukocytes rolling on the endothelium and increase the affinity of leukocyte integrins for their ligands (see Chapter 2, Fig. 2–7). This step of integrin activation is critical for the firm adherence of the leukocytes to the endothelium, as a prelude to subsequent migration into extravascular tissue. Recall that TNF and IL-1 stimulate expression of integrin ligands on endothelium, and thus these two cytokines and chemokines act cooperatively in the process of leukocyte migration. Chemokines induce movement of leukocytes and their migration toward the chemical gradient of the cytokine by stimulating alternating polymerization and depolymerization of actin filaments. Different chemokines act on different cells and, in coordina-

Table 12–4. Chemokines and Chemokine Receptors

Chemokine	Original name	Chemokine receptor	Major function
CC chemokines			
CCL1	I-309	CCR8	Monocyte recruitment and endothelial cell migration
CCL2	MCP-1	CCR2	Mixed leukocyte recruitment
CCL3	MIP-1α	CCR1, CCR5	Mixed leukocyte recruitment
CCL4	MIP-1β	CCR5	T cell, dendritic cell, monocyte, and NK recruitment; HIV coreceptor
CCL5	RANTES	CCR1, CCR3, CCR5	Mixed leukocyte recruitment
CCL7	MCP-3	CCR1, CCR2, CCR3	Mixed leukocyte recruitment
CCL8	MCP-2	CCR3, CCR5	Mixed leukocyte recruitment
CCL9/CCL10		CCR1	?
CCL11	Eotaxin	CCR3	Eosinophil, basophil, and T_H2 recruitment
CCL12	Unknown	CCR2	Mixed leukocyte recruitment
CCL13	MCP-4	CCR2, CCR3	Mixed leukocyte recruitment
CCL14	HHC-1	CCR1, CCR5	?
CCL15	MIP-1δ	CCR1, CCR3	Mixed leukocyte recruitment
CCL16	HHC-4	CCR1, CCR2	?
CCL17	TARC	CCR4	T cell and basophil recruitment
CCL18	DC-CK1	?	Lymphocyte and dendritic cell homing
CCL19	MIP-3β/ELC	CCR7	T cell and dendritic cell migration into parafollicular zones of lymph nodes
CCL20	MIP-3α	CCR6	?
CCL21	SLC	CCR7	T cell and dendritic cell migration into parafollicular zones of lymph nodes
CCL22	MDC	CCR4	T cell and basophil recruitment
CCL23	MPIF-1	CCR1	?
CCL24	Eotaxin-2	CCR3	Eosinophil, basophil, and T_H2 recruitment
CCL25	TECK	CCR9	Astrocyte migration
CCL26	Eotaxin-3	CCR3	Eosinophil, basophil, and T_H2 recruitment
CCL27	CTACK	CCR10	Dermal cell migration
CCL28	MEC	CCR10	Dermal cell migration
CXC chemokines			
CXCL1	GROα	CXCR2	Neutrophil recruitment
CXCL2	GROβ	CXCR2	Neutrophil recruitment
CXCL3	GROγ	CXCR2	Neutrophil recruitment
CXCL4	PF4	CXCR3B	Platelet aggregation
CXCL5	ENA-78	CXCR2	Neutrophil recruitment
CXCL6	GCP-2	CXCR1, CXCR2	Neutrophil recruitment
CXCL7	NAP-2	CXCR2	Neutrophil recruitment
CXCL8	IL-8	CXCR1, CXCR2	Neutrophil recruitment
CXCL9	Mig	CXCR3	Effector T cell recruitment
CXCL10	IP-10	CXCR3, CXCR3B	Effector T cell recruitment
CXCL11	I-TAC	CXCR3	Effector T cell recruitment
CXCL12	SDF-1α/β	CXCR4	Mixed leukocyte recruitment; HIV coreceptor
CXCL13	BCA-1	CXCR5	B cell migration into follicles
CXCL14	BRAK		?
CXCL16	–	CXCR6	?
C chemokines			
XCL1	Lymphotactin	XCR1	T cell and NK cell recruitment
XCL2	SCM-1β	XCL1	?
CX_3C chemokines			
CX_3CL1	Fractalkine	CX_3CR1	T cell, NK cell, and macrophage recruitment; CTL and NK cell activation

The known chemokines and the receptors they bind to are listed. Only selected major functions of the chemokines are included.

tion with the types of adhesion molecules expressed, thus control the nature of the inflammatory infiltrate. For example, in the CC family, CCL2 (MCP-1) is mainly involved in attracting monocytes in inflammatory sites, while CCL11 (eotaxin) acts mainly on eosinophils. In the CXC family, chemokines that contain a glutamate-leucine-arginine motif (CXCL-1, CXCL-2, CXCL-3, and others) are mainly involved in neutrophil recruitment to inflammatory sites, while those lacking this motif (CXCL-9, CXCL-10, and CXCL-11) act on T_H1 cells.

- ***Chemokines regulate the traffic of lymphocytes and other leukocytes through peripheral lymphoid tissues.*** Some of the most intriguing and surprising discoveries about chemokines have been their roles in the normal migration of immune cells into lymphoid organs. In Chapter 3, we mentioned the role of different chemokines in promoting the migration of T cells, B cells, and dendritic cells to different regions of peripheral lymphoid organs (see Chapter 3, Fig. 3–10). Various chemokines also promote migration of previously activated effector and memory T cells to nonlymphoid tissues, including mucosal organs and skin. The selectivity of different cell types for different anatomic sites depends to a large extent on which chemokines are produced in the sites and which chemokine receptors are expressed on the cell types.
- ***Chemokines promote angiogenesis and wound healing.*** These activities are associated mostly with CXC family chemokines, and involve both proangiogenic chemokines, expressed early after tissue injury, and anti-angiogenic chemokines, expressed later in the healing process. The angiogenic effects may be a combination of chemokine-induced production of angiogenic factors in inflammatory cells and fibroblasts, and direct effects of chemokines on vascular cells, such as endothelial cells, which express the CXCR2 receptor.
- ***Chemokines are also involved in the development of diverse nonlymphoid organs.*** Knockout mice lacking the CXCR4 receptor have fatal defects in the development of the heart and the cerebellum. These roles of chemokines raise the possibility of many other as yet undiscovered functions in morphogenesis.

Interleukin-12

IL-12 is a principal mediator of the early innate immune response to intracellular microbes and is a key inducer of cell-mediated immunity, the adaptive immune response to these microbes. IL-12 was originally identified as an activator of NK cell cytotoxic function, but its most important actions are to stimulate IFN-γ production by T cells and NK cells, and to support differentiation of naive $CD4^+$ helper T cells to the IFN-γ-producing (T_H1) subset.

Structure, Production, and Receptors

IL-12 exists as a disulfide-linked heterodimer of 35-kD (p35) and 40-kD (p40) subunits. The p35 subunit has a four-α-helical globular domain structure, which is shared by several different cytokines of the type I or hematopoietic cytokine family (see Fig. 12–3). The p40 subunit is homologous to the extracellular portion of the IL-6 receptor α chain. IL-12 belongs to a family of at least five heterodimeric cytokines whose subunits are homologous to either or both the IL-12 p35 and p40 chains. Two members of this family, IL-23 and IL-27, play important roles, along with IL-12, in protective and pathologic T cell–mediated immune responses (discussed later).

The principal sources of IL-12 are activated dendritic cells and macrophages. Many cells appear to synthesize the p35 subunit, but only phagocytes and dendritic cells produce the p40 component and therefore the biologically active cytokine. During innate immune reactions to microbes, IL-12 is produced in response to TLR signaling induced by many microbial stimuli, including LPS, infection by intracellular bacteria (such as *Listeria* and mycobacteria), and virus infections. In addition, antigen-stimulated helper T cells induce the production of IL-12 from macrophages and dendritic cells, mainly by CD40 ligand on the T cells engaging CD40 on the macrophages and dendritic cells. Thus, IL-12 is produced by APCs when they present antigens to T cells, during the induction and effector phases of cell-mediated immune responses (see Chapter 13). IFN-γ produced by NK cells or T cells also stimulates IL-12 production.

The receptor for IL-12 (IL-12R) is a member of the type I cytokine receptor family (see Fig. 12–3). It is a heterodimer composed of β1 and β2 subunits, both of which are homologous to gp130, a subunit of the IL-6 receptor. (gp130 or homologous proteins are also part of the receptors for IL-11, IL-23 and IL-27, cytokines that will be discussed later in this chapter.) IL-12 p40 binds to the IL-12Rβ1 subunit, and IL-12 p35 binds to IL-12Rβ2 subunit. Both chains are required for high-affinity binding of the cytokine, and for signaling. The IL-12 receptor signals through a Jak–STAT pathway, in which cytokine binding to the receptor activates receptor-associated protein tyrosine kinases called Janus kinases (Jaks), and ultimately leads to the activation of transcription factors called signal transducers and activators of transcription (STATs). Many cytokines use Jak–STAT pathways to induce responses in target cells, and different cytokines activate different combinations of Jaks and STATs (Box 12–2). In the case of the IL-12 receptor, the Janus kinase Tyk2 associates with the β1 subunit, Jak2 associates with the β2 subunit, and the major STAT protein involved, which is required for most of the biologic effects of IL-12, is STAT4. Expression of the β2 chain of the IL-12 receptor is itself enhanced by cytokines, mainly IFN-γ (whose production is stimulated by IL-12), and this is an example of a positive amplification loop in immune responses.

Biologic Actions

IL-12 is critical for initiating a sequence of responses involving macrophages, NK cells, and T lymphocytes that results in the eradication of intracellular microbes (Fig. 12–6).

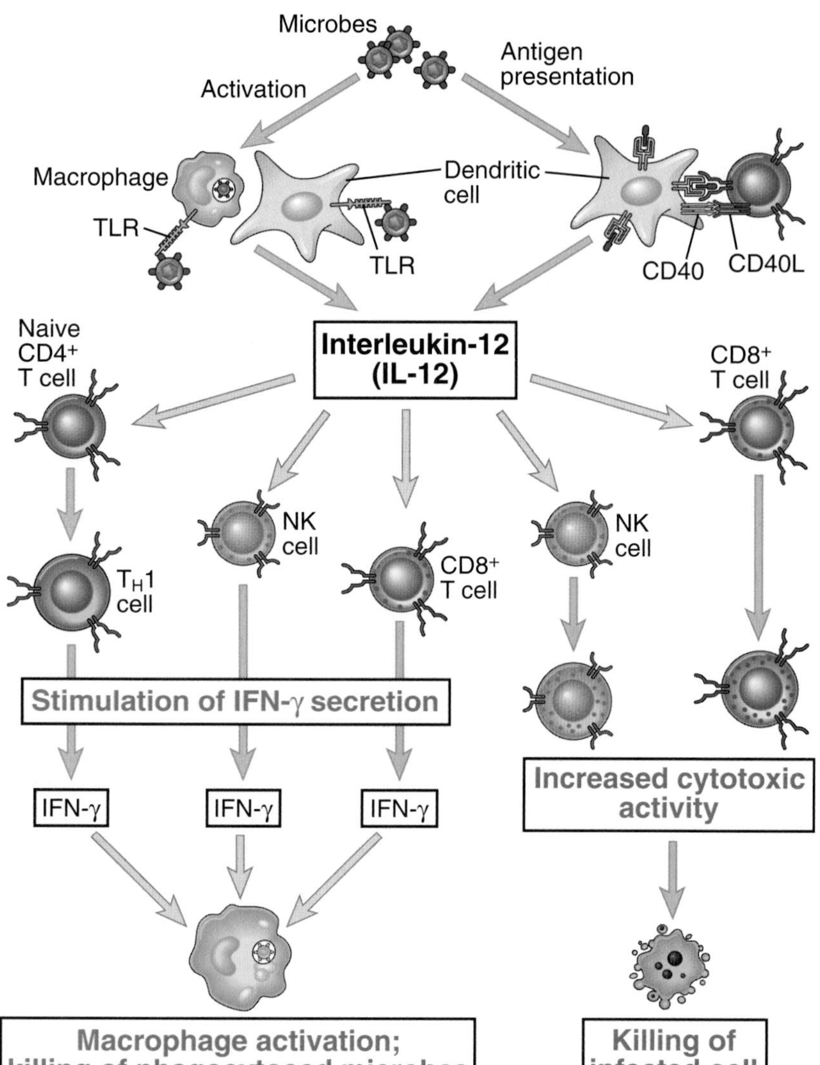

FIGURE 12–6 Biologic actions of IL-12. IL-12 is produced by macrophages and dendritic cells that respond to microbes or to T cell signals such as CD40 ligand engaging CD40. IL-12 acts on T lymphocytes and NK cells to stimulate IFN-γ production and cytotoxic activity, both of which function to eradicate intracellular microbes.

- ***IL-12 stimulates the production of IFN-γ by NK cells and T lymphocytes.*** Macrophages and dendritic cells produce IL-12 in response to many microbes. Secreted IL-12 stimulates NK cells and T cells to produce IFN-γ, which then activates the macrophages to kill the phagocytosed microbes. Thus, innate immunity against many microbes is mediated by cytokines acting in the following sequence: microbes → macrophage and dendritic cell response → IL-12 → IFN-γ → macrophage activation → killing of microbes. Large amounts of IL-12 are produced in severe gram-negative sepsis, resulting in the production of IFN-γ, which synergizes with bacterial LPS to stimulate macrophage production of TNF, the principal mediator of septic shock. IL-12 antagonists prevent lethality in some experimental models of LPS-induced septic shock. We will return to IFN-γ when we discuss the cytokines of adaptive immunity.
- ***IL-12, together with IFN-γ, promotes the differentiation of CD4⁺ helper T lymphocytes into IFN-γ-producing T_H1 cells.*** The T_H1 subset of helper T cells activates phagocytes in cell-mediated immunity. This effect of IL-12 will be discussed more fully in Chapter 13.
- ***IL-12 enhances the cytotoxic functions of activated NK cells and CD8⁺ cytotoxic T lymphocytes (CTLs).*** This action of IL-12 is also important in cell-mediated immunity (see Chapter 13).

Studies with gene knockout mice and the phenotype of rare patients with mutations in the IL-12 receptor support the conclusion that IL-12 is important for IFN-γ production, T_H1 cell differentiation, and host resistance to intracellular microbes. For example, patients with mutations in the IL-12 receptor β1 subunit have been described and they are highly susceptible to infections with intracellular bacteria, notably *Salmonella* and atypical mycobacteria. However, the interpretation of many of these genetic defects is complicated by the fact that the mutated gene products are also involved in the function of IL-23, because IL-23 contains the same p40 chain as IL-12 and the IL-23 receptor contains the IL-12Rβ1

Box 12–2 ■ IN DEPTH: CYTOKINE SIGNALING BY THE Jak-STAT PATHWAY

Cytokine receptors of the type I and type II receptor families engage signal transduction pathways that involve enzymes called Janus kinases and transcription factors called signal transducers and activators of transcription (STATs). Studies of these pathways have revealed direct links between cytokine binding to receptors and transcriptional activation of target genes.

The discovery of the Jak-STAT pathways came from biochemical and genetic analyses of IFN signaling. The promoter regions of genes responsive to IFNs contain sequences that bind cellular proteins that are phosphorylated upon IFN treatment of the cells. These proteins were shown to activate transcription of cytokine-responsive genes, and they were therefore called STAT proteins. Mutant cell lines were generated that were unresponsive to IFNs. Some of these mutant cell lines were found to lack particular STAT proteins, and introduction of the STATs by gene transfection restored cytokine responsiveness in the cells. This established the essential roles of the STATs in responses to the cytokines. Other mutant cell lines were found to be deficient in one or more related tyrosine kinases, which were called Janus kinases after the two-headed Roman god because of the presence of two kinase domains (only one of which is active). Subsequent studies, including analyses of knockout mice lacking the various STATs and Jaks, have shown that Jak-STAT pathways are involved in responses to many cytokines (see Table). There are four known Janus kinases (Jak1-3 and TYK2) and seven STATs (STAT1-4, 5a, 5b, and 6).

The sequence of events in the Jak-STAT signaling pathways is now well defined (see Figure). Inactive Jak enzymes are noncovalently attached to the cytoplasmic domains of type I and type II cytokine receptors. When two receptor molecules are brought together by binding of a cytokine molecule, the receptor-associated Jaks become active through transphosphorylation, and they phosphorylate tyrosine residues in the cytoplasmic portions of the clustered receptors. Some of these phosphotyrosine moieties of the receptors are recognized by Src homology 2 (SH2) domains of monomeric cytosolic STAT proteins, which become attached to the receptors. The STAT proteins are then phosphorylated by the receptor-associated Jak kinases. The SH2 domain of one STAT protein is able to bind to the phosphotyrosine residues of another STAT protein. As a result, two STAT proteins bind to each other and dissociate from the receptor. The STAT dimers migrate to the nucleus, where they bind to DNA sequences in the promoter regions of cytokine-responsive genes and activate gene transcription. After each round, new STAT proteins can bind to the cytokine receptor, become phosphorylated, dimerize, and again migrate to the nucleus.

An intriguing question is how the specificity of responses to many different cytokines is achieved, given the limited numbers of Jaks and STATs used by the various cytokine receptors. The likely answer is that unique amino acid sequences in the different cytokine receptors provide the scaffolding for specifically binding, and thereby activating, different combinations of Jaks and

Jak/STAT	Involved cytokine(s)	Phenotype of knockout mice
STAT1	IFN-α/β, IFN-γ	Defect in innate immunity; no reponse to IFNs
STAT2	IFN-α/β	Defective immunity to viruses
STAT3	IL-6, IL-10	Embryonic lethal
STAT4	IL-12	Defect in T_H1 development, IFN-γ production
STAT5a	Prolactin	Lactation defect
STAT5b	Growth hormone (GH)	Dwarfism
STAT5a and STAT5b	IL-2, IL-7, IL-9 (also see Prolactin and GH)	Lactation defect, dwarfism, and defective T cell proliferation in response to IL-2
STAT6	IL-4	Defect in T_H2 development, and production of IL-4-dependent Ig isotypes
Jak1	IFN-α/β, IFN-γ, cytokines using γ_c and gp130 (e.g., IL-2, IL-4, IL-6)	Perinatal lethal; defective innate immunity, possible defect in neuronal viability
Jak2	Epo, IL-3, IFN-γ	Embryonic lethal, hematopoietic failure
Jak3	Cytokines using γ_c chain (IL-7, IL-2, IL-4)	Defect in T cell maturation
Tyk2	IFN-α/β, IFN-γ, IL-10, others	Defective IL-12 response of NK cells, defective immunity to viruses

Abbreviations: IFN, interferon; IL, interleukin; Jak, Janus kinase; STAT, signal transducer and activator of transcription.

Continued on following page

Box 12–2 ■ IN DEPTH: CYTOKINE SIGNALING BY THE Jak-STAT PATHWAY (Continued)

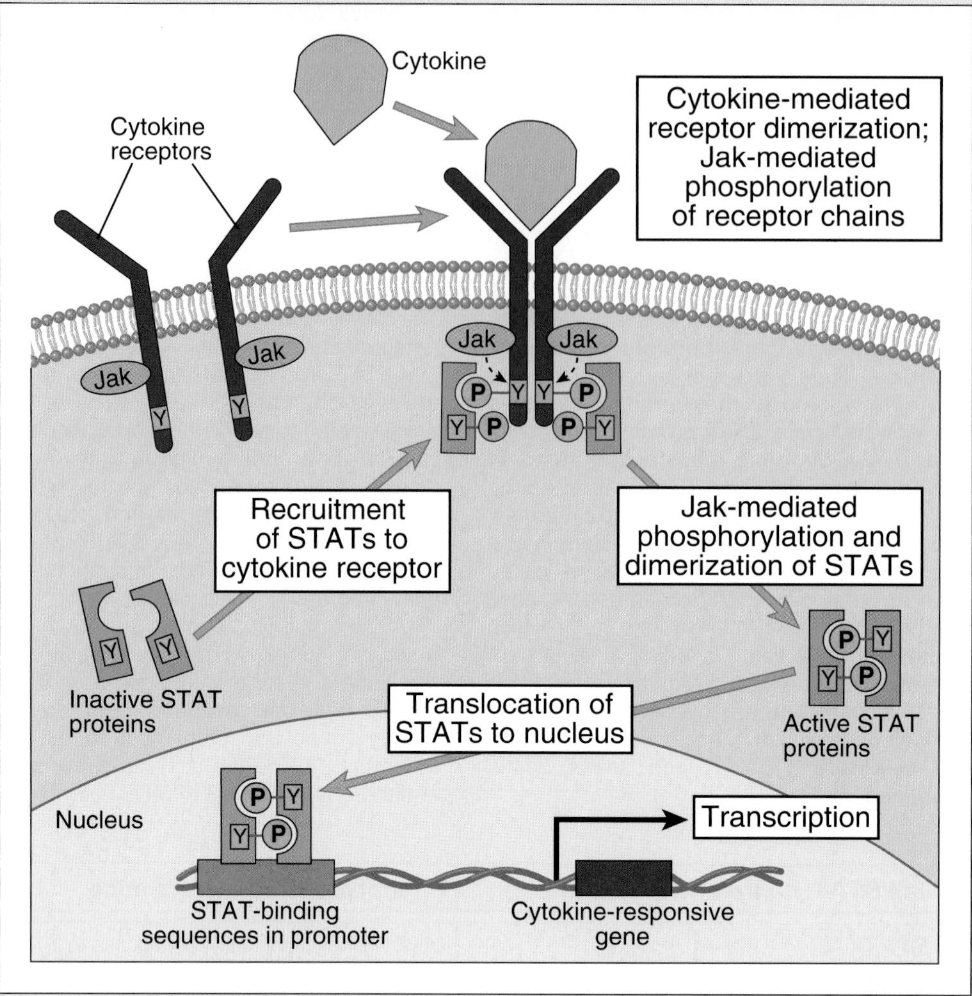

Cytokine signaling by the Jak-STAT pathway. Cytokine-induced clustering of receptors leads to Jak-mediated phosphorylation of the receptor chains, attachment of inactive STATs, phosphorylation of the bound STATs (also by the Jaks), dimerization of STATs and migration to the nucleus, and stimulation of gene transcription.

STATs. The SH2 domains of different STAT proteins selectively bind to the phosphotyrosine residues and flanking regions of different cytokine receptors. This is largely responsible for the activation of particular STATs by various cytokine receptors and therefore for the specificity of cytokine signaling. Several type I and type II cytokine receptors are heterodimers of two different polypeptide chains, each of which binds a different Jak. Furthermore, two different STATs may heterodimerize upon phosphorylation. Therefore, there is a significant amount of combinatorial diversity in the signaling that can be generated from a limited number of Jak and STAT proteins. In addition, cytokines activate signaling pathways and transcription factors other than STATs. For instance, the IL-2 receptor β chain activates Ras-dependent MAP kinase pathways that may be involved in gene transcription and growth stimulation. Other cytokine receptors may similarly activate other signaling pathways in concert with the Jak-STAT pathways to elicit biologic responses to the cytokines.

Several mechanisms of negative regulation of Jak-STAT pathways have been identified. Proteins called suppressors of cytokine signaling (SOCS) are a family of STAT pathway inhibitors. Members of this family are identified by the presence of an SH2 domain and a conserved 40–amino acid C-terminal region called a SOCS box. Eight different SOCS proteins have been identified; in addition, other SOCS box-containing proteins that do not have SH2 domains also exist. SOCS proteins inhibit cytokine actions by binding to phosphotyrosines in the cytoplasmic regions of cytokine receptors, or by binding to and inhibiting the kinase activity of Jaks. In addition, SOCS proteins facilitate E3 ubiquitin ligase targeting of Jak proteins for proteasomal degradation. SOCS genes are not

Continued on following page

expressed in resting cells, but are rapidly induced by cytokines via Jak-STAT signaling pathways. In addition, other stumuli such as TLR ligands can induce SOCS expression. In this way, SOCS serve as negative feedback regulators of the cytokine activation of cells. SOCS gene knockout mice have provided information on the physiologic role of this family of inhibitors. SOCS-1 knockout mice, for example, die at 3 weeks of age because of excessive actions of IFN-γ, and the phenotype can be corrected by crossing the mice with IFN-γ knockout mice. Other studies suggest that SOCS-2 inhibits signaling by the receptors for growth hormone and insulin-like growth factor, whereas SOCS-3 regulates IL-6 signaling. Other inhibitors of Jak-STAT signaling include tyrosine phosphatases, such as SHP-1 and -2, which can dephosphorylate and therefore deactivate Jak molecules. Another family of inhibitory proteins, called protein inhibitors of activated STAT (PIAS), were originally defined as negative regulators of STATs. PIAS proteins bind phosphorylated STATs and prevent their interaction with DNA. It is now known that PIAS proteins also interact with, and block the function of, other transcription factors associated with cytokine signaling, including IRFs, NF-κB, and SMADs.

subunit. Furthermore, IFN-γ synthesis is not completely abrogated in IL-12-deficient mice, probably because of the actions of other compensatory cytokines (notably IL-18, described later). IL-12 knockout mice also have defects in NK cell function.

IL-12 is an important link between innate and adaptive immunity, being produced during early innate immune reactions against intracellular microbes and promoting adaptive immune responses that protect the host against these microbes. This illustrates a concept, introduced in Chapter 1, that innate immune reactions stimulate and direct subsequent adaptive immune responses. IL-12 is in clinical trials to boost protective cell-mediated immune responses in patients with cancer.

Type I Interferons

Type I interferons (IFNs) are a large family of structurally related cytokines that mediate the early innate immune response to viral infections. The term *interferon* derives from the ability of these cytokines to interfere with viral infection. There are many type I IFNs, all of which have considerable structural homology and are encoded by genes in a single cluster on chromosome 9. In humans, the type I IFNs include IFN-α (which can be further subdivided into 13 different subtypes), IFN-β, IFN-ε, IFN-κ, and IFN-ω.

Structure, Production, and Receptors

Plasmacytoid dendritic cells and mononuclear phagocytes are the major sources of IFN-α. IFN-β is a single protein produced by many cells, such as fibroblasts, and it is sometimes called fibroblast IFN. The plasmacytoid dendritic cell, which circulates in human blood and is present in various tissues, is a particularly important source of type I IFNs early in the innate response to most viruses. The most potent stimuli for type I IFN synthesis are viral nucleic acids, which bind to various intracellular receptors or sensors that are linked to signaling pathway that activate the interferon regulatory factor (IRF) family of transcription factors. TLR3, TLR7, and TLR9, all in endosomal membranes, recognize dsRNA, single-stranded RNA, and unmethylated CpG DNA, respectively, leading to IRF activation and type I IFN gene expression. The cytoplasmic sensors RIG-I and MDA-5 recognize viral RNA (see Chapter 2), and also induce type I IFN expression via IRF activation. Antigen-activated T cells stimulate mononuclear phagocytes, through the CD40-CD40 ligand pathway, to synthesize type I IFNs.

All the type I IFNs bind to the same cell surface receptor and induce similar biologic responses. The type I IFN receptor is a member of the type II cytokine receptor family composed of a heterodimer of two structurally related polypeptides, IFNAR1 and IFNAR2, which are associated with the Janus family tyrosine kinases Tyk2 and Jak1, respectively. Upon type I IFN binding to the receptor, these kinases become activated and lead to STAT1 and STAT2 phosphorylation, heterodimer formation, and recruitment of IRF9 (Fig. 12–7). The resulting STAT-1/2:IRF9 complex translocates to the nucleus and binds to nucleic acid sequences called IFN-stimulated response elements (ISREs) that are present in many different genes, thereby inducing their transcription. In addition to this "classical pathway" of type I IFN receptor signaling, several other signaling pathways initiated by the type I IFN receptor also contribute to the biologic response of cells to type I IFNs. For example, STAT1 phosphorylation leads to formation of STAT1 homodimers that bind to different nucleic acid sequences, called IFN-γ-activated sites (GAS), which are present in some of the same genes containing ISREs, as well as in different genes. Type I IFN regulation of gene transcription is further regulated by several different coactivator proteins, which form complexes with STAT dimers bound to ISRE and GAS sequences. The type I IFN receptor also activates G protein–dependent mitogen-activated protein (MAP) kinase pathways and phosphatidylinositol-3 (PI-3) kinase pathways, both of which are believed to contribute to the biologic responses of cells to type I IFNs.

Biologic Actions

The actions of type I IFNs protect against viral infections and promote cell-mediated immunity against intracellular microbes (see Fig. 12–7).

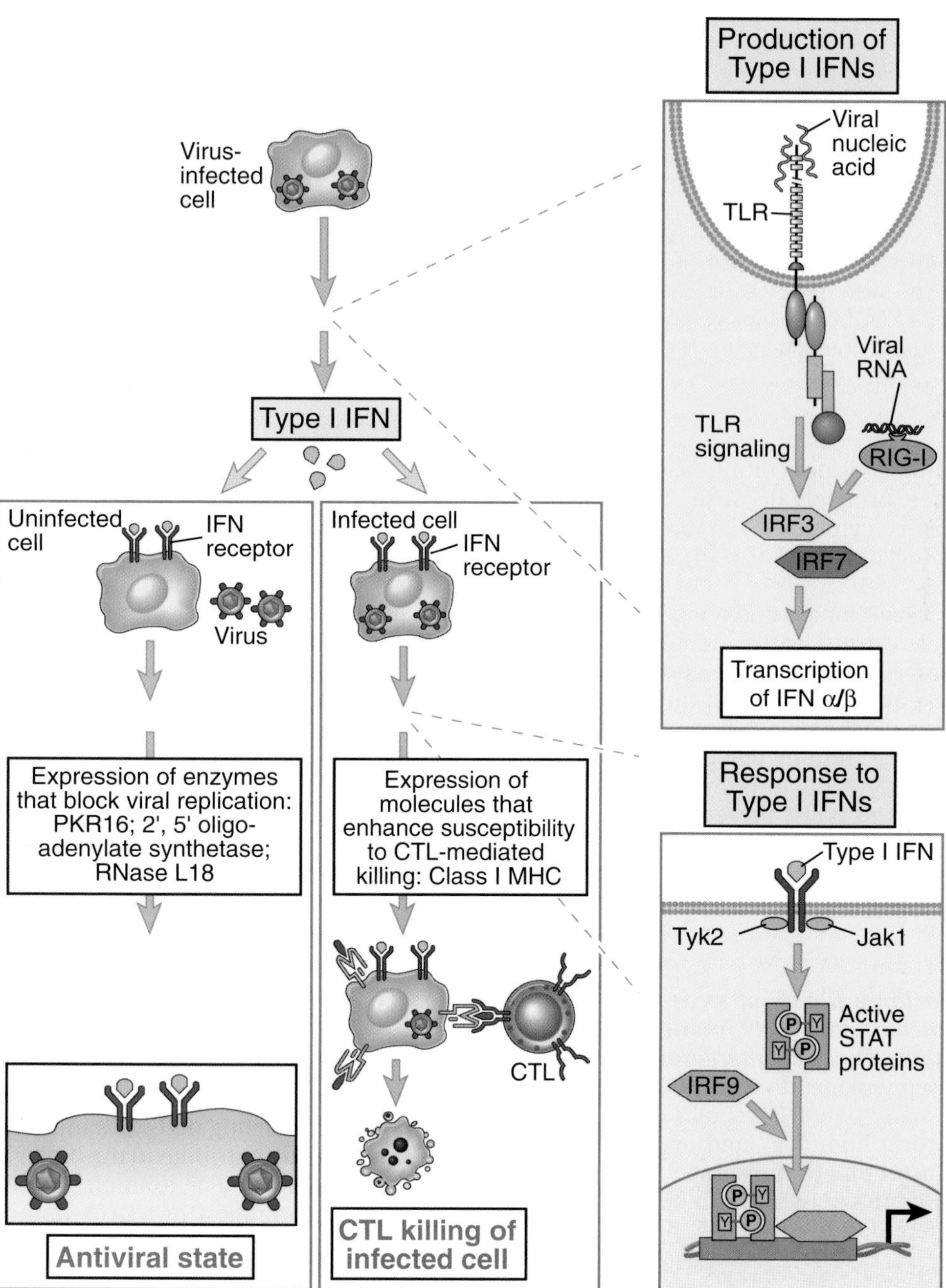

FIGURE 12–7 Biologic actions of type I IFNs. Type I IFNs (IFN-α, IFN-β) are produced by virus-infected cells in response to intracellular TLR signaling and other sensors of viral RNA. Type I IFNs bind to receptors on neighboring uninfected cells, and activate Jak-STAT signaling pathways, which induce expression of genes whose products interfere with viral replication. Type I IFNs also bind to receptors on infected cells, and induce expression of genes whose products enhance the cell's susceptibility to CTL-mediated killing.

- ***Type I IFN inhibits viral replication.*** IFN causes cells to synthesize a number of enzymes that interfere with transcription of viral RNA or DNA and viral replication. These include dsRNA-activated serine/threonine protein kinase (PKR16), which blocks viral transcriptional and translational events, and 2′,5′ oligoadenylate synthetase and RNase L18, 19, which promote viral RNA degradation. The antiviral action of type I IFN is primarily a paracrine action, in that a virally infected cell secretes IFN to protect neighboring cells that are not yet infected. A cell that has responded to IFN and is resistant to viral infection is said to be in an "antiviral state." IFN secreted by an infected cell may also act in an autocrine fashion to inhibit viral replication in that cell.
- ***Type I IFN increases expression of class I MHC molecules.*** Because CD8+ CTLs recognize foreign antigens bound to class I MHC molecules, type I IFN enhances the recognition of class I–associated viral antigens on infected cells and therefore the efficiency of CTL-mediated killing of these cells. Type I IFN also increases the cytotoxic activity of NK cells.
- Type I IFN stimulates the development of T_H1 cells in humans. This effect is mainly due to the ability of type I IFN to promote in T cells the expression of func-

tional receptors for the major T_H1-inducing cytokine IL-12.

- Type I IFNs promote sequestration of lymphocytes in lymph nodes, thus enhancing lymphocyte activation by antigens concentrated in the nodes, especially in viral infections (see Chapter 3).
- Type I IFN inhibits the proliferation of many cell types, including lymphocytes, in vitro. This is likely due to induction of the same enzymes that block viral replication, but it may also involve other enzymes that alter the metabolism of amino acids such as tryptophan.

Thus, the principal activities of type I IFN function in concert to eradicate viral infections. Knockout mice lacking the receptor for type I IFN are susceptible to viral infections. IFN-α is in clinical use as an antiviral agent in certain forms of viral hepatitis, and as a treatment for some hematologic malignancies. IFN-β is used as a therapy for multiple sclerosis, but the mechanism of its beneficial effect in this disease is not known.

Interleukin-10

IL-10 is an inhibitor of activated macrophages and dendritic cells and is thus involved in the control of innate immune reactions and cell-mediated immunity. So far, we have described cytokines that stimulate innate immunity. IL-10, in contrast, is an inhibitor of host immune responses, particularly responses involving macrophages.

Production, Structure, and Receptors

IL-10 is a member of a family of noncovalently linked dimeric cytokines, each chain of which contains a six-helix bundle domain that intercalates with that of the other chain. Other members of the family include IL-19, IL-20, IL-22, IL-24, and IL-26. The IL-10 receptor belongs to the type II cytokine receptor family and consists of two chains, which associate with Jak1 and Tyk2 Janus family kinases. STAT3 is the major downstream signaling molecule induced by IL-10. IL-10 is produced mainly by activated macrophages and regulatory T cells. Because it is both produced by and inhibits macrophage functions, it is an excellent example of a negative feedback regulator. It is not clear whether different stimuli may act on macrophages to induce the production of a regulatory cytokine like IL-10 or effector cytokines like TNF and IL-12, or whether the same stimuli elicit production of all these cytokines but with different kinetics. IL-10 is also produced by some nonlymphoid cell types (e.g., keratinocytes).

Biologic Actions

The biologic effects of IL-10 result from its ability to inhibit many of the functions of activated macrophages. As we have discussed previously, macrophages respond to microbes by secreting cytokines and by expressing costimulators that enhance T cell activation and cell-mediated immunity. IL-10 acts on the activated macrophages to terminate these responses and return the system to its resting state as the microbial infection is eradicated.

- ***IL-10 inhibits the production of IL-12 by activated macrophages and dendritic cells.*** Because IL-12 is a critical stimulus for IFN-γ secretion and is an inducer of innate and cell-mediated immune reactions against intracellular microbes, IL-10 functions to down-regulate all such reactions. In fact, IL-10 was discovered as an inhibitor of IFN-γ production.
- ***IL-10 inhibits the expression of costimulators and class II MHC molecules on macrophages and dendritic cells.*** Because of these actions, IL-10 serves to inhibit T cell activation and terminate cell-mediated immune reactions.

Knockout mice lacking IL-10 develop inflammatory bowel disease, probably as a result of uncontrolled activation of macrophages reacting to enteric microbes. These mice also show excessive inflammation and tissue injury in response to chemical irritants.

The Epstein-Barr virus contains a gene homologous to human IL-10, and viral IL-10 has the same activities as the natural cytokine. This raises the intriguing possibility that acquisition of the IL-10 gene during the evolution of the virus has given the virus the ability to inhibit host immunity and thus a survival advantage in the infected host.

Other Cytokines of Innate Immunity

IL-6 is a cytokine that functions in both innate and adaptive immunity. It is synthesized by mononuclear phagocytes, vascular endothelial cells, fibroblasts, and other cells in response to microbes and to other cytokines, notably IL-1 and TNF. It is also made by some activated T cells. The functional form of IL-6 is a homodimer, with each subunit forming a four-α-helical globular domain. The receptor for IL-6 consists of a cytokine-binding protein and a signal-transducing subunit, both of which belong to the type I cytokine receptor family. The 130-kD signal-transducing subunit is called gp130; which is also the signaling component of other cytokine receptors, as discussed earlier (see Fig. 12–3B). The major IL-6-induced signaling pathway involves Jak1 and STAT3 activation, and leads to transcription of many different genes.

IL-6 has several diverse actions. In innate immunity, it stimulates the synthesis of acute-phase proteins by hepatocytes and thus contributes to the acute-phase response. IL-6 stimulates production of neutrophils from bone marrow progenitors, usually acting in concert with colony-stimulating factors (discussed later in this chapter). In adaptive immunity, IL-6 stimulates the growth of B lymphocytes that have differentiated into antibody producers. IL-6 similarly acts as a growth factor for neoplastic plasma cells (myelomas), and many myeloma cells that grow autonomously secrete IL-6 as an autocrine growth factor. Moreover, IL-6 can promote the growth of monoclonal antibody–producing hybridomas, which are derived from myelomas. There is also emerging evidence that IL-6 promotes cell-mediated immune reactions by stimulating production of some proinflammatory cytokines (notably IL-17) and by inhibiting the generation and actions of regulatory T cells.

IL-15 is cytokine that serves important growth-stimulating and survival functions for T cells and NK cells. It is a member of the type I cytokine family and is produced by mononuclear phagocytes and probably many other cell types in response to viral infection, LPS, and other signals that trigger innate immunity. IL-15 is structurally homologous to IL-2. The receptor for IL-15 has a cytokine-binding α chain that is homologous to but distinct from the α chain of the IL-2 receptor, and the same signal-transducing IL-2/15β and γ_c chains as in the IL-2 receptor (discussed later in this chapter). The α chain alone binds IL-15 with high affinity. IL-15 binding to its receptor activates Jak3-, STAT5-, and Akt-dependent signaling pathways that promote cell survival and lead to proliferative responses. The functions of IL-15, which have been inferred from the phenotypes of IL-15 and IL-15Rα knockout mice, include the survival of memory $CD8^+$ T cells, NK cells, and NK-T cells. In addition, IL-15 appears to be required for NK cell differentiation and activation.

IL-18 is a cytokine structurally related to IL-1, but unlike IL-1, its major biologic functions are enhancing IFN-γ production by T cells and promoting differentiation of IFN-γ-producing (T_H1) $CD4^+$ T cells. These effects of IL-18 are synergistic with IL-12. The major sources of IL-18 are macrophages and dendritic cells, and production is dependent on caspase-1, as is IL-1. The IL-18 receptor is in the IL-1/TLR family, and signals through a TIR domain that recruits IRAK and TRAF proteins (see Chapter 2), leading to activation of NF-κB and AP-1 transcription factors.

IL-23 and **IL-27** are members of a family of cytokines structurally related to both IL-6 and IL-12, and their receptors are structurally related to the IL-6 and IL-12 receptors. Like IL-12, their functions bridge innate and adaptive immunity. IL-23 is a heterodimeric cytokine composed of a unique 19-kD chain (p19) paired with the p40 chain of IL-12. It is produced by macrophages and dendritic cells in response to microbial infection. The IL-23 receptor is expressed on T cells and NK cells, and consists of a heterodimer of a unique IL-23R chain and the IL-12Rβ1 chain. Studies with knockout mice lacking the p19 chain have revealed that IL-23 contributes to the inflammatory pathology of autoimmune diseases, including experimental allergic encephalomyelitis (a model of multiple sclerosis, see Chapter 18). Furthermore, IL-23 appears to be important for resistance to some bacteria, including the gram-negative organism *Klebsiella pneumoniae*. One way in which IL-23 may influence autoimmune and protective immune responses is by promoting the differentiation or maintenance of T cells that produce IL-17, a pro-inflammatory cytokine discussed later in this chapter.

IL-27 is a heterodimer composed of an α-helical subunit (IL-27 p28), bound to a subunit homologous to the extracellular domain of the IL-6 receptor. IL-27 is also produced by macrophages and dendritic cells in response to pathogens, and binds to a high-affinity heterodimeric receptor, IL-27R, composed of the IL-6 gp130 chain and a second homologous chain. IL-27R is most highly expressed by resting NK and NK-T cells, effector and memory T cells, and regulatory T cells. Studies with IL-27 knockout mice indicate that the influence of IL-27 on immune responses is complex, and includes both proinflammatory and regulatory functions. Like IL-12, IL-27 promotes T_H1 differentiation and IFN-γ production by T cells. However, IL-27R-deficent mice develop a lethal T cell–mediated inflammatory response to certain infectious pathogens, consistent with a role for IL-27 in controlling ongoing T cell responses.

Several cytokines have been identified by sequence homologies that belong to a family of IL-10–related cytokines. These include IL-19, IL-20, IL-22, IL-24, and IL-26. All of these bind to type II cytokine receptors that share various subunits. These cytokines appear to regulate inflammatory reactions in tissues, but their physiologic functions are not well understood.

Roles of Cytokines in Innate Immunity and Inflammation

Now that we have discussed the individual cytokines of innate immunity, it is useful to integrate this information and consider how these cytokines contribute to innate immune reactions against microbes. Different cytokines play key roles in innate immunity to different classes of microbes. In infections by pyogenic (pus-forming) extracellular bacteria, macrophages respond to bacterial endotoxins and perhaps to other bacterial products by producing TNF, IL-1, and chemokines (Fig. 12–8). TNF and IL-1 act on vascular endothelium at the site of the infection to induce the expression of adhesion molecules that promote stable attachment of blood neutrophils and monocytes to the endothelium at this site. Chemokines produced by the macrophages and by endothelial cells stimulate the extravasation of the leukocytes to the infection, where the innate immune reaction is mounted to eliminate the infectious microbes.

IL-12 and IFNγ are the most important cytokines in innate responses to intracellular bacteria. Macrophages and dendritic cells respond to many microbes, including intracellular bacteria and LPS-producing bacteria, by secreting IL-12, which induces the local production of IFN-γ from NK cells and T lymphocytes. IFN-γ then activates the macrophages to destroy phagocytosed microbes. IL-12 also stimulates the subsequent adaptive immune response and directs it toward T_H1 cells, which are the mediators of cellular immunity and the most effective response for destroying intracellular bacteria. These actions of IL-12 are complemented by IL-18. Cytokine-mediated leukocyte recruitment and activation are responsible for the injury to normal tissues that often accompanies innate immune reactions to infections. These macrophage-derived cytokines, especially

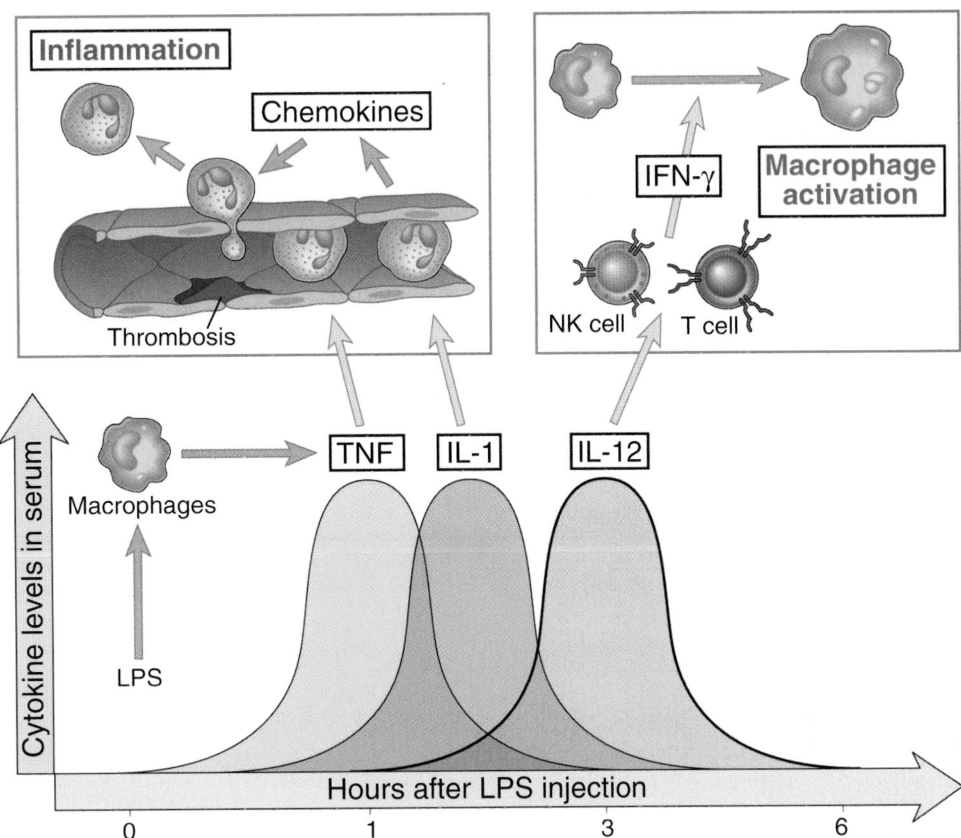

FIGURE 12–8 Roles of cytokines in innate immunity to microbes. This figure illustrates the role of cytokines in host responses to bacteria that produce LPS (endotoxin). LPS acts on macrophages to induce the secretion of multiple cytokines, including TNF, IL-1, and IL-12, which can be measured in the serum of individuals treated with LPS or infected with LPS-producing bacteria. TNF and IL-1 stimulate acute inflammation by their actions on endothelial cells and leukocytes. IL-12 stimulates the production of IFN-γ, which can also be measured in the serum. Note that chemokines may be produced by many cell populations; only endothelial cells are shown as the source in this illustration. Antagonists against TNF, IL-12, and IFN-γ reduce the pathologic complications of sepsis and decrease the mortality associated with septic shock.

TNF and IL-1, are also responsible for the systemic manifestations of infection.

In viral infections, type I IFNs are secreted by infected cells, dendritic cells, and macrophages, and function to inhibit viral replication and infection. IL-15 stimulates the development and perhaps activation of NK cells, and IL-12 enhances the cytotoxic activity of NK cells. NK cell–mediated killing of virus-infected cells eliminates the reservoir of infection.

The dominant cytokines produced in response to different microbes account for the nature of the innate immune reactions to these microbes. For instance, the early response to pyogenic bacteria consists mainly of neutrophils, the response to intracellular bacteria is dominated by activated macrophages, and the response to viruses consists of NK cells in addition to other inflammatory cells. There may be considerable overlap, however, and these varied cellular reactions may be seen to different degrees in many infections.

Cytokines That Mediate and Regulate Adaptive Immunity

Cytokines mediate the proliferation and differentiation of lymphocytes after antigen recognition in the activation phase of adaptive immune responses and mediate the activation of specialized effector cells in the effector phase of adaptive immunity. Cytokine production is one of the principal responses of T lymphocytes to antigen recognition. In the following sections, we first describe the major cytokines of adaptive immunity (Table 12–5) and conclude by describing how cytokines contribute to specialized effector cell responses against different microbes.

Interleukin-2

IL-2 is a growth, survival, and differentiation factor for T lymphocytes, and plays a major role in regulation of T cell responses through its actions on regulatory T cells. Because of its ability to support proliferation of antigen-stimulated T cells, IL-2 was originally called T cell growth factor. It acts on the same cells that produce it or on adjacent cells (i.e., it functions as an autocrine or paracrine growth and survival factor).

Production, Structure, and Receptors

IL-2 is produced mainly by $CD4^+$ T lymphocytes. Activation of T cells by antigens and costimulators stimulates transcription of the IL-2 gene and synthesis and secretion of the protein (see Chapter 9). IL-2 production is transient, with peak secretion occurring about 8 to 12 hours after activation. $CD4^+$ T cells secrete IL-2 into the immunological synapse formed between the T cell and APC (see Chapter 9). IL-2 receptors on T cells also tend to localize to the synapse, so that the cytokine and its receptor reach sufficiently high local concentrations to initiate cellular responses.

Table 12–5. Cytokines of Adaptive Immunity

Cytokine	Size (kD)	Principal cell source	Principal cellular targets and biologic effects
Interleukin-2 (IL-2)	14–17 kD	T cells	T cells: proliferation, increased cytokine synthesis; potentiates Fas-mediated apoptosis; promotes regulatory T cell development, survival NK cells: proliferation, activation B cells: proliferation, antibody synthesis (in vitro)
Interleukin-4 (IL-4)	18 kD	$CD4^+$ T cells (T_H2), mast cells	B cells: isotype switching to IgE T cells: T_H2 differentiation, proliferation Macrophages: inhibition of IFN-γ–mediated activation Mast cells: proliferation (in vitro)
Interleukin-5 (IL-5)	45–50 kD; homodimer of 20 kD subunits	$CD4^+$ T cells (T_H2)	Eosinophils: activation, increased production B cells: proliferation, IgA production (in vitro)
Interferon-γ (IFN-γ)	50 kD (glycosylated); homodimer of 21 to 24 kD subunits	T cells (T_H1, $CD8^+$ T cells), NK cells	Macrophages: activation (increased microbicidal functions) B cells: isotype switching to opsonizing and complement-fixing IgG subclasses T cells: T_H1 differentiation Various cells: increased expression of class I and class II MHC molecules, increased antigen processing and presentation to T cells
Transforming growth factor-β (TGF-β)	25 kD; homodimer of 12.5 kD subunits	T cells, macrophages, other cell types	T cells: inhibition of proliferation and effector functions B cells: inhibition of proliferation; IgA production Macrophages: inhibition of activation; stimulation of angiogenic factors Fibroblasts: increased collagen synthesis
Lymphotoxin (LT)	21–24 kD; secreted as homotrimer or associated with $LT\beta_2$ on the cell membrane	T cells	Recruitment and activation of neutrophils Lymphoid organogenesis
Interleukin-13 (IL-13)	15 kD	$CD4^+$ T cells (T_H2), NKT cells, mast cells	B cells: isotype switching to IgE Epithelial cells: increased mucus production Fibroblasts: increased collagen synthesis Macrophages: increased collagen synthesis
Interleukin-17 (IL-17)	20–30 kD	T cells	Endothelial cells: increased chemokine production Macrophages: increased chemokine and cytokine production Epithelial cells: GM-CSF and G-CSF production

Abbreviations: IgA, immunoglobulin A; kD, kilodalton; GM-CSF, granulocyte-macrophage colony stimulating factor; G-CSF, granulocyte colony stimulating factor; MHC, major histocompatibility complex; NK, natural killer.

Secreted IL-2 is a 14- to 17-kD glycoprotein that folds into a globular protein containing four α-helices. It is the prototype of the four-α-helical cytokines that interact with type I cytokine receptors (Fig. 12–9).

The expression of functional IL-2 receptors is induced upon activation of naive and effector T cells; regulatory T cells, which may be in a constant state of activation by self antigens, always express IL-2 receptors. The IL-2 receptor (IL-2R) consists of three noncovalently associated proteins including IL-2Rα (CD25), IL-2/15Rβ, and γ_c. Of the three chains, only IL-2Rα is unique to the IL-2R. IL-2 binds to the α chain alone with low affinity, and this does not lead to any detectable cytoplasmic signaling or biologic response. IL-2/15Rβ, which is also part of the IL-15 receptor, contributes to IL-2 binding and engages Jak3-STAT5–dependent signal transduction pathways. The γ chain is shared with receptors for IL-4, IL-7, and IL-15, and is therefore called the common γ

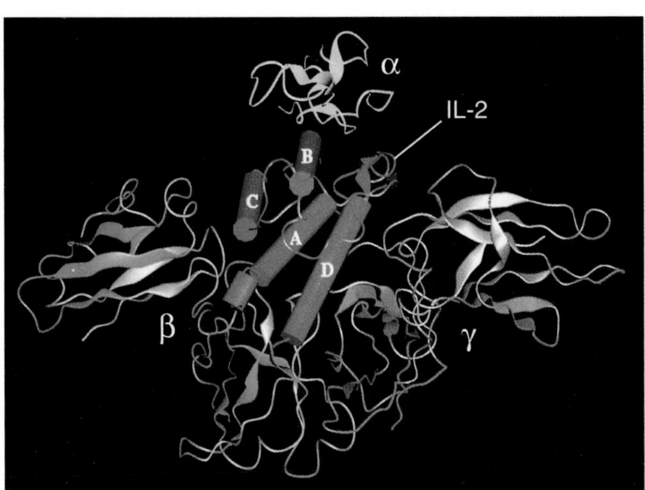

FIGURE 12–9 Model for the binding of IL-2 to its receptor. This ribbon diagram is modeled after the known x-ray crystal structure of growth hormone with its receptor and the structural similarity of growth hormone and IL-2. IL-2 is colored red, and the α, β, and γ chains of the receptor are colored yellow, green, and blue, respectively. The four α-helices of the IL-2 molecule are labeled A, B, C, and D. IL-2 interacts with all three chains of the heterotrimeric receptor, and the β and γ chains of the receptor interact with each other. (From Theze J, PM Alzari, and J Bertoglio. Interleukin 2 and its receptors: recent advances and new immunological functions. Immunology Today 17:481–486, 1996. Copyright 1996, with permission from Elsevier Science.)

chain (γ_c). Even though γ_c is not directly involved in binding IL-2, its association with the receptor complex is required for high-affinity IL-2 binding, and is also required for engagement of MAP kinase and PI-3 kinase signal transduction pathways. The IL-2R$\beta\gamma_c$ complexes are expressed at low levels on resting T cells (and on NK cells), and bind IL-2 with a K_d of approximately 10^{-9} M (Fig. 12–10). IL-2Rα expression is newly induced, and IL-2Rβ expression is up-regulated upon activation of naive CD4⁺ and CD8⁺ T cells and memory T cells. For this reason, IL-2Rα was originally called Tac (for T activation) antigen. Cells that express IL-2Rα and form IL-2R$\alpha\beta\gamma_c$ complexes can bind IL-2 more tightly, with a K_d of approximately 10^{-11} M, and growth stimulation of such cells occurs at a similarly low IL-2 concentration. In vitro studies indicate that IL-2, produced in response to antigen stimulation, is required for induction of IL-2Rα and IL-2Rβ, and therefore T cells that produce IL-2 or cells nearby to the IL-2 producers are most likely to respond to the cytokine. $CD4^+$ regulatory T cells, which play an essential role in maintaining T cell tolerance to self antigens (see Chapter 11), express IL-2Rα and IL-2Rβ, even without overt activation by antigen or IL-2. Chronic T cell stimulation leads to shedding of IL-2Rα, and an increased level of shed IL-2Rα in the serum is a clinically used marker of strong antigenic stimulation (e.g., acute rejection of a transplanted organ).

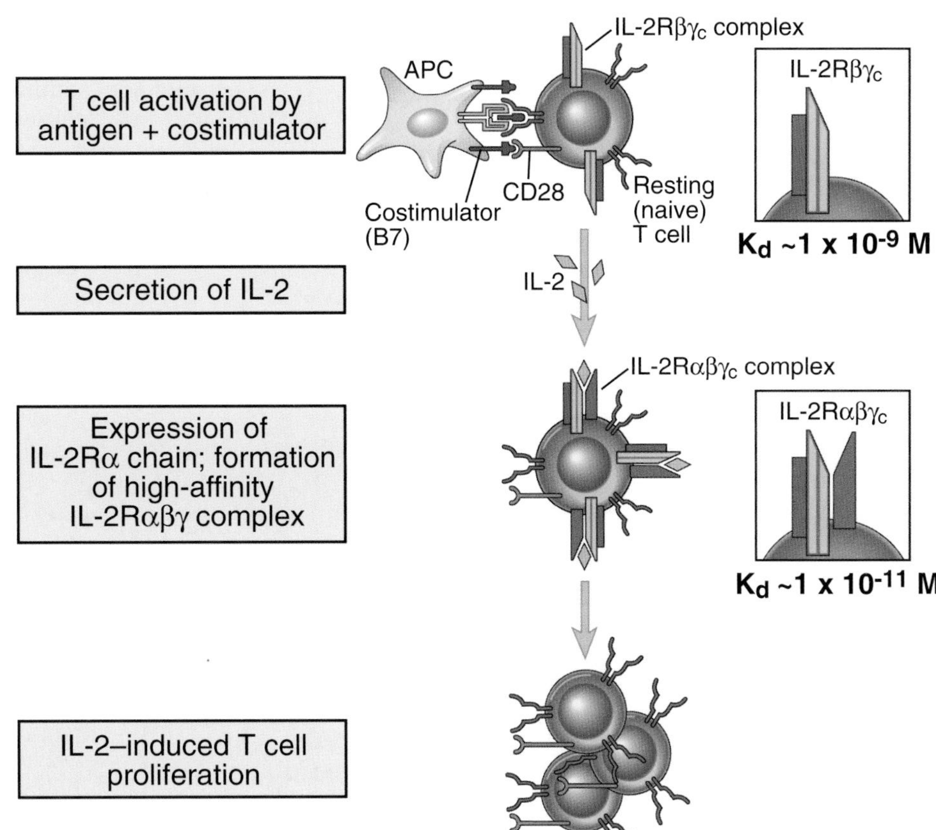

FIGURE 12–10 Regulation of IL-2 receptor expression. Resting (naive) T lymphocytes express the IL-2Rβγ complex, which has a moderate affinity for IL-2. Activation of the T cells by antigen, costimulators, and IL-2 itself leads to expression of the IL-2Rα chain and high levels of the high-affinity IL-2Rαβγ complex. APC, antigen-presenting cell.

Biologic Actions

IL-2 was originally described as a T cell growth factor, based on in vitro studies, but more recent studies indicate other roles may predominate in vivo (Fig. 12–11).

- ***IL-2 is required for the survival and perhaps function of regulatory T cells, which suppress immune responses against self and other antigens*** (see Chapter 11). The constitutive expression of IL-2 receptors on regulatory T cells is consistent with their requirement for IL-2 in order to survive.
  - Gene knockout mouse studies have provided evidence that the primary nonredundant function of IL-2 in vivo is the suppression of T responses. Mice lacking IL-2, IL-2Rα (CD25), or IL-2Rβ develop lymphadenopathy and T cell–mediated autoimmunity, and these mice lack regulatory T cells. These findings in mice indicate that other cytokines may share with IL-2 the role of growth factor for antigen-stimulated T cells, but the regulatory functions of IL-2 cannot be replaced by other cytokines. It remains to be established if IL-2 will prove to be as critical for maintenance of regulatory T cells in humans.
- ***IL-2 stimulates the survival, proliferation, and differentiation of antigen-activated T cells.*** IL-2 also promotes survival of cells by inducing the anti-apoptotic protein Bcl-2. IL-2 promotes cell cycle progression through the synthesis of cyclins and relieves a block in cell cycle progression through p27 degradation. In addition, IL-2 increases production of other effector cytokines, such as IFN-γ and IL-4, by the T cells.
- ***IL-2 promotes the proliferation and differentiation of NK cells.*** It stimulates the growth of NK cells and enhances their cytolytic function, producing so-called lymphokine-activated killer cells. Because NK cells, like resting T cells, express IL-2Rβγ_c (but not IL-2Rα), they can be stimulated only by high levels of IL-2. As mentioned earlier, in NK cells, the βγ_c complex is associated with the α chain of the IL-15 receptor, and IL-15 functions as a growth factor for these cells.
- IL-2 acts on B cells both as a growth factor and as a stimulus for antibody synthesis. This function has mainly been demonstrated in vitro.

Interleukin-4

IL-4 is the major stimulus for the production of IgE antibodies and for the development of T_H2 cells from naive CD4$^+$ helper T cells. IL-4 is the signature cytokine of the T_H2 subset and functions as both an inducer and an effector cytokine of these cells.

Structure, Production, and Receptors

IL-4 is a member of the four-α-helical cytokine family. The principal cellular sources of IL-4 are CD4$^+$ T lymphocytes of the T_H2 subset as well as activated mast cells.

The IL-4 receptor of lymphoid cells consists of a cytokine-binding α chain that is a member of the type I cytokine receptor family, associated with the γ_c chain shared by other cytokine receptors. This IL-4Rαγ_c receptor signals by the Jak–STAT pathway (Jak3- or 4-STAT6) and by a pathway that involves the insulin response substrate (IRS) called IRS-2. IL-4 is the only cytokine that activates the STAT6 protein, which induces transcription of genes that account for many of the actions of IL-4, such as T_H2 differentiation and B cell switching to IgE.

Biologic Actions

The biologic actions of IL-4 include stimulation of IgE and mast cell/eosinophil-mediated reactions (Fig. 12–12).

- ***IL-4 is the principal cytokine that stimulates B cell Ig heavy chain class switching to the IgE isotype.*** The

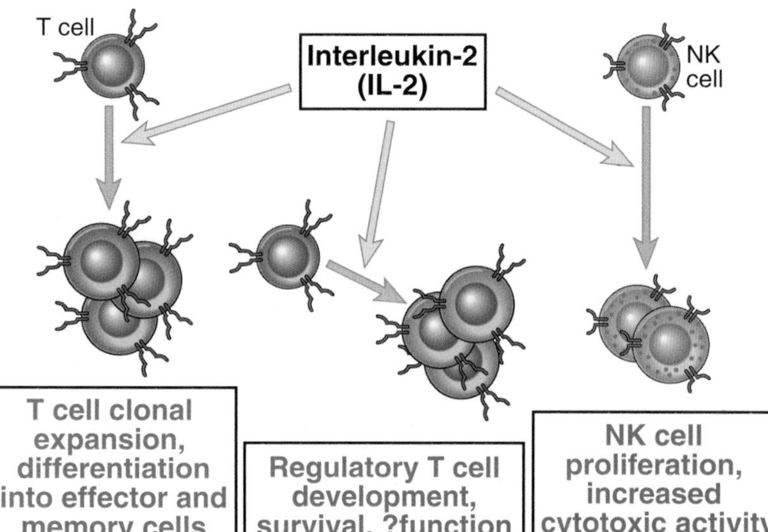

FIGURE 12–11 Biologic actions of IL-2. IL-2 stimulates the proliferation and differentiation of T and B lymphocytes and NK cells. As discussed in the text, IL-2 also functions to inhibit immune responses (e.g., against self antigens) by its effect on regulatory T cells.

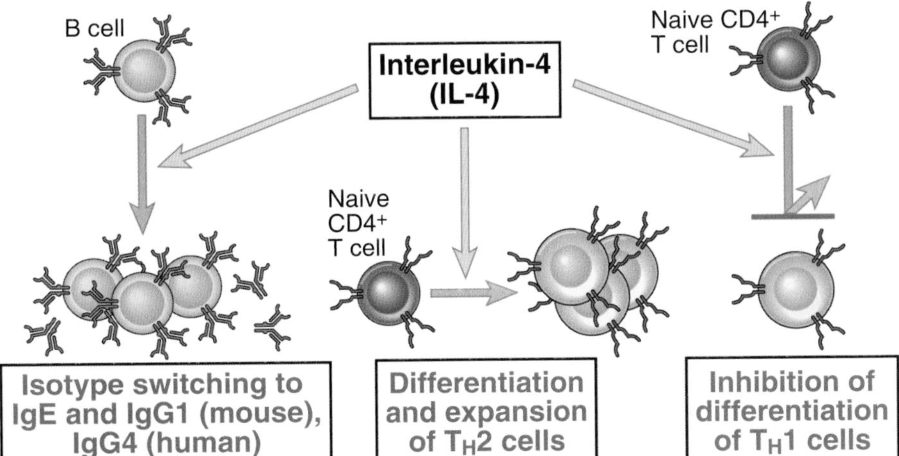

FIGURE 12–12 Biologic actions of IL-4. IL-4 stimulates B cell isotype switching to some immunoglobulin classes, notably IgE, and differentiation of naive T cells to the T_H2 subset. IL-4 also inhibits T_H1 differentiation.

mechanisms of class switching were described in Chapter 10. Knockout mice lacking IL-4 have less than 10% of normal IgE levels. IgE antibodies play a role in eosinophil-mediated defense against helminthic or arthropod infections, this being the major function of T_H2 cells in host defense. IgE is also the principal mediator of immediate hypersensitivity (allergic) reactions, and production of IL-4 is important for the development of allergies (see Chapter 19). IL-4 also enhances switching to IgG4 (in humans, or the homologous IgG1 in mice) and inhibits switching to the IgG2a and IgG3 isotypes in mice, both of which are stimulated by IFN-γ. This is one of several reciprocal antagonistic actions of IL-4 and IFN-γ.

- ***IL-4 stimulates the development of T_H2 cells from naive CD4⁺ T cells and functions as an autocrine growth factor for differentiated T_H2 cells.*** Thus, IL-4 is responsible for the induction and expansion of this subset. Knockout mice lacking IL-4 or STAT6 show a deficiency in the development and maintenance of T_H2 cells, even after stimuli (such as helminthic infections) that are normally potent inducers of this subset. This role of IL-4 is discussed in Chapter 13. IL-4 also inhibits the devleopment of T_H1 and T_H17 cells (see Chapter 13).
- IL-4, together with IL-13, contributes to an alternative form of macrophage activation that is distinct from the macrophage response to IFN-γ. The effects of IL-4 on macrophages include arginase induction leading to collagen production, and increased mannose receptor expression, which promotes the phagocytosis of microbes.

Interleukin-5

IL-5 is an activator of eosinophils and serves as the link between T cell activation and eosinophilic inflammation.

Structure, Production, and Receptors

IL-5 is a type I cytokine family member composed of a homodimer of a polypeptide containing a four-α-helical domain. It is produced by the T_H2 subset of $CD4^+$ T cells and by activated mast cells. The IL-5 receptor is a heterodimer composed of a unique α chain and a common β chain (β_c), which is also part of the IL-3 and granulocyte-macrophage colony-stimulating factor (GM-CSF) receptors. The IL-5Rα chain can bind IL-5 with low affinity, but does not signal. The β_c chain does not bind IL-5 by itself but is required for high affininty binding by the α chain, and for engaging signal transduction pathways. The major IL-5–induced signaling pathway involves Jak2 and STAT3.

Biologic Actions

The major actions of IL-5 are to activate mature eosinophils and stimulate the growth and differentiation of eosinophils. Activated eosinophils are able to kill helminths. Eosinophils express Fc receptors specific for IgG and IgA antibodies and are thereby able to bind to microbes opsonized by IgG or IgA, such as helminths. Knockout mice lacking IL-5 are defective in eosinophil responses and are susceptible to some helminthic infections. IL-5 also stimulates the proliferation of B cells and the production of IgA antibodies (see Chapter 10).

Interleukin-13

IL-13 is structurally and functionally similar to IL-4, and plays a key role in defense against helminths (see Chapter 15) and in allergic diseases (see Chapter 19).

Structure, Production, and Receptors

IL-13 is a member of the four-α-helical cytokine family, with limited sequence homology but significant structural similarity to IL-4. It is encoded by a gene in a region of human chromosome 5 that includes several other cytokine genes important to allergic disease, including IL-4, IL-5, and IL-9. IL-13 is produced mainly by $CD4^+$ helper T cells of the T_H2 subset, but other cell types, including $CD8^+$ T cells and NK-T cells, may produce significant amounts of IL-13 during the early phases of allergic responses. Other cellular sources of IL-13 include basophils and eosinophils. The functional IL-13 receptor is a heterodimer of the IL-4Rα chain and the IL-13Rα1 chain. This complex can bind both IL-4 and IL-13 with high affinity, and accounts for the fact that most of the biologic effects of IL-13 are shared with IL-4. The IL-4R/IL-13Rα1 receptor is expressed on a wide variety of cells, including B cells, mononuclear phagocytes, dendritic cells, eosinophils, basophils, fibroblasts, endothelial cells, and bronchial epithelial cells. T cells do not express the IL-13 receptor. IL-13R signaling is similar to IL-4R signaling, involving Jak1- and Tyk2-mediated phosphorylation of STAT6, as well as IRS2. Because the IL-13 receptor does not include the common γ chain, some of the downstream signaling events induced by IL-4 binding to the IL-4 receptor are not induced by either IL-4 or IL-13 binding to the IL-13 receptor. A second high affinity receptor for IL-13, called IL-13Rα2, does not appear to have any signaling functions, and may act as a dominant negative inhibitor and/or decoy receptor that blocks effects of IL-13 on certain cell types, including bronchial epithelial cells.

Biologic Actions

IL-13 works together with IL-4 in producing biologic effects associated with allergic inflammation, discussed in detail in Chapter 19, and in defense against parasites. The distinct distribution patterns of IL-4 and IL-13 receptors, the differences in signaling by these receptors, and differences in the induction and stability of IL-4 and IL-13 probably all contribute to the fact that IL-13 has biologic effects that are distinct from those of IL-4.

- ***IL-13 promotes fibrosis as part of the tissue repair phase of chronic inflammatory states.*** The fibrogenic function of IL-13, which is not shared by IL-4, is due to stimulation of fibroblasts and macrophages to synthesize collagen, in part by inducing expression of the enzyme arginase-1, and stimulation of macrophages to produce TGF-β, which itself promotes fibrosis. IL-13-induced fibrosis contributes significantly to the pathology of chronic asthma, interstitial lung diseases, and parasitic infections.
- ***IL-13 stimulates mucus production by lung epithelial cells.*** This property is also not shared by IL-4, and also contributes to the pathogenesis of asthma. IL-13–mediated mucus secretion is due to effects of the cytokine on proliferation, differentiation, and secretory function of bronchial epithelial goblet cells.
- ***IL-13 induces IgE class switching in B cells.*** This is a property shared with IL-4. IL-13 knockout mice have reduced IgE levels, even though they produce IL-4.
- ***IL-13 promotes inflammation by inducing expression of endothelial adhesion molecules (e.g., VCAM-1) and chemokines, which mediate recruitment of granulocytes and monocytes into tissues.*** The proinflammatory effects of IL-13 may be protective against parasite infections, and harmful in the case of asthma and other lung diseases.

Interferon-γ

IFN-γ is the principal macrophage-activating cytokine and serves critical functions in innate immunity and in adaptive cell-mediated immunity against intracellular microbes. IFN-γ is also called immune, or type II, IFN. Although it has some antiviral activity, it is not a potent antiviral cytokine, and it functions mainly as an activator of effector cells of the immune system.

Structure, Production, and Receptors

IFN-γ is a homodimeric protein produced by NK cells, $CD4^+$ T_H1 cells, and $CD8^+$ T cells; it is the signature cytokine of the T_H1 subset of helper T cells. NK cells secrete IFN-γ in response to activating ligands on the surface of infected or stressed host cells (see Chapter 2) or in response to IL-12; in this setting, IFN-γ functions as a mediator of innate immunity. In adaptive immunity, T cells produce IFN-γ in response to antigen recognition, and production is enhanced by IL-12 and IL-18. As we have mentioned previously and will discuss in more detail in Chapter 13, the sequence of reactions involving IL-12 and IFN-γ is central to cell-mediated immunity against intracellular microbes.

The receptor for IFN-γ is composed of two structurally homologous polypeptides belonging to the type II cytokine receptor family, called IFNγR1 and IFNγR2. IFN-γ binds to and induces the hetrodimerization of IFNγR1 and IFNγR2, which associate, respectively, with the Jak1 and Jak2 kinases. Activation of these enzymes leads to STAT1 phosphorylation and dimerization, binding of the STAT1 dimers to GAS sequences in regulatory regions of various genes, and transcription of these genes, as described for type I IFNs earlier in this chapter. IFN-γ–induced genes encode many different molecules involved in enhancing adaptive immune responses and in the effector function of macrophages, described later. Different IFN-γ–responsive genes are activated by STAT1 alone or by STAT1 acting with other transcription factors, including IFN response factor-1 (IRF-1) and class II transactivator, which are themselves induced by STAT1. STAT1 knockout mice are completely insensitive to the actions of IFN-γ.

Biologic Actions

The functions of IFN-γ are important in cell-mediated immunity against intracellular microbes (Fig. 12–13).

- ***IFN-γ activates macrophages to kill phagocytosed microbes.*** Together with CD40 ligand, IFN-γ is the means by which T_H1 helper T cells enhance macrophage function (see Chapter 13), and IFN-γ is the only way in which NK cells activate macrophages in innate immunity (see Chapter 2). IFN-γ enhances the microbicidal function of macrophages by stimu-

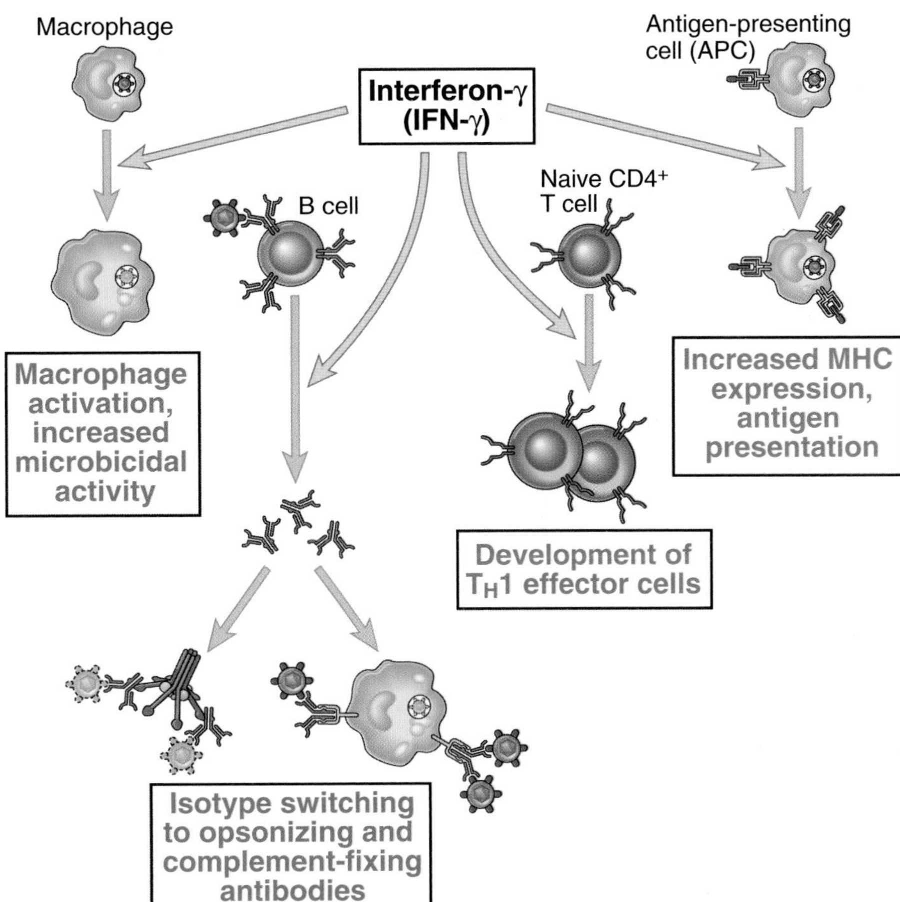

FIGURE 12–13 Biologic actions of IFN-γ. IFN-γ activates phagocytes and APCs and induces B cell switching to some immunoglobulin isotypes (which often bind complement and Fc receptors on phagocytes and are distinct from the isotypes induced by IL-4). The T_H1-inducing effect of IFN-γ may be indirect, mediated by increased IL-12 production and receptor expression.

lating the synthesis of reactive oxygen intermediates and nitric oxide. IFN-γ mediates these effects mainly by activating transcription of the genes that encode the enzymes required for generating reactive oxygen species and reactive nitrogen intermediates. These enzymes are phagocyte oxidase and inducible nitric oxide synthase, respectively. The reactive molecules are produced within lysosomes, and they destroy microbes that are contained within phagolysosomes.

- ***IFN-γ promotes the differentiation of naive CD4⁺ T cells to the T_H1 subset and inhibits the differentiation of T_H2 cells.*** IFN-γ stimulates production of a transcription factor called T-bet that directly promotes T_H1 differentiation (see Chapter 13). The T_H1-inducing effect of IFN-γ is also partly mediated indirectly by activating mononuclear phagocytes to produce IL-12, which is a major T_H1-inducing cytokine. In addition, in mice, IFN-γ enhances expression of the signaling chain of the IL-12 receptor. IFN-γ inhibition of T_H2 differentiation may involve T-bet–mediated suppression of GATA-3, a transcription factor that is required for the commitment of naive T cells to the T_H2 lineage (see Chapter 13).
- ***IFN-γ acts on B cells to promote switching to certain IgG subclasses, notably IgG2a in mice, and to inhibit switching to IL-4–dependent isotypes, such as IgE and IgG1 in mice.*** The IgG subclasses induced by IFN-γ bind to Fcγ receptors on phagocytes and activate complement, and both these mechanisms promote the phagocytosis of opsonized microbes. Thus, IFN-γ induces antibody responses that also participate in phagocyte-mediated elimination of microbes, in concert with the direct macrophage-activating effects of this cytokine.
- ***IFN-γ stimulates expression of class I and class II MHC molecules and costimulators on APCs.*** IFN-γ also stimulates the production of many proteins involved in antigen processing, including the transporter associated with antigen processing (TAP), the LMP-2 and LMP-7 components of the proteasome, and HLA-DM. Thus, IFN-γ enhances MHC-associated antigen presentation and amplifies the recognition phase of immune responses by increasing expression of the ligands that T cells recognize (see Chapter 5, Fig. 5–10). IFN-γ is also an activator of vascular endothelial cells, and it potentiates many of the actions of TNF on endothelial cells, promoting T lymphocyte adhesion and extravasation to sites of infection.

The net effect of these activities of IFN-γ is to promote macrophage-rich inflammatory reactions while inhibiting IgE-dependent eosinophil-rich reactions. Knockout mice lacking IFN-γ or the IFN-γ receptor are susceptible to infections with intracellular microbes, such as mycobacteria, because of defective macrophage activation.

Transforming Growth Factor-β

The principal action of TGF-β in the immune system is to inhibit the proliferation and activation of lymphocytes and other leukocytes. However, TGF-β can exert either anti-inflammatory or proinflammatory effects depending on the timing of its appearance, the amount produced, and systemic versus local expression. TGF-β was discovered as a tumor product that promoted the survival of cells in semisolid culture media. It is actually a family of closely related molecules encoded by distinct genes, commonly designated TGF-β1, TGF-β2, and TGF-β3. Cells of the immune system synthesize mainly TGF-β1.

Production, Structure, and Receptors

TGF-β1 is a homodimeric protein that is synthesized and secreted by antigen-stimulated T cells, LPS-activated mononuclear phagocytes, and many other cell types. Some regulatory T cells produce TGF-β, and the same cells may also produce IL-10, which, like TGF-β1, has immunosuppressive activities (see Chapter 11). TGF-β1 is synthesized as an inactive precursor that is proteolytically cleaved in the Golgi complex, and forms a homodimer. This mature TGF-β1 homodimer is secreted in a latent form in association with other polypeptides, which must be removed extracellularly by enzymatic digestion before the cytokine can bind to receptors and exert biologic effects. The TGF-β1 receptor consists of two different proteins, activin receptor-like kinase5 (ALK5) and TGF-βRII, which signal through a serine/threonine kinase domain that phosphorylates transcription factors called Smads. Upon TGF-β1 binding, ALK5 phosphorylates Smad2 and Smad3, which in complex with Smad4, translocate to the nucleus, bind to promoters of target genes, and regulate their transcription.

Biologic Actions

- ***TGF-β inhibits the proliferation and effector functions of T cells and the activation of macrophages.*** TGF-β also acts on other cells, such as neutrophils and endothelial cells, largely to counteract the effects of pro-inflammatory cytokines. By these actions, TGF-β functions to inhibit immune and inflammatory responses. Mice in which the TGF-β1 gene has been knocked out, or in which the TGF-β receptor has been selectively blocked in T cells, develop uncontrolled inflammatory lesions and lymphoproliferation.
- ***TGF-β regulates differentiation of functionally distinct subsets of T cells.*** Some studies in mice indicate that differentiation or survival of regulatory T cells depends in part on TGF-β. In addition, TGF-β produced by regulatory T cells, or perhaps dendritic cells, can block development of T_H1 and T_H2 subsets of effector $CD4^+$ T cells. Furthermore, TGF-β in combination with cytokines elicited during innate immune responses, such as IL-6, may promote the differentiation of a proinflammatory subset of $CD4^+$ T cells that secrete IL-17. Thus, TGF-β has complex effects on T cell– mediated immune responses.
- ***TGF-β stimulates production of IgA antibodies by inducing B cells to switch to this isotype.*** IgA is the antibody isotype required for mucosal immunity (see Chapter 14).
- ***TGF-β regulates tissue repair after local immune and inflammatory reactions subside.*** This function is mediated by specific actions of TGF-β on collagen synthesis and matrix-modifying enzyme production by macrophages and fibroblasts, and by contributing to angiogenesis.

Other Cytokines of Adaptive Immunity

Lymphotoxin (LT) is a cytokine produced by T lymphocytes and other cells. It is approximately 30% homologous to macrophage-derived TNF and serves many of the same functions. (For this reason, LT is also called TNF-β.) The secreted form of LT (sometimes called LTα) is a homotrimer, similar to TNF, and it binds to TNF receptors. LT is also expressed as a membrane protein in which one chain of the secreted form associates with two subunits of a structurally related membrane protein called LTβ. The LTβ membrane form binds to a different receptor also belonging to the TNF receptor family.

LT activates endothelial cells and neutrophils and is thus a mediator of the acute inflammatory response, providing a link between T cell activation and inflammation. These biologic effects of LT are the same as those of TNF, consistent with their binding to the same receptors. However, because the quantity of LT synthesized by antigen-stimulated T cells is much less than the amounts of TNF made by LPS-stimulated mononuclear phagocytes, LT is not readily detected in the circulation. Therefore, LT is usually a locally acting cytokine and not a mediator of systemic injury.

Studies in transgenic and knockout mice have shown that LT is required for the normal development of lymphoid organs (see Chapter 3). Knockout mice lacking membrane LTβ or the receptor for LTβ show various defects in the formation of lymph nodes, Peyer's patches, and splenic white pulp. In these animals, the B cell areas in the lymphoid organs do not develop normally, and no germinal centers are seen in the spleen. LT may function in lymphoid organogenesis by inducing the production of chemokines that promote lymphocyte migration into particular areas of lymphoid organs.

IL-17 includes a family of six structurally related cytokines, some of which promote tissue damage in hypersensitivity diseases and others are important for defense against bacterial infections. The structures of the IL-17 cytokines and their receptors are not shared by other cytokines discussed in this chapter, and the signal transduction pathways the receptors engage remain incompletely characterized. IL-17A and F, which are the best characterized members of the family, are produced by several cell types, including a subset of effector CD4$^+$ T cells distinct from T_H1 and T_H2 cells. The differentiation and maintenance of this IL-17-producing T cell subset are dependent on TGF-β, IL-23, and cytokines produced during innate immune reactions, such as IL-6. IL-17A and F stimulate endothelial cells and macrophages to produce IL-1, TNF, and various chemokines, which promote neutrophil recruitment. IL-17 also induces cells to produce hematopoietic cytokines, described later in this chapter, which stimulate neutrophil production by the bone marrow. IL-17 produced by T cells is thought to be responsible for the destructive inflammation characteristic of several mouse models of autoimmune disease. A role of IL-17 in human inflammatory bowel disease is also suspected.

IL-21 is a type I cytokine produced by activated CD4$^+$ T cells that has a wide variety of effects on B and T cells and NK cells. The IL-21 receptor is a type I family receptor that includes the common γ chain subunit, and activates a signaling pathway involving Jak1, Jak2, STAT1, and STAT3. The effects of IL-21 are often synergistic with or modulate the effects of other cytokines, but do not appear to be essential for immune responses. Some of the major effects of IL-21 include stimulation of proliferation and augmentation of effector function of CD8$^+$ T cells; enhancement of class switching and Ig production by B cells; and induction of differentiation and enhancement of effector function of NK cells.

Several other T cell–derived cytokines have been described, but their physiologic functions are unclear. IL-16 is a T cell–derived cytokine that acts as a specific chemoattractant of eosinophils. However, it appears to be derived from a fragment of an intracellular protein, and it is not known whether it is secreted under physiologic conditions. IL-25 is structurally homologous to IL-17 but is secreted by T_H2 cells and stimulates the production of other T_H2 cytokines, including IL-4, IL-5, and IL-13. Migration inhibition factor (MIF) is a T cell–derived substance that immobilizes mononuclear phagocytes, an effect that might cause the cells to be retained at sites of inflammation. This was the first cytokine activity to be described, but it has proved difficult to purify and biochemically characterize a cytokine with this function.

B cell activating factor belonging to the TNF family (**BAFF**) and **a proliferation-inducing ligand** (**APRIL**) are two closely related members of the TNF family of cytokines, which have important effects on B cell survival, and therefore humoral immunity. BAFF is expressed as both a membrane-bound and secreted protein, while APRIL is mainly a secreted protein. Various cell types produce BAFF, including neutrophils, monocytes, macrophages, dendritic cells, follicular dendritic cells and activated T cells. APRIL is produced mainly by monocytes, macrophages, dendritic cells, and activated T cells. BAFF and APRIL expression are upregulated by various proinflammatory cytokines. BAFF and APRIL both bind to two TNF receptor family receptors, transmembrane activator and CAML interactor (TACI), and B cell maturation antigen (BCMA). BAFF, but not APRIL, also binds to another TNF receptor family member called BAFF receptor (BAFF-R or BR3). These receptors transduce signals leading to upregulation of the anti-apoptotic protein Bcl-2 and the activation of NF-κB. Each of these receptors mediates distinct functions during B cell development, activation, and differentiation. BAFF-R is required for the survival of mature follicular B cells and facilitates the differentiation of marginal zone B cells. TACI is required for class switching particularly to IgA and IgG isotypes, and mediates the induction of AID when T-independent isotype switching occurs in responses to certain polysaccharide antigens. BCMA is required for the survival of long-lived plasma cells in the bone marrow.

Apart from their roles in B cell survival, differentiation, and activation, BAFF family cytokines and their receptors are of relevance from the viewpoint of disease. Some patients with selective IgA deficiency and with Common Variable Immunodeficiency have mutations in TACI (see Chapter 20). Enhanced secretion of BAFF may permit the survival of anergic B cells, and enhanced BAFF levels are seen in patients with humoral autoimmune disorders such as systemic lupus erythematosus. TACI, BCMA, and BAFF-R are also expressed on certain B lineage tumors, and may contribute to their malignant growth characteristics.

Roles of T Cell Cytokines in Specialized Adaptive Immune Responses

The cytokines of adaptive immunity are critical for the development of immune responses and for the activation of effector cells that serve to eliminate microbes and other antigens. In Chapter 1, we mentioned a cardinal feature of adaptive immunity, that responses are specialized to eliminate different types of microbes. Much of this specialization is due to the actions of cytokines, which may be produced by subpopulations of helper T cells. Different types of microbes stimulate naive CD4$^+$ T cells to differentiate into effector cells that produce distinct sets of cytokines and perform distinct functions. The best defined of these subsets are the T_H1 and T_H2 cells, which have been mentioned previously. We will describe the properties and functions of these subsets in Chapter 13, when we discuss the effector mechanisms of cell-mediated immunity. Many intracellular microbes (bacteria and viruses) induce the development of T_H1 cells, which produce IFN-γ, the cytokine that activates phagocytes to destroy intracellular microbes and stimulates the production of opsonizing antibodies that promote more phagocytosis. Helminthic parasites, in contrast, stimulate the development of T_H2

cells, which produce IL-4 and IL-5. IL-4 enhances production of helminth-specific IgE antibodies and IL-5 activates eosinophils, and both contribute to destruction of the parasites. In other chapters we refer to the functions of these and other cytokines at different stages of adaptive immune responses.

CYTOKINES THAT STIMULATE HEMATOPOIESIS

Cytokines are necessary for normal hematopoiesis in the bone marrow and provide a means of fine-tuning bone marrow function in response to the need for leukocytes. Several of the cytokines generated during both innate and adaptive immune responses stimulate the growth and differentiation of bone marrow progenitor cells. Thus, immune and inflammatory reactions, which consume leukocytes, also elicit production of new leukocytes.

Mature leukocytes arise from pluripotent stem cells by commitment to a particular lineage (differentiation) and progressive expansion of the progeny (Fig. 12–14). The differentiation and expansion of bone marrow progenitor cells are stimulated by cytokines, which are called **colony-stimulating factors** (CSFs) because they are often assayed by their ability to stimulate the formation of cell colonies in bone marrow cultures. Under the influence of different CSFs, these colonies acquire characteristics of specific cell lineages (e.g., granulocytes, mononuclear phagocytes, or lymphocytes). The names assigned to CSFs reflect the types of colonies that arise in these assays. In this section, we focus on cytokines that are important for the development of lymphocytes (Table 12–6).

Stem Cell Factor (c-Kit Ligand)

Pluripotent stem cells express a tyrosine kinase membrane receptor that is the protein product of the cellular proto-oncogene c-*kit*. The cytokine that interacts with

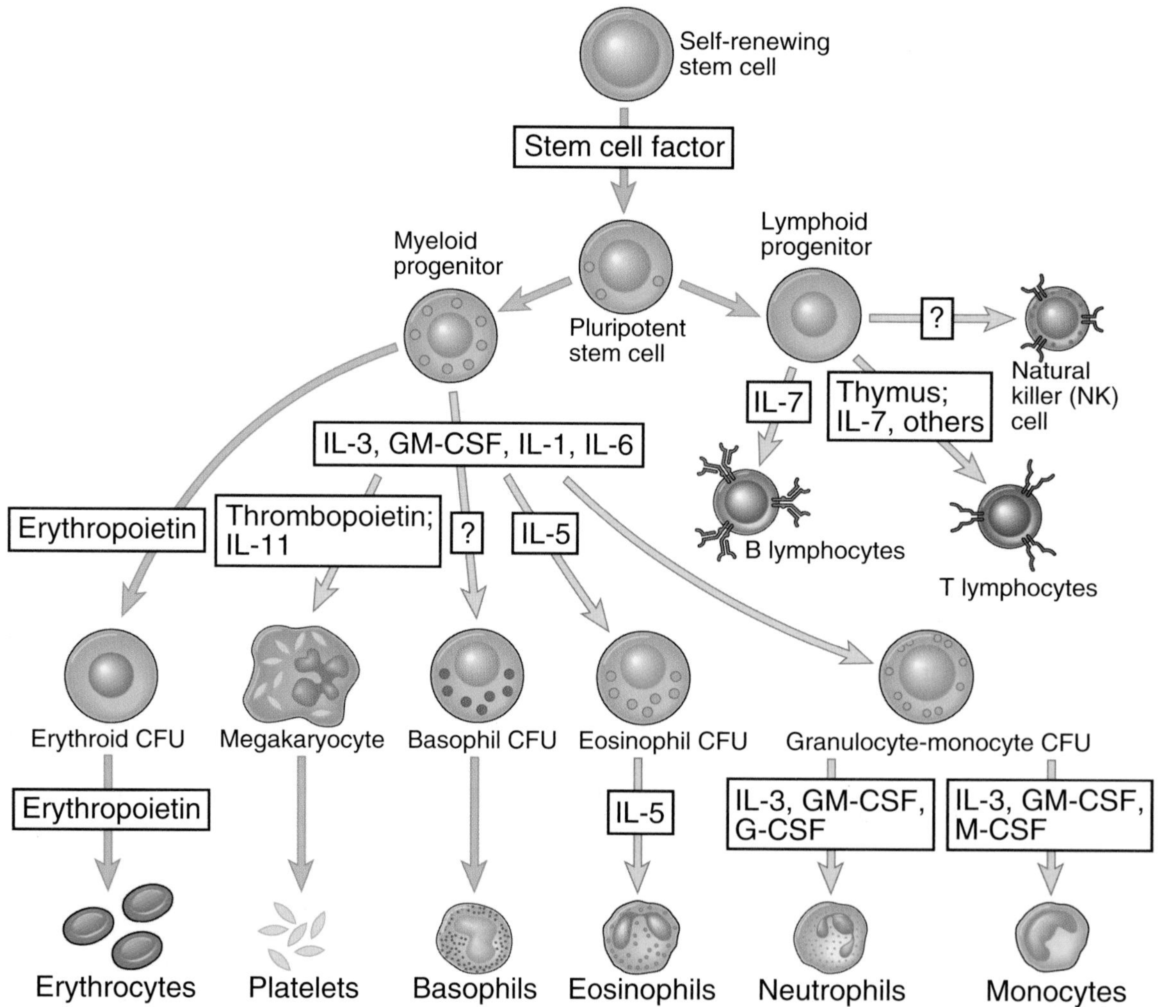

FIGURE 12–14 Roles of cytokines in hematopoiesis. Different cytokines stimulate the growth and maturation of different lineages of blood cells. CFU, colony-forming unit.

Table 12–6. Hematopoietic Cytokines

Cytokine	Size (kD)	Principal cellular sources	Principal cellular targets	Principal cell populations induced
Stem cell factor (c-Kit ligand)	24 kD	Bone marrow stromal cells	Pluripotent stem cells	All
Interleukin-7 (IL-7)	25 kD	Fibroblasts, bone marrow stromal cells	Immature lymphoid progenitors	B and T lymphocytes
Interleukin-3 (IL-3)	20–26 kD	T cells	Immature progenitors	All
Granulocyte-monocyte CSF (GM-CSF)	18–22 kD	T cells, macrophages, endothelial cells, fibroblasts	Immature and committed progenitors, mature macrophages	Granulocytes and monocytes, macrophage activity
Monocyte CSF (M-CSF)	Dimer of 70–90 kD; 40-kD subunits	Macrophages, endothelial cells, bone marrow cells, fibroblasts	Committed progenitors	Monocytes
Granulocyte CSF (G-CSF)	19 kD	Macrophages, fibroblasts, endothelial cells	Committed progenitors	Granulocytes

Abbreviations: CSF, colony-stimulating factor; kD, kilodalton.

this receptor is called c-Kit ligand, or stem cell factor, because it acts on immature stem cells. Therefore, c-Kit is also called the stem cell factor receptor. Stem cell factor is synthesized by stromal cells of the bone marrow as a transmembrane protein or a secreted protein, both produced from the same gene by alternative splicing of the RNA. It is believed that stem cell factor is needed to make bone marrow stem cells responsive to other CSFs but it does not cause colony formation by itself. It may also play a role in sustaining the viability and proliferative capacity of immature T cells in the thymus and of mast cells in mucosal tissues. The soluble form of stem cell factor is absent in a mutant mouse strain called steel. The steel mouse has defects in mast cell production but not in most other lineages, suggesting that the membrane form of the factor is more important than the soluble form for stimulating stem cells to mature into various hematopoietic lineages. Elimination of both forms of stem cell factor by gene knockout is lethal.

Interleukin-7

IL-7 is a type I family four-α-helical cytokine secreted by stromal cells in many tissues that stimulates survival and expansion of immature precursors committed to the B and T lymphocyte lineages (see Chapter 7). The IL-7 receptor consists of a unique IL-7-binding α chain associated with the γ_c chain described earlier in this chapter as part of the receptors for IL-2, IL-4, and IL-15. Knockout mice lacking IL-7 or the IL-7 receptor α chain or its associated Jak3 kinase are lymphopenic, with a decreased number of T and B cells. Knockout mice lacking γ_c, and humans with γ_c mutations, show defects in lymphocyte maturation; the human disease is called **X-linked severe combined immunodeficiency** (see Chapter 20). IL-7 is also essential for the survival of mature, naive T cells and memory cells, especially CD4$^+$ memory cells, both of which express high levels of the IL-7 receptor.

Interleukin-3

IL-3, also known as multilineage colony-stimulating factor (multi-CSF), is a product of CD4$^+$ T cells that acts on immature marrow progenitors and promotes the expansion of cells that differentiate into all known mature hematopoietic cell types. IL-3 is a member of the four-α-helical family of cytokines. In humans, the IL-3 receptor consists of a cytokine-binding component that is a member of the type I cytokine receptor family and a signal-transducing subunit that is shared with IL-5 and GM-CSF receptors. In the mouse, the signal-transducing subunit of the IL-3 receptor is unique. Signal transduction in both species involves a Jak-STAT pathway. Most functional analyses of IL-3 have been performed in mice. In addition to its effect on multiple cell lineages, IL-3 promotes the growth and development of mast cells from bone marrow–derived progenitors, an action enhanced by IL-4. However, knockout of the IL-3 receptor in mice does not cause noticeable impairment of hematopoiesis. Human IL-3 has been identified by the cDNA cloning of a molecule homologous to mouse

IL-3, but it has been difficult to establish a role for this cytokine in hematopoiesis in humans. In fact, many actions attributed to mouse IL-3 appear to be performed by human GM-CSF.

Other Hematopoietic Cytokines

GM-CSF, macrophage colony-stimulating factor (M-CSF), and granulocyte colony-stimulating factor (G-CSF) are cytokines made by activated T cells, macrophages, endothelial cells, and bone marrow stromal cells that act on bone marrow progenitors to increase production of various leukocytes. GM-CSF promotes the maturation of bone marrow cells into dendritic cells and monocytes. G-CSF is generated at sites of infection and acts as an endocrine hormone to mobilize neutrophils from the marrow to replace those consumed in inflammatory reactions. Recombinant GM-CSF and G-CSF are used to stimulate bone marrow recovery after cancer chemotherapy and bone marrow transplantation. These are some of the most successful clinical applications of cytokines.

Erythropoietin (Epo) is a member of the type I cytokine family of proteins, produced mainly in the kidney in response to low oxygen tension. Its major biologic effect is to promote production of red blood cells from already committed erythroid progenitor cells. Epo binds to a type I cytokine receptor, which signals through Jak2-STAT5, and PI-3-kinase–Akt pathways. The Epo receptor is widely expressed in many tissues, and in addition to its role in red blood cell production, Epo is involved in physiologic angiogenic responses in the developing embryo, in the uterus, and in would healing. Epo also appears to contribute to pathologic angiogenesis in the retina and in tumors. Recombinant human Epo is commonly used for the treatment of anemia in chronic renal failure.

IL-9 is a cytokine that supports the growth of some T cell lines and of bone marrow–derived mast cell progenitors. IL-9 uses the γ_c chain signaling subunit and a Jak-STAT pathway. Its physiologic role is unknown.

IL-11 is produced by bone marrow stromal cells. It uses the same gp130 signaling subunit used by IL-6 and signals by a Jak-STAT pathway. It stimulates megakaryocytopoiesis and is in clinical use to treat patients with platelet deficiencies resulting from cancer chemotherapy.

SUMMARY

- Cytokines are a family of proteins that mediate many of the responses of innate and adaptive immunity. The same cytokines may be produced by many cell types, and individual cytokines often act on diverse cell types. Cytokines are synthesized in response to inflammatory or antigenic stimuli and usually act locally, in an autocrine or a paracrine fashion, by binding to high-affinity receptors on target cells. Certain cytokines may be produced in sufficient quantity to circulate and exert endocrine actions. For many cell types, cytokines serve as growth factors.

- Cytokines mediate their actions by binding with high affinity to receptors, which belong to a limited number of structural families. Most of the receptors contain two or more subunits, and some subunits are shared between different receptors. Cytokine receptors engage several specialized signaling pathways, including Jak-STAT pathways (type I and type II receptors), TIR/IRAK pathways (IL-1 family receptors), and TRAF pathways (TNF family receptors).

- The cytokines that mediate innate immunity are produced mainly by activated macrophages and include the following: TNF and IL-1 are mediators of acute inflammatory reactions to microbes; chemokines recruit leukocytes to sites of inflammation; IL-12 and IL-18 stimulate production of the macrophage-activating cytokine IFN-γ; type I IFNs are antiviral cytokines; IL-10 is an inhibitor of macrophages and dendritic cells; IL-23 and IL-27 regulate T cell–dependent inflammatory responses. These cytokines function in innate immune responses to different classes of microbes, and some (IL-12, IL-18, IL-23, IL-27) modify adaptive immune responses that follow the innate immune response.

- The cytokines that mediate and regulate adaptive immune responses are produced mainly by antigen-stimulated T lymphocytes, and they include the following: IL-2 is a T cell growth factor and an essential regulator of T cell responses; IL-4 stimulates IgE production and the development of T_H2 cells from naive helper T cells; IL-5 activates eosinophils; IL-13 promotes IgE production, mucus secretion, and tissue fibrosis in the setting of allergic disease and parasite infections; IFN-γ is an activator of macrophages and contributes to differentiation of IFN-γ–producing helper T cells; and TGF-β inhibits the proliferation of T lymphocytes and the activation of leukocytes.

- The CSFs consist of cytokines produced by bone marrow stromal cells, T lymphocytes, and other cells that stimulate the growth of bone marrow progenitors, thereby providing a source of additional inflammatory leukocytes. Several of these (e.g., stem cell factor and IL-7) play important roles in lymphopoiesis.

- Cytokines serve many functions that are critical to host defense against pathogens and provide links between innate and adaptive immunity. Cytokines contribute to the specialization of immune responses by activating different types of effector cells. Cytokines also regulate the magnitude and nature of immune responses by influencing the growth and differentiation of lymphocytes. Finally, cytokines provide important amplification mechanisms that enable small numbers of lymphocytes specific for any one antigen to activate a variety of effector mechanisms to eliminate the antigen.

- Excessive production or actions of cytokines can lead to pathologic consequences. The administration of cytokines or their inhibitors is a potential approach for modifying biologic responses associated with immune and inflammatory diseases.

Selected Readings

Alexander WS, and DJ Hilton. The role of suppressors of cytokine signaling in regulation of the immune response. Annual Review of Immunology 22:503–529, 2004.

Brombacher F, RA Kastelein, and G Alber. Novel IL-12 family members shed light on the orchestration of Th1 responses. Trends in Immunology 24:207–212, 2003.

Charo IF, and RM Ransohoff. The many roles of chemokines and chemokine receptors in inflammation. New England Journal of Medicine. 354:610–621, 2006.

Couper KN, Blount DG, Riley EM. IL-10: the master regulator of immunity to infection. Journal of Immunology 180:5771–5777, 2008.

Hunter CA. New IL-12-family members: IL-23 and IL-27. Cytokines with divergent functions. Nature Reviews Immunology 5:521–531, 2005.

Li MO, and RA Flavell. TGF-beta: a master of all T cell trades. Cell 134:392–404, 2008.

Locksley RM, N Killeen, and MJ Lenardo. The TNF and TNF receptor superfamilies: integrating mammalian biology. Cell 104:487–501, 2001.

Ma A, R Koka, and P Burkett. Diverse functions of IL-2, IL-15, and IL-7 in lymphoid homeostasis. Annual Review of Immunology 24:657–679, 2006.

Malek TR. The biology of interleukin-2. Annual Review of Immunology 26:453–479, 2008.

Moser B, M Wolf, A Walz, and P Loetscher. Chemokines: multiple levels of leukocyte migration control. Trends in Immunology 25:75–84, 2004.

Naka T, M Fujimoto, H Tsutsui, and A Yoshimura. Negative regulation of cytokine and TLR signalings by SOCS and others. Advances in Immunology 87:61–122, 2005.

Nelson BH, and DM Willerford. Biology of the interleukin-2 receptor. Advances in Immunology 70:1–81, 1998.

O'Shea JJ, and PJ Murray. Cytokine signaling modules in inflammatory responses. Immunity 28:477–487, 2008.

Petska S, CD Krause, D Sarkaz, MR Walter, Y Shi, and PB Fisher. Interleukin-10 and related cytokines and receptors. Annual Review of Immunology 22:929–979, 2004.

Platanias LC. Mechanisms of type-I and type-II interferon-mediated signaling. Nature Reviews Immunology 5:375–386, 2005.

Rot A, and UH von Andrian. Chemokines in innate and adaptive host defense: basic chemokinese grammar for immune cells. Annual Review of Immunology 22:891–928, 2004.

Schluns KS, and L Lefrancois. Cytokine control of memory T cell development and survival. Nature Reviews Immunology 3:269–279, 2003.

Shuai K, and B Liu. Regulation of gene-activation pathways by PIAS proteins in the immune system. Nature Reviews Immunology 5:593–605, 2005.

Stark GR, IM Kerr, BR Williams, RH Silverman, and RD Schreiber. How cells respond to interferons. Annual Review of Biochemistry 67:227–264, 1998.

Sugamura KH, H Asao, M Kondo, N Tanaka, N Ishii, K Ohno, M Nakamura, and T Takeshita. The interleukin-2 receptor γ chain: its role in the multiple cytokine receptor complexes and T cell development in XSCID. Annual Review of Immunology 14:179–205, 1996.

Thelen M, and JV Stein. How chemokines invite leukocytes to dance. Nature Immunology 9:953–959, 2008.

Trinchieri G. Interleukin-12 and the regulation of innate resistance and adaptive immunity. Nature Reviews Immunology 3:133–146, 2003.

Wajant H, K Pfizenmaier, and P Scheurich. Tumor necrosis factor signaling. Cell Death and Differentiation 10:45–65, 2003.

Waldmann TA. The biology of interleukin-2 and interleukin-15: implications for cancer therapy and vaccine design. Nature Reviews Immunology 6(8):595–601, 2006.

Weaver CT, Hatton RD, Mangan PR, and Harrington LE. IL-17 family cytokines and the expanding diversity of effector T cell lineages. Annual Review of Immunology 25:821–852, 2007.

Wills-Karp M. Interleukin-13 in asthma pathogenesis. Immunological Reviews 202:175–190, 2004.

Wynn TA. Fibrotic disease and the TH1/TH2 paradigm. Nature Reviews Immunology 4:583–594, 2004.

Yoshimura A, T Naka, and M Kubo. SOCS proteins, cytokine signalling and immune regulation. Nature Reviews Immunology 7:454–465, 2007.

Zlotnik A, and O Yoshie. Chemokines: a new classification system and their role in immunity. Immunity 12:121–127, 2001.

Chapter 13

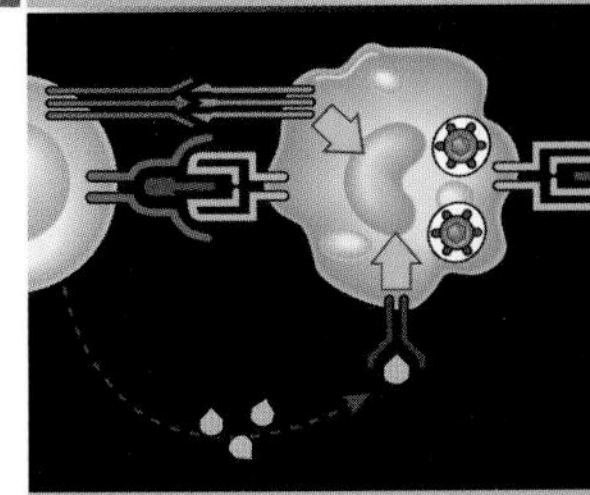

EFFECTOR MECHANISMS OF CELL-MEDIATED IMMUNITY

Cell-mediated immunity (CMI) is the effector function of T lymphocytes, and it serves as the defense mechanism against microbes that survive and replicate within phagocytes and nonphagocytic cells. Historically, immunologists have divided adaptive immunity into humoral immunity, which can be adoptively transferred from an immunized donor to a naive host by antibodies in the absence of cells, and CMI, which can be adoptively transferred only by viable T lymphocytes. The effector phase of humoral immunity is triggered by the recognition of antigen by secreted antibodies; therefore, humoral immunity neutralizes and eliminates extracellular microbes and toxins that are accessible to antibodies, but it is not effective against microbes inside infected cells. In contrast, in CMI, the effector phase is initiated by the recognition of antigens by T cells. T lymphocytes recognize protein antigens of intracellular microbes that are displayed on the surfaces of infected cells as peptides bound to self major histocompatibility complex (MHC) molecules. Defects in CMI result in increased susceptibility to infection by viruses and intracellular bacteria. T cell–mediated reactions are also important in allograft rejection (see Chapter 16), antitumor immunity (see Chapter 17), and autoimmunity (see Chapter 18). In this chapter, we discuss the properties of effector T cells and the effector mechanisms of cell-mediated immune reactions. Antigen presentation to T lymphocytes and the process of T cell activation are described in Chapters 6, 7, and 9.

TYPES OF CELL-MEDIATED IMMUNE REACTIONS

Different types of microbes elicit distinct protective T cell responses.

- ***The adaptive immune response to microbes residing within the phagosomes of phagocytes is mediated by effector CD4$^+$ T lymphocytes, called T_H1 cells, that recognize microbial antigens and activate the phagocytes to destroy the ingested microbes*** (Fig. 13–1A). Phagocytes are the major cells of host defense early after infection, i.e. during innate immune responses (see Chapter 2). The function of phagocytes is to ingest and kill microbes. Many microbes have developed mechanisms that enable them to survive and even replicate within phagocytes, so innate immunity is unable to eradicate infections by such microbes. In these situations, CMI functions to enhance the microbicidal actions of phagocytes and thus to eliminate the microbes. In CMI against phagocytosed microbes, the specificity of the response is due to T cells, but the actual effector function, that is, killing of microbes, is mediated by phagocytes. This cooperation of T lymphocytes and phagocytes illustrates an important link between adaptive and innate immunity: by means of cytokine secretion, T cells stimulate the function and focus the activity of nonspecific effector cells of innate immunity (phagocytes), thereby converting these cells into agents of adaptive immunity.

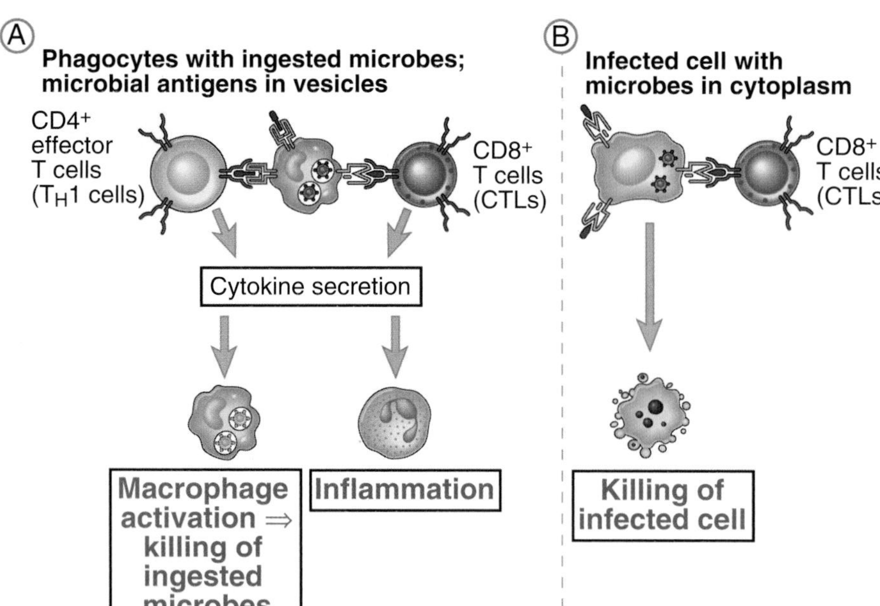

FIGURE 13–1 Types of T cell–mediated immune reactions. A. $CD4^+$ T_H1 cells and $CD8^+$ T cells recognize class II MHC-associated or class I MHC-associated peptide antigens of phagocytosed microbes, respectively, and produce cytokines that activate the phagocytes to kill the microbes and stimulate inflammation. B. $CD8^+$ CTLs recognize class I MHC-associated peptide antigens of microbes residing in the cytoplasm of infected cells and kill the cells.

- The fundamental concept that T cells are responsible for specific recognition of microbes but that phagocytes actually destroy the microbes in many cell-mediated immune responses was established with the original description of CMI to the intracellular bacterium *Listeria monocytogenes.* In the 1950s, George Mackaness showed that mice infected with a low dose of *Listeria* were protected from challenge with higher, lethal doses. Protection could be transferred to naive animals with lymphocytes (later shown to be T lymphocytes) from the infected mice, but not with serum. In vitro, the bacteria were killed not by T cells from immune animals but by activated macrophages, emphasizing the central role of macrophages in the execution of effector function (Fig. 13–2).

- ***The adaptive immune response to microbes that infect and replicate in the cytoplasm of various cell types, including nonphagocytic cells, is mediated by $CD8^+$ cytotoxic T lymphocytes (CTLs), which kill infected cells and eliminate the reservoirs of infection*** (Fig. 13–1B). CTLs are the principal defense mechanism against microbes that infect various cell types and replicate intracellularly. If the infected cells lack the capacity to kill microbes, the infection can be eradicated only by destroying these cells. CTL-mediated killing is also a mechanism for eliminating microbes that are taken up by phagocytes but escape from phagosomes into the cytosol, where they are not susceptible to the microbicidal activities of phagocytes.

- T cell–dependent macrophage activation and inflammation may damage normal tissues. This reaction is called **delayed-type hypersensitivity (DTH),** the term *hypersensitivity* referring to tissue injury caused by an immune response. DTH is a frequent accompaniment of protective CMI against microbes and the cause of much of the pathology associated with certain types of infection (see Chapter 15). DTH is also the mechanism of tissue damage in several autoimmune diseases (see Chapter 18).

- ***The adaptive immune response to helminthic parasites is mediated by T_H2 cells,*** which stimulate the production of immunoglobulin E (IgE) antibodies and activate eosinophils and mast cells to destroy the helminths. T_H2-mediated immune reactions are characterized by eosinophil-rich inflammation.

- The innate immune system also has a cellular arm, mediated by natural killer (NK) cells, which protect against viruses and other intracellular microbes. NK cells kill infected cells early in the infection (see Chapter 2).

Cell-mediated immune responses consist of the development of effector T cells from naive cells in peripheral lymphoid organs, migration of these effector T cells and other leukocytes to sites of infection, and either cytokine-mediated activation of leukocytes to destroy microbes or direct killing of infected cells (Fig. 13–3). The development of the effector T cells of CMI involves the sequence of antigen recognition, clonal expansion, and differentiation that is characteristic of all adaptive immune responses; these processes were described in Chapter 9. In the following sections, we describe the properties and functions of effector T cells.

EFFECTOR CD4+ T CELLS

One of the most exciting discoveries in immunology was the identification of subsets of $CD4^+$ T cells that differ in

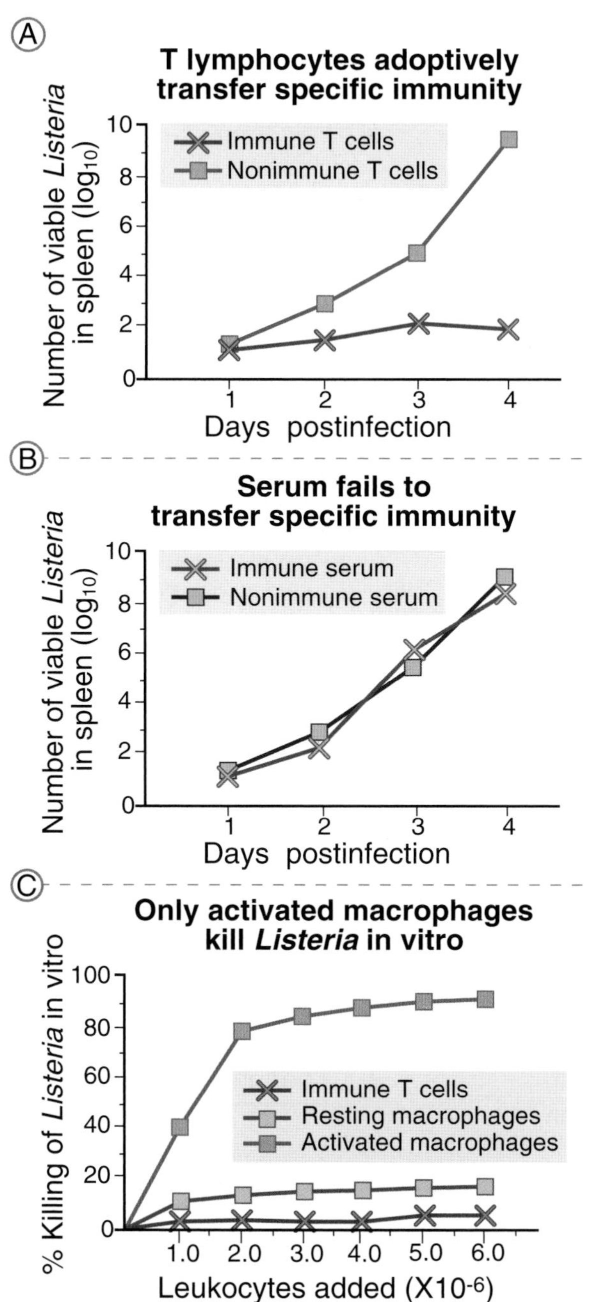

FIGURE 13–2 Cell-mediated immunity to *L. monocytogenes*. Immunity to *L. monocytogenes* is measured by inhibition of bacterial growth in the spleens of animals inoculated with a known dose of viable bacteria. Such immunity can be transferred to normal mice by T lymphocytes (A) but not by serum (B) from syngeneic mice previously immunized with killed or low doses of *L. monocytogenes*. In an in vitro assay of cell-mediated immunity, the bacteria are actually killed by activated macrophages and not by T cells (C).

the cytokines they produce and in their effector functions. These subsets are described below.

T_H1 and T_H2 Subsets of $CD4^+$ T Cells

$CD4^+$ T cells may differentiate into subsets of effector cells that produce distinct sets of cytokines and therefore perform distinct effector functions (Fig. 13–4). One of the best examples of specialization of adaptive immunity is the ability of $CD4^+$ T lymphocytes to activate diverse effector mechanisms in response to different types of microbes. The basis of this specialization is the heterogeneity of $CD4^+$ T cells, illustrated by the existence of subsets that differ in how they are induced, what cytokines they produce, and what effector mechanisms they activate. We have referred to these subpopulations in previous chapters and describe them in more detail below.

Properties of T_H1 and T_H2 Subsets

The best defined subsets of effector T cells of the $CD4^+$ helper lineage are T_H1 and T_H2 cells; interferon-γ (IFN-γ) is the signature cytokine of T_H1 cells, and IL-4 and IL-5 are the defining cytokines of T_H2 cells (see Fig. 13–4). Populations of helper T cells that could be distinguished on the basis of their secreted cytokines were discovered in the 1980s by studying large panels of cloned cell lines derived from antigen-stimulated mouse $CD4^+$ T cells. It is now clear that individual T cells may express various mixtures of cytokines, and there may be many subpopulations with heterogeneous patterns of cytokine production, especially in humans. However, chronic immune reactions are often dominated by T_H1 or T_H2 populations. The relative proportions of these subsets induced during an immune response are major determinants of the protective functions and pathologic consequences of the response.

T_H1 and T_H2 populations are distinguished most clearly by the cytokines they produce (see Fig. 13–4). The cytokines produced by these T cell subsets not only determine their effector functions but also participate in the development and expansion of the respective subsets. For instance, IFN-γ secreted by T_H1 cells promotes further T_H1 differentiation and inhibits the proliferation of T_H2 cells. Conversely, IL-4 produced by T_H2 cells promotes T_H2 differentiation, and IL-10, also produced by T_H2 cells (as well as by other cells), inhibits the development of T_H1 cells. Thus, each subset amplifies itself and cross-regulates the reciprocal subset. For this reason, once an immune response develops along one pathway, it becomes increasingly polarized in that direction, and the most extreme polarization is seen in chronic infections or in chronic exposure to environmental antigens, when the immune stimulation is persistent. T_H1 and T_H2 T cells can also be distinguished by differential expression of adhesion molecules and receptors for chemokines and other cytokines, as discussed below (see Fig. 13–4).

Development of T_H1 and T_H2 Subsets

T_H1 and T_H2 subsets develop from the same precursors, which are naive $CD4^+$ T lymphocytes, and the pattern of differentiation is determined by stimuli present early during immune responses. The most important differentiation-inducing stimuli are cytokines, with IFN-γ and IL-12 being the major inducers of T_H1 cells and IL-4 of T_H2 cells (Fig. 13–5).

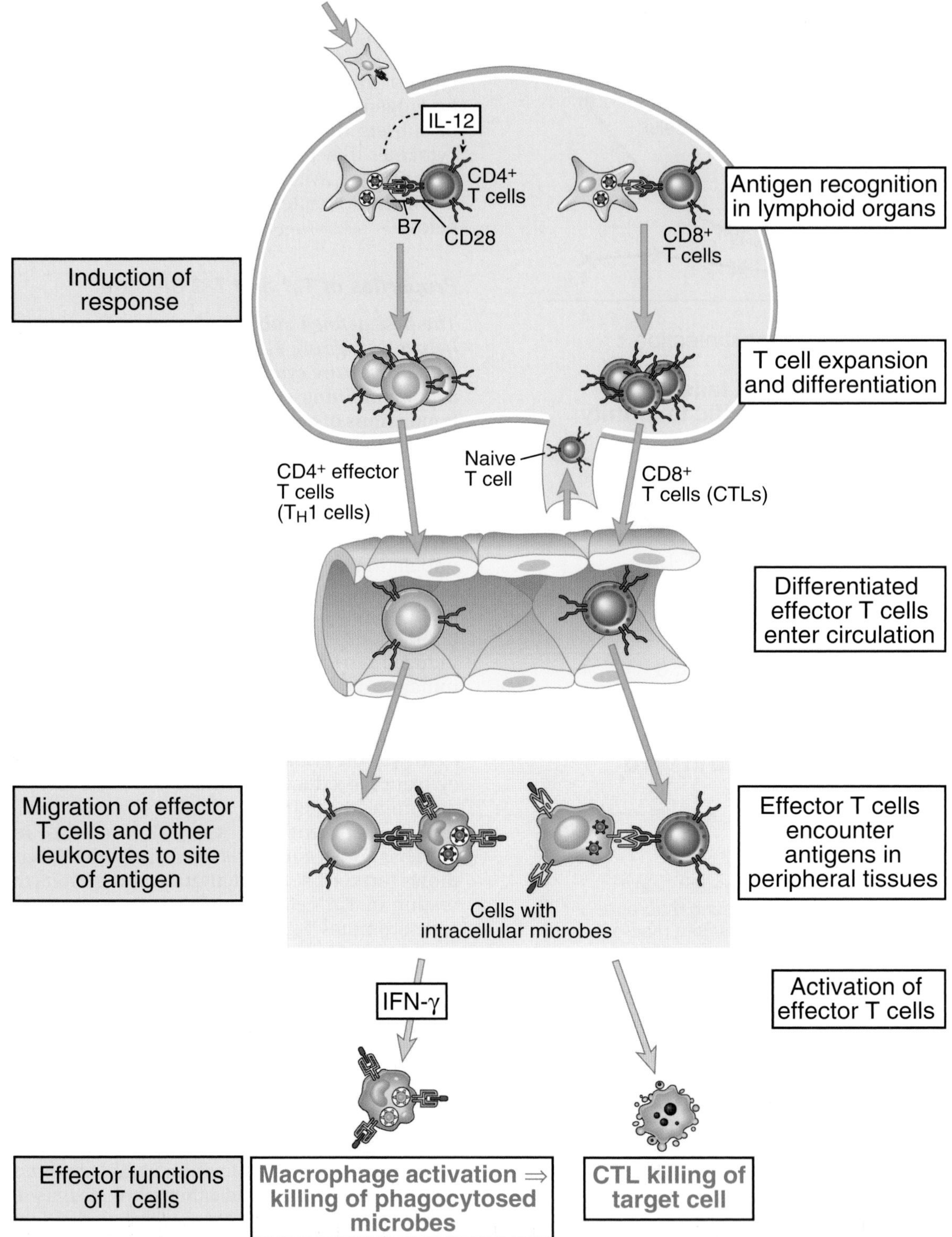

FIGURE 13–3 The induction and effector phases of cell-mediated immunity. Induction of response: $CD4^+$ T cells and $CD8^+$ T cells recognize peptides that are derived from protein antigens and presented by professional antigen-presenting cells in peripheral lymphoid organs. The T lymphocytes are stimulated to proliferate and differentiate, and effector cells enter the circulation. Migration of effector T cells and other leukocytes to the site of antigen: Effector T cells and other leukocytes migrate through blood vessels in peripheral tissues by binding to endothelial cells that have been activated by cytokines produced in response to infection in these tissues. Effector functions of T cells: Effector T cells recognize the antigen in the tissues and respond by secreting cytokines that activate phagocytes to eradicate the infection. CTLs also migrate to tissues and kill infected cells.

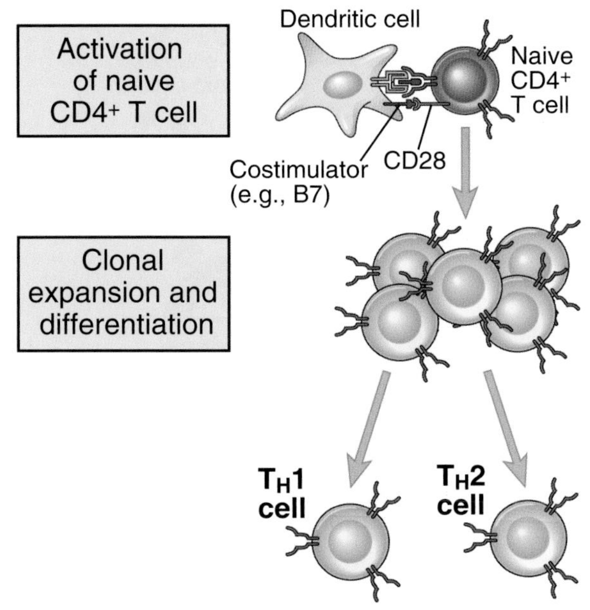

Property	T_H1 subset	T_H2 subset
Cytokines produced		
IFN-γ	+++	–
IL-4, IL-5, IL-13	–	+++
IL-10	+/–	++
IL-3, GM-CSF	++	++
Cytokine receptor expression		
IL-12R β chain	++	–
IL-18R	++	–
Chemokine receptor expression		
CCR4, CCR8, CXCR4	+/–	++
CXCR3, CCR5	++	+/–
Ligands for E- and P-selectin	++	+/–
Antibody isotypes stimulated	IgG2a (mouse)	IgE, IgG1 (mouse)/IgG4 (humans)
Macrophage activation	Classical	Alternative

FIGURE 13–4 Properties of T_H1 and T_H2 subsets of CD4+ helper T cells. Naive CD4+ T cells may differentiate into distinct subsets, such as T_H1 and T_H2 cells, in response to antigen, costimulators, and cytokines. The table lists the major differences between these two subsets.

T_H1 differentiation occurs in response to microbes that infect or activate macrophages and those that activate NK cells. The differentiation of antigen-activated CD4+ T cells to T_H1 effectors is stimulated by many intracellular bacteria, such as *Listeria* and mycobacteria, and by some parasites, such as *Leishmania,* all of which infect macrophages. It is also stimulated by viruses and by protein antigens administered with strong adjuvants. A common feature of all these infections and immunization conditions is that they elicit innate immune reactions that are associated with the production of certain cytokines, including IL-12, IL-18, and type I interferons. Some microbes engage Toll-like receptors on macrophages and dendritic cells and directly activate these cells to secrete these cytokines (Fig. 13–6). Other microbes may trigger secretion of these indirectly, for instance, by stimulating NK cells to produce IFN-γ, which in turn acts on macrophages to induce IL-12 secretion. IFN-γ produced by the NK cells, as well as by the responding T cells themselves and perhaps also by some macrophages and dendritic cells, is itself a strong T_H1-inducing cytokine. T cells may further enhance macrophage cytokine production, by virtue of CD40 ligand (CD40L) on the T cells engaging CD40 on APCs and stimulating cytokine gene transcription. IL-12 is a major cytokine responsible for differentiation of T_H1 cells and induction of CMI. Knockout mice lacking IL-12 are extremely susceptible to infections with intracellular microbes. IL-18 synergizes with IL-12, and type I interferons may be as important for T_H1 differentiation in response to viral infections in humans.

The molecular basis of T_H1 differentiation involves the interplay of signals from the T cell receptor, the cytokines IFN-γ and IL-12, and the transcription factors T-bet, STAT1, and STAT4 (see Fig. 13–5). The transcription factor T-bet, a member of the T-box family of transcription factors, is considered to be the master regulator of T_H1 differentiation. T-bet expression is induced in naive CD4+ T cells when they recognize antigen and are exposed to IFN-γ. IFN-γ activates the transcription factor STAT1, which in turn stimulates expression of T-bet. T-bet then promotes IFN-γ production through a combination of direct transcriptional activation of the IFN-γ gene and by inducing chromatin remodeling of the IFN-γ locus. The ability of IFN-γ to stimulate T-bet expression and the ability of T-bet to enhance IFN-γ transcription sets up a positive amplification loop which drives differentiation of T cells toward the T_H1 phenotype. IL-12 contributes to T_H1 lineage commitment by binding to receptors on antigen-stimulated CD4+ T cells and activating the transcription factor STAT4, which further enhances IFN-γ production (see Fig. 13–5). Mice deficient in IL-12, IL-12 receptors, or STAT4 cannot mount effective T_H1 responses to infections, and humans with genetic deficiencies in the IL-12R signaling pathway have impaired responses to infections with several kinds of intracellular bacteria.

T_H2 differentiation occurs in response to helminths and allergens, and involves the interplay of signals from the T cell receptor, the cytokine IL-4, and the transcription factors GATA-3 and STAT6 (see Fig. 13–5). Helminths and allergens cause chronic T cell stimulation, often without strong innate immune responses that are required for T_H1 differentiation. Thus, T_H2 cells may develop in response to microbes and antigens that cause persistent or repeated T cell stimulation with little

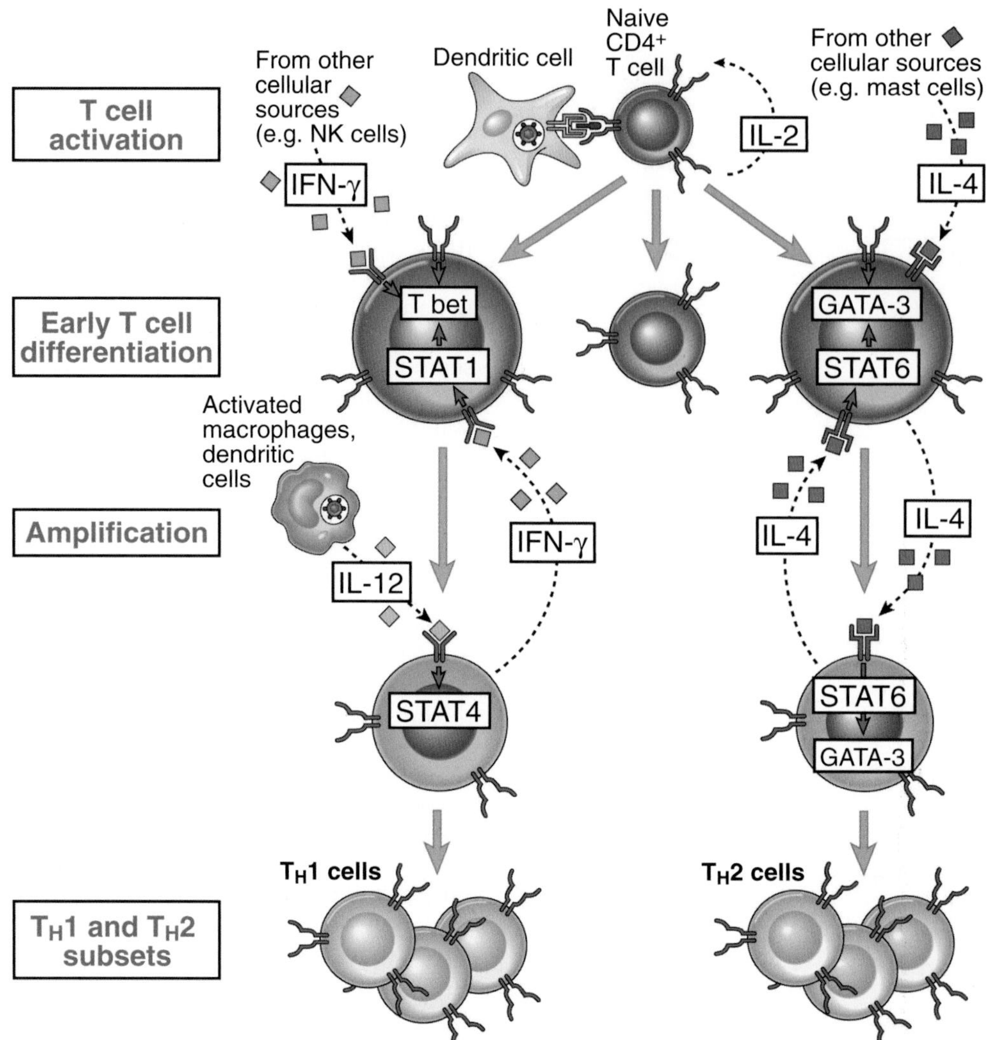

FIGURE 13–5 Development of T_H1 and T_H2 subsets. Cytokines produced in the innate immune response to microbes or early in adaptive immune responses influence the differentiation of naive CD4+ T cells into T_H1 or T_H2 cells. IL-12, made by activated macrophages and dendritic cells, induces T_H1 cell development through a STAT4-dependent pathway. IL-4, which may be produced mainly by T cells themselves, favors induction of T_H2 cells through a STAT6-dependent pathway. The transcription factor T-bet, produced in response to IFN-γ, is essential for T_H1 responses, and GATA-3 is critical for T_H2 differentiation. Other cytokines that may influence helper T cell differentiation are not shown.

inflammation or macrophage activation. The differentiation of antigen-stimulated T cells to the T_H2 subset is dependent on IL-4, which functions by activating the transcription factor STAT6 (see Fig. 13–6), and STAT6, together with TCR signals, induces expression of GATA-3. GATA-3 is a transcription factor that acts as a master regulator of T_H2 differentiation, enhancing expression of the T_H2 cytokine genes IL-4, IL-5, and IL-13, which are located in the same genetic locus. GATA-3 works by directly interacting with the promoters of these genes, and also by causing chromatin remodeling, which opens up the locus for accessibility to other transcription factors. This is similar to the way T-bet influences IFN-γ expression. GATA-3 functions to stably commit differentiating cells toward the T_H2 phenotype, enhancing its own expression via a positive feedback loop. Furthermore, GATA-3 blocks T_H1 differentiation by inhibiting expression of the signaling chain of the IL-12 receptor. Knockout mice lacking IL-4, STAT6, or GATA-3 are profoundly deficient in T_H2 responses. The obligatory role of IL-4 in T_H2 differentiation raises an interesting question: Because differentiated T_H2 cells are the major source of IL-4 during immune responses to protein antigens, where does the IL-4 come from before T_H2 cells develop? A likely explanation is that antigen-stimulated CD4+ T cells secrete small amounts of IL-4 from their initial activation. If the antigen is persistent and present at high concentrations, the local concentration of IL-4 gradually increases. If the antigen also does not trigger inflammation with attendant IL-12 production, the result is increasing differentiation of T cells to the T_H2 subset. In some situations, IL-4 produced by mast cells and,

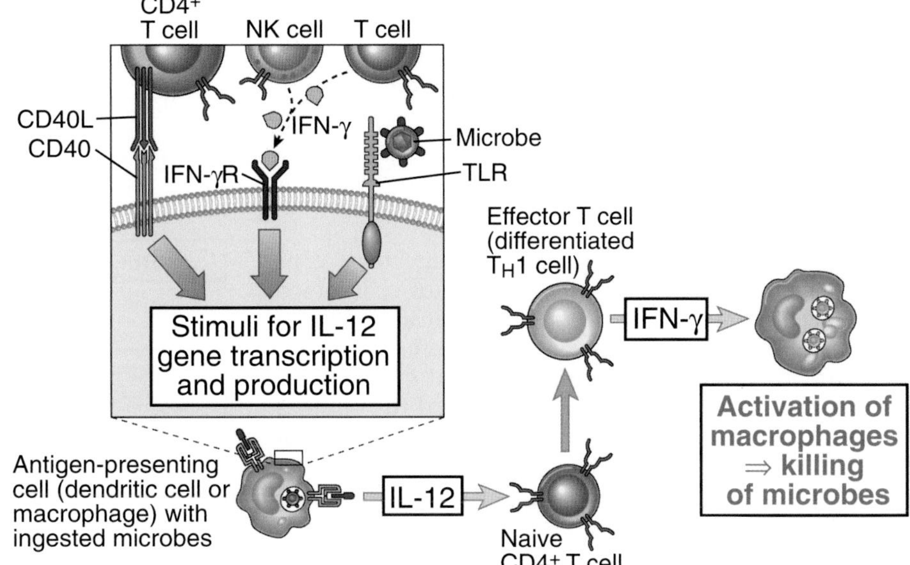

FIGURE 13–6 Role of IL-12 and IFN-γ in T_H1 differentiation and cell-mediated immunity. Antigen-presenting cells secrete IL-12 in response to microbial products such as lipopolysaccharide (LPS), IFN-γ produced by NK cells and T cells, and CD40 engagement by T cell CD40L. IL-12 stimulates the differentiation of CD4⁺ helper T cells to T_H1 effectors, which produce IFN-γ. IFN-γ then activates macrophages to kill phagocytosed microbes (and to secrete more IL-12).

possibly, other cell populations may contribute to T_H2 development.

Stimuli other than cytokines may also influence the pattern of helper T cell differentiation. In general, high doses of antigen without adjuvants favor T_H2 differentiation. Some studies indicate that different subsets of dendritic cells exist, which selectively promote either T_H1 or T_H2 differentiation. In addition, the genetic makeup of the host is an important determinant of the pattern of T cell differentiation. Inbred mice of some strains develop T_H2 responses to the same microbes that stimulate T_H1 differentiation in most other strains. Mice that develop T_H2-dominant responses are susceptible to infections by intracellular microbes (see Chapter 15).

T_H1-Mediated Immune Responses

The principal function of T_H1 cells is in phagocyte-mediated defense against infections, especially with intracellular microbes (Fig. 13–7). As we shall discuss in

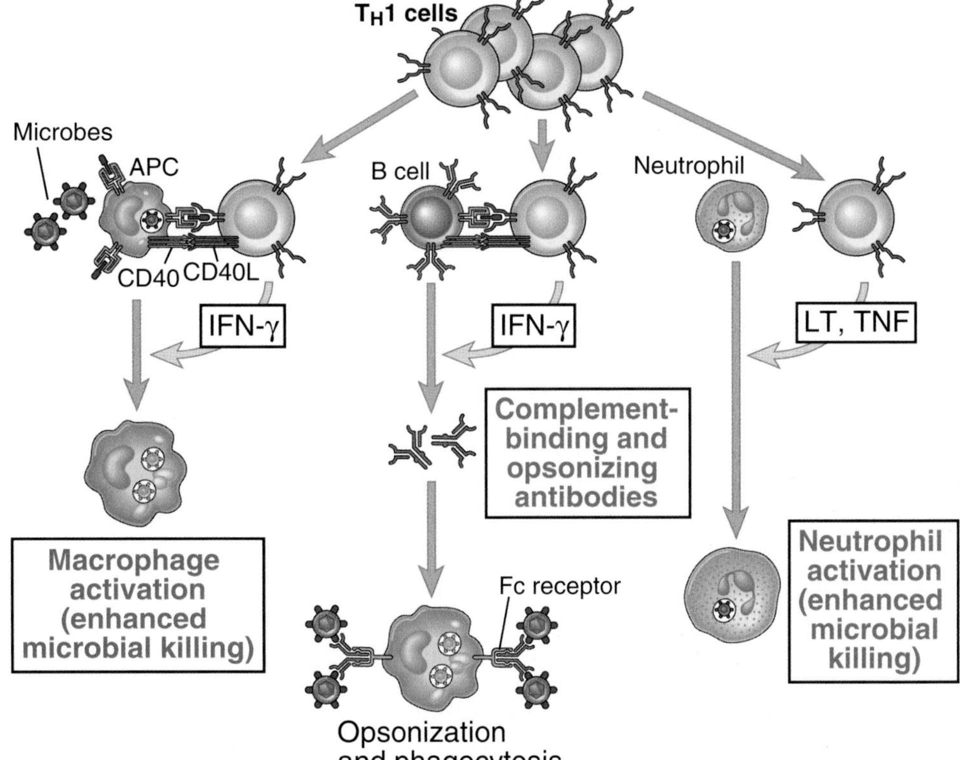

FIGURE 13–7 Effector functions of T_H1 cells. CD4⁺ T cells that differentiate into T_H1 cells secrete IFN-γ, lymphotoxin (LT) and TNF, and IL-2. IFN-γ acts on macrophages to increase phagocytosis and killing of microbes in phagolysosomes and on B lymphocytes to stimulate production of IgG antibodies that opsonize microbes for phagocytosis. LT and TNF activate neutrophils and stimulate inflammation. IL-2 is the autocrine growth factor made by this subset of T cells (not shown). APC, antigen-presenting cell.

more detail later, IFN-γ produced by T_H1 cells stimulates the microbicidal activities of phagocytes, thereby promoting the intracellular destruction of phagocytosed microbes. IFN-γ also stimulates the production of opsonizing and complement-fixing IgG antibodies, which promote the phagocytosis of microbes. Many organ-specific autoimmune diseases (see Chapter 18) and inflammatory reactions such as granulomas are due to excessive activation of T_H1 cells.

To trigger the effector phase of CMI, effector T cells have to come into contact with phagocytes or infected cells that are presenting the antigens that initiated the response. To locate microbes at any site, effector T cells that clonally expanded and differentiated in lymphoid organs, such as lymph nodes, and entered the circulation have to leave the vasculature and enter the site of infection.

Migration of T_H1 and Other Leukocytes to Sites of Antigen

T_H1 effector cells express adhesion molecules and chemokine receptors that promote their migration to and retention in sites of infection (Fig. 13–8). The directed migration of effector T lymphocytes to sites of infection is initially dependent on the innate immune response to microbes (see Chapter 2). This innate response results in an inflammatory reaction characterized by secretion of cytokines, such as tumor necrosis factor (TNF) and IL-1, by macrophages. These cytokines induce expression of endothelial selectins and integrin ligands, which bind to homing receptors on effector T cells. In addition, macrophages, NK cells, and endothelial cells elaborate chemokines, such as CXCL9, 10, and 11, and CCL2, 4, and 5, which bind to chemokine receptors on effector T cells. During differentiation from naive precursors, T_H1 cells, but not T_H2 cells, gain the capacity to produce functional ligands that bind E- and P-selectin. This aspect of T_H1 differentiation involves T-bet–dependent expression of glycosyltransferases that are required for synthesis of the carbohydrate moieties to which the selectins bind. Furthermore, the chemokine receptors CXCR3 and CCR5, which bind to chemokines elaborated in tissues during innate immune responses, are expressed by T_H1 cells but not T_H2 cells. The selective expression of selectin ligands and certain chemokine receptors on T_H1 cells ensures their efficient migration into inflammatory sites. The steps in leukocyte adhesion to endothelial cells and transmigration into tissues were discussed in detail in Chapter 2. After T_H1 cells enter the site of infection and are activated by antigen, they produce more cytokines and chemokines and stimulate much greater leukocyte migration. This later, enhanced inflammation is sometimes called immune inflammation to indicate the role of T lymphocytes (immune cells) in the process.

The migration of effector T cells from the circulation to peripheral sites of infection is largely independent of antigen, but cells that recognize antigen in extravascular tissues are preferentially retained there (see Fig. 13–8). T cell migration through blood and lymphatic vessels

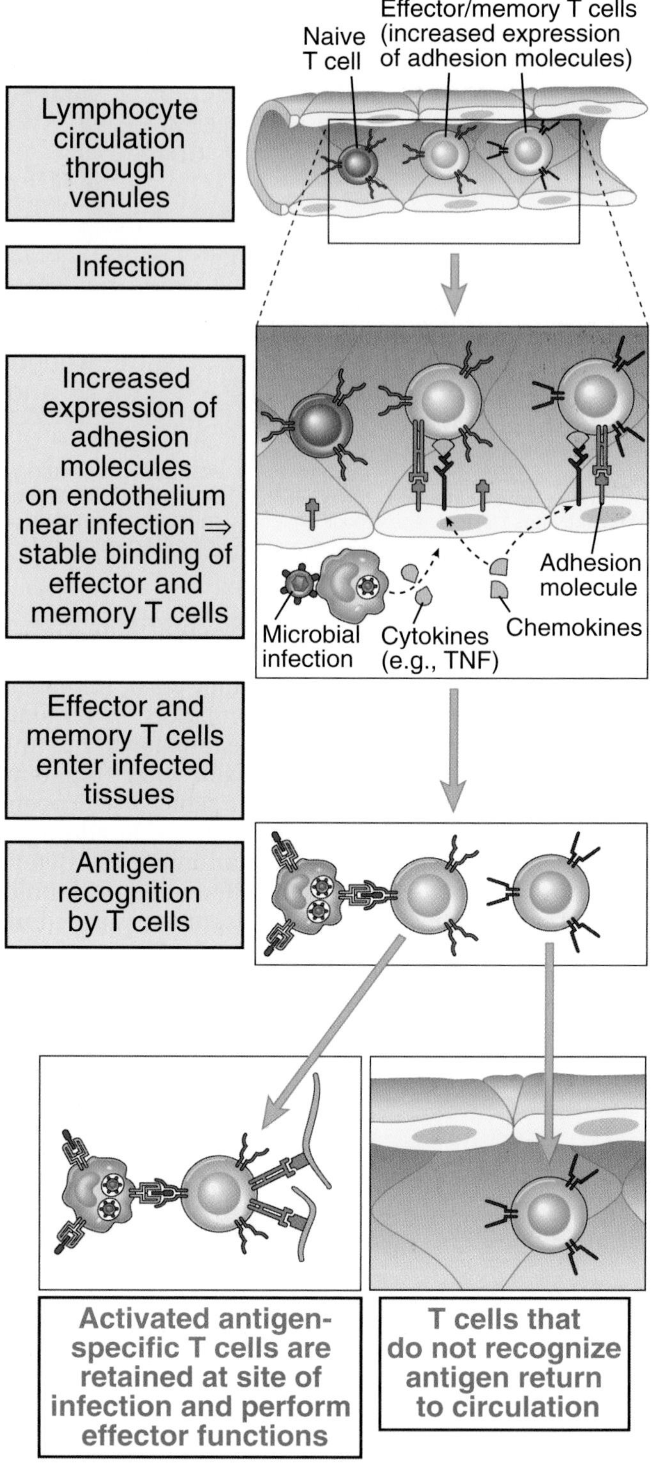

FIGURE 13–8 Migration and retention of effector and memory T cells at sites of infection. Previously activated effector and memory T cells, but not naive cells, migrate through endothelium that is activated by cytokines (e.g., TNF) produced at a site of infection. In extravascular tissue, the T cells that specifically recognize antigen are activated and retained, whereas T cells that do not encounter the antigen for which they are specific return to the circulation, largely through lymphatic vessels (not shown).

is controlled mainly by adhesion molecules and chemokines, which will engage T_H1 cells of any antigen specificity. Therefore, this process of migration results in the recruitment of circulating effector T cells to inflammatory sites, regardless of antigen specificity, ensuring that the maximum possible number of previously activated T cells have the opportunity to locate infectious microbes and eradicate the infection. Some memory T cells also migrate to peripheral tissues. Once in the tissues, the T cells encounter microbial antigens presented by macrophages and other APCs. T cells that specifically recognize antigens receive signals through their antigen receptors that increase the affinity of integrins for their ligands. Two of these integrins, VLA-4 and VLA-5, bind to fibronectin in extracellular matrices, and a third adhesion molecule, CD44, which is also expressed at high levels on effector and memory T cells, binds to hyaluronate. As a result, antigen-specific effector and memory T cells that encounter the antigen are preferentially retained at the extravascular site where the antigen is present. T cells not specific for the antigen may return through lymphatic vessels to the circulation.

T Cell–Mediated Activation of Macrophages and Other Leukocytes

T_H1 cells activate macrophages to eliminate phagocytosed microbes. Monocytes are recruited from blood into tissues and are exposed to signals from T_H1 effector cells responding to antigen in the tissues. This interaction results in conversion of the monocytes to activated macrophages that are able to kill microbes. Activation consists of increased expression of various proteins that endow activated macrophages with the capacity to perform specialized functions, such as microbial killing. In the following sections, we describe the T cell signals that activate macrophages in cell-mediated immune reactions and the effector functions of these macrophages.

$CD4^+$ T_H1 cells activate macrophages by contact-mediated signals delivered by CD40L-CD40 interactions and by the cytokine IFN-γ (Fig. 13–9). (Recall that helper T cells stimulate B lymphocyte proliferation and differentiation also by CD40-mediated signals and cytokines; see Chapter 10.) When effector T_H1 cells are

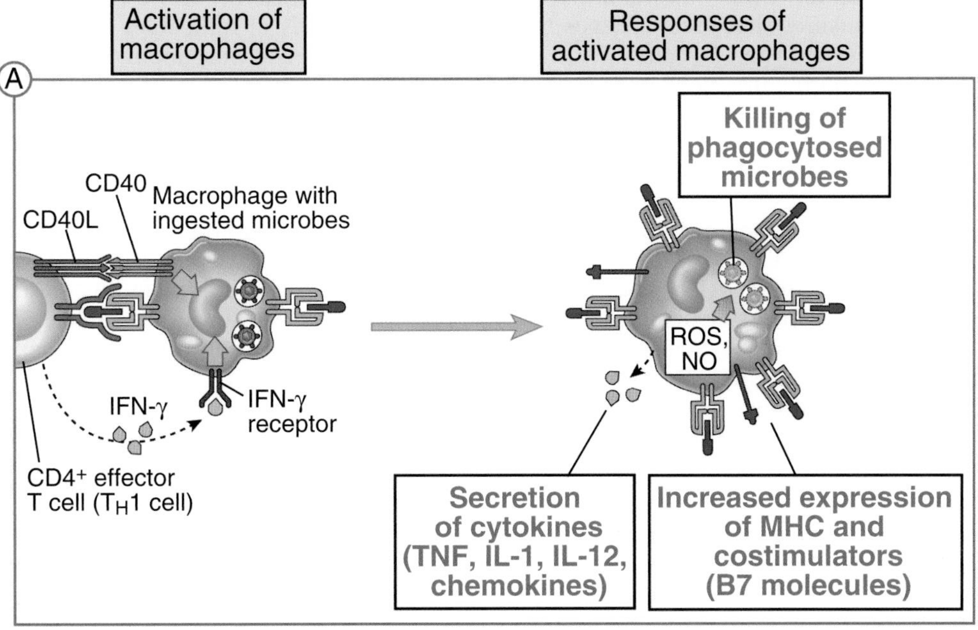

B

Macrophage response	Role in cell-mediated immunity
Production of reactive oxygen species, nitric oxide, increased lysosomal enzymes	Killing of microbes in phagolysosomes (effector function of macrophages)
Secretion of cytokines (TNF, IL-1, IL-12)	TNF, IL-1: leukocyte recruitment (inflammation) IL-12: T_H1 differentiation, IFN-γ production
Increased expression of B7 costimulators, MHC molecules	Increased T cell activation (amplification)

FIGURE 13–9 Activation and functions of macrophages in cell-mediated immunity. In cell-mediated immunity, macrophages are activated by CD40L-CD40 interactions and by IFN-γ and perform several functions that kill microbes, stimulate inflammation, and enhance the antigen-presenting capacity of the cells. Macrophages are also activated during innate immune reactions and perform the same functions (see Chapter 2).

stimulated by antigen, the cells secrete cytokines, notably IFN-γ, and they express CD40L. IFN-γ is the major macrophage-activating cytokine. It activates some macrophage responses by itself and functions together with TLR-ligands, such as bacterial lipopolysaccharide, or CD40 signals to elicit other responses. Knockout mice lacking IFN-γ or the IFN-γ receptor are extremely susceptible to infection by intracellular microbes. CD40L engages CD40 on macrophages that are presenting antigen to the T cells and activates an intracellular signal transduction pathway that is similar to the pathway activated by TNF receptors (see Chapter 12, Box 12–1). The importance of CD40 in macrophage activation is demonstrated by the immunologic defects in humans with inherited mutations in CD40L (X-linked hyper-IgM syndrome) and mice in which the gene for CD40 or CD40L is knocked out (see Chapter 20). All these disorders are characterized by severe deficiencies in CMI to intracellular microbes, and children with the X-linked hyper-IgM syndrome often succumb to infection by the intracellular pathogen *Pneumocystis jiroveci.* As expected, these patients and knockout mice also have defects in helper T cell–dependent antibody production. The requirement for CD40L-CD40 interactions for macrophage activation ensures that macrophages that are presenting antigens to the T cells (i.e., the macrophages that are harboring intracellular microbes) are also the macrophages that are most efficiently activated by the T cells.

In response to CD40 signals and IFN-γ, production of several proteins in macrophages is increased. CD40 ligation activates the transcription factors nuclear factor κB (NF-κB) and activation protein-1 (AP-1), and IFN-γ activates the transcription factors STAT1 and interferon response factor-1 (IRF-1). As a result of these signals, activated macrophages produce increased amounts of the proteins that are responsible for the effector functions of these cells in CMI (see Fig. 13–9). The effector functions of activated macrophages include the following.

- ***Activated macrophages kill phagocytosed microbes, mainly by producing microbicidal reactive oxygen species, nitric oxide, and lysosomal enzymes.*** The microbicidal mechanisms of macrophages were described in Chapter 2. To reiterate the key points, macrophage activation leads to increased synthesis of reactive oxygen species and nitric oxide, as well as lysosomal enzymes, all of which are potent microbicidal agents that are produced within the lysosomes of macrophages and kill ingested microbes after phagosomes fuse with lysosomes. These toxic substances may also be released into adjacent tissues, where they kill extracellular microbes and may cause damage to normal tissues.
- ***Activated macrophages stimulate acute inflammation through the secretion of cytokines, mainly TNF, IL-1, and chemokines, and short-lived lipid mediators such as platelet-activating factor, prostaglandins, and leukotrienes.*** The collective action of these macrophage-derived cytokines and lipid mediators is to produce a local inflammation that is rich in neutrophils, and to recruit more monocytes, which become macrophages and phagocytose and destroy infectious organisms.
- ***Activated macrophages remove dead tissues and facilitate repair after the infection is controlled.*** Activated macrophages induce the formation of repair tissue by secreting growth factors that stimulate fibroblast proliferation (platelet-derived growth factor), collagen synthesis (transforming growth factor-β [TGF-β]), and new blood vessel formation or angiogenesis (fibroblast growth factor). Thus, the activated macrophage acts as an endogenous surgeon to cauterize the wound and resolve the inflammatory reaction.

Even though macrophages can respond directly to microbes in innate immune reactions, the ability of macrophages to kill ingested microorganisms is greatly enhanced by T cells. This is why CMI is able to eradicate microbes that have evolved to survive within macrophages in the absence of adaptive immunity. In addition to these effector functions, activated macrophages become more efficient APCs because of increased levels of molecules involved in antigen processing (such as components of the proteasome and cathepsins), increased surface expression of class II MHC molecules and costimulators, and production of cytokines (such as IL-12) that stimulate T lymphocyte proliferation and differentiation. These macrophage responses function to enhance T cell activation, thus serving as amplification mechanisms for CMI.

Some tissue injury may normally accompany T_H1 cell–mediated immune reactions to microbes because the microbicidal products released by activated macrophages and neutrophils are capable of injuring normal tissue and do not discriminate between microbes and host tissue. However, this tissue injury is usually limited in extent and duration, and it resolves as the infection is cleared. In some cases, however, T_H1 responses cause significant tissue injury, as discussed below.

Delayed Type Hypersensitivity Reactions

Tissue injury and inflammation caused by T_H1 cells and activated macrophages are the hallmarks of DTH reactions. DTH reactions may occur as collateral damage during a protective T_H1 response to a microbe, or DTH may be entirely pathologic, as in the setting of certain autoimmune diseases. Many of the disorders caused by abnormal immune responses are called immune-mediated inflammatory diseases (see Chapter 18). The sequence of leukocyte migration and subsequent macrophage activation in DTH has been studied in experimental animals and in people, and this has added to our understanding of T_H1 responses.

- In the classical animal model of DTH, a guinea pig is first immunized by the administration of a protein antigen in adjuvant; this step is called the sensitiza-

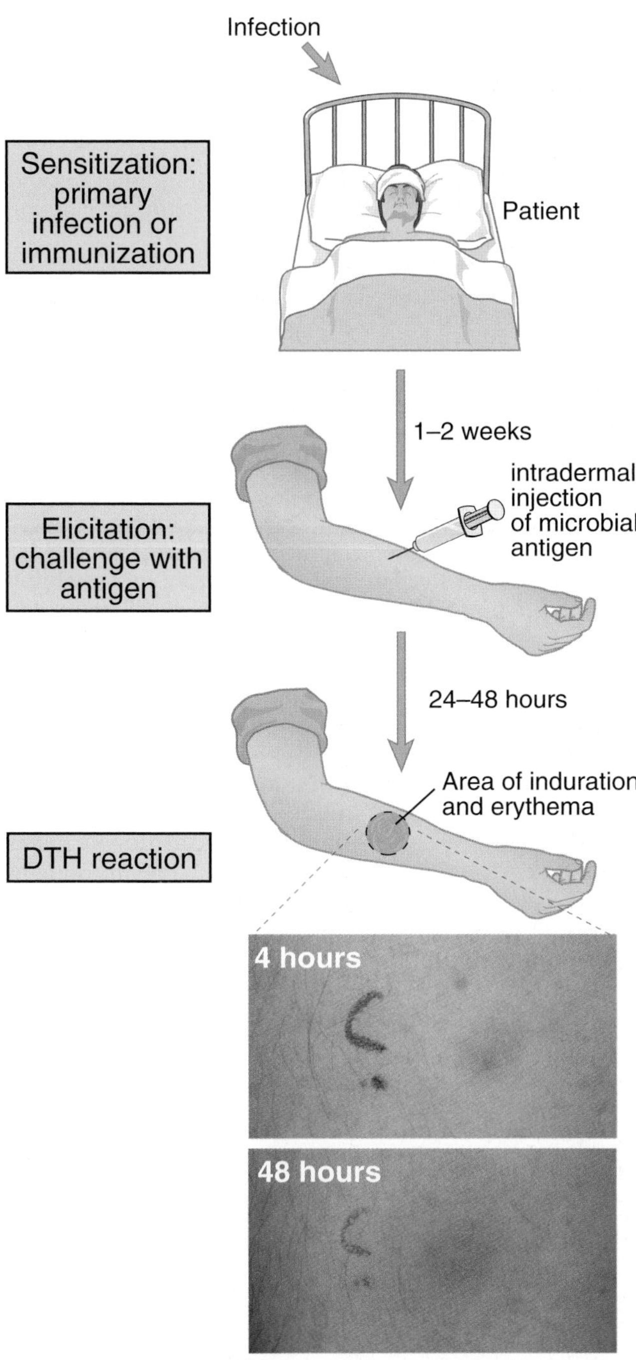

FIGURE 13–10 Delayed-type hypersensitivity reaction. Infection or immunization (vaccination) sensitizes an individual, and subsequent challenge with an antigen from the infectious agent elicits a DTH reaction. The reaction is manifested by induration with redness and swelling at the site of the challenge, which is undetectable at ~4 hours and peaks at ~48 hours. (Courtesy of Dr. J. Faix, Department of Pathology, Stanford University School of Medicine, Palo Alto, California.)

tion phase. About 2 weeks later, the animal is challenged subcutaneously with the same antigen and the subsequent reaction is analyzed; this step is called the elicitation phase.

- Humans may be sensitized for DTH reactions by microbial infection, by contact sensitization with chemicals and environmental antigens, or by intradermal or subcutaneous injection of protein antigens (Fig. 13–10). Subsequent exposure to the same antigen (also called challenge) elicits the reaction. For example, purified protein derivative (PPD), a protein antigen of *Mycobacterium tuberculosis,* elicits a DTH reaction, called the tuberculin reaction, when it is injected into individuals who have been exposed to *M. tuberculosis.*

The characteristic response of DTH evolves during 24 to 48 hours. About 4 hours after the injection of antigen, neutrophils accumulate around the postcapillary venules at the injection site. By about 12 hours, the injection site becomes infiltrated by T cells and blood monocytes, also organized in a perivenular distribution (Fig. 13–11). The endothelial cells lining these venules become plump, show increased biosynthetic organelles, and become leaky to plasma macromolecules. Fibrinogen escapes from the blood vessels into the surrounding tissues, where it is converted into fibrin. The deposition of fibrin and, to a lesser extent, the accumulation of T cells and monocytes within the extravascular tissue space around the injection site cause the tissue to swell and become firm (indurated). Induration, a diagnostic feature of DTH, is detectable by about 18 hours after the injection of antigen and is maximal by 24 to 48 hours. This lag in the onset of palpable induration is the reason for calling the response "delayed type." A positive tuberculin skin test response is a widely used clinical indicator for evidence of previous or active tuberculosis infection. In clinical practice, loss of DTH responses to universally encountered antigens (e.g., *Candida* antigens) is an indication of deficient T cell function, a condition known as anergy. (This general loss of immune responsiveness is different from lymphocyte anergy, a mechanism for maintaining tolerance to specific antigens, discussed in Chapter 11.)

Chronic DTH reactions can develop if a T_H1 response to an infection activates macrophages but fails to eradicate phagocytosed microbes. In this case, the macrophages continue to produce cytokines and growth factors, which progressively modify the local tissue environment. As a result, tissue injury is followed by replacement with connective tissue (fibrosis), and fibrosis is a hallmark of chronic DTH reactions. In chronic DTH reactions, activated macrophages also undergo changes in response to persistent cytokine signals. These macrophages develop increased cytoplasm and cytoplasmic organelles and histologically may resemble skin epithelial cells, because of which they are sometimes called epithelioid cells. Activated macrophages may fuse to form multinucleate giant cells. Clusters of activated macrophages, often surrounding particulate sources of antigen, produce nodules of inflammatory tissue called granulomas (Fig. 13–12). Granulomatous inflammation is a characteristic response to some persistent microbes, such as *M. tuberculosis* and some fungi, and represents a form of chronic DTH. Granulomatous inflammation is frequently associated with tissue fibrosis. Although fibrosis is normally a "healing reaction" to injury, it can also interfere with normal tissue function. In fact, much

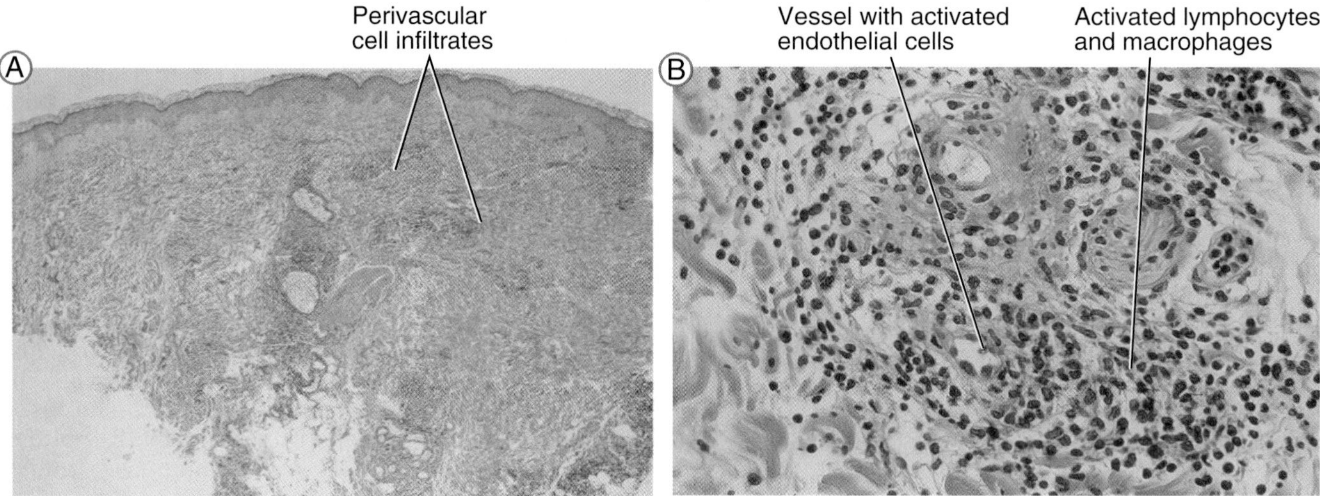

FIGURE 13–11 Morphology of a DTH reaction. Histopathologic examination of the reaction in skin illustrated in Figure 13–10 shows perivascular mononuclear cell infiltrates in the dermis (A). At higher magnification, the infiltrate is seen to consist of activated lymphocytes and macrophages surrounding small blood vessels in which the endothelial cells are also activated (B). (Courtesy of Dr. J. Faix, Department of Pathology, Stanford University School of Medicine, Palo Alto, California.)

of the respiratory difficulty associated with tuberculosis or chronic fungal infection of the lung is caused by replacement of normal lung with fibrotic tissue and not directly attributable to the microbes.

T_H2-Mediated Immune Responses

The principal effector function of T_H2 cells is to promote IgE- and eosinophil/mast cell–mediated immune reactions, which are protective against helminthic infections (Fig. 13–13). Helminths are too large to be phagocytosed and may be more resistant to the microbicidal activities of macrophages than are most bacteria and viruses. As discussed earlier, T_H2 cells secrete IL-4 and IL-13, which stimulate the production of helminth-specific IgE antibodies. These antibodies opsonize the helminths. IL-5, which is also produced by T_H2 cells, may directly activate eosinophils in the vicinity of the helminths. Activated eosinophils release their granule contents, including major basic protein and major cationic protein, which are capable of destroying even the tough integuments of helminths. Mast cells do express functional Fcε receptors, and may be activated by the IgE-coated helminths, resulting in degranulation. The granule contents of mast cells include vasoactive amines, cytokines such as TNF, and lipid mediators, all of which induce local inflammation that also functions to destroy the parasites.

The antibodies stimulated by T_H2 cytokines do not promote phagocytosis or activate complement efficiently but are capable of neutralizing microbes and toxins (see Chapter 14). IL-4 and IL-13 are also capable of activating macrophages to express mannose receptors, to express enzymes that promote collagen synthesis and fibrosis, and to produce the anti-inflammatory cytokines IL-10 and TGF-β. This process has been called "alternative macrophage activation," to distinguish it from the activation induced by IFN-γ, which results in potent microbicidal functions and has been called "classical macrophage activation." Classically and alternatively activated macrophages are also called M1 and M2 macrophages, respectively. Macrophages that are activated by the T_H2 cytokines contribute to granuloma formation and tissue remodeling in the setting of chronic parasitic infections or allergic disease, respectively. Cytokines produced by T_H2 cells are also involved in blocking entry and promoting expulsion of microbes in mucosal tissues. IL-13 stimulates mucus production, and IL-4 may stimulate peristalsis in the gastrointestinal system. Thus, T_H2 cells play an important role in "barrier immu-

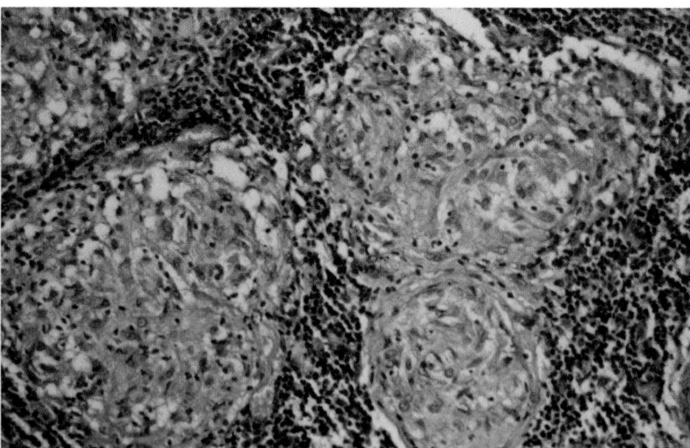

FIGURE 13–12 Granulomatous inflammation. Histopathologic examination of a lymph node shows a granuloma with activated macrophages, multinucleated giant cells, and lymphocytes. In some granulomas, there may be a central area of necrosis. Immunohistochemical studies would identify the lymphocytes as T cells. This type of inflammation is a chronic DTH reaction against persistent microbial and other antigens. (Courtesy of Dr. Henry Sanchez, Department of Pathology, University of California at San Francisco School of Medicine.)

nity" (host defense at the barriers with the external environment).

The selective homing of T_H2 cells to certain inflammatory sites is dependent on particular chemokines. T_H2 cell express chemokine receptors (i.e., CCR3, CCR4, and CCR8) that bind to chemokines (i.e., CCL11, CCL24, CCL26, CCL7, CCL13, CCL17, and CCL22) that are highly expressed at sites of helminth infection or allergic reactions; particularly in mucosal tissues.

T_H2-mediated immune responses are the underlying cause of allergic reactions (see Chapter 19), and may interfere with protective T_H1-mediated immune responses to intracellular infections (see Chapter 15).

The T_H17 Subset of $CD4^+$ T Cells

The third, and most recently identified, subset of differentiated effector $CD4^+$ T cells are called T_H17 cells, because the signature cytokine they secrete is IL-17. These cells also secrete IL-22 and other cytokines but do not produce either IFN-γ or IL-4. In fact, their differentiation from naive $CD4^+$ T cells is inhibited by the presence of either IFN-γ or IL-4, indicating that T_H17 cells are a unique subset distinct from T_H1 and T_H2 cells. The principal role of T_H17 cells appears to be protection against extracellular bacterial and fungal infections, largely through recruitment of neutrophils and other leukocytes. Studies in mice and humans suggest that T_H17 cells may be important mediators of tissue damage in immune-mediated inflammatory diseases.

T_H17 cells differentiate from naive $CD4^+$ T cells by stimulation with antigen in the presence of the cytokine TGF-β together with IL-6, IL-1, or other pro-inflammatory cytokines. The source of TGF-β in T_H17 differentiation is unknown. It is postulated that IL-6 and other inflammatory cytokines may be produced early at sites of tissue damage, and these may promote the subsequent T_H17 response. The transcription factors RORγt and STAT3 are involved in this differentiation pathway. The cytokine IL-23, which is closely related to the T_H1-inducing cytokine IL-12, promotes the survival and maintenance of differentiated T_H17 cells. Interestingly, TGF-β alone stimulates the development of regulatory T cells (see Chapter 11); thus, this cytokine can promote either pro-inflammatory (T_H17) responses or anti-inflammatory (regulatory T cell) responses, depending on which other cytokines are present in the environment.

EFFECTOR $CD8^+$ T CELLS: CYTOTOXIC T LYMPHOCYTES

$CD8^+$ CTLs are effector T cells that eliminate intracellular microbes mainly by killing infected cells. The development of a $CD8^+$ CTL response to infection proceeds through similar steps as those described for $CD4^+$ T cell responses, including primary antigen-dependent stimulation of naive $CD8^+$ T cells in lymph nodes, clonal expansion, differentiation, and migration of differentiated CTLs into tissues. These events were described in Chapter 9. Below we discuss the stimulation of differentiated CTLs and performance of effector functions at sites of infection.

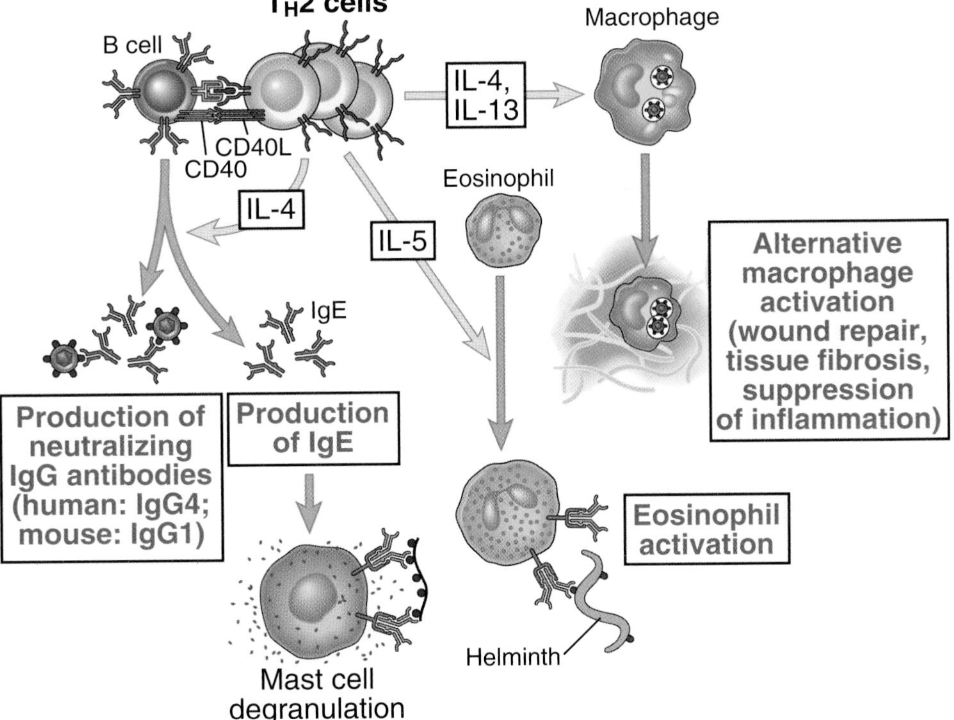

FIGURE 13–13 Effector functions of T_H2 cells. $CD4^+$ T cells that differentiate into T_H2 cells secrete IL-4 and IL-5. IL-4 acts on B cells to stimulate production of antibodies that bind to mast cells, such as IgE. IL-4 is also an autocrine growth and differentiation cytokine for T_H2 cells. IL-5 activates eosinophils, a response that is important for defense against helminthic infections. Cytokines from T_H2 cells also inhibit macrophage activation and T_H1-mediated reactions. APC, antigen-presenting cell.

CTL-Mediated Cytotoxicity

Cell killing by CTLs is antigen specific and contact dependent. CTLs kill targets that express the same class I–associated antigen that triggered the proliferation and differentiation of naive CD8$^+$ T cells from which they are derived, and do not kill adjacent uninfected cells that do not express this antigen. In fact, even the CTLs themselves are not injured during the killing of antigen-expressing targets. This specificity of CTL effector function ensures that normal cells are not killed by CTLs reacting against infected cells. The killing is highly specific because the site of contact of the CTL and the antigen-expressing target cell forms an "immunological synapse" (see Chapter 9), and the molecules that actually perform the killing are secreted into the synapse.

The process of CTL-mediated killing of targets consists of antigen recognition, activation of the CTLs, delivery of the "lethal hit" that kills the target cells, and release of the CTLs (Fig. 13–14). Each of these steps is controlled by specific proteins and molecular interactions.

Recognition of Antigen and Activation of CTLs

The CTL binds and reacts to the target cell by using its antigen receptor, coreceptor (CD8), and adhesion molecules, such as the leukocyte function–associated antigen-1 (LFA-1) integrin. To be efficiently recognized by CTLs, target cells must express class I MHC molecules complexed to a peptide (the complex serving as the ligand for the T cell receptor and the CD8 coreceptor) and intercellular adhesion molecule-1 (ICAM-1, the principal ligand for LFA-1).

- Conjugates of CTLs attached to target cells can be visualized by microscopy, and conjugate formation is the prelude to target cell lysis (Fig. 13–15).
- CTL–target cell contact results in the rapid formation of an immunological synapse, in which adhesion molecules, the TCR, and signaling molecules are reorganized in the CTL membrane and juxtaposed to ligands on the target cell membrane (see Fig. 13–15).
- Antibodies that block any of these interactions inhibit CTL-mediated lysis *in vitro,* thus indicating that all these interactions function cooperatively in the process of CTL recognition of targets.

In the CTL–target cell conjugate, the antigen receptors of the CTL recognize MHC-associated peptides on the target cell. This recognition induces clustering of T cell plasma membrane proteins, including the TCR, CD8, and LFA-1, and the clustering of the ligands for these molecules in the target cell membrane, including peptide/MHC and ICAM-1. An immunological synapse forms between the two cells, and biochemical signals are generated that activate the CTL. The biochemical signals are similar to the signals involved in the activation of helper T cells (see Chapter 9). Cytokines and other

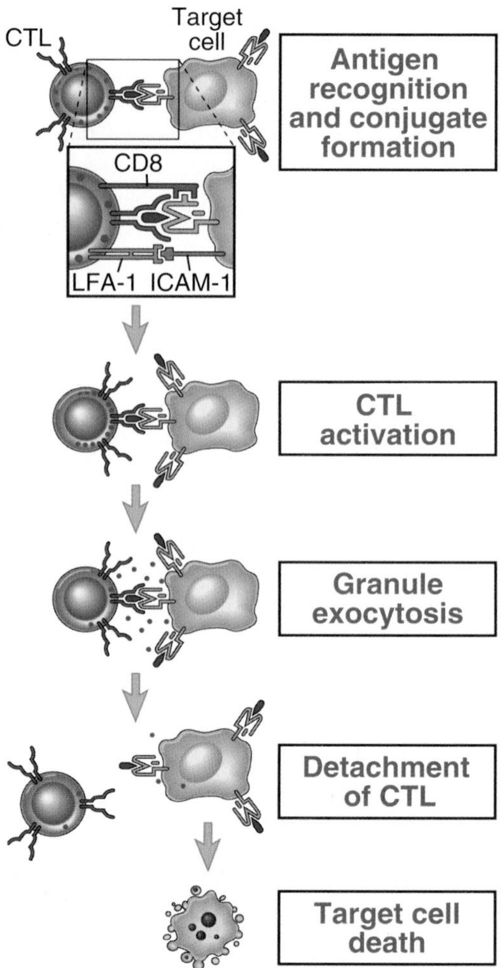

FIGURE 13–14 Steps in CTL-mediated lysis of target cells. A CTL recognizes the antigen-expressing target cell and is activated. Activation results in the release of granule contents from the CTL, which delivers a lethal hit to the target. The CTL may detach and kill another target cell while the first target goes on to die. Note that formation of conjugates between a CTL and its target and activation of the CTL also require interactions between accessory molecules (LFA-1, CD8) on the CTL and their specific ligands on the target cell; these are not shown.

signals provided by dendritic cells, which are required for the differentiation of naive CD8$^+$ T cells into CTLs, are not necessary for triggering the effector function of CTLs (i.e., target cell killing). Therefore, once CD8$^+$ T cells specific for an antigen have differentiated into fully functional CTLs, they can kill any nucleated cell that displays that antigen.

In addition to the T cell receptor, CD8$^+$ CTLs express receptors that are also expressed by NK cells, which contribute to both regulation and activation of CTL. Some of these receptors belong to the killer immunoglobulin receptor (KIR) family, discussed in Chapter 2, and recognize class I MHC molecules on target cells, but are not specific for a particular peptide-MHC complex. These KIRs transduce inhibitory signals, which may serve to prevent CTLs from killing normal cells and protect CTLs from activation-induced cell death (see Chapter 11). In addition, CTLs express the NKG2D receptor, described

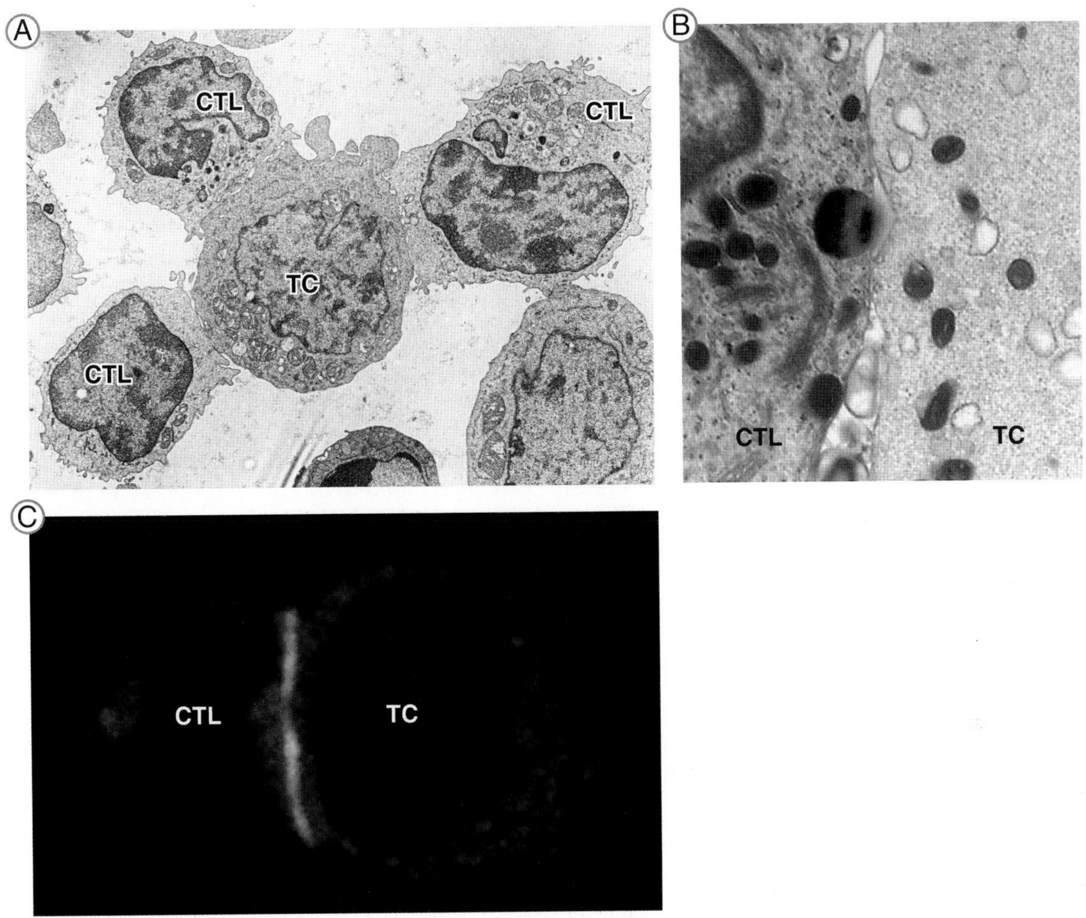

FIGURE 13–15 Immune synapse between CTLs and a target cell. A. Electron micrograph of three CTLs from a cloned cell line specific for the human MHC molecule HLA-A2 binding to an HLA-A2-expressing target cell (TC) within 1 minute after the CTLs and targets are mixed. Note that in the CTL on the upper left, the granules have been redistributed toward the target cell. (Courtesy of Dr. P. Peters, Netherlands Cancer Institute, Amsterdam.) B. Electron micrograph of the point of membrane contact between a CTL *(left)* and target cell *(right)*. Two CTL granules are near the synapse. Several mitochondria are also visible. (Reprinted from Stinchcombe JC, G Bossi, S Booth, and GM Griffiths. The immunological synapse of CTL contains a secretory domain and membrane bridges. Immunity 8:751–761, 2001, © Cell Press, with permission from Elsevier). C. Confocal fluorescence micrograph of an immune synapse between a CTL *(left)* and target cell (right) stained with antibodies against cathepsins in a secretory granule (blue), LFA-1 (green), and the cytoskeletal protein talin (red). The image demonstrates the central location of the secretory granule and the peripheral location of the adhesion molecule LFA-1 and associated cytoskeletal protein talin. (Reprinted from Stinchcombe JC and GM Griffiths. The role of the secretory immunological synapse in killing by CD8$^+$ CTL. Seminars in Immunology 15:301–305, © 2003 Elsevier Science Ltd., with permission from Elsevier.)

in Chapter 2, which recognizes class I MHC-like molecules MICA, MICB, and ULBP, expressed on infected or neoplastic cells. NKG2D may serve to deliver signals, which act together with TCR recognition of antigen, to enhance killing activity.

Killing of Target Cells by CTLs

Within a few minutes of a CTL's antigen receptor recognizing its peptide-MHC antigen on a target cell, the target cell undergoes changes that induce it to die by apoptosis. Target cell death occurs during the next 2 to 6 hours and proceeds even if the CTL detaches. Thus, the CTL is said to deliver a lethal hit to the target that results in the death of the target. The principal mechanism of CTL-mediated target cell killing is the delivery of cytotoxic proteins stored within cytoplasmic granules (also called secretory lysosomes) to the target cell, thereby triggering apoptosis of the target cell (Fig. 13–16). As discussed earlier, an immunological synapse rapidly forms between the CTL and target cell. This synapse is characterized by a ring of tight apposition between the CTL and target cell membranes, mediated by LFA-1–ICAM-1 binding, and an enclosed gap or space inside the ring. Distinct regions of the CTL membrane can be observed by immunofluorescence microscopy within the ring, including a signaling patch, which includes the TCR, protein-kinase Cθ, and Lck, and a secretory domain, which appears as a gap to one side of the signaling patch. Activation of the CTL induces cytoskeleton reorganization such that the microtubule organizing center of the CTL moves to the area of the cytoplasm near the contact with the target cell. The cytoplasmic granules of the CTL are transported along microtubules and become concentrated in the region of the synapse, and the granule membrane fuses with the plasma membrane at the secretory domain. Membrane fusion results in exocytosis of the CTL's granule contents into the confined space within the synaptic ring, between the plasma membranes of the CTL and target cell.

The granules of CTLs (and NK cells) contain several molecules that contribute to target cell apoptosis. These include **granzymes** A, B, and C, which are serine proteases that cleave proteins after aspartate residues; **perforin,** a membrane-perturbing molecule homologous to the C9 complement protein; and a sulfated proteoglycan, **serglycin,** which serves to assemble a complex containing granzymes and perforin. Both perforin and granzymes are required for efficient CTL killing of target cells, and it is known that perforin's main function is to facilitate delivery of the granzymes into the cytosol of the target cell. How this is accomplished is still not well understood. Perforin may polymerize and form aqueous pores in the target cell membrane through which granzymes enter, but there is no proof this is critical for CTL-mediated cell killing. According to another current model, complexes of granzyme B, perforin, and serglycin are discharged from the CTL onto the target cell and are internalized into endosomes by receptor-mediated endocytosis. Perforin may act on the endosomal membrane to facilitate the release of the granzymes into the target cell cytoplasm. Once in the cytoplasm, the granzymes cleave various substrates and initiate apoptotic death of the cell. Some granzyme-initiated apoptotic pathways involve caspases (see Chapter 11, Box 11–2). For example, granzyme B activates caspase-3 as well as the Bcl-2 family member, Bid, which triggers the mitochondrial pathway of apoptosis (see Chapter 11, Box 11–2). Granzymes A and C also appear to induce apoptosis in a caspase-independent manner.

CTLs use another mechanism of killing that is mediated by interactions of membrane molecules on the CTLs and target cells. On activation, CTLs express a membrane protein, called **Fas ligand (FasL),** that binds to the death receptor Fas, which is expressed on many cell types. This interaction also results in activation of caspases and apoptosis of targets (Chapter 11, Box 11–2). Studies with knockout mice lacking perforin, granzyme B, or FasL indicate that granule proteins are the principal mediators of killing by $CD8^+$ CTLs. Some $CD4^+$ T cells are also capable of killing target cells (which, of course, must express class II MHC-associated peptides to be recognized by the $CD4^+$ cells). $CD4^+$ T cells are deficient in perforin and granzymes, and FasL may be more important for their killing activity.

In infections by intracellular microbes, the killing activity of CTLs is important for eradicating the reservoir of infection. In addition, the caspases that are activated in target cells by granzymes and FasL cleave many substrates and activate enzymes that degrade DNA, but they do not distinguish between host and

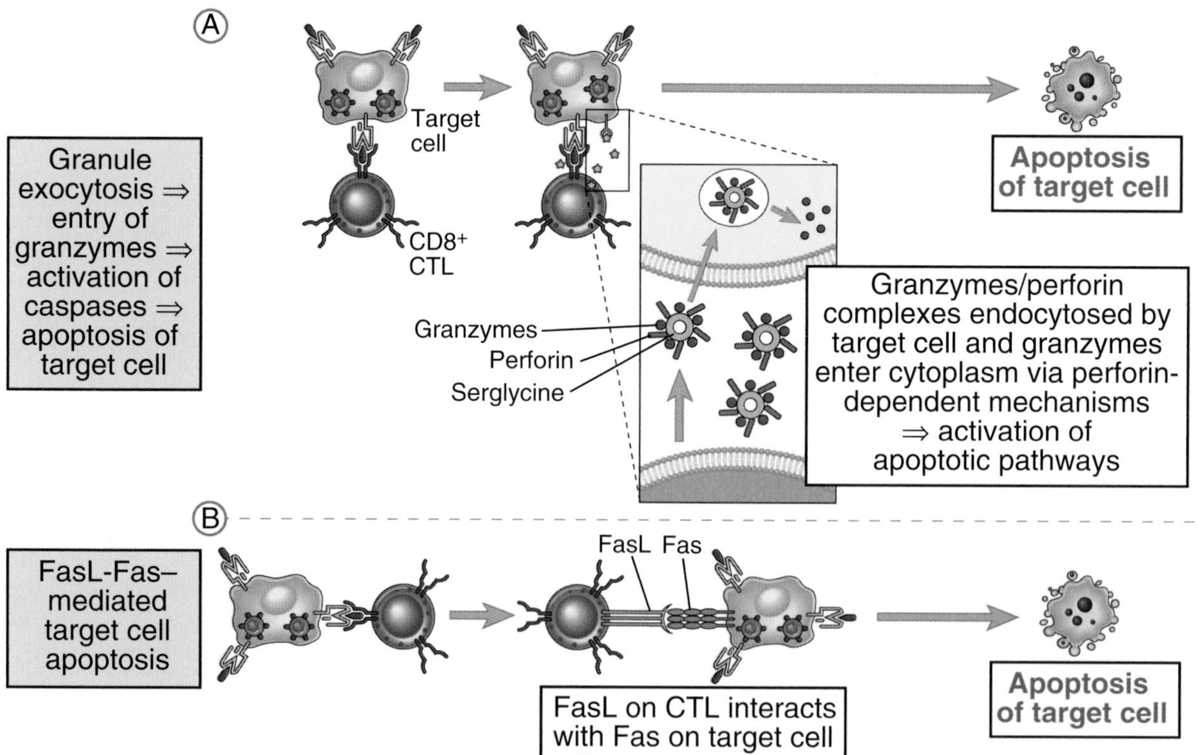

FIGURE 13–16 Mechanisms of CTL-mediated lysis of target cells. CTLs kill target cells by two main mechanisms. A. Complexes of perforin and granzymes are released from the CTL by granule exocytosis and enter target cells. The granzymes are delivered into the cytoplasm of the target cells by a perforin-dependent mechanism, and they induce apoptosis. B. FasL is expressed on activated CTLs, engages Fas on the surface of target cells, and induces apoptosis.

microbial proteins. Therefore, by activating nucleases in target cells, CTLs can initiate the destruction of microbial DNA as well as the target cell genome, thereby eliminating potentially infectious DNA. Another protein found in human CTL (and NK cell) granules, called granulysin, can alter the permeability of target cell and microbial membranes.

After delivering the lethal hit, the CTL is released from its target cell, a process that may be facilitated by decreases in the affinity of accessory molecules for their ligands. This release usually occurs even before the target cell goes on to die. CTLs themselves are not injured during target cell killing, probably because the directed granule exocytosis process during CTL-mediated killing preferentially delivers granule contents into the target cell and away from the CTL. In addition, CTL granules contain a proteolytic enzyme called cathepsin B, which is delivered to the CTL surface upon granule exocytosis, where it degrades errant perforin molecules that come into the vicinity of the CTL membrane.

Memory T Cells

T cell–mediated immune responses to an antigen usually result in the generation of memory T cells specific for that antigen, which may persist for years, even a lifetime. These memory T cells are responsible for more rapid and amplified responses when the same antigen in encountered again. Memory T cells are heterogeneous and may be derived from $CD4^+$ or $CD8^+$ T cells at various stages of differentiation from naive precursors. For example, some $CD4^+$ memory T cells may be derived from precursors before commitment to the T_H1 or T_H2 phenotype, and when activated by re-exposure to antigen, they have the potential for further differentiation into one or other subset. Other memory T cells may be derived from fully differentiated T_H1 or T_H2 precursors and retain their respective cytokine profiles upon reactivation. Memory $CD8^+$ T cells may also exist that maintain some of the phenotypic characteristics of differentiated CTL effectors.

Both $CD4^+$ and $CD8^+$ memory T cells can be further subdivided into two general subsets, based on their homing properties and effector functions. **Central memory T cells** express CCR7 and L-selectin, and home to lymph nodes. They have limited capacity to perform effector functions when they encounter antigen, but they undergo brisk proliferative responses and generate many effector cells upon antigen challenge. **Effector memory T cells**, on the other hand, do not express CCR7 or L-selectin, and home to peripheral tissues, especially mucosa. Upon antigenic stimulation, effector memory T cells produce effector cytokines such as IFN-γ, but they do not proliferate much. This effector subset, therefore, is poised for a rapid initial response to a repeat exposure to a microbe, but complete eradication of the infection may depend on the large numbers of effectors generated from the central memory T cells.

The maintenance of memory T cells is dependent on cytokines that are constitutively present in tissues, and that support low-level proliferative activity. One such cytokine is IL-7, which is required for survival and maintenance of both $CD4^+$ and $CD8^+$ memory T cells from antigen-activated cells. Predictably, memory T cells express high levels of the IL-7 receptor. (Recall from Chapter 3 that IL-7 is also important in the maintenance of naive T cells.) Maintenance of $CD8^+$ memory T cells may also require IL-15. In response to IL-7 and/or IL-15, memory T cells undergo low-level proliferation, which maintains populations of memory T cells over long time periods. This homeostatic proliferation of memory T cells does not require peptide antigen or MHC molecules.

SUMMARY

- CMI is the adaptive immune response against intracellular microbes. It is mediated by T lymphocytes and can be transferred from immunized to naive individuals by T cells and not by antibodies.

- Both $CD4^+$ and $CD8^+$ T cells contribute to CMI, but each subset has unique effector functions for the eradication of infections.

- Cell-mediated immune reactions consist of several steps: naive T cell recognition of peptide-MHC antigens in peripheral lymphoid organs, clonal expansion of the T cells and their differentiation into effector cells, migration of the effector T cells to the site of infection or antigen challenge, and elimination of the microbe or antigen.

- $CD4^+$ helper T lymphocytes may differentiate into specialized effector T_H1 cells that secrete IFN-γ, which favors phagocyte-mediated immunity, or into T_H2 cells that secrete IL-4 and IL-5, which favor IgE- and eosinophil/mast cell–mediated immune reactions. The differentiation of naive $CD4^+$ T cells into T_H1 and T_H2 populations is controlled by cytokines produced by APCs and by the T cells themselves, and is governed by transcriptions factors, including T-bet for T_H1 differentiation, and GATA-3 for T_H2 differentiation.

- $CD4^+$ T_H1 cells recognize antigens of microbes that have been ingested by phagocytes and activate the phagocytes to kill the microbes. The activation of macrophages by T_H1 cells is mediated by IFN-γ and CD40L-CD40 interactions. Activated macrophages kill phagocytosed microbes, stimulate inflammation, and repair damaged tissues. If the infection is not fully resolved, activated macrophages cause tissue injury and fibrosis.

- CD4$^+$ T_H2 cells recognize antigens produced by some extracellular microbes, including helminths, as well as certain environmental antigens associated with allergies. IL-4, secreted by activated T_H2 cells, promotes B cell isotype switching and production of IgE, which may coat helminths and mediate mast cell deregulation and inflammation. IL-5 secreted by activated T_H2 cells directly activates eosinophils to release granule contents that damage the integument of helminths, but may also damage host tissues.

- CD4$^+$ T_H17 cells comprise another subset of specialized effector T cells, which are characterized by secretion of IL-17, and which promote neutrophil-rich inflammatory responses. T_H17 cells may be important in meditating tissue damage in autoimmune diseases, and in protection against some microbial infections. Differentiation of T_H17 cells from naive precursors is stimulated by a combination of the cytokines TGF-β and IL-6.

- CD8$^+$ CTLs kill cells that express peptides derived from cytosolic antigens (e.g., viral antigens) that are presented in association with class I MHC molecules. CTL-mediated killing is mediated mainly by granule exocytosis, which releases granzymes and perforin. Perforin facilitates granzyme entry into the cytoplasm of target cells, and granzymes initiate several pathways of apoptosis. CTLs also express FasL, which engages Fas on the target cell membrane and triggers apoptosis of the target cell.

- Memory T cell are generated during CMI responses, and are maintained for years afterward by the action of cytokines such as IL-7 and IL-15. Central memory T cells home to lymphoid tissues, and respond to antigen re-exposure by proliferation and generation of effector cells. Effector memory T cells home to mucosal sites, and respond to antigen by secreting cytokines.

Selected Readings

Bettelli E, T Korn, M Oukka, and VK Kuchroo. Induction and effector functions of T_H17 cells. Nature 453:1051–1057, 2008.

Bossi G, and GM Griffiths. CTL secretory lysosomes: biogenesis and secretion of a harmful organelle. Seminars in Immunology 17:87–94, 2005.

Catalfamo M, and PA Henkart. Perforin and the granule exocytosis cytotoxicity pathway. Current Opinion in Immunology 15:522–527, 2003.

Dong C. T_H17 cells in development: an updated view of their molecular identity and genetic programming. Nature Reviews Immunology 8:337–348, 2008.

Farrar JD, H Asnagli, and KM Murphy. T helper subset development: roles of instruction, selection, and transcription. Journal of Clinical Investigation 109:431–435, 2002.

Gordon S. Alternative activation of macrophages. Nature Reviews Immunology 3:23–35, 2003.

Gourley TS, EJ Wherry, D Masopust, and R Ahmed. Generation and maintenance of immunological memory. Seminars in Immunology 16:323–333, 2004.

Korn T, E Bettelli, M Oukka, and UK Kuchroo. IL-17 and Th17 cells. Annual Review of Immunology 27, 2009.

Lanzavecchia A, and F Sallusto. Understanding the generation and function of memory T cell subsets. Current Opinion in Immunology 17:326–332, 2005.

Lee GR, ST Kim, CG Spilianakis, PE Fields, and RA Flavell. T helper cell differentiation: regulation by cis elements and epigenetics. Immunity 24:369–379, 2006.

Lieberman J. The ABCs of granule-mediated cytotoxicity: new weapons in the arsenal. Nature Reviews Immunology 3:361–370, 2003.

Martinez FO, L Helming, and S Gordon. Alternative activation of macrophages: An immunologic functional perspective. Annual Review of Immunology 27, 2009.

McGeachy MJ, and DJ Cua. Th17 cell differentiation: the long and winding road. Immunity 28:445–453, 2008.

Murphy KM, and SL Reiner. The lineage decisions of helper T cells. Nature Reviews Immunology 2:933–944, 2002.

Ouyang W, JK Kolls, and Y Zheng. The biological functions of T helper 17 cell effector cytokines in inflammation. Immunity 28:454–467, 2008.

Raja SM, SS Metkar, and CJ Froelich. Cytotoxic granule-mediated apoptosis: unraveling the complex mechanism. Current Opinion in Immunology 15:528–532, 2003.

Russell JH, and TJ Ley. Lymphocyte-mediated cytotoxicity. Annual Review of Immunology 20:323–370, 2002.

Sallusto F, J Geginat, and A Lanzavecchia. Central memory and effector memory T cell subsets: function, generation, and maintenance. Annual Review of Immunology 22:745–763, 2004.

Seder RA, and R Ahmed. Similarities and differences in CD4$^+$ and CD8$^+$ effector and memory T cell generation. Nature Immunology 4:835–842, 2003.

Steinman L. A brief history of T_H17, the first major revision in the T_H1/T_H2 hypothesis of T cell-mediated tissue damage. Nature Medicine 13:139–145, 2007.

Szabo SJ, BM Sullivan, SL Peng, and LH Glimcher. Molecular mechanisms regulating the Th1 response. Annual Review of Immunology 21:713–758, 2003.

Von Andrian UH, and CR Mackay. T-cell function and migration. New England Journal of Medicine 343:1020–1034, 2000.

Williams MA, and MJ Bevan. Effector and memory CTL differentiation. Annual Review of Immunology 25:171–192, 2007.

Wong P, and EG Pamer. CD8 T cell responses to infectious pathogens. Annual Review of Immunology 21:29–70, 2003.

Zhu J, and WE Paul. CD4 T cells: fates, functions, and faults. Blood 112:1557–1569, 2008.

Chapter 14

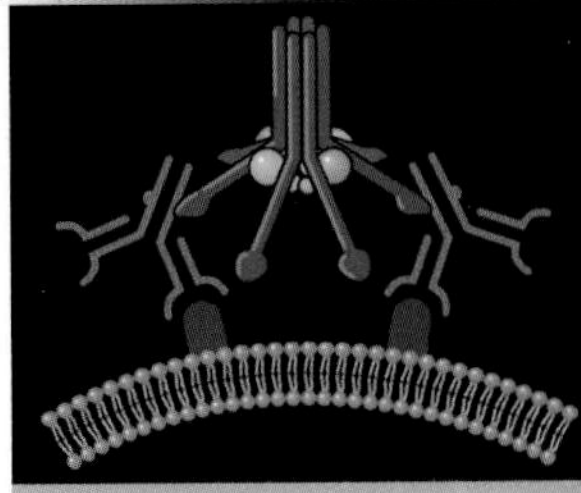

EFFECTOR MECHANISMS OF HUMORAL IMMUNITY

Humoral immunity is mediated by secreted antibodies, and its physiologic function is defense against extracellular microbes and microbial toxins. This type of immunity contrasts with cell-mediated immunity, the other effector arm of the adaptive immune system, which is mediated by T lymphocytes and functions to eradicate microbes that infect and live within host cells (see Chapter 13). Humoral immunity against microbial toxins was discovered by von Behring and Kitasato in 1890 as a form of immunity that could be conveyed from immunized to naive individuals by the transfer of serum. The types of microorganisms that are combated by humoral immunity are extracellular bacteria, fungi, and even obligate intracellular microbes such as viruses, which are targets of antibodies before they infect cells or when they are released from infected cells. Defects in antibody production result in increased susceptibility to infection with many microbes, including bacteria, fungi, and viruses. The most effective vaccines induce protection primarily by stimulating the production of antibodies. Apart from their crucial protective roles, in allergic individuals and in certain autoimmune diseases some specific antibodies can be harmful and mediate tissue injury. In this chapter, we discuss the effector mechanisms that are used by antibodies to eliminate antigens. The structure of antibodies is described in Chapter 4 and the process of antibody production in Chapter 10.

Overview of Humoral Immunity

The main function of antibodies is the neutralization and elimination of infectious microbes and microbial toxins (Fig. 14–1). As we shall see later, antibody-mediated elimination of antigens involves a number of effector mechanisms and requires the participation of various cellular and humoral components of the immune system, including phagocytes and complement proteins. Before these individual effector mechanisms are described, we will summarize the ways in which antibodies mediate protective immunity.

- ***Antibodies are produced by B lymphocytes and plasma cells in the lymphoid organs and bone marrow, but antibodies perform their effector functions at sites distant from their production.*** Antibodies produced in the lymph nodes, spleen, and bone marrow may enter the blood and then circulate to any

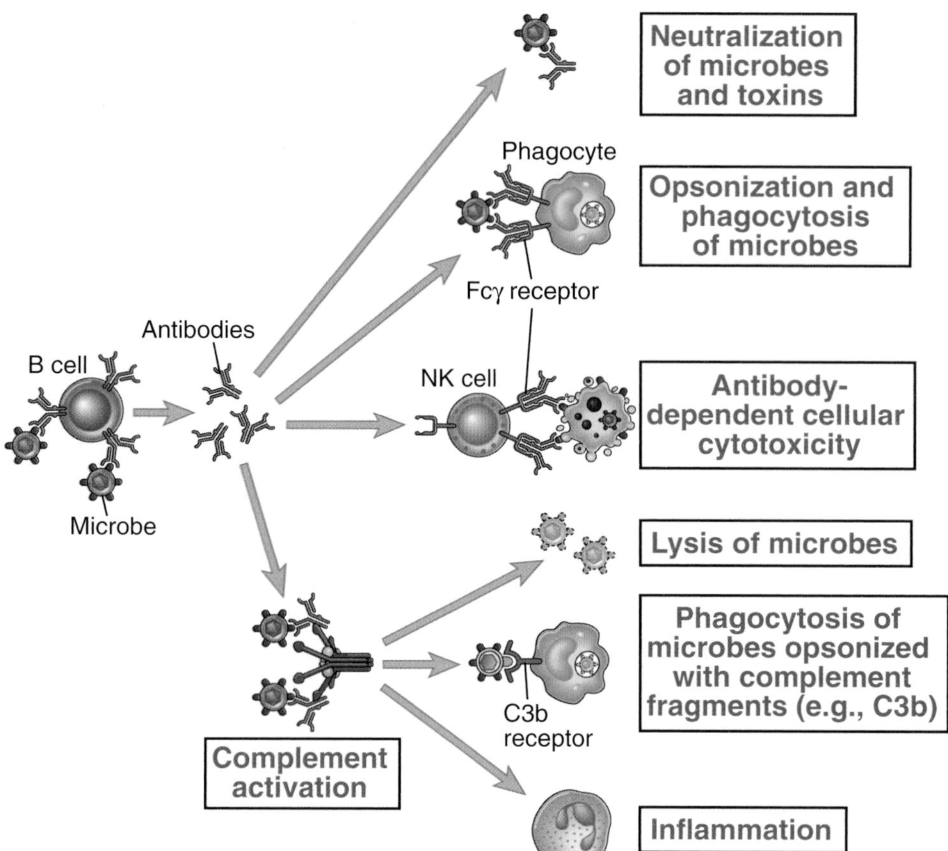

FIGURE 14–1 Effector functions of antibodies. Antibodies against microbes (and their toxins, not shown here) neutralize these agents, opsonize them for phagocytosis, sensitize them for antibody-dependent cellular cytotoxicity, and activate the complement system. These various effector functions may be mediated by different antibody isotypes.

site where antigen is located. Antibodies produced in mucosa-associated lymphoid tissues are transported across epithelial barriers into the lumens of mucosal organs; in the intestine and the airways, for instance, antibodies on the luminal surface of the epithelium inhibit the entry of ingested and inhaled microbes. Antibodies are also actively transported across the placenta into the circulation of the developing fetus. In cell-mediated immunity, activated T lymphocytes are able to migrate to peripheral sites of infection and inflammation, but they are not transported into mucosal secretions or across the placenta.

- ***The antibodies that mediate protective immunity may be derived from short-lived or long-lived antibody-producing plasma cells following the activation of naive or memory B cells*** (see Chapter 10, Fig. 10–2). The first exposure to an antigen, either by infection or by vaccination, leads to the activation of naive B lymphocytes and their differentiation into antibody-producing cells and memory cells. Subsequent exposure to the same antigens leads to the activation of memory B cells and a larger and more rapid antibody response. Plasma cells derived early in an immune response or from marginal zone or B-1 B cells tend to be short lived. In contrast, germinal center–derived class-switched antibody-secreting plasma cells migrate to the bone marrow and persist at this site, where they continue to produce antibodies for years after the antigen is eliminated. Most of the immunoglobulin G (IgG) found in the serum of normal individuals is derived from these long-lived antibody-producing plasma cells, which were induced by the exposure of naive and memory B cells to various antigens throughout the life of the individual. If an immune individual is exposed to a previously encountered microbe, the level of circulating antibody produced by persisting antibody-secreting plasma cells provides immediate protection against the infection. At the same time, activation of memory B cells generates a larger burst of antibody that provides a second and more effective wave of protection.

- ***Many of the effector functions of antibodies are mediated by the heavy chain constant regions of Ig molecules, and different Ig heavy chain isotypes serve distinct effector functions*** (Table 14–1). For instance, some IgG subclasses bind to phagocyte Fc receptors and promote the phagocytosis of antibody-coated particles, IgM and some subclasses of IgG activate the complement system, and IgE binds to the Fc receptors of mast cells and triggers their activation. Each of these effector mechanisms will be discussed later in this chapter. The humoral immune system is specialized in such a way that different microbes or antigen exposures stimulate B cell switching to the Ig isotypes

Table 14–1. Functions of Antibody Isotypes

Antibody Isotope	Isotype-specific effector functions
IgG	Opsonization of antigens for phagocytosis by macrophages and neutrophils Activation of the classical pathway of complement Antibody-dependent cell-mediated cytotoxicity mediated by natural killer cells Neonatal immunity: transfer of maternal antibody across the placenta and gut Feedback inhibition of B cell activation
IgM	Activation of the classical pathway of complement Antigen receptor of naive B lymphocytes*
IgA	Mucosal immunity: secretion of IgA into the lumens of the gastrointestinal and respiratory tracts Activation of complement by the lectin pathway or by the alternative pathway
IgE	Mast cell degranulation (immediate hypersensitivity reactions)
IgD	Antigen receptor of naive B lymphocytes*

*These functions are mediated by membrane-bound and not secreted antibodies.

that are best for combating these microbes. The major stimuli for isotype switching during the process of B cell activation are helper T cell–derived cytokines together with CD40 ligand expressed by activated helper T cells (see Chapter 10). Different types of microbes stimulate the differentiation of helper T cells into effector populations, such as T_H1 and T_H2 subsets, that produce distinct sets of cytokines and therefore induce switching of B cells to different heavy chain isotypes. For instance, viruses and many bacteria stimulate T_H1 responses and the production of T_H1-dependent IgG isotypes that bind to phagocytes and natural killer (NK) cells and activate complement. Phagocytes, NK cells, and complement are effective at eliminating many viruses and bacteria. In contrast, helminthic parasites stimulate T_H2 responses and the production of T_H2-dependent IgE antibody, which binds to and activates mast cells and basophils. Cytokines released by these cells activate eosinophils. Eosinophils are especially potent in destroying helminths. Neutralization is the only function of antibodies that is mediated entirely by binding of antigen and does not require participation of the Ig constant regions.

- ***Although many effector functions of antibodies are mediated by the Ig heavy chain constant regions, all these functions are triggered by the binding of antigens to the variable regions.*** The binding of antibodies to a multivalent antigen, such as a polysaccharide or a reiterated epitope on a microbial surface, brings the Fc regions of antibodies close together, and it is this clustering of antibody molecules that leads to complement activation and allows the antibodies to activate Fc receptors on phagocytes. The requirement for antigen binding ensures that antibodies activate various effector mechanisms only when they are needed, that is, when the antibodies encounter and specifically bind antigens, not when the antibodies are circulating in an antigen-free form.

With this introduction to humoral immunity, we proceed to a discussion of the various functions of antibodies in host defense.

NEUTRALIZATION OF MICROBES AND MICROBIAL TOXINS

Antibodies against microbes and microbial toxins block the binding of these microbes and toxins to cellular receptors (Fig. 14–2). In this way, antibodies inhibit, or "neutralize," the infectivity of microbes as well as the potential injurious effects of infection. Many microbes enter host cells by the binding of particular surface molecules to membrane proteins or lipids on the surface of host cells. For example, influenza viruses use their envelope hemagglutinin to infect respiratory epithelial cells, and gram-negative bacteria use pili to attach to and infect a variety of host cells. Antibodies that bind to these microbial structures interfere with the ability of the microbes to interact with cellular receptors, and may thus prevent infection by means of steric hindrance. In some cases, very few antibody molecules may bind to a microbe and induce conformational changes in surface molecules that prevent the microbe from interacting with cellular receptors; such interactions are examples of the allosteric effects of antibodies. Many microbial toxins mediate their pathologic effects also by binding to specific cellular receptors. For instance, tetanus toxin binds to receptors in the motor end plate of neuromuscular junctions and inhibits neuromuscular transmission, which leads to paralysis, and diphtheria toxin binds to cellular receptors and enters various cells, where it inhibits protein synthesis. Anti-toxin antibodies sterically hinder the interactions of toxins with host cells and thus prevent the toxins from causing tissue injury and disease.

Antibody-mediated neutralization of microbes and toxins requires only the antigen-binding regions of the antibodies. Therefore, such neutralization may be mediated by antibodies of any isotype in the circulation and in mucosal secretions and can experimentally also be mediated by Fab or $F(ab)_2$ fragments of specific antibodies. Most neutralizing antibodies in the blood are of the IgG isotype; in mucosal organs, they are largely of the IgA isotype. The most effective neutralizing antibodies

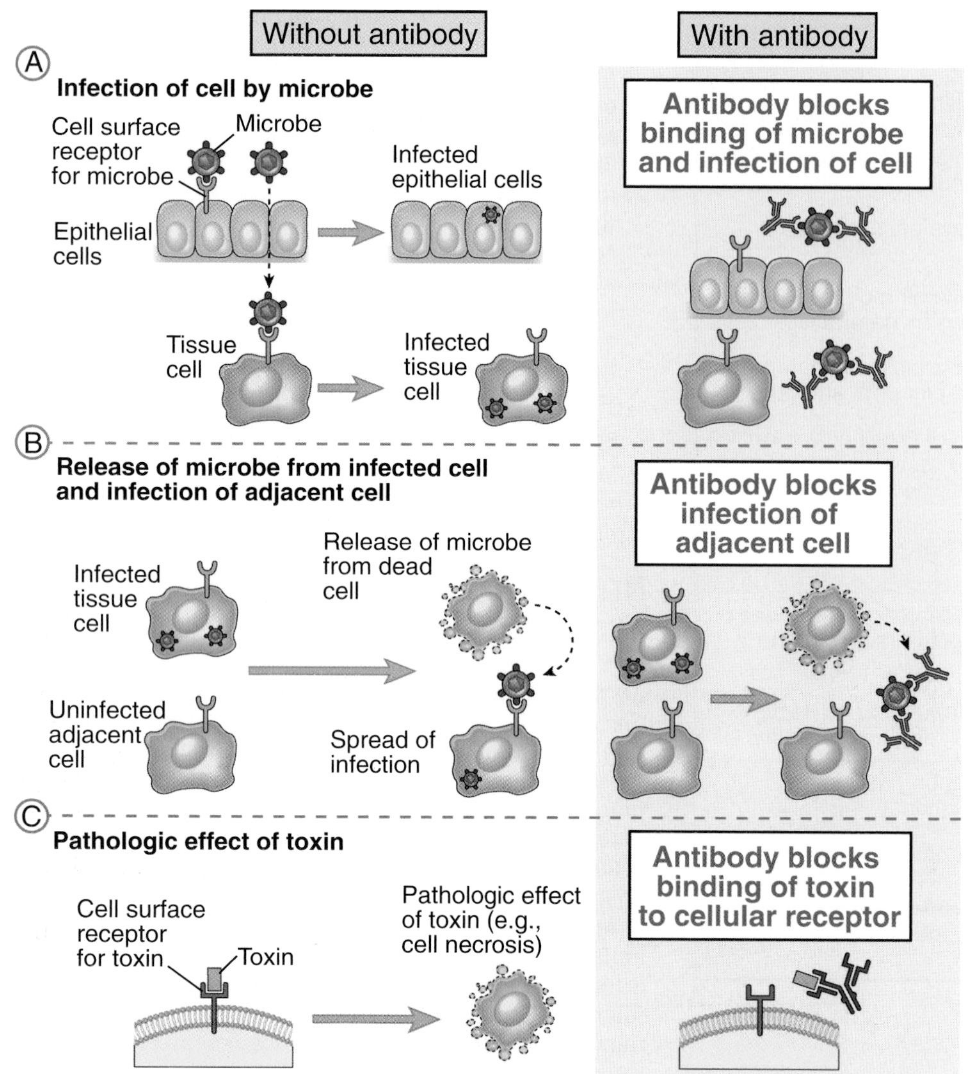

FIGURE 14–2 Neutralization of microbes and toxins by antibodies. A. Antibodies prevent the binding of microbes to cells and thus block the ability of the microbes to infect host cells. B. Antibodies inhibit the spread of microbes from an infected cell to an adjacent uninfected cell. C. Antibodies block the binding of toxins to cells and thus inhibit the pathologic effects of the toxins.

are those with high affinities for their antigens. High-affinity antibodies are produced by the process of affinity maturation (see Chapter 10). Many prophylactic vaccines work by stimulating the production of high-affinity neutralizing antibodies (Table 14–2). A mechanism that microbes have developed to evade host immunity is to mutate the genes encoding surface antigens that are the targets of neutralizing antibodies (see Chapter 15).

Antibody-Mediated Opsonization and Phagocytosis

Antibodies of the IgG isotype coat (opsonize) microbes and promote their phagocytosis by binding to Fc receptors on phagocytes. Mononuclear phagocytes and neutrophils ingest microbes as a prelude to intracellular killing and degradation. These phagocytes express a variety of surface receptors that directly bind microbes and ingest them, even without antibodies, providing one mechanism of innate immunity (see Chapter 2). The efficiency of this process is markedly enhanced if the phagocyte can bind the particle with high affinity (Fig. 14–3). Mononuclear phagocytes and neutrophils express receptors for the Fc portions of IgG antibodies that specifically bind antibody-coated (opsonized) particles. Microbes may also be opsonized by a product of complement activation called C3b and are phagocytosed by binding to a leukocyte receptor for C3b (described later in this chapter). The process of coating particles in order to promote phagocytosis is called **opsonization,** and substances that perform this function, including antibodies and complement proteins, are called specific opsonins.

Phagocyte Fc Receptors

Leukocyte Fc receptors promote the phagocytosis of opsonized particles and deliver signals that stimulate the microbicidal activities of the leukocytes. Fc receptors for different Ig heavy chain isotypes are expressed on many leukocyte populations and serve diverse func-

Table 14–2. Vaccine-Induced Humoral Immunity

Infectious disease	Vaccine	Mechanism of protective immunity
Polio	Oral attenuated polio virus	Neutralization of virus by mucosal IgA antibody
Tetanus, diphtheria	Toxoids	Neutralization of toxin by systemic IgG antibody
Hepatitis, A or B	Recombinant viral envelope proteins	Neutralization of virus by systemic IgG antibody
Pneumococcal pneumonia, Haemophilus	Conjugate vaccines composed of bacterial capsular polysaccaride and protein	Opsonization and phagocytosis mediated by IgM and IgG antibodies, directly or secondary to complement activation

Selected examples of vaccines that work by stimulating protective humoral immunity are listed.

tions in immunity (Box 14–1). Of these Fc receptors, the ones that are most important for phagocytosis of opsonized particles are receptors for the heavy chains of IgG antibodies, called Fcγ receptors. There are three types of Fcγ receptors, which have different affinities for the heavy chains of different IgG subclasses and are expressed on different cell types. The major high-affinity phagocyte Fcγ receptor is called FcγRI (CD64). It binds human IgG1 and IgG3 strongly, with a K_d of 10^{-8} to 10^{-9} M. (In mice, the high-affinity FcγRI receptor preferentially binds murine IgG2a and IgG2b antibodies.) FcγRI is composed of an Fc region–binding α chain expressed in association with a disulfide-linked homodimer of a signaling protein called the FcR γ chain, which is homologous to the signal-transducing ζ chain of the T cell receptor (TCR) complex.

Phagocytosis of IgG-coated particles is mediated by binding of the Fc portions of opsonizing antibodies to Fcγ receptors on phagocytes. Therefore, the IgG subtypes that bind best to these receptors (IgG1 and IgG3) are the most efficient opsonins for promoting phagocytosis. Antibody molecules attached to repeated determinants on the surface of a microbe, or to a polyvalent macromolecular antigen, form multivalent arrays and are bound by phagocyte Fc receptors with much higher avidity than are free circulating antibodies. For this reason, FcγRI binds antibodies attached to antigens better than it binds free antibodies. In addition, triggering of Fc receptors requires that receptors be clustered in the plane of the membrane, and clustering and consequent receptor activation can be mediated only by antigen-bound IgGs that make up a multivalent ligand for Fc receptors. Binding of Fc receptors on phagocytes to multivalent antibody-coated particles leads to the activation of phagocytes, engulfment of the particles, and their internalization in vesicles known as phagosomes. These vesicles fuse with lysosomes, and the phagocytosed particles are destroyed in phagolysosomes (see Chapter 2, Fig. 2–4).

Binding of opsonized particles to phagocyte Fc receptors, particularly FcγRI, activates phagocytes by virtue of signals transduced by the FcR γ chain. The FcR γ chain, like the TCR ζ chain, contains immunoreceptor tyrosine-based activation motifs (ITAMs) in its cytoplasmic

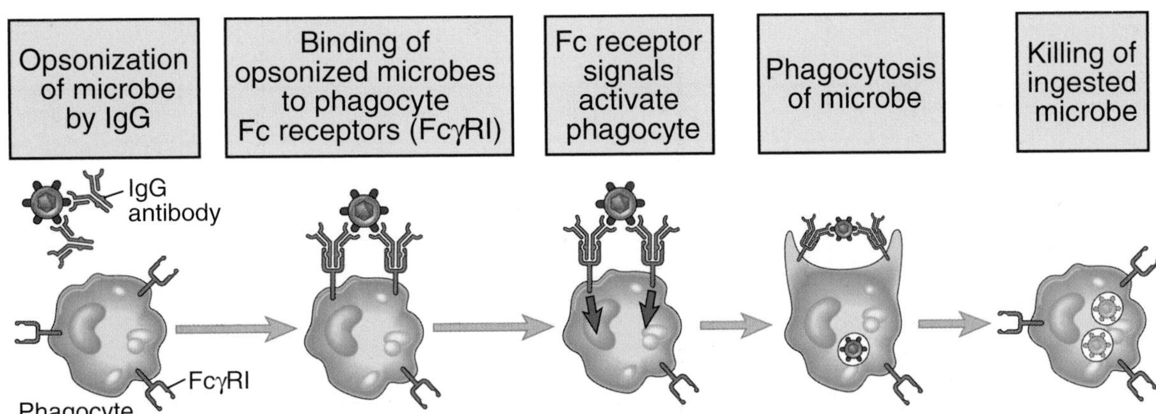

FIGURE 14–3 Antibody-mediated opsonization and phagocytosis of microbes. Antibodies of certain IgG subclasses bind to microbes and are then recognized by Fc receptors on phagocytes. Signals from the Fc receptors promote the phagocytosis of the opsonized microbes and activate the phagocytes to destroy these microbes.

Box 14–1 ■ IN DEPTH: LEUKOCYTE Fc RECEPTORS

Leukocytes express cell surface receptors that specifically bind the Fc portions of various Ig isotypes and subtypes. The Fc receptors on neutrophils and macrophages mediate the phagocytosis of opsonized particles and the activation of leukocytes to destroy phagocytosed particles. Fc receptors on NK cells are involved in activation of these cells to kill antibody-coated target cells. Fc receptors on B cells negatively regulate antibody responses. Two nonleukocyte Fc receptors are expressed on epithelial cells and mediate transepithelial transport of antibodies. Here we discuss the specific Fc receptors of leukocytes that mediate functional responses, namely, FcγRI, FcγRII, FcγRIII, FcεRI, FcεRII, and FcαR (see Table).

Each of the leukocyte FcRs contains one Fc-binding polypeptide chain, called the α chain, which is a member of the Ig superfamily. Differences in specificities or affinities of each FcR for the various IgG isotypes are based on differences in the structure of these α chains. In all the FcRs except FcγRII, the α chain is associated with one or more additional polypeptide chains involved in signal transduction, called β and γ chains (see Figure). Signaling functions of FcγRII are mediated by the cytoplasmic tail of the α chain.

There are three distinct types of Fcγ receptors, which have different affinities for heavy chains of different IgG subclasses. The major phagocyte Fcγ receptor, FcγRI (CD64), is expressed on macrophages and neutrophils and is a high-affinity receptor for IgG1 and IgG3 (in humans). The large extracellular amino-terminal region of the receptor polypeptide folds into three tandem Ig-like domains. The Fc-binding α chain of FcγRI is associated with a disulfide-linked homodimer of a signaling protein called the FcR γ chain. This γ chain is also found in the signaling complexes associated with FcγRIII, FcαR, and FcεRI. The γ chain has only a short extracellular amino terminus but a large cytoplasmic carboxyl terminus, with structural homology to the ζ chain of the TCR complex. Like the TCR ζ chain, the FcR γ chain contains an immunoreceptor tyrosine-based activation motif (ITAM) that couples receptor clustering to activation of protein tyrosine kinases. Transcription of the FcγRI gene is stimulated by the macrophage-activating cytokine IFN-γ, and for this reason activated macrophages express higher levels of the receptor than do resting monocytes.

Both humans and mice express two different classes of low-affinity receptors for IgG, called FcγRII (CD32) and FcγRIII (CD16). FcγRII is expressed on phagocytes and other cell types and binds human IgG subtypes (IgG1 and IgG3) with sufficiently low affinity (K_d 10^{-6} M) that monomeric IgG molecules are unable to occupy this receptor at physiologic antibody concentrations. Therefore, FcγRII binds IgG mainly when the antibody is in immune complexes or on opsonized microbes or cells, which display arrays of Fc regions. In humans, there are three different isoforms of FcγRII (called A, B, and C) that arise from alternative RNA splicing. These isoforms have similar intracellular domains and ligand specificities but differ in cytoplasmic tail structure, cell distribution, and functions. FcγRIIA is expressed by neutrophils and mononuclear phagocytes and probably participates in the phagocytosis of opsonized particles. FcγRIIA is also expressed by certain vascular endothelia and other cell

FcR	Affinity for immunoglobulin	Cell Distribution	Function
FcγRI (CD64)	High (K_d ~ 10^{-9} M); binds IgG1 and IgG3, can bind monomeric IgG	Macrophages, neutrophils; also eosinophils	Phagocytosis; activation of phagocytes
FcγRIIA (CD32)	Low (K_d > 10^{-7} M)	Macrophages, neutrophils; eosinophils, platelets	Phagocytosis; cell activation (inefficient)
FcγRIIB (CD32)	Low (K_d > 10^{-7} M)	B lymphocytes, dendritic cells, macrophages	Feedback inhibition of B cells, macrophages, dendritic cells
FcγRIIIA (CD16)	Low (K_d > 10^{-6} M)	NK cells	Antibody-dependent cell-mediated cytotoxicity
FcγRIIIB (CD16)	Low (K_d > 10^{-6} M); GPI-linked protein	Neutrophils, other cells	Phagocytosis (inefficient)
FcεRI	High (K_d > 10^{-10} M); binds monomeric IgE	Mast cells, basophils, eosinophils	Cell activation (degranulation)
FcεRII (CD23)	Low (K_d > 10^{-7} M)	B lymphocytes, eosinophils, Langerhans cells	Unknown
FcαR (CD89)	Low (K_d > 10^{-6} M)	Neutrophils, eosinophils, monocytes	Cell activation?

Abbreviations: NK, natural killer; GPI, glycosphosphatidylinositol

Continued on following page

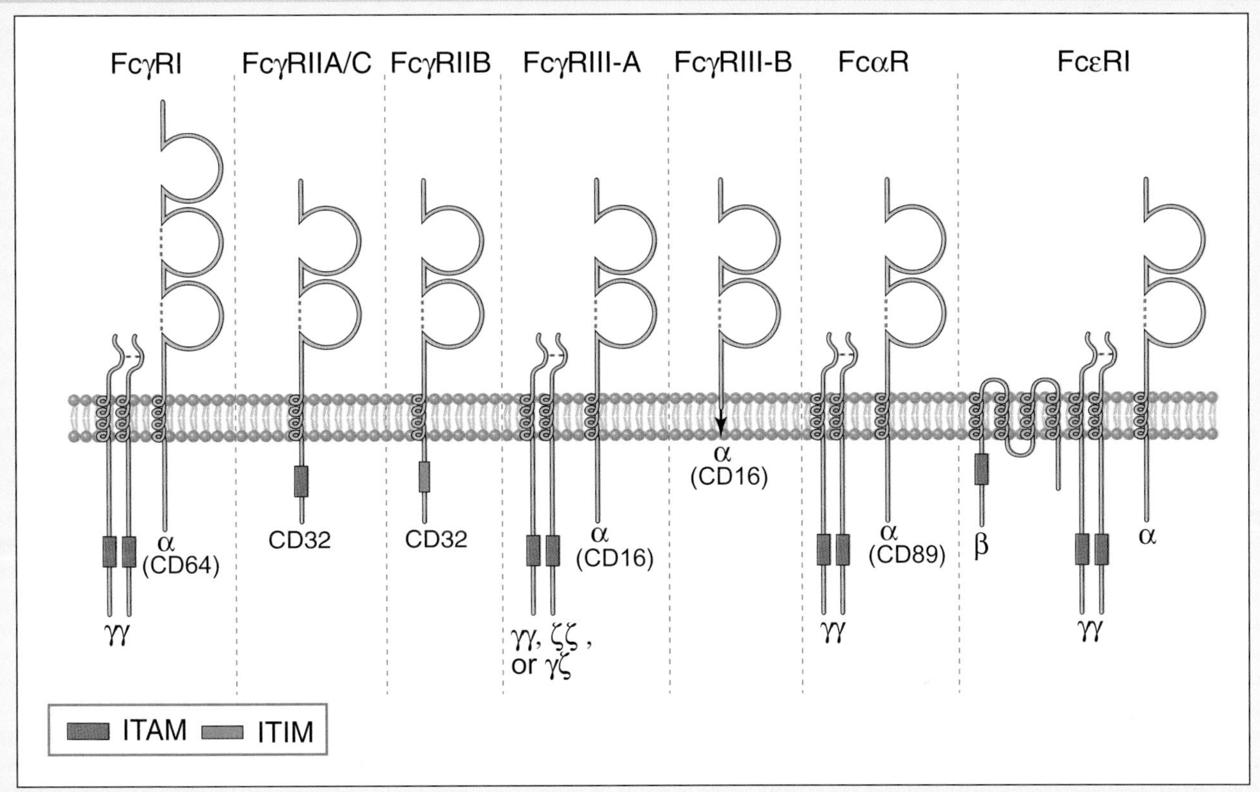

Subunit composition of Fc receptors. Schematic models of the different human Fc receptors illustrate the Fc-binding α chains and the signaling subunits.

types in which its function is unknown; it may play a role in the binding of molecules other than Ig, such as lipoproteins. The cytoplasmic tails of FcγRIIA and FcγRIIC contain ITAMs and, on clustering by IgG1- or IgG3-coated particles or cells, can deliver an activation signal to phagocytes. FcγRIIB is expressed on all immune cells, but is the only Fc receptor on B cells. The intracellular carboxy-terminal region of this isoform contains an immunoreceptor tyrosine-based inhibition motif (ITIM) that can deliver inhibitory signals, counteracting the positive signals delivered to B cells by the antigen-induced cross-linking of membrane Ig. Thus, FcγRIIB clustering, induced by occupancy with polyvalent IgG1 or IgG3, may shut off B cell activation (see Chapter 10, Fig. 10–19).

The extracellular ligand-binding portion of FcγRIII (CD16) is similar to FcγRII in structure and affinity and specificity for IgG. Two separate genes code for this molecule in humans. The FcγRIIIA isoform, the product of the A gene, is a transmembrane protein expressed mainly on NK cells. FcγRIIIA associates with homodimers of the FcR γ chain, homodimers of the TCR ζ chain, or heterodimers composed of the FcR γ chain and the ζ chain. This association is necessary for cell surface expression and, through the ITAMs in these signaling chains, can deliver intracellular activating signals. Receptor clustering induced by occupancy with IgG1 or IgG3 bound to a target cell surface activates NK cells to kill the targets, thereby mediating ADCC. The FcγRIIIB isoform, a product of the B gene, is a GPI-linked protein expressed on neutrophils; it does not mediate phagocytosis or trigger neutrophil activation.

FcεRI is an IgE receptor expressed mainly on mast cells and basophils (see Chapter 19). The affinity of this receptor for IgE is extremely high (K_d 10^{-10} M), and therefore it readily binds monomeric IgE molecules even at the low normal plasma concentrations of this antibody isotype. The IgE-binding α chain is associated with a β chain and an FcR γ chain homodimer. The β chain spans the plasma membrane four times; both its amino terminus and carboxyl terminus are intracellular, and its carboxy-terminal tail region contains an ITAM. Antigen-mediated cross-linking of IgE that is prebound to FcεRI results in activation and degranulation of the mast cells or basophils, leading to immediate hypersensitivity reactions (Chapter 19). FcεRI is also expressed on eosinophils, and on antigen-presenting cells such as monocytes, Langerhans cells, and tissue dendritic cells. The function of FcεRI on these antigen-presenting cells is not known.

Human FcεRII (CD23) is a C-type lectin that binds IgE with low affinity. It exists in two forms: CD23a is constitutively expressed on B cells, and CD23b is induced by IL-4 on T cells, Langerhans cells, monocytes, macrophages, and eosinophils. Both forms mediate endocytosis of IgE-coated particles. The physiologic function of this receptor is not known.

FcαR (CD89) is an IgA receptor expressed on neutrophils, monocytes, and eosinophils. Its ligand-binding α chain is associated with an FcR γ homodimer.

As noted before, on binding of Ig molecules, most of the FcRs serve to activate the cells on which they are expressed. Activation requires cross-linking of the

Continued on following page

Box 14–1 ▪ IN DEPTH: LEUKOCYTE Fc RECEPTORS (Continued)

FcRs by several linked Ig molecules (e.g., on Ig-coated microbes or in immune complexes). Cross-linking of the ligand-binding α chains of an FcR results in signal transduction events that are similar to those that occur after antigen-receptor cross-linking in lymphocytes (see Chapter 9). These include Src kinase–mediated tyrosine phosphorylation of the ITAMs in the signaling chains of the FcRs; SH2 domain–mediated recruitment of Syk family kinases to the ITAMs; activation of phosphatidylinositol-3 (PI-3) kinase; recruitment of adapter molecules, including SLP-76 and BLNK; and recruitment of enzymes such as phospholipase Cγ and Tec family kinases. These events lead to generation of inositol trisphosphate and diacylglycerol and sustained calcium mobilization. Responses to these mediators in leukocytes include transcription of genes encoding cytokines, inflammatory mediators, and microbicidal enzymes, and mobilization of the cytoskeleton, leading to phagocytosis, granule exocytosis, and cell migration.

Immune complex–mediated cross-linking of the inhibitory FcγRIIB on B cells leads to tyrosine phosphorylation of the ITIM in the cytoplasmic tail, recruitment and activation of the SHIP inositol phosphatase, and subsequent inhibition of B cell receptor–mediated, ITAM-dependent activation pathways. FcγRIIB may also generate ITIM-independent pro-apoptotic signals, which may be one mechanism of maintaining peripheral B cell tolerance. In addition, FcγRIIB is expressed on dendritic cells, neutrophils, macrophages, and mast cells and may play a role in regulating the responses of these cells generated by activating FcRs.

The physiologic roles of FcRs have been addressed by generating knockout mice that fail to express these molecules. Knockout of the FcR γ chain in mice results in loss of expression of FcγRI, FcγRII, and FcεRI. These animals are impaired in their ability to clear opsonized microbes and to mount inflammatory reactions to immune complexes.

portion and is required for signal transduction and surface expression of the complete Fc receptor. Clustering of FcγRI by aggregated antigen-bound IgG results in the activation of Src-family kinases that phosphorylate ITAM tyrosine residues on the cytoplasmic tail of the FcR γ chain, thus contributing to the recruitment and activation of the Syk tyrosine kinase, and subsequently of a number of downstream signaling pathways. The process of phagocyte activation is very similar in a mechanistic sense to the activation of the B cell receptor and TCR as discussed in Chapters 9 and 10. The induction of signal transduction by FcγRI in phagocytes triggers production of various microbicidal molecules. One consequence of phagocyte activation is production of the enzyme phagocyte oxidase, which catalyzes the intracellular generation of reactive oxygen intermediates that are cytotoxic for phagocytosed microbes. In addition, leukocytes that are activated by their Fc receptors secrete hydrolytic enzymes and reactive oxygen intermediates into the external milieu that are capable of killing extracellular microbes too large to be phagocytosed. The same toxic products may damage tissues; this mechanism of antibody-mediated tissue injury is important in hypersensitivity diseases (Chapter 18). Knockout mice lacking the ligand-binding chain of FcγRI, or the signal-transducing FcR γ chain, are defective in antibody-mediated defense against microbes and do not develop some forms of IgG antibody–mediated tissue injury, thus demonstrating the essential role of Fc receptors in these processes.

Expression of FcγRI on macrophages is stimulated by the macrophage-activating cytokine interferon-γ (IFN-γ). The antibody isotypes that bind best to Fcγ receptors (such as IgG2a in mice) are also produced as a result of IFN-γ-mediated isotype switching of B cells. In addition, IFN-γ directly stimulates the microbicidal activities of phagocytes (see Chapter 13). Thus, IFN-γ is an excellent example of a cytokine that has multiple actions that function synergistically in one mechanism of host defense, namely, elimination of microbes by phagocytes.

The FcγRIIB Receptor

The FcγRIIB receptor is an inhibitory Fc receptor that was described earlier in the context of inhibitory signaling in B cells (Chapter 10). This receptor is expressed on many other immune cells including phagocytes and dendritic cells and has an ITIM motif in its cytoplasmic tail. In phagocytes, engagement of FcγRIIB may attenuate signaling from other activating receptors including FcγRI. One somewhat empirical, but often useful, treatment for many autoimmune diseases has been the intravenous administration of pooled human IgG (IVIG). IVIG induces the expression of FcγRIIB on phagocytes through a poorly understood mechanism and may also engage FcγRIIB to deliver inhibitory signals to phagocytes, thus dampening inflammation. An alternative mechanism by which IVIG may ameliorate disease will be discussed later in the chapter in the context of the role of FcRn, the neonatal Fc receptor, in regulating the half-life of antibodies.

Antibody-Dependent Cell-Mediated Cytotoxicity

NK cells and other leukocytes bind to antibody-coated cells by Fc receptors and destroy these cells. This process is called antibody-dependent cell-mediated cytotoxicity (ADCC) (Fig. 14–4). It was first described as a function of

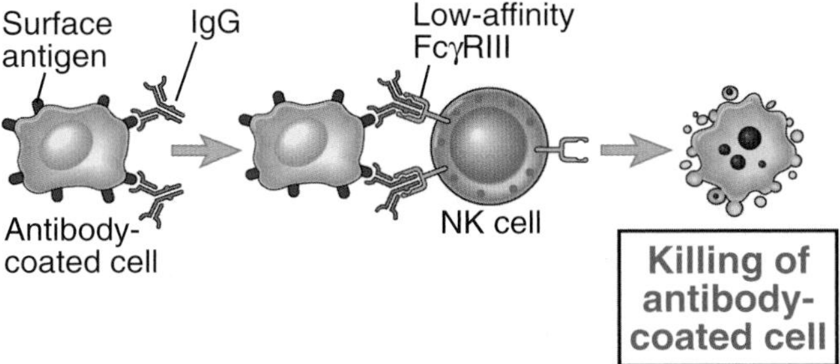

FIGURE 14–4 Antibody-dependent cell-mediated cytotoxicity. Antibodies of certain IgG subclasses bind to cells (e.g., infected cells), and the Fc regions of the bound antibodies are recognized by an Fcγ receptor on NK cells. The NK cells are activated and kill the antibody-coated cells. Presumably, NK cells can lyse even class I MHC-expressing targets when these target cells are opsonized because the Fc receptor–mediated stimulation may overcome the inhibitory actions of class I MHC-recognizing NK cell inhibitory receptors (see Chapter 12).

NK cells, which use their Fc receptor, FcγRIII, to bind to antibody-coated cells. FcγRIII/CD16 is a low-affinity receptor that binds clustered IgG molecules displayed on cell surfaces but does not bind circulating monomeric IgG. Therefore, ADCC occurs only when the target cell is coated with antibody molecules, and free IgG in plasma neither activates NK cells nor competes effectively with cell-bound IgG for binding to FcγRIII. Engagement of FcγRIII by antibody-coated target cells activates the NK cells to synthesize and secrete cytokines such as IFN-γ as well as to discharge the contents of their granules, which mediate the killing functions of this cell type (see Chapter 2). ADCC can be readily demonstrated in vitro, but its role in host defense against microbes is not definitively established.

Antibody Mediated Clearance of Helminths

Antibodies, mast cells, and eosinophils work together to mediate the expulsion and killing of some helminthic parasites. Helminths (worms) are too large to be engulfed by phagocytes, and their integuments are relatively resistant to the microbicidal products of neutrophils and macrophages. They can, however, be killed by a toxic cationic protein, known as the major basic protein, present in the granules of eosinophils. IgG and IgA antibodies that coat helminths can bind to Fc receptors on eosinophils and cause the degranulation of these cells, releasing the basic protein and other eosinophil granule contents that kill the parasites. In addition, IgE antibodies that recognize antigens on the surface of the helminths may initiate local mast cell degranulation via the high affinity IgE receptor (see Box 14–1 and Chapter 19). Mast cell mediators may contribute to bronchoconstriction, and increased local motility contributing to the expulsion of worms from sites such as the airways and the lumen of the gastrointestinal tract. Chemokines and cytokines released by activated mast cells may attract eosinophils and cause their degranulation as well. Eosinophils may also bind, via Fcε receptors, to IgE attached to parasites. However, the Fcε receptor of human eosinophils appears to lack the β chain, which is required for signaling. Therefore, IgE can bind to eosinophils but cannot activate these cells.

The Complement System

The complement system is one of the major effector mechanisms of humoral immunity and is also an important effector mechanism of innate immunity. We briefly discussed the role of complement in innate immunity in Chapter 2. Here we describe the activation and regulation of complement in more detail.

The name of the complement system is derived from experiments performed by Jules Bordet shortly after the discovery of antibodies. He demonstrated that if fresh serum containing an antibacterial antibody was added to the bacteria at physiologic temperature (37°C), the bacteria were lysed. If, however, the serum was heated to 56°C or more, it lost its lytic capacity. This loss of lytic capacity was not due to decay of antibody activity, because antibodies are relatively heat stable, and even heated serum was capable of agglutinating the bacteria. Bordet concluded that the serum must contain another heat-labile component that assists, or *complements,* the lytic function of antibodies, and this component was later given the name complement.

The complement system consists of serum and cell surface proteins that interact with one another and with other molecules of the immune system in a highly regulated manner to generate products that function to eliminate microbes. Complement proteins are plasma proteins that are normally inactive; they are activated only under particular conditions to generate products that mediate various effector functions of complement. Several features of complement activation are essential for its normal function.

- ***Activation of complement involves the sequential proteolysis of proteins to generate newly assembled enzyme complexes with proteolytic activity.*** Proteins that acquire proteolytic enzymatic activity by the action of other proteases are called zymogens. The process of sequential zymogen activation, a defining characteristic of a proteolytic enzyme cascade, is also characteristic of the coagulation and kinin systems. Proteolytic cascades allow tremendous amplification because each enzyme molecule activated at one step can generate multiple activated enzyme molecules at the next step.
- ***The products of complement activation become covalently attached to microbial cell surfaces or to antibodies bound to microbes and to other antigens.*** In the fluid phase, complement proteins are inactive or only transiently active (for seconds), and they become stably activated after they are attached to microbes or to antibodies. Many of the biologically active cleavage products of complement proteins also bind covalently to microbes, antibodies, and tissues in which the complement is activated. This characteristic ensures that the full activation and therefore the biologic functions

of the complement system are limited to microbial cell surfaces or to sites of antibodies bound to antigens and do not occur in the blood.

- ***Complement activation is inhibited by regulatory proteins that are present on normal host cells and absent from microbes.*** The regulatory proteins are an adaptation of normal cells that minimize complement-mediated damage to host cells. Microbes lack these regulatory proteins, which allows complement activation to occur on microbial surfaces.

Pathways of Complement Activation

There are three major pathways of complement activation: the classical pathway, which is activated by certain isotypes of antibodies bound to antigens; the alternative pathway, which is activated on microbial cell surfaces in the absence of antibody; and the lectin pathway, which is activated by a plasma lectin that binds to mannose residues on microbes (Fig. 14–5). The names *classical* and *alternative* arose because the classical pathway was discovered and characterized first, but the alternative pathway is phylogenetically older. Although the pathways of complement activation differ in how they are initiated, all of them result in the generation of enzyme complexes that are able to cleave the most abundant complement protein, C3. The alternative and lectin pathways are effector mechanisms of innate immunity, whereas the classical pathway is a major component of adaptive humoral immunity.

The central event in complement activation is proteolysis of the complement protein C3 to generate biologically active products and the subsequent covalent attachment of a product of C3, called C3b, to microbial cell surfaces or to antibody bound to antigen (see Fig. 14–5). Complement activation depends on the generation of two proteolytic complexes, the C3 convertase that cleaves C3 into two proteolytic fragments called C3a and C3b, and the C5 convertase that cleaves C5 into C5a and C5b. By convention, the proteolytic products of each complement protein are identified by lowercase letter suffixes, a referring to the smaller product and b to the larger one.

C3b becomes covalently attached to the microbial cell surface or to the antibody molecules at the site of complement activation. All the biologic functions of complement are dependent on the proteolytic cleavage of C3. For example, complement activation promotes phagocytosis because leukocytes and certain fixed macrophage populations express receptors for C3b. Peptides produced by proteolysis of C3 (and other complement proteins) stimulate inflammation. The C5 convertase assembles after the prior generation of C3b, and this latter convertase contributes both to inflammation (by the generation of the C5a fragment) and to the formation of pores in the membranes of microbial targets. The pathways of complement activation differ in how C3b is produced, but follow a common sequence of reactions after the cleavage of C5.

With this background, we proceed to more detailed descriptions of the alternative, classical, and lectin pathways.

The Alternative Pathway

The alternative pathway of complement activation results in the proteolysis of C3 and the stable attachment of its breakdown product C3b to microbial surfaces, without a role for antibody (Fig. 14–6 and Table 14–3). The C3 protein contains a reactive thioester bond that is buried in a relatively large domain known as the thioester domain. When C3 is cleaved, the C3b protein undergoes a major conformational change and the thioester domain flips out exposing the previously hidden reactive thioester bond. Normally, C3 in plasma is being continuously cleaved at a low rate to generate C3b in a process that is called C3 tickover. A small amount of the C3b may become covalently attached to the surfaces of cells, including microbes, via the thioester bond that reacts with the amino or hydroxyl groups of cell surface proteins or polysaccharides to form amide or ester bonds (Fig. 14–7). If these bonds are not formed, the C3b remains in the fluid phase, and the exposed and reactive thioester bond is quickly hydrolyzed, rendering the protein inactive. As a result, further complement activation cannot proceed.

When C3b undergoes its very dramatic post cleavage conformational change causing the extrusion of the thioester domain (this domain undergoes a massive shift of about 85 A^0), a binding site for a plasma protein called **factor B** is also exposed on the C3b protein that is now covalently tethered to the surface of a microbial or host cell. Bound factor B is in turn cleaved by a plasma serine protease called **factor D**, releasing a small fragment called Ba and generating a larger fragment called Bb that remains attached to C3b. The C3bBb complex is the **alternative pathway C3 convertase,** and it functions to cleave more C3 molecules, thus setting up an amplification sequence. Even when C3b is generated by the classical pathway, it can form a complex with Bb, and this complex is able to cleave more C3. Thus, the alternative pathway C3 convertase functions to amplify complement activation when it is initiated by the alternative, classical, or lectin pathways. When C3 is broken down and C3b remains attached to cells, C3a is released, and it has several biologic activities that are discussed later in this chapter.

Stable alternative pathway activation occurs on microbial cell surfaces and not on mammalian cells. If the C3bBb complex is formed on mammalian cells, it is rapidly degraded and the reaction is terminated by the action of several regulatory proteins present on these cells (discussed later in this chapter). Lack of the regulatory proteins on microbial cells allows binding and activation of the alternative pathway C3 convertase. In addition, another protein of the alternative pathway, called **properdin**, can bind to and stabilize the C3bBb complex, and the attachment of properdin is favored on microbial as opposed to normal host

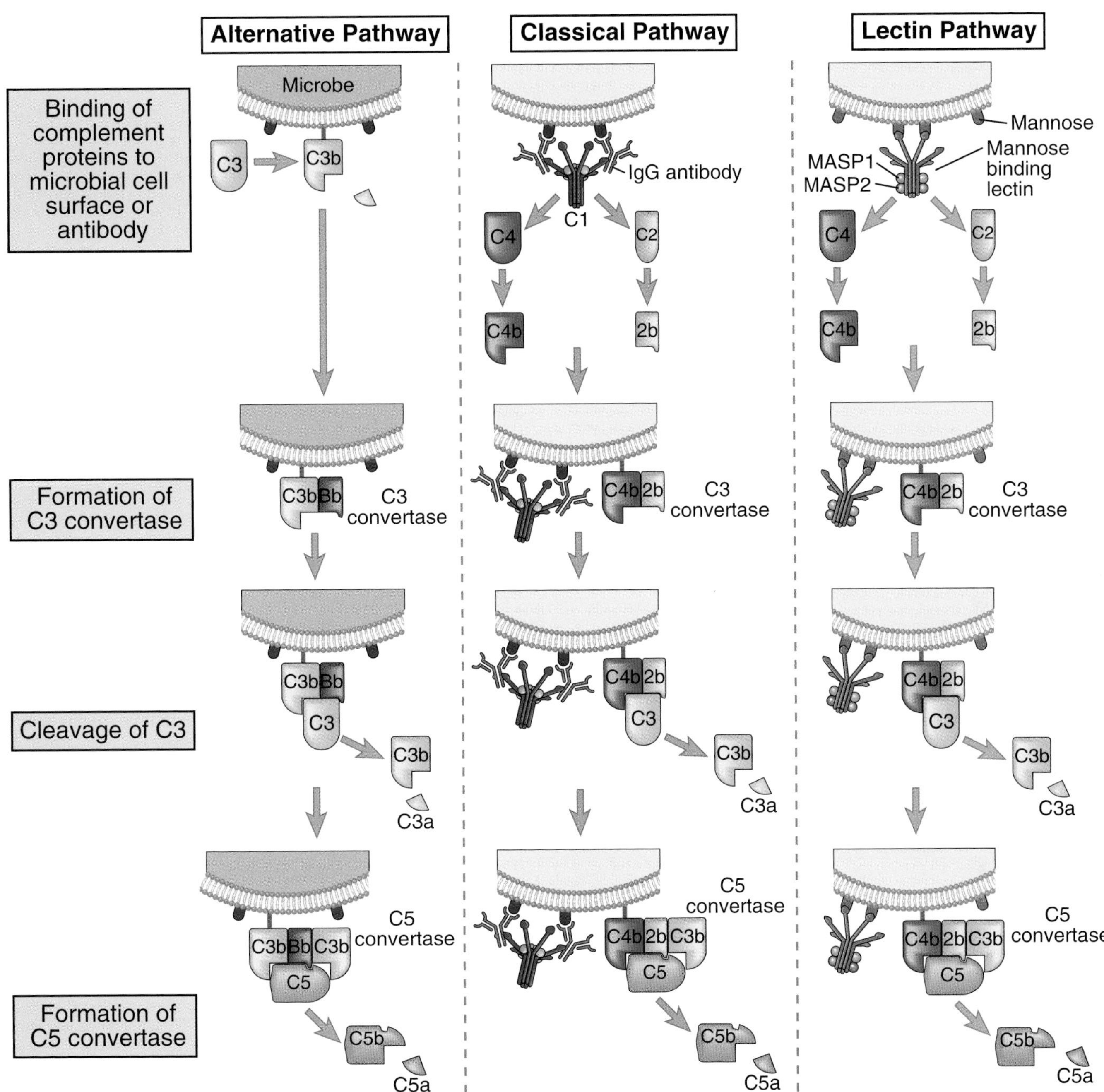

FIGURE 14–5 The early steps of complement activation by the alternative and classical pathways. The alternative pathway is activated by C3b binding to various activating surfaces, such as microbial cell walls, the classical pathway is initiated by C1 binding to antigen-antibody complexes, and the lectin pathway is activated by binding of a plasma lectin to microbes. The C3b that is generated by the action of the C3 convertase binds to the microbial cell surface or the antibody and becomes a component of the enzyme that cleaves C5 (C5 convertase) and initiates the late steps of complement activation. The late steps of all three pathways are the same (not shown here), and complement activated by all three pathways serves the same functions.

cells. Properdin is the only known positive regulator of complement.

Some of the C3b molecules generated by the alternative pathway C3 convertase bind to the convertase itself. This results in the formation of a complex containing one Bb moiety and two molecules of C3b, which functions as the **alternative pathway C5 convertase** that will cleave C5 and initiate the late steps of complement activation.

The Classical Pathway

The classical pathway is initiated by binding of the complement protein C1 to the C_H2 domains of IgG or the C_H3 domains of IgM molecules that have bound antigen (Fig. 14–8 and Table 14–4). Among IgG antibodies, IgG3 and IgG1 (in humans) are more efficient activators of complement than are other subclasses. C1 is a large, multimeric, protein complex composed of C1q, C1r, and C1s

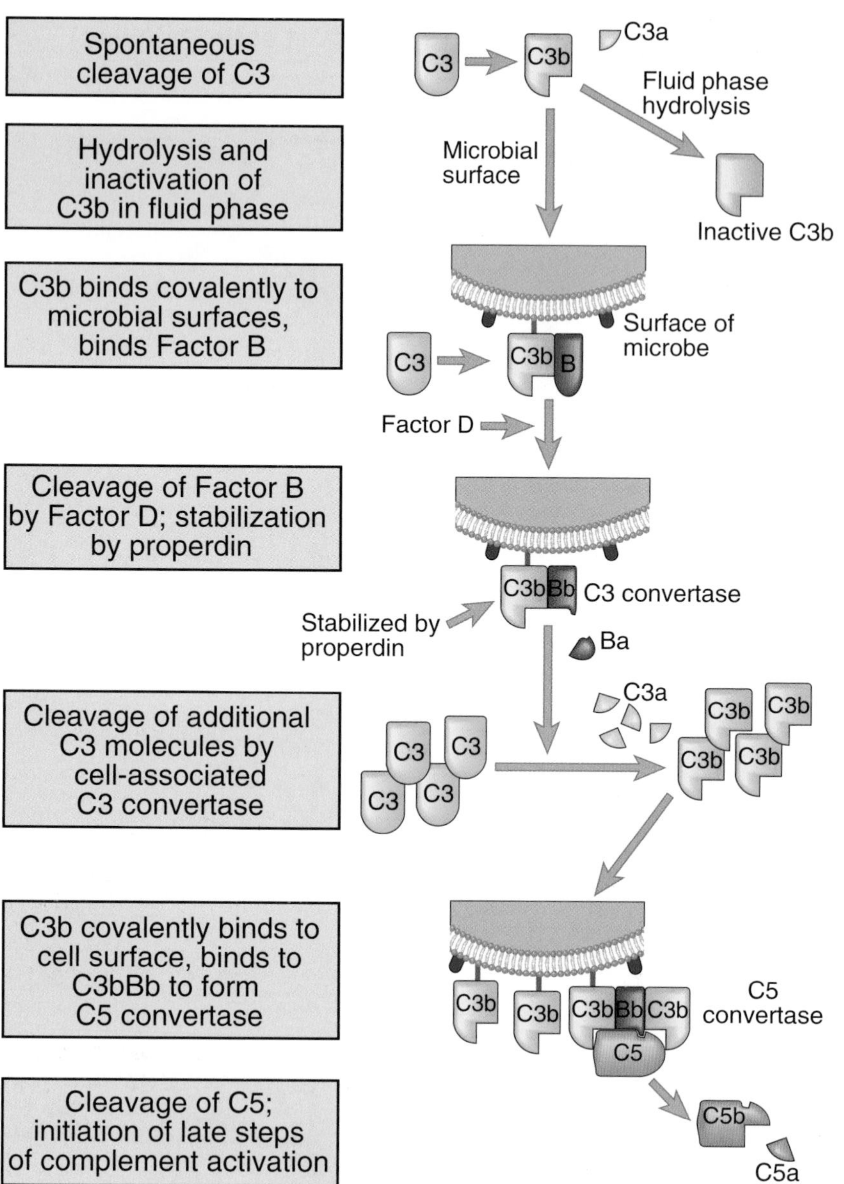
Spontaneous cleavage of C3
Hydrolysis and inactivation of C3b in fluid phase
C3b binds covalently to microbial surfaces, binds Factor B
Cleavage of Factor B by Factor D; stabilization by properdin
Cleavage of additional C3 molecules by cell-associated C3 convertase
C3b covalently binds to cell surface, binds to C3bBb to form C5 convertase
Cleavage of C5; initiation of late steps of complement activation
C3
C3b
C3a
Fluid phase hydrolysis
Microbial surface
Inactive C3b
Surface of microbe
B
Factor D
C3 convertase
Stabilized by properdin
Bb
Ba
C5 convertase
C5
C5b
C5a

FIGURE 14–6 The alternative pathway of complement activation. Soluble C3 in plasma undergoes slow spontaneous hydrolysis of its internal thioester bond, which leads to the formation of a fluid-phase C3 convertase (not shown) and the generation of C3b. If the C3b is deposited on the surfaces of microbes, it binds factor B and forms the alternative pathway C3 convertase. This convertase cleaves C3 to produce more C3b, which binds to the microbial surface and participates in the formation of a C5 convertase. The C5 convertase cleaves C5 to generate C5b, the initiating event in the late steps of complement activation.

Table 14–3. Proteins of the Alternative Pathway of Complement

Protein	Structure	Serum concentration (μg/mL)	Function
C3	185-kD (α-subunit, 110-kD; β-subunit, 75-kD)	1000-1200	C3b binds to the surface of the microbe, where it functions as an opsonin and as a component of C3 and C5 convertases C3a stimulates inflammation (anaphylatoxin)
Factor B	93-kD monomer	200	Bb is a serine protease and the active enzyme of the C3 and C5 convertases
Factor D	25-kD monomer	1-2	Plasma serine protease, cleaves factor B when it is bound to C3b
Properdin	Composed of up to four 56-kD subunits	25	Stabilizes C3 convertases (C3bBb) on microbial surfaces

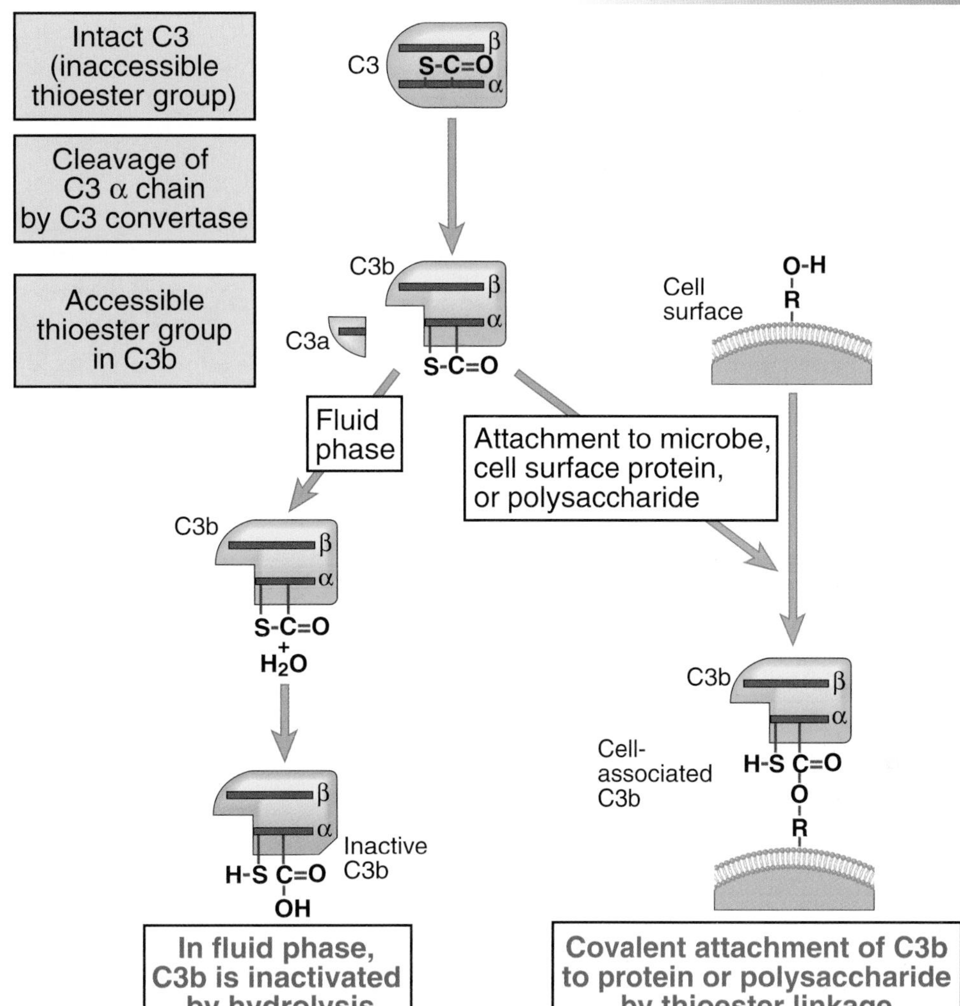

FIGURE 14–7 Internal thioester bonds of C3 molecules. A schematic view of the internal thioester groups in C3 and their role in forming covalent bonds with other molecules is shown. Proteolytic cleavage of the α chain of C3 converts it into a metastable form in which the internal thioester bonds are exposed and susceptible to nucleophilic attack by oxygen (as shown) or nitrogen atoms. The result is the formation of covalent bonds with proteins or carbohydrates on the cell surfaces. C4 is structurally homologous to C3 and has an identical thioester group.

subunits; C1q binds to the antibody, and C1r and C1s are proteases. The C1q subunit is made up of an umbrella-like radial array of six chains, each of which has a globular head connected by a collagen-like arm to a central stalk (Fig. 14–9). This hexamer performs the recognition function of the molecule and binds specifically to the Fc regions of μ and some γ heavy chains. Each Ig Fc region has a single C1q-binding site, and each C1q molecule must bind to at least two Ig heavy chains to be activated. This requirement explains why antibodies bound to antigens, and not free circulating antibodies, can initiate classical pathway activation (Fig. 14–10). Because each IgG molecule has only one Fc region, multiple IgG molecules must be brought close together before C1q can bind, and multiple IgG antibodies are brought together only when they bind to a multivalent antigen. Even though free (circulating) IgM is pentameric, it does not bind C1q, because the Fc regions of free IgM are in a planar configuration that is inaccessible to C1q. Binding of the IgM to an antigen induces a conformational change into a "staple" form that exposes the C1q binding sites in the Fc regions and allows C1q to bind. Because of its pentameric structure, a single molecule of IgM can bind two C1q molecules, and this is one reason that IgM is a more efficient complement-binding (also called complement-fixing) antibody than IgG is.

C1r and C1s are serine proteases that form a tetramer containing two molecules of each protein. Binding of two or more of the globular heads of C1q to the Fc regions of IgG or IgM leads to enzymatic activation of the associated C1r, which cleaves and activates C1s (see Fig. 14–8). Activated C1s cleaves the next protein in the cascade, C4, to generate C4b. (The smaller C4a fragment is released and has biologic activities that are described later.) C4 is homologous to C3, and C4b contains an internal thioester bond, similar to that in C3b, that forms covalent amide or ester linkages with the antigen-antibody complex or with the adjacent surface of a cell to which the antibody is bound. This attachment of C4b ensures that classical pathway activation proceeds on a cell surface or immune complex. The next complement protein, C2, then complexes with the cell surface-bound C4b and is cleaved by a nearby C1s molecule to generate a soluble C2a fragment of unknown importance and a larger C2b fragment that remains physically associated with C4b on the cell surface. (Note that in older texts, the smaller fragment is called C2b and the larger one is called C2a for historical reasons.) The resulting C4b2b complex is the **classical pathway C3 convertase**; it has the ability to bind to and proteolytically cleave C3. Binding of this enzyme complex to C3 is mediated by the C4b component, and proteolysis is catalyzed by the C2b

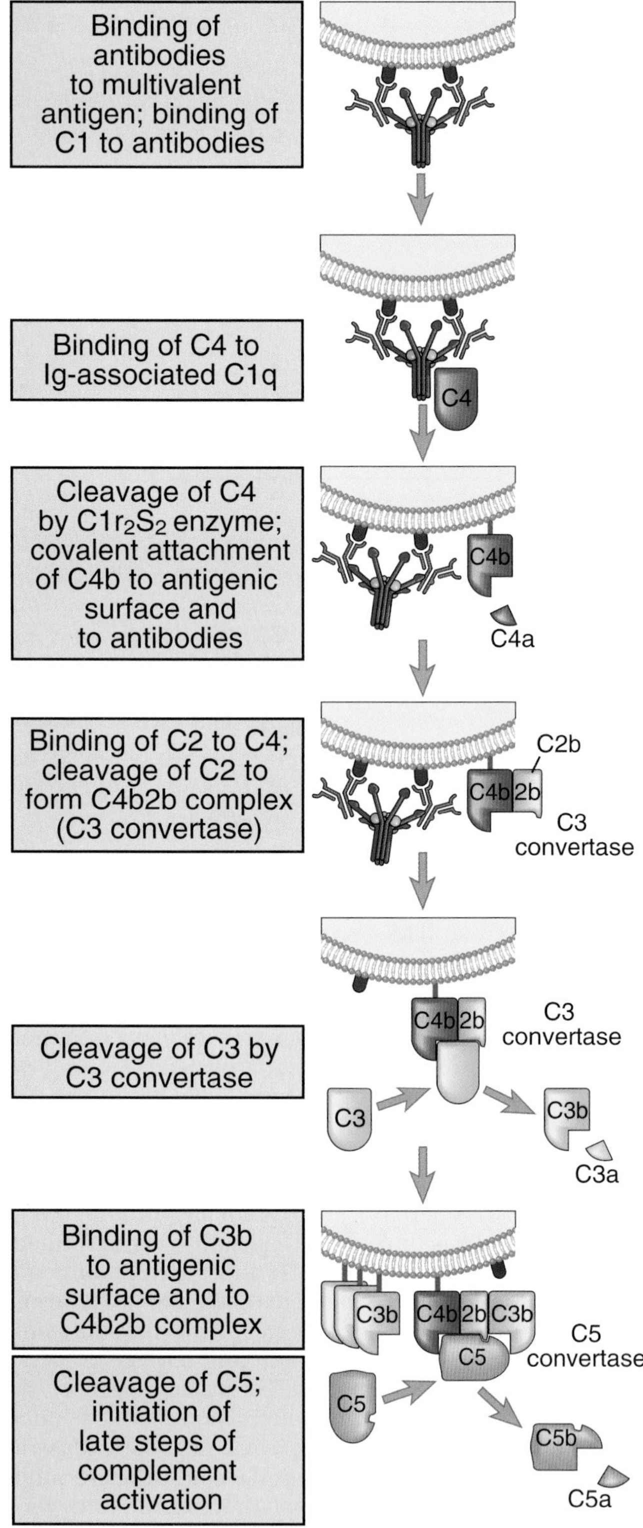

FIGURE 14–8 The classical pathway of complement activation. Antigen-antibody complexes that activate the classical pathway may be soluble, fixed on the surface of cells (as shown), or deposited on extracellular matrices. The classical pathway is initiated by the binding of C1 to antigen-complexed antibody molecules, which leads to the production of C3 and C5 convertases attached to the surfaces where the antibody was deposited. The C5 convertase cleaves C5 to begin the late steps of complement activation.

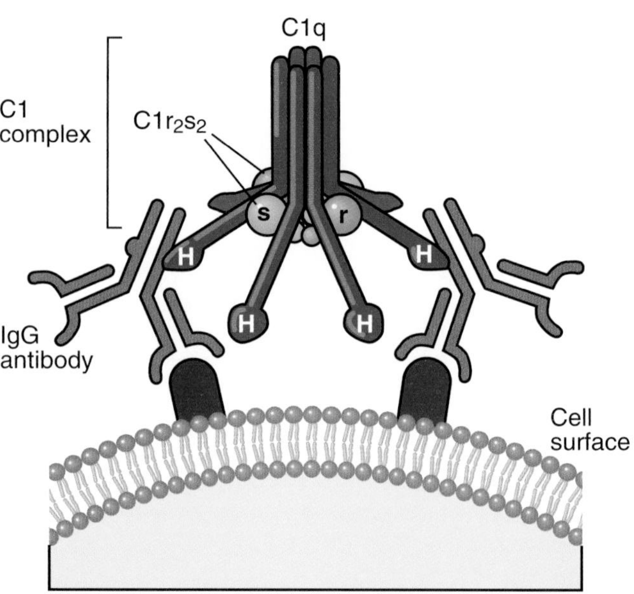

FIGURE 14–9 Structure of C1. C1q consists of six identical subunits arranged to form a central core and symmetrically projecting radial arms. The globular heads at the end of each arm, designated H, are the contact regions for immunoglobulin. C1r and C1s form a tetramer composed of two C1r and two C1s molecules. The ends of C1r and C1s contain the catalytic domains of these proteins. One $C1r_2s_2$ tetramer wraps around the radial arms of the C1q complex in a manner that juxtaposes the catalytic domains of C1r and C1s.

component. Cleavage of C3 results in the removal of the small C3a fragment, and C3b can form covalent bonds with cell surfaces or with the antibody where complement activation was initiated. Once C3b is deposited, it can bind factor B and generate more C3 convertase by the alternative pathway, as discussed before. The net effect of the multiple enzymatic steps and amplification is that a single molecule of C3 convertase can lead to the deposition of hundreds or thousands of molecules of C3b on the cell surface where complement is activated. The key early steps of the alternative and classical pathways are analogous: C3 in the alternative pathway is homologous to C4 in the classical pathway, and factor B is homologous to C2.

Some of the C3b molecules generated by the classical pathway C3 convertase bind to the convertase (as in the alternative pathway) and form a C4b2b3b complex. This complex functions as the **classical pathway C5 convertase;** it cleaves C5 and initiates the late steps of complement activation.

An unusual antibody-independent variant form of the classical pathway has been described in the context of pneumococcal infections. Splenic marginal zone macrophages express a cell surface C-type lectin called **SIGN-R1** that can recognize the pneumococcal polysaccharide and that can also bind C1q. Multivalent binding of whole bacteria or the polysaccharide to SIGN-R1 activates the classical pathway and permits the eventual coating, in a C4-dependent manner, of the pneumococcal polysaccharide with C3b. This is an example of a cell

Table 14–4. Proteins of the Classical Pathway of Complement

Protein	Structure	Serum concentration (μg/mL)	Function
C1 ($C1qr_2s_2$)	750-kD		Initiates the classical pathway
C1q	460-kD; hexamer of three pairs of chains (22, 23, 24-kD)	75–150	Binds to the Fc portion of antibody that has bound antigen, to apoptotic cells, and to cationic surfaces
C1r	85-kD dimer	50	Serine protease, cleaves C1s to make it an active protease
C1s	85-kD dimer	50	Serine protease, cleaves C4 and C2
C4	210-kD, trimer of 97-, 75-, and 33-kD chains	300–600	C4b covalently binds to the surface of a microbe or cell, where antibody is bound and complement is activated C4b binds C2 for cleavage by C1s C4a stimulates inflammation (anaphylatoxin)
C2	102-kD monomer	20	C2b is a serine protease and functions as the active enzyme of C3 and C5 convertases to cleave C3 and C5
C3	See Table 14-3		

surface lectin that mediates activation of the classical pathway but in an antibody-independent manner.

The Lectin Pathway

The **lectin pathway** of complement activation is triggered in the absence of antibody by the binding of microbial polysaccharides to circulating lectins, such as plasma mannose (or mannan)-binding lectin (MBL), or to *N*-acetylglucosamine recognizing lectins known as ficolins. These soluble lectins are members of the collectin family and structurally resemble C1q (see Chapter 2). MBL binds to mannose residues on polysaccharides, and also binds to MBL-associated serine proteases (MASPs) such as MASP-1, MASP-2, and MASP-3. Higher-order oligomers of MBL typically associate with MASP-2 and MASP-3. These two proteases form a tetrameric complex similar to the one formed by C1r and C1s, and MASP-2 cleaves C4 and C2. Subsequent events in this pathway are identical to those that occur in the classical pathway.

Late Steps of Complement Activation

C5 convertases generated by the alternative, classical, or lectin pathway initiate activation of the late components of the complement system, which culminates in formation of the cytocidal membrane attack complex (MAC) (Table 14–5 and Fig. 14–11). C5 convertases cleave C5 into a small C5a fragment that is released and a two-chain C5b fragment that remains bound to the complement proteins deposited on the cell surface. C5a has potent biologic effects on several cells that are discussed later in this chapter. The remaining components of the complement cascade, C6, C7, C8, and C9, are structurally related proteins without enzymatic activity. C5b transiently maintains a conformation capable of binding the next proteins in the cascade, C6 and C7. The C7 component of the resulting C5b,6,7 complex is hydrophobic, and it inserts into the lipid bilayer of cell membranes, where it becomes a high-affinity receptor for the C8 molecule. The C8 protein is a trimer composed of three distinct chains, one of which binds to the C5b,6,7 complex and forms a covalent heterodimer with a second chain; the third chain inserts into the lipid bilayer of the membrane. This stably inserted C5b,6,7,8 complex (C5b-8) has a limited ability to lyse cells. The formation of a fully active MAC is accomplished by the binding of C9, the final component of the complement cascades, to the C5b-8 complex. C9 is a serum protein that polymerizes at the site of the bound C5b-8 to form pores in plasma membranes. These pores are about

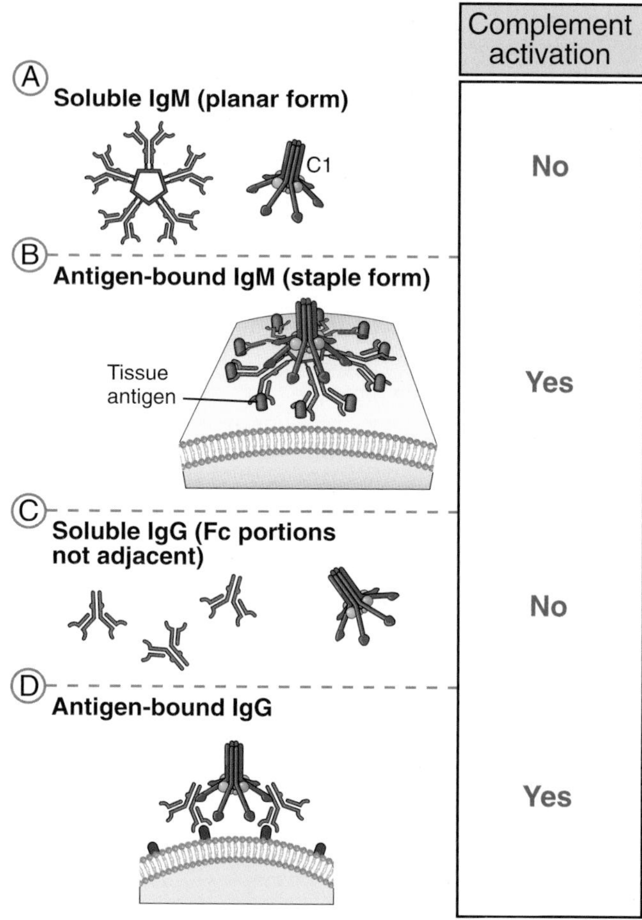

FIGURE 14–10 C1 binding to the Fc portions of IgM and IgG. C1 must bind to two or more Fc portions to initiate the complement cascade. The Fc portions of soluble pentameric IgM are not accessible to C1 (A). After IgM binds to surface-bound antigens, it undergoes a shape change that permits C1 binding and activation (B). Soluble IgG molecules will also not activate C1 because each IgG has only one Fc region (C), but after binding to cell surface antigens, adjacent IgG Fc portions can bind and activate C1 (D).

100 Å in diameter, and they form channels that allow free movement of water and ions (Fig. 14–12). The entry of water results in osmotic swelling and rupture of the cells on whose surface the MAC is deposited. The pores formed by polymerized C9 are similar to the membrane pores formed by perforin, the cytolytic granule protein found in cytotoxic T lymphocytes (CTLs) and NK cells (see Chapter 13), and C9 is structurally homologous to perforin.

Receptors for Complement Proteins

Many of the biologic activities of the complement system are mediated by the binding of complement fragments to membrane receptors expressed on various cell types. The best characterized of these receptors are specific for fragments of C3 and are described here (Table 14–6). Other receptors include those for C3a, C4a, and C5a, which stimulate inflammation, and some that regulate complement activation.

The type 1 complement receptor (CR1, or CD35) functions mainly to promote phagocytosis of C3b- and C4b-coated particles and clearance of immune complexes from the circulation. CR1 is a high-affinity receptor for C3b and C4b. It is expressed mainly on blood cells, including erythrocytes, neutrophils, monocytes, eosinophils, and T and B lymphocytes; it is also found on follicular dendritic cells in the follicles of peripheral lymphoid organs. Phagocytes use this receptor to bind and internalize particles opsonized with C3b or C4b. The binding of C3b- or C4b-coated particles to CR1 also transduces signals that activate the microbicidal mechanisms of the phagocytes, especially when the Fcγ receptor is simultaneously engaged by antibody-coated particles. CR1 on erythrocytes binds circulating immune complexes with attached C3b and C4b and transports the complexes to the liver and spleen. Here, the immune complexes are removed from the erythro-

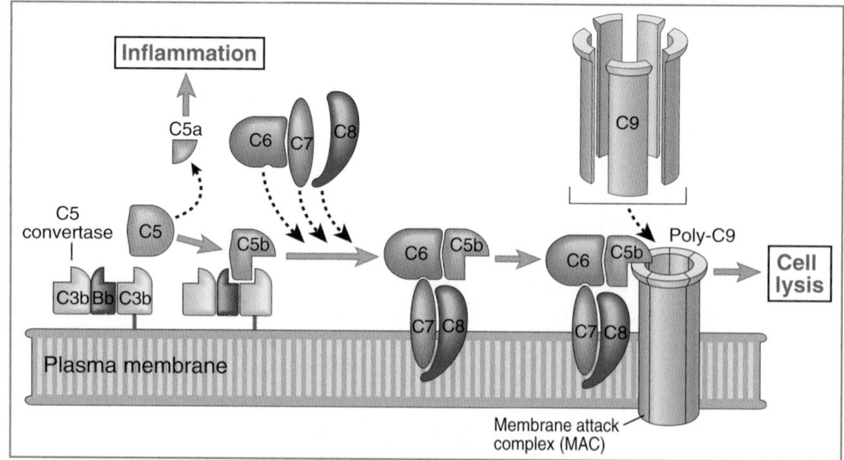

FIGURE 14–11 Late steps of complement activation and formation of the MAC. A schematic view of the cell surface events leading to formation of the MAC is shown. Cell-associated C5 convertase cleaves C5 and generates C5b, which becomes bound to the convertase. C6 and C7 bind sequentially, and the C5b,6,7 complex becomes directly inserted into the lipid bilayer of the plasma membrane, followed by stable insertion of C8. Up to 15 C9 molecules may then polymerize around the complex to form the MAC, which creates pores in the membrane and induces cell lysis. C5a released on proteolysis of C5 stimulates inflammation.

Table 14–5. Proteins of the Late Steps of Complement Activation

Protein	Structure	Serum concentration (μg/mL)	Function
C5	190-kD dimer of 115- and 75- kD chains	80	C5b initiates assembly of the membrane attack complex C5a stimulates inflammation (anaphylatoxin)
C6	110-kD monomer	45	Component of the MAC: binds to C5b and accepts C7
C7	100-kD monomer	90	Component of the MAC: binds to C5b,6 and inserts into lipid membranes
C8	155-kD trimer of 64-, 64-, 22-kD chains	60	Component of the MAC: binds to C5b,6,7 and initiates the binding and polymerization of C9
C9	79-kD monomer	60	Component of the MAC: binds to C5b,6,7,8 and polymerizes to form membrane pores

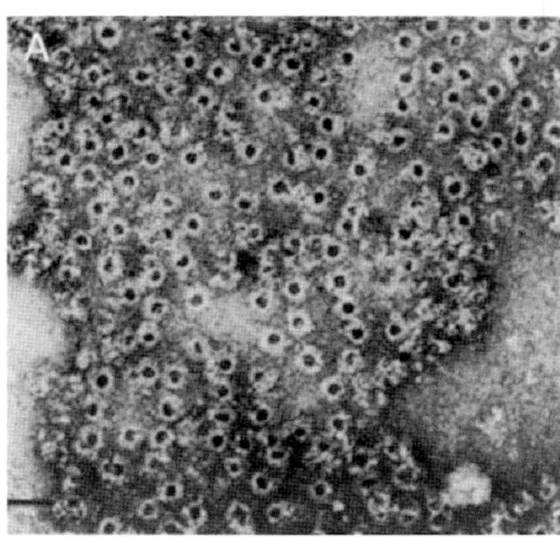

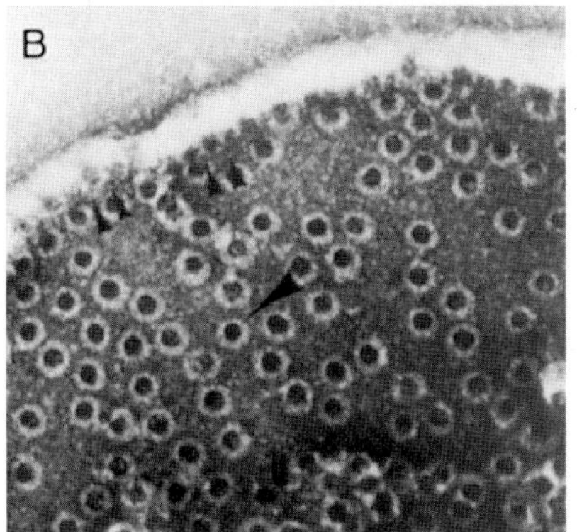

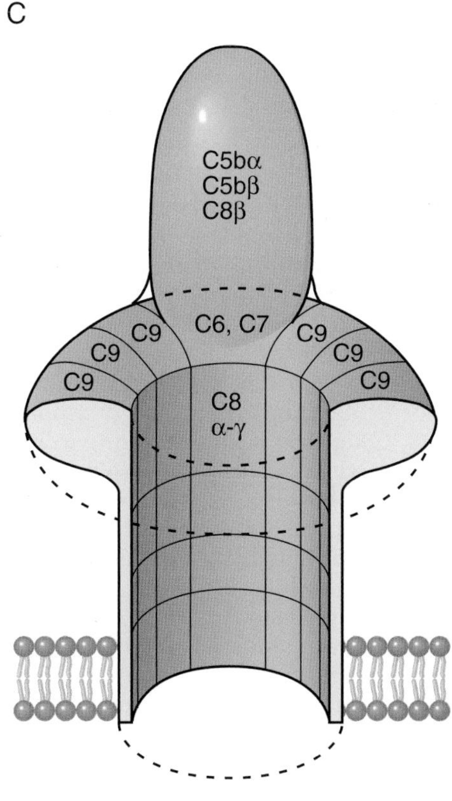

FIGURE 14–12 Structure of the MAC in cell membranes. A. Complement lesions in erythrocyte membranes are shown in this electron micrograph. The lesions consist of holes approximately 100 Å in diameter that are formed by poly-C9 tubular complexes. B. For comparison, membrane lesions induced on a target cell by a cloned CTL line are shown in this electron micrograph. The lesions appear morphologically similar to complement-mediated lesions, except for a larger internal diameter (160 Å). CTL- and NK cell–induced membrane lesions are formed by tubular complexes of a polymerized protein (perforin), which is homologous to C9 (see Chapter 13). C. A model of the subunit arrangement of the MAC is shown. The transmembrane region consists of 12 to 15 C9 molecules arranged as a tubule, in addition to single molecules of C6, C7, and C8 α and γ chains. The C5bα, C5bß, and C8ß chains form an appendage that projects above the transmembrane pore. (From Podack ER. Molecular mechanisms of cytolysis by complement and cytolytic lymphocytes. Journal of Cellular Biochemistry 30:133–170, 1986. Copyright 1986 Wiley-Liss. Reprinted by permission of Wiley-Liss, Inc., a subsidiary of John Wiley & Sons, Inc.)

Table 14–6. Receptors for Fragments of C3

Receptor	Structure	Ligands	Cell distribution	Function
Type 1 complement receptor (CR1, CD35)	160-250 kD; multiple CCPRs	C3b > C4b > iC3b	Mononuclear phagocytes, neutrophils, B and T cells, erythrocytes, eosinophils, FDCs	Phagocytosis Clearance of immune complexes Promotes dissociation of C3 convertases by acting as cofactor for cleavage of C3b,C4b
Type 2 complement receptor (CR2, CD21)	145-kD; multiple CCPRs	C3d, C3dg > iC3b	B lymphocytes, FDCs, nasopharyngeal epithelium	Coreceptor for B cell activation Trapping of antigens in germinal centers Receptor for EBV
Type 3 complement receptor (CR3, Mac-1, CD11b/ CD18)	Integrin, with 165-kD α chain and 95-kD β2 chain	iC3b, ICAM-1; also binds microbes	Mononuclear phagocytes, neutrophils, NK cells	Phagocytosis Leukocyte adhesion to endothelium (via ICAM-1)
Type 4 complement receptor (CR4, p150/95, CD11c/CD18)	Integrin, with 150-kD α chain and 95-kD β2 chain	iC3b	Mononuclear phagocytes, neutrophils, NK cells	Phagocytosis, cell adhesion?

Abbreviations: CCPR, complement control protein repeat; FDC, follicular dendritic cell; ICAM-1, intercellular adhesion molecule-1.

cyte surface by phagocytes, and the erythrocytes continue to circulate. CR1 is also a regulator of complement activation (see next section).

The type 2 complement receptor (CR2, or CD21) functions to stimulate humoral immune responses by enhancing B cell activation by antigen and by promoting the trapping of antigen-antibody complexes in germinal centers. CR2 is present on B lymphocytes, follicular dendritic cells, and some epithelial cells. It specifically binds the cleavage products of C3b, called C3d, C3dg, and iC3b (i referring to inactive), which are generated by factor I–mediated proteolysis (discussed later). On B cells, CR2 is expressed as part of a trimolecular complex that includes two other noncovalently attached proteins called CD19 and target of antiproliferative antibody-1 (TAPA-1, or CD81). This complex delivers signals to B cells that enhance the responses of B cells to antigen (see Chapter 10, Fig. 10–5). On follicular dendritic cells, CR2 serves to trap iC3b- and C3dg-coated antigen-antibody complexes in germinal centers. The functions of complement in B cell activation are described later.

In humans, CR2 is the cell surface receptor for Epstein-Barr virus, a herpesvirus that causes infectious mononucleosis and is also linked to several human malignant tumors (see Chapter 17, Box 17–2). Epstein-Barr virus infects B cells and can remain latent for life.

The type 3 complement receptor, also called Mac-1 (CR3, CD11bCD18), is an integrin that functions as a receptor for the iC3b fragment generated by proteolysis of C3b. Mac-1 is expressed on neutrophils, mononuclear phagocytes, mast cells, and NK cells. It is a member of the integrin family of cell surface receptors (see Chapter 2, Box 2–3) and consists of an α chain (CD11b) noncovalently linked to a β chain (CD18) that is identical to the β chains of two closely related integrin molecules, leukocyte function–associated antigen-1 (LFA-1) and p150,95. Mac-1 on neutrophils and monocytes promotes phagocytosis of microbes opsonized with iC3b. In addition, Mac-1 may directly recognize bacteria for phagocytosis by binding to some unknown microbial molecules (see Chapter 2). It also binds to intercellular adhesion molecule-1 (ICAM-1) on endothelial cells and promotes stable attachment of the leukocytes to endothelium, even without complement activation. This binding leads to the recruitment of leukocytes to sites of infection and tissue injury.

The **type 4 complement receptor** (CR4, p150,95, CD11cCD18) is another integrin with a different α chain (CD11c) and the same β chain as Mac-1. It also binds iC3b, and the function of this receptor is probably similar to that of Mac-1. CD11c is also abundantly expressed on dendritic cells and is used as a marker for this cell type.

The **complement receptor of the immunoglobulin family** (CRIg) is expressed on the surface of macrophages in the liver known as Kupffer cells. CRIg is an integral membrane protein with an extracellular region made up of Ig domains. It binds the complement fragments C3b and iC3b, and is a major receptor for the clearance of opsonized bacteria and other blood-borne pathogens.

SIGN-R1, discussed earlier, is a cell surface C-type lectin on marginal zone macrophages that recognizes pneumococcal polysaccharides and can also bind C1q, thus mediating the efficient activation of the classical complement pathway in an antibody-independent manner. It contributes in a major way to the opsonization and clearance of pneumococci.

Regulation of Complement Activation

Activation of the complement cascade and the stability of active complement proteins are tightly regulated to prevent complement activation on normal host cells and to limit the duration of complement activation even on microbial cells and antigen-antibody complexes. Regulation of complement is mediated by several circulating and cell membrane proteins (Table 14–7). Many of these proteins, as well as several proteins of the classical and alternative pathways, belong to a family called regulators of complement activity (RCA) and are encoded by homologous genes that are located adjacent to one another in the genome.

Complement activation needs to be regulated for two reasons. First, low-level complement activation goes on spontaneously, and if such activation is allowed to proceed, the result can be damage to normal cells and tissues. Second, even when complement is activated where needed, such as on microbial cells or antigen-antibody complexes, it needs to be controlled because degradation products of complement proteins can diffuse to adjacent cells and injure them. Different regulatory mechanisms inhibit the formation of C3 convertases in the early steps of complement activation, break

Table 14–7. Regulators of Complement Activation

Receptor	Structure	Distribution	Interacts with	Function
C1 inhibitor (C1 INH)	104-kD	Plasma protein; conc. 200 μg/mL	C1r, C1s	Serine protease inhibitor; binds to C1r and C1s and dissociates them from C1q
Factor I	88-kD dimer of 50- and 38-kD subunits	Plasma protein; conc. 35 μg/mL	C4b, C3b	Serine protease; cleaves C3b and C4b by using factor H, MCP, C4BP or CR1 as cofactors
Factor H	150-kD; multiple CCPRs	Plasma protein; conc. 480 μg/mL	C3b	Binds C3b and displaces Bb Cofactor for factor I–mediated cleavage of C3b
C4-binding protein (C4BP)	570 kD; multiple CCPRs	Plasma protein; conc. 300 μg/mL	C4b	Binds C4b and displaces C2 Cofactor for factor I–mediated cleavage of C4b
Membrane cofactor for protein (MCP CD46)	45-70 kD; four CCPRs	Leukocytes, epithelial cells endothelial cells	C3b,C4b	Cofactor for factor I–mediated cleavage of C3b and C4b
Decay-accelerating factor (DAF)	70 kD; GPI linked, four CCPRs	Blood cells, endothelial cells, epithelial cells	C4b2b, C3bBb	Displaces C2b from C4b and Bb from C3b (dissociation of C3 convertases)
CD59	18 kD; GPI linked	Blood cells, endothelial cells, epithelial cells	C7, C8	Blocks C9 binding and prevents formation of the MAC

Abbreviations: CCPR, complement control protein repeat; conc., concentration; GPI, glycophosphatidylinositol; MAC, membrane attack complex.

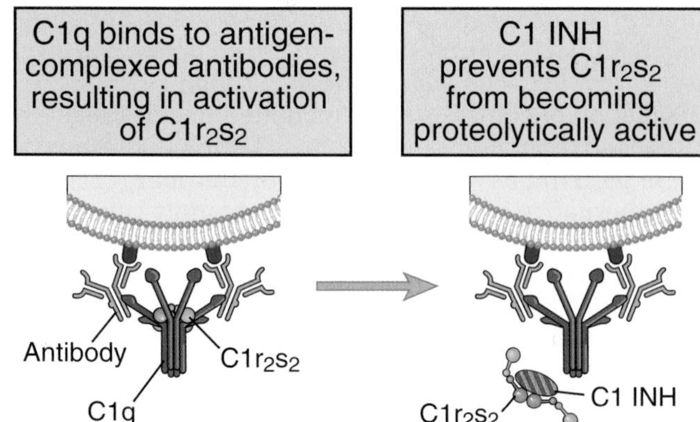
C1q binds to antigen-complexed antibodies, resulting in activation of C1r2s2
C1 INH prevents C1r2s2 from becoming proteolytically active
Antibody
C1r2s2
C1q
C1r2s2
C1 INH

FIGURE 14–13 Regulation of C1 activity by C1 INH. C1 INH displaces $C1r_2s_2$ from C1q and terminates classical pathway activation.

down and inactivate C3 and C5 convertases, and inhibit formation of the MAC in the late steps of the complement pathway.

The proteolytic activity of C1r and C1s is inhibited by a plasma protein called C1 inhibitor (C1 INH). C1 INH is a serine protease inhibitor (serpin) that mimics the normal substrates of C1r and C1s. If C1q binds to an antibody and begins the process of complement activation, C1 INH becomes a target of the enzymatic activity of the bound $C1r_2$-$C1s_2$. C1 INH is cleaved by and becomes covalently attached to these complement proteins, and as a result, the $C1r_2$-$C1s_2$ tetramer dissociates from C1q, thus stopping activation by the classical pathway (Fig. 14–13). In this way, C1 INH prevents the accumulation of enzymatically active $C1r_2$-$C1s_2$ in the plasma and limits the time for which active $C1r_2$-$C1s_2$ is available to activate subsequent steps in the complement cascade. An autosomal-dominant inherited disease called **hereditary angioneurotic edema** is due to a deficiency of C1 INH. Clinical manifestations of the disease include intermittent acute accumulation of edema fluid in the skin and mucosa, which causes abdominal pain, vomiting, diarrhea, and potentially life-threatening airway obstruction. In these patients, the plasma levels of C1 INH protein are sufficiently reduced (<20% to 30% of normal) that activation of C1 by immune complexes is not properly controlled and increased breakdown of C4 and C2 occurs. The mediators of edema formation in patients with hereditary angioneurotic edema include a proteolytic fragment of C2, called C2 kinin, and bradykinin. C1 INH is an inhibitor of other plasma serine proteases besides C1, including kallikrein and coagulation factor XII, and both activated kallikrein and factor XII can promote increased formation of bradykinin.

Assembly of the components of C3 and C5 convertases is inhibited by the binding of regulatory proteins to C3b and C4b deposited on cell surfaces (Fig. 14–14). If C3b is deposited on the surfaces of normal mammalian cells, it may be bound by several membrane proteins, including membrane cofactor protein (MCP, or CD46), type 1 complement receptor (CR1), decay-accelerating factor (DAF), and a plasma protein called factor H. C4b deposited on cell surfaces is similarly bound by DAF, CR1, and another plasma protein called C4-binding protein (C4BP). By binding to C3b or C4b, these proteins competitively inhibit the binding of other components of the C3 convertase, such as Bb of the alternative pathway and C2b of the classical pathway, thus blocking further progression of the complement cascade. (Factor H inhibits binding of only Bb to C3b and is thus a regulator of the alternative but not the classical pathway.) MCP, CR1, and DAF are produced by mammalian cells but not by microbes. Therefore, these regulators of complement selectively inhibit complement activation on host cells and allow complement activation to proceed on microbes. In addition, cell surfaces rich in sialic acid favor binding of the regulatory protein factor H over the alternative pathway protein factor B. Mammalian cells express higher levels of sialic acid than microbes do, which is another reason that complement activation is prevented on normal host cells and permitted on microbes.

DAF is a glycophosphatidylinositol-linked membrane protein expressed on endothelial cells and erythrocytes. Deficiency of an enzyme required to form such protein-lipid linkages results in failure to express many glycophosphatidylinositol-linked membrane proteins, including DAF and CD59 (see following), and causes a disease called **paroxysmal nocturnal hemoglobinuria.** This disease is characterized by recurrent bouts of intravascular hemolysis, at least partly attributable to

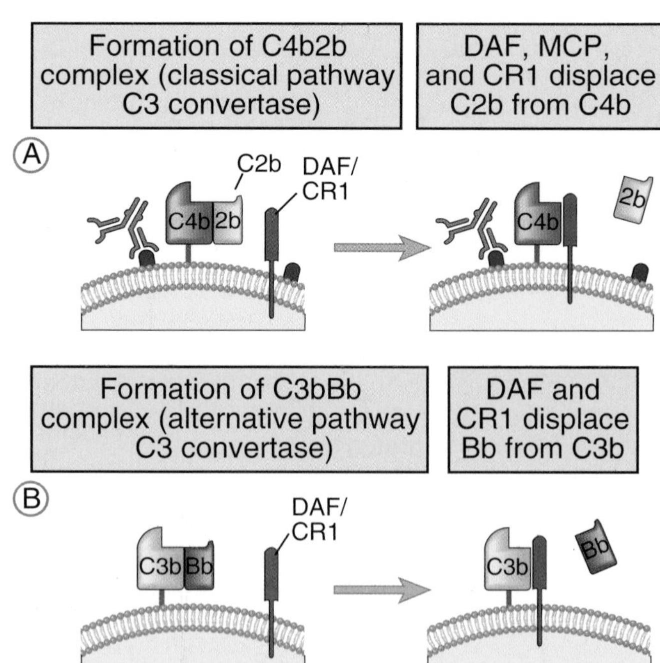
Formation of C4b2b complex (classical pathway C3 convertase)
DAF, MCP, and CR1 displace C2b from C4b
A
C2b
DAF/ CR1
C4b
2b
C4b
2b
Formation of C3bBb complex (alternative pathway C3 convertase)
DAF and CR1 displace Bb from C3b
B
DAF/ CR1
C3b
Bb
C3b
Bb

FIGURE 14–14 Inhibition of the formation of C3 convertases. Several membrane proteins present on normal cells displace either C2a from the classical pathway C3 convertase (A) or Bb from the alternative pathway C3 convertase (B) and stop complement activation.

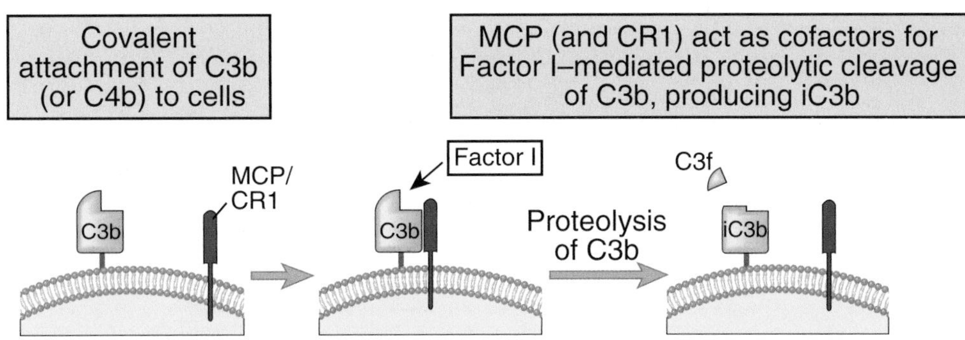

FIGURE 14–15 Factor I–mediated cleavage of C3b. In the presence of cell membrane–bound cofactors (MCP or CR1), plasma factor I proteolytically cleaves C3b attached to cell surfaces, leaving an inactive form of C3b (iC3b). Factor H and C4-binding protein can also serve as cofactors for factor I–mediated cleavage of C3b. The same process is involved in the proteolysis of C4.

unregulated complement activation on the surface of erythrocytes. Recurrent intravascular hemolysis in turn leads to chronic hemolytic anemia and venous thrombosis. An unusual feature of this disease is that the mutation in the defective gene is not inherited, but represents an acquired mutation in hematopoietic stem cells.

Cell-associated C3b is proteolytically degraded by a plasma serine protease called factor I, which is active only in the presence of regulatory proteins (Fig. 14–15). MCP, factor H, C4BP, and CR1 all serve as cofactors for factor I–mediated cleavage of C3b (and C4b). Thus, these regulatory host cell proteins promote proteolytic degradation of complement proteins; as discussed before, the same regulatory proteins cause dissociation of C3b (and C4b)-containing complexes. Factor I–mediated cleavage of C3b generates fragments called iC3b, C3d, and C3dg, which do not participate in complement activation but are recognized by receptors on phagocytes and B lymphocytes.

Formation of the MAC is inhibited by a membrane protein called CD59. CD59 is a glycophosphatidylinositol-linked protein expressed on many cell types. It works by incorporating itself into assembling MACs after the membrane insertion of C5b-8, thereby inhibiting the subsequent addition of C9 molecules (Fig. 14–16). CD59 is present on normal host cells, where it limits MAC formation, but it is not present on microbes. Formation of the MAC is also inhibited by plasma proteins such as S protein, which functions by binding to soluble C5b,6,7 complexes and thereby preventing their insertion into cell membranes near the site where the complement cascade was initiated. Growing MACs can insert into any neighboring cell membrane besides the membrane on which they were generated. Inhibitors of the MAC in the plasma and in host cell membranes ensure that lysis of innocent bystander cells does not occur near the site of complement activation.

Much of the analysis of the function of complement regulatory proteins has relied on *in vitro* experiments, and most of these experiments have focused on assays that measure MAC-mediated cell lysis as an end point. On the basis of these studies, a hierarchy of importance for inhibiting complement activation is believed to be CD59 > DAF > MCP, and this hierarchy may reflect the relative abundance of these proteins on cell surfaces.

The function of regulatory proteins may be overwhelmed by excessive activation of complement pathways. We have emphasized the importance of these regulatory proteins in preventing complement activation on normal cells. However, complement-mediated phagocytosis and damage to normal cells are important pathogenetic mechanisms in many immunologic diseases (see Chapter 18). In these diseases, large amounts of antibodies may be deposited on host cells, generating enough active complement proteins that the regulatory molecules are overwhelmed and unable to control complement activation.

Functions of Complement

The principal effector functions of the complement system in innate immunity and specific humoral immunity are to promote phagocytosis of microbes on which complement is activated, to stimulate inflammation, and to induce the lysis of these microbes. In addition, products of complement activation facilitate the activation of B lymphocytes and the production of antibodies. Phagocytosis, inflammation, and stimulation of humoral immunity are all mediated by the binding of proteolytic fragments of complement proteins to various cell surface receptors, whereas cell lysis is mediated by the MAC. In the following section, we describe each of these functions of the complement system and their role in host defense.

Opsonization and Phagocytosis

Microbes on which complement is activated by the alternative or classical pathway become coated with C3b, iC3b, or C4b and are phagocytosed by the binding of these proteins to specific receptors on macrophages and neutrophils (Fig. 14–17A). As discussed previously, activation of complement leads to the generation of C3b and iC3b covalently bound to cell surfaces. Both C3b and iC3b act as opsonins by virtue of the fact that they specifically bind to receptors on neutrophils and macrophages. C3b and C4b (the latter generated by the classical pathway only) bind to CR1, and iC3b binds to CR3 (Mac-1) and CR4. By itself, CR1 is inefficient at inducing the phagocytosis of C3b-coated microbes, but its ability to do so is enhanced if the microbes are coated with IgG antibodies that simultaneously bind to Fcγ receptors. Macrophage activation by the cytokine IFN-γ also enhances CR1-mediated phagocytosis. C3b- and

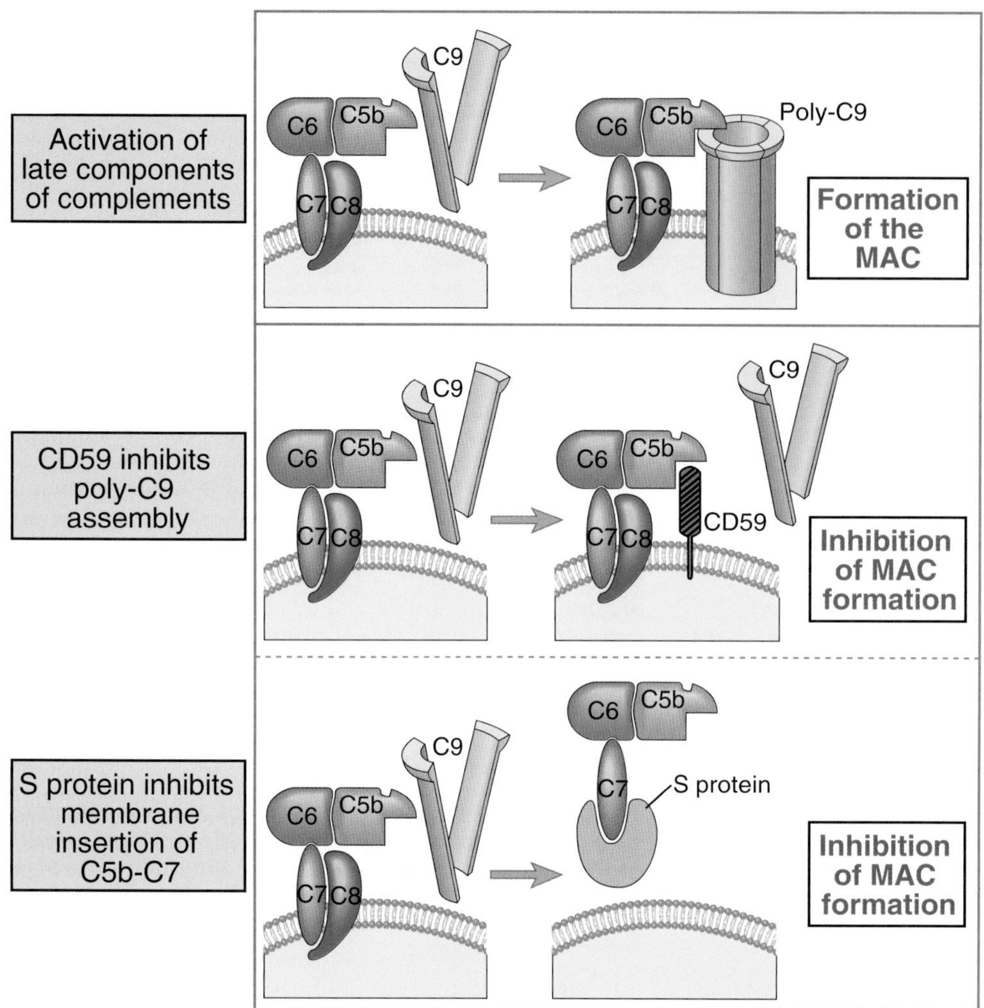

FIGURE 14–16 Regulation of formation of the MAC. The MAC is formed on cell surfaces as an end result of complement activation. The membrane protein CD59 and S protein in the plasma inhibit formation of the MAC.

iC3b-dependent phagocytosis of microorganisms is a major defense mechanism against infections in innate and adaptive immunity. One example of the importance of complement is host defense against bacteria with polysaccharide-rich capsules, such as pneumococci and meningococci, which is mediated entirely by humoral immunity. IgM antibodies against capsular polysaccharides bind to the bacteria, activate the classical pathway of complement, and cause phagocytic clearance of the bacteria in the spleen. In addition, SIGN-R1–expressing marginal zone macrophages may also bind to capsular polysaccharides and activate the classical pathway in an antibody-independent manner. This is why individuals lacking the spleen (e.g., as a result of surgical removal after traumatic rupture) are susceptible to disseminated pneumococcal and meningococcal septicemia. C3-deficient humans and mice are extremely susceptible to lethal bacterial infections.

Stimulation of Inflammatory Responses

The proteolytic complement fragments C5a, C4a, and C3a induce acute inflammation by activating mast cells and neutrophils (Fig. 14–17B). All three peptides bind to mast cells and induce degranulation, with the release of vasoactive mediators such as histamine. These peptides are also called **anaphylatoxins** because the mast cell reactions they trigger are characteristic of anaphylaxis (see Chapter 19). In neutrophils, C5a stimulates motility, firm adhesion to endothelial cells, and, at high doses, stimulation of the respiratory burst and production of reactive oxygen intermediates. In addition, C5a may act directly on vascular endothelial cells and induce increased vascular permeability and the expression of P-selectin, which promotes neutrophil binding. This combination of C5a actions on mast cells, neutrophils, and endothelial cells contributes to inflammation at sites of complement activation. C5a is the most potent mediator of mast cell degranulation, C3a is about 20-fold less potent, and C4a is about 2500-fold less. The proinflammatory effects of C5a, C4a, and C3a are mediated by binding of the peptides to specific receptors on various cell types. The C5a receptor is the most thoroughly characterized. It is a member of the seven α-helical transmembrane G-protein coupled receptor family. The C5a receptor is expressed on many cell types,

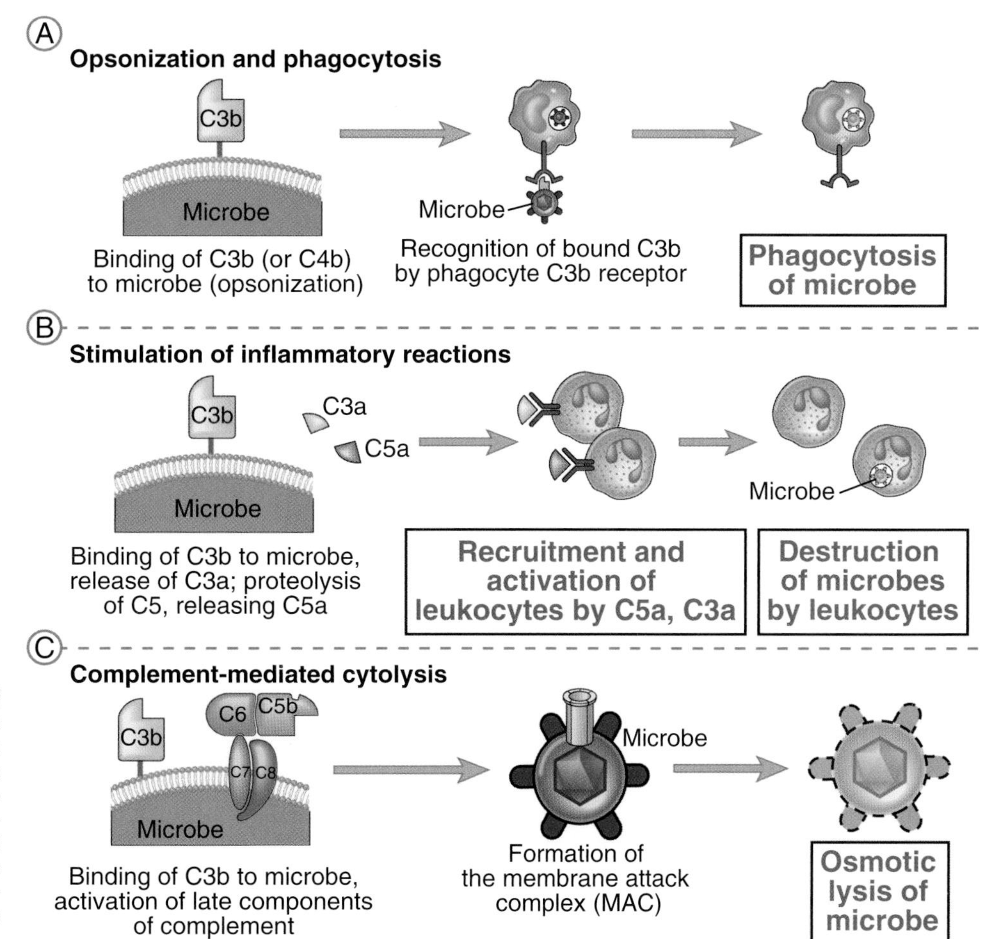

FIGURE 14–17 Functions of complement. The major functions of the complement system in host defense are shown. Cell-bound C3b is an opsonin that promotes phagocytosis of coated cells (A); the proteolytic products C5a, C3a, and (to a lesser extent) C4a stimulate leukocyte recruitment and inflammation (B); and the MAC lyses cells (C).

including neutrophils, eosinophils, basophils, monocytes, macrophages, mast cells, endothelial cells, smooth muscle cells, epithelial cells, and astrocytes. The C3a receptor is also a member of the G protein–coupled receptor family.

Complement-Mediated Cytolysis

Complement-mediated lysis of foreign organisms is mediated by the MAC (Fig. 14–17C). Most pathogens have evolved thick cell walls or capsules that impede access of the MAC to their cell membranes. Complement mediated lysis appears to be critical for defense against only a few pathogens that are unable to resist MAC insertion. Thus, genetic defects in MAC components result in increased susceptibility only to infections by bacteria of the genus *Neisseria,* all of which have very thin cell walls.

Other Functions of the Complement System

By binding to antigen-antibody complexes, complement proteins promote the solubilization of these complexes and their clearance by phagocytes. Small numbers of immune complexes are frequently formed in the circulation when an individual mounts a vigorous antibody response to a circulating antigen. If the immune complexes accumulate in the blood, they may be deposited in vessel walls and lead to inflammatory reactions that damage surrounding tissue. The formation of immune complexes may require not only the multivalent binding of Ig Fab regions to antigens but also noncovalent interactions of Fc regions of juxtaposed Ig molecules. Complement activation on Ig molecules can sterically block these Fc-Fc interactions, thereby promoting dissolution of the immune complexes. In addition, as discussed before, immune complexes with attached C3b are bound to CR1 on erythrocytes, and the complexes are cleared by phagocytes in the liver.

The C3d protein generated from C3 binds to CR2 on B cells and facilitates B cell activation and the initiation of humoral immune responses. C3d is generated when complement is activated by an antigen, either directly (e.g., when the antigen is a microbial polysaccharide) or after the binding of antibody. Complement activation results in the covalent attachment of C3b and its cleavage product C3d to the antigen. B lymphocytes can bind the antigen through their Ig receptors and simultaneously bind the attached C3d through CR2, the coreceptor for the B cell antigen receptor, thus enhancing

Box 14–2 ▪ IN DEPTH: THE COMPLEMENT SYSTEM IN DISEASE

The complement system may be involved in human disease in two general ways. First, deficiencies in any of the protein components may lead to abnormal patterns of complement activation. The absence of a component of the classical or alternative pathway or absence of the late steps may result in deficient complement activation. If regulatory components are absent, too much complement activation may occur at the wrong time or wrong site, leading to excess inflammation and cell lysis, and may also cause a deficiency in plasma complement proteins because of excessive consumption. Second, an intact, normally functioning complement system may be activated in response to abnormal stimuli such as persistent microbes, antibodies against self antigens, or immune complexes deposited in tissues. In these infectious and autoimmune diseases, the inflammatory and lytic effects of complement may significantly contribute to the pathologic changes of the disease.

COMPLEMENT DEFICIENCIES. Inherited and spontaneous deficiencies in many of the complement proteins have been described in humans.

Genetic deficiencies in classical pathway components, including C1q, C1r, C4, C2, and C3, have been described; C2 deficiency is the most commonly identified human complement deficiency. A disease that resembles the autoimmune disease systemic lupus erythematosus develops in more than 50% of patients with C2 and C4 deficiencies. The reason for this association is unknown, but defects in complement activation may lead to failure to clear circulating immune complexes. If normally generated immune complexes are not cleared from the circulation, they may be deposited in blood vessel walls and tissues, where they activate leukocytes by Fc receptor–dependent pathways and produce local inflammation. Complement may play an important role in the clearance of fragmented DNA containing apoptotic bodies. These apoptotic bodies are now considered to be key immunogens in lupus. In addition, complement proteins regulate antigen-mediated signals received by B cells; in their absence, self antigens may not induce B cell tolerance, and autoimmunity results. Somewhat surprisingly, C2 and C4 deficiencies are not usually associated with increased susceptibility to infections, which suggests that the alternative pathway and Fc receptor–mediated effector mechanisms are adequate for host defense against most microbes. Deficiency of C3 is associated with frequent serious pyogenic bacterial infections that may be fatal, illustrating the central role of C3 and its importance in opsonization, enhanced phagocytosis, and destruction of these organisms.

Deficiencies in components of the alternative pathway, including properdin and factor D, result in increased susceptibility to infection with pyogenic bacteria. C3 deficiency is mentioned above.

Mutation of the gene encoding the mannose-binding lectin (MBL) contributes to immunodeficiency in some patients; this is discussed in Chapter 20.

Deficiencies in the terminal complement components, including C5, C6, C7, C8, and C9, have also been described. Interestingly, the only consistent clinical problem in these patients is a propensity for disseminated infections by *Neisseria* bacteria, including *Neisseria meningitidis* and *Neisseria gonorrhoeae,* indicating that complement-mediated bacterial lysis is particularly important for defense against these organisms.

Deficiencies in complement regulatory proteins are associated with abnormal complement activation and a variety of related clinical abnormalities. Deficiencies in C1 inhibitor and decay-accelerating factor are mentioned in the text. In patients with factor I deficiency, plasma C3 is depleted as a result of the unregulated formation of fluid-phase C3 convertase (by the normal "tickover" mechanism). The clinical consequence is increased infections with pyogenic bacteria. Factor H deficiency is rare and is characterized by excess alternative pathway activation, consumption of C3, and glomerulonephritis caused by inadequate clearance of immune complexes and renal deposition of complement by-products. Specific allelic variants of factor H are strongly associated with age-related macular degeneration. The effects of a lack of factor I or factor H are similar to the effects of an autoantibody called C3 nephritic factor (C3NeF), which is specific for alternative pathway C3 convertase (C3bBb). C3NeF stabilizes C3bBb and protects the complex from factor H–mediated dissociation, which results in unregulated consumption of C3. Patients with this antibody often have glomerulonephritis, possibly caused by inadequate clearing of circulating immune complexes.

Deficiencies in complement receptors include the absence of CR3 and CR4, both resulting from rare mutations in the β chain (CD18) gene common to the CD11CD18 family of integrin molecules. The congenital disease caused by this gene defect is called leukocyte adhesion deficiency (see Chapter 20). This disorder is characterized by recurrent pyogenic infections and is caused by inadequate adherence of neutrophils to endothelium at tissue sites of infection and perhaps by impaired iC3b-dependent phagocytosis of bacteria.

PATHOLOGIC EFFECTS OF A NORMAL COMPLEMENT SYSTEM. Even when it is properly regulated and appropriately activated, the complement system can cause significant tissue damage. Some of the pathologic effects associated with bacterial infections may be due to complement-mediated acute inflammatory responses to infectious organisms. In some situations, complement activation is associated with intravascular thrombosis and can lead to ischemic injury to tissues. For instance, antiendothelial antibodies against vascularized organ transplants and the immune complexes produced in autoimmune diseases may bind to vascular endothelium and activate complement, thereby leading to inflammation and generation of the MAC with damage to the endothelial surface, which favors coagulation. There is also evidence that some of the late complement proteins may activate prothrombinases in the circulation that initiate thrombosis independent of MAC-mediated damage to endothelium.

It has long been believed that the clearest example of complement-mediated pathology is immune complex disease. Systemic vasculitis and immune complex glomerulonephritis result from the deposition of antigen-antibody complexes in the walls of vessels and kidney glomeruli (see Chapter 18). Complement activated by the immunoglobulin in these deposited immune complexes initiates the acute inflammatory responses that destroy the vessel walls or glomeruli and lead to thrombosis, ischemic damage to tissues, and scarring. However, as mentioned in the text, studies with knockout mice lacking the complement proteins C3 or C4 or lacking Fcγ receptors suggest that Fc receptor–mediated leukocyte activation may cause inflammation and tissue injury as a result of IgG deposition even in the absence of complement activation.

antigen-induced signaling in B cells (see Chapter 10, Fig. 10–5). Opsonized antigens are also bound by follicular dendritic cells in the germinal centers of lymphoid organs. Follicular dendritic cells display antigens to B cells in the germinal centers, and this process is important for the selection of high-affinity B cells (see Chapter 10, Fig. 10–12). The importance of complement in humoral immune responses is illustrated by the severe impairment in antibody production and germinal center formation seen in knockout mice lacking C3 or C4 or the CR2 protein.

Although our discussion has emphasized the physiologic functions of complement as an effector mechanism of host defense, the complement system is also involved in several pathologic conditions (Box 14–2). Some autoimmune diseases are associated with the production of autoantibodies specific for self proteins expressed on cell surfaces (see Chapter 18). Binding of these antibodies results in complement-dependent lysis and phagocytosis of the cells. In other diseases, immune complexes deposit in tissues and induce inflammation by complement-mediated recruitment and activation of leukocytes. Genetic deficiencies of complement proteins and regulatory proteins are the causes of various human diseases.

The similarities in the roles of complement and Fc receptors in phagocytosis and inflammation raise the question of which is the more important effector mechanism of humoral immunity. Surprisingly, knockout mice lacking C3 or C4 show virtually no defects in IgG antibody–mediated phagocytosis of opsonized erythrocytes or in immune complex–mediated vasculitis. Both these reactions are abolished in knockout mice lacking the high-affinity Fcγ receptor. These results suggest that in IgG antibody–mediated phagocytosis and inflammation, Fc receptor–dependent reactions may be more important than complement-mediated reactions. Whether this phenomenon is true in humans remains to be established. Also, IgM antibody–mediated protective immunity and pathologic reactions are dependent only on the complement system because IgM is an efficient activator of complement but does not bind to leukocyte Fc receptors.

Evasion of Complement by Microbes

Pathogens have evolved diverse mechanisms for evading the complement system. Some microbes express thick cell walls that prevent the binding of complement proteins, such as the MAC. Gram-positive bacteria and some fungi are examples of microbes that use this relatively non-specific evasion strategy. A few of the more specific mechanisms employed by a small subset of pathogens will be considered here. These evasion mechanisms may be divided into three groups.

- ***Microbes can evade the complement system by recruiting host complement regulatory proteins.*** Many pathogens express sialic acids which can inhibit the alternative pathway of complement by recruiting factor H, which displaces C3b from Bb. Some pathogens, like schistosomes, *Neisseria gonorrheae,* and certain *Hemophilus* species, scavenge sialic acids from the host and enzymatically transfer the sugar to their cell surfaces. Others, including *Escherichia coli K1* and some meningococci, have evolved special biosynthetic routes for sialic acid generation. Some microbes synthesize proteins that can recruit the regulatory protein factor H to the cell surface. Gp41 on HIV can bind to factor H, and this property of the virus is believed to contribute to virion protection. Many other pathogens have evolved proteins that facilitate the recruitment of factor H to their cell walls. These include bacteria such as *Streptococcus pyogenes, Borrelia burgdorferi* (the causative agent of Lyme disease), *Neisseria gonorrhea, Neisseria meningitides,* the fungal pathogen *Candida albicans,* and nematodes such as *Echinococcus granulosus.* Other microbes, such as HIV, incorporate multiple host regulatory proteins into their envelopes. For instance, HIV incorporates the GPI-anchored complement regulatory proteins DAF and CD59 when it buds from an infected cell.

- ***A number of pathogens produce specific proteins that mimic human complement regulatory proteins.*** *Escherichia coli* makes a C1q binding protein (C1qBP) that inhibits the formation of a complex between C1q and C1r and C1s. *Staphylococcus aureus* makes a protein called SCIN (Staphylococcal complement inhibitor) that binds to and stably inhibits both the classical and alternative pathway C3 convertases and thus inhibits all three complement pathways. Glycoprotein C-1 of the Herpes simplex viruses destabilizes the alternative pathway convertase by preventing its C3b component from binding to properdin. GP160, a membrane protein on *Trypanosoma cruzi,* the causative agent of Chagas' disease, binds to C3b and prevents the formation of the C3 convertase, and also accelerates its decay. VCP-1 (vaccinia virus complement inhibitory protein-1), a protein made by the vaccinia virus, structurally resembles human C4bp, but can bind to both C4b and C3b and accelerate the decay of both C3 and C5 convertases.

- ***Complement-mediated inflammation can also be inhibited by microbial gene products.*** *Staphylococcal aureus* synthesizes a protein called CHIPS (Chemokine Inhibitory Protein of Staphylococci), which is an antagonist of the C5a anaphylatoxin.

These examples illustrate how microbes have acquired the ability to evade the complement system, presumably contributing to their pathogenicity.

Functions of Antibodies at Special Anatomic Sites

So far, we have described the effector functions of antibodies that are systemic and do not show any particular features related to location. Antibodies serve special defense functions as a result of active transport into two anatomic compartments, the lumens of mucosal organs and the developing fetus. In these sites, the principal mechanism of protective immunity against microbes is antibody-mediated neutralization because lymphocytes and other effector cells do not pass through mucosal epithelia or the placenta.

Mucosal Immunity

IgA is the major class of antibody that is produced in the mucosal immune system. The gastrointestinal and respiratory tracts are two of the most common portals of entry of microbes. Defense against microbes that enter by these routes is provided by antibody, largely IgA, that is produced in mucosal lymphoid tissues and secreted through the mucosal epithelium into the lumens of the organs. In mucosal secretions, IgA binds to microbes and toxins present in the lumen and neutralizes them by blocking their entry into the host (see Fig. 14–2). Secretory immunity is the mechanism of protective immunity induced by oral vaccines such as the polio vaccine.

The mucosal immune system is a collection of lymphocytes and other cell types, often organized into discrete anatomic structures with definable lymphoid follicles that are located underneath the epithelia of the gastrointestinal and respiratory tracts (see Chapter 3). IgA is produced in larger amounts than any other antibody isotype, mainly because of the size of the mucosal immune system. It is estimated that a normal 70-kg adult secretes about 2 g of IgA per day, which accounts for 60% to 70% of the total output of antibodies. Because IgA synthesis occurs mainly in mucosal lymphoid tissue and transport into the mucosal lumen is efficient, this isotype constitutes less than one quarter of the antibody in plasma and is a minor component of systemic humoral immunity compared with IgG and IgM. Antibody responses to antigens encountered by ingestion or inhalation are typically dominated by IgA. In antigen-stimulated B cells, switching to the IgA isotype is stimulated by transforming growth factor-β (which may be produced by T cells as well as by nonlymphoid stromal cells) and cytokines of the TNF family, including BAFF (see Chapter 10). The reason why larger amounts of IgA are produced in the mucosal immune system than in other tissues is that isotype switching to IgA occurs most efficiently in mucosal lymphoid tissue, particularly in Peyer's patches and mesenteric lymph nodes, and class-switched IgA plasmablasts have a special propensity to home to the lamina propria of the intestine and to other mucosal sites.

Secreted IgA is transported through epithelial cells into the intestinal lumen by an IgA-specific Fc receptor called the poly-Ig receptor. IgA is produced by plasma cells in the lamina propria and secreted in the form of a dimer that is held together by the coordinately produced J chain. (In contrast, serum IgA is usually a monomer lacking the J chain.) From the lamina propria, the IgA must be transported across the epithelium into the lumen, by a process known as transcytosis, and this function is mediated by the **poly-Ig receptor**. This receptor is synthesized by mucosal epithelial cells and expressed on their basal and lateral surfaces. It is an integral membrane glycoprotein with five extracellular domains homologous to Ig domains and is thus a member of the Ig superfamily. The secreted, dimeric IgA containing the J chain binds to the poly-Ig receptor on mucosal epithelial cells (Fig. 14–18). This complex is endocytosed into the epithelial cell and actively transported in vesicles to the luminal surface. Here the poly-Ig receptor is proteolytically cleaved, its transmembrane and cytoplasmic domains are left attached to the epithelial cell, and the extracellular domain of the receptor, which carries the IgA molecule, is released into the intestinal lumen. The soluble IgA-associated component of the receptor is called the **secretory component.** The poly-Ig receptor is also responsible for the secretion of IgA into bile, milk, sputum, saliva, and sweat. Although its ability to transport IgA has been studied most extensively, the receptor is capable of transporting IgM into intestinal secretions as well. (Note that secreted IgM is also a polymer associated with the J chain.) This is why this receptor is called the poly-Ig receptor.

Neonatal Immunity

Neonatal mammals are protected from infection by maternally produced antibodies transported across the placenta into the fetal circulation and by antibodies in ingested milk transported across the gut epithelium of newborns by a specialized process known as transcyto-

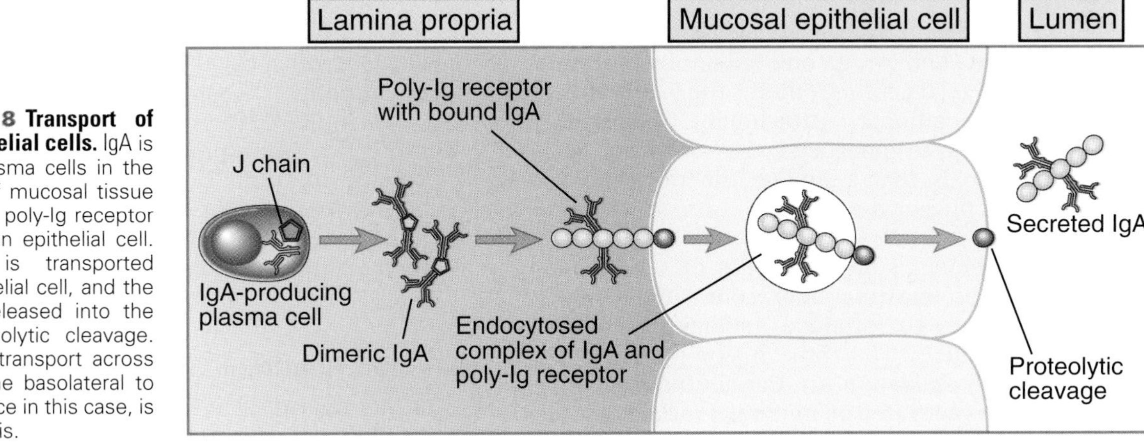

FIGURE 14–18 Transport of IgA across epithelial cells. IgA is produced by plasma cells in the lamina propria of mucosal tissue and binds to the poly-Ig receptor at the base of an epithelial cell. The complex is transported across the epithelial cell, and the bound IgA is released into the lumen by proteolytic cleavage. The process of transport across the cell, from the basolateral to the luminal surface in this case, is called transcytosis.

sis. Neonates lack the ability to mount effective immune responses against microbes, and for several months after birth, their major defense against infection is passive immunity provided by maternal antibodies. Maternal IgG is transported across the placenta, and maternal IgA and IgG in breast milk are ingested by the nursing infant. Ingested IgA and IgG can neutralize pathogenic organisms that attempt to colonize the infant's gut, and ingested IgG antibodies are also transported across the gut epithelium into the circulation of the newborn. Thus, a newborn contains essentially the same IgG antibodies as the mother.

Transport of maternal IgG across the placenta and across the neonatal intestinal epithelium is mediated by an IgG-specific Fc receptor called the **neonatal Fc receptor** (FcRn). The FcRn is unique among Fc receptors in that it resembles a class I major histocompatibility complex (MHC) molecule containing a transmembrane heavy chain that is noncovalently associated with β_2-microglobulin. However, the interaction of IgG with FcRn does not involve the portion of the molecule analogous to the peptide-binding cleft used by class I MHC molecules to display peptides for T cell recognition.

Adults also express the FcRn in the endothelium and in many epithelial tissues. In the post-neonatal period, this receptor functions to protect plasma IgG antibodies from catabolism. It binds circulating IgG, promotes endocytosis of the IgG complexes with the receptor in a form that protects the internalized antibody from intracellular degradation, and recycles the bound antibody to the cell surface before releasing it back into the circulation. This process of repeated sequestering and release of IgG contributes to its enhanced half-life. Knockout mice lacking β_2-microglobulin have 10-fold lower levels of serum IgG than normal mice do because of increased catabolism of antibodies resulting from the failure to express this protective β_2-microglobulin–associated Fc receptor. The contribution of the Fc portion of IgG to enhancing the half-life of antibodies has been utilized to generate therapeutically useful fusion proteins that include the Fc portion of human IgG, and consequently survive for extended periods of time in the circulation. One such example of a long-lived fusion protein is a chimeric protein that contains the extracellular domains of the TNF receptor fused to the Fc portion of human IgG. This protein competitively inhibits TNF–TNFR interactions and is used to treat patients with rheumatoid arthritis and Crohn disease.

The FcRn contributes to the long half-life of all IgG molecules including pathogenic autoantibodies. While the efficacy of IVIG in autoimmune diseases may depend on inhibitory signals derived from FcγRIIB (see above), large amounts of infused exogenous IgG antibodies might compete with endogenous and pathogenic IgG autoantibodies for recognition by the FcRn and thus attenuate the half-lives of disease-associated antibodies.

SUMMARY

- Humoral immunity is mediated by antibodies and is the effector arm of the adaptive immune system responsible for defense against extracellular microbes and microbial toxins. The antibodies that provide protection against infection may be produced by long-lived antibody-secreting cells generated by the first exposure to microbial antigen or by reactivation of memory B cells by the antigen.

- The effector functions of antibodies include neutralization of antigens, Fc receptor–dependent phagocytosis of opsonized particles, and activation of the complement system.

- Antibodies block, or neutralize, the infectivity of microbes by binding to the microbes and sterically hindering interactions of the microbes with cellular receptors. Antibodies similarly block the pathologic actions of toxins by preventing binding of the toxins to host cells.

- Antibody-coated (opsonized) particles are phagocytosed by binding of the Fc portions of the antibodies to phagocyte Fc receptors. There are several types of Fc receptors specific for different subclasses of IgG and for IgA and IgE antibodies, and different Fc receptors bind the antibodies with varying affinities. Attachment of antigen-complexed Ig to phagocyte Fc receptors also delivers signals that stimulate the microbicidal activities of phagocytes.

- The complement system consists of serum and membrane proteins that interact in a highly regulated manner to produce biologically active protein products. The three major pathways of complement activation are the alternative pathway, which is activated on microbial surfaces in the absence of antibody, the classical pathway, which is activated by antigen-antibody complexes, and the lectin pathway, initiated by collectins binding to antigens. These pathways generate enzymes that cleave the C3 protein, and cleaved products of C3 become covalently attached to microbial surfaces or antibodies, so subsequent steps of complement activation are limited to these sites. All pathways converge on a common pathway that involves the formation of a membrane pore following the proteolytic cleavage of C5.

- Complement activation is regulated by various plasma and cell membrane proteins that inhibit different steps in the cascades.

- The biologic functions of the complement system include opsonization of organisms and immune complexes by proteolytic fragments of C3, followed by binding to phagocyte receptors for complement fragments and phagocytic clearance, activation of inflammatory cells by proteolytic fragments of complement proteins called anaphylatoxins (C3a, C4a, C5a), cytolysis mediated by MAC formation on cell surfaces, solubilization and clearance of immune complexes, and enhancement of humoral immune responses.

- Defense against microbes and toxins in the lumens of mucosal organs is provided by IgA antibody that is produced in mucosal lymphoid tissue and actively transported through epithelial cells into the lumen.

- Protective immunity in neonates is a form of passive immunity provided by maternal antibodies transported across the placenta or ingested and transported across gut epithelium by a specialized neonatal Fc receptor.

Selected Readings

Carroll MC. The complement system in regulation of adaptive immunity. Nature Immunology 5:981–986, 2004.

Fagarasan S. Evolution, development, mechanism and function of IgA in the gut. Current Opinion in Immunology 20:170–177, 2008.

Gould HJ, and BJ Sutton. IgE in allergy and asthma today. Nature Reviews Immunology 8:205–217, 2008.

Gros P, FJ Milder, and BJ Janssen. Complement driven by conformational changes. Nature Reviews Immunology 8:48–58, 2008.

Lencer WI, and RS Blumberg. A passionate kiss, then run: exocytosis and recycling of IgG by FcRn. Trends in Cell Biology 15:5–9, 2005.

Manderson AP, M Botto, and MJ Walport. The role of complement in the development of systemic lupus erythematosus. Annual Review of Immunology 22:431–456, 2004.

Nimmerjahn F, Ravetch JV. Fcgamma receptors as regulators of immune responses. Nature Reviews Immunology 8:34–47, 2008.

Parren PW, and DR Burton. The antiviral activity of antibodies in vitro and in vivo. Advances in Immunology 77:195–262, 2001.

Petersen SV, S Thiel, and JC Jensenius. The mannan-binding lectin pathway of complement activation: biology and disease association. Molecular Immunology 38:133–149, 2001.

Roozendaal R, and MC Carroll. Emerging patterns in complement-mediated pathogen recognition. Cell 125:29–32, 2006.

Smith GP, and RA Smith. Membrane-targeted complement inhibitors. Molecular Immunology 38:249–255, 2001.

Walport MJ. Complement. New England Journal of Medicine 344:1058–1066, 1141–1144, 2001.

Section V

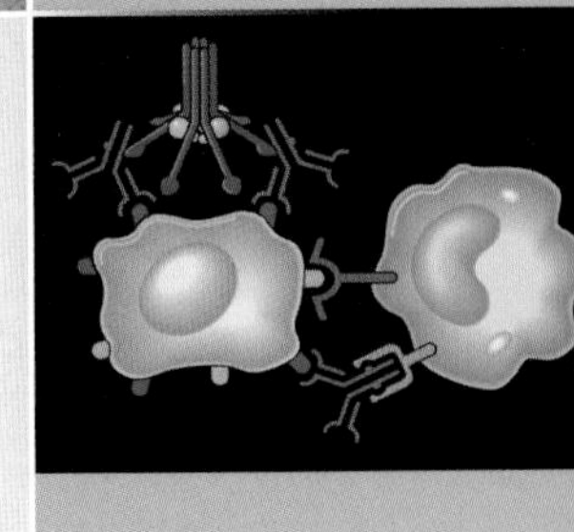

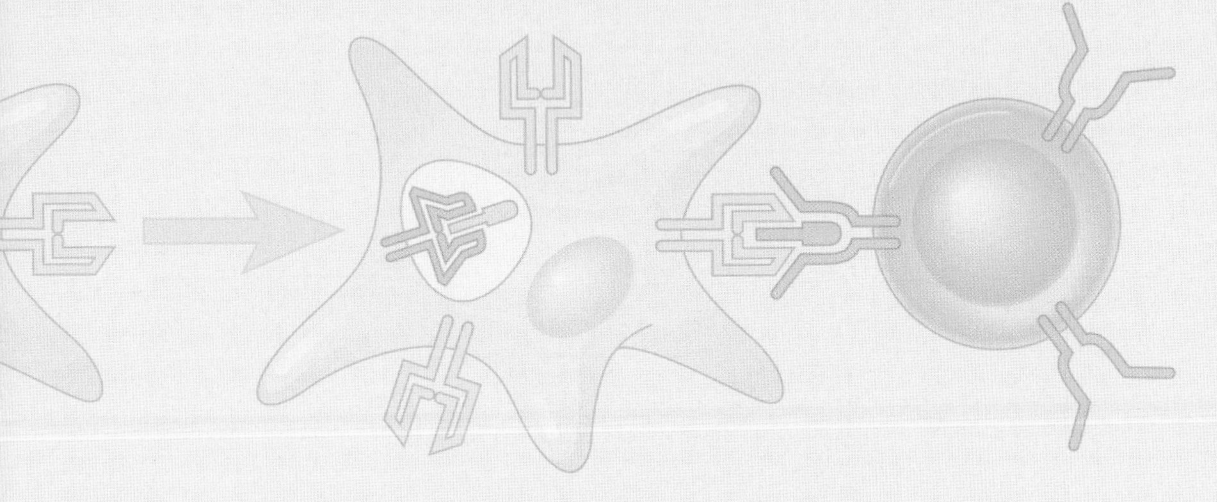

Immunity in Defense and Disease

In this final section of the book, we apply our knowledge of the basic mechanisms of innate and adaptive immunity to understanding immunological defenses against microbes and tumors, reactions against transplants, and diseases caused by abnormal immune responses. Chapter 15 is an overview of the mechanisms of innate and adaptive immunity against different types of microbes, and the interplay between microbes and the immune system. Chapter 16 is devoted to the immunology of tissue transplantation, a promising therapy for a variety of diseases whose success is limited in large part by the immunologic rejection response. Chapter 17 describes immune responses to tumors and immunological approaches for cancer therapy. Chapter 18 deals with the mechanisms of diseases caused by aberrant immune responses, so-called hypersensitivity diseases, and emphasizes the pathogenesis of autoimmune disorders. In Chapter 19 we describe immediate hypersensitivity and allergy, the most common group of diseases caused by immune responses. In Chapter 20 we discuss the cellular and molecular bases of congenital and acquired immunodeficiencies, including the acquired immunodeficiency syndrome.

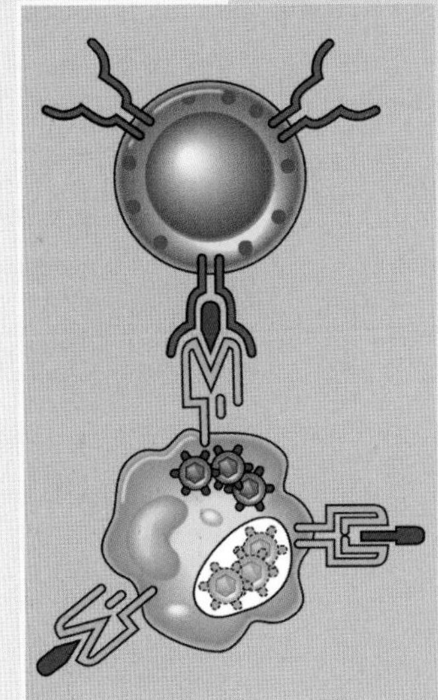

Chapter 15

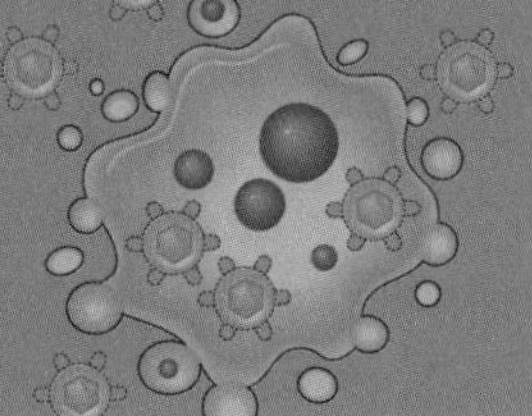

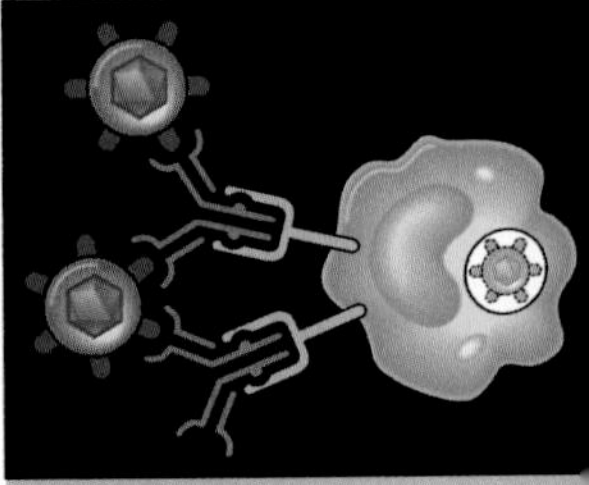

IMMUNITY TO MICROBES

In the preceding chapters, we have described the components of the immune system and the generation and functions of immune responses. In this chapter, we integrate the information and discuss how the immune system performs its major physiologic function, which is to protect the host against microbial infections. We illustrate the physiologic relevance of various aspects of immune system function by describing the main features of immunity to different types of pathogenic microorganisms and how microbes try to resist the mechanisms of host defense.

The development of an infectious disease in an individual involves complex interactions between the microbe and the host. The key events during infection include entry of the microbe, invasion and colonization of host tissues, evasion of host immunity, and tissue injury or functional impairment. Microbes produce disease by killing host cells or by liberating toxins, even without extensive colonization of host tissues, and in some infections the host response is the culprit, being the main cause of tissue damage and disease. Many features of microorganisms determine their virulence, and many diverse mechanisms contribute to the pathogenesis of infectious diseases. The topic of microbial pathogenesis is beyond the scope of this book and will not be discussed in detail. Rather, our discussion focuses on host immune responses to pathogenic microorganisms.

General Features of Immune Responses to Microbes

Although antimicrobial host defense reactions are numerous and varied, there are several important general features of immunity to microbes.

- ***Defense against microbes is mediated by the effector mechanisms of innate and adaptive immunity.*** The innate immune system provides early defense, and the adaptive immune system provides a more sustained and stronger response. Many pathogenic microbes have evolved to resist innate defense mechanisms, and protection against such microbes is critically dependent on adaptive immune responses. Adaptive immune responses are generally more potent than innate immunity for several reasons, including expansion of the pool of antigen-specific lymphocytes and specialization (see below). Adaptive immune responses to microbes induce effector cells that eliminate the microbes and memory cells that protect the individual from subsequent infections.
- ***The immune system responds in distinct and specialized ways to different types of microbes to most effectively combat these infectious agents.*** Because microbes differ greatly in patterns of host invasion and colonization, their elimination requires diverse effector systems. The specialization of adaptive immunity allows the host to respond optimally to each type of microbe.
- ***The survival and pathogenicity of microbes in a host are critically influenced by the ability of the microbes to evade or resist the effector mechanisms of immunity.*** Infectious microbes and their hosts are engaged in a constant struggle for survival, and the balance between host immune responses and microbial strategies for resisting immunity often determines the outcome of infections. As we shall see later in this chapter, microorganisms have developed a variety of mechanisms for surviving in the face of powerful immunologic defenses.
- ***In many infections, tissue injury and disease may be caused by the host response to the microbe and its products rather than by the microbe itself.*** Immunity, like many other defense mechanisms, is necessary for host survival but also has the potential for causing injury to the host.

This chapter considers five categories of pathogenic microorganisms that illustrate the main features of immunity to microbes: extracellular bacteria, intracellular bacteria, fungi, viruses, and protozoan and multicellular parasites (Table 15–1). Our discussion of the immune responses to these microbes illustrates the diversity of antimicrobial immunity and the physiologic significance of the effector functions of lymphocytes discussed in earlier chapters.

Immunity to Extracellular Bacteria

Extracellular bacteria are capable of replicating outside host cells, for example, in the circulation, in connective tissues, and in tissue spaces such as the lumens of the airways and gastrointestinal tract. Many different species of extracellular bacteria are pathogenic, and disease is caused by two principal mechanisms. First, these bacteria induce inflammation, which results in tissue destruction at the site of infection. This is how pyogenic (pus-forming) cocci cause a large number of suppurative infections in humans. Second, many of

Table 15–1. Examples of Pathogenic Microbes

Microbe	Examples of human diseases	Mechanisms of pathogenicity
Extracellular bacteria		
Staphylococcus aureus	Skin and soft tissue infections, lung abscess; systemic: toxic shock syndrome, food poisoning	Skin infections; acute inflammation induced by toxins; cell death caused by pore-forming toxins Systemic: enterotoxin ("superantigen")-induced cytokine production by T cells causing skin necrosis, shock, diarrhea
Streptococcus pyogenes (group A)	Pharyngitis Skin infections: impetigo, erysipelas; cellulitis Systemic: scarlet fever	Acute inflammation induced by various toxins, e.g., streptolysin O damages cell membranes (antiphagocytic action of capsular polysaccharides)
Streptococcus pyogenes (pneumococcus)	Pneumonia, meningitis	Acute inflammation induced by cell wall constituents; pneumolysin is similar to streptolysin O
Escherichia coli	Urinary tract infections, gastroenteritis, septic shock	Toxins act on intestinal epithelium and cause increased chloride and water secretion; endotoxin (LPS) stimulates cytokine secretion by macrophages

Table 15–1. *Continued*

Microbe	Examples of human diseases	Mechanisms of pathogenicity
Vibrio cholerae	Diarrhea (cholera)	Cholera toxin ADP ribosylates G protein subunit, which leads to increased cyclic AMP in intestinal epithelial cells and results in chloride secretion and water loss
Clostridium tetani	Tetanus	Tetanus toxin binds to the motor end-plate at neuromuscular junctions and causes irreversible muscle contraction
Neisseria meningitidis (meningococcus)	Meningitis	Acute inflammation and systemic disease caused by potent endotoxin
Corynebacterium diphtheriae	Diphtheria	Diphtheria toxin ADP ribosylates elongation factor-2 and inhibits protein synthesis
Intracellular bacteria		
Mycobacteria	Tuberculosis, leprosy	Macrophage activation resulting in granulomatous inflammation and tissue destruction
Listeria monocytogenes	Listeriosis	Listeriolysin damages cell membranes
Legionella pneumophila	Legionnaires' disease	Cytotoxin lyses cells and causes lung injury and inflammation
Fungi		
Candida albicans	Candidiasis	Unknown; binds complement proteins
Aspergillus fumigatus	Aspergillosis	Invasion and thrombosis of blood vessels causing ischemic necrosis and cell injury
Histoplasma capsulatum	Histoplasmosis	Lung infection caused by granulomatous inflammation
Viruses		
Polio	Poliomyelitis	Inhibits host cell protein synthesis (tropism for motor neurons in the anterior horn of the spinal cord)
Influenza	Influenza pneumonia	Inhibits host cell protein synthesis (tropism for ciliated epithelial cells)
Rabies	Rabies encephalitis	Inhibits host cell protein synthesis (tropism for peripheral nerves)
Herpes simplex	Various herpes infections (skin, systemic)	Inhibits host cell protein synthesis; functional impairment of immune cells
Hepatitis B	Viral hepatitis	Host CTL response to infected hepatocytes
Epstein-Barr virus	Infectious mononucleosis; B cell proliferation, lymphomas	Acute infection: cell lysis (tropism for B lymphocytes) Latent infection: stimulates B cell proliferation
Human immunodeficiency virus (HIV)	Acquired immunodeficiency syndrome (AIDS)	Multiple: killing of $CD4^+$ T cells, functional impairment of immune cells (see Chapter 20)

Abbreviations: ADP, adenosine diphosphate; AMP, adenosine monophosphate; CTL, cytotoxic T lymphocyte; LPS, lipopolysaccaride.

Examples of pathogenic microbes of different classes are listed, with brief summaries of known or postulated mechanisms of tissue injury and disease. Examples of parasites are in Table 15–4.

This table was compiled with the assistance of Dr. Arlene Sharpe, Department of Pathology, Harvard Medical School and Brigham and Women's Hospital, Boston, Massachusetts.

these bacteria produce **toxins,** which have diverse pathologic effects. Such toxins may be endotoxins, which are components of bacterial cell walls, or exotoxins, which are actively secreted by the bacteria. The endotoxin of gram-negative bacteria, also called lipopolysaccharide (LPS), has been mentioned in earlier chapters as a potent activator of macrophages. Many exotoxins are cytotoxic, and they kill cells by various biochemical mechanisms. Other exotoxins interfere with normal cellular functions without killing cells, and yet other exotoxins stimulate the production of cytokines that cause disease.

Innate Immunity to Extracellular Bacteria

The principal mechanisms of innate immunity to extracellular bacteria are complement activation, phagocytosis, and the inflammatory response. Gram-positive bacteria contain a peptidoglycan in their cell walls that activates the alternative pathway of complement by promoting formation of the alternative pathway C3 convertase (see Chapter 14). LPS in the cell walls of gram-negative bacteria also activates the alternative complement pathway in the absence of antibody. Bacteria that express mannose on their surface may bind mannose-binding lectin, thereby leading to complement activation by the lectin pathway. One result of complement activation is opsonization and enhanced phagocytosis of the bacteria. In addition, the membrane attack complex lyses bacteria, especially *Neisseria* species, and complement by-products stimulate inflammatory responses by recruiting and activating leukocytes. Phagocytes use various surface receptors, including mannose receptors and scavenger receptors, to recognize extracellular bacteria, and use Fc receptors and complement receptors to recognize appropriately opsonized bacteria. Toll-like receptors (TLRs) of phagocytes participate in the activation of the phagocytes as a result of encounter with microbes. These various receptors promote the phagocytosis of the microbes and stimulate the microbicidal activities of the phagocytes (see Chapter 2). In addition, activated phagocytes secrete cytokines, which induce leukocyte infiltration into sites of infection (inflammation). Injury to normal tissue is a pathologic side effect of inflammation. Cytokines also induce the systemic manifestations of infection, including fever and the synthesis of acute-phase proteins.

Adaptive Immunity to Extracellular Bacteria

Humoral immunity is the principal protective immune response against extracellular bacteria, and it functions to block infection, eliminate the microbes, and neutralize their toxins (Fig. 15–1). Antibody responses against extracellular bacteria are directed against cell wall antigens and secreted and cell-associated toxins, which may be polysaccharides or proteins. The polysaccharides are prototypic thymus-independent antigens, and a major function of humoral immunity is defense against polysaccharide-rich encapsulated bacteria. The effector mechanisms used by antibodies to combat these infections include neutralization, opsonization and phagocytosis, and activation of complement by the classical pathway (see Chapter 14). Neutralization is mediated by high-affinity immunoglobulin G (IgG) and IgA isotypes, opsonization by some subclasses of IgG, and complement activation by IgM and subclasses of IgG. The protein antigens of extracellular bacteria also activate $CD4^+$ helper T cells, which produce cytokines that stimulate antibody production, induce local inflammation, and enhance the phagocytic and microbicidal activities of macrophages and neutrophils (see Fig. 15–1). Interferon-γ (IFN-γ) is the T cell cytokine responsible for macrophage activation, and tumor necrosis factor (TNF) and lymphotoxin trigger inflammation. Recent work, done mainly in mice, has shown that IL-17 produced by "T_H17" cells is responsible for neutrophil-rich inflammation and defense against some bacterial infections.

Injurious Effects of Immune Responses

The principal injurious consequences of host responses to extracellular bacteria are inflammation and septic shock. The same reactions of neutrophils and macrophages that function to eradicate the infection also cause tissue damage by local production of reactive oxygen species and lysosomal enzymes. These inflammatory reactions are usually self-limited and controlled. **Septic shock** is a severe pathologic consequence of disseminated infection by gram-negative and some gram-positive bacteria. It is a syndrome characterized by circulatory collapse and disseminated intravascular coagulation (Box 15–1). The early phase of septic shock is caused by cytokines produced by macrophages that are activated by microbial components, particularly LPS. TNF is the principal cytokine mediator of septic shock, but IFN-γ and interleukin-12 (IL-12) may also contribute. In fact, serum levels of TNF are predictive of the outcome of severe gram-negative bacterial infections. This early burst of deadly amounts of cytokines is sometimes called a "cytokine storm." There is some evidence that the progression of septic shock is associated with defective immune responses, perhaps related to depletion of T cells, resulting in unchecked microbial spread. Certain bacterial toxins stimulate all the T cells in an individual that express a particular family of V_β T cell receptor genes. Such toxins are called **superantigens** (Box 15–2). Their importance lies in their ability to activate many T cells, with the subsequent production of large amounts of cytokines that also cause septic shock.

A late complication of the humoral immune response to bacterial infection may be the generation of disease-producing antibodies. The best defined examples are two rare sequelae of streptococcal infections of the throat or skin that are manifested weeks or even months after the infections are controlled. Rheumatic fever is a sequel to pharyngeal infection with some serologic types of β-hemolytic streptococci. Infection leads to the production of antibodies against a bacterial cell wall protein (M protein). Some of these antibodies cross-react with myocardial sarcolemmal proteins and myosin and are deposited in the heart and subsequently cause inflammation (carditis). Poststreptococcal glomerulonephritis is a sequel to infection of the skin or throat with other

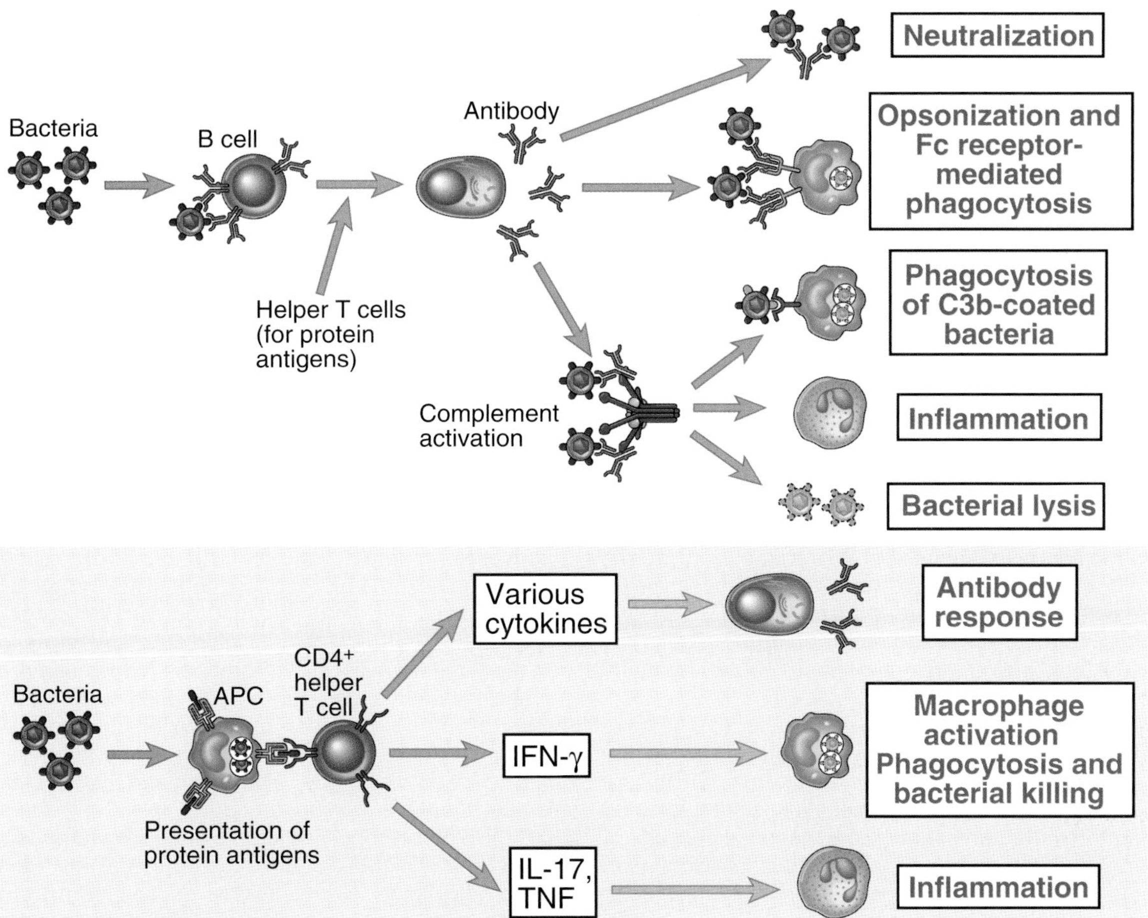

FIGURE 15–1 Adaptive immune responses to extracellular microbes. Adaptive immune responses to extracellular microbes, such as bacteria, and their toxins consist of antibody production and the activation of CD4+ helper T cells. Antibodies neutralize and eliminate microbes and toxins by several mechanisms. Helper T cells produce cytokines that stimulate B cell responses, macrophage activation, and inflammation. APC, antigen-presenting cell.

serotypes of β-hemolytic streptococci. Antibodies produced against these bacteria form complexes with bacterial antigen, which may be deposited in kidney glomeruli and cause nephritis.

Immune Evasion by Extracellular Bacteria

The virulence of extracellular bacteria has been linked to a number of mechanisms that resist innate immunity (Table 15–2), including antiphagocytic mechanisms and inhibition of complement or inactivation of complement products. Bacteria with polysaccharide-rich capsules resist phagocytosis and are therefore much more virulent than homologous strains lacking a capsule. The capsules of many gram-positive and gram-negative bacteria contain sialic acid residues that inhibit complement activation by the alternative pathway.

The major mechanism used by bacteria to evade humoral immunity is genetic variation of surface antigens. Some surface antigens of bacteria such as gonococci and *Escherichia coli* are contained in their pili, which are the structures responsible for bacterial adhesion to host cells. The major antigen of the pili is a protein called pilin. The pilin genes of gonococci undergo extensive gene conversion, because of which the progeny of one organism can produce up to 10^6 antigenically distinct pilin molecules. This ability to alter antigens helps the bacteria evade attack by pilin-specific antibodies, although its principal significance for the bacteria may be to select for pili that are more adherent to host cells so that the bacteria are more virulent. In other bacteria, such as *Haemophilus influenzae,* changes in the production of glycosidases lead to chemical alterations in surface LPS and other polysaccharides, which enable the bacteria to evade humoral immune responses against these antigens.

Immunity to Intracellular Bacteria

A characteristic of facultative intracellular bacteria is their ability to survive and even replicate within phagocytes. Because these microbes are able to find a niche where they are inaccessible to circulating antibodies, their elimination requires the mechanisms of cell-mediated immunity (Fig. 15–2). As we shall discuss later

Box 15–1 ▪ IN DEPTH: PHYSIOLOGIC AND PATHOLOGIC RESPONSES TO BACTERIAL LIPOPOLYSACCHARIDE

Bacterial LPS (or endotoxin) is a product of gram-negative bacteria, and a potent stimulator of innate immune responses. LPS is present in the outer cell walls of gram-negative bacteria and contains both lipid components and polysaccharide moieties. The polysaccharide groups can be highly variable and are the major antigens of gram-negative bacteria recognized by the adaptive immune system. The lipid moiety, by contrast, is highly conserved and is an example of a molecular pattern recognized by the innate immune system.

LPS is a potent activator of macrophages. LPS binds to a plasma LPS-binding protein (LBP) and the complex then binds to CD14 on macrophages and dendritic cells. The LPS moiety is then recognized by TLR4 (see Chapter 2). Macrophages, which synthesize and express CD14, can respond to minute quantities of LPS, as little as 10 pg/mL, and cells that lack CD14 are generally unresponsive to LPS. The genes that are induced by LPS encode cytokines, costimulators, and enzymes of the respiratory burst. The functions of these proteins in innate immunity are described in Chapter 2.

The systemic changes observed in patients who have disseminated bacterial infections, sometimes called the systemic inflammatory response syndrome (SIRS), are reactions to cytokines whose production is stimulated by LPS. In mildly affected patients, the response consists of neutrophilia, fever, and a rise in acute-phase reactants in the plasma. Neutrophilia is a response of the bone marrow to circulating cytokines, especially G-CSF, resulting in increased production and release of neutrophils to replace those consumed during inflammation. An elevated circulating neutrophil count, especially one accompanied by the presence of immature neutrophils prematurely released from the bone marrow, is a clinical sign of infection. Fever is produced in response to substances called pyrogens that act to elevate prostaglandin synthesis in the vascular and perivascular cells of the hypothalamus. Bacterial products such as LPS (called exogenous pyrogens) stimulate leukocytes to release cytokines such as IL-1 and TNF (called endogenous pyrogens) that increase the enzyme called cyclooxygenase that converts arachidonic acid into prostaglandins. Nonsteroidal anti-inflammatory drugs, including aspirin, reduce fever by inhibiting cyclooxygenase-2 and thus blocking prostaglandin synthesis. An elevated body temperature has been shown to help amphibians ward off microbial infections, and it is assumed that fever does the same for mammals, although the mechanism is unknown. Acute-phase reactants are plasma proteins, mostly synthesized in the liver, whose plasma concentrations increase as part of the response to LPS. Three of the best known examples of these proteins are c-reactive protein, (CRP) fibrinogen, and serum amyloid A protein. Synthesis of these molecules by hepatocytes is up-regulated by cytokines, especially IL-6 (for CRP and fibrinogen) and IL-1 or TNF (for serum amyloid A protein). The rise in fibrinogen causes erythrocytes to form stacks (rouleaux) that sediment more rapidly at unit gravity than do individual erythrocytes. This is the basis for measuring erythrocyte sedimentation rate as a simple test for the systemic inflammatory response due to any number of stimuli, including LPS.

When a severe bacterial infection leads to the presence of organisms and LPS in the blood, a condition called sepsis, circulating cytokine levels increase and the form of the host response changes. High levels of cytokines produced in response to LPS can result in disseminated intravascular coagulation (DIC), caused by increased expression of pro-coagulant proteins (e.g. tissue factor) and reduced anti-coagulant activity on TNF-activated endothelial cells. Multiple organs show inflammation and intravascular thrombosis, which can produce organ failure. Tissue injury in response to LPS can also result from the activation of neutrophils before they exit the vasculature, thus causing damage to endothelial cells and reduced blood flow. The lungs and liver are particularly susceptible to injury by neutrophils. Lung damage in the SIRS is commonly called the adult respiratory distress syndrome (ARDS) and results when neutrophil-mediated endothelial injury allows fluid to escape from the blood into the airspace. Liver injury and impaired liver function result in a failure to maintain normal blood glucose levels due to a lack of gluconeogenesis from stored glycogen. The kidney and the bowel are also injured, largely as a result of reduced perfusion. Overproduction of nitric oxide by cytokine-activated cardiac myocytes and vascular smooth muscle cells leads to heart failure and loss of perfusion pressure, respectively, resulting in hemodynamic shock. The clinical triad of DIC, hypoglycemia, and cardiovascular failure is described as **septic shock.** This condition is often fatal.

TNF produced by LPS-activated macrophages is a major mediator of LPS-induced injury. This is known because many of the effects of LPS can be mimicked by TNF, and in mice, anti-TNF antibodies or soluble TNF receptors can attenuate or completely block responses to LPS. IL-12 and IFN-γ also contribute to LPS-induced injury because IL-12 stimulates IFN-γ production by NK cells and T cells, and IFN-γ increases TNF secretion by LPS-activated macrophages and synergizes with TNF in effects on endothelium. Clinical trials of TNF and IL-1 antagonists in septic shock have not been successful, perhaps because several cytokines may contribute to this disorder.

Box 15–2 ▪ IN DEPTH: BACTERIAL SUPERANTIGENS

Some microbial toxins are called superantigens because they stimulate large numbers of T cells (more than conventional antigens), but not all T cells (which distinguishes them from polyclonal activators). Staphylococcal enterotoxins are exotoxins produced by the gram-positive bacterium *Staphylococcus aureus* and consist of five serologically distinct groups of proteins: SEA, SEB, SEC, SED, and SEE. These toxins are the most common cause of food poisoning in humans. A related toxin, TSST, causes a disease called toxic shock syndrome (TSS), which has been associated with tampon use and surgical wounds. Pyrogenic exotoxins of streptococci and exotoxins produced by mycoplasmas may be structurally and functionally related to these enterotoxins.

The potency of superantigens as T cell activators is related to the way these molecules interact with APCs and with T cells. Importantly, most superantigens work by bringing T cells and APCs into direct contact, by simultaneously binding to both MHC molecules and T cell receptors (TCRs).

- Enterotoxins bind to the V_β region of TCRs, and each toxin stimulates T cells that express antigen receptors whose V_β regions are encoded by a single V_β gene or gene family. In other words, the specificity of T cells for different enterotoxins is encoded in the V_β region and is not related to other components of the TCR, such as the V_α, J, or D segments, because enterotoxins bind directly to the β chains of TCR molecules close to but outside the antigen-binding (complementarity-determining) regions. Different enterotoxins stimulate T cells expressing V_β genes from different families (see Table). The specificity of enterotoxins for V_β regions explains why they stimulate many but not all T cells.
- Enterotoxins bind to class II MHC molecules on APCs at a site distinct from the peptide-binding cleft. Enterotoxins do not need to undergo intracellular processing, as do conventional protein antigens, to bind to these MHC molecules. The same enterotoxin binds to class II molecules of different alleles, indicating that the polymorphism of the MHC does not influence the binding of these toxins. Each staphylococcal enterotoxin molecule possesses two binding sites for class II MHC molecules. This characteristic allows each enterotoxin molecule to cross-link MHC molecules on APCs, and the enterotoxin-MHC molecule dimer may cross-link two antigen receptors on each T cell and thus initiate T cell responses.

Enterotoxin	Mice	Humans
SEB	V_β7, 8.1-8.3,17	V_β3,12,14,15,17,20
SEC 2	V_β8.2,10	V_β12,13,14,15,17,20
SEE	V_β11,15,17	V_β5.1,6.1-6.3,8,18
TSST-1	V_β15,16	V_β2

Abbreviations: SE, staphylococcal enterotoxin; TSST, toxic shock syndrome toxin.

Staphylococcal enterotoxins are among the most potent naturally occurring T cell mitogens known. They are capable of stimulating the proliferation of naive T lymphocytes at concentrations of 10^{-9} M or less. As many as one in five T cells in mouse lymphoid tissue or human peripheral blood may respond to a particular enterotoxin. The high frequency of staphylococcal enterotoxin-responding T cells, particularly $CD4^+$ cells, has several functional implications. Acutely, exposure to high concentrations of enterotoxin leads to systemic reactions such as fever, disseminated intravascular coagulation, and cardiovascular shock. These abnormalities are probably mediated by cytokines, such as TNF, produced directly by the T cells or by macrophages that are activated by the T cells. These reactions resemble systemic reactions to endotoxin (LPS), as in septic shock, which are also mediated by cytokines (see Box 15–1). Prolonged administration of enterotoxins to mice results in wasting, thymic atrophy, and profound immunodeficiency, also probably secondary to chronic high levels of TNF.

Staphylococcal enterotoxins are useful tools for analyzing T lymphocyte maturation, activation, and tolerance. Administration of SEB to neonatal mice leads to intrathymic deletion of all immature T cells that express the $V_\beta3$ and $V_\beta8$ TCR genes. This deletion mimics self antigen-induced negative selection of self-reactive T cells during thymic maturation. Superantigens also induce apoptotic death of mature $CD4^+$ and $CD8^+$ T cells. This type of cell death is postulated to be a model of deletion of mature T cells that are exposed to self antigens.

Viral gene products may also function as superantigens. In certain inbred strains of mice, different mouse mammary tumor virus genes have become incorporated into the genome. Viral antigens produced by the cells of one strain are capable of activating T lymphocytes from other strains that express particular V_β segments in their antigen receptors. The result is a form of "mixed lymphocyte reaction" that is not caused by MHC disparity. This was discovered long before viral superantigens were identified, and the interstrain reactions were attributed to minor lymphocyte-stimulating (Mls) loci. We now know that Mls "loci" are actually different retroviral superantigen genes that are stably incorporated into the genome and inherited in different inbred strains.

Table 15–2. Mechanisms of Immune Evasion by Bacteria

Mechanism of immune evasion	Examples
Extracellular bacteria	
Antigenic variation	*Neisseria gonorrhoeae, Escherichia coli, Salmonella typhimurium*
Inhibition of complement activation	Many bacteria
Resistance to phagocytosis	Pneumococcus
Scavenging of reactive oxygen intermediates	Catalase-positive staphylococci
Intracellular bacteria	
Inhibition of phagolysosome formation	*Mycobacterium tuberculosis, Legionella pneumophila*
Inactivation of reactive oxygen and nitrogen species	*Mycobacterium leprae* (phenolic glycolipid)
Disruption of phagosome membrane, escape into cytoplasm	*Listeria monocytogenes* (hemolysin protein)

in this section, the pathologic consequences of infection by many intracellular bacteria are due to the host response to these microbes.

Innate Immunity to Intracellular Bacteria

The innate immune response to intracellular bacteria is mainly mediated by of phagocytes and natural killer (NK) cells. Phagocytes, initially neutrophils and later macrophages, ingest and attempt to destroy these microbes, but pathogenic intracellular bacteria are resistant to degradation within phagocytes. Intracellular bacteria activate NK cells by inducing expression of NK cell–activating ligands on infected cells or by stimulating dendritic cell and macrophage production of IL-12, a powerful NK cell–activating cytokine. The NK cells produce IFN-γ, which in turn activates macrophages and promotes killing of the phagocytosed bacteria. Thus, NK cells provide an early defense against these microbes, before the development of adaptive immunity. In fact, mice with severe combined immunodeficiency, which lack T and B cells, are able to transiently control infection with the intracellular bacterium *Listeria monocytogenes* by NK cell–derived IFN-γ production. However, innate immunity usually fails to eradicate these infections, and eradication requires adaptive cell-mediated immunity.

Adaptive Immunity to Intracellular Bacteria

The major protective immune response against intracellular bacteria is T cell–mediated immunity. Individuals with deficient cell-mediated immunity, such as patients with acquired immunodeficiency syndrome

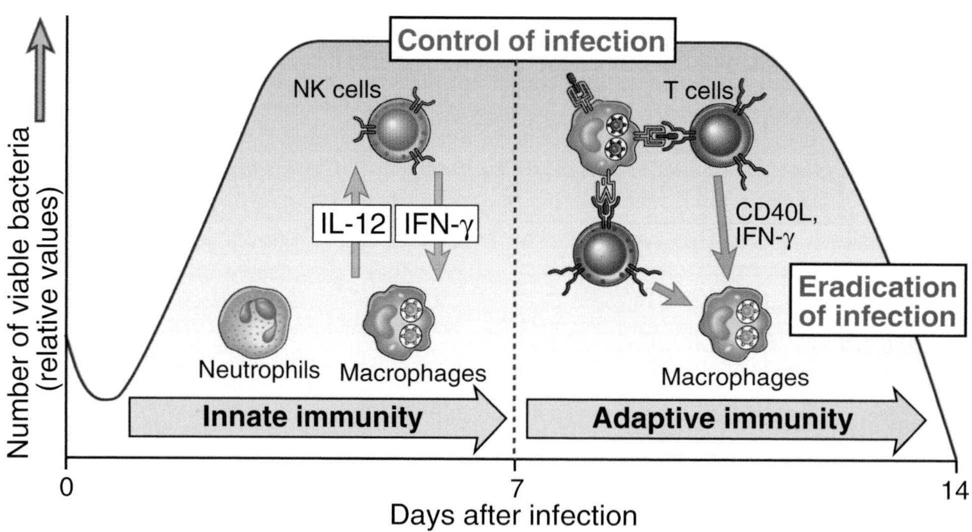

FIGURE 15–2 Innate and adaptive immunity to intracellular bacteria. The innate immune response to intracellular bacteria consists of phagocytes and NK cells, interactions among which are mediated by cytokines (IL-12 and IFN-γ). The typical adaptive immune response to these microbes is cell-mediated immunity, in which T cells activate phagocytes to eliminate the microbes. Innate immunity may control bacterial growth, but elimination of the bacteria requires adaptive immunity. These principles are based largely on analysis of *Listeria monocytogenes* infection in mice; the numbers of viable bacteria shown on the y-axis are relative values of bacterial colonies that can be grown from the tissues of infected mice. (From Unanue ER. Studies in listeriosis show the strong symbiosis between the innate cellular system and the T-cell response. Immunological Reviews 158: 11–25, 1997.)

(AIDS), are extremely susceptible to infections with intracellular bacteria (and viruses). Cell-mediated immunity was first identified by George Mackaness in the 1950s as protection against the intracellular bacterium *L. monocytogenes.* This form of immunity could be adoptively transferred to naive animals with lymphoid cells but not with serum from infected or immunized animals (see Chapter 13, Fig. 13–2).

As we discussed in Chapter 13, cell-mediated immunity consists of two types of reactions: macrophage activation by the T cell–derived signals CD40 ligand and IFN-γ, which results in killing of phagocytosed microbes, and lysis of infected cells by cytotoxic T lymphocytes (CTLs). Both $CD4^+$ T cells and $CD8^+$ T cells respond to protein antigens of phagocytosed microbes, which are displayed as peptides associated with class II and class I major histocompatibility complex (MHC) molecules, respectively. $CD4^+$ T cells differentiate into T_H1 effectors under the influence of IL-12, which is produced by macrophages and dendritic cells. The T cells express CD40 ligand and secrete IFN-γ, and these two stimuli activate macrophages to produce several microbicidal substances, including reactive oxygen species, nitric oxide, and lysosomal enzymes. IFN-γ also stimulates the production of antibody isotypes (e.g., IgG2a in mice) that activate complement and opsonize bacteria for phagocytosis, thus aiding the effector functions of macrophages.

- The importance of IL-12 and IFN-γ in immunity to intracellular bacteria has been demonstrated in several experimental models. For instance, knockout mice lacking either of these cytokines are extremely susceptible to infection with intracellular bacteria such as *Mycobacterium tuberculosis* and *L. monocytogenes* (Fig. 15–3).

Phagocytosed bacteria stimulate $CD8^+$ T cell responses if bacterial antigens are transported from phagosomes into the cytosol or if the bacteria escape from phagosomes and enter the cytoplasm of infected cells. In the cytoplasm, the microbes are no longer susceptible to the microbicidal mechanisms of phagocytes, and the infection is eradicated by the killing of infected cells by CTLs. Thus, the effectors of cell-mediated immunity, namely, $CD4^+$ T cells that activate macrophages and $CD8^+$ CTLs, function cooperatively in defense against intracellular bacteria (Fig. 15–4).

- The role of different T cell populations in defense against intracellular bacteria has been analyzed by adoptively transferring T cells from *L. monocytogenes*–infected mice to normal mice and chal-

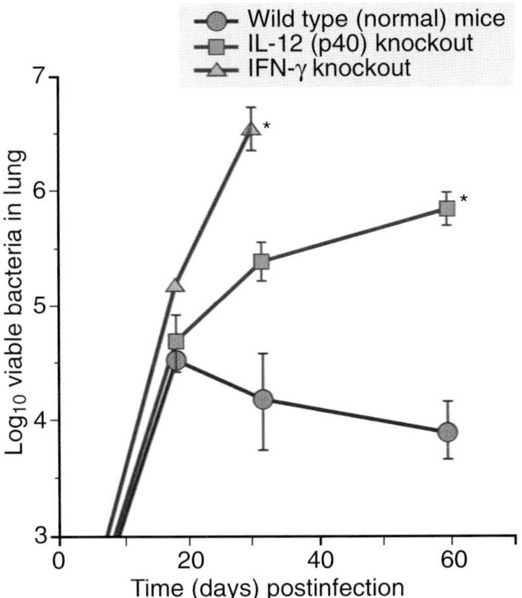

FIGURE 15–3 Role of IL-12 and IFN-γ in defense against an intracellular bacterial infection. In this experiment, wild-type (normal control) mice and knockout mice lacking the p40 subunit of IL-12 or IFN-γ were infected with the intracellular bacterium *M. tuberculosis* by aerosol. Lungs were examined at different times after infection for the number of bacteria capable of forming colonies in culture. Normal mice control bacterial growth, mice lacking IL-12 have a reduced ability to control the infection (and die by day 60), and IFN-γ knockout mice are incapable of limiting bacterial growth (and die by day 30 to 35). Asterisks indicate the time of death. (Data courtesy of Dr. Andrea Cooper, Department of Microbiology, Colorado State University, Fort Collins.)

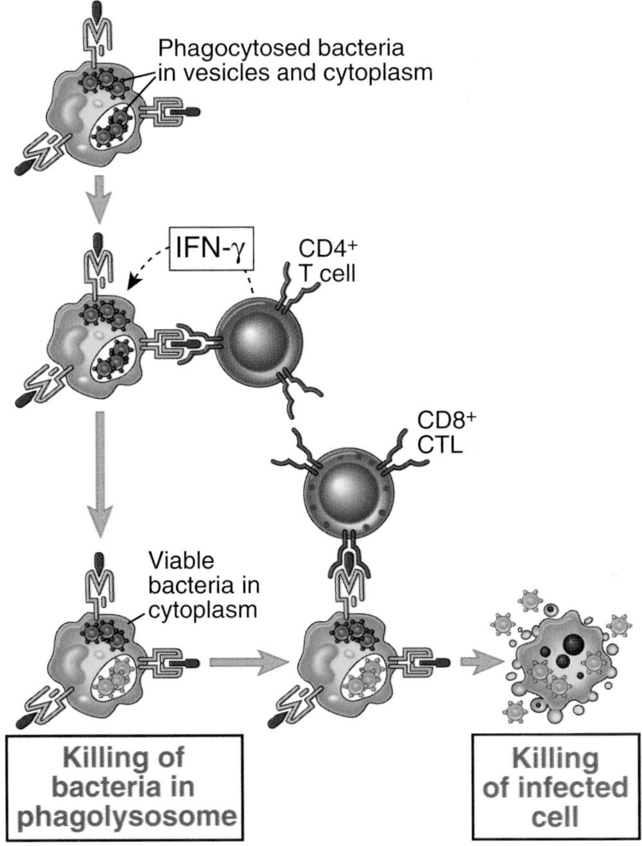

FIGURE 15–4 Cooperation of $CD4^+$ and $CD8^+$ T cells in defense against intracellular microbes. Intracellular bacteria such as *L. monocytogenes* are phagocytosed by macrophages and may survive in phagosomes and escape into the cytoplasm. $CD4^+$ T cells respond to class II MHC-associated peptide antigens derived from the intravesicular bacteria. These T cells produce IFN-γ, which activates macrophages to destroy the microbes in phagosomes. $CD8^+$ T cells respond to class I–associated peptides derived from cytosolic antigens and kill the infected cells.

lenging the recipients with the bacteria. By depleting particular cell types, it is possible to determine which effector population is responsible for protection. Such experiments have shown that both $CD4^+$ T cells and $CD8^+$ T cells function cooperatively to eliminate infection by wild-type *L. monocytogenes.* The $CD4^+$ cells produce large amounts of IFN-γ, which activates macrophages to kill phagocytosed microbes. However, *L. monocytogenes* produces a protein called listeriolysin that allows bacteria to escape from the phagolysosomes of macrophages into the cytoplasm. In their cytoplasmic haven, the bacteria are protected from the microbicidal mechanisms of macrophages, such as reactive oxygen species, which are produced mainly within phagolysosomes. $CD8^+$ T cells are then activated and function by killing any macrophages that may be harboring bacteria in their cytoplasm. A mutant of *L. monocytogenes* that lacks listeriolysin remains confined to phagolysosomes. Such mutant bacteria can be completely eradicated by $CD4^+$ T cell–derived IFN-γ production and macrophage activation.

The macrophage activation that occurs in response to intracellular microbes is also capable of causing tissue injury. This injury may be the result of delayed-type hypersensitivity (DTH) reactions to microbial protein antigens (see Chapter 13). Because intracellular bacteria have evolved to resist killing within phagocytes, they often persist for long periods and cause chronic antigenic stimulation and T cell and macrophage activation, which may result in the formation of **granulomas** surrounding the microbes (see Chapter 13, Fig. 13–12). The histologic hallmark of infection with some intracellular bacteria is granulomatous inflammation. This type of inflammatory reaction may serve to localize and prevent spread of the microbes, but it is also associated with severe functional impairment caused by tissue necrosis and fibrosis. The concept that protective immunity and pathologic hypersensitivity may coexist because they are manifestations of the same type of adaptive immune response is clearly exemplified in mycobacterial infections (Box 15–3).

Differences among individuals in the patterns of T cell responses to intracellular microbes are important determinants of disease progression and clinical outcome (Fig. 15–5). An example of this relationship between the type of T cell response and disease outcome is leprosy, which is caused by *Mycobacterium leprae.* There are two polar forms of leprosy, the lepromatous and tuberculoid forms, although many patients fall into less clear intermediate groups. In lepromatous leprosy, patients have high specific antibody titers but weak cell-mediated responses to *M. leprae* antigens. Mycobacteria proliferate within macrophages and are detectable in large numbers. The bacterial growth and persistent, but inadequate, macrophage activation result in destructive lesions in the skin and underlying tissue. In contrast, patients with tuberculoid leprosy have strong cell-mediated immunity but low antibody levels. This pattern of immunity is reflected in granulomas that form around nerves and produce peripheral sensory nerve defects and secondary traumatic skin lesions but less tissue destruction and a paucity of bacteria in the lesions. One possible reason for the differences in these two forms of disease caused by the same organism may be that there are different patterns of T cell differentiation and cytokine production in individuals. Some studies indicate that patients with the tuberculoid form of the disease produce IFN-γ and IL-2 in lesions (indicative of T_H1 cell activation), whereas patients with lepromatous leprosy produce less IFN-γ

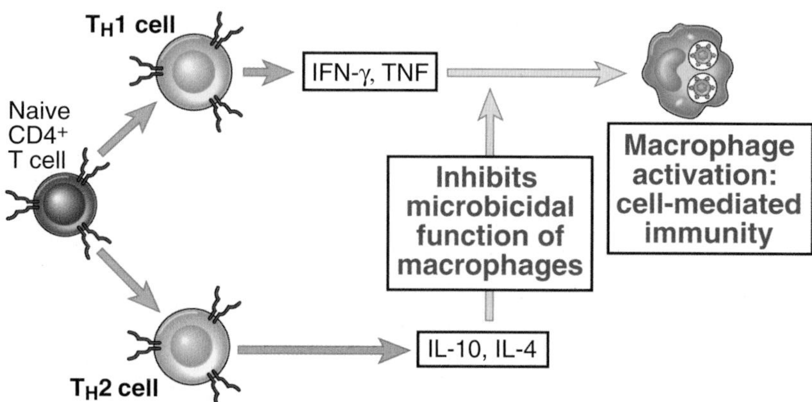

Infection	Response	Outcome
Leishmania major	Most mouse strains: T_H1	⇒ Recovery
	BALB/c mice: T_H2	⇒ Disseminated infection
Mycobacterium leprae	Some patients: T_H1	⇒ Tuberculoid leprosy
	Some patients: Defective T_H1 or dominant T_H2	⇒ Lepromatous leprosy (high bacterial count)

FIGURE 15–5 Role of T cells and cytokines in determining outcome of infections. Naive $CD4^+$ T lymphocytes may differentiate into T_H1 cells, which activate phagocytes to kill ingested microbes, and T_H2 cells, which inhibit macrophage activation. The balance between these two subsets may influence the outcome of infections, as illustrated by *Leishmania* infection in mice and leprosy in humans.

Box 15–3 ■ IN DEPTH: IMMUNITY TO *MYCOBACTERIUM TUBERCULOSIS*

Mycobacteria are slow-growing, aerobic, facultative intracellular bacilli whose cell walls contain high concentrations of lipids. These lipids are responsible for the acid-resistant staining of the bacteria with the red dye carbol fuchsin, because of which these organisms are also called acid-fast bacilli. Two common human pathogens in this class of bacteria are *Mycobacterium tuberculosis* and *Mycobacterium leprae;* in addition, atypical mycobacteria such as *Mycobacterium avium-intracellulare* cause opportunistic infections in immunodeficient hosts (e.g., AIDS patients). *Mycobacterium bovis* infects cattle and may infect humans, and bacillus Calmette-Guérin (BCG) is an attenuated, nonvirulent strain of *M. bovis* that is used as a vaccine against tuberculosis.

Tuberculosis is an example of an infection with an intracellular bacterium in which protective immunity and pathologic hypersensitivity coexist, and the lesions are caused mainly by the host response. *M. tuberculosis* does not produce any known exotoxin or endotoxin. Infection usually occurs by the respiratory route and is transmitted from person to person. It is estimated that almost 2 billion people worldwide are infected with *M. tuberculosis.* In a primary infection, bacilli multiply slowly in the lungs and cause only mild inflammation. The infection is contained by alveolar macrophages (and probably dendritic cells). More than 90% of infected patients remain asymptomatic, but bacteria survive in lungs, mainly in macrophages. By 6 to 8 weeks after infection, the macrophages have traveled to the draining lymph nodes, and $CD4^+$ T cells are activated; $CD8^+$ T cells may also be activated later. These T cells produce IFN-γ, which activates macrophages and enhances their ability to kill phagocytosed bacilli. TNF produced by T cells and macrophages also plays a role in local inflammation and macrophage activation, and TNF receptor knockout mice are highly susceptible to mycobacterial infections. The T cell reaction is adequate to control bacterial spread. However, *M. tuberculosis* is capable of surviving within macrophages because components of its cell wall inhibit the fusion of phagocytic vacuoles with lysosomes.

Continuing T cell activation leads to the formation of granulomas, which attempt to wall off the bacteria, and are often associated with central necrosis, called caseous necrosis, that is caused by macrophage products such as lysosomal enzymes and reactive oxygen species. Granulomatous inflammation is a form of DTH reaction to the bacilli. It is postulated that necrosis serves to eliminate infected macrophages and provides an anoxic environment in which the bacilli cannot divide. Thus, even the tissue injury may serve a protective function. Caseating granulomas and the fibrosis (scarring) that accompanies granulomatous inflammation are the principal causes of tissue injury and clinical disease in tuberculosis. Previously infected persons show cutaneous DTH reactions to skin challenge with a bacterial antigen preparation (purified protein derivative, or PPD). Bacilli may survive for many years and are contained without any pathologic consequences, but may be reactivated at any time, especially if the immune response becomes unable to control the infection. Although the prevalence of tuberculosis has been greatly reduced with the use of antibiotics, the incidence of the disease has recently been increasing. This is mainly because of the emergence of antibiotic-resistant strains and the increased incidence of immunodeficiency caused by HIV infection and immunosuppressive therapies. In immunodeficient individuals, lesions may result from continued, and inadequate, macrophage activation and are typically not associated with well-formed granulomas. The efficacy of BCG as a prophylactic vaccine remains controversial. In rare cases, *M. tuberculosis* may cause lesions in extrapulmonary sites. In chronic tuberculosis, sustained production of TNF leads to cachexia.

Different inbred strains of mice vary in their susceptibility to infection with *M. tuberculosis* (and with other intracellular microbes, such as the protozoan *L. major*). Susceptibility or resistance to *M. tuberculosis* has been mapped to a gene originally called *bcg* or *lsh* that has been identified as a polymorphic *NRAMP1* (NRAMP, natural resistance-associated macrophage protein) gene. *NRAMP1* is expressed on phagolysosomal membranes in macrophages and is involved in divalent cation transport. It is hypothesized that *NRAMP1* contributes to microbial killing by depleting the phagosome of divalent cations, and allelic variants of *NRAMP1* are defective in this function. Studies in humans also suggest that some variants of *NRAMP1* are associated with increased susceptibility to mycobacterial infection.

M. tuberculosis also stimulates unusual populations of T cells, including $\gamma\delta$ cells and NK-T cells. The $\gamma\delta$ T cells may be reacting to mycobacterial antigens that are homologous to heat shock proteins. NK-T cells respond to bacterial lipid antigens displayed by the CD1 class I MHC–like molecule. It is postulated that the response of unconventional T cells is a primitive defense mechanism against mycobacteria and other microbes. However, the effector functions of these cells and their roles in protective immunity against mycobacteria are not clearly established.

M. leprae is the cause of leprosy. The nature of the T cell response and specifically the types of cytokines produced by activated T cells are important determinants of the lesions and clinical course of *M. leprae* infection (see text).

and perhaps more IL-4 and IL-10 (typical of T_H2 cells). In lepromatous leprosy, both the deficiency of IFN-γ and the macrophage-suppressive effects of IL-10 and possibly IL-4 may result in weak cell-mediated immunity and failure to control bacterial spread. The role of T_H1- and T_H2-derived cytokines in determining the outcome of infection has been most clearly demonstrated in infection by the protozoan parasite *Leishmania major* in different strains of inbred mice (discussed later in this chapter).

Immune Evasion by Intracellular Bacteria

Different intracellular bacteria have developed various strategies to resist elimination by phagocytes (see Table 15–2). These include inhibiting phagolysosome fusion or escaping into the cytosol, thus hiding from the microbicidal mechanisms of lysosomes, and directly scavenging or inactivating microbicidal substances such as reactive oxygen species. The outcome of infection by these organisms often depends on whether the T cell–stimulated antimicrobial mechanisms of macrophages or microbial resistance to killing gains the upper hand. Resistance to phagocyte-mediated elimination is also the reason that such bacteria tend to cause chronic infections that may last for years, often recur after apparent cure, and are difficult to eradicate.

IMMUNITY TO FUNGI

Fungal infections, also called mycoses, are important causes of morbidity and mortality in humans. Some fungal infections are endemic, and these infections are usually caused by fungi that are present in the environment and whose spores are inhaled by humans. Other fungal infections are said to be opportunistic because the causative agents cause mild or no disease in healthy individuals but may infect and cause severe disease in immunodeficient persons. Compromised immunity is the most important predisposing factor for clinically significant fungal infections. Neutrophil deficiency as a result of bone marrow suppression or damage is frequently associated with such infections. A recent increase has been noted in opportunistic fungal infections secondary to an increase in immunodeficiencies caused mainly by AIDS and by therapy for disseminated cancer and transplant rejection, which inhibits bone marrow function and suppresses immune responses. A dreaded opportunistic fungal infection associated with AIDS is *Pneumocystis jiroveci* pneumonia, but many others contribute to the morbidity and mortality caused by immune deficiencies.

Different fungi infect humans and may live in extracellular tissues and within phagocytes. Therefore, the immune responses to these microbes are often combinations of the responses to extracellular and intracellular bacteria. However, much less is known about antifungal immunity than about immunity against bacteria and viruses. This lack of knowledge is partly due to the paucity of animal models for mycoses and partly due to the fact that these infections typically occur in individuals who are incapable of mounting effective immune responses.

Innate and Adaptive Immunity to Fungi

The principal mediators of innate immunity against fungi are neutrophils and macrophages. Patients with neutropenia are extremely susceptible to opportunistic fungal infections. Neutrophils presumably liberate fungicidal substances, such as reactive oxygen intermediates and lysosomal enzymes, and phagocytose fungi for intracellular killing. Virulent strains of *Cryptococcus neoformans* inhibit the production of cytokines such as TNF and IL-12 by macrophages and stimulate production of IL-10, thus inhibiting macrophage activation.

Cell-mediated immunity is the major mechanism of adaptive immunity against fungal infections. *Histoplasma capsulatum,* a facultative intracellular parasite that lives in macrophages, is eliminated by the same cellular mechanisms that are effective against intracellular bacteria. $CD4^+$ and $CD8^+$ T cells cooperate to eliminate the yeast forms of *C. neoformans,* which tend to colonize the lungs and brain in immunodeficient hosts. *Candida* infections often start at mucosal surfaces, and cell-mediated immunity is believed to prevent spread of the fungi into tissues. In many of these situations, T_H1 responses are protective and T_H2 responses are detrimental to the host. Not surprisingly, granulomatous inflammation is an important cause of host tissue injury in some intracellular fungal infections, such as histoplasmosis. Fungi often elicit specific antibody responses that are of protective value. Antibody-dependent cellular cytotoxicity, mediated via Fc receptors, plays a role in clearing some fungi, such as *C. neoformans.*

IMMUNITY TO VIRUSES

Viruses are obligatory intracellular microorganisms that replicate within cells, using components of the nucleic acid and protein synthetic machinery of the host. Viruses typically infect a wide variety of cell populations by using normal cell surface molecules as receptors to enter the cells. After entering cells, viruses can cause tissue injury and disease by any of several mechanisms. Viral replication interferes with normal cellular protein synthesis and function and leads to injury and ultimately death of the infected cell. This result is one type of cytopathic effect of viruses, and the infection is said to be "lytic" because the infected cell is lysed. Viruses may also cause latent infections, during which viral DNA persists in host cells and produces proteins that may or may not alter cellular functions. Latency is often a state of balance between persistent infection and an immune response that can control the infection but not eradicate it. Predictably, some of these latent infections become widespread and even lytic if the immune response is compromised. Innate and adaptive immune responses to viruses are aimed at blocking infection and eliminating infected cells (Fig. 15–6).

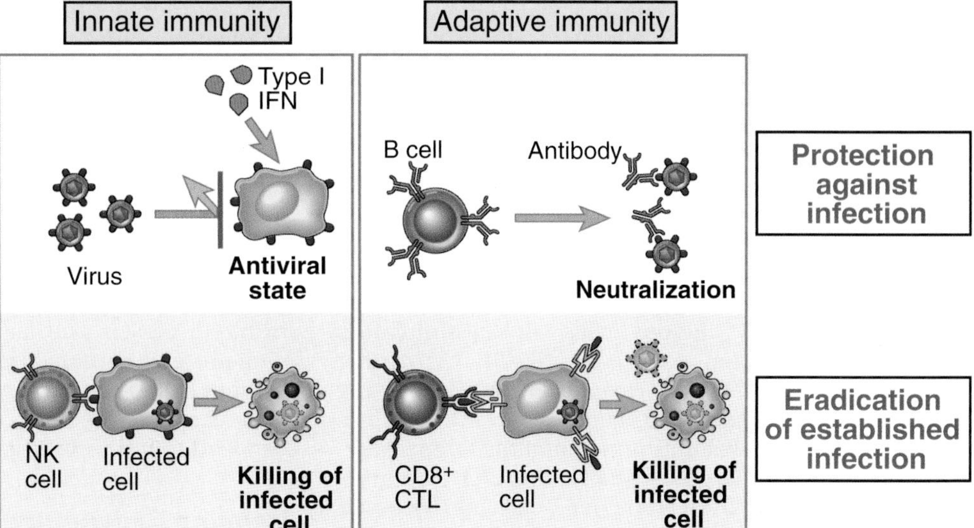

FIGURE 15–6 Innate and adaptive immune responses against viruses. Immunity against viruses functions to prevent infection and to eradicate established infection. Innate immunity is mediated by type I IFNs, which prevent infection, and NK cells, which eliminate infected cells. Adaptive immunity is mediated by antibodies and CTLs, which also block infection and kill infected cells, respectively.

Innate Immunity to Viruses

The principal mechanisms of innate immunity against viruses are inhibition of infection by type I IFNs and NK cell-mediated killing of infected cells. Infection by many viruses is associated with production of type I IFN by infected cells, especially dendritic cells of the plasmacytoid type (see Box 6–1, Chapter 6). Several biochemical pathways trigger IFN production (see Chapters 2 and 12). These include recognition of viral RNA and DNA by endosomal Toll-like receptors (TLRs), and activation of cytoplasmic kinases by viral RNA. Cytoplasmic sensors of viruses provide TLR-independent pathways of IFN production. These sensors include RNA helicases, such as RIG-I (retinoid-inducible gene-I) and MDA-5, that recognize RNAs produced in virus-infected cells. The TLR- and cytoplasmic sensor-initiated pathways converge on the activation of protein kinases, which in turn activate transcription factors that stimulate IFN gene transcription. Type I IFNs function to inhibit viral replication in both infected and uninfected cells by inducing an "antiviral state" (see Chapter 12). One of the key molecules induced by IFNs is PKR, a protein kinase that must bind dsRNA in order to be activated, and is therefore functional only in virus-infected cells. Active PKR shuts off protein synthesis, causing infected cells to die. NK cells kill cells infected with a variety of viruses and are an important mechanism of immunity against viruses early in the course of infection, before adaptive immune responses have developed. NK cells also recognize infected cells in which the virus has shut off class I MHC expression (discussed later) because the absence of class I releases NK cells from a normal state of inhibition (see Chapter 2, Fig. 2–10).

Adaptive Immunity to Viruses

Adaptive immunity against viral infections is mediated by antibodies, which block virus binding and entry into host cells, and by CTLs, which eliminate the infection by killing infected cells (see Fig. 15–6). Antibodies are produced and are effective against viruses only during the extracellular stage of the lives of these microbes. Viruses may be extracellular early in the course of infection, before they enter host cells, or when they are released from infected cells by virus budding or if the cells are killed. Antiviral antibodies function mainly as neutralizing antibodies to prevent virus attachment and entry into host cells. These neutralizing antibodies bind to viral envelope or capsid antigens. Secreted antibodies of the IgA isotype are important for neutralizing viruses that enter through the respiratory and intestinal mucosa. Oral immunization against poliomyelitis works by inducing mucosal immunity. In addition to neutralization, antibodies may opsonize viral particles and promote their clearance by phagocytes. Complement activation may also participate in antibody-mediated viral immunity, mainly by promoting phagocytosis and possibly by direct lysis of viruses with lipid envelopes.

The importance of humoral immunity in defense against viral infections is supported by the observation that resistance to a particular virus, induced by either infection or vaccination, is often specific for the serologic (antibody-defined) type of the virus. An example is influenza virus, in which exposure to one serologic type does not confer resistance to other serotypes of the virus. Neutralizing antibodies block viral infection of cells and spread of viruses from cell to cell, but once the viruses enter cells and begin to replicate intracellularly, they are inaccessible to antibodies. Therefore, humoral immunity induced by previous infection or vaccination is able to protect individuals from viral infection but cannot by itself eradicate established infection.

Elimination of viruses that reside within cells is mediated by CTLs, which kill the infected cells. As we have mentioned in previous chapters, the principal physiologic function of CTLs is surveillance against viral infection. Most virus-specific CTLs are $CD8^+$ T cells that recognize cytosolic, usually endogenously synthesized, viral antigens in association with class I MHC molecules on any nucleated cell. If the infected cell is a tissue cell and not a professional antigen-presenting cell (APC), the infected cell may be phagocytosed by a professional APC, such as a dendritic cell, which processes the viral antigens and presents them to naive $CD8^+$ T cells. This process of cross-presentation, or cross-priming, was described in Chapter 9 (see Fig. 9–3). Full differentiation of $CD8^+$ CTLs requires innate immunity or cytokines produced by $CD4^+$ helper cells or costimulators expressed on infected cells (Chapter 9). Cytopathic viruses, especially RNA viruses, tend to stimulate strong innate immune responses and are able to induce CTLs without T cell help, whereas noncytopathic latent infections, often by DNA viruses, usually elicit CTL responses only in the presence of $CD4^+$ helper T cells. As discussed in Chapters 9 and 13, $CD8^+$ T cells undergo massive proliferation during viral infection, and most of the proliferating cells are specific for a few viral peptides. Some of the activated T cells differentiate into effector CTLs, which can kill any infected nucleated cell. The antiviral effects of CTLs are mainly due to killing of infected cells, but other mechanisms include activation of nucleases within infected cells that degrade viral genomes, and secretion of cytokines such as IFN-γ, which has some antiviral activity.

The importance of CTLs in defense against viral infection is demonstrated by the increased susceptibility to such infections seen in patients and animals that are deficient in T lymphocytes, and by the experimental observation that mice can be protected against some virus infections by adoptive transfer of virus-specific, class I–restricted CTLs. Furthermore, many viruses are able to alter their surface antigens, such as envelope glycoproteins, and thus escape attack by antibodies. However, infected cells produce viral proteins that are often invariant, so that CTL-mediated defense remains effective against such viruses.

In some viral infections, especially with noncytopathic viruses, tissue injury may be caused by CTLs. An experimental model of a disease in which the pathology is due to the host immune response is lymphocytic choriomeningitis virus (LCMV) infection in mice, which induces inflammation of the spinal cord meninges. LCMV infects meningeal cells, but it is noncytopathic and does not injure the infected cells directly. The virus stimulates the development of virus-specific CTLs that kill infected meningeal cells during a physiologic attempt to eradicate the infection. Therefore, T cell–deficient mice infected with LCMV become chronic carriers of the virus, but pathologic lesions do not develop, whereas in normal mice, meningitis develops. This observation appears to contradict the usual situation, in which immunodeficient individuals are more susceptible to infectious diseases than normal individuals are. Hepatitis B virus infection in humans shows some similarities to murine LCMV in that immunodeficient persons who become infected do not develop the disease but become carriers who can transmit the infection to otherwise healthy persons. The livers of patients with acute and chronic active hepatitis contain large numbers of $CD8^+$ T cells, and hepatitis virus–specific, class I MHC–restricted CTLs can be isolated from liver biopsy specimens and propagated in vitro.

Immune responses to viral infections may be involved in producing disease in other ways. A consequence of persistent infection with some viruses, such as hepatitis B, is the formation of circulating immune complexes composed of viral antigens and specific antibodies (see Chapter 18). These complexes are deposited in blood vessels and lead to systemic vasculitis. Some viral proteins contain amino acid sequences that are also present in some self antigens. It has been postulated that because of this "molecular mimicry," antiviral immunity can lead to immune responses against self antigens.

Immune Evasion by Viruses

Viruses have evolved numerous mechanisms for evading host immunity (Table 15–3).

- ***Viruses can alter their antigens and are thus no longer targets of immune responses.*** The antigens affected are most commonly surface glycoproteins that are recognized by antibodies, but T cell epitopes may also undergo variation. The principal mechanisms of antigenic variation are point mutations and

Table 15–3. Mechanisms of Immune Evasion by Viruses

Mechanism of immune evasion	Examples
Antigenic variation	Influenza, rhinovirus, HIV
Inhibition of antigen processing	
Blockade of TAP transporter	Herpes simplex
Removal of class I molecules from the ER	Cytomegalovirus
Production of cytokine receptor homologs	Vaccinia, poxviruses (IL-1, IFN-γ) Cytomegalovirus (chemokine)
Production of immunosuppressive cytokine	Epstein-Barr virus (IL-10)
Infection of immunocompetent cells	HIV

Abbreviations: ER, endoplasmic reticulum; HIV, human immunodeficiency virus; TAP, transporter associated with antigen processing.

Representative examples of different mechanisms used by viruses to resist host immunity are listed.

reassortment of RNA genomes (in RNA viruses). Because of antigenic variation, a virus may become resistant to immunity generated in the population by previous infections. The influenza pandemics that occurred in 1918, 1957, and 1968 were due to different strains of the virus, and subtler variants arise more frequently. There are so many serotypes of rhinovirus that specific immunization against the common cold may not be a feasible preventive strategy. Human immunodeficiency virus 1 (HIV-1), the virus that causes AIDS, is also capable of tremendous antigenic variation (see Chapter 20). In these situations, prophylactic vaccination may have to be directed against invariant viral proteins.

- ***Some viruses inhibit class I MHC–associated presentation of cytosolic protein antigens.*** Several mechanisms that inhibit antigen presentation have been described with different viruses (Box 15–4). Inhibition of antigen processing and presentation blocks the assembly and expression of stable class I MHC molecules and the display of viral peptides. As a result, cells infected by such viruses cannot be recognized or killed by $CD8^+$ CTLs. NK cells may have evolved as an adaptation to this viral evasion strategy because NK cells are activated by infected cells, especially in the absence of class I MHC molecules.

- ***Some viruses produce molecules that inhibit the immune response.*** Poxviruses encode molecules that are secreted by infected cells and bind to several cytokines, including IFN-γ, TNF, IL-1, IL-18, and chemokines. The secreted cytokine-binding proteins may function as competitive antagonists of the cytokines. Some cytomegaloviruses produce a molecule that is homologous to class I MHC proteins and may compete for binding and presentation of peptide antigens. Epstein-Barr virus produces a protein that is homologous to the cytokine IL-10, which inhibits activation of macrophages and dendritic cells and may thus suppress cell-mediated immunity. These examples probably represent a small fraction of immunosuppressive viral molecules. Identification of these molecules raises the intriguing possibility that viruses have acquired genes encoding endogenous inhibitors of immune responses during their passage through human hosts and have thus evolved to infect and colonize humans.

- ***Some chronic viral infections are associated with failure of CTL responses,*** which allows viral persistence. Studies of a chronic infection with lymphocytic choriomeningitis in mice have shown that this type of immune deficit may result from activation of inhibitory T cell pathways, such as the PD-1 pathway, which normally functions to maintain T cell tolerance to self antigens (see Chapter 11). Reduced T cell responses resulting from HIV infection may also be partly because of PD-1–mediated T cell unresponsiveness. Thus, viruses may have learned to exploit normal mechanisms of immune regulation and to activate these pathways in T cells.

- ***Viruses may infect and either kill or inactivate immunocompetent cells.*** The obvious example is HIV, which survives by infecting and eliminating $CD4^+$ T cells, the key inducers of immune responses to protein antigens.

IMMUNITY TO PARASITES

In infectious disease terminology, parasitic infection refers to infection with animal parasites such as protozoa, helminths, and ectoparasites (e.g., ticks and mites). Such parasites currently account for greater morbidity and mortality than any other class of infectious organisms, particularly in developing countries. It is estimated that about 30% of the world's population suffers from parasitic infestations. Malaria alone affects more than 100 million people worldwide and is responsible for about 1 million deaths annually. The magnitude of this public health problem is the principal reason for the great interest in immunity to parasites and for the development of immunoparasitology as a distinct branch of immunology.

Most parasites go through complex life cycles, part of which occurs in humans (or other vertebrates) and part of which occurs in intermediate hosts, such as flies, ticks, and snails. Humans are usually infected by bites from infected intermediate hosts or by sharing a particular habitat with an intermediate host. For instance, malaria and trypanosomiasis are transmitted by insect bites, and schistosomiasis is transmitted by exposure to water in which infected snails reside. Most parasitic infections are chronic because of weak innate immunity and the ability of parasites to evade or resist elimination by adaptive immune responses. Furthermore, many antiparasite antibiotics are not effective at killing the organisms. Individuals living in endemic areas require repeated chemotherapy because of continued exposure, and such treatment is often not possible because of expense and logistic problems. Therefore, the development of prophylactic vaccines for parasites has long been considered an important goal for developing countries.

Innate Immunity to Parasites

Although different protozoan and helminthic parasites have been shown to activate different mechanisms of innate immunity, these organisms are often able to survive and replicate in their hosts because they are well adapted to resisting host defenses. The principal innate immune response to protozoa is phagocytosis, but many of these parasites are resistant to phagocytic killing and may even replicate within macrophages. Some protozoa may express surface molecules that are recognized by TLRs and activate phagocytes. Phagocytes also attack helminthic parasites and secrete microbicidal substances to kill organisms that are too large to be phagocytosed. Many helminths have thick teguments that make them resistant to the cytocidal mechanisms of neutrophils and macrophages. Some helminths may

Box 15–4 ▪ IN DEPTH: INHIBITION OF ANTIGEN PROCESSING BY VIRUSES

As viruses have co-evolved with their hosts, they have developed many strategies to evade immune responses. Several viral genes have been identified that encode proteins that modulate host immune responses. Some of these viral proteins inhibit the presentation of viral antigens to T cells. CD8$^+$ class I MHC-restricted CTLs are the major mechanisms of defense against viral infections of cells. If a virus could inhibit the class I–restricted antigen presentation pathway, that virus would become invisible to CTLs and would be able to replicate in infected cells. In Chapter 6, we described the steps in the processing of cytosolic antigens and the presentation of antigenic peptides bound to class I molecules (see Fig. 6–13). Each of these steps may be targeted for inhibition by a viral product. Some examples are shown in the figure below and listed here:

- The transcription of class I MHC genes is inhibited by the E1A protein of pathogenic strains of adenovirus.
- Herpes simplex viruses 1 and 2 produce a protein, called ICP-47, that binds to the peptide-binding site of the TAP transporter and prevents the transporter from capturing cytosolic peptides and transporting them into the endoplasmic reticulum for binding to class I molecules.
- The adenovirus E3 19-kD protein binds to and retains class I molecules in the endoplasmic reticulum, preventing these molecules from exiting with their peptide cargo.
- The human cytomegalovirus (CMV) US3 protein sequesters class I molecules in the endoplasmic reticulum, and murine CMV gp40 (40-kD glycoprotein) retains class I molecules in the cis-Golgi compartment.
- Human CMV produces two proteins, US2 and US11, which bind to class I molecules in the endoplasmic reticulum and actively carry, or "dislocate," these molecules into the cytosol, where they cannot be loaded with antigenic peptides and are degraded in the proteasome.
- Kaposi sarcoma herpes virus (KSHV) K3 and K5 proteins induce rapid internalization of class I MHC molecules from the cell surface.
- Two proteins of HIV, Vpu and Nef, also inhibit class I expression in infected cells; Nef appears to do this by forcing internalization of class I molecules from the surface of infected cells, and Vpu destabilizes newly synthesized class I molecules.

The consequence of blocking class I–peptide association in all these cases is that infected cells show reduced expression of stable class I molecules on the surface and do not display viral peptides for T cell recognition. However, it is difficult to prove that the viral genes encoding proteins that inhibit antigen presentation are actually virulence genes, required for the infectivity or pathogenicity of the viruses.

An excellent example of the constant struggle between microbes and their hosts is the adaptation of the mammalian immune system to recognize class I–deficient cells. Thus, viruses try to evade recognition by CTLs by inhibiting class I MHC expression, but NK cells have evolved to respond specifically to the absence of class I MHC on virus-infected cells (see Chapter 2). Not surprisingly, there is emerging evidence that some viruses may produce proteins that act as ligands for NK cell inhibitory receptors and thus inhibit NK cell activation.

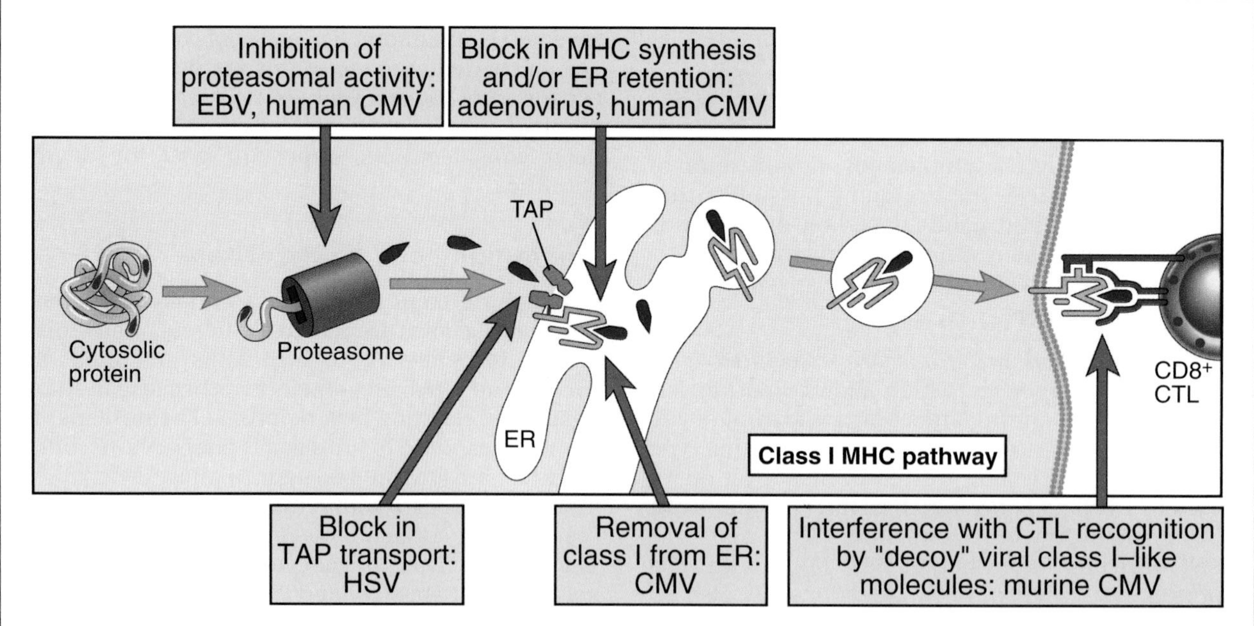

The pathway of class I MHC-associated antigen presentation is shown, with examples of viruses that block different steps in this pathway. CMV, cytomegalovirus; EBV, Epstein-Barr virus; ER, endoplasmic reticulum; HSV, herpes simplex virus; TAP, transporter associated with antigen processing.

also activate the alternative pathway of complement, although as we shall discuss later, parasites recovered from infected hosts appear to have developed resistance to complement-mediated lysis.

Adaptive Immunity to Parasites

Different protozoa and helminths vary greatly in their structural and biochemical properties, life cycles, and pathogenic mechanisms. It is therefore not surprising that different parasites elicit distinct adaptive immune responses (Table 15–4). Some pathogenic protozoa have evolved to survive within host cells, so protective immunity against these organisms is mediated by mechanisms similar to those that eliminate intracellular bacteria and viruses. In contrast, metazoa such as helminths survive in extracellular tissues, and their elimination is often dependent on special types of antibody responses.

The principal defense mechanism against protozoa that survive within macrophages is cell-mediated immunity, particularly macrophage activation by T_H1 cell–derived cytokines. Infection of mice with *Leishmania major,* a protozoan that survives within the endosomes of macrophages, is the best documented example of how dominance of T_H1 or T_H2 responses determines disease resistance or susceptibility (see Fig. 15–5). Resistance to the infection is associated with activation of *Leishmania*-specific T_H1 $CD4^+$ T cells, which produce IFN-γ and thereby activate macrophages to destroy intracellular parasites. Conversely, activation of T_H2 cells by the protozoa results in increased parasite survival and exacerbation of lesions because of the macrophage-suppressive actions of T_H2 cytokines, notably IL-4.

- Most inbred strains of mice are resistant to infection with *L. major,* but inbred BALB/c mice are highly susceptible and die if they are infected with large numbers of parasites. After infection, the resistant strains produce large amounts of IFN-γ in response to leishmanial antigens, whereas the strains that are susceptible to fatal leishmaniasis produce more IL-4 in response to the parasite. IFN-γ activates macrophages and enhances intracellular killing of *Leishmania,* and high levels of IL-4 inhibit the activation of macrophages by IFN-γ. Treatment of resistant mice with anti-IFN-γ antibody makes them susceptible, and conversely, treatment of susceptible mice with anti-IL-4 antibody induces resistance. The same results are seen in knockout mice lacking IFN-γ or IL-4. Treatment of susceptible mice with IL-12 at the time of infection also induces resistance to the infection. IL-12 enhances the production of IFN-γ and the development of T_H1 cells. This result is the basis for the suggested use of IL-12 as a vaccine adjuvant, not only for leishmaniasis but also for other infections that are combated by cell-mediated immunity.

Multiple genes appear to control the balance of protective and harmful immune responses to intracellular parasites in inbred mice and presumably in humans as well. Attempts to identify these genes are ongoing in many laboratories.

Protozoa that replicate inside various host cells and lyse these cells stimulate specific antibody and CTL

Table 15–4. Immune Responses to Disease-Causing Parasites

Parasite	Diseases	Principal mechanisms of protective immunity
Protozoa		
Plasmodium species	Malaria	Antibodies and $CD8^+$ CTLs
Leishmania donovani	Leishmaniasis (mucocutaneous, disseminated)	$CD4^+$ T_H1 cells activate macrophages to kill phagocytosed parasites
Trypanosoma brucei	African trypanosomiasis	Antibodies
Entamoeba histolytica	Amebiasis	Antibodies, phagocytosis
Metazoa		
Schistosoma species	Schistosomiasis	ADCC mediated by eosinophils, macrophages
Filaria, e.g., *Wuchereria bancrofti*	Filariasis	Cell-mediated immunity; role of antibodies?

Abbreviations: ADCC, antibody-dependent cell-mediated cytotoxicity; CTLs, cytotoxic T lymphocytes.

Selected examples of parasites and immune responses to them are listed.

responses, similar to cytopathic viruses. An example of such an organism is the malaria parasite. It was thought for many years that antibodies were the major protective mechanism against malaria, and early attempts at vaccinating against this infection focused on generating antibodies. It is now apparent that the CTL response is an important defense against the spread of this intracellular protozoan (Box 15–5).

Defense against many helminthic infections is mediated by the activation of T_H2 cells, which results in production of IgE antibodies and activation of eosinophils. IgE antibodies that bind to the surface of the helminths may activate mast cells, and IgG and IgA antibodies bring eosinophils to the helminths and activate the eosinophils to release granule contents. The combined actions of mast cells and eosinophils lead to expulsion and destruction of the parasites (see Chapter 14). Production of specific IgE antibody and eosinophilia are frequently observed in infections by helminths. These responses are attributed to the propensity of helminths to stimulate differentiation of naive $CD4^+$ helper T cells to the T_H2 subset of effector cells, which secrete IL-4 and IL-5. IL-4 stimulates the production of IgE, and IL-5 stimulates the development and activation of eosinophils. Eosinophils may be more effective at killing helminths than other leukocytes are because the major basic protein of eosinophil granules may be more toxic for helminths than the proteolytic enzymes and reactive oxygen intermediates produced by neutrophils and macrophages. The expulsion of some intestinal nematodes may be due to IL-4–dependent mechanisms such as increased peristalsis that do not require IgE.

Adaptive immune responses to parasites can also contribute to tissue injury. Some parasites and their products induce granulomatous responses with concomitant fibrosis. *Schistosoma mansoni* eggs deposited in the liver stimulate $CD4^+$ T cells, which in turn activate macrophages and induce DTH reactions. DTH reactions result in the formation of granulomas around the eggs; an unusual feature of these granulomas, especially in mice, is the association with T_H2 responses. (Recall that granulomas are generally induced by T_H1 responses against persistent antigens; see Chapter 13.) Such T_H2-induced granulomas may result from the process of "alternative" macrophage activation induced by IL-4 and IL-13 (see Chapter 13). The granulomas serve to contain the schistosome eggs, but severe fibrosis associated with this chronic cell-mediated immune response leads to disruption of venous blood flow in the liver, portal hypertension, and cirrhosis. In lymphatic filariasis, lodging of the parasites in lymphatic vessels leads to chronic cell-mediated immune reactions and ultimately to fibrosis. Fibrosis results in lymphatic obstruction and severe lymphedema. Chronic and persistent parasitic infestations are often associated with the formation of complexes of parasite antigens and specific antibodies. The complexes can be deposited in blood vessels and kidney glomeruli and produce vasculitis and nephritis, respectively (see Chapter 20). Immune complex disease is a complication of schistosomiasis and malaria.

Immune Evasion by Parasites

Parasites evade protective immunity by reducing their immunogenicity and by inhibiting host immune responses. Different parasites have developed remarkably effective ways of resisting immunity (Table 15–5).

- Parasites change their surface antigens during their life cycle in vertebrate hosts. Two forms of antigenic variation are well defined. The first is a stage-specific change in antigen expression, such that the mature tissue stages of parasites produce different antigens than the infective stages do. For example, the infective sporozoite stage of malaria parasites is antigenically distinct from the merozoites that reside in the host and are responsible for chronic infection. By the time the immune system has responded to infection by sporozoites, the parasite has differentiated, expresses new antigens, and is no longer a target for immune elimination. The second and more remarkable example of antigenic variation in parasites is the continuous variation of major surface antigens seen in African trypanosomes such as *Trypanosoma brucei* and *Trypanosoma rhodesiense.* Continuous antigenic variation in trypanosomes is probably due to programmed variation in expression of the genes encoding the major surface antigen. Infected individuals show waves of blood parasitemia, and each wave consists of parasites expressing a surface antigen that is different from the previous wave (Fig. 15–7). Thus, by the time the host produces antibodies against the parasite, an antigenically different organism has grown out. More than a hundred such waves of parasitemia can occur in an infection. One consequence of antigenic variation in parasites is that it is difficult to effectively vaccinate individuals against these infections.
- Parasites become resistant to immune effector mechanisms during their residence in vertebrate hosts. Perhaps the best examples are schistosome larvae, which travel to the lungs of infected animals and

Table 15–5. Mechanisms of Immune Evasion by Parasites

Mechanism of immune evasion	Examples
Antigenic variation	Trypanosomes, *Plasmodium*
Acquired resistance to complement, CTLs	Schistosomes
Inhibition of host immune responses	Filaria (secondary to lymphatic obstruction), trypanosomes
Antigen shedding	Entamoeba

Abbreviation: CTL, cytotoxic T lymphocyte.

Box 15–5 ■ IN DEPTH: IMMUNITY TO MALARIA

Malaria is a disease caused by a protozoan parasite *(Plasmodium)* that infects more than 100 million people and causes 1 to 2 million deaths annually. Infection is initiated when sporozoites are inoculated into the blood stream by the bite of an infected mosquito *(Anopheles).* The sporozoites rapidly disappear from the blood and invade the parenchymal cells of the liver. In the hepatocytes, sporozoites develop into merozoites by a multiple-fission process termed *schizogony.* One to 2 weeks after infection, the infected hepatocytes burst and release thousands of merozoites, thereby initiating the erythrocytic stage of the life cycle. The merozoites invade red blood cells by a process that involves multiple ligand-receptor interactions, such as binding of the *Plasmodium falciparum* protein EBA-175 to glycophorin A on erythrocytes. Merozoites develop sequentially into ring forms, trophozoites, and schizonts, each of which expresses both shared and unique antigens. The erythrocytic cycle continues when schizont-infected red blood cells burst and release merozoites that invade other erythrocytes. Sexual stage gametocytes develop in some cells and are taken up by mosquitoes during a blood meal, after which they fertilize and develop into oocysts. Immature sporozoites develop in the mosquitoes within 2 weeks and travel to the salivary glands, where they mature and become infective.

The clinical features of malaria caused by the four species of *Plasmodium* that infect humans include fever spikes, anemia, and splenomegaly. Many pathologic manifestations of malaria may be due to the activation of T cells and macrophages and production of TNF. The development of cerebral malaria in a murine model is prevented by depletion of $CD4^+$ T lymphocytes or by injection of neutralizing anti-TNF antibody.

The immune response to malaria is complex and stage specific; that is, immunization with antigens derived from sporozoites, merozoites, or gametocytes protects only against the particular stage. On the basis of this observation, it is postulated that a vaccine consisting of combined immunogenic epitopes from each of these stages should stimulate more effective immunity than a vaccine that incorporates antigens from only one stage. The best characterized malaria vaccines are directed against sporozoites. Because of the stage-specific nature of sporozoite antigens, such vaccines must provide sterilizing immunity to be effective. Protective immunity may be induced in humans by injection of radiation-inactivated sporozoites. This type of protection is partly mediated by antibodies that inhibit sporozoite invasion of liver cells *in vitro.* Such antibodies recognize the circumsporozoite (CS) protein, which mediates the binding of parasites to liver cells. The CS protein contains a central region of about 40 tandem repeats of the sequence Asn-Ala-Asn-Pro (NANP), which makes up the immunodominant B cell epitope of the protein. Anti-(NANP)n antibodies neutralize sporozoite infectivity, but such antibodies provide only partial protection against infection. The antibody response to CS protein is dependent on helper T cells. Most CS-specific helper T cells recognize epitopes outside the NANP region, and some of these T cell epitopes correspond to the most variable residues of the CS protein, which suggests that variation of the antigens of the surface coat may have arisen in response to selective pressures imposed by specific T cell responses.

$CD8^+$ T cells play an important role in immunity to the hepatic stages of infection. If sporozoite-immunized mice are depleted of $CD8^+$ T cells by injection of anti-CD8 antibodies, they are unable to resist a challenge infection. The protective effects of $CD8^+$ T cells may be mediated by direct killing of sporozoite-infected hepatocytes or indirectly by the secretion of IFN-γ and activation of hepatocytes to produce nitric oxide and other agents that kill parasites. IL-12 induces resistance to sporozoite challenge in rodents and nonhuman primates, presumably by stimulating IFN-γ production. Conversely, resistance of *Plasmodium berghei* sporozoite-immunized mice to a challenge infection is abrogated by treatment with anti-IFN-γ antibodies.

The sexual blood stage of malaria is an important target for vaccine development. The major goal of this form of immunization is to generate antibodies that kill infected erythrocytes or block merozoite invasion of new red cells. Although infected individuals mount strong immune responses against blood stage antigens during natural malaria infections, most of these responses do not appear to affect parasite survival or to result in the selection of new antigenic variants. Nevertheless, some merozoite proteins may be good vaccine candidates. Of particular interest is the major merozoite surface antigen MSP-1, which contains a highly conserved carboxy-terminal region. Immunization with recombinant DNA-derived carboxy-terminal peptides has been shown to confer significant protection against malaria in rodents and has shown promising results in primate trials with human malaria parasite strains. The resistance induced by MSP-1 vaccination appears to involve antibody-dependent mechanisms.

Transmission-blocking vaccines are being developed to act on stages of the parasite life cycle that are found in mosquitoes. Such vaccines provide no protection for an immunized individual but act to reduce the number of parasites available for development in the mosquito vector. One such vaccine is an antigen, Pfs25, that is located on the surface of zygotes and ookinetes and is involved in parasite invasion of mosquito gut epithelium. In individuals immunized against this parasite antigen, the antibodies that develop are ingested by the mosquito during a blood meal and block the ability of the parasite to infect and mature in the mosquito. These parasite stages are found only in the mosquito vector and are not exposed to host immune responses. Therefore, the antigens expressed in the mosquito do not undergo the high rates of variation that are typical of immunodominant parasite antigens in the vertebrate host.

This box was written with the assistance of Drs. Alan Sher and Louis Miller, National Institutes of Health, Bethesda, Maryland.

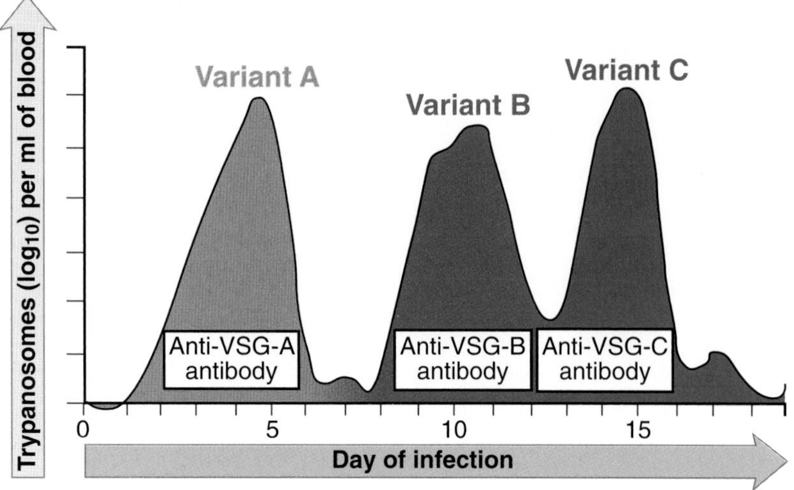

FIGURE 15–7 Antigenic variation in trypanosomes. In a mouse infected experimentally with a single clone of *T. rhodesiense,* the blood parasite counts show cyclic waves. Each wave is due to a new antigenic variant of the parasite (labeled variants A, B, and C) that expresses a new variable surface glycoprotein (VSG, the immunodominant antigen of the parasite), and each decline is a result of a specific antibody response to that variant. (Courtesy of Dr. John Mansfield, University of Wisconsin, Madison.)

during this migration develop a tegument that is resistant to damage by complement and by CTLs. The biochemical basis of this change is not known.

- Protozoan parasites may conceal themselves from the immune system either by living inside host cells or by developing cysts that are resistant to immune effectors. Some helminthic parasites reside in intestinal lumens and are sheltered from cell-mediated immune effector mechanisms. Parasites may also shed their antigenic coats, either spontaneously or after binding specific antibodies. Shedding of antigens renders the parasites resistant to subsequent antibody-mediated attack.
- Parasites inhibit host immune responses by multiple mechanisms. T cell anergy to parasite antigens has been observed in severe schistosomiasis involving the liver and spleen and in filarial infections. The mechanisms of immunologic unresponsiveness in these infections are not well understood. In lymphatic filariasis, infection of lymph nodes with subsequent architectural disruption may contribute to deficient immunity. Some parasites, such as *Leishmania,* stimulate the development of $CD25^+$ regulatory T cells, which suppress the immune response enough to allow persistence of the parasites. More nonspecific and generalized immunosuppression is observed in malaria and African trypanosomiasis. This immune deficiency has been attributed to the production of immunosuppressive cytokines by activated macrophages and T cells and defects in T cell activation.

The worldwide implications of parasitic infestations for health and economic development are well appreciated. Attempts to develop effective vaccines against these infections have been actively pursued for many years. Although the progress has been slower than one would have hoped, elucidation of the fundamental mechanisms of immune responses to and immune evasion by parasites holds promise for the future.

STRATEGIES FOR VACCINE DEVELOPMENT

The birth of immunology as a science dates from Edward Jenner's successful vaccination against smallpox in 1796. The importance of prophylactic immunization against infectious diseases is best illustrated by the fact that worldwide programs of vaccination have led to the complete or nearly complete eradication of many of these diseases in developed countries (see Chapter 1, Table 1–1).

The success of active immunization in eradicating infectious disease is dependent on numerous factors:

- Vaccines are effective if the infectious agent does not establish latency, if it does not undergo much or any antigenic variation, and if it does not interfere with the host immune response. It is difficult to effectively vaccinate against microbes such as HIV, which establishes latent infection, is highly variable, and disables key components of the immune system.
- Vaccines are most effective against infections that are limited to human hosts, and do not have animal reservoirs.

Vaccines induce protection against infections by stimulating the development of antibodies, long-lived effector cells, and memory cells. Most vaccines in routine use today work by inducing humoral immunity, and attempts to stimulate cell-mediated immune responses by vaccination are ongoing.

In the following section, we summarize the approaches to vaccination that have been tried (Table 15–6) and their major value and limitations.

Attenuated and Inactivated Bacterial and Viral Vaccines

Vaccines composed of intact nonpathogenic microbes are made by treating the microbe in such a way that it can no longer cause disease (i.e., its virulence is attenu-

Table 15–6. Vaccine Approaches

Type of vaccine	Examples
Live attenuated or killed bacteria	BCG, cholera
Live attenuated viruses	Polio, rabies
Subunit (antigen) vaccines	Tetanus toxoid, diphtheria toxoid
Conjugate vaccines	*Haemophilus influenzae*, pneumococcus
Synthetic vaccines	Hepatitis (recombinant proteins)
Viral vectors	Clinical trials of HIV antigens in canarypox vector
DNA vaccines	Clinical trials ongoing for several infections

Abbreviations: BCG, bacillus Calmette-Guérin, HIV, human immunodeficiency virus.

ated) or by killing the microbe while retaining its immunogenicity. The great advantage of attenuated microbial vaccines is that they elicit all the innate and adaptive immune responses (both humoral and cell-mediated) that the pathogenic microbe would, and they are therefore the ideal way of inducing protective immunity. Live, attenuated bacteria were first shown by Louis Pasteur to confer specific immunity. The attenuated or killed bacterial vaccines in use today generally induce limited protection and are effective for only short periods. Live, attenuated viral vaccines are usually more effective; polio, measles, and yellow fever are three good examples. The most frequently used approach for producing such attenuated viruses is repeated passage in cell culture. More recently, temperature-sensitive and deletion mutants have been generated with the same goal in mind. Viral vaccines often induce long-lasting specific immunity, so immunization of children is sufficient for lifelong protection. Some attenuated viral vaccines (e.g., polio) may cause disease in immune-compromised hosts, and for this reason inactivated poliovirus vaccines are now more commonly used.

Purified Antigen (Subunit) Vaccines

Subunit vaccines are composed of antigens purified from microbes or inactivated toxins and are usually administered with an adjuvant. One effective use of purified antigens as vaccines is for the prevention of diseases caused by bacterial toxins. Toxins can be rendered harmless without loss of immunogenicity, and such "toxoids" induce strong antibody responses. Diphtheria and tetanus are two infections whose life-threatening consequences have been largely controlled because of immunization of children with toxoid preparations. Vaccines composed of bacterial polysaccharide antigens are used against *Pneumococcus* and *H. influenzae.* Because polysaccharides are T-independent antigens, they tend to elicit low-affinity antibody responses, and may be poorly immunogenic in infants (who do not mount strong T cell–independent antibody responses). High-affinity antibody responses may be generated against polysaccharide antigens even in infants by coupling the polysaccharides to proteins to form **conjugate vaccines.** Such vaccines work like hapten-carrier conjugates and are an excellent practical application of the principle of T-B cell cooperation (see Chapter 10). The currently used *H. influezae*, pneumococcal, and meningococcal vaccines are conjugate vaccines. Purified protein vaccines stimulate helper T cells and antibody responses, but they do not generate potent CTLs. The reason for poor CTL development is that exogenous proteins (and peptides) are inefficient at entering the class I MHC pathway of antigen presentation and cannot readily displace peptides from surface class I molecules. As a result, protein vaccines are not recognized efficiently by class I–restricted $CD8^+$ T cells.

Synthetic Antigen Vaccines

A goal of vaccine research has been to identify the most immunogenic microbial antigens or epitopes, to synthesize these in the laboratory, and to use the synthetic antigens as vaccines. It is possible to deduce the protein sequences of microbial antigens from nucleotide sequence data and to prepare large quantities of proteins by recombinant DNA technology. Vaccines made of recombinant DNA-derived antigens are now in use for hepatitis virus, herpes simplex virus, and foot-and-mouth disease virus (a major pathogen for livestock), and are being tested for human papilloma virus and rotavirus.

Live Viral Vectors

Another approach for vaccine development is to introduce genes encoding microbial antigens into a noncytopathic virus and to infect individuals with this virus. Thus, the virus serves as a source of the antigen in an inoculated individual. The great advantage of viral vectors is that they, like other live viruses, induce the full complement of immune responses, including strong CTL responses. This technique has been used most commonly with vaccinia virus vectors. Inoculation of such recombinant viruses into many species of animals induces both humoral and cell-mediated immunity against the antigen produced by the foreign gene (and, of course, against vaccinia virus antigens as well). A potential problem with viral vectors is that the viruses may infect various host cells, and even though they are not pathogenic, they may produce antigens that stimulate CTL responses that kill the infected host cells. These and other safety concerns have limited widespread use of viral vectors for vaccine delivery.

DNA Vaccines

An interesting method of vaccination was developed on the basis of an unexpected observation. Inoculation of a plasmid containing complementary DNA (cDNA) encoding a protein antigen leads to strong and long-lived humoral and cell-mediated immune responses to the antigen. It is likely that APCs, such as dendritic cells, are transfected by the plasmid and the cDNA is transcribed and translated into immunogenic protein that elicits specific responses. The unique feature of DNA vaccines is that they provide the only approach, other than live viruses, for eliciting strong CTL responses because the DNA-encoded proteins are synthesized in the cytosol of transfected cells. Furthermore, bacterial plasmids are rich in unmethylated CpG nucleotides and are recognized by a TLR (TLR9) on macrophages and other cells, thereby eliciting an innate immune response that enhances adaptive immunity (see Chapter 2). Therefore, plasmid DNA vaccines are effective even when they are administered without adjuvants. The ease of manipulating cDNAs to express many diverse antigens, the ability to store DNA without refrigeration for use in the field, and the ability to co-express other proteins that may enhance immune responses (such as cytokines and costimulators) make this technique promising. However, DNA vaccines have not been as effective as hoped in clinical trials, and the factors that determine the efficacy of these vaccines, especially in humans, are still not fully defined.

Adjuvants and Immunomodulators

The initiation of T cell–dependent immune responses against protein antigens requires that the antigens be administered with adjuvants. Most adjuvants elicit innate immune responses, with increased expression of costimulators and production of cytokines such as IL-12 that stimulate T cell growth and differentiation. Heat-killed bacteria are powerful adjuvants that are commonly used in experimental animals. However, the severe local inflammation that such adjuvants trigger precludes their use in humans. Much effort is currently being devoted to development of safe and effective adjuvants for use in humans. Several are in clinical practice, including aluminum hydroxide gel (which appears to promote B cell responses) and lipid formulations that are ingested by phagocytes. An alternative to adjuvants is to administer natural substances that stimulate T cell responses together with antigens. For instance, IL-12 incorporated in vaccines promotes strong cell-mediated immunity and is being tested in early clinical trials. As mentioned, plasmid DNA has intrinsic adjuvant-like activities, and it is possible to incorporate costimulators (e.g., B7 molecules) or cytokines into plasmid DNA vaccines.

Passive Immunization

Protective immunity can also be conferred by passive immunization, for instance, by transfer of specific antibodies. In the clinical situation, passive immunization is most commonly used for rapid treatment of potentially fatal diseases caused by toxins, such as tetanus, and for protection from rabies and hepatitis. Antibodies against snake venom can be lifesaving treatments of poisonous snakebites. Passive immunity is short-lived because the host does not respond to the immunization and protection lasts only as long as the injected antibody persists. Moreover, passive immunization does not induce memory, so an immunized individual is not protected against subsequent exposure to the toxin or microbe.

SUMMARY

- The interaction of the immune system with infectious organisms is a dynamic interplay of host mechanisms aimed at eliminating infections and microbial strategies designed to permit survival in the face of powerful defense mechanisms. Different types of infectious agents stimulate distinct types of immune responses and have evolved unique mechanisms for evading immunity. In some infections, the immune response is the cause of tissue injury and disease.
- Innate immunity against extracellular bacteria is mediated by phagocytes and the complement system (the alternative and lectin pathways).
- The principal adaptive immune response against extracellular bacteria consists of specific antibodies that opsonize the bacteria for phagocytosis and activate the complement system. Toxins produced by such bacteria are also neutralized by specific antibodies. Some bacterial toxins are powerful inducers of cytokine production, and cytokines account for much of the systemic disease associated with severe, disseminated infections with these microbes.
- Innate immunity against intracellular bacteria is mediated mainly by macrophages. However, intracellular bacteria are capable of surviving and replicating within host cells, including phagocytes, because they have developed mechanisms for resisting degradation within phagocytes.
- Adaptive immunity against intracellular bacteria is principally cell mediated and consists of activation of macrophages by $CD4^+$ T cells (as in DTH) as well as killing of infected cells by $CD8^+$ CTLs. The characteristic pathologic response to infection by intracellular bacteria is granulomatous inflammation.
- Protective responses to fungi consist of innate immunity, mediated by neutrophils and macrophages, and adaptive cell-mediated and humoral immunity. Fungi are usually readily eliminated

by phagocytes and a competent immune system, because of which disseminated fungal infections are seen mostly in immunodeficient persons.

- Innate immunity against viruses is mediated by type I IFNs and NK cells. Neutralizing antibodies protect against virus entry into cells early in the course of infection and later if the viruses are released from killed infected cells. The major defense mechanism against established infection is CTL-mediated killing of infected cells. CTLs may contribute to tissue injury even when the infectious virus is not harmful by itself. Viruses evade immune responses by antigenic variation, inhibition of antigen presentation, and production of immunosuppressive molecules.

- Parasites such as protozoa and helminths give rise to chronic and persistent infections because innate immunity against them is weak and parasites have evolved multiple mechanisms for evading and resisting specific immunity. The structural and antigenic diversity of pathogenic parasites is reflected in the heterogeneity of the adaptive immune responses that they elicit. Protozoa that live within host cells are destroyed by cell-mediated immunity, whereas helminths are eliminated by IgE antibody and eosinophil-mediated killing as well as by other leukocytes. Parasites evade the immune system by varying their antigens during residence in vertebrate hosts, by acquiring resistance to immune effector mechanisms, and by masking and shedding their surface antigens.

Selected Readings

Antoniou AN, and SJ Powis. Pathogen evasion strategies for the major histocompatibility complex class I assembly pathway. Immunology 124:1–12, 2008.

Baker MD, and KR Acharya. Superantigens: structure-function relationships. International Journal of Medical Microbiology 293:529–537, 2004.

Burton DR. Antibodies, viruses and vaccines. Nature Reviews Immunology 2:706–713, 2002.

Casanova J-L, and L Abel. The human model: a genetic dissection of immunity to infection in natural conditions. Nature Reviews Immunology 4:55–66, 2004.

Doherty PC, and JP Christensen. Accessing complexity: the dynamics of virus-specific T cell responses. Annual Review of Immunology 18:561–592, 2000.

Donnelly JJ, B Wahren, and MA Liu. DNA vaccines: progress and challenges. Journal of Immunology 175:633–639, 2005.

Finlay BB, and G McFadden. Anti-immunology: evasion of the host immune system by bacterial and viral pathogens. Cell 124:767–782, 2006.

Flynn JL, and J Chan. Immune evasion by *Mycobacterium tuberculosis:* living with the enemy. Current Opinion in Immunology 15:450–455, 2003.

Good MF, H Xu, M Wykes, and CR Engwerda. Development and regulation of cell-mediated immune responses to the blood stages of malaria: implications for vaccine research. Annual Review of Immunology 23:69–99, 2005.

Guidotti LG, and FV Chisari. Noncytolytic control of viral infections by the innate and adaptive immune response. Annual Review of Immunology 19:65–91, 2001.

Kaufmann SHE. Tuberculosis: back on the immunologists' agenda. Immunity 24:351–357, 2006.

Kaufmann SHE, and AJ McMichael. Annulling a dangerous liaison: vaccination strategies against AIDS and tuberculosis. Nature Medicine 11:S33–44, 2005.

Kawai T, and S Akira. Innate immune recognition of viral infection. Nature Immunology 7:131–137, 2006.

Klenerman P, and A Hill. T cells and viral persistence: lessons from diverse infections. Nature Immunology 6:873–879, 2005.

Langhorne J, FM Ndungu, A-M Sponaas, and K Marsh. Immunity to malaria: more questions than answers. Nature Immunology 9:725–732, 2008.

Lybarger L, X Wang, MR Harris, HW Virgin, and TH Hansen. Virus subversion of the MHC class I peptide-loading complex. Immunity 18:121–130, 2003.

McCulloch R. Antigenic variation in African trypanosomes: monitoring progress. Trends in Parasitology 20:117–121, 2004.

Munford RS. Severe sepsis and septic shock: the role of gram-negative bacteria. Annual Review of Pathology: Mechanisms of Disease 1:467–495, 2006.

North RJ, and Y-J Jung. Immunity to tuberculosis. Annual Review of Immunology 22:599–623, 2004.

Pearce EJ, and AS MacDonald. The immunobiology of schistosomiasis. Nature Reviews Immunology 2:499–511, 2002.

Perry AK, G Chen, D Zheng, H Tang, and G Cheng. The host type I interferon response to viral and bacterial infections. Cell Research 15:407–422, 2005.

Romani L. Immunity to fungal infections. Nature Reviews Immunology 4:1–23, 2004.

Sacks D, and N Noben-Trauth. The immunology of susceptibility and resistance to *Leishmania major* in mice. Nature Reviews Immunology 2:845–858, 2002.

Seet BT, JB Johnston, CR Brunetti, JW Barrett, H Everett, C Cameron, J Sypula, SH Nazarian, A Lucas, and G McFadden. Poxviruses and immune evasion. Annual Review of Immunology 21:377–423, 2003.

Van Lier RAW, IJM ten Berge, and LE Gamadia. Human $CD8^+$ T cell differentiation in response to viruses. Nature Reviews Immunology 3:931–939, 2003.

Wong P, and EG Pamer. CD8 T-cell responses to infectious pathogens. Annual Review of Immunology 21:29–70, 2003.

Zinkernagel RM. On natural and artificial vaccinations. Annual Review of Immunology 21:515–546, 2003.

Chapter 16

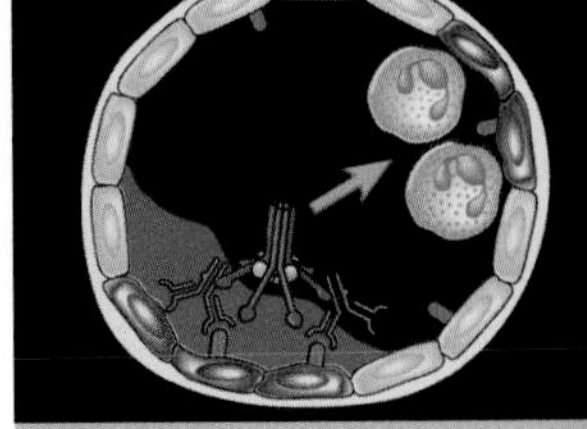

TRANSPLANTATION IMMUNOLOGY

Transplantation is the process of taking cells, tissues, or organs, called a **graft,** from one individual and placing them into a (usually) different individual. The individual who provides the graft is called the **donor,** and the individual who receives the graft is called either the **recipient** or the host. If the graft is placed into its normal anatomic location, the procedure is called orthotopic transplantation; if the graft is placed in a different site, the procedure is called heterotopic transplantation. **Transfusion** refers to the transfer of circulating blood cells or plasma from one individual to another. In clinical practice, transplantation is used to overcome a functional or anatomic deficit in the recipient. This approach to treatment of human diseases has increased steadily during the past 40 years, and transplantation of kidneys, hearts, lungs, livers, pancreata, and bone marrow is widely used today. More than 30,000 kidney, heart, lung, liver, and pancreas transplantations are currently performed in the United States each year. In addition, transplantation of many other organs or cells is now being attempted.

A major factor limiting the success of transplantation is the immune response of the recipient to the donor tissue. This problem was first appreciated when attempts to replace damaged skin on burn patients with skin from unrelated donors proved to be uniformly unsuccessful. During a matter of 1 to 2 weeks, the transplanted skin would undergo necrosis and fall off. The failure of the grafts led Peter Medawar and many other investigators to study skin transplantation in animal models. These experiments established that the failure of skin grafting was caused by an inflammatory reaction called **rejection.** Several lines of experimental evidence indicated that rejection is caused by an adaptive immune response (Fig. 16–1).

- A skin graft transplanted between genetically unrelated individuals, for example, from a strain A mouse to a strain B mouse, is rejected by a naive recipient in 7 to 10 days. This process is called first-set rejection and is due to a primary immune response to the graft. A subsequent skin graft transplanted from the same donor to the original recipient is rejected more rapidly, in only 2 or 3 days. This accelerated response, called second-set rejection, is due to a secondary immune response. Thus, grafts that are genetically disparate from the recipients induce immunologic memory, one of the cardinal features of adaptive immune responses.

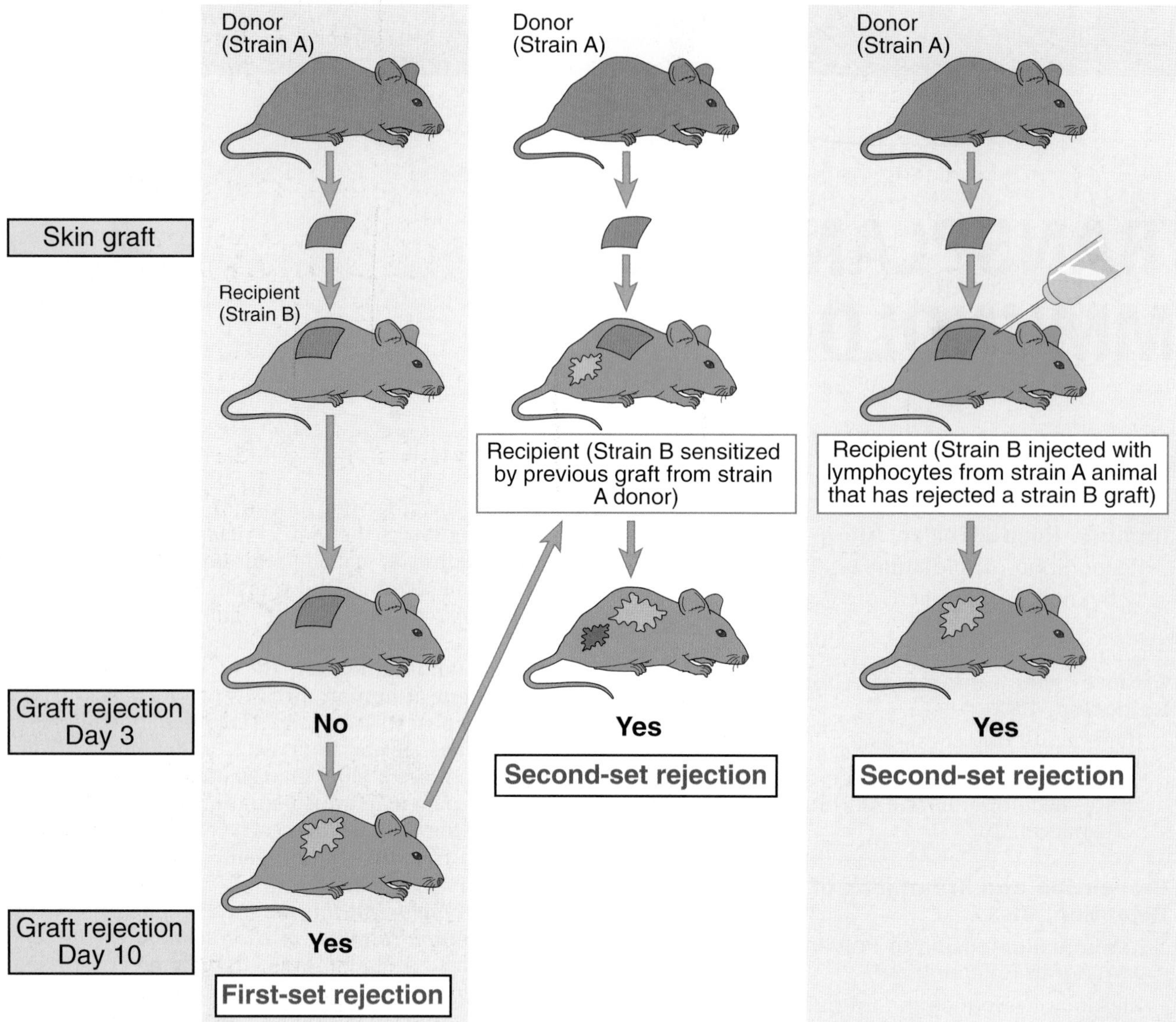

FIGURE 16–1 First- and second-set allograft rejection. Results of the experiments shown indicate that graft rejection displays the features of adaptive immune responses, namely, memory and mediation by lymphocytes. An inbred strain B mouse will reject a graft from an inbred strain A mouse with first-set kinetics *(left panel)*. An inbred strain B mouse sensitized by a previous graft from an inbred strain A mouse will reject a second graft from an inbred strain A mouse with second-set kinetics *(middle panel)*, demonstrating memory. An inbred strain B mouse injected with lymphocytes from another strain B mouse that has rejected a graft from a strain A mouse will reject a graft from a strain A mouse with second-set kinetics *(right panel)*, demonstrating the role of lymphocytes in mediating rejection and memory. An inbred strain B mouse sensitized by a previous graft from a strain A mouse will reject a graft from a third unrelated strain with first-set kinetics, thus demonstrating another feature of adaptive immunity, specificity (not shown). Syngeneic grafts are never rejected (not shown).

- Second-set rejection ensues if the first and second skin grafts are derived from the same donor or from genetically identical donors, for example, strain A mice. However, if the second graft is derived from an individual unrelated to the donor of the first graft, for example, strain C, no second-set rejection occurs; the new graft elicits only a first-set rejection. Thus, the phenomenon of second-set rejection shows specificity, another cardinal feature of adaptive immune responses.

- The ability to mount second-set rejection against a graft from strain A mice can be adoptively transferred to a naive strain B recipient by lymphocytes taken from a strain B animal previously exposed to a graft from strain A mice. This experiment demonstrated that second-set rejection is mediated by sensitized lymphocytes and provided the definitive evidence that rejection is the result of an adaptive immune response.

Transplant immunologists have developed a special vocabulary to describe the kinds of cells and tissues encountered in the transplant setting. A graft transplanted from one individual to the same individual is called an **autologous graft** (shortened to autograft). A graft transplanted between two genetically identical or syngeneic individuals is called a **syngeneic graft**. A graft transplanted between two genetically different individuals of the same species is called an **allogeneic graft** (or **allograft**). A graft transplanted between individuals of different species is called a **xenogeneic graft** (or **xenograft**). The molecules that are recognized as foreign on allografts are called **alloantigens,** and those on xenografts are called **xenoantigens**. The lymphocytes and antibodies that react with alloantigens or xenoantigens are described as being **alloreactive** or **xenoreactive,** respectively.

The immunology of transplantation is important for two reasons. First, the immunologic rejection response is still one of the major barriers to transplantation today. Second, although an encounter with alloantigens is unlikely in the normal life of an organism, the immune response to allogeneic molecules is strong and has therefore been a useful model for studying the mechanisms of lymphocyte activation. Most of this chapter focuses on allogeneic transplantation because it is far more commonly practiced and better understood than xenogeneic transplantation, which is discussed briefly at the end of the chapter. We consider both the basic immunology and some aspects of the clinical practice of transplantation. We conclude the chapter with a discussion of bone marrow transplantation, which raises special issues not usually encountered with solid organ transplants.

IMMUNE RESPONSES TO ALLOGRAFTS

Alloantigens elicit both cell-mediated and humoral immune responses. In this section of the chapter, we discuss the molecular and cellular mechanisms of allorecognition, with an emphasis on the nature of graft antigens that stimulate allogeneic responses and the features of the responding lymphocytes.

Recognition of Alloantigens

Recognition of transplanted cells as self or foreign is determined by polymorphic genes that are inherited from both parents and are expressed codominantly. This conclusion is based on the results of experimental transplantation between inbred strains of mice. The basic rules of transplantation immunology are derived from such animal experiments (Fig. 16–2).

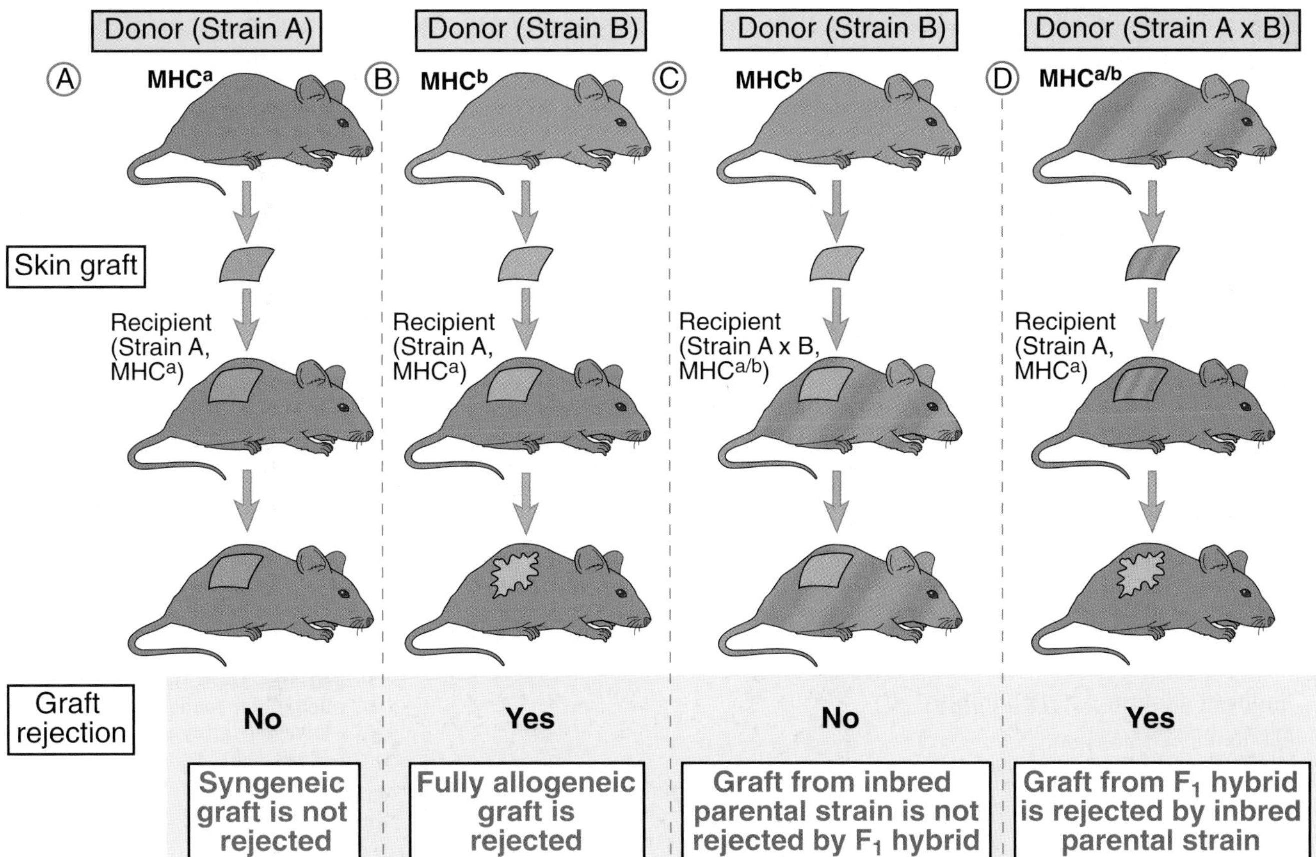

FIGURE 16–2 The genetics of graft rejection. In the illustration, the two different mouse colors represent inbred strains with different MHC haplotypes. Inherited MHC alleles from both parents are codominantly expressed in the skin of an A × B offspring, and therefore these mice are represented by both colors. Syngeneic grafts are not rejected (A). Allografts are always rejected (B). Grafts from a parent of an A × B mating will not be rejected by the offspring (C), but grafts from the offspring will be rejected by either parent (D). These phenomena are due to the fact that MHC gene products are responsible for graft rejection; grafts are rejected only if they express an MHC type (represented by a color) that is not expressed by the recipient mouse.

- Cells or organs transplanted between individuals of the same inbred strain of a species are never rejected.
- Cells or organs transplanted between individuals of different inbred strains of a species are almost always rejected.
- The offspring of a mating between two different inbred strains will typically not reject grafts from either parent. In other words, an $(A \times B)F_1$ animal will not reject grafts from an A or B strain animal. (This rule is violated by bone marrow transplantation, which we will discuss later in the chapter.)
- A graft derived from the offspring of a mating between two different inbred strains will almost always be rejected by either parent. In other words, a graft from an $(A \times B)F_1$ animal will be rejected by either an A or a B strain animal.

Such experimental results suggested that polymorphic, codominantly expressed molecules in the grafts were responsible for eliciting rejection. Polymorphism refers to the fact that these graft antigens differed among individuals of a species or between different inbred strains of animals, for example, between strain A and strain B mice. Codominant expression means that an $(A \times B)F_1$ animal expresses both A strain and B strain alleles. $(A \times B)F_1$ animals see both A and B tissues as self, and A or B animals see $(A \times B)F_1$ tissues as partly foreign. This is why an $(A \times B)F_1$ animal does not reject either A or B strain grafts and why both A and B strain recipients reject an $(A \times B)F_1$ graft.

Major histocompatibility complex (MHC) molecules are responsible for almost all strong (rapid) rejection reactions. George Snell and colleagues used congenic strains of inbred mice to identify the MHC complex as the locus of polymorphic genes that encode the molecular targets of allograft rejection (see Chapter 5, Fig. 5–2). Because MHC molecules, the targets of allograft rejection, are widely expressed, many different kinds of tissues evoke responses from alloreactive T cells. As discussed in Chapters 5 and 6, MHC molecules play a critical role in normal immune responses to foreign antigens, namely, the presentation of peptides derived from protein antigens in a form that can be recognized by T cells. The role of MHC molecules as alloantigens is incidental, as discussed later.

Allogeneic MHC molecules are presented for recognition by the T cells of a graft recipient in two fundamentally different ways (Fig. 16–3). The first way, called **direct presentation,** involves recognition of an intact MHC molecule displayed by donor antigen-presenting cells (APCs) in the graft and is a consequence of the similarity in structure of an intact foreign (allogeneic) MHC molecule and self MHC molecules. Therefore, direct presentation is unique to foreign MHC molecules. The second way, called **indirect presentation,** involves processing of donor MHC molecules by recipient APCs and presentation of peptides derived from the allogeneic MHC molecules in association with self MHC molecules. In this case, the foreign MHC molecule is handled as though it were any foreign protein antigen, and the mechanisms of indirect antigen presentation are the same as the mechanisms of presentation of a microbial protein antigen. Alloantigens other than MHC molecules in a graft can also be presented to host T cells by the indirect pathway. We discuss the molecular basis of direct and indirect presentation separately.

Direct Recognition of Alloantigens

Direct recognition of foreign MHC molecules is a cross-reaction of a normal T cell receptor (TCR), which was selected to recognize a self MHC molecule plus foreign

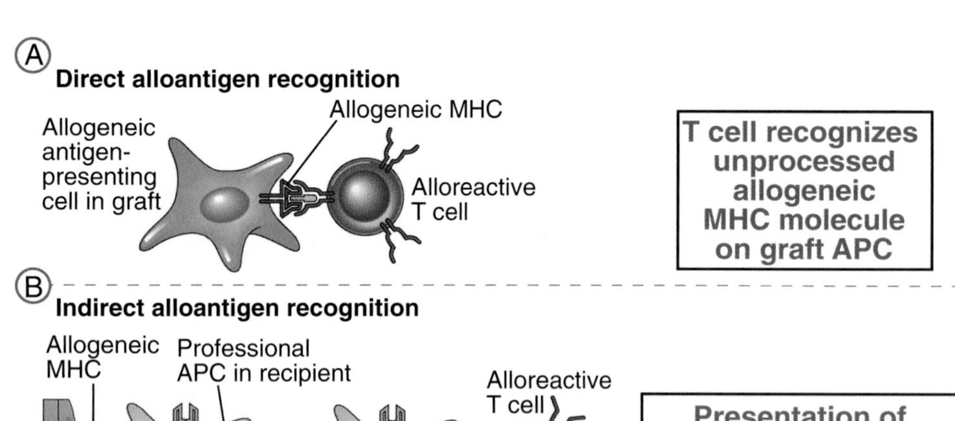

FIGURE 16–3 Direct and indirect alloantigen recognition. A. Direct alloantigen recognition occurs when T cells bind directly to an intact allogeneic MHC molecule on a graft (donor) antigen-presenting cell (APC). B. Indirect alloantigen recognition occurs when allogeneic MHC molecules from graft cells are taken up and processed by recipient APCs, and peptide fragments of the allogeneic MHC molecules containing polymorphic amino acid residues are bound and presented by recipient (self) MHC molecules.

peptide, with an allogeneic MHC molecule plus peptide. On face value, it seems puzzling that T cells that are normally selected to be self MHC restricted are capable of recognizing foreign MHC molecules. The explanation for this apparent paradox is related to the fact that the repertoire of TCR specificities is already biased to recognize any MHC molecule, even before selection. In other words, the TCR genes have evolved to encode a protein structure that has intrinsic affinity for MHC molecules. During T cell development in the thymus, positive selection results in survival of T cells with weak self-MHC reactivity, but does not eliminate T cells with strong reactivity to allogenic MHC molecules. Negative selection in the thymus efficiently eliminates T cells with high affinity for self MHC, but again does not necessarily eliminate T cells that bind strongly to allogeneic MHC molecules, unless they also happen to bind strongly to self MHC. The result is a mature repertoire that has an intrinsic affinity for self MHC molecules, which includes many T cells that bind allogeneic MHC molecules with high affinity. Many of these mature T cells will strongly bind both self MHC–foreign peptide complexes and allogeneic MHC molecules. By chance, some may be useless T cells that bind allogenic MHC molecules but do not bind strongly to self-MHC–foreign peptide complexes.

An allogeneic MHC molecule with a bound peptide can mimic the determinant formed by a self MHC molecule plus a particular foreign peptide (Fig. 16–4). MHC molecules that are expressed on cell surfaces normally contain bound peptides. The peptides bound to allogeneic MHC molecules may play several roles in the recognition of these molecules. Peptides may simply be required for stable cell surface expression of the allogeneic MHC molecules. However, some alloreactive T cell clones have been shown to recognize allogeneic MHC molecules with some, but not other, bound peptides. This observation suggests that the peptide contributes to the determinant recognized by the alloreactive T cell, exactly like the role of peptides in the normal recognition of antigen by self MHC–restricted T cells. Many of the peptides associated with allogeneic MHC molecules that are involved in direct presentation are derived from proteins that are identical in the donor and recipient. In other words, they are self peptides. The mechanisms of tolerance induction, described in Chapter 11, work only to eliminate or to inactivate T cells that respond to complexes of self peptides plus self MHC molecules. Therefore, T cells specific for self peptide plus

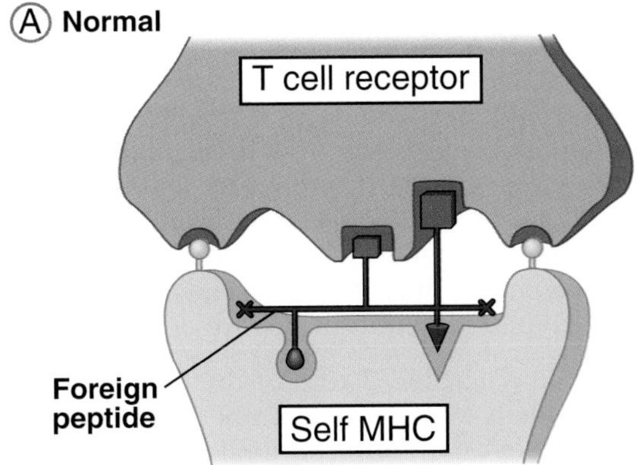

Self MHC molecule presents foreign peptide to T cell selected to recognize self MHC weakly, but may recognize self MHC–foreign peptide complexes well

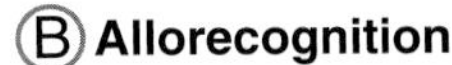

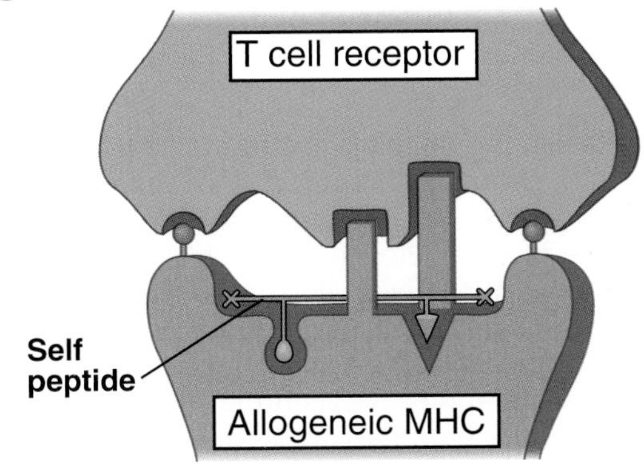

The self MHC–restricted T cell recognizes the allogeneic MHC molecule whose structure resembles a self MHC–foreign peptide complex

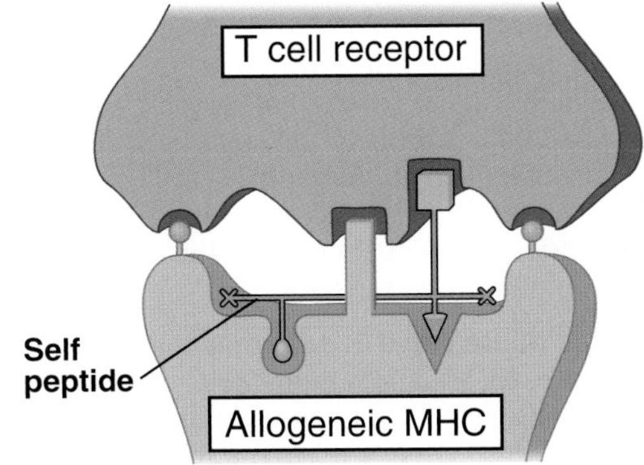

The self MHC–restricted T cell recognizes a structure formed by both the allogeneic MHC molecule and the bound peptide

FIGURE 16–4 Molecular basis of direct recognition of allogeneic MHC molecules. Direct recognition of allogeneic MHC molecules may be thought of as a cross-reaction in which a T cell specific for a self MHC molecule–foreign peptide complex (A) also recognizes an allogeneic MHC molecule (B, C). Nonpolymorphic donor peptides, labeled "self peptide," may not contribute to allorecognition (B), or they may (C).

allogeneic MHC are not removed from the repertoire and are available to respond to allografts.

As many as 2% of an individual's T cells are capable of directly recognizing and responding to a single foreign MHC molecule, and this high frequency of T cells reactive with allogeneic MHC molecules is one reason that allografts elicit strong immune responses in vivo. The fact that each allogeneic MHC molecule is directly recognized by so many different TCRs, each selected for different foreign peptides, may be due to several factors.

- The highly polymorphic nature of the MHC implies that an allogeneic MHC molecule will differ from self MHC molecules at multiple amino acid residues. Because many of the polymorphic residues are concentrated in the regions that bind to the TCR, each different residue may contribute to a distinct determinant recognized by a different clone of self MHC–restricted T cells. Thus, each allogeneic MHC molecule can be recognized by multiple T cell clones. In this case, the cross-reactive T cell allorecognition is entirely attributable to differences in amino acid sequences between self MHC and allogeneic MHC molecules, and bound peptide serves only to ensure stable expression of the allogeneic MHC molecule.
- Many different peptides may combine with one allogeneic MHC gene product to produce determinants that are recognized by different cross-reactive T cells. The surface of each allogeneic cell has 10^5 or more copies of each allogeneic MHC molecule, and each MHC molecule can form a complex with a different peptide. Thus, any cell in an allograft may express many distinct peptide-MHC complexes composed of different peptides bound to one or a few alleles of the foreign MHC molecules. Because only a few hundred peptide-MHC complexes are needed to activate a particular T cell clone, many different clones may be activated by the same allogeneic cell.
- All of the MHC molecules on an allogeneic APC are foreign to a recipient and can therefore be recognized by T cells. In contrast, on self APCs, most of the self MHC molecules are displaying self peptides, and any foreign peptide probably occupies 1% or less of the total MHC molecules expressed. As a result, the density of allogeneic determinants on allogeneic APCs is much higher than the density of foreign peptide–self MHC complexes on self APCs. The abundance of recognizable allogeneic MHC molecules may allow activation of T cells with low affinities for the determinant, thereby increasing the numbers of T cells that can respond.
- Many of the alloreactive T cells that respond to the first exposure to an allogeneic MHC molecule are memory T cells that were generated during previous exposure to other foreign (e.g., microbial) antigens. Thus, in contrast to the initial naive T cell response to microbial antigens, the initial response to alloantigens is mediated in part by already expanded clones of memory T cells.

Because of the high frequency of alloreactive T cells, primary responses to alloantigens are the only primary responses that can readily be detected *in vitro.*

Indirect Presentation of Alloantigens

Allogeneic MHC molecules may be processed and presented by recipient APCs that enter grafts, and the processed MHC molecules are recognized by T cells like conventional foreign protein antigens (see Fig. 16–3). Because allogeneic MHC molecules differ structurally from those of the host, they can be processed and presented in the same way that any foreign protein antigen is, generating foreign peptides associated with self MHC molecules on the surface of host APCs. Indirect presentation may result in allorecognition by $CD4^+$ T cells because alloantigen is acquired by host APCs primarily through the endosomal vesicular pathway (i.e., as a consequence of phagocytosis) and is therefore presented by class II MHC molecules. Some antigens of phagocytosed graft cells appear to enter the class I MHC pathway of antigen presentation and are indirectly recognized by $CD8^+$ T cells. This phenomenon is an example of cross-presentation or cross-priming (see Chapter 9, Fig. 9–3), in which professional APCs, usually dendritic cells, present antigens of another cell, from the graft, to activate, or "prime," $CD8^+$ T lymphocytes. Because MHC molecules are the most polymorphic proteins in the genome, each allogeneic MHC molecule may give rise to multiple foreign peptides, each recognized by different T cells.

- One of the first indications that T cell responses to allogeneic MHC molecules can occur by indirect presentation was the demonstration of cross-priming of alloreactive $CD8^+$ cytotoxic T lymphocytes (CTLs) by self APCs that had been exposed to allogeneic cells.
- Evidence that indirect presentation of allogeneic MHC molecules occurs in graft rejection was obtained from studies with knockout mice lacking class II MHC expression. For example, skin grafts from donor mice lacking class II MHC are able to induce recipient $CD4^+$ (i.e., class II–restricted) T cell responses to the donor alloantigens, including peptides derived from donor class I MHC molecules. This result implies that the donor class I MHC molecules are processed and presented by class II molecules on the recipient's APCs and stimulate the recipient's helper T cells.
- More recently, evidence has been obtained from human transplant recipients that indirect antigen presentation may contribute to late rejection of allografts. For example, $CD4^+$ T cells from heart and liver allograft recipients can be activated *in vitro* by peptides derived from donor MHC and presented by host APCs.

There may be polymorphic antigens other than MHC molecules that differ between the donor and the recipient. These antigens induce weak or slower (more gradual) rejection reactions than do MHC molecules and are called **minor histocompatibility antigens.** Most minor histocompatibility antigens are proteins that are processed and presented to host T cells in association with self MHC molecules on host APCs (i.e., by the indirect pathway).

Activation of Alloreactive Lymphocytes

The activation of alloreactive T cells in vivo requires presentation of alloantigens by donor-derived APCs in the graft (direct presentation of alloantigens) or by host APCs that pick up and present graft alloantigens (indirect presentation). Most organs contain resident APCs such as dendritic cells. Transplantation of these organs into an allogeneic recipient provides APCs that express donor MHC molecules as well as costimulators. Presumably, these donor APCs migrate to regional lymph nodes and are recognized by the recipient's T cells that circulate through the peripheral lymphoid organs (the direct pathway). Dendritic cells from the recipient may also migrate into the graft, or graft alloantigens may traffic into lymph nodes, where they are captured and presented by recipient APCs (the indirect pathway). Alloreactive T cells in the recipient may be activated by both pathways, and these T cells migrate into the grafts and cause graft rejection. Alloreactive $CD4^+$ helper T cells differentiate into cytokine-producing effector cells that damage grafts by reactions that resemble delayed-type hypersensitivity (DTH). Alloreactive $CD8^+$ T cells activated by the direct pathway differentiate into CTLs that kill nucleated cells in the graft, which express the allogeneic class I MHC molecules. The $CD8^+$ CTLs that are generated by the indirect pathway are self MHC restricted, and they cannot directly kill the foreign cells in the graft. Therefore, when alloreactive T cells are stimulated by the indirect pathway, the principal mechanism of rejection is probably DTH mediated by $CD4^+$ effector T cells that infiltrate the graft and recognize donor alloantigens being displayed by host APCs that have also entered the graft. The relative importance of the direct and indirect pathways in graft rejection is still unclear. It has been suggested that $CD8^+$ CTLs induced by direct recognition of alloantigens are most important for acute rejection of allografts, whereas $CD4^+$ effector T cells stimulated by the indirect pathway play a greater role in chronic rejection.

The importance of MHC molecules in the rejection of tissue allografts has been established by studies with inbred animals showing that rapid rejection usually requires class I or class II MHC differences between the graft donor and the recipient. In clinical transplantation, minimizing MHC differences between the donor and the recipient improves graft survival, as we shall discuss later.

The response of alloreactive T cells to foreign MHC molecules has also been analyzed in an *in vitro* reaction called the **mixed lymphocyte reaction** (MLR). The MLR is a model of direct T cell recognition of allogeneic MHC molecules and is used as a predictive test of T cell–mediated graft rejection. Studies of the MLR were among the first to establish the role of class I and class II MHC molecules in activating distinct populations of T cells ($CD8^+$ and $CD4^+$, respectively).

- The MLR is induced by culturing mononuclear leukocytes (which include T cells, B cells, natural killer [NK] cells, mononuclear phagocytes, and dendritic cells) from one individual with mononuclear leukocytes derived from another individual. Clinically, these cells are typically isolated from peripheral blood; in mouse or rat experiments, mononuclear leukocytes are usually purified from the spleen or lymph nodes. If the two individuals have differences in the alleles of the MHC genes, a large proportion of the mononuclear cells will proliferate during a period of 4 to 7 days. This proliferative response is called the allogeneic MLR (Fig. 16–5). In this experiment, the cells from each donor react and proliferate against the other, thus resulting in a two-way MLR. To simplify the analysis, one of the two leukocyte populations can be rendered incapable of proliferation before culture, either by γ-irradiation or by treatment with the antimitotic drug mitomycin C. In this one-way MLR, the treated cells serve exclusively as stimulators, and the untreated cells, still capable of proliferation, serve as the responders.
- Among the T cells that have responded in an MLR, any one cell is specific for only one allogeneic MHC molecule, and the entire population of activated T lymphocytes contains cells that recognize all the MHC differences between stimulators and responders. $CD8^+$ CTLs are generated only if the class I MHC alleles of the stimulators and responders are different. Similarly, $CD4^+$ effector T cells are generated only if the class II molecules are different.
- Stimulator cells lacking MHC molecules cannot activate responder cells in an MLR. Transfection of MHC genes into the stimulators makes these cells capable of inducing an MLR.
- $CD8^+$ CTLs generated in an MLR will kill cells from other donors only if these cells share some class I alleles with the original stimulators. Similarly, $CD4^+$ T cells generated in an MLR recognize APCs from other donors only if these APCs share class II alleles with the stimulators. Such experiments demonstrate that alloreactive T cells are specific for allogeneic MHC molecules, and activation of alloreactive T cells in the MLR occurs mainly by the direct pathway.

In addition to recognition of alloantigen, costimulation of T cells by B7 molecules on APCs is important for activating alloreactive T cells.

- Rejection of allografts, and stimulation of alloreactive T cells in an MLR, can be inhibited by agents that bind to and block B7 molecules. Most studies indicate that B7 antagonists are more effective at blocking acute rejection of allografts and activation of alloreactive T cells by the direct pathway. In contrast, chronic rejection and activation of alloreactive T cells by the indirect pathway are often insensitive to such agents, for unknown reasons.

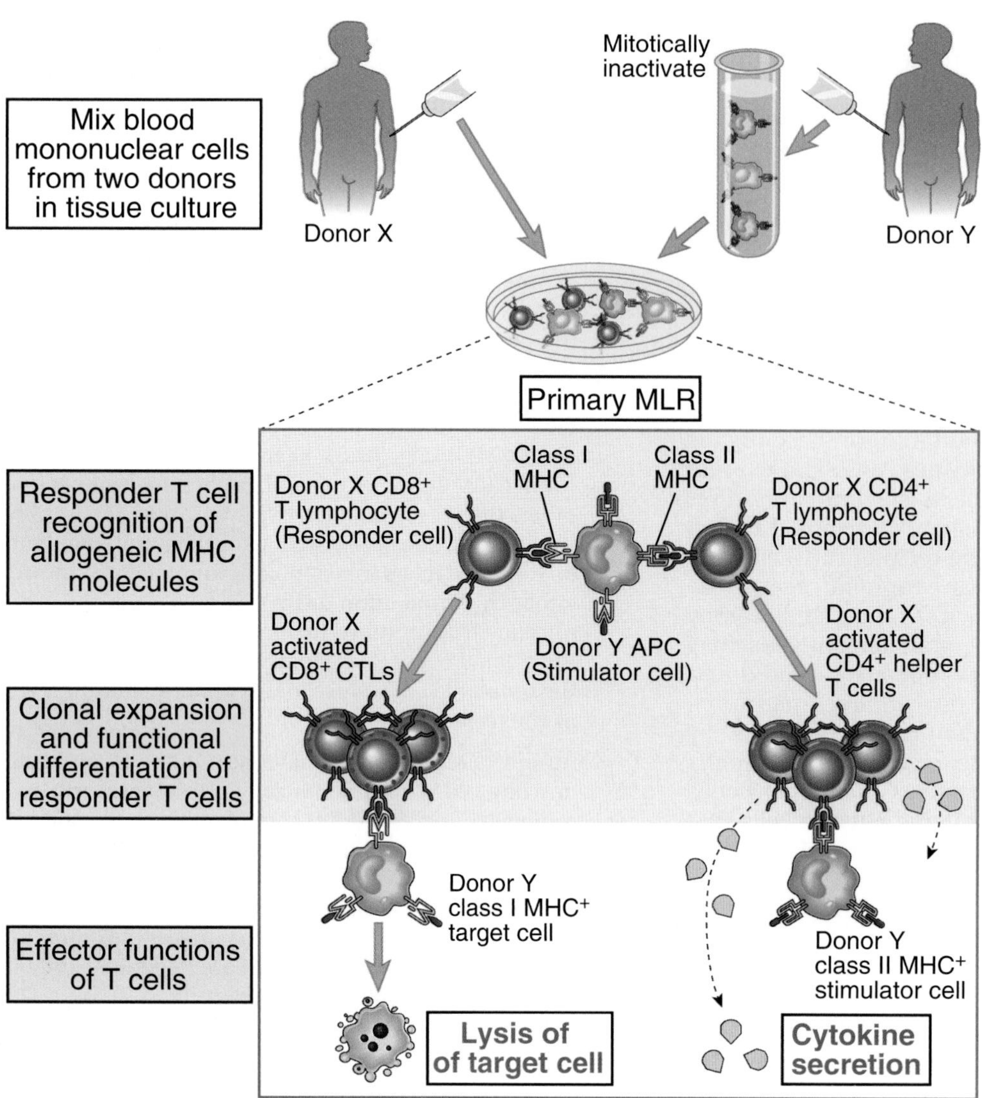

FIGURE 16–5 The mixed lymphocyte reaction (MLR). In a one-way primary MLR, stimulator cells (from donor Y) activate and cause the expansion of two types of responder T cells (from donor X). $CD4^+$ T cells from donor X react to donor Y class II molecules, and $CD8^+$ T lymphocytes from donor X react to donor Y class I MHC molecules. The $CD4^+$ T cells differentiate into cytokine-secreting helper T cells, and the $CD8^+$ T cells differentiate into CTLs. APC, antigen-presenting cell.

- Allografts survive for longer periods when they are transplanted into knockout mice lacking B7-1 (CD80) and B7-2 (CD86) compared with transplants into normal recipients. Both acute rejection and graft vasculopathy are reduced in this model.

In contrast to T cell alloreactivity, much less is known about the mechanisms that lead to the production of alloantibodies against foreign MHC molecules. The helper T cell-dependent production of antibodies against MHC molecules must involve indirect allorecognition. In this case, B lymphocytes recognize foreign MHC molecules, internalize and process these proteins, and present peptides derived from them to helper T cells that were previously activated by the same peptides presented by dendritic cells. Therefore, both the dendritic cells and B cells process and present the allogeneic MHC protein to host T cells, and helper T cells "indirectly" recognize foreign MHC molecules presented by host APCs. This sequence of events is, of course, the same as in any B cell response to foreign protein antigens (see Chapter 10).

Many of the issues that arise in discussions of alloreactivity and graft rejection are also relevant to maternal-fetal interactions. The fetus expresses paternal MHC molecules and is therefore semiallogeneic to the mother. Nevertheless, the fetus is not rejected by the maternal immune system. Many possible mechanisms have been proposed to account for this lack of rejection, and it is not yet clear which of these mechanisms is the most significant (Box 16–1).

EFFECTOR MECHANISMS OF ALLOGRAFT REJECTION

Thus far, we have described the molecular basis of alloantigen recognition and the cells involved in the recognition of and responses to allografts. We now turn to a consideration of the effector mechanisms used by the immune system to reject allografts. In different experimental models in animals and in clinical transplantation, alloreactive $CD4^+$ or $CD8^+$ T cells or alloanti-

Box 16–1 ▪ IN DEPTH: IMMUNE RESPONSES TO AN ALLOGENEIC FETUS

The mammalian fetus, except in instances in which the mother and father are syngeneic, will express paternally inherited antigens that are allogeneic to the mother. In essence, the fetus is a naturally occurring allograft. Nevertheless, fetuses are not normally rejected by the mother. It is clear that the mother is exposed to fetal antigens during pregnancy since maternal antibodies against paternal MHC molecules are easily detectable. Protection of the fetus from the maternal immune system probably involves several mechanisms including special molecular and barrier features of the placenta and local immunosuppression.

Several experimental observations indicate that the anatomic location of the fetus is a critical factor in the absence of rejection. For example, pregnant animals are able to recognize and reject allografts syngeneic to the fetus placed at extrauterine sites without compromising fetal survival. Wholly allogeneic fetal blastocysts that lack maternal genes can successfully develop in a pregnant or pseudopregnant mother. Thus, neither specific maternal nor paternal genes are necessary for survival of the fetus. Hyperimmunization of the mother with cells bearing paternal antigens does not compromise placental and fetal growth.

The failure to reject the fetus has focused attention on the region of physical contact between the mother and fetus. The fetal tissues of the placenta that most intimately contact the mother are composed of either vascular trophoblast, which is exposed to maternal blood for purposes of mediating nutrient exchange, or implantation site trophoblast, which diffusely infiltrates the uterine lining (decidua) for purposes of anchoring the placenta to the mother.

One simple explanation for fetal survival is that trophoblast cells fail to express paternal MHC molecules. So far, class II molecules have not been detected on trophoblast. In mice, cells of implantation trophoblast, but not of vascular trophoblast, do express paternal class I MHC molecules. In humans, the situation may be more complex in that trophoblast cells express only a nonpolymorphic class IB molecule called HLA-G. This molecule may be involved in protecting trophoblast cells from maternal NK cell–mediated lysis. A specialized subset of NK cells called uterine NK cells are the major type of lymphocyte present at implantation sites, and IFN-γ production by these cells is essential for decidual development. The way uterine NK cells are stimulated and their role in maternal responses to fetal alloantigens are not known. Even if trophoblast cells do express classical MHC molecules, they may lack costimulator molecules and fail to act as APCs.

A second explanation for lack of rejection is that the uterine decidua may be an **immunologically privileged site.** These anatomic sites are tissues where immune responses generally fail to occur and include brain, eye, and testis. Several factors may contribute to immune privilege. For example, the brain vasculature limits lymphocyte access to the brain tissue, and the anterior chamber of the eye may contain high concentrations of immunosuppressive cytokines such as TGF-β. In support of the idea that the decidua is an immune-privileged site is the observation that mouse decidua is highly susceptible to infection by *Listeria monocytogenes* and cannot support a DTH response. The basis of immunologic privilege is clearly not a simple anatomic barrier because maternal blood is in extensive contact with trophoblast. Rather, the barrier is likely to be created by functional inhibition. Cultured decidual cells directly inhibit macrophage and T cell functions, perhaps by producing inhibitory cytokines, such as TGF-β. Some of these inhibitory decidual cells may be resident regulatory T cells, although the evidence for this proposal is limited. Some experiments have led to the suggestion that T_H2 cytokines are produced at the maternal-fetal interface and are responsible for local suppression of T_H1 responses to fetal antigens. However, this idea is not supported by the data that IL-4 and IL-10 knockout mice have normal pregnancies. There is also evidence that the fetus contains abundant regulatory T cells, but their significance is unclear.

There is evidence that immune responses to the fetus may be regulated by local concentrations of tryptophan and its metabolites in the decidua. The enzyme indolamine 2,3-dioxygenase (IDO) catabolizes tryptophan, and the IDO-inhibiting drug 1-methyl-tryptophan induces abortions in mice in a T cell–dependent manner. These observations led to the hypothesis that T cell responses to the fetus are normally blocked because decidual tryptophan levels are kept low or the levels of toxic metabolites are high.

Trophoblast and decidua may also be relatively resistant to complement-mediated damage because they express high levels of a C3 and C4 inhibitor called Crry. Crry-deficient embryos die before birth and show evidence of complement activation on trophoblast cells. Thus, this inhibitor may block maternal alloantibody-mediated damage through the classical pathway of complement activation.

bodies are capable of mediating allograft rejection. These different immune effectors cause graft rejection by different mechanisms.

For historical reasons, graft rejection is classified on the basis of histopathologic features or the time course of rejection after transplantation rather than on the basis of immune effector mechanisms. Based on the experience of renal transplantation, the histopathologic patterns are called hyperacute, acute, and chronic (Fig. 16–6).

Hyperacute Rejection

Hyperacute rejection is characterized by thrombotic occlusion of the graft vasculature that begins within

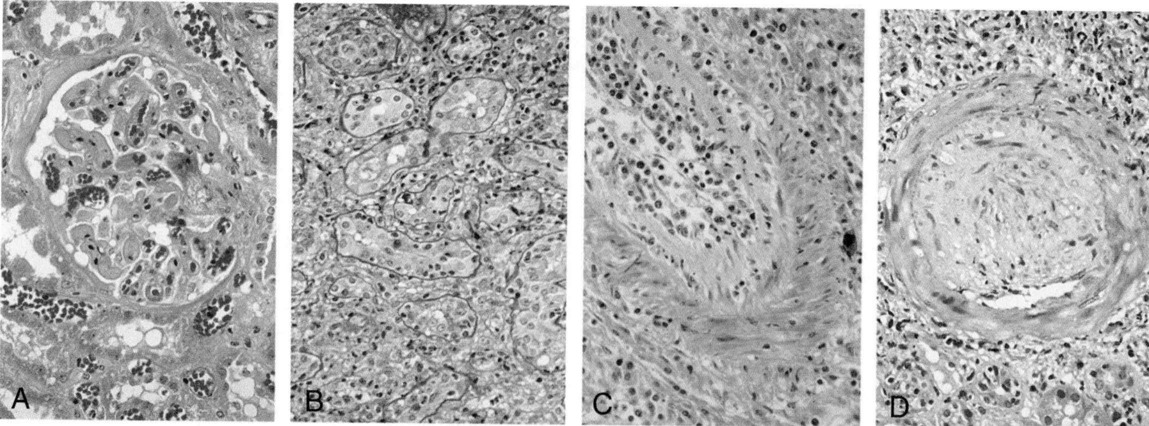

FIGURE 16–6 Histopathology of different forms of graft rejection. A. Hyperacute rejection of a kidney allograft with endothelial damage, platelet and thrombin thrombi, and early neutrophil infiltration in a glomerulus. B. Acute rejection of a kidney with inflammatory cells in the connective tissue around the tubules and between epithelial cells of the tubules. C. Acute rejection of a kidney allograft with destructive inflammatory reaction destroying the endothelial layer of an artery. D. Chronic rejection in a kidney allograft with graft arteriosclerosis. The vascular lumen is replaced by an accumulation of smooth muscle cells and connective tissue in the vessel intima. (Courtesy of Dr. Helmut Rennke, Department of Pathology, Brigham and Women's Hospital and Harvard Medical School, Boston.)

minutes to hours after host blood vessels are anastomosed to graft vessels and is mediated by preexisting antibodies in the host circulation that bind to donor endothelial antigens (Fig. 16–7). Binding of antibody to endothelium activates complement, and antibody and complement induce a number of changes in the graft endothelium that promote intravascular thrombosis. Complement activation leads to endothelial cell injury and exposure of subendothelial basement membrane proteins that activate platelets. The endothelial cells are stimulated to secrete high molecular weight forms of von Willebrand factor that mediate platelet adhesion and aggregation. Both endothelial cells and platelets undergo membrane vesiculation, leading to shedding of lipid particles that promote coagulation. Endothelial cells lose the cell surface heparan sulfate proteoglycans that normally interact with antithrombin III to inhibit coagulation. These processes contribute to thrombosis and vascular occlusion (see Fig. 16–6A), and the grafted organ suffers irreversible ischemic damage.

In the early days of transplantation, hyperacute rejection was often mediated by preexisting IgM alloantibodies, which are present at high titer before transplantation. Such "natural antibodies" are believed to arise in response to carbohydrate antigens expressed by bacteria that normally colonize the intestine. The best known examples of such alloantibodies are those directed against the ABO blood group antigens expressed on red blood cells (Box 16–2). ABO antigens are also expressed on vascular endothelial cells. Today, hyperacute rejection by anti-ABO antibodies is extremely rare because all donor and recipient pairs are selected so that they have the same ABO type. However, as we shall discuss later in this chapter, hyperacute rejection caused by natural antibodies is the major barrier to xenotransplantation and limits the use of animal organs for human transplantation.

Currently, hyperacute rejection of allografts, when it occurs, is usually mediated by IgG antibodies directed against protein alloantigens, such as foreign MHC molecules, or against less well defined alloantigens expressed on vascular endothelial cells. Such antibodies generally arise as a result of previous exposure to alloantigens through blood transfusion, previous transplantation, or multiple pregnancies. If the titer of these alloreactive antibodies is low, hyperacute rejection may develop slowly, over several days. In this case, it is sometimes referred to as accelerated allograft rejection because the onset is still earlier than that typical for acute rejection. As we will discuss later in this chapter, patients in need of allografts are routinely screened before grafting for the presence of antibodies that bind to cells of a potential organ donor to avoid hyperacute rejection.

Acute Rejection

Acute rejection is a process of vascular and parenchymal injury mediated by T cells and antibodies that usually begins after the first week of transplantation. Effector T cells and antibodies that mediate acute rejection develop over a few days or weeks in response to the graft, accounting for the time of onset of acute rejection.

T lymphocytes play a central role in acute rejection by responding to alloantigens, including MHC molecules, present on vascular endothelial and parenchymal cells (see Fig. 16–7B). The activated T cells cause direct killing of graft cells or produce cytokines that recruit and activate inflammatory cells, which injure the graft. In vascularized grafts such as kidney grafts, endothelial cells are the earliest targets of acute rejection. Microvascular endothelialitis is a frequent early finding in acute rejection episodes. Endothelialitis or intimal arteritis in medium sized arteries also occurs at an early stage of acute rejection and is indicative of severe rejection, which, if left untreated, will likely result in acute graft failure.

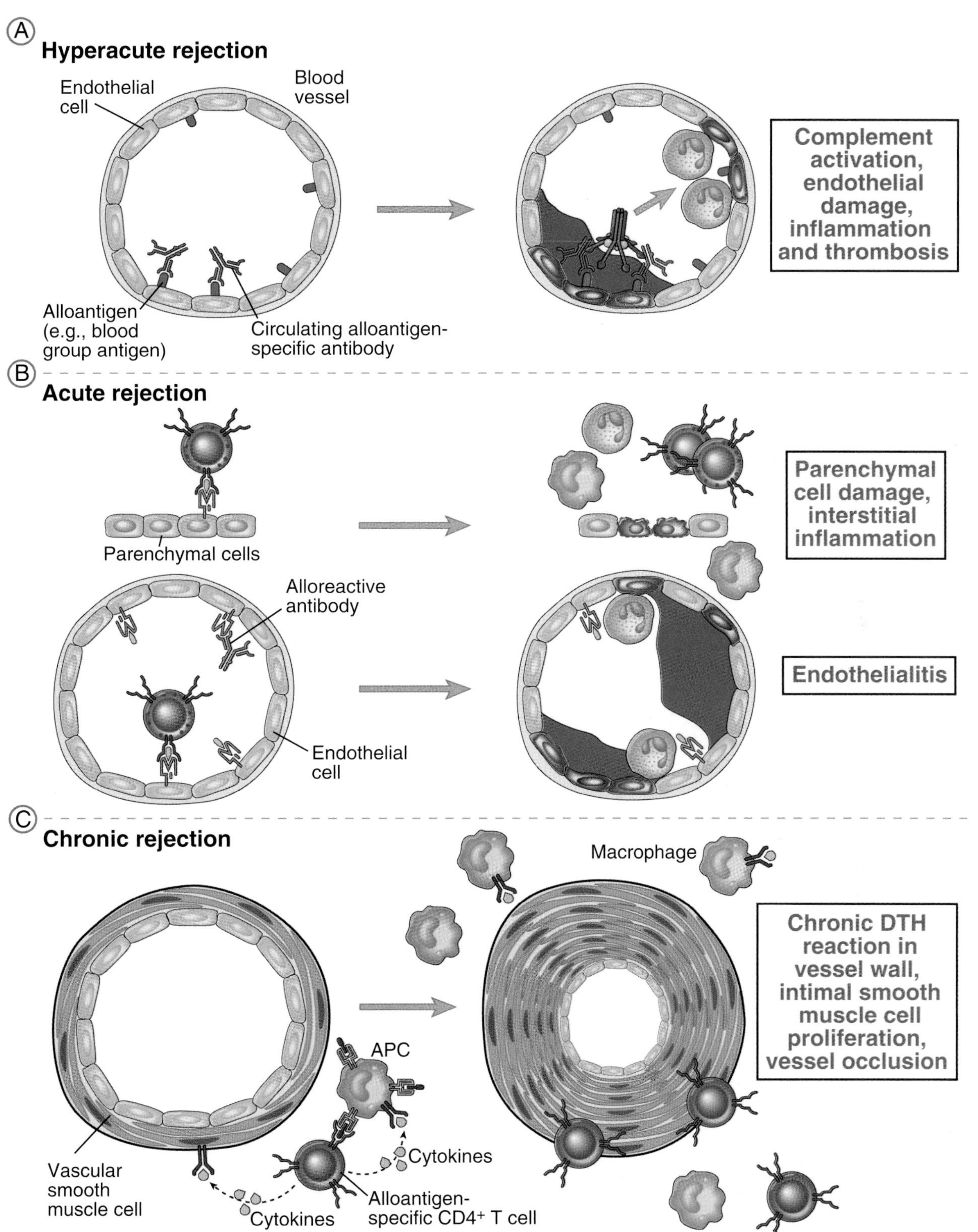

FIGURE 16–7 Immune mechanisms of graft rejection. A. In hyperacute rejection, preformed antibodies reactive with vascular endothelium activate complement and trigger rapid intravascular thrombosis and necrosis of the vessel wall. B. In acute rejection, $CD8^+$ T lymphocytes reactive with alloantigens on endothelial cells and parenchymal cells mediate damage to these cell types. Alloreactive antibodies formed after engraftment may also contribute to vascular injury. C. In chronic rejection with graft arteriosclerosis, injury to the vessel wall leads to intimal smooth muscle cell proliferation and luminal occlusion. This lesion may be caused by a chronic DTH reaction to alloantigens in the vessel wall.

Box 16–2 ■ IN DEPTH: ABO AND RH BLOOD GROUP ANTIGENS

The first alloantigen system to be defined in mammals was a family of red blood cell surface antigens called ABO, which are the targets of blood transfusion reactions (see text). The antigens in this system are cell surface glycosphingolipids. All normal individuals synthesize a common core glycan, called the O antigen, that is attached to a sphingolipid. Most individuals possess a fucosyltransferase that adds a fucose moiety to a nonterminal sugar residue of the O antigen, and the fucosylated glycan is called the H antigen. A single gene on chromosome 9 encodes a glycosyltransferase enzyme, which further modifies the H antigen. There are three allelic variants of this gene. The O allele gene product is devoid of enzymatic activity. The A allele-encoded enzyme transfers a terminal *N*-acetylgalactosamine moiety, and the B allele gene product transfers a terminal galactose moiety. Individuals who are homozygous for the O allele cannot attach terminal sugars to the H antigen and express only the H antigen. In contrast, individuals who possess an A allele (AA homozygotes, AO heterozygotes, or AB heterozygotes) form the A antigen by adding terminal *N*-acetylgalactosamine to some of their H antigens. Similarly, individuals who express a B allele (BB homozygotes, BO heterozygotes, or AB heterozygotes) form the B antigen by adding terminal galactose to some of their H antigens. AB heterozygotes form both A and B antigens from some of their H antigens. The terminology has been simplified so that OO individuals are said to be blood type O; AA and AO individuals are blood type A; BB and BO individuals are blood type B; and AB individuals are blood type AB. Mutations in the gene encoding the fucosyltransferase that produces the H antigen are rare; people who are homozygous for such a mutation cannot produce H, A, or B antigens. These individuals make antibodies against H, A, and B antigens and cannot receive type O, A, B, or AB blood.

The same glycosphingolipid that carries the ABO determinants can be modified by other glycosyltransferases to generate minor blood group antigens that may elicit milder transfusion reactions than the ABO antigens. For example, addition of fucose moieties at other nonterminal positions can be catalyzed by different fucosyltransferases and results in epitopes of the Lewis antigen system. Lewis antigens have recently received much attention from immunologists because these carbohydrate groups serve as ligands for E-selectin and P-selectin.

The Rhesus (Rh) antigens, named after the monkey species in which they were originally identified, is another clinically important group of blood group antigens. Rh antigens are nonglycosylated, hydrophobic cell surface proteins found in the red blood cell membranes and are structurally related to other red cell membrane glycoproteins with transporter functions. Rh proteins are encoded by two tightly linked and highly homologous genes, but only one of them, called RhD, is commonly considered in clinical blood typing. This is because up to 15% of the population have a deletion or other alterations of the RhD allele. These people, called Rh negative, are not tolerant to the RhD antigen and will make antibodies to the antigen if they are exposed to Rh-positive blood cells. The major clinical significance of anti-Rh antibodies is related to problems with pregnancy, as discussed in the text.

Both $CD4^+$ T cells and $CD8^+$ T cells may contribute to acute rejection. Several lines of evidence suggest that recognition and killing of graft cells by alloreactive $CD8^+$ CTLs is an important mechanism of acute rejection.

- The cellular infiltrates present in grafts undergoing acute cellular rejection (Fig. 16–6B) are markedly enriched for $CD8^+$ CTLs specific for graft alloantigens.
- The presence of CTLs in renal graft biopsy specimens, as indicated by sensitive reverse-transcriptase polymerase chain reaction assays for RNAs encoding CTL-specific genes (e.g., perforin and granzyme B), is a specific and sensitive indicator of clinical acute rejection.
- Alloreactive $CD8^+$ CTLs can be used to adoptively transfer acute cellular graft rejection.
- The destruction of allogeneic cells in a graft is highly specific, a hallmark of CTL killing. The best evidence for this specificity has come from mouse skin graft experiments using chimeric grafts that contain two distinct cell populations, one syngeneic to the host and one allogeneic to the host. When these skin grafts are transplanted, the allogeneic cells are killed without injury to the "bystander" syngeneic cells.

$CD4^+$ T cells may be important in mediating acute graft rejection by secreting cytokines and inducing DTH-like reactions in grafts, and some evidence indicates that $CD4^+$ T cells are sufficient to mediate acute rejection.

- Acute rejection of allografts does occur in knockout mice lacking $CD8^+$ T cells or perforin, suggesting that other effector mechanisms also contribute.
- Adoptive transfer of alloreactive $CD4^+$ T cells into a mouse can cause rejection of an allograft.

Antibodies can also mediate acute rejection if a graft recipient mounts a humoral immune response to vessel wall antigens and the antibodies that are produced bind to the vessel wall and activate complement. The histologic pattern of this form of acute rejection is one of transmural necrosis of graft vessel walls with acute inflammation (see Fig. 16–6C), which is different from the thrombotic occlusion without vessel wall necrosis seen in hyperacute rejection. Immunohistochemical identification of the C4d complement fragment in capillaries of renal allografts is used clinically as an indicator of activation of the classical complement pathway and humoral rejection.

Graft Vasculopathy and Chronic Rejection

Vascularized grafts that survive for more than 6 months slowly develop arterial occlusion as a result of the proliferation of intimal smooth muscle cells, and eventually fail due to ischemic damage. The arterial changes are called graft vasculopathy or accelerated graft arteriosclerosis (see Fig. 16–6D). Graft vasculopathy is frequently seen in failed cardiac and renal allografts and can develop in any vascularized organ transplant within 6 months to a year after transplantation. The pathogenesis of the lesions likely involves a combination of processes, including a response of the vessel to injury caused by perioperative ischemia and acute rejection episodes, in combination with a chronic DTH-like reaction of host lymphocytes to donor alloantigens in the graft vessel. The smooth muscle cell accumulation in the graft arterial intima appears to be stimulated by growth factors and chemokines secreted by endothelial cells, smooth muscle cells, and macrophages in response to interferon-γ (IFN-γ) and tumor necrosis factor (TNF) produced by alloreactive T cells (see Fig. 16–7C).

- Knockout mice lacking different components of the adaptive immune system have been used as graft recipients and show varying resistance to graft arteriosclerosis. For instance, accelerated graft arteriosclerosis does not develop in IFN-γ-deficient recipients, consistent with the hypothesis that DTH is involved in lesion formation. Other studies with knockout mice indicate that $CD4^+$ T cells and B lymphocytes are more important for the development of graft arteriosclerosis than are $CD8^+$ T cells.

As the arterial lesions of graft arteriosclerosis progress, blood flow to the graft parenchyma is compromised, and the parenchyma is slowly replaced by nonfunctioning fibrous tissue. In addition, fibrosis in older grafts may also reflect the final outcome of parenchymal injury caused by episodes of acute rejection. Several growth factors and cytokines have been implicated in graft fibrosis, including fibroblast growth factor, transforming growth factor-β (TGF-β), and interleukin-13 (IL-13). Often, the process of graft fibrosis is called **chronic rejection**. As therapy for controlling acute rejection has improved, graft vasculopathy and chronic rejection have emerged as the major cause of allograft loss.

Chronic rejection of different transplanted organs is associated with distinct pathologic changes. Lung transplants undergoing chronic rejection show thickened small airways (bronchiolitis obliterans), and liver transplants show fibrotic and nonfunctional bile ducts (the vanishing bile duct syndrome).

Prevention and Treatment of Allograft Rejection

If the recipient of an allograft has a fully functional immune system, transplantation almost invariably results in some form of rejection. The strategies used in clinical practice and in experimental models to avoid or delay rejection are general immunosuppression and minimizing the strength of the specific allogeneic reaction. An important goal in transplantation is to induce donor-specific tolerance, which would allow grafts to survive without nonspecific immunosuppression.

Immunosuppression to Prevent or to Treat Allograft Rejection

Immunosuppression is the major approach for the prevention and management of transplant rejection. Several methods of immunosuppression are commonly used (Table 16–1).

Immunosuppressive drugs that inhibit or kill T lymphocytes are the principal treatment regimen for graft rejection. The most important immunosuppressive agents in current clinical use are the calcineurin inhibitors, including cyclosporine and FK-506 (tacrolimus). The major action of these drugs is to inhibit T cell transcription of certain genes, most notably those encoding cytokines such as IL-2. Cyclosporine is a cyclic peptide made by a species of fungus, which binds with high affinity to a ubiquitous cellular protein called cyclophilin. As discussed in Chapter 9, the complex of

Table 16–1. Methods of Immunosuppression in Clinical Use

Drug	Mechanism of action
Cyclosporine and FK-506	Block T cell cytokine production by inhibiting activation of the NFAT transcription factor
Azathioprine	Blocks proliferation of lymphocyte precursors
Mycophenolate mofetil	Blocks lymphocyte proliferation by inhibiting guanine nucleotide synthesis in lymphocytes
Rapamycin	Blocks lymphocyte proliferation by inhibiting IL-2 signaling
Corticosteroids	Reduce inflammation by inhibiting macrophage cytokine secretion
Anti-CD3 monoclonal antibody	Depletes T cells by binding to CD3 and promoting phagocytosis or complement-mediated lysis (used to treat acute rejection)
Anti–IL-2 receptor (CD25) antibody	Inhibits T cell proliferation by blocking IL-2 binding and depletes activated T cells that express CD25
CTLA-4-Ig	Inhibits T cell activation by blocking B7 costimulator binding to T cell CD28; in clinical trials
Anti-CD40 ligand	Inhibits macrophage and endothelial activation by blocking T cell CD40 ligand binding to CD40; in clinical trials

cyclosporine and cyclophilin binds to and inhibits the enzymatic activity of the calcium/calmodulin-activated protein phosphatase calcineurin. Because calcineurin is required to activate the transcription factor NFAT (nuclear factor of activated T cells), cyclosporine blocks NFAT activation and the transcription of IL-2 and other cytokine genes. The net result is that cyclosporine blocks the IL-2–dependent growth and differentiation of T cells. FK-506 is a macrolide lactone made by a bacterium that functions like cyclosporine. FK-506 and its binding protein (called FKBP) share with the cyclosporine-cyclophilin complex the ability to bind calcineurin and inhibit its activity.

The introduction of cyclosporine into clinical practice ushered in the modern era of transplantation. Before the use of cyclosporine, the majority of transplanted hearts and livers were rejected. Now the majority of these allografts survive for more than 5 years (Fig. 16–8). Nevertheless, cyclosporine is not a panacea for transplantation. Drug levels needed for optimal immunosuppression cause kidney damage, and some rejection episodes are refractory to cyclosporine treatment. FK-506 has been used most frequently in liver transplant recipients and in cases of kidney allograft rejection that are not adequately controlled by cyclosporine.

Another class of immunosuppressive agents that are used frequently to control allograft rejection are the inhibitors of the cellular enzyme called mammalian target of rapamycin (mTOR). The first drug discovered in this class is **rapamycin,** whose principal effect is to inhibit T cell proliferation. Like FK-506, rapamycin also

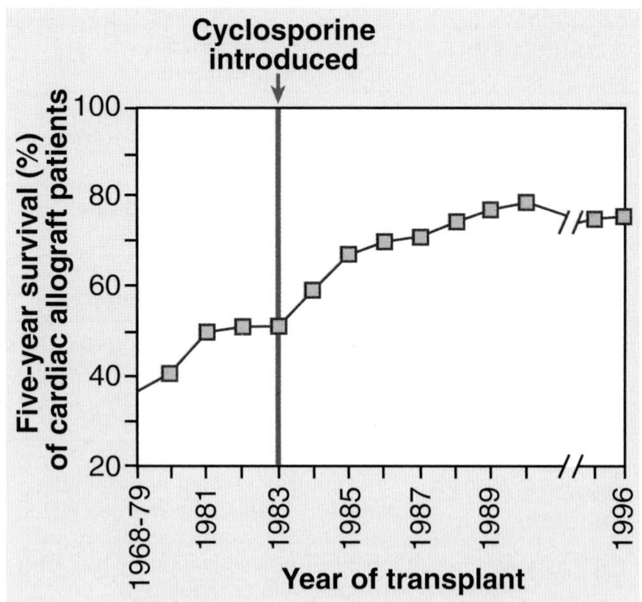

FIGURE 16–8 Influence of cyclosporine on graft survival. Five-year survival rates for patients receiving cardiac allografts increased significantly beginning when cyclosporine was introduced in 1983. (Data from Transplant Patient DataSource, United Network for Organ Sharing, Richmond, Va. Retrieved February 16, 2000, from http://207.239.150.13/tpd/.)

binds to FKBP, but the rapamycin-FKBP complex does not inhibit calcineurin. Instead, this complex binds to mTOR, which is a serine/threonine protein kinase required for translation of proteins that promote cell proliferation. Interaction of the rapamycin-FKBP complex with mTOR inhibits the function of mTOR and thus blocks cellular proliferation. Combinations of cyclosporine (which blocks IL-2 synthesis) and rapamycin (which blocks IL-2-driven proliferation) are potent inhibitors of T cell responses. In addition to rapamycin, other mTOR inhibitors have been developed for immunosuppression of allograft recipients and for cancer therapy.

Metabolic toxins that kill proliferating T cells are also used to treat graft rejection. These agents inhibit the maturation of lymphocytes from immature precursors and also kill proliferating mature T cells that have been stimulated by alloantigens. The first such drug to be developed for the prevention and treatment of rejection was azathioprine. This drug is still used, but it is toxic to precursors of leukocytes in the bone marrow and enterocytes in the gut. The newest and most widely used drug in this class is **mycophenolate mofetil (MMF).** MMF is metabolized to mycophenolic acid, which blocks a lymphocyte-specific isoform of inosine monophosphate dehydroxygenase, an enzyme required for de novo synthesis of guanine nucleotides. Because MMF selectively inhibits the lymphocyte-specific isoform of this enzyme, it has relatively few toxic effects on other cells. MMF is now routinely used, often in combination with cyclosporine, to prevent acute allograft rejection.

Antibodies that react with T cell surface structures and deplete or inhibit T cells are used to treat acute rejection episodes. The most widely used antibody is a mouse monoclonal antibody called OKT3 that is specific for human CD3. It may seem surprising that one would use a potential polyclonal activator such as anti-CD3 antibody to reduce T cell reactivity. In vivo, however, OKT3 either acts as a lytic antibody by activating the complement system to eliminate T cells or opsonizes T cells for phagocytosis. T cells that escape elimination probably do so by endocytosing ("modulating") CD3 off their surface, but such cells may be rendered nonfunctional. Another antibody now in clinical use is specific for CD25, the α-subunit of the IL-2 receptor. This reagent, which is administered at the time of transplantation, may prevent T cell activation by blocking IL-2 binding to activated T cells, and it may deplete CD25-expressing activated T cells by mechanisms similar to those described for OKT3. The major limitation on the use of mouse monoclonal antibodies is that humans given these agents produce anti-mouse immunoglobulin (Ig) antibodies that eliminate the injected mouse Ig. For this reason, human-mouse chimeric ("humanized") antibodies to CD3 and CD25 that may be less immunogenic have been developed.

Drugs that block T cell costimulatory pathways are now used to prevent acute allograft rejection. The rationale for the use of these types of drugs is to prevent the delivery of second signals required for activation of

T cells (see Chapter 9). A soluble form of CTLA-4 fused to an IgG Fc domain (called CTLA-4-Ig) prevents B7 molecules on APCs from interacting with T cell CD28, and is approved for use in allograft recipients.

- Clinical studies have shown that CTLA-4-Ig can be as effective as cyclosporine in preventing acute rejection. Studies with experimental animals show that graft rejection is reduced or delayed by CTLA-4-Ig, and as well as by an antibody that binds to T cell CD40 ligand and prevents its interactions with CD40 on APCs (see Chapters 7 and 9). In some experimental protocols, simultaneous blockade of both B7 and CD40 appears to be more effective than either alone in promoting graft survival. Antibody to CD40 ligand also delays the rejection of kidney and pancreatic islet allografts in primates. It is likely that these treatments inhibit the activation of alloreactive T cells and do not induce long-lived tolerance in these cells.

Acute antibody-mediated rejection can be treated with drugs that inhibit antibody production. Several new immunosuppressive agents, including rapamycin and brequinar, inhibit antibody synthesis and are therefore potentially useful in preventing acute vascular rejection.

Anti-inflammatory agents are also routinely used for the prevention and treatment of graft rejection. The most potent anti-inflammatory agents available are corticosteroids. The proposed mechanism of action of these natural hormones and their synthetic analogues is to block the synthesis and secretion of cytokines, including TNF and IL-1, and other inflammatory mediators by macrophages. Lack of TNF and IL-1 synthesis reduces graft endothelial cell activation and recruitment of leukocytes (see Chapters 2 and 13). Corticosteroids may also block the generation of prostaglandins, reactive oxygen species, and nitric oxide. Very high doses of corticosteroids may inhibit T cell secretion of cytokines or even kill T cells, but it is unlikely that the levels of corticosteroids achieved in vivo act in this way. Newer anti-inflammatory agents are in clinical trials, including soluble cytokine receptors, anti-cytokine antibodies, and antibodies that block leukocyte-endothelial adhesion (e.g., anti-intercellular adhesion molecule-1 [anti-ICAM-1]).

A new therapeutic agent, called FTY720, works by binding to and blocking sphingosine 1-phosphate receptors on lymphocytes. This phospholipid is involved in the egress of lymphocytes from lymphoid organs (see Chapter 3), and blocking its action leads to the sequestration of lymphocytes in lymph nodes. This inhibits immune responses to transplants. This drug is now in clinical trials for preventing graft rejection and treating some autoimmune diseases.

Current immunosuppressive protocols have dramatically improved graft survival. Before the use of cyclosporine, the 1-year survival rate of unrelated cadaveric kidney grafts was between 50% and 60%, with a 90% rate for grafts from living related donors (which are better matched with the recipients). Since cyclosporine and MMF have been introduced, the survival rate of unrelated cadaveric kidney grafts has approached about 90% at 1 year. The use of rapamycin promises to improve early survival of grafts even more. Heart transplantation, for which human leukocyte antigen (HLA) matching (discussed later) is not practical, has significantly improved with the use of cyclosporine and now has a similar 90% 1-year survival rate. Experience with other organs is more limited, but survival rates for liver and lung transplants have also benefited from modern immunosuppressive therapy.

Acute rejection, when it occurs, is managed by rapidly intensifying immunosuppressive therapy. In modern transplantation, chronic rejection has become a more common cause of allograft failure, especially in cardiac transplantation. Chronic rejection is more insidious than acute rejection, and it is much less reversible by immunosuppression.

Sustained immunosuppression required for prolonged graft survival leads to increased susceptibility to viral infections and virus-associated tumors. The major thrust of transplant-related immunosuppression is to reduce the generation and function of helper T cells and CTLs, which mediate acute cellular rejection. It is therefore not surprising that defense against viruses, the physiologic function of CTLs, is also undermined in immunosuppressed transplant recipients. Reactivation of latent cytomegalovirus, a herpesvirus, is particularly common in immunosuppressed patients. For this reason, transplant recipients are now given prophylactic antiviral therapy for cytomegalovirus infections. Two malignant tumors commonly seen in allograft patients are B cell lymphomas and squamous cell carcinoma of the skin. The B cell lymphomas are thought to be sequelae of unchecked infection by Epstein-Barr virus, another herpesvirus (see Chapter 17, Box 17–2). The squamous cell carcinomas of the skin are associated with human papillomavirus.

Methods to Reduce the Immunogenicity of Allografts

In human transplantation, the major strategy to reduce graft immunogenicity has been to minimize alloantigenic differences between the donor and recipient . To avoid hyper-acute rejection, the ABO blood group antigens of the graft donor are selected to be identical to those of the recipient. Patients in need of allografts are also tested for the presence of preformed antibodies against donor cells. This type of testing is called crossmatching. It is done by mixing recipient serum with leukocytes from potential donors and adding complement to promote classical pathway–mediated lysis of donor cells. If preformed antibodies, usually against donor MHC molecules, are present in the recipient's serum, the donor cells are lysed (called a positive crossmatch), and such lysis indicates that the donor is not suitable for that recipient. For kidney transplantation from living related donors, attempts are made to minimize both class I and class II MHC allelic differences between the donor and recipient. All potential kidney donors and recipients are "tissue typed" to determine the identity of the HLA molecules that are expressed (Box 16–3).

In kidney transplantation, the larger the number of MHC alleles that are matched between the donor and recipient, the better the graft survival, especially in the first year after transplantation (Fig. 16–9). MHC matching had a more profound influence on graft survival

Box 16–3 ■ IN DEPTH: TESTING FOR DONOR-RECIPIENT COMPATIBILITY IN TRANSPLANTATION

Several clinical laboratory tests are routinely performed to reduce the risk for immunologic rejection in transplantation. These include ABO blood typing; the determination of HLA alleles expressed on donor and recipient cells, called tissue typing; the detection of preformed antibodies in the recipient that recognize HLA and other antigens representative of the donor population; and the detection of preformed antibodies in the recipient that bind to antigens of an identified donor's leukocytes, called crossmatching. Not all of these tests are done in all types of transplantation.

ABO BLOOD TYPING. This test is uniformly used in all transplantation because no type of graft will survive if there are ABO incompatibilities between the donor and recipient. Natural IgM antibodies specific for allogeneic ABO blood group antigens (see Box 16–2) will cause hyperacute rejection. Blood typing is performed by mixing a patient's red blood cells with standardized sera containing anti-A or anti-B antibodies. If the patient expresses either blood group antigen, the serum specific for that antigen will agglutinate the red cells.

TISSUE TYPING: HLA MATCHING. For living related kidney transplantation, attempts are made to reduce the number of differences in HLA alleles expressed on donor and recipient cells, which will have a modest effect in reducing the chance of rejection. In bone marrow transplantation, HLA matching is essential to reduce the risk for GVHD. Routine HLA typing focuses only on HLA-A, HLA-B, and HLA-DR because these are the only loci that appear to predict the likelihood of rejection or GVHD. Until recently, most HLA haplotype determinations were performed by serologic testing. This procedure relies on standardized collections of sera from multiple donors previously sensitized to different HLA molecules by pregnancy or transfusions. Each of these sera is mixed with a person's lymphocytes in separate wells of a tissue culture plate. A source of complement is added to the wells, as is a fluorescent dye that will enter only dead cells. After an incubation time, the wells are examined under a fluorescence microscope for the presence of dead cells. B lymphocytes are used as target cells because they normally express both class I and class II MHC molecules. On the basis of which antisera cause lysis, the HLA haplotype of the individual can be determined. Since the typing sera may not be absolutely specific for a single allelic product, serologic typing cannot always resolve exactly which alleles are present.

The polymerase chain reaction (PCR) has recently been used for more detailed typing of the MHC, replacing serologic methods. MHC genes can be amplified by PCR methods with use of primers that bind to conserved sequences within the 5′ and 3′ ends of exons encoding the polymorphic regions of class I and class II MHC molecules. The amplified segment of DNA can then readily be sequenced. Thus, the actual nucleotide sequence, and therefore the predicted amino acid sequence, can be directly determined for the alleles of any cell, providing precise molecular tissue typing. Based on these DNA sequencing efforts, the nomenclature of HLA alleles has changed to reflect the identification of many alleles not distinguished by previous serologic methods. Each allele defined by sequence has at least a four-digit number, but some alleles require 6 or 8 digits for precise definition. The first two digits usually correspond to the serologically defined allotype. The third and fourth digits indicate the subtypes. Alleles with differences in the first four digits encode proteins with different amino acids. For example, HLA-DRB1*1301 is a sequence-defined allele that is one of many alleles previously called HLA-DRB1 based on serologic techniques.

SCREENING FOR THE PRESENCE OF PREFORMED ANTIBODIES. Patients waiting for organ transplants are screened for the presence of preformed antibodies reactive with allogeneic HLA molecules. These antibodies, which may be produced as a result of previous pregnancies, transfusions, or transplantation, can identify risk for hyperacute or acute vascular rejection. Small amounts of the patient's serum are mixed, in separate wells, with cells from a panel of 40 to 60 different donors representative of the organ donor population. Binding of the patient's antibodies to cells of each donor of the panel is determined by complement-mediated lysis, as described before, or by flow cytometry with use of fluorescent-labeled secondary antibodies to human IgG. The results are reported as percent reactive antibody (PRA), which is the percentage of the donor cell pool with which the patient's serum reacts. The PRA is determined on multiple occasions while a patient waits for an organ allograft. This is because the PRA can vary, since each panel is chosen at random, and the patient's serum antibody titers may change over time.

CROSSMATCHING. If a potential donor is identified, the crossmatching test will determine whether the patient has antibodies that react specifically with the donor cells. The test is performed in a way similar to the antibody screening assays, but in this case, the recipient's serum is tested for reactivity against only the particular donor's cells (typically lymphocytes). Cytotoxic and flow cytometric assays can be used.

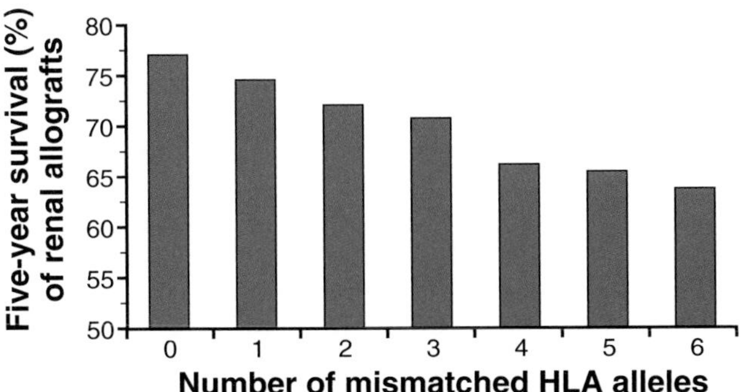

FIGURE 16–9 Influence of MHC matching on graft survival. Matching of MHC alleles between the donor and recipient significantly improves renal allograft survival. The data shown are for living donor grafts. HLA matching has even more of an impact on survival of renal allografts from cadaver donors, and some MHC alleles are more important than others in determining outcome. (Data from Organ Procurement and Transplantation Network/Scientific Registry annual report, 2003.)

before modern immunosuppressive drugs were routinely used. Clinical experience has shown that of all the class I and class II loci, matching only HLA-A, HLA-B, and HLA-DR is important for predicting outcome. (HLA-C is not as polymorphic as HLA-A or HLA-B, and HLA-DR and HLA-DQ are in strong linkage disequilibrium, so matching at the DR locus often also matches at the DQ locus. DP typing is not in common use, and its importance is unknown.) Because two codominantly expressed alleles are inherited for each of these MHC genes, it is possible to have zero to six MHC antigen mismatches between the donor and recipient. Zero-antigen mismatches predict the best survival of living related donor grafts, and one-antigen–matched grafts do slightly worse. The survival of grafts with two to six MHC mismatches all are significantly worse than zero- or one-antigen mismatches. MHC matching has an even greater impact on nonliving (unrelated) donor renal allografts.

HLA matching in renal transplantation is possible because donor kidneys can be stored in organ banks before transplantation until a well-matched recipient can be identified, and because patients needing a kidney allograft can be maintained on dialysis until a well-matched organ is available. In the case of heart and liver transplantation, organ preservation is more difficult, and potential recipients are often in critical condition. For these reasons, HLA typing is not considered in pairing of potential donors and recipients, and the choice of donor and recipient is based only on ABO blood group matching and anatomic compatibility.

Methods to Induce Donor-Specific Tolerance

Allograft rejection may be prevented by making the host tolerant to the alloantigens of the graft. Tolerance in this setting means that the host does not injure the graft despite the absence or withdrawal of immunosuppressive and anti-inflammatory agents. It is presumed that tolerance to an allograft will involve the same mechanisms that are involved in tolerance to self antigens (see Chapter 11), namely peripheral anergy, deletion, or active suppression of alloreactive T cells. Tolerance is desirable in transplantation because it is alloantigen specific and will therefore avoid the major problem associated with nonspecific immunosuppression, namely, increased susceptibility to infection and to virus-induced tumors. In addition, achieving graft tolerance may reduce chronic rejection, which has to date been unaffected by the commonly used immunosuppressive agents that prevent and reverse acute rejection episodes.

Several experimental approaches and clinical observations have suggested that it should be possible to achieve tolerance to allografts.

- In experiments with skin grafts in mice, Medawar and colleagues showed that if neonatal mice of one strain (the recipient) are given spleen cells of another strain (the donor), the recipients will subsequently accept grafts from the donor. Such tolerance is alloantigen specific because the recipients will reject grafts from mouse strains that express MHC alleles that differ from the donor's (see Chapter 11, Fig. 11–2).
- Renal transplant patients who have received blood transfusions containing allogeneic leukocytes have a lower incidence of acute rejection episodes than do those who have not been transfused. The postulated explanation for this effect is that the introduction of allogeneic leukocytes by transfusion produces tolerance to alloantigens. Indeed, pretreatment of potential recipients with blood transfusions is now used as prophylactic therapy to reduce rejection.
- Animals given bone marrow transplants who subsequently contain both donor and recipient cells in the circulation (called mixed chimerism) are tolerant to organ allografts derived from the same donor as the bone marrow graft. Human allogeneic bone marrow transplantation to establish mixed chimerism has been tried in a small number of patients before solid organ transplantation, but this approach may be limited by the problem of graft-versus-host disease (GVHD), which is discussed later in this chapter. More benign methods to establish mixed chimerism in humans are under investigation.

Strategies are also being developed for inducing regulatory T lymphocytes specific for graft alloantigens. Although the best approaches for inducing tolerance need to be established in clinical trials, it is hoped that tolerance induction will become a standard part of transplantation therapy in the near future.

Xenogeneic Transplantation

The use of solid organ transplantation as a clinical therapy is greatly limited by the lack of availability of donor organs. For this reason, the possibility of transplantation of organs from other mammals, such as pigs, into human recipients has kindled great interest.

A major immunologic barrier to xenogeneic transplantation is the presence of natural antibodies that cause hyperacute rejection. More than 95% of primates have natural IgM antibodies that are reactive with the carbohydrate determinants expressed by the cells of members of species that are evolutionarily distant, such as the pig. The vast majority of human anti-pig natural antibodies are directed at one particular carbohydrate determinant formed by the action of a pig α-galactosyltransferase enzyme. This enzyme places an α-linked galactose moiety on the same substrate that in human and other primate cells is fucosylated to form the blood group H antigen (see Box 16–2). Species combinations that give rise to natural antibodies against each other are said to be discordant. Natural antibodies are rarely produced against carbohydrate determinants of closely related, concordant species, such as humans and chimpanzees. Thus, chimpanzees or other higher primates technically can and have been used as organ donors for humans. However, ethical and logistic concerns have limited such procedures. For reasons of anatomic compatibility, pigs are the preferred xenogeneic species for organ donation to humans.

Natural antibodies against xenografts induce hyperacute rejection by the same mechanisms as those seen in hyperacute allograft rejection. These mechanisms include the generation of endothelial cell procoagulants and platelet-aggregating substances, coupled with the loss of endothelial anticoagulant mechanisms. However, the consequences of activating human complement on pig cells are typically more severe than the consequences of activation of complement by natural antibodies on human allogeneic cells, possibly because some of the complement regulatory proteins made by pig cells, such as decay accelerating factor, are not able to interact with human complement proteins and thus cannot limit the extent of complement-induced injury (see Chapter 14). A strategy under exploration for reducing hyperacute rejection in xenotransplantation is to breed transgenic pigs expressing human proteins that inhibit complement activation or fail to express enzymes that synthesize pig antigens. Such pigs could, for example, overexpress human H group fucosyltransferase and overexpress human complement regulatory proteins such as decay accelerating factor.

Even when hyperacute rejection is prevented, xenografts are often damaged by a form of acute vascular rejection that occurs within 2 to 3 days of transplantation. This form of rejection has been called delayed xenograft rejection, accelerated acute rejection, or acute vascular rejection and is characterized by intravascular thrombosis and fibrinoid necrosis of vessel walls. The mechanisms of delayed xenograft rejection are incompletely understood, but it is likely to be caused by natural antibodies to various endothelial antigens and by T cell activation and cytokine-mediated endothelial damage.

Xenografts can also be rejected by T cell-mediated immune responses to xenoantigens. The mechanisms of cell-mediated rejection of xenografts are believed to be similar to those that we have described for allograft rejection, and T cell responses to xenoantigens can be as strong as or even stronger than responses to alloantigens. Human T cell recognition of pig MHC molecules may involve both direct and indirect pathways. Furthermore, several intercellular molecular interactions required for T cell responses, such as CD4/class II MHC, CD8/class I MHC, CD2/LFA-3, CD28/B7, CD40L/CD40, and VLA-4/vascular cell adhesion molecule-1 (VCAM-1), are functional even when one member of these pairs is from a pig and the other from a human.

Cell-mediated responses to xenografts may be too strong to be adequately controlled by the immunosuppressive protocols used for allograft rejection, and research is therefore focused on inducing specific tolerance to xenografts. The methods of tolerance induction that are being considered include those we have discussed for allografts, such as mixed hematopoietic chimerism, costimulation blockade, and administration of peptides from xenogeneic MHC molecules to induce specific tolerance.

Blood Transfusion

Blood transfusion is a form of transplantation in which whole blood or blood cells from one or more individuals are transferred intravenously into the circulation of a host. Blood transfusions are performed to replace blood lost by hemorrhage or to correct defects caused by inadequate production of blood cells, which may occur in a variety of diseases. The major barrier to successful blood transfusions is the immune response to cell surface molecules that differ between individuals. The most important alloantigen system in blood transfusion is the ABO system (see Box 16–2). ABO antigens are expressed on all cells, including red blood cells. Individuals lacking a particular blood group antigen may produce natural IgM antibodies against that antigen, probably as a result of responses to cross-reactive antigens expressed on bacteria that colonize the gut. If such individuals are given blood cells expressing the missing antigen, the preexisting antibodies bind to the transfused cells, activate complement, and lyse the transfused cells. Lysis of the foreign red blood cells results in **transfusion reactions,** which can be life threatening. Transfusion across an ABO barrier may trigger an immediate hemolytic reaction, resulting in both intravascular lysis of red blood cells, probably mediated by the complement system, and extensive phagocytosis of antibody- and complement-coated erythrocytes by macrophages of the liver and spleen. Hemoglobin is liberated from the lysed red cells in quantities that may be toxic for kidney cells, producing acute renal tubular cell necrosis and kidney failure. High fevers, shock, and disseminated intravascular coagulation may also develop, suggestive of massive cytokine release (e.g., of TNF or IL-1; see Chapter 15, Box 15–1). The disseminated intravascular coagulation consumes clotting factors faster than they can be synthesized, and the patient may paradoxically die of bleeding in the presence of widespread clotting. More delayed hemolytic reactions may result from incompatibilities of minor blood group antigens. These result in progressive loss of the transfused red cells, leading to anemia, and jaundice, a consequence of overloading the liver with hemoglobin-derived pigments.

The choice of blood donors for a particular recipient is based on our understanding of blood group antigens. Virtually all individuals express the H antigen, and therefore they are tolerant to this antigen and do not produce anti-H antibodies. Individuals who express A or B antigens are tolerant to these molecules and do not produce anti-A or anti-B antibodies, respectively. However, OO and AO individuals (see Box 16–2) produce anti-B IgM antibodies, and OO and BO individuals produce anti-A IgM antibodies. If a patient receives a transfusion of red blood cells from a donor who expresses the antigen not expressed on self red blood cells, a transfusion reaction may result (described above). It follows that AB individuals can tolerate transfusions from all potential donors and are therefore called universal recipients; similarly, OO individuals can tolerate transfusions only from OO donors but can provide blood to all recipients and are therefore called universal donors. In general, differences in minor blood groups lead to red cell lysis only after repeated transfusions trigger a secondary antibody response.

ABO antigens are expressed on many other cell types in addition to blood cells, including endothelial cells. For this reason, ABO typing is critical to avoid hyperacute rejection of solid organ allografts, as discussed earlier in the chapter.

The Rhesus (Rh) antigen is another important red blood cell antigen that may be responsible for transfusion reactions (see Box 16–2). Although there are no natural antibodies to Rh antigens, individuals who do not express the RhD antigen (approximately 15% of the population) can be sensitized to this antigen and produce anti-Rh antibodies if they receive blood transfusions from an RhD-expressing donor. Transfusion reactions can arise after a second transfusion of Rh-positive blood. In addition, Rh-negative mothers carrying an Rh-positive fetus can be sensitized by fetal red blood cells that enter the maternal circulation, usually during childbirth. Subsequent pregnancies in which the fetus is Rh positive are at risk because the maternal anti-Rh antibodies can cross the placenta and mediate the destruction of the fetal red blood cells. This causes **erythroblastosis fetalis** (hemolytic disease of the newborn) and can be lethal for the fetus. This disease can be prevented by administration of anti-RhD (RhD-immune) antibodies to the mother within 72 hours of birth of the first Rh-positive baby. The treatment prevents the baby's Rh-positive red blood cells that entered the mother's circulation from inducing the production of anti-Rh antibodies in the mother. The exact mechanisms of action of the antibodies are not clear, but may include phagocytic clearance or complement-mediated lysis of the baby's red cells, or Fc receptor–dependent feedback inhibition of the mother's RhD-specific B cells (see Chapter 10).

Bone Marrow Transplantation

Bone marrow transplantation is the transplantation of pluripotent hematopoietic stem cells, most commonly in an inoculum of bone marrow cells collected by aspiration. Hematopoietic stem cells can also be purified from the blood of donors after treatment with colony-stimulating factors, which mobilize stem cells from the bone marrow. After transplantation, stem cells repopulate the recipient's bone marrow and differentiate into all the hematopoietic lineages. We consider bone marrow transplantation separately in this chapter because several unique features of this type of grafting are not encountered with solid organ transplantation.

Bone marrow transplantation may be used clinically to remedy acquired defects in the hematopoietic system or in the immune system because blood cells and lymphocytes develop from a common stem cell. It has also been proposed as a means of correcting inherited deficiencies or abnormalities of enzymes or other proteins (e.g., abnormal hemoglobin) by providing a self-renewing source of normal stem cells. Some stem cells in the bone marrow may also have the potential to differentiate into various nonhematopoietic tissue cell types, which is an area of active investigation for the possible treatment of diseases of many organ systems. In addition, allogeneic bone marrow transplantation may be used as part of the treatment of bone marrow malignant disease (i.e., leukemias) and disseminated solid tumors. In this case, the chemotherapeutic agents needed to destroy cancer cells also destroy normal marrow elements, and bone marrow transplantation is used to "rescue" the patient from the side effects of chemotherapy. In addition, in some forms of leukemia, the grafted cells can be effective in destroying residual leukemia cells by a process analogous to the graft-versus-host responses discussed later. For other malignant tumors, when the marrow is not involved by tumor or when it can be purged of tumor cells, the patient's own bone marrow may be harvested and reinfused after chemotherapy. This procedure, called autologous bone marrow transplantation, does not elicit the immune responses associated with allogeneic bone marrow transplantation and will not be discussed further.

Before bone marrow is transplanted, recipients must often be "prepared" with radiation and chemotherapy to deplete their own marrow cells and vacate these sites to allow the transplanted stem cells to "home" to the marrow and establish themselves in the appropriate environment. Allogeneic stem cells are readily rejected by even a minimally immunocompetent host, and therefore the donor and recipient must be carefully matched at all polymorphic MHC loci. In addition, it is often necessary to greatly suppress the recipient's immune system to permit successful bone marrow transplantation. Such suppression is accomplished by radiation and chemotherapy. The mechanisms of rejection of bone marrow cells are not completely known, but in addition to adaptive immune mechanisms, hematopoietic stem cells may also be rejected by NK cells. The role of NK cells in bone marrow rejection has been studied in experimental animals.

- Irradiated F_1 hybrid mice reject bone marrow donated by either inbred parent. This phenomenon, called hybrid resistance, is in distinction to the classical laws of solid tissue transplantation (see Fig. 16–2). Hybrid resistance is seen in T cell–deficient mice, and depletion of recipient NK cells with anti–NK cell antibodies prevents the rejection of parental bone marrow. Hybrid resistance is probably due to host NK cells reacting against bone marrow precursors that lack class I MHC molecules expressed by the host.

Even after successful engraftment, two additional problems are frequently associated with bone marrow transplantation, namely, GVHD and immunodeficiency.

Graft-Versus-Host Disease

GVHD is caused by the reaction of grafted mature T cells in the marrow inoculum with alloantigens of the host. It occurs when the host is immunocompromised and therefore unable to reject the allogeneic cells in the graft. In most cases, the reaction is directed against minor histocompatibility antigens of the host because bone marrow transplantation is not performed when the donor and recipient have differences in MHC molecules. GVHD may also develop when solid organs that contain significant numbers of T cells are transplanted, such as the small bowel, lung, or liver.

GVHD is the principal limitation to the success of bone marrow transplantation. As in solid organ transplantation, GVHD may be classified on the basis of histologic patterns into acute and chronic forms.

Acute GVHD is characterized by epithelial cell death in the skin, liver (mainly the biliary epithelium), and gastrointestinal tract (Fig. 16–10). It is manifested clinically by rash, jaundice, diarrhea, and gastrointestinal hemorrhage. When the epithelial cell death is extensive, the skin or lining of the gut may slough off. In this circumstance, acute GVHD may be fatal.

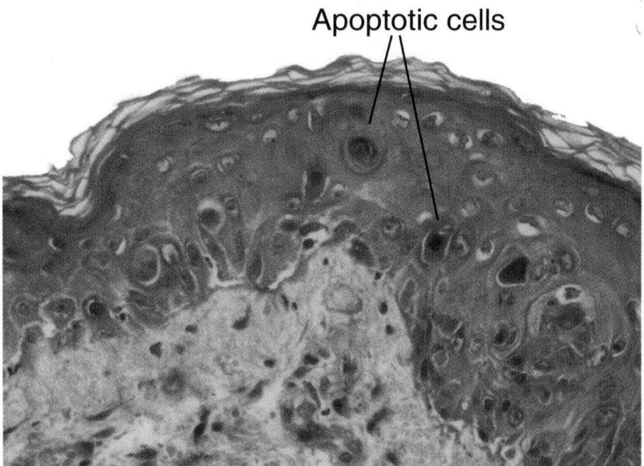

FIGURE 16–10 Histopathology of acute GVHD in the skin. A sparse lymphocytic infiltrate can be seen at the dermal-epidermal junction, and damage to the epithelial layer is indicated by spaces at the dermal-epidermal junction (vacuolization), cells with abnormal keratin staining (dyskeratosis), apoptotic keratinocytes, and disorganization of maturation of keratinocytes from the basal layer to the surface. (Courtesy of Dr. Scott Grantor, Department of Pathology, Brigham and Women's Hospital and Harvard Medical School, Boston.)

Chronic GVHD is characterized by fibrosis and atrophy of one or more of the same organs, without evidence of acute cell death. Chronic GVHD may also involve the lungs and produce obliteration of small airways. When it is severe, chronic GVHD leads to complete dysfunction of the affected organ.

In animal models, acute GVHD is initiated by mature T cells present in the bone marrow inoculum, and elimination of mature donor T cells from the graft can prevent the development of GVHD. Efforts to eliminate T cells from the marrow inoculum have reduced the incidence of GVHD but also reduce the efficiency of engraftment, probably because mature T cells produce colony-stimulating factors that aid in stem cell repopulation. A current approach is to combine removal of T cells with supplemental granulocyte-macrophage colony-stimulating factor treatment to promote engraftment. Elimination of T cells from the donor marrow also decreases the graft-versus-leukemia effect that is often critical in treating leukemias by bone marrow transplantation.

Although GVHD is initiated by grafted T cells recognizing host alloantigens, the effector cells that cause epithelial cell injury are less well defined. On histologic examination, NK cells are often attached to the dying epithelial cells, suggesting that NK cells are important effector cells of acute GVHD. $CD8^+$ CTLs and cytokines also appear to be involved in tissue injury in acute GVHD.

The relationship of chronic GVHD to acute GVHD is not known and raises issues similar to those of relating chronic allograft rejection to acute allograft rejection. For example, chronic GVHD may represent the fibrosis of wound healing secondary to loss of epithelial cells. However, chronic GVHD can arise without evidence of prior acute GVHD. An alternative explanation is that chronic GVHD represents a response to ischemia caused by vascular injury.

Both acute and chronic GVHD are commonly treated with intense immunosuppression. It is not clear that either condition responds very well. A possible explanation for this therapeutic failure is that conventional immunosuppression is targeted against T lymphocytes, especially CTLs, but is less effective in controlling NK cell–mediated responses. Agents that suppress cytokine production, such as the drug thalidomide, or that antagonize cytokine action have been used for treating GVHD in clinical trials. Much effort has focused on prevention of GVHD, and HLA typing is important in this regard. Cyclosporine and the metabolic toxin methotrexate are also used for prophylaxis against GVHD.

Immunodeficiency after Bone Marrow Transplantation

Bone marrow transplantation is often accompanied by clinical immunodeficiency. Several factors may contribute to defective immune responses in recipients. Bone marrow transplant recipients may be unable to regenerate a complete new lymphocyte repertoire. Radiation and chemotherapy used to prepare recipients for transplantation are likely to deplete the patient's memory cells and long-lived plasma cells, and it can take a long time to regenerate these populations.

The consequence of immunodeficiency is that bone marrow transplant recipients are susceptible to viral infections, especially cytomegalovirus infection, and to many bacterial infections. They are also susceptible to Epstein-Barr virus–provoked B cell lymphomas. The immunodeficiencies of bone marrow transplant recipients can be more severe than those of conventionally immunosuppressed patients. Therefore, bone marrow transplant recipients commonly receive prophylactic antibiotics and anticytomegalovirus therapy and are often actively immunized against capsular bacteria such as *Pneumococcus* prior to transplantation.

SUMMARY

- Transplantation of tissues from one individual to a genetically nonidentical recipient leads to a specific immune response called rejection that can destroy the graft. The major molecular targets in transplant rejection are allogeneic class I and class II MHC molecules.

- Many different, normally present T cell clones specific for different foreign peptides plus self MHC molecules may cross-react with an individual allogeneic MHC molecule. This high frequency of T cells capable of directly recognizing allogeneic MHC molecules explains why the response to alloantigens is much stronger than the response to conventional foreign antigens.

- Allogeneic MHC molecules may be presented on donor APCs to recipient T cells (the direct pathway), or the alloantigens may be picked up by host APCs that enter the graft or reside in draining lymphoid organs and be processed and presented to T cells as peptides associated with self MHC molecules (the indirect pathway).

- Graft rejection is mediated by T cells, including CTLs that kill graft cells and helper T cells that cause DTH reactions, and by antibodies.

- Several effector mechanisms cause rejection of solid organ grafts, and each mechanism may lead to a histologically characteristic reaction. Preexisting antibodies cause hyperacute rejection characterized by thrombosis of graft vessels. Alloreactive T cells and antibodies produced in response to the graft cause blood vessel wall damage and parenchymal cell death, called acute rejection. Chronic rejection is characterized by fibrosis and vascular abnormalities (accelerated arteriosclerosis), which may represent a chronic DTH reaction in the walls of arteries.

- Rejection may be prevented or treated by immunosuppression of the host and by minimizing the immunogenicity of the graft (by limiting MHC allelic differences). Most immunosuppression is directed at T cell responses and entails the use of cytotoxic drugs, specific immunosuppressive agents, or anti-T cell antibodies. The most widely used immunosuppressive agent is cyclosporine, which blocks T cell cytokine synthesis. Immunosuppression is often combined with anti-inflammatory drugs such as corticosteroids that inhibit cytokine synthesis by macrophages.

- Patients receiving solid organ transplants may become immunodeficient because of their therapy and are susceptible to viral infections and virus-related malignant tumors.

- Xenogeneic transplantation of solid organs is limited by the presence of natural antibodies to carbohydrate antigens on the cells of discordant species that cause hyperacute rejection, antibody-mediated acute vascular rejection, and a strong T cell–mediated immune response to xenogeneic MHC molecules.

- Bone marrow transplants are susceptible to rejection, and recipients require intense preparatory immunosuppression. In addition, T lymphocytes in the bone marrow graft may respond to alloantigens of the host and cause GVHD. Acute GVHD is characterized by epithelial cell death in the skin, intestinal tract, and liver; it may be fatal. Chronic GVHD is characterized by fibrosis and atrophy of one or more of these same target organs as well as the lungs and may also be fatal. Bone marrow transplant recipients also often develop severe immunodeficiency, rendering them susceptible to infections.

Selected Readings

Akl A, S Luo, and KJ Wood. Induction of transplantation tolerance—the potential of regulatory T cells. Transplantation Immunology 14:225–230, 2005.

Brinkman V, JG Cyster, and T Hla. FTY720: sphingosine 1-phosphate receptor-1 in the control of lymphocyte egress and endothelial barrier function. American Journal of Transplantation 4:1019–1025, 2004.

Cascalho M, and JL Platt. Xenotransplantation and other means of organ replacement. Nature Reviews Immunology 1:154–160, 2001.

Chidgey AP, D Layton, A Trounson, and RL Boyd. Tolerance strategies for stem-cell-based therapies. Nature 453:330–377, 2008.

Clarkson MR, and MH Sayegh. T-cell costimulatory pathways in allograft rejection and tolerance. Transplantation 80:555–563, 2005.

Cobbold SP. Regulatory T cells and transplantation tolerance. Journal of Nephrology 21:485–496, 2008.

Colvin RB, and RN Smith. Antibody-mediated organ-allograft rejection. Nature Review Immunology 5:807–817, 2005.

Cornell LD, RN Smith, and RB Colvin. Kidney transplantation: mechanisms of rejection and acceptance. Annual Review of Pathology 3:189–220, 2008.

Erlebacher A. Why isn't the fetus rejected? Current Opinion in Immunology 13:590–593, 2001.

Felix NJ, and PM Allen. Specificity of T-cell alloreactivity. Nature Reviews Immunology 7:942–953, 2007.

Gibbons C, and M Sykes. Manipulating the immune system for anti-tumor responses and transplant tolerance via mixed hematopoietic chimerism. Immunological Reviews 223:334–360, 2008.

Halloran PF. Immunosuppressive drugs for kidney transplantation. New England Journal of Medicine 351:2715–2729, 2004.

Heeger PS. T-cell allorecognition and transplant rejection: a summary and update. American Journal of Transplantation 3:525–533, 2003.

Jiang, S, O Herrera, and RI Lechler. New spectrum of allorecognition pathways: implications for graft rejection and transplantation tolerance. Current Opinions in Immunology 16:550–557, 2004.

LaRosa DF, AH Rahman, and LA Turka. The innate immune system in allograft rejection and tolerance. Journal of Immunology 178:7503–7509, 2007.

Lechler RI, M Sykes, AW Thomson, and LA Turka. Organ transplantation—how much of the promise has been realized? Nature Medicine 11:605–613, 2005.

Newell KA, CP Larsen, and AD Kirk. Transplant tolerance: converging on a moving target. Transplantation 81:1–6, 2006.

Pascual M, T Theruvath, T Kawai, N Tolkoff-Rubin, and AB Cosimi. Strategies to improve long-term outcomes after renal transplantation. New England Journal of Medicine 346:580–590, 2002.

Ricordi C, and TB Strom. Clinical islet transplantation: advances and immunological challenges. Nature Reviews Immunology 4:259–268, 2004.

Trowsdale J, and AG Betz. Mother's little helpers: mechanisms of maternal-fetal tolerance. Nature Immunology 7:241–246, 2006.

Wood KJ, and S Sakaguchi. Regulatory T cells in transplantation tolerance. Nature Reviews Immunology 3:199–210, 2003.

Yamada A, AD Salama, and MH Sayegh. The role of novel costimulatory pathways in autoimmunity and transplantation. Journal of the American Society of Nephrology 13:559–575, 2002.

Yang YG, M Sykes. Xenotransplantation: current status and a perspective on the future. Nature Reviews Immunology 7:519–531, 2007.

Chapter 17

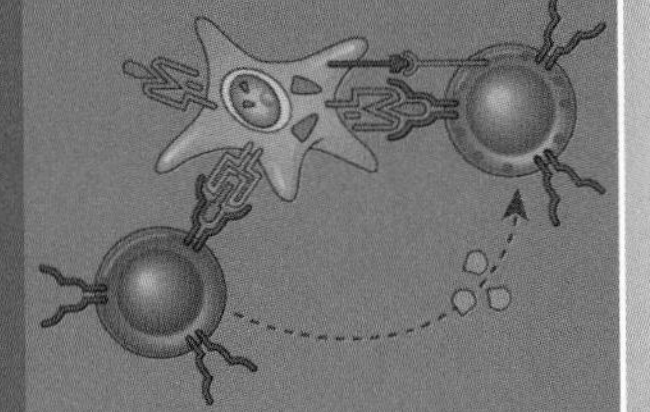

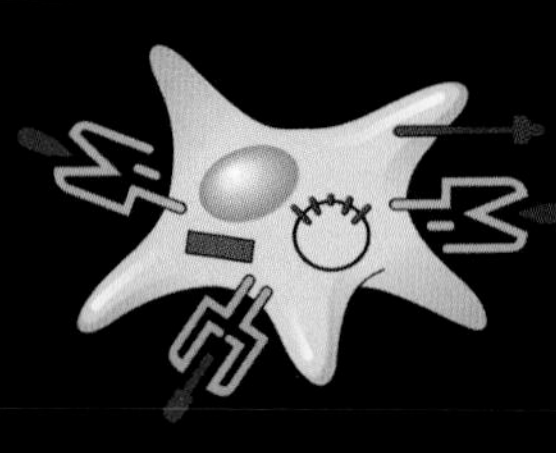

IMMUNITY TO TUMORS

Cancer is a major health problem worldwide and one of the most important causes of morbidity and mortality in children and adults. Cancers arise from the uncontrolled proliferation and spread of clones of transformed cells. The growth of malignant tumors is determined in large part by the proliferative capacity of the tumor cells and by the ability of these cells to invade host tissues and metastasize to distant sites. The possibility that cancers can be eradicated by specific immune responses has been the impetus for a large body of work in the field of tumor immunology. The concept of **immune surveillance,** which was proposed by Macfarlane Burnet in the 1950s, states that a physiologic function of the immune system is to recognize and destroy clones of transformed cells before they grow into tumors and to kill tumors after they are formed. The existence of immune surveillance has been demonstrated by the increased incidence of some types of tumors in immunocompromised experimental animals and humans. Although the overall importance of immune surveillance has been controversial, it is now clear that the immune system does react against many tumors, and exploiting these reactions to specifically destroy tumors remains an important goal of tumor immunologists. In addition, one of the factors in the growth of malignant tumors is the ability of these cancers to evade or overcome the mechanisms of host defense. In this chapter, we describe the types of antigens that are expressed by malignant tumors, how the immune system recognizes and responds to these antigens, and the application of immunologic approaches to the treatment of cancer.

GENERAL FEATURES OF TUMOR IMMUNITY

Several characteristics of tumor antigens and immune responses to tumors are fundamental to understanding tumor immunity and developing strategies for cancer immunotherapy.

- ***Tumors express antigens that are recognized as foreign by the immune system of the tumor-bearing host.*** Clinical observations and animal experiments have established that although tumor cells are derived from host cells, the tumors elicit immune responses.
  - Histopathologic studies show that many tumors are surrounded by mononuclear cell infiltrates composed of T lymphocytes, natural killer (NK) cells, and macrophages, and activated lymphocytes and macrophages are present in lymph nodes draining the sites of tumor growth. The presence of lymphocytic infiltrates in some types of melanoma and breast cancer is predictive of a better prognosis.

- The first experimental demonstration that tumors can induce protective immune responses came from studies of transplanted tumors performed in the 1950s (Fig. 17–1). A sarcoma may be induced in an inbred mouse by painting its skin with the chemical carcinogen methylcholanthrene (MCA). If the MCA-induced tumor is excised and transplanted into other syngeneic mice, the tumor grows. In contrast, if the tumor is transplanted back into the original host, the mouse rejects the tumor. The same mouse that had become immune to its tumor is incapable of rejecting MCA-induced tumors produced in other mice. Furthermore, T cells from the tumor-bearing animal can transfer protective immunity to the tumor to another tumor-free animal. Thus, immune responses to tumors exhibit the defining characteristics of adaptive immunity, namely, specificity and memory, and are mediated by lymphocytes.

The immunogenicity of tumors implies that tumor cells express antigens that are recognized as foreign by the adaptive immune system. As predicted from the transplantation experiments, defense against tumors is mediated mainly by T lymphocytes.

- ***Immune responses frequently fail to prevent the growth of tumors.*** There may be several reasons that anti-tumor immunity is unable to eradicate transformed cells. First, tumor cells are derived from host cells and therefore resemble normal cells in many respects. In other words, most tumors express only a few antigens that may be recognized as nonself, and as a result, most tumors tend to be weakly immunogenic. Tumors that elicit strong immune responses include those induced by oncogenic viruses, in which the viral proteins are foreign antigens, and tumors induced in animals by potent carcinogens, which often cause mutations in normal cellular genes. Many spontaneous tumors induce weak or even undetectable immunity, and studies of such tumors led to considerable skepticism about the concept of immune surveillance. In fact, the importance of immune surveillance and tumor immunity is likely to vary with the type of tumor. Second, the rapid growth and spread of tumors may overwhelm the capacity of the immune system to eradicate tumor cells, and control of a tumor requires that all the malignant cells be eliminated. Third, many tumors have specialized mechanisms for evading host

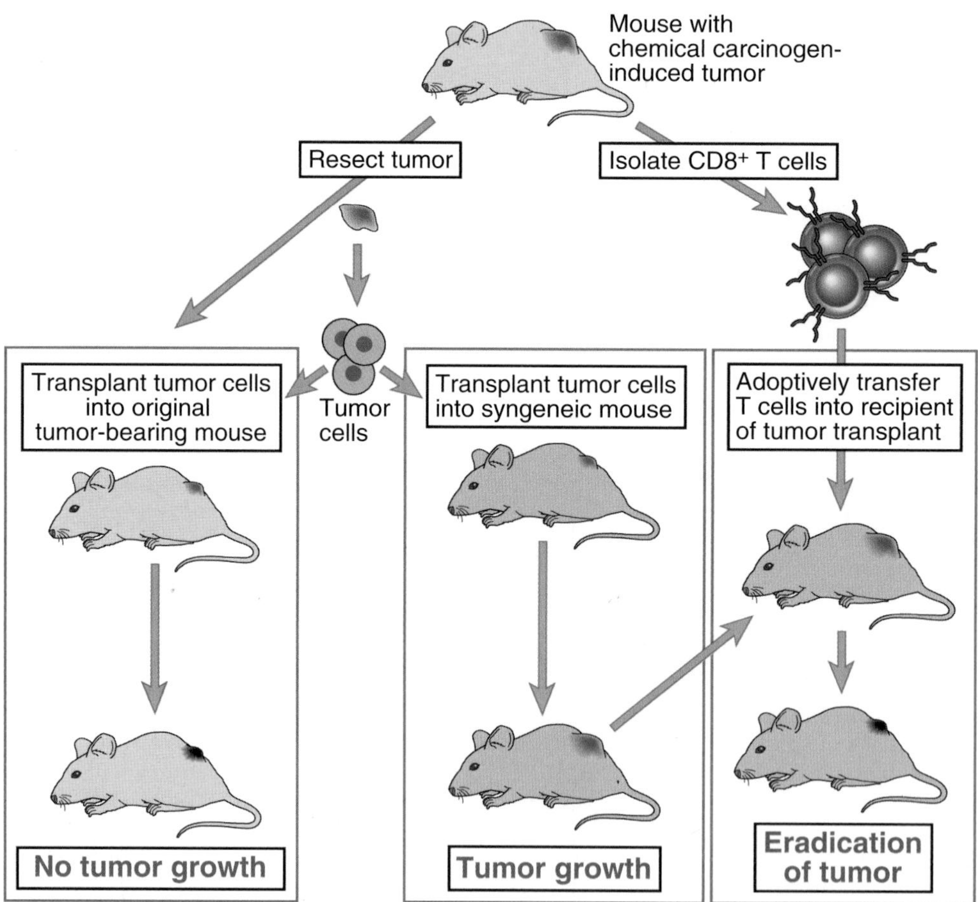

FIGURE 17–1 Experimental demonstration of tumor immunity. Mice that have been surgically cured of a chemical carcinogen (MCA)-induced tumor reject subsequent transplants of the same tumor, whereas the transplanted tumor grows in normal syngeneic mice. The tumor is also rejected in normal mice that are given adoptive transfer of T lymphocytes from the original tumor-bearing animal.

immune responses. We will return to these mechanisms later in the chapter.

- ***The immune system can be activated by external stimuli to effectively kill tumor cells and eradicate tumors.*** As we shall see at the end of the chapter, this realization has spurred new directions in tumor immunotherapy in which augmentation of the host anti-tumor response is the goal of treatment.

TUMOR ANTIGENS

A variety of tumor antigens that may be recognized by T and B lymphocytes have been identified in human and animal cancers. In the experimental situation, as in MCA-induced mouse sarcomas, it is often possible to demonstrate that these antigens elicit adaptive immune responses and are the targets of such responses. Tumor antigens have also been identified in humans, but the methods used in this case are generally not suitable for proving that these antigens can elicit protective immunity to tumors. Nevertheless, it is important to identify tumor antigens in humans because they may be used as components of tumor vaccines, and antibodies and effector T cells generated against these antigens may be used for immunotherapy.

The earliest classification of tumor antigens was based on their patterns of expression. Antigens that are expressed on tumor cells but not on normal cells are called tumor-specific antigens; some of these antigens are unique to individual tumors, whereas others are shared among tumors of the same type. Tumor antigens that are also expressed on normal cells are called tumor-associated antigens; in most cases, these antigens are normal cellular constituents whose expression is aberrant or dysregulated in tumors. The modern classification of tumor antigens relies on the molecular structure and source of the antigens, which is how we will discuss tumor antigens.

The existence of tumor antigens was first established by transplantation experiments in animals, as described earlier. The initial attempts to purify and characterize these antigens were based on producing monoclonal antibodies specific for tumor cells and defining the antigens that these antibodies recognized. The antibodies were made by immunizing mice with tumors from other species, and most of the anti-tumor antibodies recognized antigens that are shared by different tumors arising from the same types of cells and that are also found on some normal cells and benign tumor cells. A more recently developed approach for identification of tumor antigens specifically recognized by antibodies in the serum of cancer patients is called serologic analysis of recombinant complementary DNA expression (SEREX). In this method, expression libraries of complementary DNA (cDNA) derived from a patient's tumor RNA are screened using the cancer patient's serum immunoglobulins. In this way, gene sequences are obtained, and predicted protein products are identified.

Anti-tumor antibodies do not recognize the major histocompatibility complex (MHC)-associated peptides that are the antigens seen by T cells. Tumor antigens that are recognized by T cells are likely to be the major inducers of tumor immunity and the most promising candidates for tumor vaccines. An important breakthrough in tumor immunology was the development of techniques for identifying antigens that are recognized by tumor-specific T lymphocytes (Box 17–1). Much of our knowledge of these antigens is limited to antigens recognized by $CD8^+$ cytotoxic T lymphocytes (CTLs), and only recently have attempts been made to identify antigens that are recognized by $CD4^+$ helper cells. Tumor antigens that are recognized by $CD8^+$ T cells are peptides derived from proteins processed in the cytosol and displayed on the tumor cell surface bound to class I MHC molecules (see Chapter 5). In the following section, we describe the main classes of tumor antigens (Fig. 17–2 and Table 17–1) and use selected examples of human and animal tumors to illustrate the importance of these antigens in tumor immunity and their potential as therapeutic targets.

Products of Mutated Genes

Some tumor antigens are produced by oncogenic mutants of normal cellular genes. Many tumors express genes whose products are required for malignant transformation or for maintenance of the malignant phenotype. Often, these genes are produced by point mutations, deletions, chromosomal translocations, or viral gene insertions affecting cellular proto-oncogenes or tumor suppressor genes. The products of these altered proto-oncogenes and tumor suppressor genes are synthesized in the cytoplasm of the tumor cells, and like any cytosolic protein, they may enter the class I antigen-processing pathway. In addition, these proteins may enter the class II antigen-processing pathway in antigen-presenting cells (APCs) that have phagocytosed dead tumor cells. Because these altered genes are not present in normal cells, peptides derived from them do not induce self-tolerance and may stimulate T cell responses in the host. Some patients with cancer have circulating $CD4^+$ and $CD8^+$ T cells that can respond to the products of mutated oncogenes such as Ras and Bcr-Abl proteins and mutated tumor supressor genes such as *p53*. Furthermore, in animals, immunization with mutated Ras or p53 proteins induces CTLs and rejection responses against tumors expressing these mutants. However, these proteins do not appear to be major targets of tumor-specific CTLs in most patients with a variety of tumors.

Tumor antigens may be produced by randomly mutated genes whose products are not related to the transformed phenotype. Tumor antigens that were defined by the transplantation of carcinogen-induced tumors in animals, called tumor-specific transplantation antigens (TSTAs), are mutants of various host cellular proteins. Studies with chemically induced rodent sarcomas, such as those illustrated in Figure 17–1, established that different rodent tumors, all induced by the

Box 17–1 ■ IN DEPTH: IDENTIFICATION OF TUMOR ANTIGENS RECOGNIZED BY T LYMPHOCYTES

Tumor antigens recognized by T cells have been identified by two main approaches: transplantation of tumors in rodents and the identification of peptides recognized by tumor-specific CTLs or identification of the genes encoding these peptides.

TUMOR TRANSPLANTATION. Studies of transplanted tumors in rodents were the first experiments to indicate the existence of tumor antigens recognized by T cells. Initial studies of this type used chemically induced rodent sarcomas (see Fig. 17–1 and the text), and they demonstrated the existence of tumor-specific transplantation antigens (TSTAs) that elicited highly specific immune responses. Another, more recent approach to characterize antigens that stimulate tumor rejection by CTLs relies on the *in vitro* mutagenesis of an established tumorigenic

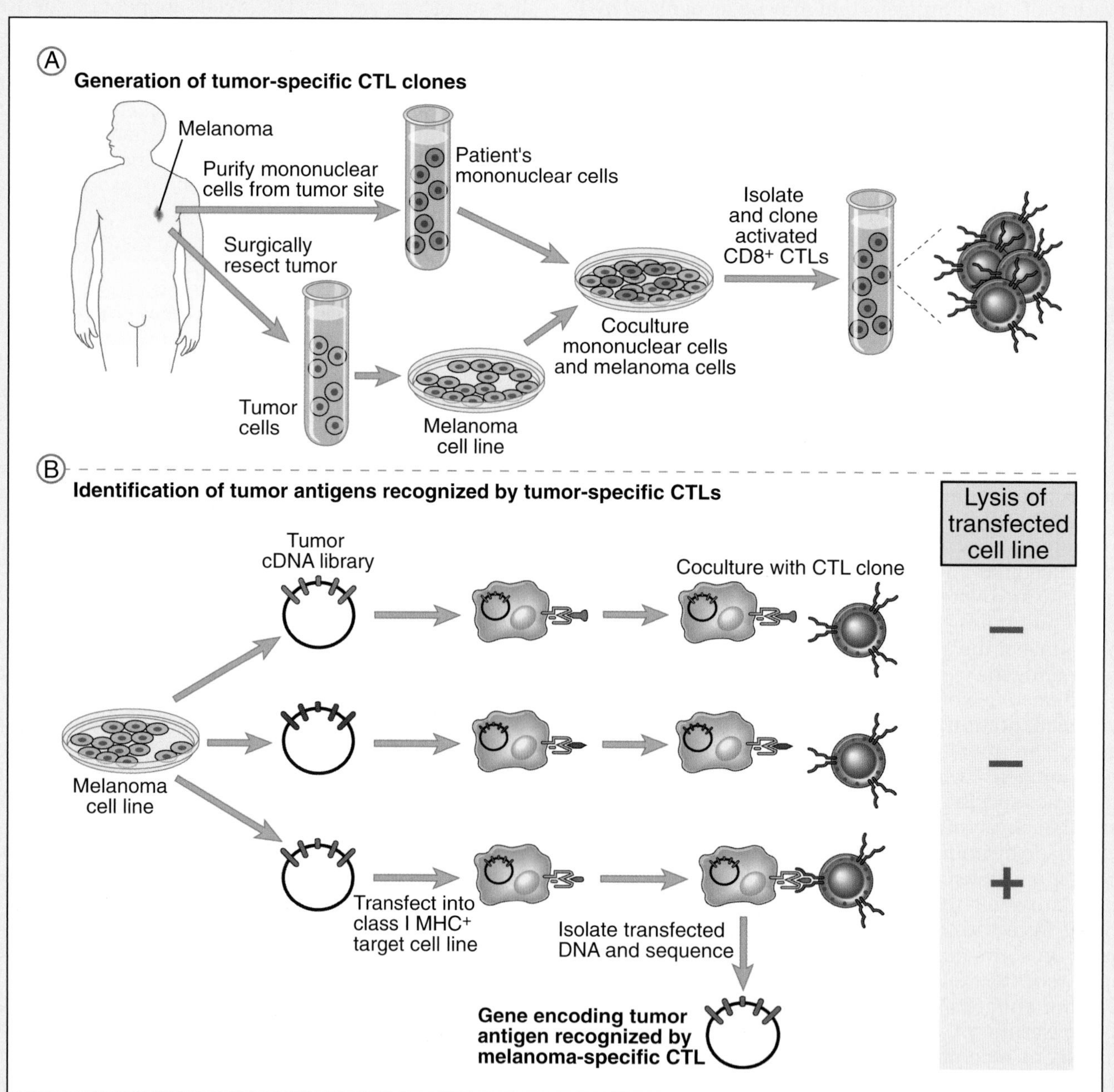

Cloned CTL lines specific for human tumors are used to identify specific tumor antigens. A. $CD8^+$ T cells isolated from blood, lymph nodes, or tumors of patients with melanoma are propagated in culture by stimulating them with melanoma cell lines derived from the patient's tumor. Single T cells from these cultures are expanded into clonal CTL lines. B. DNA from melanoma gene libraries is transfected into class I MHC-expressing target cells. Genes that sensitize the target cells for lysis by the melanoma-specific CTL clones are analyzed to identify the melanoma protein antigens recognized by the patient's CTLs.

Continued on following page

mouse cell line and isolation of nontumorigenic variants that are rejected on transplantation into syngeneic mice. In this system, the tumorigenic cell line does not express TSTAs and therefore grows unchecked when it is injected into a host animal, but the mutagenized cell line does express mutant protein antigens that induce its rejection. The role of CTLs in the rejection process in this model has been established by adoptive transfer experiments and by the propagation of CTL clones that recognize the tumor, as discussed below. The actual genes encoding the rejection antigens in a few of these tumor variants have been cloned, by methods described below.

GENERATION OF TUMOR-SPECIFIC CTL CLONES. The establishment of cloned CTL lines that recognize tumor antigens has been a key advance in the identification of tumor antigens because such clones provide sensitive probes for identifying tumor antigens that are likely to be important targets of host anti-tumor immune responses. This approach is particularly valuable for human tumors, whose immunogenicity cannot easily be studied by transplantation in animals. Many cloned CTL lines specific for human tumors, particularly melanomas, have been generated from the T cells of patients. Melanomas, which are malignant tumors of melanocytes, are often readily accessible, surgically resectable tumors that may be grown in tissue culture. CTLs specific for these tumors may be propagated and subsequently cloned by culturing T cells from a melanoma patient with cells derived from the patient's melanoma. The T cells can be isolated from peripheral blood, lymph nodes draining the tumor, or cells that have actually infiltrated the tumor *in vivo*. Because the T cells and the tumor are from the same individual, the MHC restriction of the T cells matches the MHC alleles expressed by the tumor. In these cocultures, CTLs that recognize peptide antigens displayed by the tumor cells are stimulated to grow, and single-cell clones are propagated in IL-2 by limiting dilution techniques (see Figure).

IDENTIFICATION OF TUMOR ANTIGENS RECOGNIZED BY T CELLS. Identification of the peptide antigens that induce CTL responses in patients with tumors and identification of the genes encoding the proteins from which the peptides are derived have relied on cloned tumor-specific CTL lines. These tumor antigens have been identified by two methods. First, a direct biochemical approach is used in which peptides bound to tumor cell class I MHC molecules are eluted by acid treatment and fractionated by reverse-phase high-performance liquid chromatography (HPLC). The fractions are tested for their ability to sensitize MHC-matched nontumor target cells for lysis by a tumor-specific CTL clone. This strategy relies on having a target cell that expresses the class I MHC molecules for which the CTL clone is specific but does not normally express the tumor antigen, and on the ability to load these cell surface MHC molecules with the exogenous HPLC-purified peptides. Peptide fractions that do sensitize the target cells are then analyzed by mass spectroscopy to determine their amino acid sequences. Once the peptide sequence is known, it may be possible to compare it with databases of protein sequences to see whether it matches with any previously characterized protein and to determine whether any point mutations are present in the normal sequences.

The second method of identifying tumor antigens is molecular cloning of the genes encoding these antigens (see Figure). This method relies on preparing a cDNA library from a tumor cell line that contains genes encoding all the tumor proteins. The library is prepared in molecular constructs that will allow constitutive expression of the genes when they are introduced into cell lines. Pools of DNA from such a library are transfected into a cell line expressing a class I MHC allele also expressed by the tumor, and the transfected cells are tested for sensitivity to lysis by an anti-tumor CTL clone. The DNA pools that sensitize the target cell line contain the gene that encodes the protein antigen recognized by the CTL clone. Multiple rounds of transfections using smaller and smaller subfractions of the DNA pool can lead to isolation of the single relevant gene. The sequence of the gene can then be determined, and comparisons can be made with known genes. Synthetic peptides corresponding to different regions of the encoded protein can be tested for their ability to sensitize target cells in much the same way as in the peptide elution approach. Both the biochemical and genetic approaches have been used successfully to identify human melanoma antigens that stimulate CTL responses in the patients with melanoma.

same carcinogen, expressed different transplantation antigens. For example, an MCA-induced sarcoma will induce protective immunity against itself but not against another MCA-induced sarcoma, even if both tumors are derived from the same normal cell type and in the same mouse. We now know that the tumor antigens identified by such experiments are peptides derived from mutated self proteins and presented in the form of peptide–class I MHC complexes capable of stimulating CTLs. These antigens are extremely diverse because the carcinogens that induce the tumors may randomly mutagenize virtually any host gene, and the class I MHC antigen-presenting pathway can display peptides from any mutated cytosolic protein in each tumor. Mutated cellular proteins are found more frequently in chemical carcinogen- or radiation-induced animal tumors than in spontaneous human cancers, probably because chemical carcinogens and radiation mutagenize many cellular genes. Nevertheless, TSTAs of experimental animal tumors are relevant to the study of human cancers in two ways. First, the finding of TSTAs was the first result to prove that adaptive immune responses may be able to control tumors. Second, the general principle that mutated host proteins can function as tumor antigens, which also came from studies of animal TSTAs, has been demonstrated in human cancers as well.

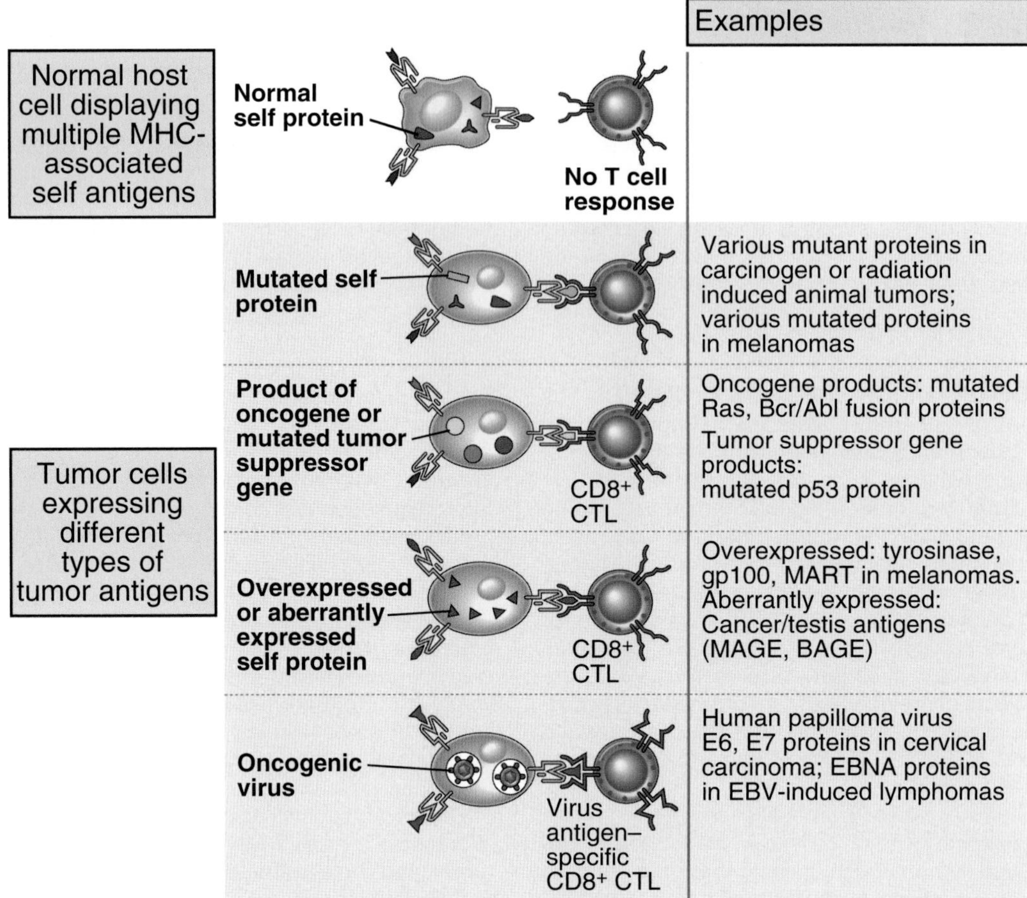

FIGURE 17–2 Types of tumor antigens recognized by T cells. Tumor antigens that are recognized by tumor-specific $CD8^+$ T cells may be mutated forms of normal self proteins, products of oncogenes, overexpressed or aberrantly expressed self proteins, or products of oncogenic viruses.

Abnormally Expressed Cellular Proteins

Tumor antigens may be normal cellular proteins that are abnormally expressed in tumor cells and elicit immune responses. Many such antigens have been identified in human tumors, such as melanomas, by the molecular cloning of antigens that are recognized by T cells from tumor-bearing patients (see Box 17–1). One of the surprises that emerged from these studies was that some tumor antigens are normal proteins that are produced at low levels in normal cells and overexpressed in tumor cells (see Table 17–1). One such antigen is tyrosinase, an enzyme involved in melanin biosynthesis that is expressed only in normal melanocytes and melanomas. Both class I MHC-restricted $CD8^+$ CTL clones and class II MHC-restricted $CD4^+$ T cell clones from melanoma patients recognize peptides derived from tyrosinase. On face value, it is surprising that these patients are able to respond to a normal self antigen. The likely explanation is that tyrosinase is normally produced in such small amounts and in so few cells that it is not recognized by the immune system and fails to induce tolerance. The finding of tyrosinase-specific T cell responses in patients raises the possibility that tyrosinase vaccines may stimulate such responses to melanomas; clinical trials with these vaccines are ongoing.

Cancer/testis antigens are proteins expressed in gametes and trophoblasts, and in many types of cancers, but not in normal somatic tissues. The first cancer/testis antigens were identified by cloning genes from human melanomas that encoded cellular protein antigens recognized by melanoma-specific CTL clones derived from the melanoma-bearing patients. These were called MAGE proteins, and they were subsequently found to be expressed in other tumors in addition to melanomas, including carcinomas of the bladder, breast, skin, lung, and prostate, and some sarcomas, as well as in normal testes. Subsequent to identification of the MAGE genes, several other unrelated gene families have been identified that encode melanoma antigens recognized by CTL clones derived from melanoma patients. Like the MAGE proteins, these other melanoma antigens are silent in most normal tissues, except the testes or trophoblasts in the placenta, but they are expressed in a variety of malignant tumors. There are now over 44 different

Table 17–1. Tumor Antigens

Type of antigen	Examples of human tumor antigens
Products of oncogenes, tumor suppressor genes	Oncogenes: Ras mutations (~10% of human carcinomas), p210 product of Bcr/Abl rearrangements (CML), overexpressed Her-2/neu (breast and other carcinomas)
	Tumor supressor genes: mutated p53 (present in ~50% of human tumors)
Mutants of cellular genes not involved in tumorigenesis	p91A mutation in mutagenized murine mastocytoma; various mutated proteins in melanomas recognized by CTLs
Products of genes that are silent in most normal tissues	Cancer/testis antigens expressed in melanomas and many carcinomas; normally expressed mainly in the testis and placenta
Products of overexpressed genes	Tyrosinase, gp100, MART in melanomas (normally expressed in melanocytes)
Products of oncogenic viruses	Papillomavirus E6 and E7 proteins (cervical carcinomas)
	EBNA-1 protein of EBV (EBV-associated lymphomas, nasopharyngeal carcinoma)
	SV40 T antigen (SV40-induced rodent tumors)
Oncofetal antigens	Carcinoembryonic antigen (CEA) on many tumors, also expressed in liver and other tissues during inflammation
	Alpha-fetoprotein (AFP)
Glycolipids and glycoproteins	GM_2, GD_2 on melanomas
Differentiation antigens normally present in tissue of origin	Prostate-specific antigen
	Markers of lymphocytes: CD10, CD20, Ig idiotypes on B cells

Abbreviations: CML, chronic myelogenous leukemia; CTL, cytotoxic T lymphocyte; EBNA, Epstein-Barr nuclear antigen; EBV, Epstein-Barr virus; Ig, immunoglobulin; MART, melanoma antigen recognized by T cells.

cancer/testis antigen families identified. About half are encoded by genes on the X-chromosome, while the rest are encoded by genes distributed throughout the genome. Although some cancer/testis antigens have been shown to regulate transcription or translation of other genes, the functions of most cancer/testis antigens are unknown. In general, they are not required for the malignant phenotype of the cells, and their sequences are identical to the corresponding genes in normal cells; that is, they are not mutated. Several X-linked cancer/testis antigens are currently being used in tumor vaccine trials.

Antigens of Oncogenic Viruses

The products of oncogenic viruses function as tumor antigens and elicit specific T cell responses that may serve to eradicate the tumors. DNA viruses are implicated in the development of a variety of tumors in humans and experimental animals. Examples in humans include the Epstein-Barr virus (EBV), which is associated with B cell lymphomas and nasopharyngeal carcinoma (Box 17–2), and human papillomavirus (HPV), which is associated with cervical carcinoma. Papovaviruses, including polyomavirus and simian virus 40 (SV40), and adenoviruses induce malignant tumors in neonatal or immunodeficient adult rodents. In most of these DNA virus–induced tumors, virus-encoded protein antigens are found in the nucleus, cytoplasm, or plasma membrane of the tumor cells. These endogenously synthesized proteins can be processed, and complexes of processed viral peptides with class I MHC molecules may be expressed on the tumor cell surface. Because the viral peptides are foreign antigens, DNA virus–induced tumors are among the most immunogenic tumors known.

The ability of adaptive immunity to prevent the growth of DNA virus–induced tumors has been established by many observations.

- EBV-associated lymphomas and HPV-associated skin and cervical cancers arise more frequently in immunosuppressed individuals, such as allograft recipients receiving immunosuppressive therapy and patients with acquired immunodeficiency syndrome (AIDS), than in normal individuals.

Box 17–2 ▪ IN DEPTH: THE RELATIONSHIPS BETWEEN EPSTEIN-BARR VIRUS, MALIGNANCY, AND IMMUNODEFICIENCY

EBV is a double-stranded DNA virus of the herpesvirus family. The virus is transmitted by saliva, infects nasopharyngeal epithelial cells and B lymphocytes, and is ubiquitous in human populations worldwide. It infects human B cells by binding specifically to complement receptor type 2 (CR2, or CD21), followed by receptor-mediated endocytosis and fusion of the viral envelope with the endosomal membrane. Two types of cellular infections can occur. In a lytic infection, viral DNA, RNA, and protein are synthesized, followed by assembly of viral particles and lysis of the infected cell. Alternatively, a latent nonlytic infection can occur in which the viral DNA is maintained as an episome in infected cells. Various virally encoded antigens are detectable in infected cells. At least six Epstein-Barr nuclear antigens (EBNAs) are expressed early in lytic infections and may also be expressed by some latently infected cells. Two other proteins, called latent membrane proteins (LMPs), are expressed on the surface of latently infected cells. Viral antigens are typically expressed in infected naive and recently activated B cells but not in memory B cells. Other viral structural protein antigens, including viral capsid antigens (VCAs), are expressed within infected cells and on released viral particles during lytic infections.

EBV has profound effects on B lymphocyte growth in vitro. The virus is a T cell–independent polyclonal activator of B cell proliferation. EBV immortalizes human B cells so that they proliferate in culture indefinitely. The resulting long-term B lymphoblastoid cell lines are latently infected with the virus, express EBNAs and LMPs, and have a malignant phenotype as demonstrated by transplantation into immunodeficient mice. Five EBNAs and LMP-1 have been shown to be critical for transforming B lymphocytes into immortal cells. The cytoplasmic tail of LMP-1 binds the physiologic signaling molecules called TRAFs, which normally transduce signals resulting from engagement of TNF receptors and the important B cell activation molecule CD40 (see Chapter 12, Box 12–1). By this mechanism, EBV appears to have co-opted a normal B cell activation pathway to promote proliferation of the cells that the virus infects and lives in.

The spectrum of clinical sequelae to EBV infection is wide. Most people are infected during childhood; they do not experience any symptoms, and viral replication is apparently controlled by humoral and T cell–mediated immune responses. In previously uninfected young adults, infectious mononucleosis typically develops after EBV infection. This disease is characterized by sore throat, fever, and generalized lymphadenopathy. Large morphologically atypical lymphocytes are abundant in the peripheral blood of patients with infectious mononucleosis. Most of these cells are CTLs; in fact, in acute infections, up to 10% of all the $CD8^+$ T cells in the blood may be EBV specific, and small numbers of these CTLs may persist for life. Previously infected, healthy individuals harbor the virus for the rest of their lives in latently infected B cells and often in nasopharyngeal epithelium. An estimated one of every million B cells in a previously infected individual is latently infected. Importantly, EBV infection is one of the etiologic factors for the development of certain malignant tumors, including nasopharyngeal carcinoma in Chinese populations, Burkitt's lymphoma in equatorial Africa, and B cell lymphomas in immunosuppressed patients.

The evidence is compelling that T cell–mediated immunity is required for control of EBV infections and, in particular, for killing of EBV-infected B cells. First, individuals with deficiencies in T cell–mediated immunity are susceptible to uncontrolled, widely disseminated, and lethal acute EBV infections. Second, EBV-infected B cells isolated from patients with infectious mononucleosis can be propagated in vitro indefinitely, but only if the patient's T cells are removed or inactivated by drugs such as cyclosporine. In fact, immortalization of normal peripheral blood B cells by in vitro infection with EBV is successful only if the donor's T cells are removed or inactivated. Third, CTLs specific for EBV-encoded antigens, including EBNAs and LMP, are present in patients suffering from acute infectious mononucleosis and recovered patients. Cloned CTL lines have been established in vitro that specifically lyse EBV-infected B cells, and these CTLs most often recognize peptide fragments of EBNA or LMP proteins in association with class I MHC molecules. EBV-specific T cells are required in vivo to limit the number of infected B cells, but latently infected B cells can be found in up to 90% of people worldwide. A loss of normal T cell–mediated immunity allows these infected B cells to progress toward malignant transformation. Infusion of EBV-specific CTLs restores the normal balance and provides protection against the growth of malignant B cell tumors.

The epidemiology and molecular genetics of Burkitt's lymphoma and other EBV-associated lymphomas have been the subject of intense investigation, and they offer fascinating insight into various aspects of viral oncogenesis and tumor immunity. Burkitt's lymphoma is a histologic type of malignant B cell tumor composed of monotonous small malignant B cells. The African form of the disease is endemic in regions where both EBV and malaria infection are common. In these regions, the tumor occurs frequently in young children, often beginning in the jaw. Virtually 100% of patients with African Burkitt's lymphoma have evidence of previous EBV infection, and their tumors usually carry the EBV genome and express EBV-encoded antigens. Malarial infections in this population are known to cause T cell immunodeficiencies, and this association may be the link between EBV infection and the development of lymphoma. Sporadic Burkitt's lymphoma occurs less frequently in other parts of the world, and although these B cell tumors are histologically similar to the endemic form, only about 20% carry the EBV genome. Both endemic and sporadic Burkitt's lymphoma cells have reciprocal chromosomal translocations involving Ig gene loci and the cellular *MYC* gene on chromosome 8.

Continued on following page

B cell lymphomas occur at a high frequency in T cell–immunodeficient individuals, including individuals with congenital immunodeficiencies, patients with AIDS, and kidney or heart allograft recipients receiving immunosuppressive drugs. Only some of these tumors can be called Burkitt's lymphomas on the basis of histology. Regardless of their histologic appearance, many of these tumors are latently infected with EBV, like Burkitt's lymphoma. A smaller subset also contains *MYC* translocations to Ig loci.

These observations can be synthesized into a hypothesis about the pathogenesis of EBV-associated B cell tumors. African children with malaria, allograft recipients, congenitally immunodeficient children, and AIDS patients all have abnormalities in T cell function. Because of a deficiency of EBV-specific T cells, EBV-induced polyclonal proliferation of B cells is uncontrolled. This exuberant proliferation of B cells increases the chances of errors made during DNA replication, including translocations of oncogenes. The Ig loci are accessible sites for translocations compared with other loci in B cells. Translocation of the *MYC* gene to the Ig locus leads to transcriptional deregulation and abnormal expression of MYC, and this alteration appears to be causally related to malignant transformation and outgrowth of a neoplastic clone of cells. Many EBV-positive tumors in immunosuppressed patients do not have *MYC* translocations, and the proteins encoded by the integrated EBV genome may be sufficient to cause lymphomas. This proposed scheme predicts that early in their course, EBV-associated B cell tumors may be polyclonal because they arise from a polyclonally stimulated population of normal B cells. Later, one or a few clones may obtain selective growth advantages, perhaps because of deregulation of *MYC* or other cellular or viral genes. As a result, the polyclonal proliferation evolves into a monoclonal or oligoclonal tumor. In fact, such has been shown to be the case by Southern blot analysis of Ig gene rearrangements in some EBV-positive B cell tumors from immunosuppressed patients.

- Adenovirus infection induces tumors much more frequently in neonatal or T cell–deficient mice than in normal adult mice.
- Tumor transplantation experiments of the kind illustrated in Figure 17–1 have shown that animals may be specifically immunized against DNA virus–induced tumors and will reject transplants of these tumors. Unlike MCA-induced tumor antigens, which are the products of randomly mutated cellular genes, virus-encoded tumor antigens are not unique for each tumor but are shared by all tumors induced by the same type of virus.
- Immunization of experimental animals with SV40 virus and adenovirus produces protective immunity against the development of tumors induced by each virus, and immunity is mediated by class I MHC-restricted CTLs specific for the antigens of that virus.
- Immunization of women with human papillomavirus (HPV) coat proteins prevents the development of precancerous lesions in the uterine cervix.

Thus, a competent immune system may play a role in surveillance against virus-induced tumors because of its ability to recognize and kill virus-infected cells. In fact, the concept of immune surveillance against tumors is better established for DNA virus–induced tumors than for any other type of tumor.

RNA tumor viruses (retroviruses) are important causes of tumors in animals. Retroviral oncogene products theoretically have the same potential antigenic properties as mutated cellular oncogenes, and humoral and cell-mediated immune responses to retroviral gene products on tumor cells can be observed experimentally. The only well-defined human retrovirus that is known to cause tumors is human T cell lymphotropic virus 1 (HTLV-1), the etiologic agent for adult T cell leukemia/lymphoma (ATL), a malignant tumor of $CD4^+$ T cells. Although immune responses specific for HTLV-1–encoded antigens have been demonstrated in individuals infected with the virus, it is not clear whether they play any role in protective immunity against the development of tumors. Furthermore, patients with ATL are often profoundly immunosuppressed, probably because the virus infects $CD4^+$ T cells and induces functional abnormalities in these cells.

Oncofetal Antigens

Oncofetal antigens are proteins that are expressed at high levels in cancer cells and in normal developing fetal but not adult tissues. It is believed that the genes encoding these proteins are silenced during development and are derepressed with malignant transformation. Oncofetal antigens are identified with antibodies raised in other species, and their main importance is that they provide markers that aid in tumor diagnosis. As techniques for detecting these antigens have improved, it has become clear that their expression in adults is not limited to tumors. The proteins are increased in tissues and in the circulation in various inflammatory conditions and are found in small quantities even in normal tissues. There is no evidence that oncofetal antigens are important inducers or targets of anti-tumor immunity. The two most thoroughly characterized oncofetal antigens are carcinoembryonic antigen (CEA) and α-fetoprotein (AFP).

CEA (CD66) is a highly glycosylated integral membrane protein that is a member of the immunoglobulin (Ig) superfamily. It is an intercellular adhesion molecule that functions to promote the binding of tumor cells to one another. High CEA expression is normally restricted to cells in the gut, pancreas, and liver during the first two trimesters of gestation, and low expression is seen in normal adult colonic mucosa and the lactating breast. CEA expression is increased in many carcinomas of the colon, pancreas, stomach, and breast, and serum levels are increased in these patients. The level of serum CEA is used to monitor the persistence or recurrence of the tumors after treatment. The usefulness of CEA as a diagnostic marker for cancer is limited by the fact that serum CEA can also be elevated in the setting of non-neoplastic diseases, such as chronic inflammatory conditions of the bowel or liver.

AFP is a circulating glycoprotein normally synthesized and secreted in fetal life by the yolk sac and liver. Fetal serum concentrations can be as high as 2 to 3 mg/mL, but in adult life, the protein is replaced by albumin, and only low levels are present in serum. Serum levels of AFP can be significantly elevated in patients with hepatocellular carcinoma, germ cell tumors, and, occasionally, gastric and pancreatic cancers. An elevated serum AFP level is a useful indicator of advanced liver or germ cell tumors or of recurrence of these tumors after treatment. Furthermore, the detection of AFP in tissue sections by immunohistochemical techniques can help in the pathologic identification of tumor cells. The diagnostic value of AFP as a tumor marker is limited by the fact that elevated serum levels are also found in non-neoplastic diseases, such as cirrhosis of the liver.

Altered Glycolipid and Glycoprotein Antigens

Most human and experimental tumors express higher than normal levels or abnormal forms of surface glycoproteins and glycolipids, which may be diagnostic markers and targets for therapy. These altered molecules include gangliosides, blood group antigens, and mucins. Some aspects of the malignant phenotype of tumors, including tissue invasion and metastatic behavior, may reflect altered cell surface properties that result from abnormal glycolipid and glycoprotein synthesis. Many antibodies have been raised in animals that recognize the carbohydrate groups or peptide cores of these molecules. Although most of the epitopes recognized by these antibodies are not specifically expressed on tumors, they are present at higher levels on cancer cells than on normal cells. This class of tumor-associated antigen is a target for cancer therapy with specific antibodies.

Among the glycolipids expressed at high levels in melanomas are the gangliosides GM_2, GD_2, and GD_3. Clinical trials of anti-GM_2 and anti-GD_3 antibodies and immunization with vaccines containing GM_2 are under way in patients with melanoma. Mucins are high molecular weight glycoproteins containing numerous O-linked carbohydrate side chains on a core polypeptide. Tumors often have dysregulated expression of the enzymes that synthesize these carbohydrate side chains, which leads to the appearance of tumor-specific epitopes on the carbohydrate side chains or on the abnormally exposed polypeptide core. Several mucins have been the focus of diagnostic and therapeutic studies, including CA-125 and CA-19-9, expressed on ovarian carcinomas, and MUC-1, expressed on breast carcinomas. Unlike many mucins, MUC-1 is an integral membrane protein that is normally expressed only on the apical surface of breast ductal epithelium, a site that is relatively sequestered from the immune system. In ductal carcinomas of the breast, however, the molecule is expressed in an unpolarized fashion and contains new, tumor-specific carbohydrate and peptide epitopes detectable by mouse monoclonal antibodies. The peptide epitopes induce both antibody and T cell responses in cancer patients and are therefore being considered as candidates for tumor vaccines.

Tissue-Specific Differentiation Antigens

Tumors express molecules that are normally present on the cells of origin. These antigens are called differentiation antigens because they are specific for particular lineages or differentiation stages of various cell types. Their importance is as potential targets for immunotherapy and for identifying the tissue of origin of tumors. For example, several melanoma antigens that are targets of CTLs in patients are melanocyte differentiation antigens, such as tyrosinase, mentioned earlier. Lymphomas may be diagnosed as B cell–derived tumors by the detection of surface markers characteristic of this lineage, such as CD10 (previously called common acute lymphoblastic leukemia antigen, or CALLA) and CD20. Antibodies against these molecules are also used for tumor immunotherapy. The idiotypic determinants of the surface Ig of a clonal B cell population are markers for that B cell clone because all other B cells express different idiotypes. Therefore, the Ig idiotype is a highly specific tumor antigen for B cell lymphomas and leukemias. These differentiation antigens are normal self molecules, and therefore they do not usually induce strong immune responses in tumor-bearing hosts.

Immune Responses to Tumors

The effector mechanisms of both innate and adaptive immunity have been shown to kill tumor cells in vitro. The challenge for tumor immunologists is to determine which of these mechanisms may contribute to protective immune responses against tumors in vivo, and to enhance these effector mechanisms in ways that are tumor specific. In this section, we review the evidence for tumor killing by various immune effector mechanisms and discuss which are the most likely to be relevant to human tumors.

Innate Immune Responses to Tumors

Much of the early research on functions of effector cells of the innate immune system, including NK cells and macrophages, focused on the ability of these cells to kill cultured tumor cells.

NK Cells

NK cells kill many types of tumor cells, especially cells that have reduced class I MHC expression but do express ligands for NK cell activating receptors. In vitro, NK cells can kill virally infected cells and certain tumor cell lines, especially hematopoietic tumors. NK cells also respond to the absence of class I MHC molecules because the recognition of class I MHC molecules delivers inhibitory signals to NK cells (see Chapter 2, Fig. 2–10). As we shall see later, some tumors lose expression of class I MHC molecules, perhaps as a result of selection against class I MHC-expressing cells by CTLs. This loss of class I MHC molecules makes the tumors particularly good targets for NK cells. Some tumors also express MICA, MICB, and ULB, which are ligands for the NKG2D activating receptor on NK cells. In addition, NK cells can be targeted to IgG antibody–coated cells by Fc receptors (FcγRIII or CD16). The tumoricidal capacity of NK cells is increased by cytokines, including interferons and interleukins (IL-2 and IL-12), and the anti-tumor effects of these cytokines are partly attributable to stimulation of NK cell activity. IL-2-activated NK cells, called lymphokine-activated killer (LAK) cells, are derived by culturing peripheral blood cells or tumor-infiltrating lymphocytes (TILs) from tumor patients with high doses of IL-2. The use of LAK cells in adoptive immunotherapy for tumors is discussed later.

The role of NK cells in tumor immunity in vivo is unclear. It has been suggested that T cell–deficient mice do not have a high incidence of spontaneous tumors because they have normal numbers of NK cells that serve an immune surveillance function. A few patients have been described with deficiencies of NK cells and an increased incidence of EBV-associated lymphomas.

Macrophages

The role of macrophages in anti-tumor immunity is largely inferred from the demonstration that, in vitro, activated macrophages can kill many tumor cells more efficiently than they can kill normal cells. How macrophages are activated by tumors is not known. Possible mechanisms include direct recognition of some surface antigens of tumor cells and activation of macrophages by interferon-γ (IFN-γ) produced by tumor-specific T cells. Macrophages can kill tumor cells by several mechanisms, probably the same as the mechanisms of macrophage killing of infectious organisms. These mechanisms include the release of lysosomal enzymes, reactive oxygen species, and nitric oxide. Activated macrophages also produce the cytokine tumor necrosis factor (TNF), which was first characterized, as its name implies, as an agent that can kill tumors mainly by inducing thrombosis in tumor blood vessels.

Adaptive Immune Responses to Tumors

Both T cell–mediated and humoral immune responses occur spontaneously to tumors, and some evidence suggests that the T cell responses play a protective role. Particular efforts are now being made to enhance these T cell responses in immunotherapeutic protocols.

T Lymphocytes

The principal mechanism of tumor immunity is killing of tumor cells by CD8⁺ CTLs. The ability of CTLs to provide effective anti-tumor immunity in vivo is most clearly seen in animal experiments using carcinogen-induced and DNA virus–induced tumors. As discussed previously, CTLs may perform a surveillance function by recognizing and killing potentially malignant cells that express peptides derived from mutant cellular proteins or oncogenic viral proteins and presented in association with class I MHC molecules. The role of immune surveillance in preventing common, non–virally induced tumors remains controversial because the frequency of such tumors in T cell–deficient animals or people is not clearly greater than the frequency in immunocompetent individuals. However, tumor-specific CTLs can be isolated from animals and humans with established tumors, such as melanomas. Furthermore, mononuclear cells derived from the inflammatory infiltrate in human solid tumors, called TILs, also include CTLs with the capacity to kill the tumor from which they were derived.

$CD8^+$ T cell responses specific for tumor antigens may require cross-presentation of the tumor antigens by professional APCs, such as dendritic cells. Most tumor cells are not derived from APCs and therefore do not express the costimulators needed to initiate T cell responses or the class II MHC molecules needed to stimulate helper T cells that promote the differentiation of $CD8^+$ T cells. A likely possibility is that tumor cells or their antigens are ingested by host APCs, particularly dendritic cells; the tumor antigens are then processed inside the APCs, and peptides derived from these antigens are displayed bound to class I MHC molecules for recognition by $CD8^+$ T cells. The APCs express costimulators that may provide the signals needed for differentiation of $CD8^+$ T cells into anti-tumor CTLs, and the APCs express class II MHC molecules that may present internalized tumor antigens and activate $CD4^+$ helper T cells as well (Fig. 17–3). This process of cross-presentation, or cross-priming, has been described in earlier chapters (see Chapter 9, Fig. 9–3). Once effector CTLs are generated, they are able to recognize and kill the tumor cells without a requirement for costimulation. A practical application of the concept of cross-priming is to grow dendritic cells from a patient with cancer, incubate the APCs with the cells or antigens from that patient's tumor, and use these antigen-pulsed APCs as vaccines to stimulate anti-tumor T cell responses.

The importance of $CD4^+$ helper T cells in tumor immunity is less clear. $CD4^+$ cells may play a role in anti-tumor immune responses by providing cytokines for effective CTL development (see Chapter 13). In addition, helper T cells specific for tumor antigens may secrete cytokines, such as TNF and IFN-γ, that can increase tumor cell class I MHC expression and sensitivity to lysis by CTLs. IFN-γ may also activate macrophages to kill

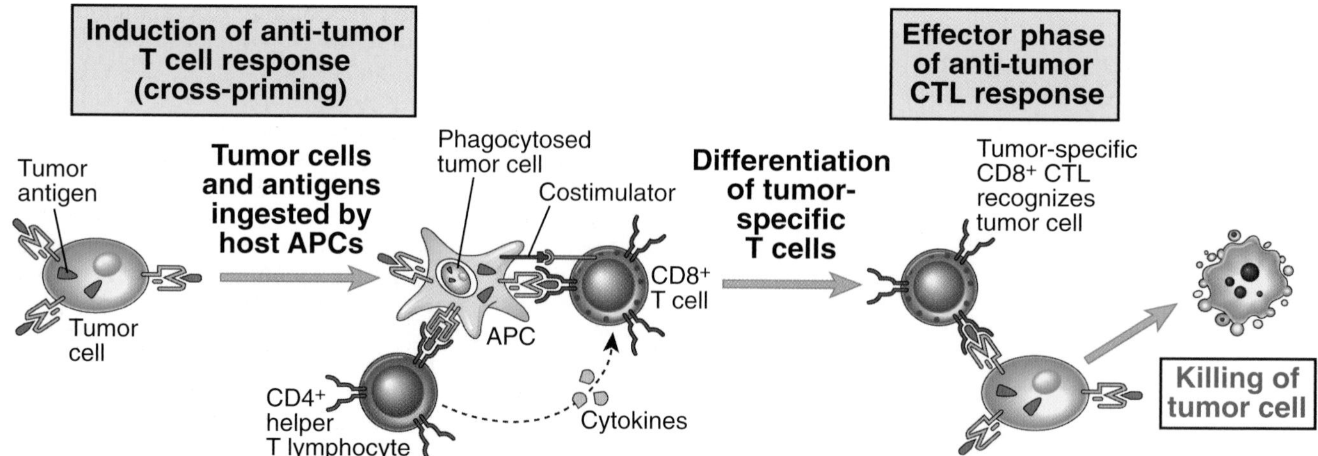

FIGURE 17–3 Induction of T cell responses to tumors. $CD8^+$ T cell responses to tumors may be induced by cross-priming (cross-presentation), in which the tumor cells or tumor antigens are taken up, processed, and presented to T cells by professional antigen-presenting cells (APCs). In some cases, B7 costimulators expressed by the APCs provide the second signals for differentiation of $CD8^+$ T cells. The APCs may also stimulate $CD4^+$ helper T cells, which provide the second signals for CTL development. Differentiated CTLs kill tumor cells without a requirement for costimulation or T cell help. (The roles of cross-presentation and $CD4^+$ helper T cells in CTL responses are discussed in Chapter 9).

tumor cells. The importance of IFN-γ in tumor immunity is demonstrated by the finding of increased incidence of tumors in knockout mice lacking this cytokine, the IFN-γ receptor, or components of the IFN-γ receptor signaling cascade.

Antibodies

Tumor-bearing hosts may produce antibodies against various tumor antigens. For example, patients with EBV-associated lymphomas have serum antibodies against EBV-encoded antigens expressed on the surface of the lymphoma cells. Antibodies may kill tumor cells by activating complement or by antibody-dependent cell-mediated cytotoxicity, in which Fc receptor–bearing macrophages or NK cells mediate the killing. However, the ability of antibodies to eliminate tumor cells has been demonstrated largely in vitro, and there is little evidence for effective humoral immunity against tumors.

Antibodies specific for oncogenic viruses, such as HPV, can prevent infection by these viruses and thereby prevent virally induced tumors.

EVASION OF IMMUNE RESPONSES BY TUMORS

Many malignant tumors possess mechanisms that enable them to evade or resist host immune responses (Fig. 17–4). A major focus of tumor immunology is to understand the ways in which tumor cells evade immune destruction, with the hope that interventions can be designed to increase the immunogenicity of tumors and the responses of the host. The process of evasion may involve many different mechanisms. Experimental evidence in mouse models indicates that immune responses to tumor cells impart selective pressures that result in the survival and outgrowth of variant tumor cells with reduced immunogenicity, a process that has been called "tumor editing."

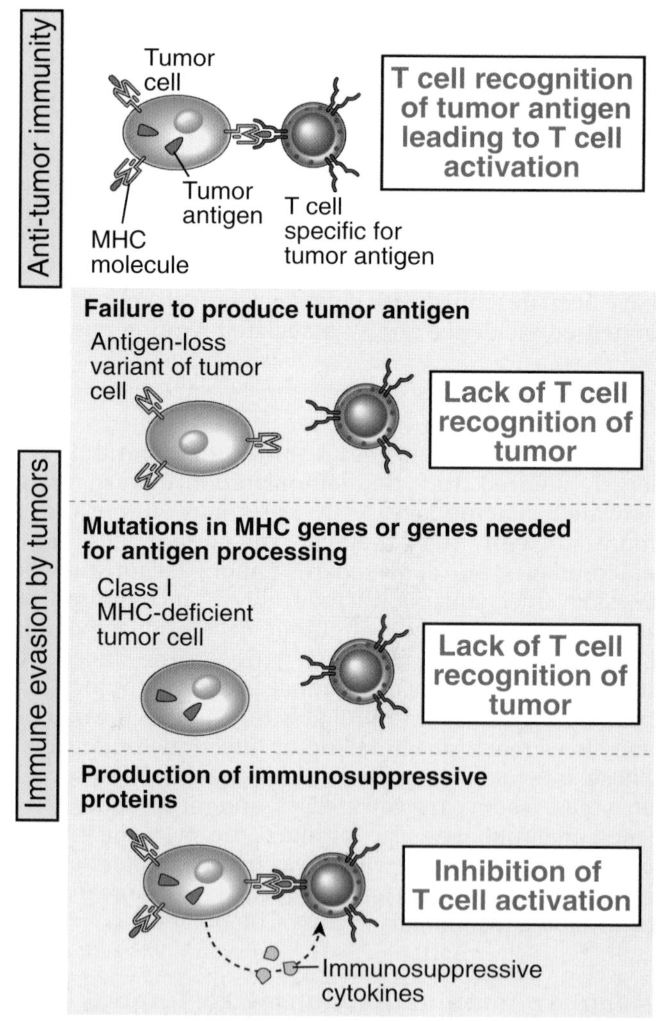

FIGURE 17–4 Mechanisms by which tumors escape immune defenses. Anti-tumor immunity develops when T cells recognize tumor antigens and are activated. Tumor cells may evade immune responses by losing expression of antigens or MHC molecules or by producing immunosuppressive cytokines.

- When tumors are induced by carcinogen-treatment in either immunodeficient or immunocompetent mice, and the tumors are then transplanted into new immunocompetent mice, the tumors that were derived from the immunodeficient mice are more frequently rejected by the recipient animal's immune system than are the tumors derived from the immunocompetent mice. This result indicates that tumors developing in the setting of a normal immune system become less immunogenic over time.

Tumor editing is thought to underlie the emergence of tumors that "escape" immunosurveillance. Tumor editing and escape may be a result of several mechanisms.

- ***Tumor antigens may induce specific immunological tolerance.*** Tolerance may occur because tumor antigens are self antigens encountered by the developing immune system or because the tumor cells present their antigens in a tolerogenic form to mature lymphocytes. Several experimental studies have shown that tolerance to tumor antigens promotes the outgrowth of tumors expressing these antigens.
  - Neonatal mice may acquire the mouse mammary tumor virus from their mothers during nursing. The mice become tolerant to the virus and carry it for life. When these mice become adults, mammary cancers induced by the virus often develop, and the tumors do not elicit immune responses. However, the tumors are potentially immunogenic because they are rejected when they are transplanted into syngeneic, virus-free (uninfected) adult mice.
  - Transgenic mice expressing the SV40 T antigen throughout their lives develop tumors when they are infected with the SV40 virus, and the high incidence of these tumors correlates with tolerance to the SV40 T antigen. In contrast, other SV40 T antigen transgenic mice in which expression of the transgene is delayed until later in life are not tolerant to the T antigen and have a low incidence of tumors.
  - In some experimental models, tumor cells transplanted into adult mice induce anergy in T cells specific for antigens expressed in these tumors. Immunity against the tumors may be stimulated by blocking CTLA-4, the inhibitory T cell receptor for B7 molecules. This result suggests that the tumor antigens may be presented to host T cells by APCs that induce T cell tolerance, in part as a result of B7 : CTLA-4 interactions (see Chapter 11).
- ***Regulatory T cells may suppress T cell responses to tumors.*** Evidence from mouse model systems and cancer patients indicates that the numbers of regulatory T cells are increased in tumor-bearing individuals, and these cells can be found in the cellular infiltrates in certain tumors. Depletion of regulatory T cells in tumor-bearing mice enhances antitumor immunity and reduces tumor growth.
- ***Tumors lose expression of antigens that elicit immune responses.*** Such "antigen loss variants" are common in rapidly growing tumors and can readily be induced in tumor cell lines by culture with tumor-specific antibodies or CTLs. Given the high mitotic rate of tumor cells and their genetic instability, mutations or deletions in genes encoding tumor antigens are common. If these antigens are not required for growth of the tumors or maintenance of the transformed phenotype, the antigen-negative tumor cells have a growth advantage in the host. Analysis of tumors that are serially transplanted from one animal to another has shown that the loss of antigens recognized by tumor-specific CTLs correlates with increased growth and metastatic potential. Apart from tumor-specific antigens, class I MHC expression may be down-regulated on tumor cells so that they cannot be recognized by CTLs. Various tumors show decreased synthesis of class I MHC molecules, β_2-microglobulin, or components of the antigen-processing machinery, including the transporter associated with antigen processing and some subunits of the proteasome. These mechanisms are presumably adaptations of the tumors that arise in response to the selection pressures of host immunity, and they may allow tumor cells to evade T cell–mediated immune responses. However, when the level of MHC expression on a broad range of experimental or human tumor cells is compared with the in vivo growth of these cells, there is no clear correlation.
- ***Tumors may fail to induce CTLs because most tumor cells do not express costimulators or class II MHC molecules.*** Costimulators are required for initiating T cell responses, and class II molecules are needed for the activation of helper T cells, which are required, in some circumstances, for the differentiation of CTLs. Therefore, the induction of tumor-specific T cell responses often requires cross-priming by dendritic cells, which express costimulators and class II molecules. If such APCs do not adequately take up and present tumor antigens and activate helper T cells, CTLs specific for the tumor cells may not develop. Tumor cells transfected with genes encoding the costimulators B7-1 (CD80) and B7-2 (CD86) are able to elicit strong cell-mediated immune responses. Predictably, CTLs induced by B7-transfected tumors are effective against the parent (B7-negative) tumor as well because the effector phase of CTL-mediated killing does not require costimulation (see Fig. 17–3). As we shall see later, these experimental results are being extended to the clinical situation as immunotherapy for tumors.
- ***The products of tumor cells may suppress anti-tumor immune responses.*** An example of an immunosuppressive tumor product is transforming growth factor-β, which is secreted in large quantities by many tumors and inhibits the proliferation and effector functions of lymphocytes and macrophages (see Chapter 12). Some tumors express Fas ligand (FasL), which recognizes the death receptor Fas on leukocytes that attempt to attack the tumor; engagement of Fas by FasL may result in apoptotic death of the leukocytes. The importance of this mechanism of

tumor escape is not established because FasL has been detected on only a few spontaneous tumors, and when it is expressed in tumors by gene transfection, it is not always protective.

- The cell surface antigens of tumors may be hidden from the immune system by glycocalyx molecules, such as sialic acid–containing mucopolysaccharides. This process is called antigen masking and may be a consequence of the fact that tumor cells often express more of these glycocalyx molecules than normal cells do.

IMMUNOTHERAPY FOR TUMORS

The potential for treating cancer patients by immunologic approaches has held great promise for oncologists and immunologists for many years. The main reason for interest in an immunologic approach is that current therapies for cancer rely on drugs that kill dividing cells or block cell division, and these treatments have severe effects on normal proliferating cells. As a result, the treatment of cancers causes significant morbidity and mortality. Immune responses to tumors may be specific for tumor antigens and will not injure most normal cells. Therefore, immunotherapy has the potential of being the most tumor-specific treatment that can be devised. Advances in our understanding of the immune system and in defining antigens on tumor cells have encouraged many new strategies. Immunotherapy for tumors aims to augment the weak host immune response to the tumors (active immunity) or to administer tumor-specific antibodies or T cells, a form of passive immunity. In this section, we describe some of the modes of tumor immunotherapy that have been tried in the past or are currently being investigated.

Stimulation of Active Host Immune Responses to Tumors

The earliest attempts to boost anti-tumor immunity relied on nonspecific immune stimulation. More recently, vaccines composed of killed tumor cells or tumor antigens have been administered to patients, and strategies for enhancing immune responses against the tumor are being developed.

Vaccination with Tumor Cells and Tumor Antigens

Immunization of tumor-bearing individuals with killed tumor cells or tumor antigens may result in enhanced immune responses against the tumor (Table 17–2 and

Table 17–2. Tumor Vaccines

Type of vaccine	Vaccine preparation	Animal models	Clinical trials
Killed tumor vaccine	Killed tumor cells + adjuvants	Melanoma, colon cancer, others	Melanoma, colon cancer
	Tumor cell lysates + adjuvants	Sarcoma	Melanoma
Purified tumor antigens	Melanoma antigens	Melanoma	Melanoma
	Heat shock proteins	Various	Melanoma, renal cancer, sarcoma
Professional APC-based vaccines	Dendritic cells pulsed with tumor antigens	Melanoma, B cell lymphoma, sarcoma	Melanoma, non-Hodgkin's lymphoma, prostate cancer, others
	Dendritic cells transfected with genes encoding tumor antigens	Melanoma, colon cancer	Various carcinomas
Cytokine- and costimulator-enhanced vaccines	Tumor cells transfected with cytokine or B7 genes	Renal cancer, sarcoma, B cell leukemia, lung cancer	Melanoma, sarcoma, others
	APCs transfected with cytokine genes and pulsed with tumor antigens		Melanoma, renal cancer, others
DNA vaccines	Immunization with plasmids encoding tumor antigens	Melanoma	Melanoma
Viral vectors	Adenovirus, vaccinia virus encoding tumor antigen ± cytokines	Melanoma, sarcoma	Melanoma

Abbreviations: APC, antigen-presenting cell.

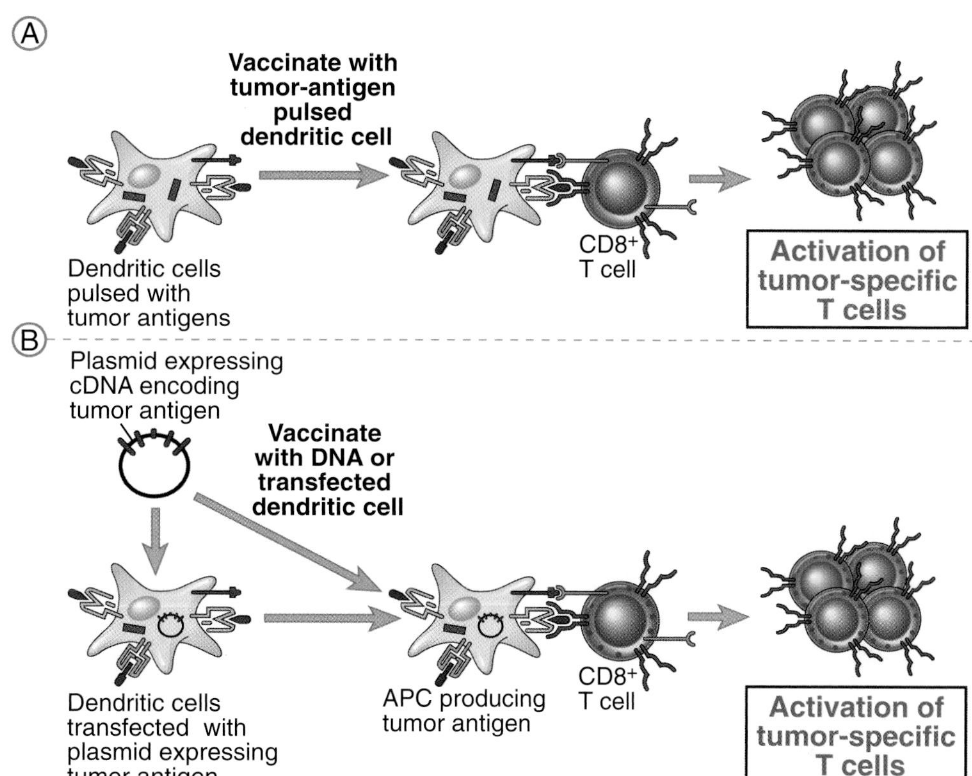

FIGURE 17–5 Tumor vaccines. The types of tumor vaccines that have shown efficacy in animal models are illustrated. Many vaccine approaches are undergoing clinical testing.

Fig. 17–5). The identification of peptides recognized by tumor-specific CTLs and the cloning of genes that encode tumor-specific antigens recognized by CTLs have provided many candidates for tumor vaccines. One of the earliest vaccine approaches, immunization with purified tumor antigens plus adjuvants, is still being tried. More recently, attempts to immunize patients with cancer have been made with dendritic cells purified from the patients and either incubated with tumor antigens or transfected with genes encoding these antigens and by injection of plasmids containing cDNAs encoding tumor antigens (DNA vaccines). The cell-based and DNA vaccines may be the best ways to induce CTL responses because the encoded antigens are synthesized in the cytoplasm and enter the class I MHC pathway of antigen presentation. For antigens that are unique to individual tumors, such as antigens produced by random point mutations in cellular genes, these vaccination methods are impractical because they would require identification of the antigens from every tumor. On the other hand, tumor antigens shared by many tumors, such as the MAGE, tyrosinase, and gp100 antigens on melanomas and mutated Ras and p53 proteins in various tumors, are potentially useful immunogens for all patients with certain types of cancer. In fact, clinical trials of such cancer vaccines are under way for a variety of tumors. A limitation of treating established tumors with vaccines is that these vaccines need to be therapeutic and not simply preventive, and it is often difficult to induce a strong enough immune response that will eradicate all the cells of growing tumors.

The development of virally induced tumors can be blocked by preventive vaccination with viral antigens or attenuated live viruses. This approach is successful in reducing the incidence of feline leukemia virus–induced hematologic malignant tumors in cats and in preventing the herpesvirus-induced lymphoma called Marek's disease in chickens. In humans, the ongoing vaccination program against hepatitis B virus may reduce the incidence of hepatocellular carcinoma, a liver cancer associated with hepatitis B virus infection. As mentioned earlier, newly developed HPV vaccines promise to reduce the incidence of HPV-induced tumors, including uterine cervical carcinoma.

Augmentation of Host Immunity to Tumors with Costimulators and Cytokines

Cell-mediated immunity to tumors may be enhanced by expressing costimulators and cytokines in tumor cells and by treating tumor-bearing individuals with cytokines that stimulate the proliferation and differentiation of T lymphocytes and NK cells. As discussed earlier in this chapter, tumor cells may induce weak immune responses because they lack costimulators and usually do not express class II MHC molecules, so they do not activate helper T cells. Two potential approaches for boosting host responses to tumors are to artificially provide costimulation for tumor-specific T cells and to provide cytokines that can enhance the activation of tumor-specific T cells, particularly $CD8^+$ CTLs (Fig. 17–6). Many cytokines also have the potential to induce

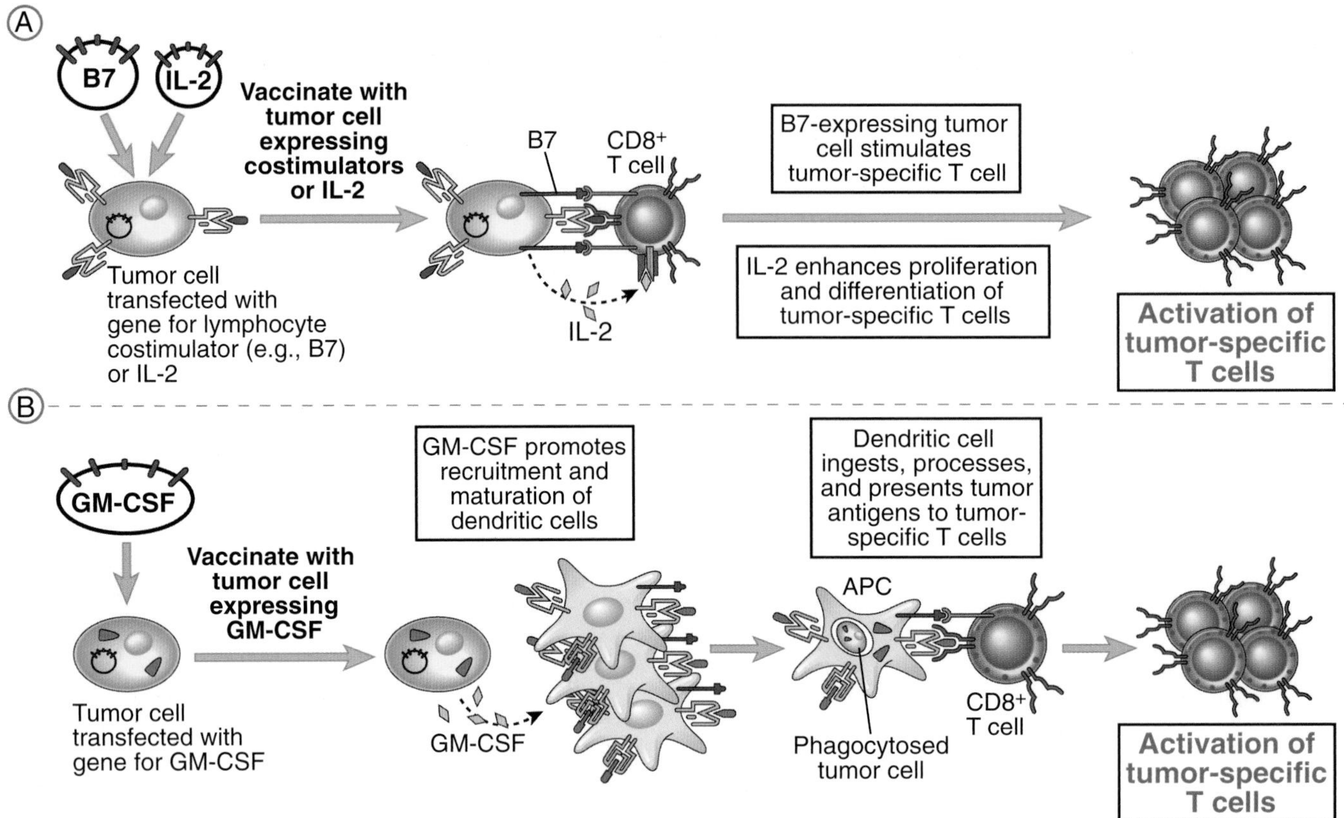

FIGURE 17–6 Enhancement of tumor cell immunogenicity by transfection of costimulator and cytokine genes. Tumor cells that do not adequately stimulate T cells on transplantation into an animal will not be rejected and will therefore grow into tumors. Vaccination with tumor cells transfected with genes encoding costimulators or IL-2 (A) can lead to enhanced activation of T cells, and tumors transfected with GM-CSF (B) activate professional APCs, notably dendritic cells. These transfected tumor cell vaccines stimulate tumor-specific T cells, leading to T cell–mediated rejection of the tumor (even untransfected tumor cells).

nonspecific inflammatory responses, which by themselves may have anti-tumor activity.

The efficacy of enhancing T cell costimulation for anti-tumor immunotherapy has been demonstrated by animal experiments in which tumor cells were transfected with genes that encode B7 costimulatory molecules and used to vaccinate animals. These B7-expressing tumor cells induce protective immunity against unmodified tumor cells injected at a distant site. The successes with experimental tumor models have led to therapeutic trials in which a sample of a patient's tumor is propagated in vitro, transfected with costimulator genes, irradiated, and reintroduced into the patient. Such approaches may succeed even if the immunogenic antigens expressed on tumors are not known.

It is possible to use cytokines to enhance adaptive and innate immune responses against tumors. Tumor cells may be transfected with cytokine genes to localize the cytokine effects to where they are needed (Table 17–3). For instance, when rodent tumors transfected with IL-2, IL-4, IFN-γ, or granulocyte-macrophage colony-stimulating factor (GM-CSF) genes are injected into animals, the tumors are rejected or begin to grow and then regress. In some cases, intense inflammatory infiltrates accumulate around the cytokine-secreting tumors, and the nature of the infiltrate varies with the cytokine. Different cytokines may stimulate anti-tumor immunity by different mechanisms (see Fig. 17–6). Importantly, in several of these studies, the injection of cytokine-secreting tumors induced specific, T cell–mediated immunity to subsequent challenges by unmodified tumor cells. Thus, the local production of cytokines may augment T cell responses to tumor antigens, and cytokine-expressing tumors may act as effective tumor vaccines. Several clinical trials with cytokine gene–transfected tumors are under way in patients with advanced cancer.

Cytokines may also be administered systemically for the treatment of various human tumors (Table 17–4). The largest clinical experience is with IL-2 administered in high doses alone or in combination with adoptive cellular immunotherapy (discussed later). IL-2 presumably works by stimulating the proliferation and anti-tumor activity of NK cells and CTLs. The limitation of this treatment is that it can be highly toxic and induces fever, pulmonary edema, and vascular shock. These side effects occur because IL-2 stimulates the production of other cytokines by T cells, such as TNF and IFN-γ, and these cytokines act on vascular endothelium and other cell types. IL-2 has been effective in inducing measurable tumor regression responses in about 10% of patients

Table 17–3. Immunotherapy with Cytokine Gene-Transfected Tumor Cells

Cytokine	Tumor rejection in animals	Inflammatory infiltrate	Immunity against parental tumor (animal models)	Clinical trials
Interleukin-2	Yes; mediated by T cells	Lymphocytes, neutrophils	In some cases of renal cancer, melanoma	Renal cancer, melanoma
Interleukin-4	Yes	Eosinophils, macrophages	No long-lasting immunity in human trials	Melanoma, renal cancer
Interferon-γ	Variable	Macrophages, other cells	Sometimes	
TNF	Variable	Neutrophils and lymphocytes	No	
GM-CSF	Yes	Macrophages, other cells	Yes (long-lived T cell immunity)	Renal cancer
Interleukin-3	Sometimes	Macrophages, other cells	Sometimes	

Abbreviations: GM-CSF, granulocyte-macrophage colony-stimulating factor; TNF, tumor necrosis factor.

with advanced melanoma and renal cell carcinoma and is currently an approved therapy for these cancers. IFN-α may be effective against tumors because it increases the cytotoxic activity of NK cells and increases class I MHC expression on various cell types (see Chapter 12). Clinical trials of this cytokine indicate that it can induce the regression of renal carcinomas, melanomas, Kaposi's sarcoma, various lymphomas, and hairy cell leukemia (a B cell lineage tumor). IFN-α is currently used in combination with chemotherapy for the treatment of melanoma. Other cytokines, such as TNF and IFN-γ, are effective anti-tumor agents in animal models, but their use in patients is limited by serious toxic side effects. The potential of IL-12 to enhance anti-tumor T cell– and NK cell–mediated immune responses has aroused great interest, and early trials in patients with advanced cancer are now under way. Hematopoietic growth factors, including GM-CSF, G-CSF, and IL-11, are used in cancer treatment protocols to shorten periods of neutropenia and thrombocytopenia after chemotherapy or autologous bone marrow transplantation.

Blocking Inhibitory Pathways to Promote Tumor Immunity

Another immunotherapy strategy is based on the idea that T cells exploit various normal pathways of immune regulation or tolerance to evade the host immune response. One series of studies in mice and humans has targeted the inhibitory receptor for B7, called CTLA-4, which functions normally to shut off responses (see Chapter 11). If tumor-bearing mice are vaccinated with

Table 17–4. Systemic Cytokine Therapy for Tumors

Cytokine	Tumor rejection in animals	Clinical trials	Toxicity
Interleukin-2	Yes	Melanoma, renal cancer, colon cancer; limited success (<15% response rate)	Vascular leak, shock, pulmonary edema
Interferon-α	No	Approved for melanoma	Fever, fatigue
TNF	Only with local administration	Sarcoma, melanoma (isolated limb perfusion)	Septic shock syndrome
Interleukin-12	Variable	Toxicity trials (phase I) in melanoma, others	Abnormal liver function
GM-CSF	No	In routine use to promote bone marrow recovery	Bone pain

Abbreviations: GM-CSF, granulocyte-macrophage colony-stimulating factor; TNF, tumor necrosis factor.

the tumor and also treated with an antibody that blocks CTLA-4, the mice develop strong anti-tumor T cell responses and destroy the tumor. The potential of such approaches for tumor immunotherapy in humans is being evaluated. In clinical trials, a common complication of this treatment has been the development of autoimmune reactions. This is predictable in light of the known role of CTLA-4 in maintaining self-tolerance. The depletion of regulatory T cells may also enhance anti-tumor immunity, and this approach is being tested in animal models.

Nonspecific Stimulation of the Immune System

Immune responses to tumors may be stimulated by the local administration of inflammatory substances or by systemic treatment with agents that function as polyclonal activators of lymphocytes. Nonspecific immune stimulation of patients with tumors by injection of inflammatory substances such as bacillus Calmette-Guérin (BCG) at the sites of tumor growth has been tried for many years. The BCG mycobacteria activate macrophages and thereby promote macrophage-mediated killing of the tumor cells. In addition, the bacteria function as adjuvants and may stimulate T cell responses to tumor antigens. Another approach for immune stimulation is to administer low doses of activating anti-CD3 antibodies. In animal studies of transplantable tumors, this treatment results in polyclonal activation of T cells and, concomitantly, prevention of tumor growth. Early clinical trials with specific antibodies directed at tumor antigens and CD3 are ongoing. Cytokine therapies, discussed before, represent another method of enhancing immune responses in a nonspecific manner.

Passive Immunotherapy for Tumors with T Cells and Antibodies

Passive immunotherapy involves the transfer of immune effectors, including tumor-specific T cells and antibodies, into patients. Passive immunization against tumors is rapid but does not lead to long-lived immunity. Several approaches to passive immunotherapy are being tried, with variable success.

Adoptive Cellular Therapy

Adoptive cellular immunotherapy is the transfer of cultured immune cells that have anti-tumor reactivity into a tumor-bearing host. The cells to be transferred are expanded from the lymphocytes of patients with the tumor. One protocol for adoptive cellular immunotherapy is to generate LAK cells by removing peripheral blood leukocytes from patients with the tumor, culturing the cells in high concentrations of IL-2, and injecting the LAK cells back into the patients (Fig. 17–7). As discussed previously, LAK cells are derived mainly from NK cells. Adoptive therapy with autologous LAK cells, in conjunction with in vivo administration of IL-2 or chemotherapeutic drugs, has yielded impressive results in mice, with regression of solid tumors. Human LAK cell therapy trials have thus far been largely restricted to advanced cases of metastatic tumors, and the efficacy of this approach appears to vary from patient to patient. A variation of this approach is to isolate TILs from the inflammatory infiltrate present in and around solid tumors, obtained from surgical resection specimens, and to expand the TILs by culture in IL-2. The rationale for this approach is that TILs may be enriched for tumor-specific CTLs and for activated NK cells. Human trials with TIL therapy are ongoing.

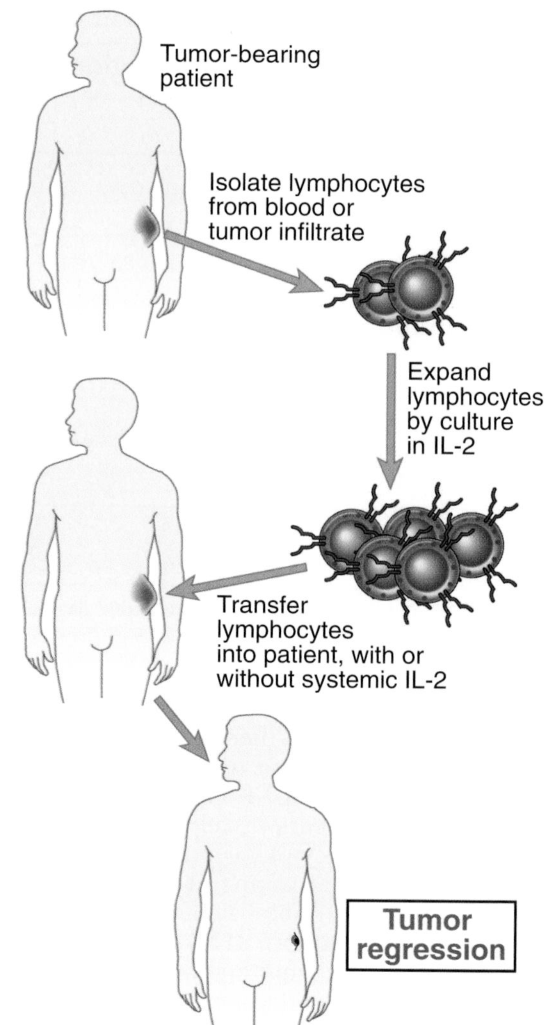

FIGURE 17–7 Adoptive cellular therapy. In a commonly used approach for adoptive cellular therapy, lymphocytes isolated from the blood or tumor infiltrate of a patient are expanded by culture in IL-2 and are infused back into the patient. This treatment, often combined with systemic IL-2 administration, leads to tumor regression in some patients.

Graft-versus-Leukemia Effect

In leukemia patients, administration of alloreactive T cells together with hematopoietic stem cell transplants

can contribute to eradication of the tumor. This graft-versus-leukemia effect is directed at the allogeneic MHC molecules present on the recipient's hematopoietic cells, including the leukemia cells. The challenge in using this treatment to improve clinical outcome is to minimize the dangerous graft-versus-host disease that may be mediated by the same donor T cells (see Chapter 16).

Therapy with Anti-tumor Antibodies

Tumor-specific monoclonal antibodies may be useful for specific immunotherapy for tumors. The potential of using antibodies as "magic bullets" has been alluring to investigators for many years and is still an active area of research. Currently there are over 100 different monoclonal antibodies being considered, either in experimental animal studies or in human trials, as therapeutic agents for cancer, and a few have been approved for clinical use (Table 17–5). Anti-tumor antibodies may eradicate tumors by the same effector mechanisms that are used to eliminate microbes, including opsonization and phagocytosis and activation of the complement system (see Chapter 14). In addition, some antibodies may directly activate intrinsic apoptosis pathways in tumor cells; this is the proposed mechanism for the use of anti-CD30 to treat lymphomas, currently in clinical trials. A monoclonal antibody specific for the oncogene product Her-2/Neu, which is expressed at high levels in some tumors, is effective in patients with breast cancer and is approved for clinical use. In addition to eliciting immune effector mechanisms, the anti-Her-2/Neu antibody interferes with growth-signaling functions of the Her-2/Neu molecule.

Because the anti-tumor antibodies used in the early human trials were mouse monoclonal antibodies, an immune response frequently occurred against the mouse Ig, resulting in anti-mouse Ig antibodies that caused increased clearance of the anti-tumor antibodies or blocked binding of the therapeutic agent to its target. This problem has been diminished by use of "humanized" antibodies consisting of the variable regions of a mouse monoclonal antibody specific for the tumor antigen combined with human Fc portions. One of the most difficult problems with the use of anti-tumor antibodies is the outgrowth of antigen loss variants of the tumor cells that no longer express the antigens that the antibodies recognize. One way to avoid this problem may be to use cocktails of antibodies specific for different antigens expressed on the same tumor.

Many variations on anti-tumor antibodies have been tried in attempts to improve their effectiveness. Tumor-specific antibodies may be coupled to toxic molecules, radioisotopes, and anti-tumor drugs to promote the delivery of these cytotoxic agents specifically to the tumor. Toxins such as ricin and diphtheria toxin are potent inhibitors of protein synthesis and can be effective at extremely low doses if they are carried to tumors attached to anti-tumor antibodies; such conjugates are called immunotoxins. This approach requires covalent coupling of the toxin (lacking its cell-binding component) to an anti-tumor antibody molecule without loss of toxicity or antibody specificity. The systemically injected **immunotoxin** is endocytosed by tumor cells, and the toxin part is delivered to its intracellular site of action. Several practical difficulties must be overcome for this technique to be successful. The specificity of the antibody must be such that it does not bind to non-tumor cells. A sufficient amount of antibody must reach the appropriate tumor target before it is cleared from the blood by Fc receptor–bearing phagocytic cells. The toxins, drugs, or radioisotopes attached to the antibody may have systemic effects as a result of circulation through normal tissues. For example, hepatotoxicity and

Table 17–5. Anti-tumor Monoclonal Antibodies Approved for Clinical Use

Specificity of antibody	Form of antibody used	Clinical trials
Her-2/Neu	Humanized mouse monoclonal	Breast cancer (approved for clinical use)
CD20 (B cell marker)	Humanized mouse monoclonal	B cell lymphoma
CD10	Humanized mouse monoclonal, immunotoxin	B cell lymphoma; in routine use to purge bone marrow of residual tumor cells
CEA	Humanized mouse monoclonal	Gastrointestinal cancers, lung cancer
CA-125	Mouse monoclonal	Ovarian cancer
GD3 ganglioside	Humanized mouse monoclonal	Melanoma

Abbreviation: CEA, carcinoembryonic antigen.

vascular leak syndromes are common problems with immunotoxin therapy. Administration of immunotoxins may result in antibody responses against the toxins and the injected antibodies. Because of these practical difficulties, clinical trials of immunotoxins have had variable and modest success.

Anti-idiotypic antibodies have been used to treat B cell lymphomas that express surface Ig with particular idiotypes. The idiotype is a highly specific tumor antigen because it is expressed only on the neoplastic clone of B cells, and it was once hoped that anti-idiotypic antibodies would be effective therapeutic reagents with absolute tumor specificity. (Anti-idiotypic antibodies are raised by immunizing rabbits with a patient's B cell tumor and depleting the serum of reactivity against all other human immunoglobulins.) The approach has not proved generally successful, largely because of the selective outgrowth of tumor cells with altered idiotypes that do not bind the anti-idiotypic antibody. In part, this result may reflect the high rate of somatic mutation in Ig genes and the fact that the surface Ig is dispensable for tumor growth.

Tumor growth is usually dependent on growth factors, which are potential targets for therapy. Antibodies that block the epidermal growth factor receptor (EGFR) are approved for the treatment of colorectal tumors. Tumors depend on the formation of new blood vessels that supply the tumor with oxygen and nutrients. This process, called tumor angiogenesis, is dependent on other specialized growth factors, including vascular endothelial growth factor (VEGF). Various inhibitors of these angiogenic factors can block tumor growth. Anti-VEGF antibodies are now approved for clinical use, in combination with chemotherapeutic agents, to treat metastatic tumors.

Anti-tumor antibodies are also used to remove cancer cells from the bone marrow before autologous marrow transplantation. In this protocol, some of the patient's bone marrow is removed, and the patient is given doses of radiation and chemotherapy lethal enough to destroy tumor cells as well as the remaining normal marrow cells. The bone marrow cells removed from the patient are treated with antibodies or immunotoxins specific for tumor antigens to kill any tumor cells. The treated marrow, having been purged of tumor cells, is transplanted back into the patient to reconstitute the hematopoietic system destroyed by irradiation and chemotherapy.

The Role of the Immune System in Promoting Tumor Growth

In addition to protection against cancer, the immune system may contribute to the development of some tumors. In fact, chronic inflammation has long been recognized as a risk factor for development of tumors in many different tissues. Some cancers associated with infections are considered to be an indirect result of the carcinogenic effects of the chronic inflammatory states that are induced by the infectious organisms. These include gastric cancer in the setting of chronic *Helicobacter pylori* infection and hepatocellular carcinomas associated with chronic hepatitis B and C virus infections. Although the mechanisms by which chronic inflammation can promote tumor development are not well understood, there are several possibilities, supported by data in rodent models. Cells of the innate immune system are considered the most direct tumor-promoting culprits among immune cells. Chronic activation of innate immune cells, notably macrophages, is characterized by angiogenesis and tissue remodeling, both of which favor tumor formation. Innate immune cells can also contribute to malignant transformation of cells by generating free radicals that cause DNA damage and lead to mutations in tumor suppressor genes and oncogenes. Some data suggest that cells of the innate immune system, including mast cells, neutrophils, and macrophages, secrete soluble factors that promote cell-cycle progression and survival of tumor cells. The adaptive immune system can promote chronic activation of innate immune cells in several ways, including T cell mediated activation of macrophages in the setting of persistent intracellular microbial infections. Thus, the adaptive immune system may indirectly enhance the tumor-promoting activities of the innate immune system. The tumor-promoting effects of the immune system are paradoxical, and a topic of active investigation at present. These effects of chronic inflammation are theoretically also excellent targets for pharmacologic intervention, because there are a large variety of effective anti-inflammatory drugs already available. The challenge for oncologists is to achieve a beneficial balance in which protective anti-tumor adaptive immune responses are not compromised, while potentially dangerous chronic inflammatory conditions are controlled.

SUMMARY

- Tumors express antigens that are recognized by the immune system, but most tumors are weakly immunogenic, and immune responses often fail to prevent the growth of tumors. The immune system can be stimulated to effectively kill tumors.

- Tumor antigens recognized by CTLs are the principal inducers of and targets for antitumor immunity. These antigens include mutants of oncogenes and other cellular proteins, normal proteins whose expression is dysregulated or increased in tumors, and products of oncogenic viruses.

- Antibodies specific for tumor cells recognize antigens that are used for diagnosis and are potential targets for antibody therapy. These antigens include oncofetal antigens, which are expressed normally during fetal life and whose expression is dysregulated in some tumors; altered surface glycoproteins and glycolipids; and molecules that are normally expressed on the cells from which the tumors arise and are thus differentiation antigens for particular cell types.

- Immune responses that are capable of killing tumor cells consist of CTLs, NK cells, and activated macrophages. The role of these immune effector mechanisms in protecting individuals from tumors is not well defined.
- Tumors evade immune responses by several mechanisms, including down-regulating the expression of MHC molecules, selecting cells that do not express tumor antigens, producing immunosuppressive substances, and inducing tolerance to tumor antigens.
- Immunotherapy for tumors is designed to augment active immune responses against these tumors or to administer tumor-specific immune effectors to patients. Immune responses may be actively enhanced by vaccination with tumor cells or antigens, administration of tumors modified to express high levels of costimulators or cytokines that stimulate T cell proliferation and differentiation, and systemic administration of cytokines. Anti-tumor immunity may also be enhanced by blocking inhibitory pathways of immunoregulation. Approaches for passive immunotherapy include the administration of anti-tumor antibodies, antibodies conjugated with toxic drugs (immunotoxins), and tumor-reactive T cells and NK cells isolated from patients and expanded by culture with growth factors.

Selected Readings

Berzofsky JA, M Terabe, S Oh, IM Belyakov, JD Ahlers, JE Janik, and JC Morris. Progress on new vaccine strategies for the immunotherapy and prevention of cancer. Journal of Clinical Investigation 113:1515–1525, 2004.

Bleakley M, and SR Riddell. Molecules and mechanisms of the graft-versus-leukaemia effect. Nature Reviews Cancer 4:371–380, 2004.

Boon T, PG Coulie, BJ Van den Eynde, and P van der Bruggen. Human T cell responses against melanoma. Annual Review of Immunology 24:175–208, 2006.

Burnet FM. The concept of immunological surveillance. Progress in Experimental Tumor Research 13:1–27, 1970.

Cook HT, and M Botto. Mechanisms of disease: the complement system and the pathogenesis of systemic lupus erythematosus. Nature Clinical Practice Rheumatology 2:330–337, 2006.

Coulie PG, and T Connerotte. Human tumor-specific T lymphocytes: does function matter more than number? Current Opinion in Immunology 17:320–325, 2005.

Curiel TJ. Regulatory T cells and treatment of cancer. Current Opinions in Immunology 20:241–246, 2008.

de Visser KE, A Eichten, and LM Coussens. Paradoxical roles of the immune system during cancer development. Nature Reviews Cancer 6:24–37, 2006.

Dranoff G. Cytokines in cancer pathogenesis and cancer therapy. Nature Reviews Cancer 4:11–22, 2004.

Dunn GP, LJ Old, and RD Schreiber. The three Es of cancer immunoediting. Annual Review of Immunology 22:329–360, 2004.

Dunn GP, CM Koebel, and RD Schreiber. Interferons, immunity and cancer immunoediting. Nature Reviews Immunology 6:836–848, 2006.

Finn OJ. Cancer immunology. New England Journal of Medicine 358:2704–2715, 2008.

Fong L, and EG Engelman. Dendritic cells in cancer immunotherapy. Annual Review of Immunology 18:245–273, 2000.

Gattinoni L, DJ Powell, Jr., SA Rosenberg, and NP Restifo. Adoptive immunotherapy for cancer: building on success. Nature Reviews Immunology 6:383–393, 2006.

Gilboa E. DC-based cancer vaccines. Journal of Clinical Investigation 117:1195–1203, 2007.

Harris M. Monoclonal antibodies as therapeutic agents for cancer. Lancet Oncology 5:292–302, 2004.

Laheru DA, DM Pardoll, and EM Jaffee. Genes to vaccines for immunotherapy: how the molecular biology revolution has influenced cancer immunology. Molecular Cancer Therapy 4:1645–1652, 2005.

Pardoll DM. Does the immune system see tumors as foreign or self? Annual Review of Immunology 21:807–839, 2003.

Peggs KS, SA Quezada, AJ Korman, and JP Allison. Principles and use of anti-CTLA4 antibody in human cancer immunotherapy. Current Opinions in Immunology 18:206–213, 2006.

Reiter Y. Recombinant immunotoxins in targeted cancer cell therapy. Advances in Cancer Research 81:93–124, 2001.

Simpson AJ, OL Caballero, A Jungbluth, YT Chen, and LJ Old. Cancer/testis antigens, gametogenesis and cancer. Nature Reviews Cancer 5:615–625, 2005.

Smyth MJ, Y Hayakawa, K Takeda, and H Yagita. New aspects of natural killer cell surveillance and therapy of cancer. Nature Reviews Cancer 2:850–861, 2002.

Steinman RM, and J Banchereau. Taking dendritic cells into medicine. Nature 449:419–426, 2007.

Stevanovic S. Identification of tumour-associated T-cell epitopes for vaccine development. Nature Reviews Cancer 2:514–520, 2002.

Terme M, E Ullrich, NF Delahaye, N Chaput, and L Zitvogel. Natural killer cell-directed therapies: moving from unexpected results to successful strategies. Nature Immunology 9:486–494, 2008.

Thorley-Lawson DA, and A Gross. Persistence of the Epstein-Barr virus and the origins of associated lymphomas. New England Journal of Medicine 350:1328–1337, 2004.

Waldmann TA. Effective cancer therapy through immunomodulation. Annual Review of Medicine 57:65–81, 2006.

Zou W. Regulatory T cells, tumour immunity and immunotherapy. Nature Reviews Immunology 6:295–307, 2006.

Chapter 18

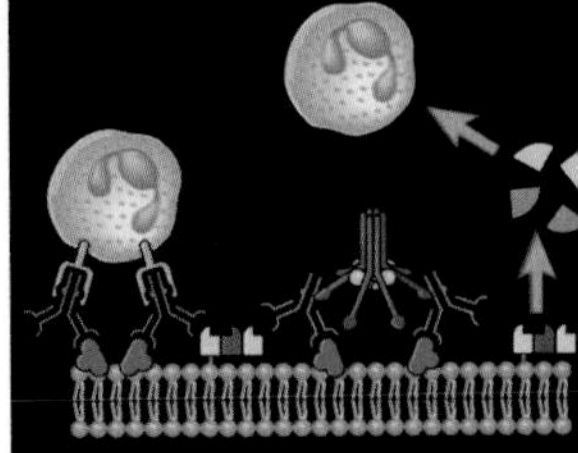

DISEASES CAUSED BY IMMUNE RESPONSES: HYPERSENSITIVITY AND AUTOIMMUNITY

Adaptive immunity serves the important function of host defense against microbial infections, but immune responses are also capable of causing tissue injury and disease. Disorders caused by immune responses are called **hypersensitivity diseases.** This term arose from the clinical definition of immunity as "sensitivity," which is based on the observation that an individual who has been exposed to an antigen exhibits a detectable reaction, or is "sensitive," to subsequent encounters with that antigen. Normally, the immune response eradicates infecting organisms without serious injury to host tissues. However, sometimes these responses are inadequately controlled or inappropriately targeted to host tissues, and in these situations, the normally beneficial response is the cause of disease.

In this chapter, we describe the pathogenesis of different types of hypersensitivity diseases, with an emphasis on the effector mechanisms that cause tissue injury and on the mechanisms of autoimmunity. Throughout the chapter, we use examples of clinical and experimental diseases to illustrate important principles. We conclude with a brief consideration of the treatment of immunologic diseases.

CAUSES AND TYPES OF HYPERSENSITIVITY DISEASES

Immune responses may be pathologic because of several different abnormalities.

- *Autoimmunity.* Failure of the normal mechanisms of self-tolerance (see Chapter 11) results in reactions against one's own cells and tissues that are called *autoimmunity.* The diseases caused by autoimmunity are referred to as *autoimmune diseases.* We will return to the mechanisms of autoimmunity later in this chapter.
- *Reactions against microbes.* Immune responses against microbial antigens may cause disease if the reactions are excessive or the microbes are unusually persistent. If antibodies are produced against such

antigens, the antibodies may bind to the microbial antigens to produce immune complexes, which deposit in tissues and trigger inflammation. T cell responses against persistent microbes may give rise to severe inflammation, sometimes with the formation of granulomas; this is the cause of tissue injury in tuberculosis and other infections. Rarely, antibodies or T cells reactive with a microbe may cross-react with a host tissue. Sometimes the disease-causing immune response may be entirely normal, but in the process of eradicating the infection host tissues are injured. In *viral hepatitis,* the virus that infects liver cells is not cytopathic, but it is recognized as foreign by the immune system. Cytotoxic T lymphocytes (CTLs) try to eliminate infected cells, and this normal immune response damages liver cells. This type of normal reaction is not considered hypersensitivity.

- *Reactions against environmental antigens.* Most healthy individuals do not react against common, generally harmless, environmental substances, but almost 20% of the population is "abnormally responsive" to these substances. Reactions against these environmental substances may be caused by immediate or delayed-type hypersensitivity (DTH) reactions (see below).

In all these conditions, the mechanisms of tissue injury are the same as those that normally function to eliminate infectious pathogens, namely, antibodies, T lymphocytes, and various other effector cells. The problem in hypersensitivity diseases is that the response is triggered and maintained inappropriately. Because the stimuli for these abnormal immune responses are difficult or impossible to eliminate (e.g., self antigens and persistent microbes), and the immune system has many built-in positive feedback loops (amplification mechanisms), once a pathologic immune response starts it is difficult to control or terminate it. Therefore, these hypersensitivity diseases tend to be chronic, often debilitating, and therapeutic challenges. Since inflammation, typically chronic inflammation, is a major component of the pathology of these disorders, they are sometimes grouped under the rubric *immune-mediated inflammatory diseases.*

Hypersensitivity diseases are commonly classified according to the type of immune response and the effector mechanism responsible for cell and tissue injury (Table 18–1). Immediate hypersensitivity caused by immunoglobulin E (IgE) antibodies and mast cells, which is also called type I hypersensitivity, is the most prevalent type of hypersensitivity disease and will be described separately in Chapter 19. Antibodies other than IgE can cause tissue injury by activating the complement system, recruiting inflammatory cells, and by interfering with normal cellular functions. Some of these antibodies are specific for antigens of particular cells or the extracellular matrix and are found either attached to these cells or tissues or as unbound antibodies in the circulation; the diseases induced by such antibodies are called type II hypersensitivity disorders. Other antibodies may form immune complexes in the circulation, and the complexes are subsequently deposited in tissues, particularly in blood vessels, and cause injury. Immune complex diseases are also called type III hypersensitivity. Finally, tissue injury may be due to T lymphocytes that activate the effector mechanisms of DTH or directly kill target cells; such conditions are called type IV hypersensitivity disorders. We now realize that many hyper-

Table 18–1. Classification of Immunological Diseases

Type of hypersensitivity	Pathologic immune mechanisms	Mechanisms of tissue injury and disease
Immediate hypersensitivity: Type I	IgE antibody	Mast cells and their mediators (vasoactive amines, lipid mediators, cytokines)
Antibody mediated: Type II	IgM, IgG antibodies against cell surface or extracellular matrix antigens	Opsonization and phagocytosis of cells Complement- and Fc receptor–mediated recruitment and activation of leukocytes (neutrophils, macrophages) Abnormalities in cellular functions, e.g., hormone receptor signaling
Immune complex mediated: Type III	Immune complexes of circulating antigens and IgM or IgG antibodies	Complement- and Fc receptor–mediated recruitment and activation of leukocytes
T cell mediated: Type IV	1. $CD4^+$ T cells (delayed-type hypersensitivity) 2. $CD8^+$ CTLs (T cell–mediated cytolysis)	1. Macrophage activation, cytokine-mediated inflammation 2. Direct target cell killing, cytokine-mediated inflammation

sensitivity diseases are T_H1 mediated, in which the T cells either directly cause inflammation or stimulate the production of antibodies that damage tissues and induce inflammation. Other T cell populations that promote inflammation are the IL-17–producing "T_H17" cells. In contrast, immediate hypersensitivity (allergic) diseases are the prototypes of T_H2-mediated diseases, in which the T cells stimulate the production of IgE antibodies (see Chapter 19).

In our discussion, we use descriptions that identify the pathogenic mechanisms rather than the less informative numerical designations. This classification is useful because distinct types of pathologic immune responses show different patterns of tissue injury and may vary in their tissue specificity. As a result, they produce disorders with distinct clinical and pathologic features. However, immunologic diseases in the clinical situation are often complex and due to combinations of humoral and cell-mediated immune responses and multiple effector mechanisms. This complexity is not surprising given that a single antigen may normally stimulate both humoral and cell-mediated immune responses.

DISEASES CAUSED BY ANTIBODIES

Antibody-mediated diseases are produced either by antibodies that bind to antigens in particular cells or extracellular tissues or by antigen-antibody complexes that form in the circulation and are deposited in vessel walls (Fig. 18–1). To prove that a particular disease is caused by antibodies, one would need to demonstrate that the lesions can be induced in a normal animal by the adoptive transfer of immunoglobulin purified from the blood or affected tissues of individuals with the disease. An experiment of nature is occasionally seen in children of mothers suffering from antibody-mediated diseases. These infants may be born with transient manifestations of such diseases because of transplacental passage of antibodies. However, in clinical situations, the diagnosis of diseases caused by antibodies or immune complexes is usually based on the demonstration of antibodies or immune complexes in the circulation or deposited in tissues, as well as clinicopathologic similarities with experimental diseases that are proved to be antibody mediated by adoptive transfer.

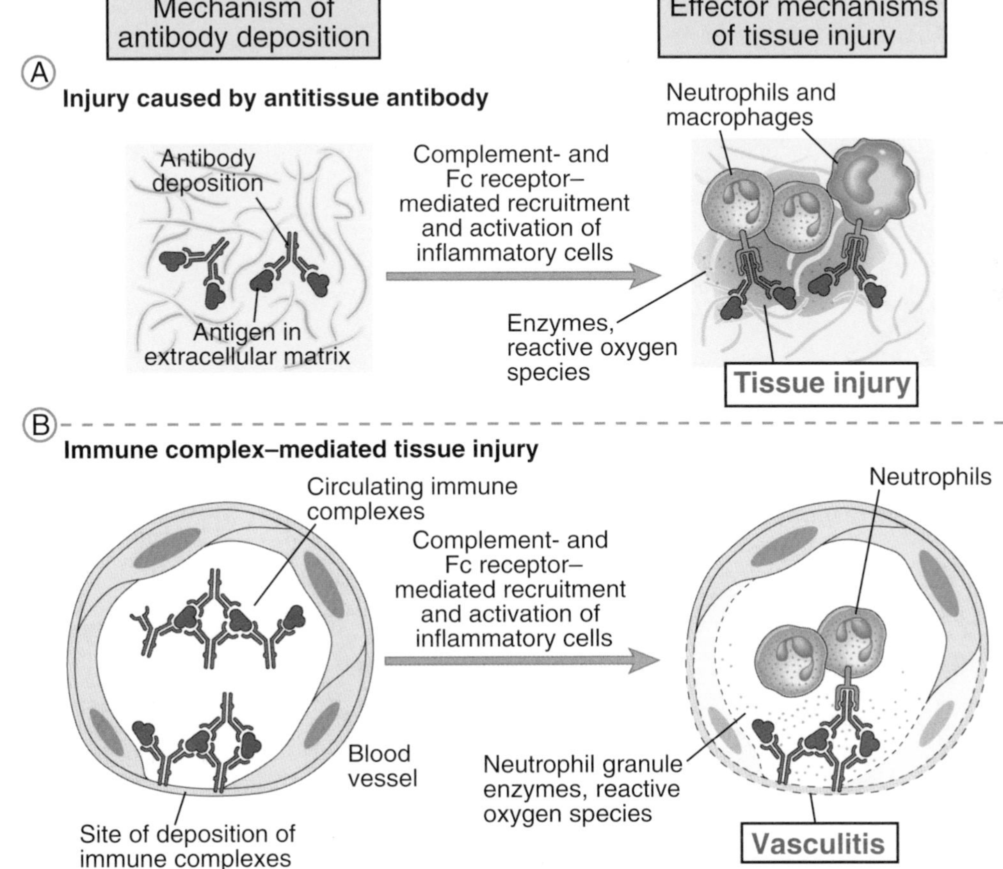

FIGURE 18–1 Types of antibody-mediated diseases. Antibodies may bind specifically to tissue antigens (A), or they may be deposited as immune complexes that are formed in the circulation (B). In both cases, the deposited antibodies induce inflammation, leading to tissue injury.

Diseases Caused by Antibodies Against Fixed Cell and Tissue Antigens

Antibodies against cellular or matrix antigens cause diseases that specifically affect the cells or tissues where these antigens are present, and these diseases are often not systemic. In most cases, such antibodies are autoantibodies, but they may occasionally be produced against a foreign antigen that is immunologically cross-reactive with a component of self tissues. Antibodies against tissue antigens cause disease by three main mechanisms (Fig. 18–2). First, antibodies may directly opsonize cells, or they may activate the complement system, resulting in the production of complement proteins that opsonize cells. These cells are phagocytosed and destroyed by phagocytes that express receptors for the Fc portions of antibodies and receptors for complement proteins. This is the principal mechanism of cell destruction in autoimmune hemolytic anemia and autoimmune thrombocytopenic purpura. The same mechanism is responsible for hemolysis in transfusion reactions. Second, antibodies deposited in tissues recruit neutrophils and macrophages, which bind to the antibodies or attached complement proteins by Fc and complement receptors. These leukocytes are activated and their products induce acute inflammation and tissue injury. This is the mechanism of injury in antibody-mediated glomerulonephritis and many other diseases. Third, antibodies that bind to normal cellular receptors or other proteins may interfere with the functions of these receptors or proteins and cause disease without inflammation or tissue damage. Antibody-mediated functional abnormalities are the cause of Graves' disease (hyperthyroidism) and myasthenia gravis. Examples of hypersensitivity diseases in humans that are caused by autoantibodies against self antigens

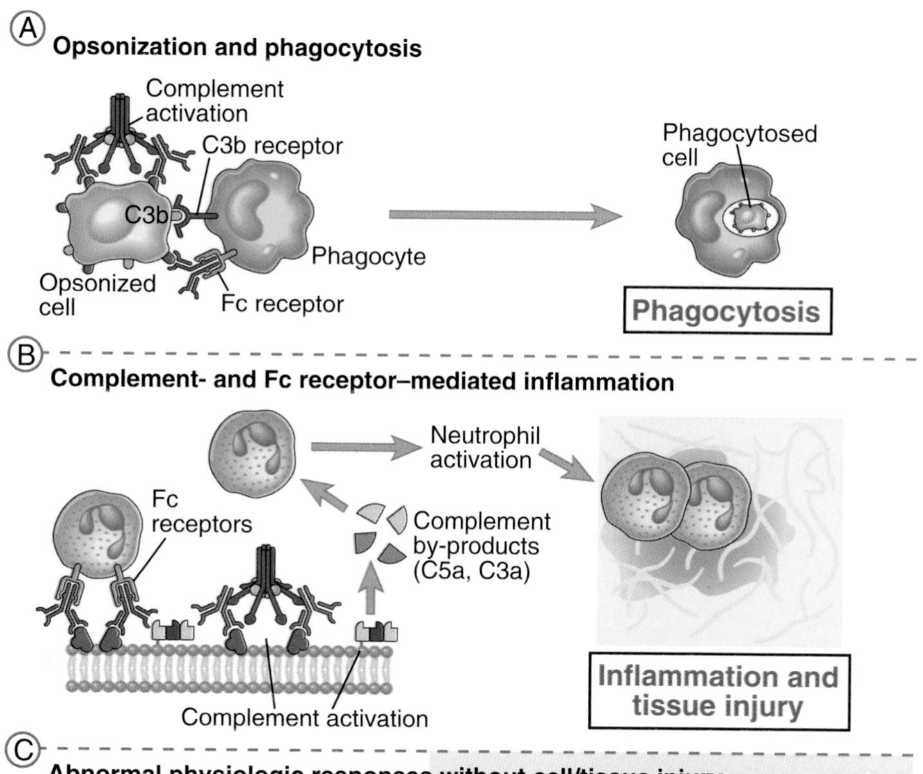

FIGURE 18–2 Effector mechanisms of antibody-mediated disease. A. Antibodies opsonize cells and may activate complement, generating complement products that also opsonize cells, leading to phagocytosis of the cells through phagocyte Fc receptors or C3 receptors. B. Antibodies recruit leukocytes by binding to Fc receptors or by activating complement and thereby releasing by-products that are chemotactic for leukocytes. C. Antibodies specific for cell surface receptors for hormones or neurotransmitters may stimulate the activity of the receptors even in the absence of the hormone *(left panel)* or may inhibit binding of the neurotransmitter to its receptor *(right panel)*. TSH, thyroid-stimulating hormone.

Table 18–2. Examples of Diseases Caused by Cell- or Tissue-Specific Antibodies

Disease	Target antigen	Mechanisms of disease	Clinicopathologic manifestations
Autoimmune hemolytic anemia	Erythrocyte membrane proteins (Rh blood group antigens, I antigen)	Opsonization and phagocytosis of erythrocytes	Hemolysis, anemia
Autoimmune thrombocytopenic purpura	Platelet membrane proteins (gpIIb:IIIa integrin)	Opsonization and phagocytosis of platelets	Bleeding
Pemphigus vulgaris	Proteins in intercellular junctions of epidermal cells (epidermal cadherin)	Antibody-mediated activation of proteases, disruption of intercellular adhesions	Skin vesicles (bullae)
Vasculitis caused by ANCA	Neutrophil granule proteins, presumably released from activated neutrophils	Neutrophil degranulation and inflammation	Vasculitis
Goodpasture's syndrome	Noncollagenous protein in basement membranes of kidney glomeruli and lung alveoli	Complement- and Fc receptor–mediated inflammation	Nephritis, lung hemorrhage
Acute rheumatic fever	Streptococcal cell wall antigen; antibody cross-reacts with myocardial antigen	Inflammation, macrophage activation	Myocarditis, arthritis
Myasthenia gravis	Acetylcholine receptor	Antibody inhibits acetylcholine binding, down-modulates receptors	Muscle weakness, paralysis
Graves' disease (hyperthyroidism)	TSH receptor	Antibody-mediated stimulation of TSH receptors	Hyperthyroidism
Insulin-resistant diabetes	Insulin receptor	Antibody inhibits binding of insulin	Hyperglycemia, ketoacidosis
Pernicious anemia	Intrinsic factor of gastric parietal cells	Neutralization of intrinsic factor, decreased absorption of vitamin B_{12}	Abnormal erythropoiesis, anemia

Abbreviations: ANCA, antineutrophil cytoplasmic antibodies; TSH, thyroid-stimulating hormone.

are listed in Table 18–2. Tissue deposits of antibodies may be detected by morphologic examination in some of these diseases, and the deposition of antibody is often associated with local complement activation, inflammation, and tissue injury (Fig. 18–3).

Immune Complex–Mediated Diseases

Immune complexes that cause disease may be composed of antibodies bound to either self antigens or foreign antigens. The pathologic features of diseases caused by immune complexes reflect the site of immune complex deposition and are not determined by the cellular source of the antigen. Therefore, immune complex–mediated diseases tend to be systemic, with little or no specificity for a particular tissue or organ.

The occurrence of diseases caused by immune complexes was suspected as early as 1911 by an astute physician named Clemens von Pirquet. At that time, diphtheria infections were being treated with serum from horses immunized with the diphtheria toxin, which is an example of passive immunization against the toxin by the transfer of serum containing antitoxin antibodies. von Pirquet noted that joint inflammation (arthritis), rash, and fever developed in patients injected with the antitoxin-containing horse serum. Two clinical features of this reaction suggested that it was not due to the infection or a toxic component of the serum itself. First, these symptoms appeared even after the injection of horse serum not containing the antitoxin, so the lesions could not be attributed to the anti-diphtheria antibody. Second, the symptoms appeared at least a week after the first injection of horse serum and more rapidly with each repeated injection. von Pirquet concluded that this disease was due to a host response to some component of the serum. He suggested that the host made antibodies to horse serum proteins, these antibodies formed complexes with the

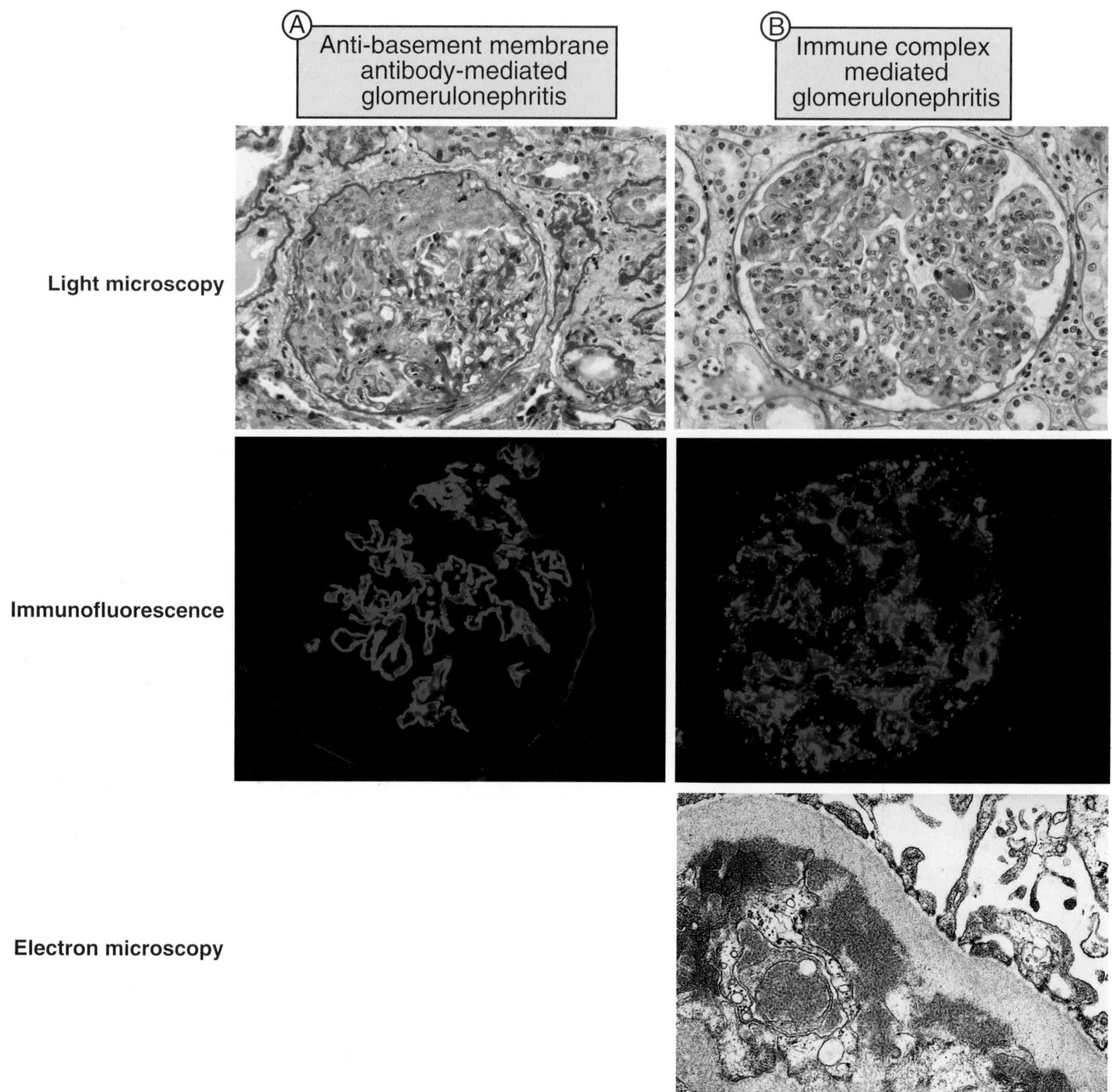

FIGURE 18–3 Pathologic features of antibody-mediated glomerulonephritis. A. Glomerulonephritis induced by an antibody against the glomerular basement membrane (Goodpasture's syndrome): the light micrograph shows glomerular inflammation and severe damage, and immunofluorescence shows smooth (linear) deposits of antibody along the basement membrane. B. Glomerulonephritis induced by the deposition of immune complexes (SLE): the light micrograph shows neutrophilic inflammation, and the immunofluorescence and electron micrograph show coarse (granular) deposits of antigen-antibody complexes along the basement membrane. (Immunofluorescence micrographs are courtesy of Dr. Jean Olson, Department of Pathology, University of California San Francisco, and the electron micrograph is courtesy of Dr. Helmut Rennke, Department of Pathology, Brigham and Women's Hospital, Boston.)

injected proteins, and the disease was due to the antibodies or immune complexes. We now know that his conclusions were entirely accurate. He called this disease serum disease; it is now more commonly known as **serum sickness** and is the prototype for systemic immune complex–mediated disorders.

- Much of our current knowledge of immune complex diseases is based on analyses of experimental models of serum sickness. Immunization of an animal such as a rabbit with a large dose of a foreign protein antigen leads to the formation of antibodies against the antigen (Fig. 18–4). These antibodies complex with circulating antigen and initially lead to enhanced phagocytosis and clearance of the antigen by macrophages in the liver and spleen. As more and more antigen-antibody complexes are formed, some of them are deposited in vascular beds. In these tissues, the antibodies in the complexes may activate complement, with a concomitant fall in serum com-

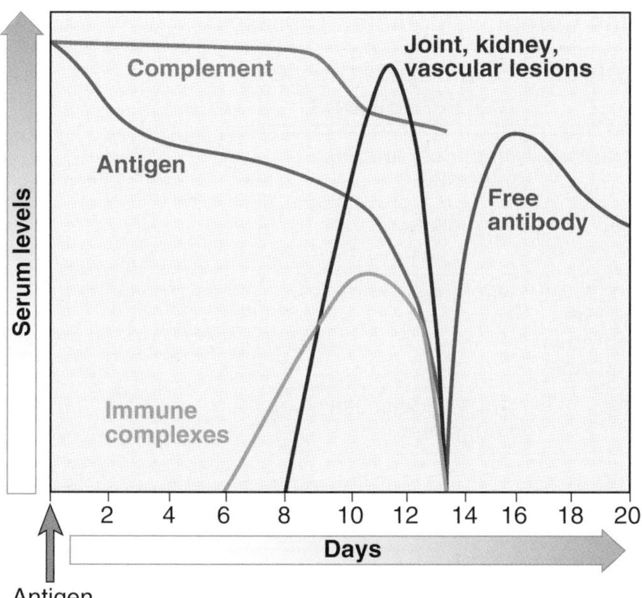

FIGURE 18–4 Sequence of immunological responses in experimental acute serum sickness. Injection of bovine serum albumin into a rabbit leads to the production of specific antibody and the formation of immune complexes. These complexes are deposited in multiple tissues, activate complement (leading to a fall in serum complement levels), and cause inflammatory lesions, which resolve as the complexes and the remaining antigen are removed. (Adapted from Cochrane CG. Immune complex-mediated tissue injury. *In* Cohen S, PA Ward, and RT McCluskey [eds]. Mechanisms of Immunopathology. Werbel & Peck, New York, 1979, pp 29–48. Copyright 1979, Wiley-Liss, Inc.)

plement levels. Complement activation leads to recruitment and activation of inflammatory cells, predominantly neutrophils, at the sites of immune complex deposition, and the neutrophils cause tissue injury. Neutrophils also bind to the immune complexes by their Fcγ receptors. Because the complexes are deposited mainly in small arteries, renal glomeruli, and the synovia of joints, the clinical and pathologic manifestations are vasculitis, nephritis, and arthritis. The clinical symptoms are usually short lived, and the lesions heal unless the antigen is injected again. This type of disease is an example of **acute serum sickness.** A more indolent and prolonged disease, called **chronic serum sickness,** is produced by multiple injections of antigen, which lead to the formation of smaller complexes that are deposited most often in the kidneys, arteries, and lungs.

- A localized form of experimental immune complex–mediated vasculitis is called the **Arthus reaction.** It is induced by injecting an antigen subcutaneously into a previously immunized animal or an animal that has been given intravenous antibody specific for the antigen. Circulating antibodies rapidly bind to the injected antigen and form immune complexes that are deposited in the walls of small arteries at the injection site. This deposition gives rise to a local cutaneous vasculitis with tissue necrosis.

Antigen-antibody complexes are produced during normal immune responses, but they cause disease only when they are produced in excessive amounts, are not efficiently cleared, and become deposited in tissues. The amount of immune complex deposition in tissues is determined by the nature of the complexes and the characteristics of the blood vessels. Small complexes are often not phagocytosed and tend to be deposited in vessels more than large complexes, which are usually cleared by phagocytes. Complexes containing cationic antigens bind avidly to negatively charged components of the basement membranes of blood vessels and kidney glomeruli. Such complexes typically produce severe and long-lasting tissue injury. Capillaries in the renal glomeruli and synovia are vessels in which plasma is ultrafiltered (to form urine and synovial fluid, respectively) by passing through the capillary wall at high hydrostatic pressure, and these locations are among the most common sites of immune complex deposition. Immune complexes may also bind to Fc receptors of mast cells and leukocytes and activate these cells to secrete cytokines and vasoactive mediators. These mediators may enhance immune complex deposition by increasing vascular permeability and blood flow.

The deposition of immune complexes in vessel walls leads to complement- and Fc receptor–mediated inflammation and injury to the vessels and adjacent tissues. Deposits of antibody and complement may be detected in the vessels, and if the antigen is known, it is possible to identify antigen molecules in the deposits as well (see Fig. 18–3). Many systemic immunologic diseases in humans are caused by the deposition of immune complexes in blood vessels (Table 18–3). A prototype of such diseases is **systemic lupus erythematosus** (SLE), an autoimmune disease in which numerous autoantibodies are produced. Its clinical manifestations include glomerulonephritis and arthritis, which are attributed to the deposition of immune complexes composed of self DNA or nucleoprotein antigens and specific antibodies (Box 18–1).

DISEASES CAUSED BY T LYMPHOCYTES

T lymphocytes injure tissues either by triggering DTH reactions or by directly killing target cells (Fig. 18–5). DTH reactions are elicited by $CD4^+$ T cells of the T_H1 subset and $CD8^+$ cells, both of which secrete cytokines that activate macrophages (interferon-γ [IFN-γ]) and induce inflammation (such as tumor necrosis factor [TNF]). The inflammatory reaction associated with T cell–mediated diseases is typically chronic inflammation. Because inflammation plays a central role in many T cell–mediated diseases, these are often referred to as "immune-mediated inflammatory diseases." In some T cell–mediated disorders, $CD8^+$ cytotoxic T lymphocytes (CTLs) kill target cells bearing class I major histocompatibility complex (MHC)-associated antigens. The T cells that cause tissue injury may be autoreactive, or they may be specific for

Table 18–3. Examples of Human Immune Complex–Mediated Diseases

Disease	Antigen involved	Clinicopathologic manifestations
Systemic lupus erythematosus	DNA, nucleoproteins, others	Nephritis, arthritis, vasculitis
Polyarteritis nodosa	Hepatitis B virus surface antigen	Vasculitis
Poststreptococcal glomerulonephritis	Streptococcal cell wall antigen(s); may be "planted" in glomerular basement membrane	Nephritis
Serum sickness	Various proteins	Arthritis, vasculitis, nephritis

foreign protein antigens that are present in or bound to cells or tissues. T lymphocyte–mediated tissue injury may also accompany strong protective immune responses against persistent microbes, especially intracellular microbes that resist eradication by phagocytes and antibodies.

A role for T cells in causing a particular immunologic disease is suspected largely based on the demonstration of T cells in lesions and the isolation of T cells specific for self or microbial antigens from the tissues or blood of patients. Animal models have also been very useful for elucidating the pathogenesis of these disorders.

Diseases Caused by Delayed-Type Hypersensitivity

In DTH reactions, tissue injury results from the products of activated macrophages, such as lysosomal enzymes, reactive oxygen intermediates, nitric oxide, and proinflammatory cytokines (see Chapter 13). Vascular endothelial cells in the lesions may express enhanced levels of cytokine-regulated surface proteins such as adhesion molecules and class II MHC molecules. Chronic DTH reactions often produce fibrosis as a result of the secretion of cytokines and growth factors by the macrophages.

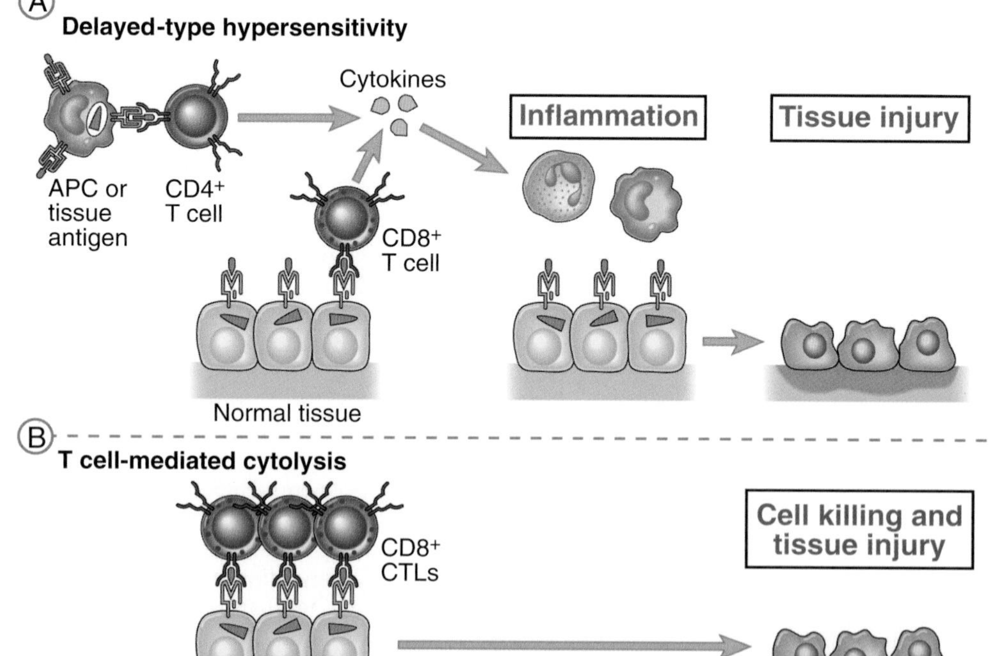

FIGURE 18–5 Mechanisms of T cell–mediated diseases. A. In delayed-type hypersensitivity reactions, $CD4^+$ T cells (and sometimes $CD8^+$ cells) respond to tissue antigens by secreting cytokines that stimulate inflammation and activate phagocytes, leading to tissue injury. APC, antigen-presenting cell. B. In some diseases, $CD8^+$ CTLs directly kill tissue cells.

Box 18–1 ▪ IN DEPTH: SYSTEMIC LUPUS ERYTHEMATOSUS

CLINICAL FEATURES. SLE is a chronic, remitting and relapsing, multisystem autoimmune disease that affects predominantly women, with an incidence of 1 in 700 among women between the ages of 20 and 60 years (about 1 in 250 among black women) and a female-to-male ratio of 10:1. The principal clinical manifestations are rashes, arthritis, and glomerulonephritis, but hemolytic anemia, thrombocytopenia, and CNS involvement are also common. Many different autoantibodies are found in patients with SLE. The most frequent are antinuclear, particularly anti-DNA, antibodies; others include antibodies against ribonucleoproteins, histones, and nucleolar antigens. Immune complexes formed from these autoantibodies and their specific antigens are responsible for glomerulonephritis, arthritis, and vasculitis involving small arteries throughout the body. Hemolytic anemia and thrombocytopenia are due to autoantibodies against erythrocytes and platelets, respectively. The principal diagnostic test for the disease is the presence of antinuclear antibodies; antibodies against double-stranded native DNA are specific for SLE.

PATHOGENESIS. The pathogenic antibodies in the disease are high-affinity, helper T cell–dependent antibodies specific for nuclear components. It is not known whether the primary pathogenic defect is failure of central or peripheral tolerance in B lymphocytes, in helper T cells, or in both. It is thought that the antigens that elicit autoantibody production are released from apoptotic cells, which is one reason that exposure to ultraviolet light (which promotes apoptosis) exacerbates disease. A current model for the pathogenesis of the disease is that apoptotic cells are not cleared efficiently, resulting in persistence of nuclear antigens. Together with failure of self-tolerance, this results in the production of antibodies against nuclear proteins and the formation of immune complexes. Genetic factors also contribute to the disease. The relative risk for individuals with HLA-DR2 or HLA-DR3 is 2 to 3, and if both haplotypes are present, the relative risk is about 5. Deficiencies of classical pathway complement proteins, especially C1q, C2, or C4, are seen in about 10% of patients with SLE. The complement deficiencies may result in defective clearance of immune complexes and apoptotic cells. Studies with mice also suggest a role of complement proteins in displaying self antigens and maintaining B cell tolerance. Interestingly, the peripheral blood lymphocytes of patients show evidence of excessive production and response to type I IFNs. What this cytokine has to do with the development of the disease remains unknown. Recent studies suggest that engagement of Toll-like recepters by RNA and DNA may play a role in activating B cells to produce antibodies against these nucleic acids and nucleoproteins. A duplication in TLR7 may be a susceptibility gene for lupus in the BXSB mouse strain, described below.

ANIMAL MODELS. Several inbred mouse strains in which lupus-like autoimmune diseases spontaneously develop have provided valuable experimental systems for analyzing the pathogenesis of this disorder. The first to be described and the ones most like SLE are the NZB strain and (NZB × NZW)F_1. Kidney lesions and hemolytic anemia develop in female mice, and anti-DNA autoantibodies are produced spontaneously. The B cells of (NZB × NZW)F_1 mice are hyperresponsive to foreign antigens as well as to polyclonal activators and cytokines, and autoantibody production is dependent on pathogenic helper T cells reactive with nucleosomal peptides. The activation of B cells may also involve engagement of Toll-like receptors (TLR-9) by nuclear DNA, perhaps complexed with antibody. Extensive breeding studies have shown that MHC genes from the NZW parent and non-MHC genes inherited from both parental strains contribute to development of the disease. Attempts are being made to define the susceptibility genes in these mice.

Mice with mutations in either the Fas or Fas ligand genes develop an autoimmune disease with some resemblance to SLE. The *lpr* and *gld* genes are mutant alleles of the Fas and Fas ligand genes, respectively, and the mouse strains that are homozygous for these mutant alleles have greatly reduced expression of Fas or nonfunctional Fas ligand. Both *lpr* and *gld* mice produce multiple autoantibodies, especially anti-DNA antibodies, and develop immune complex nephritis. Severe lymphadenopathy also develops in these inbred strains because of the accumulation of an unusual population of functionally inert $CD3^+CD4^-CD8^-$ T cells. Because of the defect in Fas or Fas ligand in these mice, anergic B cells cannot be eliminated by Fas-mediated killing, and self-reactive helper T cells may survive for abnormally long times, as well. The disease of *lpr* and *gld* mice is also influenced by background genes in that it is more severe in an inbred strain called MRL than in any other. A phenotypically similar human disease called the autoimmune lymphoproliferative syndrome is caused by mutations in the gene encoding Fas that abolish the ability of this death receptor to deliver apoptotic signals. No evidence for Fas or Fas ligand abnormalities has been demonstrated in typical SLE.

A third inbred strain in which a lupus-like disease develops is a recombinant strain called BXSB; disease susceptibility in this strain is linked to the Y chromosome, and only males are affected. These mice produce anti-antibodies against nuclear antigens, and severe nephritis and vasculitis develop.

Another mutant mouse strain, called the viable moth-eaten mouse (because of skin lesions), also produces high levels of autoantibodies. The moth-eaten mouse carries a mutation of the tyrosine phosphatase SHP-1, which associates with several receptors that serve negative regulatory functions in cells of the immune system. The signal transduction abnormalities caused by the phosphatase mutation and the mechanism of autoantibody production in moth-eaten mice are not well defined. Knockout of the inhibitory Fc receptor, FcγRIIb, also causes a lupus-like disease in mice.

Transgenic mouse models of lupus have been created in which an antibody against self DNA is expressed in B cells as a transgene. These models are useful for studying the control of self-reactive B cells.

Many organ-specific autoimmune diseases are caused by DTH reactions induced by autoreactive T cells (Table 18–4). In **type 1 diabetes mellitus** (T1D) (Box 18–2), infiltrates of lymphocytes and macrophages are found around the islets of Langerhans in the pancreas, with destruction of insulin-producing β cells in the islets and a resultant deficiency in insulin production. In animal models of T1D, the disease can be transferred to young, prediseased animals by injecting T cells from older diseased animals. **Multiple sclerosis** (MS) is an autoimmune disease of the central nervous system (CNS) in which $CD4^+$ T cells of the T_H1 and/or T_H17 subset react against self myelin antigens (Box 18–3). The DTH reaction results in the activation of macrophages around nerves in the brain and spinal cord, destruction of the myelin, abnormalities in nerve conduction, and neurologic deficits. An animal model of MS is **experimental autoimmune encephalomyelitis** (EAE), induced by immunization with protein antigens of CNS myelin in adjuvant. Such immunization leads to an autoimmune T cell response against myelin. EAE can be transferred to naive animals with myelin antigen-specific $CD4^+$ T cells, and the disease can be prevented by treating immunized animals with antibodies specific for class II MHC or for CD4 molecules, indicating that $CD4^+$ class II MHC-restricted T cells play an obligatory role in this disorder. **Rheumatoid arthritis** (Box 18–4) is a systemic disease affecting the small joints and many other tissues. A role for T cell–mediated inflammation is suspected in this disease because of its similarity to animal models in which arthritis is known to be caused by T cells specific for joint collagen. Antibodies may also contribute to joint inflammation in this disease. Antagonists against the inflammatory cytokine TNF have a beneficial effect in rheumatoid arthritis.

Cell-mediated immune responses to microbes and other foreign antigens may also lead to tissue injury at the sites of infection or antigen exposure. Intracellular bacteria such as *Mycobacterium tuberculosis* induce strong T cell and macrophage responses that result in granulomatous inflammation and fibrosis; the inflammation and fibrosis may cause extensive tissue destruction and functional impairment, in this case in the lungs. Tuberculosis is a good example of an infectious disease in which tissue injury is mainly due to the host immune response (see Chapter 15). A variety of skin diseases that result from topical exposure to chemicals and environmental antigens, called **contact sensitivity,** are due to DTH reactions, presumably against neoantigens formed by the binding of the chemicals to self proteins.

Inflammatory bowel disease (IBD) consists of a group of disorders, including Crohn disease and ulcerative colitis, in which an immunologic etiology has been suspected for many years. Crohn disease is an inflammatory disease caused by T cells that presumably react against intestinal microbes as well as self antigens. About 25% of patients with this disease have mutations in NOD2, an intracellular sensor of microbial products (see Chapter 2). The pathogenetic link between NOD2 mutations and the disease is still not understood. Recent

Table 18–4. Examples of T Cell–Mediated Immunological Diseases

Disease	Specificity of pathogenic T cells	Human disease	Animal models
Type I (insulin-dependent) diabetes mellitus	Islet cell antigens (insulin, glutamic acid decarboxylase, others)	Yes; specificity of T cells not established	NOD mouse, BB rat, transgenic mouse models
Rheumatoid arthritis	Unknown antigen in joint synovium	Yes; specificity of T cells and role of antibody not established	Collagen-induced arthritis, others
Multiple sclerosis, experimental autoimmune encephalomyelitis	Myelin basic protein, proteolipid protein	Yes; T cells recognize myelin antigens	EAE induced by immunization with CNS myelin antigens; TCR transgenic models
Inflammatory bowel disease (Crohn's, ulcerative colitis)	Unknown	Yes	Colitis induced by depletion of regulatory T cells, knockout of IL-10
Peripheral neuritis	P2 protein of peripheral nerve myelin	Guillain-Barre syndrome	Induced by immunization with peripheral nerve myelin antigens
Autoimmune myocarditis	Myocardial proteins	Yes (post-viral myocarditis); specificity of T cells not established	Induced by immunization with myosin or infection by Coxsackie virus

Abbreviations: CNS, central nervous system; NOD nonobese diabetic; TCR, T cell receptor

Box 18–2 ■ IN DEPTH: TYPE 1 DIABETES MELLITUS

T1D, previously called insulin-dependent diabetes mellitus (IDDM), is a multisystem metabolic disease resulting from impaired insulin production. The disease is characterized by hyperglycemia and ketoacidosis. Chronic complications of T1D include progressive atherosclerosis of arteries, which can lead to ischemic necrosis of limbs and internal organs, and microvascular obstruction causing damage to the retina, renal glomeruli, and peripheral nerves. The relationship of abnormal glucose metabolism and vascular lesions is not known. Type 1 diabetes affects about 0.2% of the U.S. population, with a peak age at onset of 11 to 12 years, and the incidence is increasing. These patients have a deficiency of insulin resulting from destruction of the insulin-producing β cells of the islets of Langerhans in the pancreas, and continuous hormone replacement therapy is needed.

Several mechanisms may contribute to β cell destruction, including DTH reactions mediated by $CD4^+$ T_H1 cells reactive with islet antigens (including insulin), CTL-mediated lysis of islet cells, local production of cytokines (TNF and IL-1) that damage islet cells, and autoantibodies against islet cells. In the rare cases in which the pancreatic lesions have been examined at the early active stages of the disease, the islets show cellular necrosis and lymphocytic infiltration. This lesion is called insulitis. The infiltrates consist of both $CD4^+$ and $CD8^+$ T cells. Surviving islet cells often express class II MHC molecules, probably an effect of local production of IFN-γ by the T cells. Autoantibodies against islet cells and insulin are also detected in the blood of these patients. These antibodies may participate in causing the disease or may be a result of T cell–mediated injury and release of normally sequestered antigens. In susceptible children who have not developed diabetes (such as relatives of patients), the presence of antibodies against islet cells is predictive of the development of T1D. This suggests that the anti–islet cell antibodies contribute to injury to the islets.

Multiple genes are involved in T1D. A great deal of attention has been devoted to the role of HLA genes. Ninety percent to 95% of whites with T1D have HLA-DR3, or DR4, or both, in contrast to about 40% of normal subjects, and 40% to 50% of patients are DR3/DR4 heterozygotes, in contrast to 5% of normal subjects. Interestingly, susceptibility to T1D is actually associated with alleles of DQ2 and DQ8 that are often in linkage disequilibrium with DR3 and DR4. Sequencing of DQ molecules associated with diabetes has led to the hypothesis that development of T1D is influenced by the structure of the DQ peptide-binding cleft, with one particular residue (residue 57) playing a significant role. Despite the high relative risk for T1D in individuals with particular class II alleles, most persons who inherit these alleles do not develop the disease.

Non-HLA genes also contribute to the disease. The first of these to be identified is insulin, with tandem repeats in the promoter region being associated with disease susceptibility. The mechanism of this association is unknown; it may be related to the level of expression of insulin in the thymus, which determines whether or not insulin-specific T cells will be deleted (negatively selected) during maturation. Several polymorphisms have been identified in the NOD mouse model, including one believed to be in the IL-2 gene. The functional consequences of this polymorphism are not known. Some studies have suggested that viral infections (e.g., with coxsackievirus B4) may precede the onset of T1D, perhaps by initiating cell injury, inducing inflammation and the expression of costimulators, and triggering an autoimmune response. However, epidemiologic data suggest that repeated infections protect against T1D, and this is similar to the NOD model. In fact, it has been postulated that one reason for the increased incidence of T1D in developed countries is the control of infectious diseases.

ANIMAL MODELS OF SPONTANEOUS T1D. The NOD mouse strain develops a spontaneous T cell–mediated insulitis, which is followed by overt diabetes. Disease can be transferred to young NOD mice with T cells from older, affected animals. As mentioned earlier, the linkage of this disease with the MHC is remarkably similar to the HLA linkage of T1D in humans. In NOD mice, disease is induced by diabetogenic T cells that may recognize various islet antigens, including insulin and an islet cell enzyme called glutamic acid decarboxylase. Induction of T cell tolerance to these antigens retards the onset of diabetes in NOD mice. The underlying abnormalities in NOD mice that lead to autoimmunity include defective negative selection of self-reactive T cells in the thymus and reduced numbers of regulatory T cells in peripheral tissues. Another animal model of the disease is the BB rat, in which insulitis and diabetes are associated with lymphopenia.

TRANSGENIC MOUSE MODELS OF T1D. Several different transgenic models have been created by expressing transgenes in pancreatic islet β cells by introducing these genes into mice under the control of insulin promoters. Allogeneic class I and class II MHC molecules can be expressed in islet cells to test the hypothesis that this will create an endogenous "allograft" that should be attacked by the immune system. Insulitis does not develop in these mice because T cells specific for the allogeneic MHC molecules become tolerant, in part because the insulin promoter is leaky and the alloantigens are expressed in the thymus. Expression of the costimulator B7-1 in islet cells increases susceptibility to insulitis (see text). In some models, if both allogeneic MHC molecules and IL-2 are expressed in islets, insulitis does develop, probably because local IL-2 production breaks T cell anergy and initiates an allogeneic reaction against the islets. Other model protein antigens have also been expressed in islet β cells, and the reaction of T cells to these antigens has been studied as a model for T1D.

A different transgenic model involves expressing in T cells a T cell receptor (TCR) specific for an islet β cell antigen. As these mice age, they develop insulitis and diabetes. A variation of this approach is to express a model protein antigen in the islets and introduce into these antigen-expressing mice T cells from TCR transgenic mice expressing receptors specific for that antigen. These models are valuable for studying T cell tolerance and responses to tissue antigens.

Box 18–3 ▪ IN DEPTH: MULTIPLE SCLEROSIS AND EXPERIMENTAL AUTOIMMUNE ENCEPHALOMYELITIS

MS is the most common neurologic disease of young adults. On pathologic examination, there is inflammation in the CNS white matter with secondary demyelination. The disease is characterized clinically by weakness, paralysis, and ocular symptoms with exacerbations and remissions; CNS imaging suggests that in patients with active disease, there is frequent new lesion formation. The disease is modeled by EAE in mice, rats, guinea pigs, and nonhuman primates, and this is one of the best characterized experimental models of an organ-specific autoimmune disease mediated mainly by T lymphocytes. EAE is induced by immunizing animals with antigens normally present in CNS myelin, such as myelin basic protein (MBP), proteolipid protein (PLP), and myelin oligodendrocyte glycoprotein (MOG), with an adjuvant containing heat-killed mycobacterium, which is necessary for eliciting a strong T cell response. About 1 to 2 weeks after immunization, animals develop an encephalomyelitis, characterized by perivascular infiltrates composed of lymphocytes and macrophages in the CNS white matter, followed by demyelination. The severity of the lesions depends on the animal species, antigen, and adjuvant. The neurologic lesions can be mild and self-limited or chronic and relapsing.

In mice, EAE is caused by activated, $CD4^+$ T cells specific for MBP, PLP, or MOG. This has been established by many lines of experimental evidence. Mice immunized with MBP or PLP contain $CD4^+$ T cells that secrete IL-2 and IFN-γ and proliferate in response to that antigen *in vitro.* The disease can be transferred to naive animals by $CD4^+$ T cells from MBP- or PLP-immunized syngeneic animals or with MBP- or PLP-specific cloned $CD4^+$ T cell lines. Although it has been accepted for many years that the pathogenic T cells are T_H1 cells, recent studies have indicated that IL-17–producing T_H17 cells also contribute to the devleopment of EAE in mice. In humans, T cells specific for myelin proteins can be isolated from the peripheral blood of normal subjects as well as from patients with MS; however, as predicted by the EAE model, the myelin-reactive T cells derived from patients with MS are in an activated state compared with those from normal subjects, which appear to be naive.

Disease-causing T cells in EAE express high levels of the β_1 integrin very late antigen-4 (VLA-4). The infiltration of T cells into the CNS is thought to depend on the binding of VLA-4 to its ligand, vascular cell adhesion molecule-1 (VCAM-1), on microvascular endothelium. Studies in EAE have demonstrated that monoclonal antibodies blocking the VLA-4–VCAM interaction block the onset of EAE. Similarly, blocking VLA-4 can significantly prevent the onset of new lesions in MS patients. However, in rare patients, blocking T cell traffic into the brain has allowed secondary viral infections to occur in the CNS, with serious consequences.

The sequence of events in the development of EAE, and by analogy MS, is thought to be the following. Potentially autoreactive T cells specific for myelin proteins are present in the circulation of normal individuals. Immunization with a myelin antigen together with an adjuvant leads to T cell activation against epitopes of autologous myelin proteins. Activated T cells traffic into the CNS more readily than do naive cells. In the CNS, the activated T cells encounter myelin proteins and release cytokines that recruit and activate macrophages and other T cells, leading to myelin destruction. The disease is propagated by the process known as epitope spreading. Within weeks after the onset of EAE, there is tissue breakdown with release of new protein epitopes; local antigen-presenting cells in the CNS itself express high levels of class II MHC and costimulatory molecules. Thus, the immunologically activated brain tissue induces the activation of autoreactive T cells recognizing many myelin proteins other than the antigen that triggered the disease. The clinical relevance of the phenomenon is that by the time patients present to the clinic, there is unlikely to be a single antigen driving the disease.

EAE has been used to analyze the fine specificity of myelin-reactive encephalitogenic T cells and to help define immunodominant regions of myelin proteins that may be relevant to MS in humans. Mutational analysis of various MBP and PLP peptides has shown that some amino acid residues are critical for binding to MHC molecules and others for recognition by T cells. Altered peptide ligands may be produced by introducing conservative substitutions in the TCR contact residues of MBP or PLP. Administration of such mutant peptides blocks the induction of EAE. It is thought that the altered peptide ligands induce anergy in T cells specific for native MBP or PLP or stimulate the development of anti-inflammatory T_H2 cells specific for these myelin antigens. This approach has recently been tried in patients with MS. TCR contact residues identified in an immunodominant MBP peptide were modified to produce an APL, and the APL was injected into patients. At high antigen doses, a subset of patients experienced a flare-up of the disease associated with very high frequencies of MBP-reactive T cells that were cross-reactive with the native self antigen. These unfortunate results provide strong evidence that flare-ups of MS are related to T cell responses to myelin proteins.

Both EAE and MS have strong genetic components and occur only in genetically susceptible hosts. Identical twins have a 25% to 40% concordance rate for development of MS, whereas nonidentical twins have a 1% concordance rate. In both mice and humans, certain MHC haplotypes have been linked to the disease.

Box 18–4 ▪ IN DEPTH: RHEUMATOID ARTHRITIS

Rheumatoid arthritis is an inflammatory disease involving small joints of the extremities, particularly of the fingers, as well as larger joints including shoulders, elbows, knees, and ankles. Rheumatoid arthritis is characterized by inflammation of the synovium associated with destruction of the joint cartilage and bone, with a morphologic picture suggestive of a local immune response. Both cell-mediated and humoral immune responses may contribute to development of synovitis. $CD4^+$ T cells, activated B lymphocytes, plasma cells, and macrophages, as well as other inflammatory cells, are found in the inflamed synovium, and in severe cases, well-formed lymphoid follicles with germinal centers may be present. Numerous cytokines, including IL-1, IL-8, TNF, and IFN-γ, have been detected in the synovial (joint) fluid. Cytokines, especially TNF, are believed to activate resident synovial cells to produce proteolytic enzymes, such as collagenase, that mediate destruction of the cartilage, ligaments, and tendons of the joints. Many of the cytokines thought to play a role in initiating joint destruction are probably produced as a result of local T cell and macrophage activation. Antagonists against TNF have proved to be of benefit in patients, and soluble TNF receptor as well as anti-TNF antibody are now approved for treatment of the disease. The bone destruction in rheumatoid arthritis is due to increased osteoclast activity in the joints, and this may be related to the production of the TNF family cytokine RANK (receptor activator of nuclear factor κB) ligand by activated T cells. RANK ligand binds to RANK, a member of the TNF receptor family that is expressed on osteoclast precursors, and induces their differentiation and activation. The specificity of the T cells that may be involved in the pathogenesis of arthritis and the nature of the initiating antigen are not known. Significant numbers of T cells expressing the $\gamma\delta$ antigen receptor have also been detected in the synovial fluid of some patients with rheumatoid arthritis. However, the pathogenic role of this subset of T cells, like their physiologic function, is obscure.

Systemic complications of rheumatoid arthritis include vasculitis, presumably caused by immune complexes, and lung injury. The nature of the antigen or the antibodies in these complexes is not known. Patients with the adult form of rheumatoid arthritis frequently have circulating antibodies, which may be IgM or IgG, reactive with the Fc (and rarely Fab) portions of their own IgG molecules. These autoantibodies are called rheumatoid factors, and their presence is used as a diagnostic test for rheumatoid arthritis. Rheumatoid factors may participate in the formation of injurious immune complexes, but their pathogenic role is not established. Although activated B cells and plasma cells are often present in the synovia of affected joints, the specificities of the antibodies produced by these cells or their roles in causing joint lesions are not known. Susceptibility to rheumatoid arthritis is linked to the HLA-DR4 haplotype and less so to DR1 and DRW1D. In all these alleles, the amino acid sequences from positions 65 to 75 of the β chain are nearly identical. These residues are located in or close to the peptide-binding clefts of the HLA molecules, suggesting that they influence antigen presentation or T cell recognition.

There are several experimental models of arthritis. MRL/lpr mice develop spontaneous arthritis and have high serum levels of rheumatoid factors. The immune mechanisms of joint disease in MRL/lpr mice are not known. T cell–mediated arthritis can be induced in susceptible strains of mice and rats by immunization with type II collagen (the type found in cartilage), and the disease can be adoptively transferred to unimmunized animals with collagen-specific T cells. However, in the human disease, there is no convincing evidence for collagen-specific autoimmunity. An antibody-mediated arthritis that mimics some aspects of rheumatoid arthritis is seen in a TCR transgenic strain of mice called K/B × N. In this model, autoantibodies that recognize the ubiquitous cytoplasmic enzyme glucose-6-phosphate isomerase mediate inflammation specifically on articular surfaces. Experimental arthritis can also be produced by immunization with various bacterial antigens, including mycobacterial and streptococcal cell wall proteins. However, such diseases bear little resemblance to human rheumatoid arthritis.

studies suggest that a mutation in the gene encoding the IL-23 receptor is strongly associated with IBD. IL-23 is the cytokine that enhances T_H17 responses, and T_H17 cells may be involved in the inflammatory lesions of IBD. It is not known if the IL-23R mutation influences this reaction. Several mouse models of IBD suggest that deficiency of regulatory T cells may be involved in the excessive reactions to enteric bacteria.

Although T cell–induced chronic inflammation is believed to be the common pathogenetic basis for all these diseases, recent therapeutic trials suggest that there may be subtle differences in the pathogenesis of these diseases. For instance, TNF antagonists are beneficial in patients with rheumatoid arthritis and Crohn's disease but not multiple sclerosis. Also, as mentioned earlier in the chapter, T cells may play an indirect role in antibody-mediated diseases by activating self-reactive B lymphocytes.

Diseases Caused by Cytotoxic T Lymphocytes

CTL responses to viral infection can lead to tissue injury by killing infected cells, even if the virus itself has no cytopathic effects. The principal physiologic function of CTLs is to eliminate intracellular microbes, primarily viruses, by killing infected cells. Some viruses directly injure infected cells and are said to be cytopathic, whereas others are not. Because CTLs cannot distinguish *a priori* between cytopathic and noncytopathic viruses, they kill virally infected cells regardless of whether the infection itself is harmful to the host. Examples of viral infections in which the lesions are due to the host CTL response and not the virus itself include lymphocytic choriomeningitis in mice and certain forms of viral hepatitis in humans (see Chapter 15).

Few examples of autoimmune diseases mediated only by CTLs have been documented. Myocarditis with infiltration of the heart by $CD8^+$ T cells develops in mice, and sometimes in humans, infected with coxsackievirus B. The infected animals contain virus-specific, class I MHC-restricted CTLs as well as CTLs that kill uninfected myocardial cells. It is postulated that the heart lesions are initiated by the virus infection and virus-specific CTLs, and myocardial injury leads to the exposure or alteration of self antigens and the subsequent development of autoreactive CTLs. CTLs may also contribute to tissue injury in disorders that are caused primarily by $CD4^+$ T cells, such as type 1 diabetes.

Pathogenesis of Autoimmunity

The possibility that an individual's immune system may react against autologous antigens and cause tissue injury was appreciated by immunologists from the time that the specificity of the immune system for foreign antigens was recognized. In the early 1900s, Paul Ehrlich coined the rather melodramatic phrase "horror autotoxicus" for harmful ("toxic") immune reactions against self. When Macfarlane Burnet proposed the clonal selection hypothesis about 50 years later, he added the corollary that clones of autoreactive lymphocytes were deleted during development to prevent autoimmune reactions. We now know that the key events in the development of autoimmunity are the recognition of self antigens by autoreactive lymphocytes, the activation of these cells to proliferate and differentiate into effector cells, and the tissue injury caused by the effector cells and their products. How self-tolerance fails and self-reactive lymphocytes are activated are the fundamental issues in autoimmunity and likely to be the basis for understanding the pathogenesis of these diseases.

Autoimmunity is an important cause of disease in humans and is estimated to affect 2% to 5% of the U.S. population. The term *autoimmunity* is often erroneously used for any disease in which immune reactions accompany tissue injury, even though it may be difficult or impossible to establish a role for immune responses to self antigens in causing these disorders. Our understanding of autoimmunity has improved greatly during the past two decades, mainly because of the development of a variety of animal models of these diseases and the identification of genes that may predispose to autoimmunity. Nevertheless, the etiology of most human autoimmune diseases remains obscure, and understanding these disorders is a major challenge in immunology.

Several important general concepts have emerged from analyses of autoimmunity.

- ***Autoimmunity results from a failure or breakdown of the mechanisms normally responsible for maintaining self-tolerance in B cells, T cells, or both.*** The potential for autoimmunity exists in all individuals because during their development, lymphocytes may express receptors specific for self antigens, and many self antigens are readily accessible to the immune system. As discussed in Chapter 11, tolerance to self antigens is normally maintained by selection processes that prevent the maturation of some self antigen–specific lymphocytes and by mechanisms that inactivate or delete self-reactive lymphocytes that do mature. Loss of self-tolerance may result from abnormal selection or regulation of self-reactive lymphocytes and by abnormalities in the way that self antigens are presented to the immune system.

  Much recent attention has focused on the role of T cells in autoimmunity, for two main reasons. First, helper T cells are the key regulators of all immune responses to proteins. Second, several autoimmune diseases are genetically linked to the MHC (the HLA complex in humans), and the function of MHC molecules is to present peptide antigens to T cells. Therefore, it is believed that failure of T cell tolerance is an important mechanism of autoimmune diseases. Failure of self-tolerance in T lymphocytes may result in autoimmune diseases in which the lesions are caused by cell-mediated immune reactions. Helper T cell abnormalities may also lead to autoantibody production because helper T cells are necessary for the production of high-affinity antibodies against protein antigens.

- ***The major factors that contribute to the development of autoimmunity are genetic susceptibility and environmental triggers, such as infections.*** Susceptibility genes and infections both contribute to the breakdown of self-tolerance, and infections in tissues promote the influx of autoreactive lymphocytes and activation of these cells, resulting in tissue injury (Fig. 18–6). Infections and tissue injury may also alter the way in which self antigens are displayed to the immune system, leading to failure of self-tolerance. The roles of these factors in the development of autoimmunity are discussed later.

- ***Autoimmune diseases may be either systemic or organ specific.*** For instance, the formation of circulating immune complexes composed of self antigens and specific antibodies typically produces systemic diseases, such as SLE. In contrast, autoantibody or T cell responses against self antigens with restricted tissue distribution lead to organ-specific diseases, such as myasthenia gravis, T1D, and MS.

- ***Various effector mechanisms are responsible for tissue injury in different autoimmune diseases.*** These mechanisms include immune complexes, circulating autoantibodies, and autoreactive T lymphocytes and are discussed earlier in the chapter.

- Autoimmune reactions initiated against one self antigen that injure tissues may result in the release

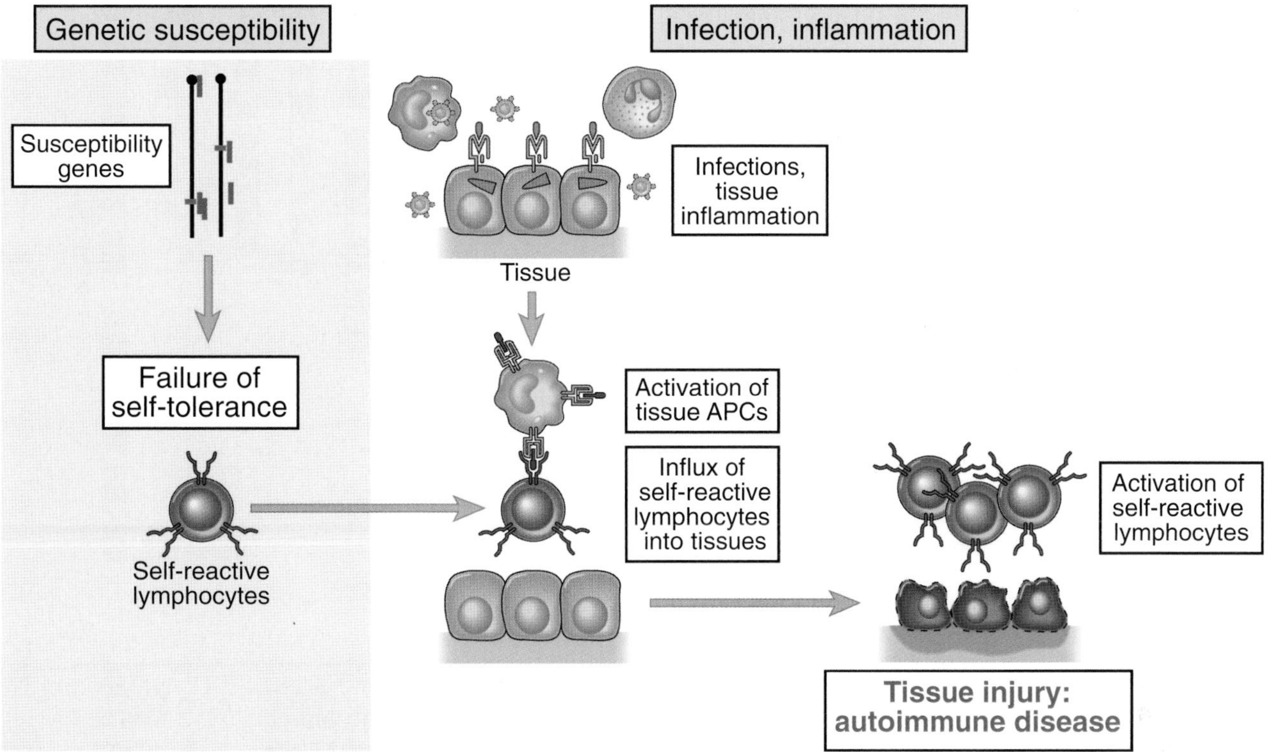

FIGURE 18–6 Postulated mechanisms of autoimmunity. In this proposed model of an organ-specific T cell–mediated autoimmune disease, various genetic loci may confer susceptibility to autoimmunity, in part by influencing the maintenance of self-tolerance. Environmental triggers, such as infections and other inflammatory stimuli, promote the influx of lymphocytes into tissues and the activation of self-reactive T cells, resulting in tissue injury.

and alterations of other tissue antigens, activation of lymphocytes specific for these other antigens, and exacerbation of the disease. This phenomenon is called **epitope spreading**, and it may explain why once an autoimmune disease has developed, it tends to be chronic and often progressive.

In the following section, we describe the general principles of the pathogenesis of autoimmune diseases, with an emphasis on susceptibility genes, infections, and other factors that contribute to the development of autoimmunity.

Genetic Susceptibility to Autoimmunity

From the earliest studies of autoimmune diseases in patients and experimental animals, it has been appreciated that these diseases have a strong genetic component. For instance, T1D (see Box 18–2) shows a concordance of 35% to 50% in monozygotic twins and 5% to 6% in dizygotic twins. Much more has been learned about the genes involved in autoimmune diseases by linkage analyses in families, breeding studies in animal models, and genome scanning methods exploiting the large amount of information that has been developed about human and mouse genome sequences.

Most autoimmune diseases are polygenic, and affected individuals inherit multiple genetic polymorphisms that contribute to disease susceptibility. Some of these polymorphisms are associated with several autoimmune diseases, suggesting that the causative genes influence general mechanisms of immune regulation and self-tolerance. Other loci are associated with particular diseases, suggesting that they affect end-organ damage (Fig. 18–7). It is believed that the products of many of these polymorphic genes influence the development of self-tolerance, and affected individuals express products of the genes that are defective in the maintenance of tolerance. However, most of the susceptibility loci identified to date span large chromosomal segments that have been shown to be disease associated by family and linkage studies. These loci may contain tens or hundreds of genes, and the actual disease-associated genes or their causal associations with the disease are often not known. Furthermore, the mechanistic links between suspected genes and failure of self-tolerance are not defined. An illustrative example is T1D (see Box 18–2). In both the human disease and the mouse model, the nonobese diabetic (NOD) strain, more than 20 susceptibility loci have been identified; several of these are also susceptibility loci for other autoimmune diseases. The first disease-associated gene to be identified in T1D, and the only one that is common to both humans and mice, is a class II MHC gene, consistent with the fact that the disease is caused by class II–restricted $CD4^+$ T lymphocytes.

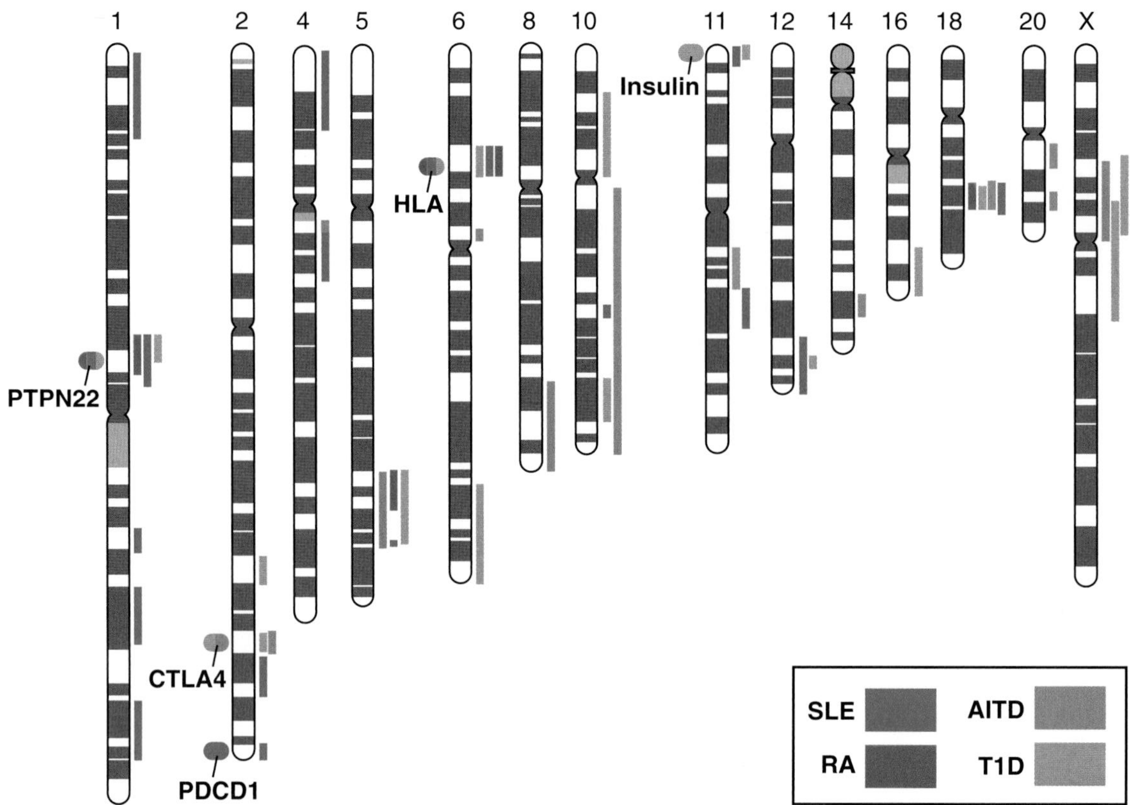

FIGURE 18–7 Susceptibility loci for autoimmune diseases. The chromosomal loci associated with some autoimmune diseases are shown. The location of candidate genes of immunologic interest are indicated as ovals on the left of the chromosomes. These ovals are color coded to indicate the diseases to which the genes are linked. SLE, systemic lupus erythematosus; AITD, autoimmune thyroid disease; RA, rheumatoid arthritis; T1D, type 1 diabetes. (Modified from Yamada R and K Ymamoto. Recent findings on genes associated with inflammatory diseases. Mutation Research 573:136–151, Copyright 2005 with permission from Elsevier.)

Among the genes that are associated with autoimmunity, the strongest associations are with MHC genes, especially class II MHC genes. HLA typing of large groups of patients with various autoimmune diseases has shown that some HLA alleles occur at higher frequency in these patients than in the general population. From such studies, one can calculate the relative risk for development of a disease in individuals who inherit various HLA alleles (Table 18–5). The strongest such association is between ankylosing spondylitis, an inflammatory, presumably autoimmune, disease of vertebral joints, and the class I HLA allele B27. Individuals who are HLA-B27 positive have a 90- to 100-fold greater chance for developing ankylosing spondylitis than do individuals lacking B27. Neither the mechanism of this disease nor the basis of its association with HLA-B27 is known. The association of class II HLA-DR and HLA-DQ alleles with autoimmune diseases has received great attention, mainly because class II MHC molecules are involved in the selection and activation of $CD4^+$ T cells, and $CD4^+$ T cells regulate both humoral and cell-mediated immune responses to protein antigens.

Several features of the association of HLA alleles with autoimmune diseases are noteworthy. First, an HLA-disease association may be identified by serologic typing of one HLA locus, but the actual association may be with other alleles that are linked to the typed allele and inherited together. For instance, individuals with a particular HLA-DR allele (hypothetically, DR1) may show a higher probability of inheriting a particular HLA-DQ allele (hypothetically DQ2) than the probability of inheriting these alleles separately and randomly (i.e., at equilibrium) in the population. Such inheritance is an example of linkage disequilibrium. A disease may be found to be DR1 associated by HLA typing, but the causal association may actually be with the co-inherited DQ2. This realization has emphasized the concept of "extended HLA haplotypes," which refers to sets of linked genes, both classical HLA and adjacent non-HLA genes, that tend to be inherited together as a single unit. Second, in many autoimmune diseases, the disease-associated HLA molecules differ from HLA molecules that are not disease associated in their peptide-binding clefts. This finding is not surprising because polymorphic residues of MHC molecules are located within and adjacent to the clefts, and the structure of the clefts is the key determinant of both functions of MHC molecules, namely, antigen presentation and recognition by T cells (see Chapters 5 and 6). These results support the general concept that MHC molecules influence the development of autoimmunity by controlling T cell selection and activation. Third, disease-associated HLA sequences are found in healthy individuals. In fact, if all individuals bearing a particular disease-associated HLA allele are monitored prospectively, most will never acquire the disease. Therefore, expression of a particular HLA gene is not by itself the cause of any autoimmune disease, but it may be one of several factors that contribute to autoimmunity.

The mechanisms underlying the association of particular HLA alleles with various autoimmune diseases are still not clear. The disease-associated MHC molecule may present a particular self peptide and activate pathogenic T cells, or it may influence negative selection of developing T cells.

Studies with knockout mice and patients have identified several non-MHC genes that influence the maintenance of tolerance to self antigens. Many of these genes were mentioned in Chapter 11, when we discussed the molecular pathways of self-tolerance. The known mutations that predispose to autoimmunity have provided valuable information about the importance of various mechanisms of self-tolerance (Table 18–6).

- Knockout of the gene encoding CTLA-4, the inhibitory T cell receptor for B7 molecules, results in fatal autoimmunity with T cell infiltrates and tissue destruction involving the heart, pancreas, and other organs. Blocking CTLA-4 with specific antibodies also greatly exacerbates the severity of autoimmune tissue injury in mouse models of encephalomyelitis and diabetes. Because CTLA-4 may function normally to induce and maintain T cell anergy to self antigens, eliminating this function leads to autoimmunity. A polymorphism of *CTLA4* has been shown to be associated with autoimmune thyroid disease and T1D. This polymorphism affects production of a splice variant of the protein that is believed to inhibit T cell activation.

Table 18–5. Examples of HLA-Linked Immunological Diseases

Disease	HLA allele	Relative risk*
Rheumatoid arthritis	DR4	4
Insulin-dependent diabetes mellitus	DR3	5
	DR4	5–6
	DR3/DR4 heterozygote	25
Multiple sclerosis	DR2	4
Systemic lupus erythematosus	DR2/DR3	5
Pemphigus vulgaris	DR4	14
Ankylosing spondylitis	B27	90–100

*Relative risk is defined as the probability of development of a disease in individuals with a particular HLA allele versus individuals lacking that HLA allele. The numbers given are approximations.

- Mutations in the autoimmune regulator *(AIRE)* gene in humans and mice result in the autoimmune polyendocrine syndrome (APS), characterized by destruction of several endocrine organs. *AIRE* is required for expression or presentation of tissue-specific proteins in thymic epithelial cells, and hence for deletion (negative selection) of T cells that recognize these self proteins (see Chapter 11).
- Mutations in the gene encoding the transcription factor FoxP3 cause deficiencies of regulatory T cells and systemic autoimmunity. The human disease associated with these mutations is called IPEX (immune dysregulation, polyendocrinopathy, enteropathy, X-linked), and the mouse strain that develops systemic autoimmunity because of mutations in *FoxP3* is called the scurfy mouse. FoxP3 is required for the development of regulatory T cells.
- Mice lacking interleukin-2 (IL-2) or the α or β chain of the IL-2 receptor develop splenomegaly, lymphadenopathy, autoimmune hemolytic anemia, anti-DNA autoantibodies, and IBD. These mice are deficient in $CD4^+CD25^+$ regulatory T cells, which need IL-2 for their survival and function.
- Genetic deficiencies of several complement proteins, including C1q, C2, and C4 (see Chapter 14, Box 14–2), are associated with lupus-like autoimmune diseases. The postulated mechanism of this association is that complement activation promotes the clearance of circulating immune complexes and apoptotic cell bodies, and in the absence of complement proteins, these complexes accumulate in the blood and are deposited in tissues and the antigens of dead cells persist.
- As mentioned above, mutations in the intracellular microbial sensor NOD2 are associated with Crohn's disease, and mice in which the *NOD2* gene is knocked out develop IBD. It is not clear if these mutations reduce host defense against microbes and allow infections to become chronic and elicit inflammatory reactions, or if the mutations lead to excessive host reactions to intestinal microbes.
- Several autoimmune diseases (RA, T1D, autoimmune thyroid disease) are associated with particular variants of the protein tyrosine phosphatase PTPN22, especially in white populations. Because RA is the most prevalent autoimmune disease, *PTPN22* is the most common autoimmunity-associated gene. One explanation for this association is that the disease-associated variants have reduced function, and decreased phosphatase activity allows uncontrolled lymphocyte stimulation by self antigens. However, some of the variants are thought to be gain of function, and could promote autoimmunity by altering selection of self-reactive lymphocytes during maturation.
- Mice carrying homozygous mutations of the *fas* or *fas ligand* gene provided the first clear evidence that failure of apoptotic cell death results in autoimmunity (see Box 18–1). These mice die by the age of 6

Table 18–6. Examples of Gene Mutations that Result in Autoimmunity

Gene	Phenotype of mutant or knockout mouse	Mechanism of failure of tolerance	Human disease?
AIRE	Destruction of endocrine organs by antibodies, lymphocytes	Failure of central tolerance	Autoimmune polyendocrine syndrome (APS)
C4	SLE	Defective clearance of immune complexes; failure of B cell tolerance?	SLE
CTLA-4	Lymphoproliferation; T cell infiltrates in multiple organs, especially heart; lethal by 3-4 weeks	Failure of anergy in $CD4^+$ T cells	CTLA-4 polymorphisms associated with several autoimmune diseases
Fas/FasL	Anti-DNA and other autoantibodies; immune complex nephritis; arthritis; lymphoproliferation	Defective deletion of anergic self-reactive B cells; reduced deletion of mature $CD4^+$ T cells	Autoimmune lymphoproliferative syndrome (ALPS)
FoxP3	Multi-organ lymphocytic infiltrates, wasting	Deficiency of regulatory T cells	IPEX
IL-2; IL-2Rα/β	Inflammatory bowel disease; anti-erythrocyte and anti-DNA autoantibodies	Defective development, survival or function of regulatory T cells	None known
SHP-1	Multiple autoantibodies	Failure of negative regulation of B cells	None known
PTPN22	Increased lymphocyte proliferation, antibody production	Reduced inhibition by tyrosine phosphatase?	PTPN22 polymorphisms are associated with several autoimmune diseases

Abbreviations: AIRE, autoimmune regulator gene; IL-2, interleukin-2; IPEX, immune dysregulation, polyendocrinopathy, enteropathy, X-linked syndrome; SHP-1, SH2-containing phosphatase-1.

months of a systemic autoimmune disease with multiple autoantibodies and nephritis. The lpr/lpr (for "lymphoproliferation") mouse strain produces low levels of Fas protein, and the gld/gld (for "generalized lymphoproliferative disease") strain produces Fas ligand with a point mutation that interferes with its signaling function. A principal cause of autoimmunity is believed to be accumulation of autoreactive B cells, because these B cells are normally eliminated by Fas-dependent death resulting from interactions with T cells, and this pathway of B cell deletion is defective in lpr and gld mice. In addition, defects in Fas or Fas ligand may result in an inability to delete mature $CD4^+$ T cells by activation-induced cell death. Children with a phenotypically similar disease have been identified and shown to carry mutations in the gene encoding Fas or in genes encoding proteins in the Fas-mediated death pathway that result in a failure of activation-induced cell death. These diseases are the only ones known in which genetic abnormalities in one apoptosis-inducing ligand-receptor pair lead to phenotypically complex autoimmune diseases.

Role of Infections in Autoimmunity

Viral and bacterial infections may contribute to the development and exacerbation of autoimmunity. In patients, the onset of autoimmune diseases is often associated with or preceded by infections, and in several animal models, autoimmune tissue injury is reduced when the animals are free of infections. (One notable and unexplained exception is the NOD mouse, in which infections tend to ameliorate insulitis and diabetes.) In most of these cases, the infectious microorganism is not present in lesions and is not even detectable in the individual when autoimmunity develops. Therefore, the lesions of autoimmunity are not due to the infectious agent itself but result from host immune responses that may be triggered or dysregulated by the microbe.

Infections may promote the development of autoimmunity by two principal mechanisms (Fig. 18–8).

- Infections of particular tissues may induce local innate immune responses that recruit leukocytes into the tissues and result in the activation of tissue APCs. These APCs express costimulators and secrete T cell–activating cytokines, resulting in the breakdown of T cell tolerance. Thus, the infection results in the activation of T cells that are not specific for the infectious pathogen; this type of response is called bystander activation. The importance of aberrant expression of costimulators has been demonstrated by several types of experiments.
    - Experimental T cell–mediated autoimmune diseases, such as encephalomyelitis (see Box 18–3) and thyroiditis, develop only if the self antigens (myelin pro-

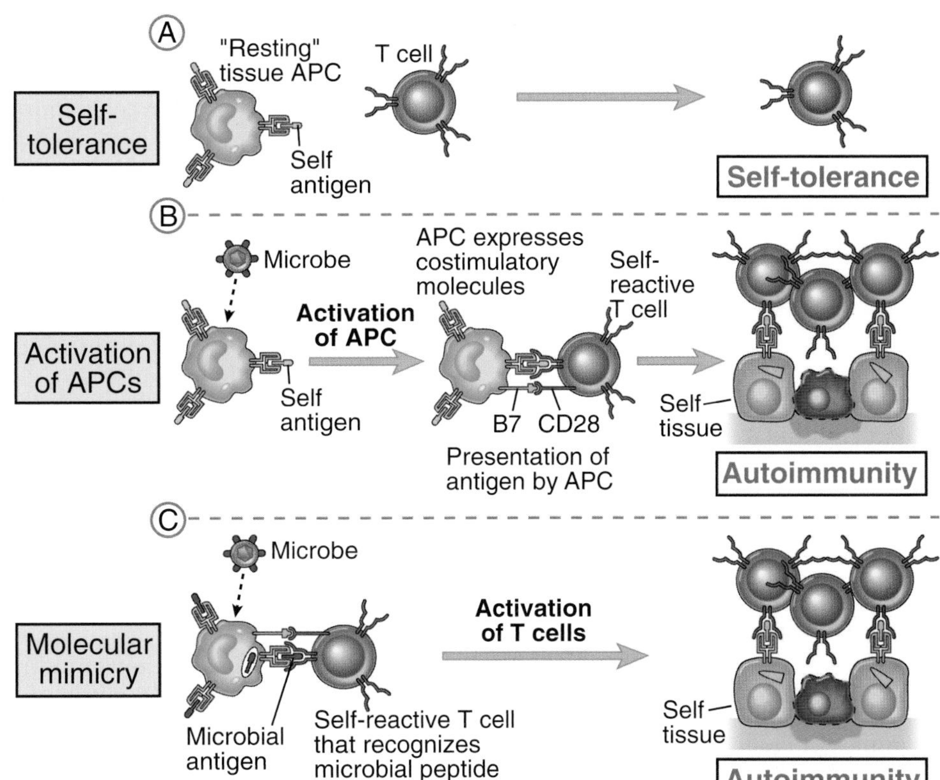

FIGURE 18–8 Role of infections in the development of autoimmunity. A. Normally, encounter of a mature self-reactive T cell with a self antigen presented by a costimulator-deficient resting tissue antigen-presenting cell (APC) results in peripheral tolerance by anergy. (Other possible mechanisms of self-tolerance are not shown.) B. Microbes may activate the APCs to express costimulators, and when these APCs present self antigens, the self-reactive T cells are activated rather than rendered tolerant. C. Some microbial antigens may cross-react with self antigens (molecular mimicry). Therefore, immune responses initiated by the microbes may activate T cells specific for self antigens.

teins and thyroglobulin, respectively) are administered with strong adjuvants. Such adjuvants may function like infectious agents to activate tissue dendritic cells and macrophages, leading to the expression of the costimulators B7-1 and B7-2, the breakdown of T cell anergy, and the development of effector T cells reactive with the self antigen.

- More formal demonstration of autoimmune tissue injury resulting from the abnormal expression of costimulators and breakdown of T cell anergy has come from transgenic mouse models of type 1 diabetes (see Box 18–2). Various genes can be expressed selectively in pancreatic islet β cells as transgenes under the control of insulin promoters. If a foreign antigen such as a viral protein is expressed as a transgene in islet β cells, this antigen effectively becomes "self" and does not elicit an autoimmune reaction (see Chapter 11, Fig. 11–5). However, coexpression of the viral antigen and B7-1 breaks peripheral tolerance in viral antigen–specific T cells, triggers a response to the antigen in the islets, and results in insulitis and diabetes. In this model, transgene-encoded expression of the costimulator is equivalent to converting resting tissue APCs to activated APCs, much like what happens in infections.

- Infectious microbes may contain antigens that cross-react with self antigens, so immune responses to the microbes may result in reactions against self antigens. This phenomenon is called **molecular mimicry,** because the antigens of the microbe cross-react with, or mimic, self antigens.

  - One example of an immunologic cross-reaction between microbial and self antigens is rheumatic fever, which develops after streptococcal infections and is caused by antistreptococcal antibodies that cross-react with myocardial proteins. These antibodies are deposited in the heart and cause myocarditis. Molecular sequencing has revealed numerous short stretches of homologies between myocardial proteins and streptococcal protein.

- Microbes may engage Toll-like receptors (TLRs) on dendritic cells, leading to the production of lymphocyte-activating cytokines, or on autoreactive B cells, leading to autoantibody production. A role of TLR signaling in autoimmunity has been demonstrated in mouse models of SLE, but its significance in human autoimmune diseases is unclear.

The significance of limited homologies between microbial and self antigens remains to be established, and it has been difficult to prove that a microbial protein can actually cause a disease that resembles a spontaneous autoimmune disease. On the basis of transgenic mouse models, it has been suggested that molecular mimicry is involved in triggering autoimmunity when the frequency of autoreactive lymphocytes is low; in this situation, the microbial mimic of the self antigen serves to expand the number of self-reactive lymphocytes above some pathogenic threshold. When the frequency of self-reactive lymphocytes is high, the role of microbes may be to induce tissue inflammation, to recruit self-reactive lymphocytes into the tissue, and to provide second signals for the activation of these bystander lymphocytes.

Some infections may protect against the development of autoimmunity. Epidemiologic studies suggest that reducing infections increases the incidence of T1D and MS, and experimental studies show that the disease of NOD mice (the mouse model of type 1 diabetes) is greatly retarded if the mice are infected. It seems paradoxical that infections can be triggers of autoimmunity and also inhibit autoimmune diseases. How they may reduce the incidence of autoimmune diseases is unknown.

Other Factors in Autoimmunity

The development of autoimmunity is related to several factors in addition to susceptibility genes and infections.

Anatomic alterations in tissues, caused by inflammation (possibly secondary to infections), ischemic injury, or trauma, may lead to the exposure of self antigens that are normally concealed from the immune system. Such sequestered antigens may not have induced self-tolerance. Therefore, if previously hidden self antigens are released, they can interact with immunocompetent lymphocytes and induce specific immune responses. Examples of anatomically sequestered antigens include intraocular proteins and sperm. Posttraumatic uveitis and orchitis are thought to be due to autoimmune responses to self antigens that are released from their normal locations by trauma.

Hormonal influences play a role in some autoimmune diseases. Many autoimmune diseases have a higher incidence in females than in males. For instance, SLE affects women about 10 times more frequently than men. The SLE-like disease of (NZB × NZW)F_1 mice develops only in females and is retarded by androgen treatment. Whether this predominance results from the influence of sex hormones or other gender-related factors is not known.

Autoimmune diseases are among the most challenging scientific and clinical problems in immunology. The current knowledge of pathogenetic mechanisms remains incomplete, so theories and hypotheses continue to outnumber facts. The application of new technical advances and the rapidly improving understanding of self-tolerance will, it is hoped, lead to clearer and more definitive answers to the enigmas of autoimmunity.

Therapeutic Approaches for Immunologic Diseases

Strategies for treatment of immune-mediated diseases are similar to the approaches used to prevent graft rejection, another form of injurious immune response (see Chapter 16). The mainstay of therapy for hypersensitivity diseases is anti-inflammatory drugs, particularly corticosteroids. Such drugs are targeted at reducing tissue injury, specifically, the effector phases of the pathologic immune responses. Biologic agents that inhibit immune responses and inflammation have become important treatment options for many immune-mediated inflammatory diseases. Many of these newer therapies are based on our improving understanding of immune response, and are remarkable examples of rational drug design. A soluble form of the TNF receptor and anti-TNF antibodies that bind to and neutralize TNF are of great benefit in many patients with rheumatoid arthritis and Crohn's disease. Antagonists of other proinflammatory cytokines, such as IL-1, and agents that block leukocyte emigration into tissues, such as antibodies against integrins, are also being tested for their anti-inflammatory effects. Agents that block B7 costimulators are approved for treatment of rheumatoid arthritis and psoriasis. These antagonists are now in clinical trials for SLE, psoriasis, and other diseases. Depletion of B cells with anti-CD20 antibody is being tested in rheumatoid arthritis and other diseases. In severe cases, immunosuppressive drugs such as cyclosporine are used to block T cell activation, or anti-proliferative drugs such as methotrexate are used to reduce the generation and expansion of lymphocytes. Plasmapheresis has been used during exacerbations of antibody-mediated diseases to reduce circulating levels of antibodies or immune complexes. Large doses of intravenous IgG have beneficial effects in some hypersensitivity diseases. It is not clear how this agent suppresses immune inflammation; one possibility is that the IgG binds to inhibitory Fc receptors on B lymphocytes and shuts off antibody production, similar to the phenomenon of antibody feedback (see Chapter 10, Fig. 10–19). There are ongoing attempts at more specific treatment, such as inducing tolerance in disease-producing lymphocyte clones, or inducing regulatory T cells specific for self antigens.

SUMMARY

- Disorders caused by abnormal immune responses are called hypersensitivity diseases. Pathologic immune responses may be autoimmune responses directed against self antigens or uncontrolled and excessive responses to foreign antigens.

- Hypersensitivity diseases may result from antibodies that bind to cells or tissues, circulating immune complexes that are deposited in tissues, or T lymphocytes reactive with antigens in tissues.

- The effector mechanisms of antibody-mediated tissue injury are complement activation and Fc receptor-mediated inflammation. Some antibodies cause disease by interfering with normal cellular functions without producing tissue injury. The effector mechanisms of T cell–mediated tissue injury are DTH reactions and cell lysis by CTLs.

- Autoimmunity results from a failure of self-tolerance. Autoimmune reactions may be triggered by environmental stimuli, such as infections, in genetically susceptible individuals.

- Most autoimmune diseases are polygenic, and numerous susceptibility genes contribute to disease development. The greatest contribution is from MHC genes; other genes are believed to influence the selection of self-reactive lymphocytes and the development of self-tolerance.
- Infections may predispose to autoimmunity by several mechanisms, including enhanced expression of costimulators in tissues and cross-reactions between microbial antigens and self antigens.
- The current treatment of autoimmune diseases is targeted at reducing immune activation and the injurious consequences of the autoimmune reaction. A future goal of therapy is to inhibit the responses of lymphocytes specific for self antigens and to induce tolerance in these cells.

Selected Readings

Bach J-F. Infections and autoimmune diseases. Journal of Autoimmunity 25 suppl 1:74–80, 2005.

Crow MK, and KA Kirou. Interferon-alpha in systemic lupus erythematosus. Current Opinion in Rheumatology 16: 541–547, 2004.

Davidson A, and B Diamond. Autoimmune diseases. New England Journal of Medicine 345:340–350, 2001.

Deng L, and RA Mariuzza. Recognition of self-peptide-MHC complexes by autoimmune T-cell receptors. Trends in Biochemical Sciences 32:500–508, 2007.

Eckmann L, and M Karin. NOD2 and Crohn's disease: loss or gain of function? Immunity 22:661–667, 2005.

Fernando MM, et al. Defining the role of the MHC in autoimmunity: a review and pooled analysis. PLoS Genetics 4:e1000024, 2008.

Fourneau JM, JM Bach, PM van Endert, and JF Bach. The elusive case for a role of mimicry in autoimmune diseases. Molecular Immunology 40:1095–1102, 2004.

Frohman EM, MK Racke, and CS Raine. Multiple sclerosis—the plague and its pathogenesis. New England Journal of Medicine 354:942–955, 2006.

Goodnow CC, J Sprent, BF de St Groth, and CG Vinuesa. Cellular and genetic mechanisms of self tolerance and autoimmunity. Nature 435:590–597, 2005.

Gregersen PK. Gaining insight into PTPN22 and autoimmunity. Nature Genetics 37:1300–1302, 2005.

Hill NJ, C King, and M Flodstrom-Tullberg. Recent acquisitions on the genetic basis of autoimmune disease. Frontiers in Bioscience 13:4838–4851, 2008.

Kuchroo VK, AC Anderson, H Waldner, E Bettelli, and LB Nicholson. T cell response in experimental autoimmune encephalomyelitis (EAE): role of self and cross-reactive antigens in shaping, tuning, and regulating the autopathogenic T cell repertoire. Annual Review of Immunology 20:101–123, 2002.

Marrack P, J Kappler, and BL Kotzin. Autoimmune disease: why and where it occurs. Nature Medicine 7:899–905, 2001.

Marshak-Rothstein A. Toll-like receptors in systemic autoimmune disease. Nature Reviews Immunology 6:823–835, 2006.

Melanitou E, P Fain, and GS Eisenbarth. Genetics of type 1A (immune mediated) diabetes. Journal of Autoimmunity 21:93–98, 2003.

Nicholson MJ, M Hahn, and KW Wucherpfennig. Unusual features of self-peptide/MHC binding by autoimmune T cell repertoires. Immunity 23:351–360, 2005.

O'Shea JJ, A Ma, and P Lipsky. Cytokines and autoimmunity. Nature Reviews Immunology 2:37–45, 2002.

Plotz PH. The autoantibody repertoire: searching for order. Nature Reviews Immunology 3:73–78, 2003.

Rioux JD, and AK Abbas. Paths to understanding the genetic basis of autoimmune disease. Nature 435:584–589, 2005.

Rose NR, and C Bona. Defining criteria for autoimmune diseases (Witebsky's postulates revisited). Immunology Today 14:426–430, 1993.

Shlomchik MJ. Sites and stages of autoreactive B cell activation and regulation. Immunity 28:18–28, 2008.

Todd JA, and LS Wicker. Genetic protection from the inflammatory disease type 1 diabetes in humans and animal models. Immunity 15:387–395, 2001.

Vanderlugt CL, and SD Miller. Epitope spreading in immune-mediated diseases: implications for immunotherapy. Nature Reviews Immunology 2:85–95, 2002.

von Herrath MG, RS Fujinami, and JL Whitton. Microorganisms and autoimmunity: making the barren field fertile? Nature Reviews Microbiology 1:151–157, 2003.

Wakeland EW, K Liu, RR Graham, and TW Behrens. Delineating the genetic basis of systemic lupus erythematosus. Immunity 15:397–408, 2001.

Xavier RJ, and JD Rioux. Genome-wide association studies: a new window into immune-mediated diseases. Nature Reviews Immunology 8:631–643, 2008.

Yamada R, and K Ymamoto. Recent findings on genes associated with inflammatory diseases. Mutation Research 573:136–151, 2005.

Chapter 19

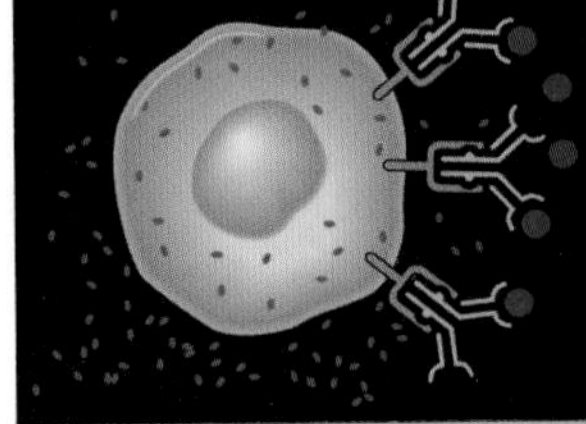

IMMEDIATE HYPERSENSITIVITY

A variety of human diseases are caused by immune responses to environmental antigens that lead to $CD4^+$ T_H2 differentiation and production of immunoglobulin E (IgE) antibodies that are specific for the antigens and bind to Fc receptors on mast cells and basophils. When these cell-associated IgE antibodies are cross-linked by antigen, the cells are activated to rapidly release a variety of mediators. These mediators collectively cause increased vascular permeability, vasodilation, and bronchial and visceral smooth muscle contraction. This reaction is called **immediate hypersensitivity** because it begins rapidly, within minutes of antigen challenge (immediate), and has major pathologic consequences (hypersensitivity). In clinical medicine, these reactions are commonly called **allergy** or **atopy,** and the associated diseases are called allergic or immediate hypersensitivity diseases. These diseases also have a major inflammatory component, which is triggered by cytokines produced by $CD4^+$ T_H2 cells and mast cells, as well as by lipid mediators secreted by mast cells. Although atopy originally meant "unusual," we now realize that allergy is the most common disorder of immunity and affects 20% of all individuals in the United States. This chapter focuses on immune reactions mediated by T_H2 cells and IgE and mast cells. We begin by summarizing some important general features of immediate hypersensitivity and proceed to describe the production of IgE, the structure and functions of IgE-specific Fc receptors, and the cellular mediators of immediate hypersensitivity, including mast cells, basophils, and eosinophils. We then describe selected clinical syndromes associated with immediate hypersensitivity and the principles of therapy for these diseases. We conclude with a discussion of the physiologic role of IgE-mediated immune reactions in host defense.

General Features of Immediate Hypersensitivity Reactions

All immediate hypersensitivity reactions share common features, although they differ greatly in the types of antigens that elicit these reactions and their clinical and pathologic manifestations.

- ***The hallmarks of allergic diseases are the activation of T_H2 cells and the production of IgE antibody.*** Whereas healthy individuals either do not respond or have harmless T cell and antibody responses to common environmental antigens, atopic individuals develop strong T_H2 responses and produce IgE upon exposure to these potentially allergenic substances.
- ***The typical sequence of events in immediate hypersensitivity consists of exposure to an antigen, activation of T_H2 cells and B cells specific for the antigen, production of IgE antibody, binding of the antibody to Fc receptors of mast cells, and triggering of the mast cells by re-exposure to the antigen, resulting in the release of mediators from the mast cells and the subsequent pathologic reaction*** (Fig. 19–1). Binding of IgE to mast cells is also called **sensitization** because IgE-coated mast cells are ready to be activated on antigen encounter (i.e., they are sensitive to the antigen). We describe each of these steps in the following sections.
- ***There is a strong genetic predisposition for the development of immediate hypersensitivity.*** Many susceptibility genes are associated with atopy. These genes are thought to influence different steps in the development and reactions of immediate hypersensitivity. We will discuss some of the major known susceptibility genes and their likely roles later in the chapter.
- ***The antigens that elicit immediate hypersensitivity, also called allergens, are usually common environmental proteins and chemicals.*** Many structurally distinct antigens can be allergenic. It is still not established if allergens share particular chemical features that are the basis for stimulation of T_H2 responses in genetically susceptible individuals.
- ***The cytokines produced by T_H2 cells are responsible for many of the features of immediate hypersensitivity.*** Thus, immediate hypersensitivity is the prototypic T_H2-mediated disorder, in contrast to delayed-type hypersensitivity, which is the classical T_H1-mediated immune reaction.

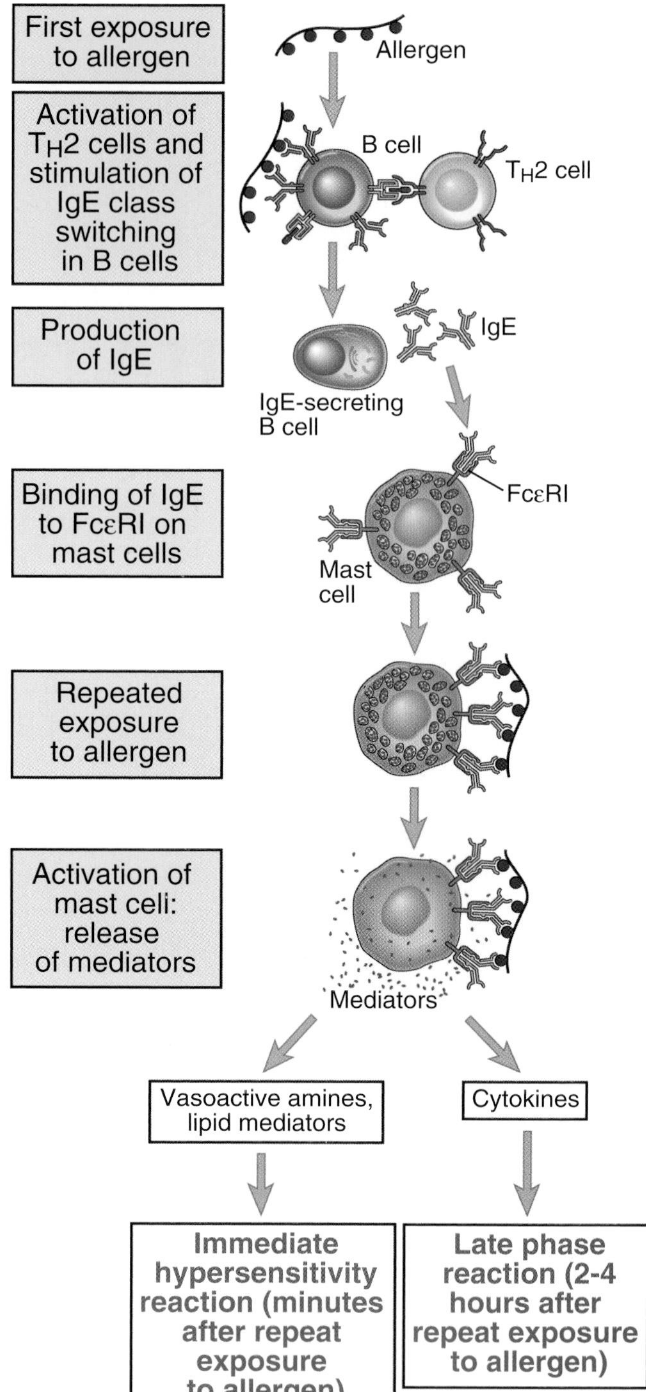

FIGURE 19–1 Sequence of events in immediate hypersensitivity reactions. Immediate hypersensitivity diseases are initiated by the introduction of an allergen, which stimulates T_H2 reactions and IgE production. IgE sensitizes mast cells by binding to FcεRI, and subsequent exposure to the allergen activates the mast cells to secrete the mediators that are responsible for the pathologic reactions of immediate hypersensitivity.

- ***The clinical and pathologic manifestations of immediate hypersensitivity consist of the vascular and smooth muscle reaction that develops rapidly after repeat exposure to the allergen (the immediate reaction) and a delayed late-phase reaction consisting mainly of inflammation.*** These reactions may be triggered by IgE-mediated mast cell activation, but different mediators are responsible for different components of the immediate and late-phase reactions. Since mast cells are present in all connective tissues and under all epithelia, these are the most common sites of immediate hypersensitivity reactions. Some immediate hypersensitivity reactions may be triggered by nonimmunologic stimuli, such as exercise and exposure to cold. Such stimuli presumably induce mast cell degranulation and the release of mediators without antigen exposure or IgE production. Such reactions are said to be nonatopic.

- ***Immediate hypersensitivity reactions are manifested in different ways, including skin and mucosal allergies, food allergies, asthma, and systemic anaphylaxis.*** In the most extreme systemic form, called anaphylaxis, mast cell–derived mediators can restrict airways to the point of asphyxiation and produce cardiovascular collapse leading to death. (The term **anaphylaxis** was coined to indicate that antibodies, especially IgE antibodies, could confer the opposite of protection [prophylaxis] on an unfortunate individual.) We will return to the pathogenesis of these reactions later in the chapter.

With this introduction, we proceed to a description of the steps in the development and reactions of immediate hypersensitivity.

Production of IgE

IgE antibody is responsible for sensitizing mast cells and provides recognition of antigen for immediate hypersensitivity reactions. IgE is the antibody isotype that contains the ε heavy chain (see Chapter 4), and of all the Ig isotypes, IgE is the most efficient at binding to Fc receptors on mast cells and activating these cells. We will describe the experimental evidence demonstrating the essential role of IgE in immediate hypersensitivity later in the chapter.

Atopic individuals produce high levels of IgE in response to environmental allergens, whereas normal individuals generally synthesize other Ig isotypes, such as IgM and IgG, and only small amounts of IgE. Regulation of IgE synthesis depends on the propensity of an individual to mount a T_H2 response to allergens because T_H2 cell–derived cytokines stimulate heavy chain isotype switching to the IgE class in B cells. This propensity toward T_H2 responses against particular antigens may be influenced by a variety of factors, including inherited genes, the nature of the antigens, and the history of antigen exposure.

The Nature of Allergens

Antigens that elicit immediate hypersensitivity reactions (allergens) are proteins or chemicals bound to proteins to which the atopic individual is chronically exposed. Typical allergens include proteins in pollen, house dust mites, animal dander, foods, and chemicals like the antibiotic penicillin. It is not known why some antigens induce strong T_H2 responses and allergic reactions whereas others do not. Two important characteristics of allergens are that individuals are exposed to them repeatedly and, unlike microbes, they do not stimulate the innate immune responses that would promote macrophage activation and secretion of the T_H1-inducing cytokines interleukin-12 (IL-12) and IL-18. Chronic or repeated T cell activation in the absence of innate immunity may drive $CD4^+$ T cells toward the T_H2 pathway, as the T cells themselves make IL-4, the major T_H2-inducing cytokine (see Chapter 13).

The property of being allergenic may also reside in the chemical nature of the antigen itself. Although no structural characteristics of proteins can definitively predict whether they will be allergenic, some features are typical of many common allergens. These features include low molecular weight, glycosylation, and high solubility in body fluids. Anaphylactic responses to foods typically involve highly glycosylated small proteins. These structural features probably protect the antigens from denaturation and degradation in the gastrointestinal tract and allow them to be absorbed intact. Curiously, many allergens, such as the cysteine protease of the house dust mite *Dermatophagoides pteronyssinus* and phospholipase A_2 in bee venom, are enzymes, but the importance of the enzymatic activity in triggering immediate hypersensitivity reactions is not known.

Because immediate hypersensitivity reactions are dependent on T cells, T cell–independent antigens such as polysaccharides cannot elicit such reactions unless they become attached to proteins. Some drugs such as penicillin often do elicit strong IgE responses. These drugs react chemically with amino acid residues in self proteins to form hapten-carrier conjugates, which stimulate T_H2 responses and IgE production.

The natural history of antigen exposure is an important determinant of the amount of specific IgE antibodies produced. Repeated exposure to a particular antigen is necessary for development of an allergic reaction to that antigen because switching to the IgE isotype and sensitization of mast cells with IgE must happen before a hypersensitivity reaction to an antigen can occur. Individuals with allergic rhinitis or asthma often benefit from a geographic change of residence with a change in indigenous plant pollens, although environmental antigens in the new residence may trigger an eventual return of the symptoms. The most dramatic examples of the importance of repeated exposure to antigen in allergic disease are seen in cases of bee stings. The proteins in the insect venoms are not usually of concern on the first encounter because an atopic individual has no preexisting specific IgE antibodies. However, an IgE response may occur after a single encounter with antigen, and a second sting by an insect of the same species may induce fatal anaphylaxis!

Activation of T_H2 Cells

IgE synthesis is dependent on the activation of $CD4^+$ helper T cells of the T_H2 subset and their secretion of IL-4 and IL-13. It is likely that dendritic cells in epithelia through which allergens enter capture the antigens, transport them to draining lymph nodes, process them, and present peptides to naive T cells. The T cells then differentiate into the T_H2 subset of effector cells. Differentiated T_H2 cells promote switching to IgE mainly through the secretion of IL-4 and IL-13. T_H2 cells are involved in other components of the immediate hypersensitivity reaction in addition to promoting switching to IgE. IL-5 secreted by T_H2 cells activates eosinophils, a cell type that is abundant in many immediate hypersensitivity reactions. IL-13 stimulates epithelial cells (e.g., in the airways) to secrete increased amounts of mucus, and excessive mucus production is also a common feature of these reactions. Consistent with a central role of T_H2 cells in immediate hypersensitivity, atopic individuals contain larger numbers of allergen-specific IL-4-secreting T cells in their circulation than do non-atopic persons. In atopic patients, the allergen-specific T cells also produce more IL-4 per cell than in normal individuals.

- The role of T_H2 cells in allergic reactions is demonstrated by experiments in which mice are made to inhale a model protein antigen, such as chicken egg albumin, and are injected with T cells specific for the antigen. The adoptive transfer of T_H2 cells induces airway hyperresponsiveness, resembling asthma. In the same model, blocking T_H2 responses reduces the severity of the allergic reaction.
- Knockout mice lacking the T_H1 transcription factor T-bet (see Chapter 13) show defective T_H1 responses and a compensatory increase in T_H2 responses. Such mice develop spontaneous airway allergic reactions.

In addition to stimulating IgE production, T_H2 cells contribute to the inflammation of the late-phase reaction. Accumulations of T_H2 cells are found at sites of immediate hypersensitivity reactions in the skin and bronchial mucosa. These T cells are recruited to sites of immediate hypersensitivity, mainly in response to chemokines. T_H2 cells express the chemokine receptors CCR4 and CCR3, and the chemokines that bind to these receptors are produced by many cell types at sites of immediate hypersensitivity reactions, including epithelial cells.

Activation of B Cells and Switching to IgE

B cells specific for allergens are activated by T_H2 cells, as in other T cell–dependent B cell responses (see Chapter 10). Under the influence of CD40 ligand and cytokines, mainly IL-4, produced by the T_H2 cells, the B cells undergo heavy chain isotype switching and produce IgE. IgE circulates as a bivalent antibody and is normally present in plasma at a concentration of less than 1 μg/mL. In pathologic conditions such as helminthic infections and severe atopy, this level can rise to more than 1000 μg/mL. Allergen-specific IgE produced by B cells enters the circulation and binds to Fc receptors on tissue mast cells, so that these cells are sensitized and poised to react to a subsequent encounter with the allergen. Circulating basophils are also capable of binding IgE. We will first describe the Fc receptors used by these cell types to bind IgE and then the properties and reactions of the cells.

Binding of IgE to Mast Cells and Basophils

Mast cells and basophils express a high-affinity Fc receptor specific for ε heavy chains, called FcεRI that binds IgE. IgE, like all other antibody molecules, is made exclusively by B cells, yet IgE functions as an antigen receptor on the surface of the cells of immediate hypersensitivity. This function is accomplished by IgE binding to FcεRI on these cells. The affinity of FcεRI for IgE is very high (dissociation constant [K_d] of about 1×10^{-10} M); this binding is much stronger than that of any other Fc receptor for its ligand (see Chapter 14, Box 14–1). Therefore, the normal serum concentration of IgE, although low in comparison to other Ig isotypes (less than 5×10^{-10} M), is sufficiently high to allow occupancy of FcεRI receptors. Tissue mast cells in all individuals are normally coated with IgE, which is bound to the FcεRI. In atopic individuals, enough of this bound IgE is specific for one or a few antigens that exposure to that antigen or antigens is able to cross-link the Fc receptors and activate the cells (discussed later). In addition to mast cells and basophils, FcεRI, usually lacking the β chain, has been detected on eosinophils, epidermal Langerhans cells, some dermal macrophages, and activated monocytes; its function on these cells is not known.

Each FcεRI molecule is composed of one α chain that mediates ligand binding and a β chain and two γ chains that are responsible for signaling (Fig. 19–2). The amino-terminal extracellular portion of the α chain includes two Ig-like domains that form the binding site for IgE. The β chain of FcεRI contains a single immunoreceptor tyrosine-based activation motif (ITAM) in the cytoplasmic carboxyl terminus. The two identical γ chain polypeptides are linked by a disulfide bond and are homologous to the ζ chain of the T cell antigen receptor complex (see Chapter 6). The cytoplasmic portion of each γ chain contains one ITAM. The γ chain of FcεRI serves as the signaling subunit for FcγRI, FcγRIIIA, and FcαR and is called the FcR γ chain (see Chapter 14, Box 14–1). Tyrosine phosphorylation of the ITAMs of the β and γ chains initiates the signals from the receptor that are required for mast cell activation. We will return to the nature of these signals when we discuss mast cells later in the chapter.

- The importance of FcεRI in IgE-mediated immediate hypersensitivity reactions has been demonstrated in FcεRI α chain knockout mice. When these mice are given intravenous injections of IgE specific for a known antigen followed by that antigen, anaphylaxis does not develop, whereas it does in wild-type mice treated in the same way.

FcεRI expression on the surface of mast cells and basophils is up-regulated by IgE, thereby providing a mechanism for the amplification of IgE-mediated reactions. The relationship between the levels of IgE and FcεRI expression is supported by several observations.

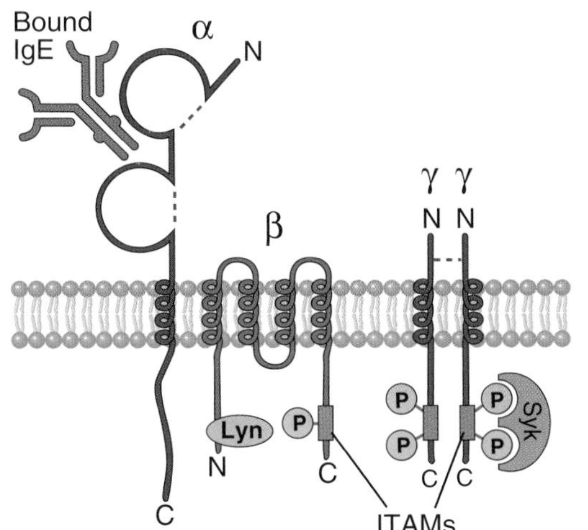

FIGURE 19–2 Polypeptide chain structure of the high-affinity IgE Fc receptor (FcεRI). IgE binds to the Ig-like domains of the α chain. The β chain and the γ chains mediate signal transduction. The boxes in the cytoplasmic region of the β and γ chains are ITAMs, similar to those found in the T cell receptor complex (see Fig. 6–5). A model structure of FcεRI is shown in Chapter 14, Box 14–1.

- A positive correlation between FcεRI expression on human blood basophils and circulating IgE levels has been observed.
- Treatment of mast cells in vitro with IgE induces increased expression of FcεRI.
- Mast cells from knockout mice lacking IgE have very low levels of FcεRI.

Another IgE receptor called FcεRII, also known as CD23, is a protein related to C-type mammalian lectins, whose affinity for IgE is much lower than that of FcεRI. The biologic roles of FcεRII are not known.

Role of Mast Cells, Basophils, and Eosinophils in Immediate Hypersensitivity

Mast cells, basophils, and eosinophils are the effector cells of immediate hypersensitivity reactions and allergic disease. Although each of these cell types has unique characteristics, all three contain cytoplasmic granules whose contents are the major mediators of allergic reactions, and all three cell types produce lipid mediators and cytokines that induce inflammation. T_H2 cells also function as effector cells of immediate hypersensitivity; their role has been discussed earlier. In this section of the chapter, we discuss the properties and functions of mast cells, basophils, and eosinophils (Table 19–1). Because mast cells are the major cell type responsible for immediate hypersensitivity reactions in tissues, much of our subsequent discussion focuses on mast cells.

Properties of Mast Cells and Basophils

All mast cells are derived from progenitors in the bone marrow. Normally, mature mast cells are not found in

Table 19–1. Properties of Mast Cells, Basophils, and Eosinophils

Characteristic	Mast cells	Basophils	Eosinophils
Major site of maturation	Connective tissue	Bone marrow	Bone marrow
Major cells in circulation	No	Yes (0.5% of blood leukocytes)	Yes (~2% of blood leukocytes)
Mature cells recruited into tissues from circulation	No	Yes	Yes
Mature cells residing in connective tissue	Yes	No	Yes
Proliferative ability of mature cells	Yes	No	No
Life span	Weeks to months	Days	Days to weeks
Major development factor (cytokine)	Stem cell factor, IL-3	IL-3	IL-5
Expression of FcεRI	High levels	High levels	Low levels (function unclear)
Major granule contents	Histamine, heparin and/or chondroitin sulfate, proteases	Histamine, chondroitin sulfate, protease	Major basic protein, eosinophil cationic protein, peroxidases, hydrolases, lysophospholipase

Abbreviations: FcεRI, Fcε receptor type I; IL-3, interleukin-3.

the circulation. Progenitors migrate to the peripheral tissues as immature cells and undergo differentiation *in situ.* Mature mast cells are found throughout the body, predominantly near blood vessels and nerves and beneath epithelia. They are also present in lymphoid organs. Human mast cells vary in shape and have round nuclei, and the cytoplasm contains membrane-bound granules and lipid bodies (Fig. 19–3). The granules contain acidic proteoglycans that bind basic dyes.

There are two major subsets of mast cells that differ in their anatomic locations, granule contents, and activities (Table 19–2). In rodents, one subset of mast cells is found in the mucosa of the gastrointestinal tract. These mucosal mast cells have abundant chondroitin sulfate and little histamine in their granules. The development of mucosal mast cells in vivo depends on the cytokine IL-3 produced by T cells. Mast cells may be cultured from rodent bone marrow in the presence of IL-3, and such cultured mast cells resemble mucosal mast cells on the basis of the high granule content of chondroitin sulfate and low histamine concentration. The human counterpart of mucosal mast cells is most often identified by the presence of tryptase and the absence of other neutral proteases in the granules. In humans, the mucosal type of mast cells predominate in intestinal mucosa and alveolar spaces in the lung, and their presence is also T cell dependent. A second subset of mast cells, also first identified in rodents, is found in the lung and in the serosa of body cavities, and these cells are called connective tissue mast cells. Their major

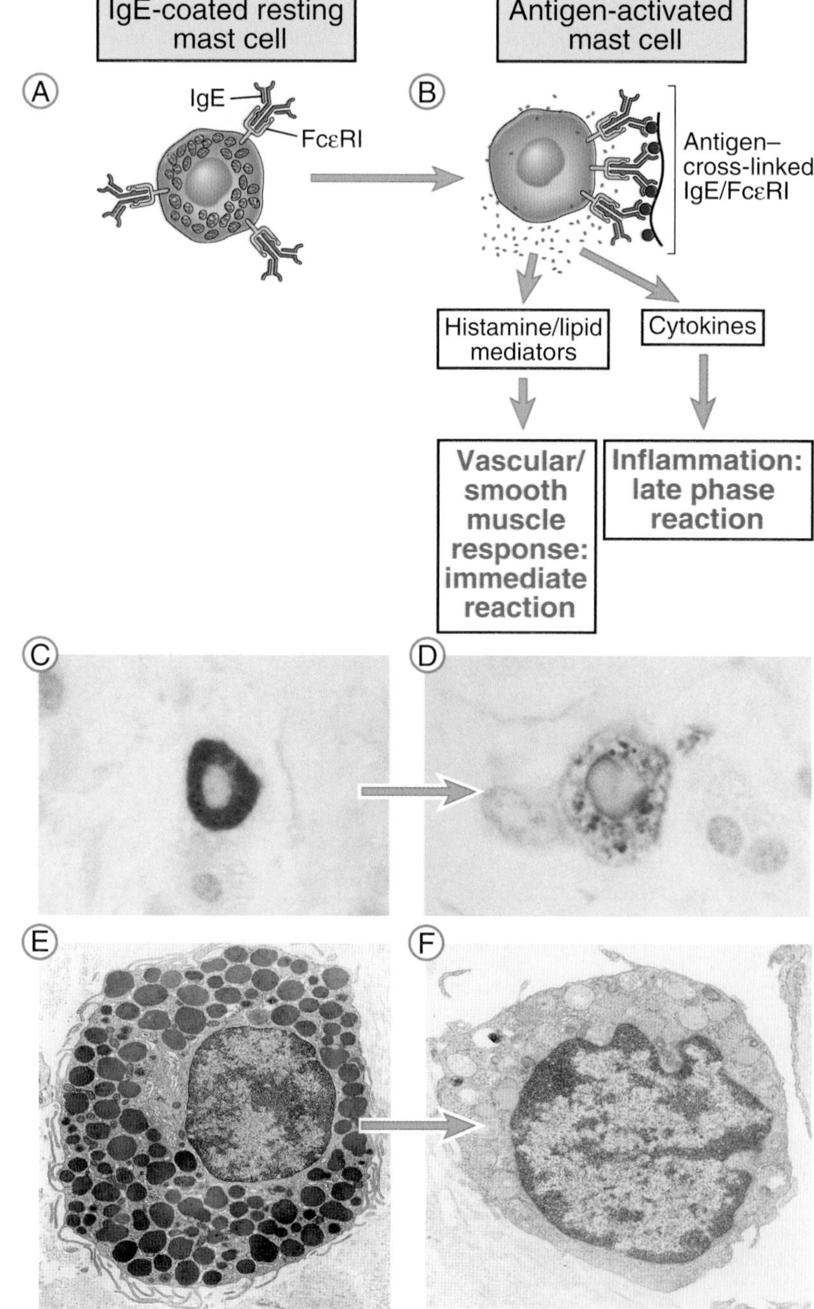

FIGURE 19–3 Mast cell activation. Antigen binding to IgE cross-links FcεRI molecules on mast cells, which induces the release of mediators that cause the hypersensitivity reaction (A, B). Other stimuli, including the complement fragment C5a, can also activate mast cells. A light photomicrograph of a resting mast cell with abundant purple-staining cytoplasmic granules is shown in C. These granules are also seen in the electron micrograph of a resting mast cell shown in E. In contrast, the depleted granules of an activated mast cell are shown in the light photomicrograph (D) and electron micrograph (F). (Courtesy of Dr. Daniel Friend, Department of Pathology, Brigham and Women's Hospital and Harvard Medical School, Boston, Massachusetts.)

Table 19–2. Mast Cell Subsets

Characteristic	Connective tissue mast cells		Mucosal mast cells	
	Rodent	Human	Rodent	Human
Location	Peritoneal cavity	Skin, intestinal submucosa	Intestinal mucosa	Alveoli, intestinal mucosa
T cell dependence for development of phenotype in tissues	No	No	Yes	Yes
Granule contents	High levels of histamine, heparin	Major neutral proteases: tryptase, chymase, carboxypeptidase, cathepsin G	Low levels of histamine; high levels of chondroitin sulfate	Major neutral protease: tryptase

granule proteoglycan is heparin, and they also produce large quantities of histamine. Unlike mucosal mast cells, connective tissue mast cells show little T cell dependence. In humans, the corresponding subset is identified by the presence of several neutral proteases in the granules, including tryptase, chymase, cathepsin G-like protease, and carboxypeptidase. Human connective tissue mast cells are found in the skin and intestinal submucosa.

Although we do not know if these mast cell subsets serve distinct functions, their locations, granule contents, and relative T cell dependence suggest that each subset may be important in a different set of disease processes. It is likely that mucosal mast cells are involved in T cell– and IgE-dependent immediate hypersensitivity diseases involving the airways, such as bronchial asthma, and other mucosal tissues. Conversely, connective tissue mast cells mediate immediate hypersensitivity reactions in the skin. The phenotype of a mast cell is not fixed and may vary in response to cytokines and growth factors. For example, bone marrow–derived mucosal mast cells can be changed to a connective tissue mast cell phenotype by coculture with fibroblasts or incubation with c-Kit ligand (stem cell factor) (see Chapter 12). Repopulation experiments in mast cell–deficient mice further suggest that the mucosal and connective tissue phenotypes are not distinct lineages and that bidirectional changes occur in different microenvironments.

Basophils are blood granulocytes with structural and functional similarities to mast cells. Like other granulocytes, basophils are derived from bone marrow progenitors (a lineage different from that of mast cells), mature in the bone marrow, and circulate in the blood (Fig. 19–4). Basophils constitute less than 1% of blood leukocytes. Although they are normally not present in tissues, basophils may be recruited to some inflammatory sites. Basophils contain granules that bind basic dyes, and they are capable of synthesizing many of the same mediators as mast cells (see Table 19–3). Like mast cells, basophils express FcεRI, bind IgE, and can be triggered by antigen binding to the IgE. Therefore, basophils that are recruited into tissue sites where antigen is present may contribute to immediate hypersensitivity reactions.

Activation of Mast Cells

Mast cells are activated by cross-linking of FcεRI molecules, which occurs by binding of multivalent antigens to the IgE molecules that are attached to the Fc receptors (see Fig. 19–3). In an individual allergic to a particular antigen, a large proportion of the IgE bound to mast cells is specific for that antigen. Exposure to the antigen will cross-link sufficient IgE molecules to trigger mast cell activation. In contrast, in nonatopic individuals, the mast cell-associated IgE is specific for many different antigens, all of which may have induced low levels of IgE production. Therefore, no single antigen will cross-link

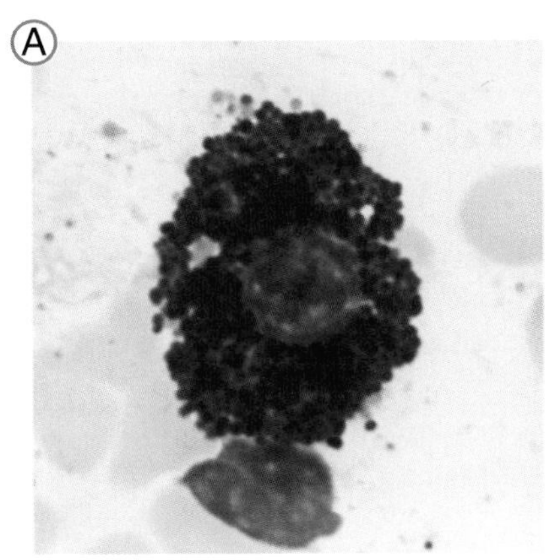

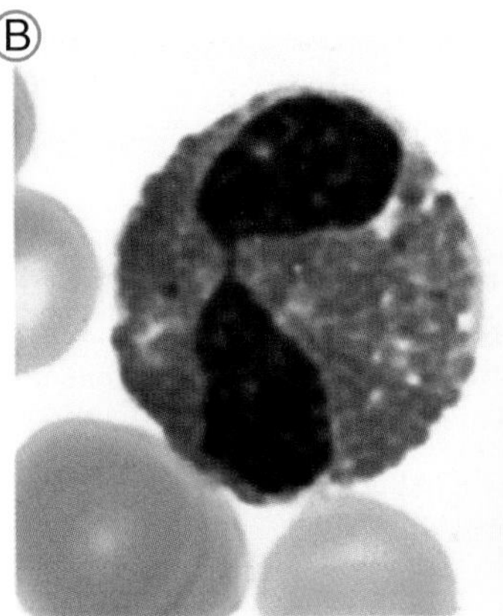

FIGURE 19–4 Morphology of basophils and eosinophils. Photomicrographs of a Wright-Giemsa-stained peripheral blood basophil (A) and eosinophil (B) are presented. Note the characteristic red staining of the cytoplasmic granules in the eosinophil and blue-staining cytoplasmic granules of the basophil. (Courtesy of Dr. Jonathan Hecht, Department of Pathology, Brigham and Women's Hospital, Boston, Massachusetts.)

enough of the IgE molecules to cause mast cell activation. Experimentally, antigen binding can be mimicked by polyvalent anti-IgE or by anti-FcεRI antibodies. In fact, anti-IgE antibodies can cross-link IgE molecules regardless of antigen specificity and lead to comparable triggering of mast cells from both atopic and nonatopic individuals.

Activation of mast cells results in three types of biologic response: secretion of the preformed contents of their granules by a regulated process of exocytosis, synthesis and secretion of lipid mediators, and synthesis and secretion of cytokines. These responses result from the cross-linking of FcεRI, which initiates a signaling cascade in mast cells involving protein tyrosine kinases (Fig. 19–5). The signaling cascade is similar to the proximal signaling events initiated by antigen binding to lymphocytes (see Chapters 9 and 10). The Lyn tyrosine kinase is constitutively associated with the cytoplasmic tail of the FcεRI β chain. On cross-linking of FcεRI molecules by antigen, Lyn tyrosine kinase phosphorylates the ITAMs in the cytoplasmic domains of FcεRI β and γ chains. The Syk tyrosine kinase is then recruited to the ITAMs of the γ chain, becomes activated, and phosphorylates and activates other proteins in the signaling cascade, including

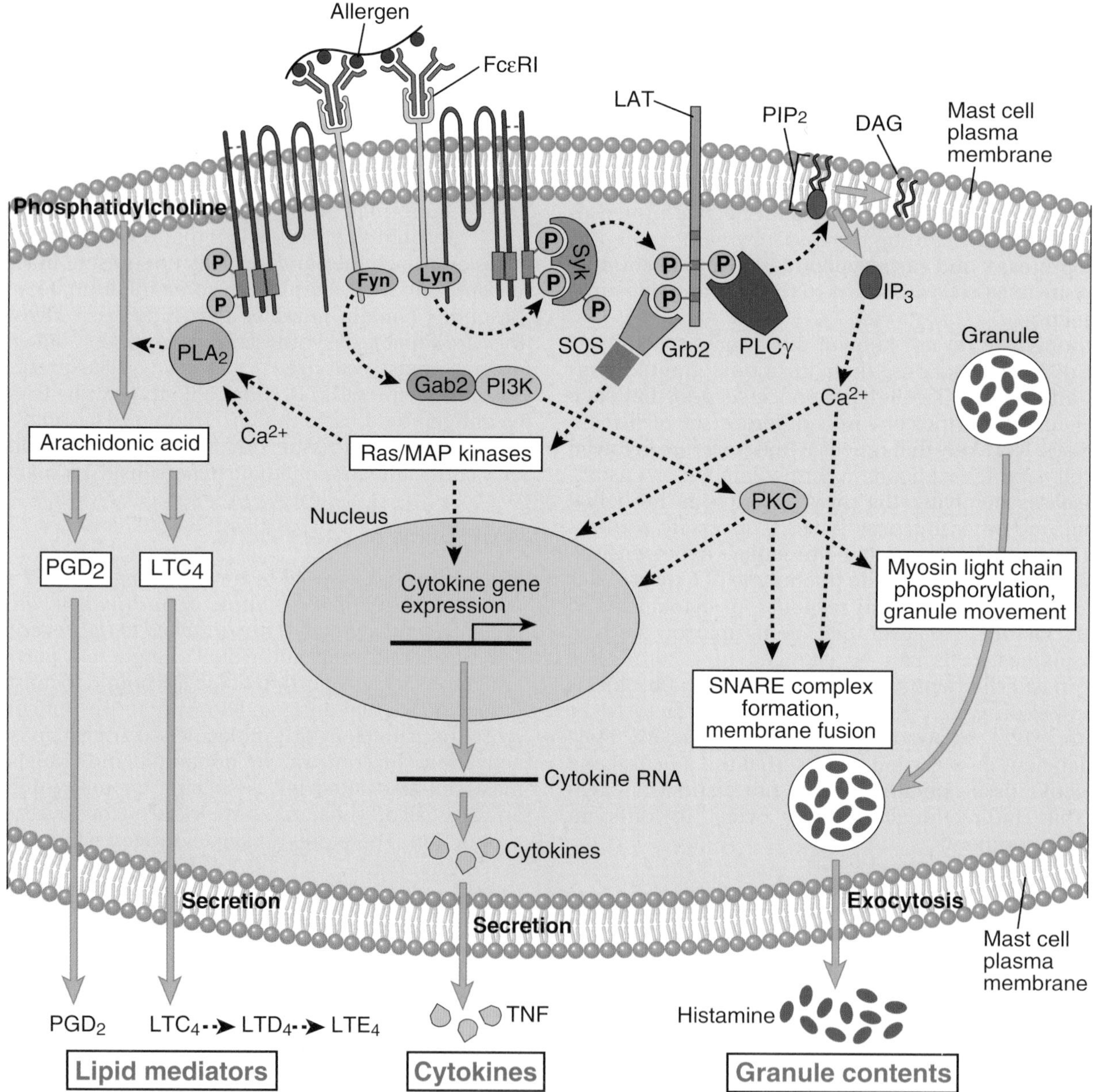

FIGURE 19–5 Biochemical events of mast cell activation. Cross-linking of bound IgE by antigen is thought to activate protein tyrosine kinases (Syk and Lyn), which in turn cause activation of a MAP kinase cascade and a phosphatidylinositol-specific phospholipase C (PI-PLCγ). PI-PLCγ catalyzes the release of IP_3 and DAG from membrane PIP_2. IP_3 causes release of intracellular calcium from the endoplasmic reticulum. Calcium and DAG activate PKC, which phosphorylates substrates such as myosin light chain protein and thereby leads to the degradation and release of preformed mediators. Calcium and MAP kinases combine to activate the enzyme cytosolic phospholipase A_2 ($cPLA_2$), which initiates the synthesis of lipid mediators.

several adapter molecules and enzymes that participate in the formation of multicomponent signaling complexes, as described in T cells. Linker for activation of T cells (LAT) is one of the essential adapter proteins involved in mast cell activation, and one of the enzymes recruited to LAT is the γ isoform of a phosphatidylinositol-specific phospholipase C (PLCγ). Once bound to LAT, PLCγ is phosphorylated and then catalyzes phosphatidylinositol bisphosphate breakdown to yield inositol triphosphate (IP_3) and diacylglycerol (DAG) (see Chapter 9). IP_3 causes elevation of cytoplasmic calcium levels and DAG activates protein kinase C (PKC). Another adapter protein essential for mast cell degranulation is Grb-2-associated binder-like protein 2 (Gab2). Phosphorylation of Gab2 by the tyrosine kinase Fyn leads to binding and activation of phosphoinositide 3 (PI-3) kinase, which also leads to activation of PKC. Phosphorylation of the myosin light chains by activated protein kinase C leads to disassembly of the actin-myosin complexes beneath the plasma membrane, thereby allowing granules to come in contact with the plasma membrane.

Fusion of the mast cell granule membrane with the plasma membrane is mediated by members of the SNARE protein family, which are involved in many other membrane fusion events. Different SNARE proteins present on the granule and plasma membranes interact to form a multimeric complex that catalyzes fusion. The formation of SNARE complexes is regulated by several accessory molecules, including Rab3 guanosine triphosphatases, and Rab-associated kinases and phosphatases. In resting mast cells, these regulatory molecules inhibit mast cell granule membrane fusion with the plasma membrane. Upon FcεRI cross-linking, the resulting increased cytoplasmic calcium concentrations and the activation of PKC block the regulatory functions of the accessory molecules. In addition, calcium-sensor proteins, called synaptotagmins, respond to the elevated calcium concentrations by promoting SNARE complex formation and membrane fusion.

Synthesis of lipid mediators is controlled by activation of the cytosolic enzyme phospholipase A_2 (PLA_2) (see Fig. 19–5). This enzyme is activated by two signals: elevated cytoplasmic calcium and phosphorylation catalyzed by a mitogen-activated protein (MAP) kinase such as extracellular receptor–activated kinase (ERK). ERK is activated as a consequence of a kinase cascade initiated through the receptor ITAMs, probably using the same intermediates as in T cells (see Chapter 9). Once activated, PLA_2 hydrolyzes membrane phospholipids to release substrates that are converted by enzyme cascades into the ultimate mediators. The major substrate is arachidonic acid, which is converted by cyclooxygenase or lipoxygenase into different mediators (discussed later).

Cytokine production by activated mast cells is a consequence of newly induced cytokine gene transcription. The biochemical events that regulate cytokine gene transcription in mast cells appear to be similar to the events that occur in T cells. Recruitment and activation of various adapter molecules and kinases in response to FcεRI cross-linking lead to nuclear translocation of nuclear factor of activated T cells (NFAT) and nuclear factor κB (NF-κB), as well as activation of activation protein-1 (AP-1) by protein kinases such as c-Jun N-terminal kinase. These transcription factors stimulate transcription of several cytokines (IL-4, IL-5, IL-6, IL-13, and tumor necrosis factor [TNF], among others) but, in contrast to T cells, not IL-2.

Mast cell activation through the FcεRI pathway is regulated by various inhibitory receptors, which contain an immunoreceptor tyrosine-based inhibition motif (ITIM) within their cytoplasmic tails (see Chapter 2, Box 2–4). One such inhibitory receptor is FcγRIIb, which coaggregates with FcεRI during mast cell activation, and the ITIM is phosphorylated by Lyn. This leads to recruitment of the phosphatase called SH2 domain-containing inositol 5-phosphatase (SHIP) and inhibition of FcεRI signaling. Experiments in mice indicate that FcγRIIb can regulate mast cell degranulation in vivo. Several other inhibitory receptors are also expressed on mast cells, but their relative importance in vivo is not yet known.

Mast cells can be directly activated by a variety of biologic substances independent of allergen-mediated cross-linking of FcεRI, including polybasic compounds, peptides, chemokines, and complement-derived anaphylatoxins. These additional modes of mast cell activation may be important in non-immune-mediated immediate hypersensitivity reactions, or they may amplify IgE-mediated reactions. Certain types of mast cells or basophils may respond to mononuclear phagocyte-derived chemokines, such as macrophage inflammatory protein-1α (MIP-1α), produced as part of innate immunity, and to T cell–derived chemokines, produced as part of adaptive cell-mediated immunity. The complement-derived anaphylatoxins, especially C5a, bind to specific receptors on mast cells and stimulate degranulation. These chemokines and complement fragments are likely to be produced at sites of inflammation. Therefore, mast cell activation and release of mediators may amplify even IgE-independent reactions. Polybasic compounds, such as compound 48/40 and mastoparan, are used as pharmacologic triggers for mast cells. These agents contain a cationic region adjacent to a hydrophobic moiety, and they work by activating G proteins.

Many neuropeptides, including substance P, somatostatin, and vasoactive intestinal peptide, induce mast cell histamine release and may mediate neuroendocrine-linked mast cell activation. The nervous system is known to modulate immediate hypersensitivity reactions, and neuropeptides may be involved in this effect. The flare produced at the edge of the wheal in elicited immediate hypersensitivity reactions is in part mediated by the nervous system, as shown by the observation that it is markedly diminished in skin sites lacking innervation. Cold temperatures and intense exercise may also trigger mast cell degranulation, but the mechanisms involved are not known.

Mast cells also express activating Fc receptors for IgG heavy chains, and these cells can be activated by cross-linking bound IgG. This IgG-mediated reaction is the likely explanation for the finding that ε chain knockout mice remain susceptible to antigen-induced mast cell–

mediated anaphylaxis. However, IgE is by far the major antibody isotype involved in most immediate hypersensitivity reactions.

Mast cell activation is not an all-or-nothing phenomenon, and different types or levels of stimuli may elicit partial responses, with production of some mediators but not others. Such variations in activation and mediator release may account for variable clinical presentations.

Mediators Derived from Mast Cells

The effector functions of mast cells are mediated by soluble molecules released from the cells on activation (Fig. 19–6 and Table 19–3). These mediators may be divided into preformed mediators, which include biogenic amines and granule macromolecules, and newly synthesized mediators, which include lipid-derived mediators and cytokines.

Biogenic Amines

Many of the biologic effects of mast cell activation are mediated by biogenic amines that are stored in and released from cytoplasmic granules. Biogenic amines, sometimes called vasoactive amines, are low molecular weight compounds that contain an amine group. In human mast cells, the major mediator of this class is histamine, but in some rodents, serotonin may be of equal or greater import. Histamine acts by binding to target cell receptors, and different cell types express distinct classes of histamine receptors (e.g., H_1, H_2, H_3) that can be distinguished by their sensitivity to pharmacologic inhibitors. The actions of histamine are short lived because histamine is rapidly removed from the extracellular milieu by amine-specific transport systems. On binding to cellular receptors, histamine initiates intracellular events, such as phosphatidylinositol breakdown to IP_3 and DAG,

Table 19–3. Mediators Produced by Mast Cells, Basophils, and Eosinophils

Cell type	Mediator category	Mediator	Function/pathologic effects
Mast cells and basophils			
	Stored preformed in cytoplasmic granules	Histamine	Increases vascular permeability; stimulates smooth muscle cell contraction
		Enzymes: neutral proteases (tryptase and/or chymase), acid hydrolases, cathepsin G, carboxypeptidase	Degrade microbial structures; tissue damage/remodeling
	Major lipid mediators produced on activation	Prostaglandin D_2	Vasodilation, bronchoconstriction, neutrophil chemotaxis
		Leukotrienes C_4, D_4, E_4	Prolonged bronchoconstriction, mucus secretion, increased vascular permeability
		Platelet-activating factor	Chemotaxis and activation of leukocytes, bronchoconstriction, increased vascular permeability
	Cytokines produced on activation	IL-3	Mast cell proliferation
		TNF, MIP-1α	Inflammation/late phase reaction
		IL-4, IL-13	IgE production, mucus secretion
		IL-5	Eosinophil production and activation
Eosinophils			
	Stored performed in cytoplasmic granules	Major basic protein, eosinophil cationic protein	Toxic to helminths, bacteria, host cells
		Eosinophil peroxidase, lysosomal hydrolases, lysophospholipase	Degrades helminthic and protozoan cell walls; tissue damage/remodeling
	Major lipid mediators produced on activation	Leukotrienes C_4, D_4, E_4	Prolonged bronchoconstriction; mucus secretion, increased vascular permeability
	Cytokines produced on activation	IL-3, IL-5, GM-CSF	Eosinophil production and activation
		IL-8, IL-10, RANTES, MIP-1α, eotaxin	Chemotaxis of leukocytes

Abbreviations: GM-CSF, granulocyte-monocyte colony-stimulating factor; IL-3, interleukin-3, MIP-1α, monocyte inflammatory protein-1α; RANTES, regulated by activation, normal T cell expressed and secreted; TNF, tumor necrosis factor.

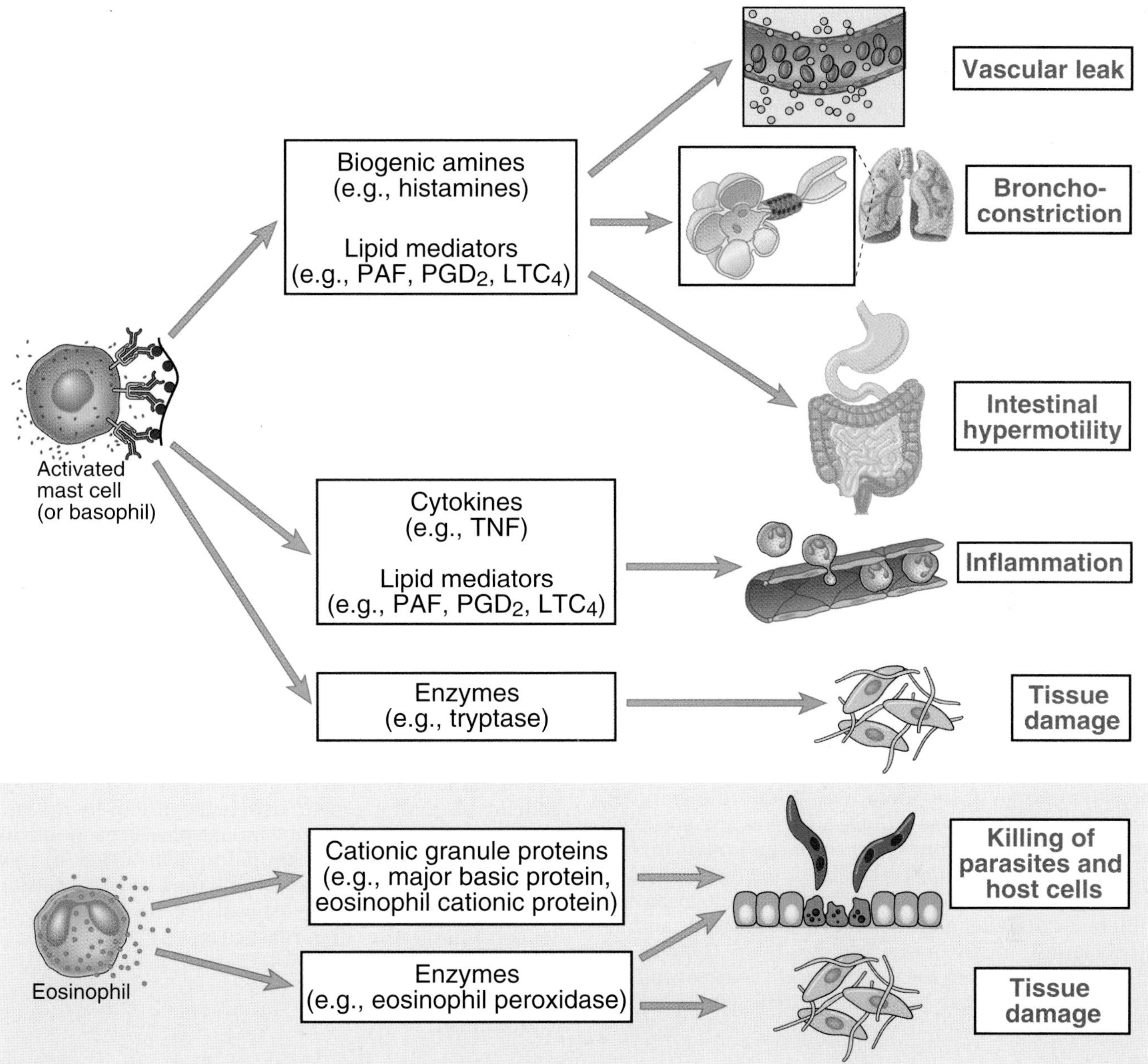

FIGURE 19–6 Biologic effects of mediators of immediate hypersensitivity. Mast cells and basophil mediators include biogenic amines and enzymes stored preformed in granules as well as cytokines and lipid mediators, which are largely newly synthesized on cell activation. The biogenic amines and lipid mediators induce vascular leakage, bronchoconstriction, and intestinal hypermotility, all components of the immediate response. Cytokines and lipid mediators contribute to inflammation, which is part of the late-phase reaction. Enzymes probably contribute to tissue damage. Activated eosinophils release preformed cationic proteins as well as enzymes that are toxic to parasites and host cells. Some eosinophil granule enzymes probably contribute to tissue damage in chronic allergic diseases.

and these products cause different changes in different cell types. Binding of histamine to endothelium causes cell contraction, leading to increased interendothelial spaces, increased vascular permeability, and leakage of plasma into the tissues. Histamine also stimulates endothelial cells to synthesize vascular smooth muscle cell relaxants, such as prostacyclin (PGI_2) and nitric oxide, which cause vasodilation. These actions of histamine produce the wheal and flare response of immediate hypersensitivity (described later). H_1 histamine receptor antagonists (commonly called antihistamines) can inhibit the wheal and flare response to intradermal allergen or anti-IgE antibody. Histamine also causes constriction of intestinal and bronchial smooth muscle. Thus, histamine may contribute to the increased peristalsis and bronchospasm associated with ingested and inhaled allergens, respectively. However, in some allergic disorders, and especially in asthma, antihistamines are not effective at blocking the reaction. Moreover, bronchoconstriction in asthma is more prolonged than are the effects of histamine, suggesting that other mast cell–derived mediators are important in some forms of immediate hypersensitivity.

Granule Enzymes and Proteoglycans

Neutral serine proteases, including tryptase and chymase, are the most abundant protein constituents of mast cell secretory granules and contribute to tissue damage in immediate hypersensitivity reactions. Tryptase is present in all human mast cells and is not known to be present in any other cell type. Consequently, the presence of tryptase in human biologic fluids is interpreted as a marker of mast cell activation. Chymase is found in some human mast cells, and its presence or absence is one criterion for characterizing human mast cell subsets, as discussed earlier. The functions of these enzymes in vivo are not known; however, several activities demonstrated in vitro suggest important biologic effects. For example, tryptase cleaves fibrinogen and activates collagenase, thereby causing tissue damage, whereas chymase can convert angiotensin I to angiotensin II, degrade epidermal basement membrane, and stimulate mucus secretion. Other enzymes found within mast cell granules include carboxypeptidase A and cathepsin G. Basophil granules also contain several enzymes, some of which are the same as those in mast cell granules, such as neutral proteases, and others are found in eosinophil granules, such as major basic protein and lysophospholipase.

Proteoglycans, including heparin and chondroitin sulfate, are also major constituents of both mast cell and basophil granules. These molecules are composed of a polypeptide core and multiple unbranched glycosaminoglycan side chains that impart a strong net negative charge to the molecules. Within the granules, proteoglycans serve as storage matrices for positively charged biogenic amines, proteases, and other mediators and prevent their accessibility to the rest of the cell. The mediators are released from the proteoglycans at different rates after granule exocytosis, biogenic amines dissociating much more rapidly than tryptase or chymase. In this way, the proteoglycans may control the kinetics of immediate hypersensitivity reactions.

Lipid Mediators

Mast cell activation results in the rapid **de novo** ***synthesis and release of lipid-derived mediators that have a variety of effects on blood vessels, bronchial smooth muscle, and leukocytes.*** The most important of these mediators are metabolites of arachidonic acid generated by the actions of cyclooxygenase and lipoxygenase.

The major arachidonic acid–derived mediator produced by the cyclooxygenase pathway in mast cells is **prostaglandin D_2** (PGD_2). Released PGD_2 binds to receptors on smooth muscle cells and acts as a vasodilator and a bronchoconstrictor. PGD_2 also promotes neutrophil chemotaxis and accumulation at inflammatory sites. PGD_2 synthesis can be prevented by inhibitors of cyclooxygenase, such as aspirin and other nonsteroidal anti-inflammatory agents. These drugs may paradoxically exacerbate asthmatic bronchoconstriction, because they shunt arachidonic acid toward production of leukotrienes, discussed next.

The major arachidonic acid–derived mediators produced by the lipoxygenase pathway are the **leukotrienes,** especially LTC_4 and its degradation products LTD_4 and LTE_4. LTC_4 is made by mucosal mast cells and basophils, but not by connective tissue mast cells. Mast cell–derived leukotrienes bind to specific receptors on smooth muscle cells, different from the receptors for PGD_2, and cause prolonged bronchoconstriction. When injected into the skin, these leukotrienes produce a characteristic long-lived wheal and flare reaction. Collectively, LTC_4, LTD_4, and LTE_4 constitute what was once called slow-reacting substance of anaphylaxis (SRS-A) and are thought to be major mediators of asthmatic bronchoconstriction. Pharmacologic inhibitors of 5-lipoxygenase also block anaphylactic reactions in experimental systems.

A third type of lipid mediator produced by mast cells is called **platelet-activating factor** (PAF) for its original bioassay as an inducer of rabbit platelet aggregation. In mast cells and basophils, PAF is synthesized by acylation of lysoglyceryl ether phosphorylcholine, a derivative of PLA_2-mediated hydrolysis of membrane phospholipids. PAF has direct bronchoconstricting actions. It also causes retraction of endothelial cells and can relax vascular smooth muscle. However, PAF is hydrophobic and is rapidly destroyed by a plasma enzyme called PAF hydrolase, which limits its biologic actions. Pharmacologic inhibitors of PAF receptors ameliorate some aspects of immediate hypersensitivity in the rabbit lung. Recent genetic evidence has pointed to PAF as a mediator of asthma. Asthma develops in early childhood in individuals with a genetic deficiency of PAF hydrolase. PAF may also be important in late-phase reactions, in which it can activate inflammatory leukocytes. In this situation, the major source of PAF may be basophils or vascular endothelial cells (stimulated by histamine or leukotrienes) rather than mast cells.

Cytokines

Mast cells (and basophils) produce many different cytokines that contribute to allergic inflammation (the late-phase reaction). These cytokines include TNF, IL-1, IL-4, IL-5, IL-6, IL-13, MIP-1α, MIP-1β, and various colony-stimulating factors such as IL-3 and granulocyte-monocyte colony-stimulating factor (GM-CSF). As mentioned before, mast cell activation induces transcription and synthesis of these cytokines, but preformed TNF may also be stored in granules and rapidly released on FcεRI cross-linking. T_H2 cells that are recruited into the sites of allergic reactions also produce some of these cytokines. The cytokines that are released on IgE-mediated mast cell or basophil activation or on T_H2 cell activation are mainly responsible for the late-phase reaction. TNF activates endothelial expression of adhesion molecules and, together with chemokines, accounts for neutrophil and monocyte infiltrates (see Chapter 2). In addition to allergic inflammation, mast cell cytokines also apparently contribute to the innate immune responses to infections. For example, as we will discuss later, mouse models indicate that mast cells are required for effective defense against some bacterial infections, and this effector function is mediated largely by TNF.

Properties of Eosinophils

Eosinophils are bone marrow–derived granulocytes that are abundant in the inflammatory infiltrates of late-phase reactions and contribute to many of the pathologic processes in allergic diseases. Eosinophils develop in the bone marrow, and after maturation they circulate in the blood. GM-CSF, IL-3, and IL-5 promote eosinophil maturation from myeloid precursors. Eosinophils are normally present in peripheral tissues, especially in mucosal linings of the respiratory, gastrointestinal, and genitourinary tracts, and their numbers can increase by recruitment in the setting of inflammation. The granules of eosinophils contain basic proteins that bind acidic dyes such as eosin (see Fig. 19–5).

Cytokines produced by T_H2 cells promote the activation of eosinophils and their recruitment to late-phase reaction inflammatory sites. IL-5 is a potent eosinophil-activating cytokine. It enhances the ability of eosinophils to release granule contents. IL-5 also increases maturation of eosinophils from bone marrow precursors, and in the absence of this cytokine (e.g., in IL-5 knockout mice), there is a deficiency of eosinophil numbers and functions. Eosinophils are recruited into late-phase reaction sites as well as sites of helminthic infection, and their recruitment is mediated by a combination of adhesion molecule interactions and chemokines. Eosinophils bind to endothelial cells expressing E-selectin and the ligand for the VLA-4 integrin. IL-4 produced by T_H2 cells may enhance expression of adhesion molecules for eosinophils. Eosinophil recruitment and infiltration into tissues also depend on the chemokine eotaxin (CCL11), which is produced by epithelial cells at sites of allergic reactions and binds to the chemokine receptor CCR3 expressed constitutively by eosinophils. In addition, the complement product C5a and the lipid mediators PAF and LTB_4, which are produced by mast cells, also function as chemoattractants for eosinophils.

Eosinophils release granule proteins that are toxic to parasitic organisms and may injure normal tissue. Little is known about the mechanisms involved in eosinophil degranulation and mediator production. Although eosinophils express Fc receptors for IgG, IgA, and IgE, they do not appear to be as sensitive to activation by antigen-mediated cross-linking of these receptors as are mast cells and basophils. The granule contents of eosinophils include lysosomal hydrolases found in other granulocytes as well as eosinophil-specific proteins that are particularly toxic to helminthic organisms, including major basic protein and eosinophil cationic protein. These two cationic polypeptides have no known enzymatic activities, but they are toxic to helminths, bacteria, and normal tissue. In addition, eosinophilic granules contain eosinophil peroxidase, which is distinct from the myeloperoxidase found in neutrophils and catalyzes the production of hypochlorous or hypobromous acid. These products are also toxic to helminths, protozoa, and host cells.

Activated eosinophils, like mast cells and basophils, produce and release lipid mediators, including PAF, prostaglandins, and leukotrienes (LTC_4 and its derivatives LTD_4 and LTE_4). The importance of eosinophil-derived lipid mediators in immediate hypersensitivity is not completely known, but it is likely that they contribute to the pathologic processes of allergic diseases. Eosinophils also produce a variety of cytokines that may promote inflammatory responses, but the biologic significance of eosinophil cytokine production is not known.

Reactions of Immediate Hypersensitivity

The IgE- and mast cell–mediated reactions of immediate hypersensitivity consist of the immediate reaction, in which vascular and smooth muscle responses to mediators are dominant, and the late-phase reaction, characterized by leukocyte recruitment and inflammation (Fig. 19–7).

The Immediate Reaction

The early vascular changes that occur during immediate hypersensitivity reactions are demonstrated by the wheal and flare reaction to the intradermal injection of an allergen (Fig. 19–8). When an individual who has previously encountered an allergen and produced IgE antibody is challenged by intradermal injection of the same antigen, the injection site becomes red from locally dilated blood vessels engorged with red blood cells. The site then rapidly swells as a result of leakage of plasma from the venules. This soft swelling is called a wheal and can involve an area of skin as large as several centimeters in diameter. Subsequently, blood vessels at the margins of the wheal dilate and become engorged with red blood cells and produce a characteristic red rim called a flare. The full wheal and flare reaction can appear within 5 to 10 minutes after administration of antigen and usually subsides in less than an hour. By electron microscopy, the venules in the area of the wheal show slight separation of the endothelial cells, which accounts for the escape of macromolecules and fluid, but not cells, from the vascular lumen.

The wheal and flare reaction is dependent on IgE and mast cells. Histologic examination shows that mast cells in the area of the wheal and flare have released preformed mediators; that is, their cytoplasmic granules have been discharged. A causal association of IgE and mast cells with immediate hypersensitivity was deduced from three kinds of experiments.

- Immediate hypersensitivity reactions against an allergen can be elicited in unresponsive individuals if the local skin site is first injected with IgE from an allergic individual. Thus, IgE is responsible for specific recognition of antigen and can be used to adoptively transfer immediate hypersensitivity. Such adoptive transfer experiments were first performed with serum from immunized individuals, and the serum factor

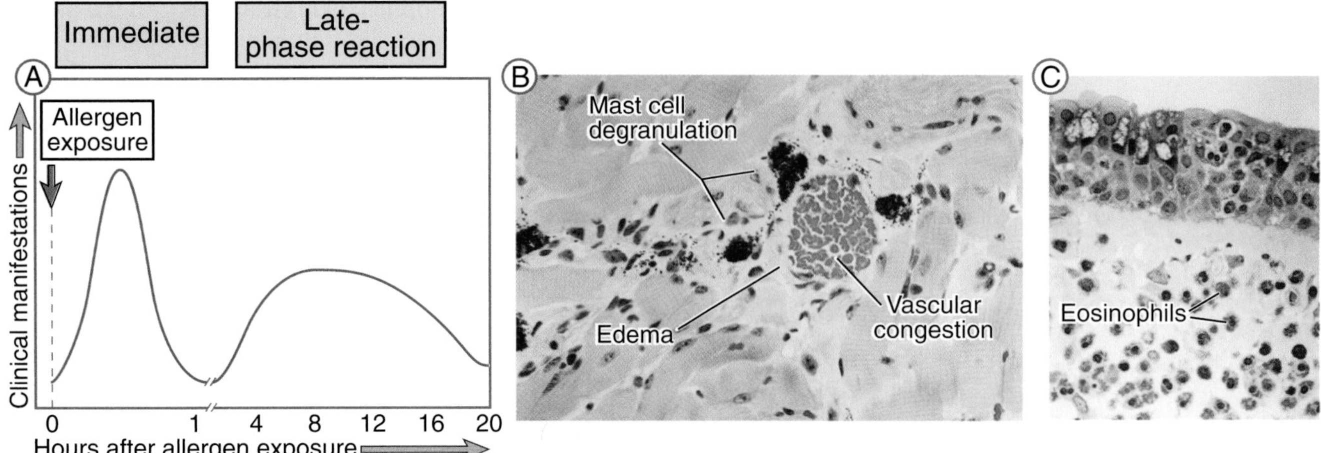

FIGURE 19–7 The immediate and late-phase reactions. A. Kinetics: The immediate vascular and smooth muscle reaction to allergen develops within minutes after challenge (allergen exposure in a previously sensitized individual), and the late-phase reaction develops 2 to 24 hours later. B, C. Morphology: The immediate reaction (B) is characterized by vasodilation, congestion, and edema, and the late-phase reaction (C) is characterized by an inflammatory infiltrate rich in eosinophils, neutrophils, and T cells. (Courtesy of Dr. Daniel Friend, Department of Pathology, Brigham and Women's Hospital, Boston, Massachusetts.)

responsible for the reaction was originally called reagin. For this reason, IgE molecules are still sometimes called reaginic antibodies. The antigen-initiated skin reaction that follows adoptive transfer of IgE is called passive cutaneous anaphylaxis.

- Immediate hypersensitivity reactions can be mimicked by injecting anti-IgE antibody instead of antigen. Anti-IgE antibodies act as an analogue of antigen and directly activate mast cells that have bound IgE on their surface. This use of anti-IgE to activate mast cells is similar to the use of anti-IgM antibodies as analogues of antigen to activate B cells (see Appendix III), except that in the case of mast cells, secreted IgE, made by B cells, is bound to high-affinity Fc receptors on the cell surface rather than being synthesized as membrane IgE. Anti-IgE antibodies activate mast cells even in normal (nonatopic) individuals because, as mentioned earlier, mast cells are normally coated with IgE that can be cross-linked by the anti-IgE. In contrast, an antigen will activate mast cells only in individuals who are allergic to that antigen because only these individuals will produce enough specific IgE to be cross-linked by the antigen.
- Immediate hypersensitivity reactions can be mimicked by the injection of other agents that directly activate mast cells, such as the complement fragments C5a, C4a, and C3a, called anaphylatoxins, or by local trauma, which also causes degranulation of mast cells. Conversely, these reactions can be inhibited by agents that prevent mast cell activation.

The wheal and flare reaction results from sensitization of dermal mast cells by IgE bound to FcεRI, cross-linking of the IgE by the antigen, and activation of mast cells with release of mediators, notably histamine. Histamine binds to histamine receptors on venular endothelial cells; the endothelial cells synthesize and release PGI_2, nitric oxide, and PAF; and these mediators cause vasodilation and vascular leak, as described earlier in the chapter. Skin mast cells appear to produce only small amounts of long-acting mediators such as leukotrienes, and the wheal and flare response typically subsides after about 15 to 20 minutes. Allergists often test patients for allergies to different antigens by examining the ability of these antigens applied in skin patches to elicit wheal and flare reactions.

The Late-Phase Reaction

The immediate wheal and flare reaction is followed 2 to 4 hours later by a late-phase reaction consisting of the accumulation of inflammatory leukocytes, including neutrophils, eosinophils, basophils, and T_H2 cells (see Fig. 19–7). The inflammation is maximal by about 24 hours and then gradually subsides. The capacity to mount a late-phase reaction can be adoptively transferred with IgE, and the reaction can be mimicked by anti-IgE antibodies or mast cell–activating agents, like the immediate wheal and flare reaction. Mast cells produce cytokines, including TNF, that can up-regulate endothelial expression of leukocyte adhesion molecules, such as E-selectin and intercellular adhesion molecule-1 (ICAM-1), and chemokines that recruit blood leukocytes. Thus, mast cell activation promotes the recruitment of leukocytes into tissues. The types of leukocytes that are typical of late-phase reactions are eosinophils and T_H2 cells; in addition, neutrophils are often present in these reactions. Eosinophils and T_H2 cells express receptors for many of the same chemokines, such as eotaxin, and this is why both cell types are recruited to sites of production of these chemokines. The late-phase reaction differs from delayed-type hypersensitivity reactions, in which macrophages and T_H1 cells are dominant.

The late-phase reaction may occur without a detectable preceding immediate hypersensitivity reac-

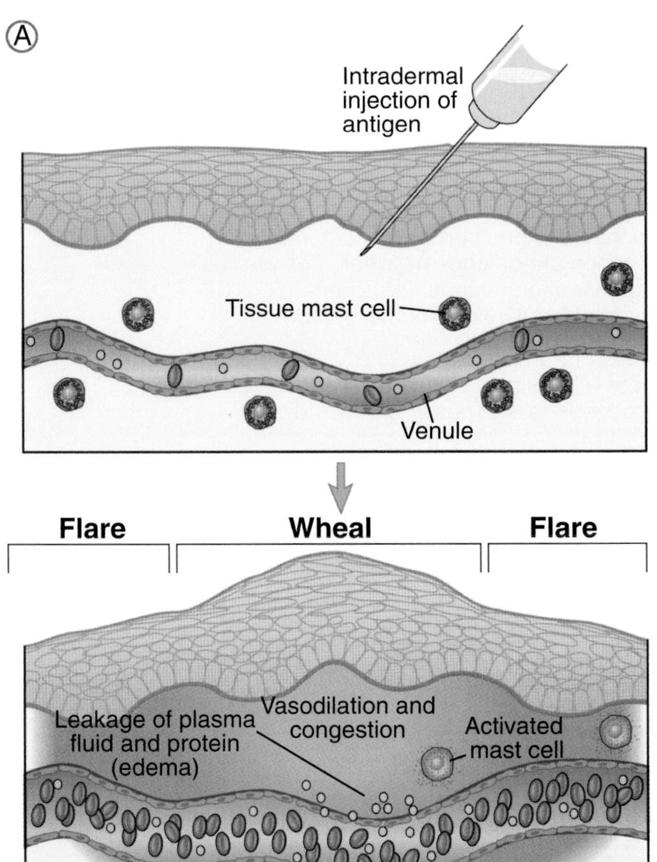

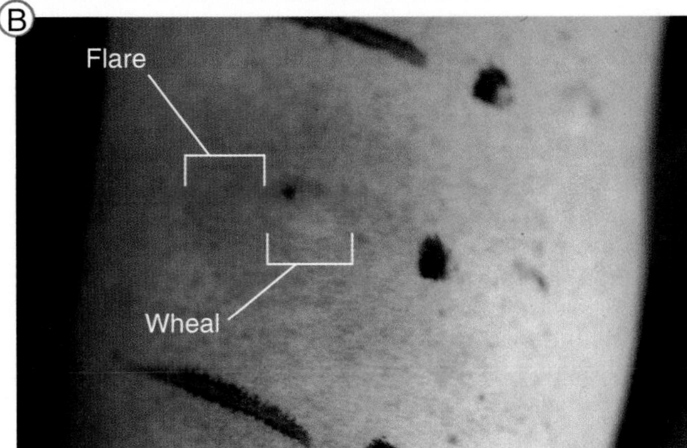

FIGURE 19–8 The wheal and flare reaction in the skin. A. In response to antigen-stimulated release of mast cell mediators, local blood vessels first dilate and then become leaky to fluid and macromolecules, which produces redness and local swelling (a wheal). Subsequent dilation of vessels on the edge of the swelling produces the appearance of a red rim (the flare). B. Photograph of a typical wheal and flare reaction in the skin in response to injection of an allergen. (Courtesy of Dr. James D. Faix, Department of Pathology, Stanford University School of Medicine, Palo Alto, California.)

tion. Bronchial asthma is a disease in which there may be repeated bouts of inflammation with accumulations of eosinophils and T_H2 cells without the vascular changes that are characteristic of the immediate response. In such disorders, there may be little mast cell activation, and the cytokines that sustain the late-phase reaction may be produced mainly by T cells.

Genetic Susceptibility to Immediate Hypersensitivity

The propensity to produce IgE is influenced by the inheritance of several genes. Abnormally high levels of IgE synthesis and associated atopy often run in families. Family studies have shown clear autosomal transmission of atopy, although the full inheritance pattern is multigenic. Within the same family, the target organ of atopic disease is variable. Thus, hay fever, asthma, and eczema can be present to various degrees in different members of the same kindred. All these individuals, however, will show higher than average plasma IgE levels.

Genome-wide linkage analyses for atopy/asthma susceptibility loci have identified several chromosomal regions of importance in allergic disease (Table 19–4). Each of these loci may contain several genes of potential importance to disease. Some of the genes in these loci may regulate T_H2 responses and IgE production. Other genes may have tissue-specific influences, such as airway remodeling in the asthmatic lung. One of these susceptibility loci for atopy is on chromosome 5q, near the site of the gene cluster encoding the cytokines IL-3, IL-4, IL-5, IL-9, and IL-13 and the IL-4 receptor. This region is of great interest because of the connection between several of the genes located here and the mechanisms of IgE regulation and mast cell and eosinophil growth and differentiation. Furthermore, the homologous chromosomal region in mice has been linked to a propensity for $CD4^+$ T cells in some inbred strains of mice to differentiate into T_H2 cells in response to model protein antigens. Among the genes in this cluster, polymorphisms in the IL-13 gene appear to have the strongest associations with asthma. The tendency to produce IgE antibodies against some but not all antigens, such as ragweed pollen, may be linked to particular class II major histocompatibility complex (MHC) alleles. This linkage may be an example of an "immune response gene" (*Ir* gene) effect in which atopic individuals inherit class II MHC alleles that can bind and display dominant epitopes of certain allergens (see Chapter 4). Several other chromosomal regions have been shown to be associated with high serum IgE levels, atopy, and asthma. In addition to these linkage studies, individual asthma-associated genes have been identified by positional cloning. These include *ADAM33*, *DPP10*, and *PHF11* (see Table 19–4). Although there are highly significant associations of polymorphisms of these genes with asthma, the way in which the products of the genes contribute to disease are not yet understood.

Some genes whose products regulate the innate immune response to infections have been associated with allergy and asthma. These include CD14, a component of the lipopolysaccharide receptor, and Tim-1, a protein thought to influence helper T cell differentiation.

Table 19–4. Examples of Chromosomal Locations and Genes Associated with Atopy and Asthma

Chromosomal location	Candidate genes	Putative role of gene products in disease
5q	Cytokine gene cluster (IL-4, IL-5, IL-13), CD14, β_2-adrenergic receptor	IL-4 and IL-13 promote IgE switching, IL-5 promotes eosinophil growth and activation; CD14 is a component of the LPS receptor which, via interaction with TLR4, may influence the balance between T_H1 vs. T_H2 responses to antigens; β2-adrenergic receptor regulates bronchial smooth muscle contraction
6p	Class II MHC	Some alleles may regulate T cell responses to allergens
11q	FcεRI β chain	Mediates mast cell activation
12q	Stem cell factor, interferon-γ, STAT6	Stem cell factor regulates mast cell growth and differentiation; interferon-γ opposes actions of IL-4; STAT6 mediates IL-4 signal transduction
16	IL-4 receptor α chain	Subunit of both IL-4 and IL-13 receptors
20p	*ADAM33*	Metalloproteinase involved in airway remodeling
2q	*DPP10*	Peptidase that may regulate chemokine and cytokine activity
13q	*PHF11*	Transcriptional regulator involved in B cell clonal expansion and Ig expression

Abbreviations: FcεRI, Fcε receptor type I; IL-4, interleukin-4.

Strong innate responses to infections generally favor development of T_H1 responses, and inhibit T_H2 responses (see Chapter 13). Therefore, polymorphisms or mutations in genes that result in diminished innate responses to common infectious organisms may increase the risk for development of atopy.

Allergic Diseases in Humans: Pathogenesis and Therapy

Mast cell degranulation is a central component of all allergic diseases, and the clinical and pathologic manifestations of the diseases depend on the tissues in which the mast cell mediators have effects as well as the chronicity of the resulting inflammatory process. Atopic individuals may have one or more manifestations of atopic disease. The most common forms of atopic disease are allergic rhinitis (hay fever), bronchial asthma, atopic dermatitis (eczema), and food allergies. The clinical and pathologic features of allergic reactions vary with the anatomic site of the reaction, for several reasons. The point of contact with the allergen determines the organs or tissues that are involved. For example, inhaled antigens cause rhinitis or asthma, ingested antigens often cause vomiting and diarrhea, and injected antigens cause systemic effects on the circulation. The concentrations of mast cells in various target organs influence the severity of responses. Mast cells are particularly abundant in the skin and the mucosa of the respiratory and gastrointestinal tracts, and these tissues frequently suffer the most injury in immediate hypersensitivity reactions. The local mast cell phenotype may influence the characteristics of the immediate hypersensitivity reaction. For example, connective tissue mast cells with abundant histamine are responsible for wheal and flare reactions in the skin. In the following section, we discuss the major features of allergic diseases manifested in different tissues.

Systemic Anaphylaxis

Anaphylaxis is a systemic immediate hypersensitivity reaction characterized by edema in many tissues and a fall in blood pressure, secondary to vasodilation. These effects usually result from the systemic presence of antigen introduced by injection, an insect sting, or absorption across an epithelial surface such as the skin or gut mucosa. The allergen activates mast cells in many tissues, resulting in the release of mediators that gain access to vascular beds throughout the body. The decrease in vascular tone and leakage of plasma caused by the released mediators can lead to a fall in blood pressure or shock, called anaphylactic shock, which is often fatal. The cardiovascular effects are accompanied by constriction of the upper and lower airways, laryngeal edema, hypermotility of the gut, outpouring of mucus in the gut and respiratory tract, and urticarial lesions (hives) in the skin. It is not known which mast cell mediators are the most important in anaphylactic shock. The mainstay of treatment is systemic epinephrine, which can be lifesaving by reversing the bronchoconstrictive and vasodilatory effects of the various mast cell mediators. Epinephrine also improves cardiac output, further aiding survival from threatened circulatory collapse. Antihistamines may also be beneficial in anaphylaxis, suggesting a role for histamine in this reaction. In some animal models, PAF receptor antagonists offer partial protection.

Bronchial Asthma

Asthma is an inflammatory disease caused by repeated immediate hypersensitivity and late-phase reactions in the lung leading to the clinicopathologic triad of intermittent and reversible airway obstruction, chronic bronchial inflammation with eosinophils, and bronchial smooth muscle cell hypertrophy and hyperreactivity to bronchoconstrictors (Fig. 19–9). Patients suffer paroxysms of bronchial constriction and increased production of thick mucus, which leads to bronchial obstruction and exacerbates respiratory difficulties. Asthma frequently coexists with bronchitis or emphysema, and the combination of diseases can cause severe damage to lung tissue. Affected individuals may suffer considerable morbidity, and asthma can be fatal. Asthma affects about 10 million people in the United States, and the frequency of this disease has increased significantly in recent years. The prevalence rate is similar to that in other industrialized countries, but it may be lower in less developed areas of the world. One possible explanation for the increased prevalence of asthma and other atopic diseases in industrialized countries is that the frequency of infections in these countries is generally lower. As we discussed earlier, the innate immune responses associated with most infections promote T_H1 responses and suppress T_H2 responses required for development of atopy. A variety of epidemiologic data are consistent with the idea that reducing infections leads to increased prevalence of allergic disease. This idea has been given the catchy name *the hygiene hypothesis.*

About 70% of cases of asthma are due to IgE-mediated immediate hypersensitivity. In the remaining 30% of patients, asthma may not be associated with atopy and may be triggered by nonimmune stimuli such as drugs, cold, and exercise. Even among nonatopic asthmatics, the pathophysiologic process of airway constriction is similar, which suggests that alternative mechanisms of mast cell degranulation (e.g., by locally produced neurotransmitters) may underlie the disease.

The pathophysiologic sequence in atopic asthma is probably initiated by mast cell activation in response to allergen binding to IgE as well as by T_H2 cells reacting to allergens (Fig. 19–10). The cytokines produced by the mast cells and T cells lead to the recruitment of eosinophils, basophils, and more T_H2 cells. The chronic inflammation in this disease may continue without mast cell activation. Smooth muscle cell hypertrophy and hyperreactivity are thought to result from leukocyte-derived mediators and cytokines. Mast cells, basophils, and eosinophils all produce mediators that constrict airway smooth muscle. The most important of the bronchoconstricting mediators are LTC_4, its breakdown products LTD_4 and LTE_4, and PAF. In clinical experiments, antagonists of LTC_4 synthesis or leukotriene receptor antagonists prevent allergen-induced airway constriction. Increased mucus secretion results from the action of cytokines, mainly IL-13, on bronchial epithelial cells.

Current therapy for asthma has two major targets: prevention and reversal of inflammation and relaxation

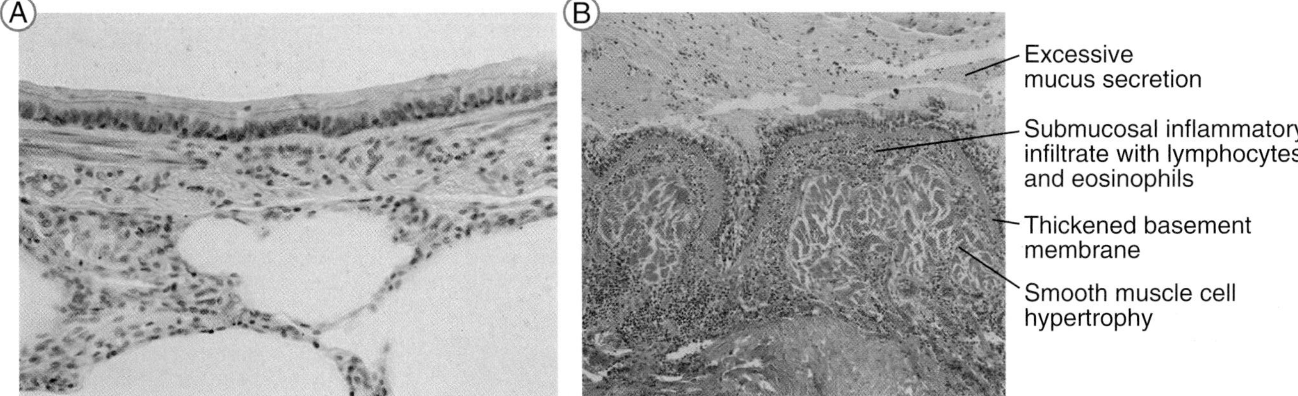

FIGURE 19–9 Histopathologic features of bronchial asthma. Atopic bronchial asthma results from repeated immediate hypersensitivity reactions in the lungs with chronic late-phase reactions. A cross-section of a normal bronchus is shown in A; a bronchus from a patient with asthma is shown in B. The diseased bronchus has excessive mucus production, many submucosal inflammatory cells (including eosinophils), and smooth muscle hypertrophy. (Courtesy of Dr. James D. Faix, Department of Pathology, Stanford University School of Medicine, Palo Alto, California.)

of airway smooth muscle. In recent years, the balance of therapy has shifted toward anti-inflammatory agents as the primary mode of treatment. Several classes of drugs are in current use to treat asthma. Corticosteroids block the production of inflammatory cytokines. Sodium cromolyn appears to antagonize IgE-induced release of mediators. Both agents can be used prophylactically as inhalants. Corticosteroids may also be given systemically, especially once an attack is under way, to reduce inflammation. Leukotriene inhibitors block the binding of bronchoconstricting leukotrienes to airway smooth muscle cells. Humanized monoclonal anti-IgE antibody is a recently approved therapy that effectively reduces serum IgE levels in patients. Because histamine has little role in airway constriction, antihistamines (H_1 receptor antagonists) are not useful in the treatment of asthma. Indeed, because many antihistamines are also anticholinergics, these drugs may worsen airway obstruction by causing thickening of mucus secretions.

Bronchial smooth muscle cell relaxation has principally been achieved by elevating intracellular cyclic adenosine monophosphate (cAMP) levels in smooth muscle cells, which inhibits contraction. The major drugs used are activators of adenylate cyclase, such as epinephrine and related β_2-adrenergic agents. Theophylline is a commonly used anti-asthma drug, which inhibits phosphodiesterase enzymes that degrade cAMP. However, theophylline may also have anti-inflammatory effects unrelated to its effects on smooth muscle cell relaxation, which contribute to its effectiveness.

Immediate Hypersensitivity Reactions in the Upper Respiratory Tract, Gastrointestinal Tract, and Skin

Allergic rhinitis, also called hay fever, is perhaps the most common allergic disease and is a consequence of immediate hypersensitivity reactions to common allergens such as plant pollen or house dust mites localized to the upper respiratory tract by inhalation. The pathologic and clinical manifestations include mucosal edema, leukocyte infiltration with abundant eosinophils, mucus secretion, coughing, sneezing, and difficulty breathing. Allergic conjunctivitis with itchy eyes is commonly associated with the rhinitis. Focal protrusions of the nasal mucosa, called nasal polyps, filled with edema fluid and eosinophils may develop in patients who suffer frequent repetitive bouts of allergic rhinitis. Antihistamines are the most common drugs used to treat allergic rhinitis.

Food allergies are immediate hypersensitivity reactions to ingested foods that lead to the release of mediators from intestinal mucosal and submucosal mast cells. Clinical manifestations include enhanced peristal-

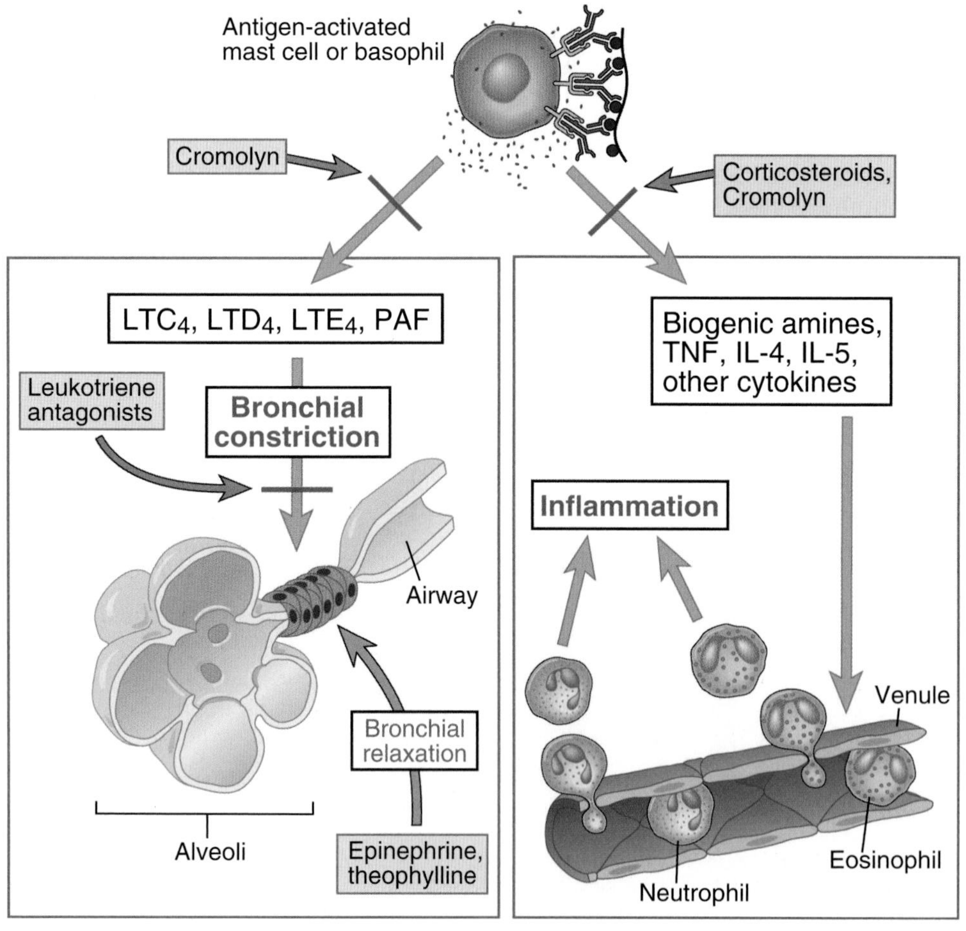

FIGURE 19–10 Mediators and treatment of asthma. Mast cell–derived leukotrienes and PAF are thought to be the major mediators of acute bronchoconstriction. Therapy is targeted both at reducing mast cell activation with inhibitors such as cromolyn and at countering mediator actions on bronchial smooth muscle by bronchodilators such as epinephrine and theophylline. These drugs also inhibit mast cell activation. Mast cell–derived cytokines are thought to be the major mediators of sustained airway inflammation, which is an example of a late-phase reaction, and corticosteroid therapy is used to inhibit cytokine synthesis. Cytokines are also produced by T_H2 cells (not shown).

sis, increased fluid secretion from intestinal lining cells, and associated vomiting and diarrhea. Urticaria is often associated with allergic reactions to food, and systemic anaphylaxis may occasionally ensue. Allergic reactions to many different types of food have been described, but some of the most common are peanuts and shellfish. Individuals may be so sensitive to these allergens that severe systemic reactions can occur in response to minute contaminants of the allergen introduced accidentally during food preparation.

Allergic reactions in the skin are manifested as **urticaria** and **eczema.** Urticaria, which is essentially an acute wheal and flare reaction induced by mast cell mediators, occurs in response to direct contact with the allergen or after an allergen enters the circulation through the intestinal tract or by injection. Because the reaction that ensues is mediated largely by histamine, antihistamines (H_1 receptor antagonists) can block this response almost completely. The urticaria may persist for several hours, probably because antigen persists in the plasma. Chronic eczema is a common skin disorder that may be caused by a late-phase reaction to an allergen in the skin. In the cutaneous late-phase reaction, TNF, IL-4, and other cytokines, probably derived from T_H2 cells and mast cells, act on the venular endothelial cells to promote inflammation. As may be expected for a cytokine-mediated response, the late-phase inflammatory reaction is not inhibited by antihistamines. It can be blocked by treatment with corticosteroids, which inhibit cytokine synthesis.

Immunotherapy for Allergic Diseases

In addition to therapy aimed at the consequences of immediate hypersensitivity, clinical immunologists often try to limit the onset of allergic reactions by treatments aimed at reducing the quantity of IgE present in the individual. Several empirical protocols have been developed to diminish specific IgE synthesis. In one approach, called **desensitization,** small quantities of antigen are repeatedly administered subcutaneously. As a result of this treatment, specific IgE levels decrease and IgG titers often rise, perhaps further inhibiting IgE production by neutralizing the antigen and by antibody feedback (see Chapter 10). It is also possible that desensitization may work by inducing specific T cell tolerance or by changing the predominant phenotype of antigen-specific T cells from T_H2 to T_H1; however, there is no clear evidence to support any of these hypotheses. The beneficial effects of desensitization may occur in a matter of hours, much earlier than changes in IgE levels. Although the precise mechanism is unknown, this approach has been successful in preventing acute anaphylactic responses to protein antigens (e.g., insect venom) or vital drugs (e.g., penicillin). It is more variable in its effectiveness for chronic atopic conditions such as hay fever and asthma.

Other approaches being used to reduce IgE levels include systemic administration of humanized monoclonal anti-IgE antibodies mentioned earlier.

The Protective Roles of IgE- and Mast Cell–Mediated Immune Reactions

Although most of our understanding of mast cell– and basophil-mediated responses comes from analysis of hypersensitivity diseases, it is logical to assume that these responses have evolved because they provide protective functions. In fact, some evidence shows that IgE- and mast cell–mediated responses are important for defense against certain types of infection.

A major protective function of IgE-initiated immune reactions is the eradication of parasites. Eosinophil-mediated killing of helminths is an effective defense against these organisms. The activities of IL-4, IL-5, and IL-13 in IgE production and eosinophil activation contribute to a coordinated defense against helminths. It has also been speculated that IgE-dependent mast cell activation in the gastrointestinal tract promotes the expulsion of parasites by increasing peristalsis and by an outpouring of mucus. Studies in mice have highlighted the beneficial roles of IgE and mast cells.

- Mice treated with anti-IL-4 antibody and IL-4 knockout mice do not make IgE and appear to be more susceptible than normal animals to some helminthic infections. IL-5 knockout mice, which are unable to activate eosinophils, also show increased susceptibility to some helminths.
- Genetically mast cell–deficient mice show increased susceptibility to infection by tick larvae, and immunity can be provided to these mice by adoptive transfer of specific IgE and mast cells (but not by either component alone). The larvae are eradicated by the late-phase reaction.

Mast cells play an important protective role as part of the innate immune response to bacterial infections. Studies in mice have indicated that mast cells can be activated by IgE-independent mechanisms in the course of an acute bacterial infection and that the mediators they release are critical for clearing the infection.

- Mast cell–deficient mice are less capable of clearing, and are more likely to die of, acute bacterial infection of the peritoneum than are normal mice. The protective role of mast cells in this setting is mediated by TNF and depends on TNF-stimulated influx of neutrophils to the peritoneum, specifically, the late-phase reaction. The mechanisms by which mast cells are activated during innate immune responses to bacterial infection are not known but may involve complement activation by the alternative pathway, leading to the release of C5a, which directly triggers mast cell degranulation. It is also possible that the classical pathway of complement could be activated by natural antibodies that are produced by B-1 B cells and that recognize common microbial pathogens.

Mast cell-derived proteases have been shown to destroy some snake and insect venoms in mice. This is an unusual form of "innate immunity" against a potentially lethal encounter with non-microbial organisms.

SUMMARY

- Immediate hypersensitivity is an immune reaction that is triggered by antigen binding to IgE preattached to mast cells and that leads to inflammatory mediator release.

- The steps in the development of immediate hypersensitivity are exposure to an antigen (allergen) that stimulates T_H2 responses and IgE production, binding of the IgE to Fcε receptors on mast cells, cross-linking of the IgE and the Fcε receptors by the allergen, activation of mast cells, and release of mediators.

- Individuals susceptible to immediate hypersensitivity reactions are called atopic and often have more IgE in the blood and more IgE-specific Fc receptors per mast cell than do nonatopic individuals. IgE synthesis is induced by exposure to antigen and T_H2 cytokines, particularly IL-4.

- Mast cells are derived from the bone marrow and mature in the tissues. They express high-affinity receptors for IgE (FcεRI) and contain cytoplasmic granules in which are stored various inflammatory mediators. Subsets of mast cells, including mucosal and connective tissue mast cells, may produce different mediators. Basophils are a type of circulating granulocyte that expresses high-affinity Fcε receptors and contains granules with contents similar to mast cells.

- Eosinophils are a special class of granulocyte; they are recruited into inflammatory reactions by chemokines and IL-4 and are activated by IL-5. Eosinophils are effector cells that are involved in killing parasites. In allergic reactions, eosinophils contribute to tissue injury.

- On binding of antigen to IgE on the surface of mast cells or basophils, the high-affinity Fcε receptors become cross-linked and activate intracellular second messengers that lead to granule release and new synthesis of mediators. Activated mast cells and basophils produce three important classes of mediators: biogenic amines, such as histamine; lipid mediators, such as prostaglandins, leukotrienes, and PAF; and cytokines, such as TNF, IL-4, IL-13, and IL-5.

- Biogenic amines and lipid mediators cause the rapid vascular and smooth muscle reactions of immediate hypersensitivity, such as vascular leakage, vasodilation, and bronchoconstriction. Cytokines mediate the late-phase reaction.

- Various organs show distinct forms of immediate hypersensitivity involving different mediators and target cell types. Any allergen may lead to a systemic reaction called anaphylactic shock. Asthma is a manifestation of immediate hypersensitivity and late-phase reactions in the lung. Allergic rhinitis (hay fever) is the most common allergic disease of the upper respiratory tract. Food allergens can cause diarrhea and vomiting. In the skin, immediate hypersensitivity is manifested as wheal and flare and late-phase reactions and may lead to chronic eczema.

- Drug therapy is aimed at inhibiting mast cell mediator production and at blocking or counteracting the effects of released mediators on target organs. The goal of immunotherapy is to prevent or to reduce T_H2 cell responses to specific allergens and the production of IgE.

- Immediate hypersensitivity reactions provide protection against helminthic infections by promoting IgE- and eosinophil-mediated ADCC and gut peristalsis. Furthermore, mast cells may play an important role in innate immune responses to bacterial infections.

Selected Readings

Blank U, and J Rivera. The ins and outs of IgE-dependent mast-cell exocytosis. Trends in Immunology 25:266–273, 2004.

Bufford JD, and JE Gern. The hygiene hypothesis revisited. Immunology and Allergy Clinics of North America 25:247–262, v–vi, 2005.

Cohn L, JA Elias, and GL Chupp. Asthma: mechanisms of disease persistence and progression. Annual Review of Immunology 22:789–815, 2004.

Galli SJ, M Grimbaldeston, and M Tsai. Immunomodulatory mast cells: negative, as well as positive, regulators of immunity. Nature Reviews Immunology 8:478–486, 2008.

Galli SJ, M Tsai, and AM Piliponsky. The development of allergic inflammation. Nature 454:445–454, 2008.

Geha RS, HH Jabara, and SR Brodeur. The regulation of immunoglobulin E class-switch recombination. Nature Reviews Immunology 3:721–732, 2003.

Gilfillan AM, and C Tkaczyk. Integrated signalling pathways for mast-cell activation. Nature Reviews Immunology 6:218–230, 2006.

Gould HJ, and BJ Sutton. IgE in allergy and asthma today. Nature Reviews Immunology 8:205–217, 2008.

Herrick CA, and K Bottomly. To respond or not to respond: T cells in allergic asthma. Nature Reviews Immunology 3:405–412, 2003.

Kalesnikoff J, and SJ Galli. New developments in mast cell biology. Nature Immunology 9:1215–1223, 2008.

Kay AB. Allergy and allergic diseases. New England Journal of Medicine 344:30–37, 109–113, 2001.

Lambrecth BN, and H Hammad. Taking our breath away: dendritic cells in the pathogenesis of asthma. Nature Reviews Immunology 3:994–1003, 2003.

Maddox L, and DA Schwartz. The pathophysiology of asthma. Annual Review of Medicine 53:477–498, 2002.

Medoff BD, SY Thomas, and AD Luster. T cell trafficking in allergic asthma: the ins and outs. Annual Review of Immunology 26:205–232, 2008.

Nadler MJ, SA Matthews, H Turner, and J-P Kinet. Signal transduction by the high affinity immunoglobulin E receptor FcεRI: coupling form to function. Advances in Immunology 76:325–355, 2000.

Piccinni MP, E Maggi, and S Romagnani. Environmental factors favoring the allergen-specific Th2 response in allergic subjects. Annals of the New York Academy of Sciences 917:844–852, 2000.

Rivera J, NA Fierro, A Olivera, and R Suzuki. New insights on mast cell activation via the high affinity receptor for IgE. Advances in Immunology 98:85–120, 2008.

Rothenberg ME, and SP Hogan. The Eosinophil. Annual Review of Immunology 24:147–174, 2006.

Sullivan BM and RM Locksley. Basophils: A nonredundant contributor to host immunity. Immunity 30:12–20, 2009.

Vercelli D. Discovering susceptibility genes for asthma and allergy. Nature Reviews Immunology 8:169–182, 2008.

Wills-Karp M, and SL Ewart. Time to draw breath: asthma-susceptibility genes are identified. Nature Reviews Genetics 5:376–387, 2004.

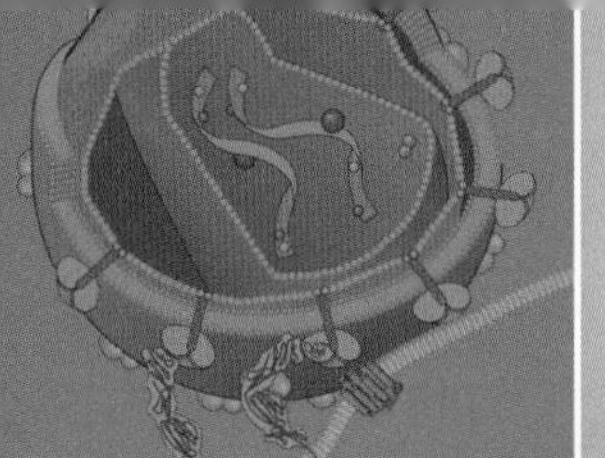

Chapter 20

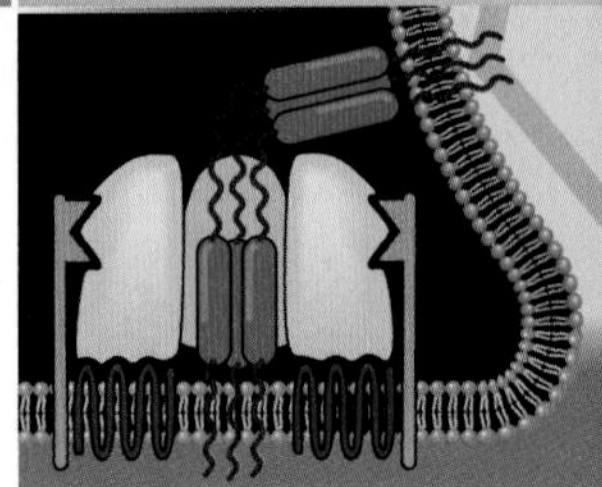

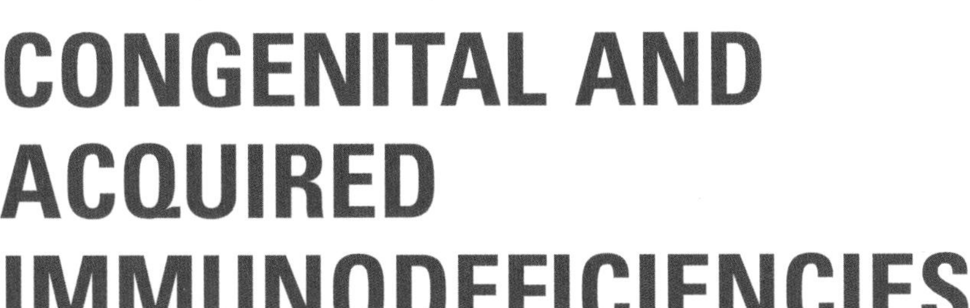

CONGENITAL AND ACQUIRED IMMUNODEFICIENCIES

Integrity of the immune system is essential for defense against infectious organisms and their toxic products and therefore for the survival of all individuals. Defects in one or more components of the immune system can lead to serious and often fatal disorders, which are collectively called immunodeficiency diseases. These diseases are broadly classified into two groups. The **congenital** or **primary immunodeficiencies** are genetic defects that result in an increased susceptibility to infection that is frequently manifested early in infancy and childhood but is sometimes clinically detected later in life. It is estimated that in the United States, approximately 1 in 500 individuals is born with a defect in some component of the immune system, although only a small proportion are affected severely enough for development of life-threatening complications. **Acquired** or **secondary immunodeficiencies** develop as a consequence of malnutrition, disseminated cancer, treatment with immunosuppressive drugs, or infection of cells of the immune system, most notably with the human immunodeficiency virus (HIV), the etiologic agent of acquired immunodeficiency syndrome (AIDS). This chapter describes the major types of congenital and acquired immunodeficiencies, with an emphasis on their pathogenesis and the components of the immune system that are involved in each.

GENERAL FEATURES OF IMMUNODEFICIENCY DISEASES

Before beginning our discussion of individual diseases, it is important to summarize some general features of immunodeficiencies.

- ***The principal consequence of immunodeficiency is an increased susceptibility to infection.*** The nature of

Table 20–1. Features of Immunodeficiencies Affecting T or B Lymphocytes

Feature	B cell deficiency	T cell deficiency
Diagnosis		
Serum Ig levels	Reduced	Normal or reduced
DTH reactions to common antigens	Normal	Reduced
Morphology of lymphoid tissues	Absent or reduced follicles and germinal centers (B cell zones)	Usually normal follicles, may be reduced parafollicular cortical regions (T cell zones)
Susceptibility to infection	Pyogenic bacteria (otitis, pneumonia, meningitis, osteomyelitis), enteric bacteria and viruses, some parasites	Many viruses, atypical mycobacteria and other intracellular bacteria, fungi

Abbreviations: DTH, delayed-type hypersensitivity.

the infection in a particular patient depends largely on the component of the immune system that is defective (Table 20–1). Deficient humoral immunity usually results in increased susceptibility to infection by pyogenic bacteria, whereas defects in cell-mediated immunity lead to infection by viruses and other intracellular microbes. Combined deficiencies in both humoral and cell-mediated immunity make patients susceptible to infection by all classes of microorganisms.

- ***Patients with immunodeficiencies are also susceptible to certain types of cancer.*** Many of these cancers appear to be caused by oncogenic viruses, such as the Epstein-Barr virus (EBV). An increased incidence of cancer is most often seen in T cell immunodeficiencies because, as discussed in Chapter 17, T cells play an important role in surveillance against oncogenic viruses and the tumors they cause.
- ***Immunodeficiency may result from defects in lymphocyte maturation or activation or from defects in the effector mechanisms of innate and adaptive immunity.*** Immunodeficiency diseases are clinically and pathologically heterogeneous, in part because different diseases involve different components of the immune system.
- Paradoxically, certain immunodeficiencies are associated with an increased incidence of autoimmunity. The mechanism underlying this association is not known; it may reflect a deficiency of regulatory T lymphocytes that normally serve to maintain self-tolerance.

In this chapter, we first describe congenital immunodeficiencies, including defects in the humoral and cell-mediated arms of the adaptive immune system and defects in components of the innate immune system. We conclude with a discussion of acquired immunodeficiencies, with an emphasis on AIDS.

CONGENITAL (PRIMARY) IMMUNODEFICIENCIES

The first inherited immunodeficiency to be described, in 1952, was a disease called X-linked agammaglobulinemia that affects boys and is now known to be caused by a defect in B lymphocyte development (see below). Since then, a large number of other congenital immunodeficiencies have been described, and the genetic bases of many of these disorders are now known. This understanding has led to an increased hope for gene replacement as therapy for these diseases.

In different immunodeficiencies, the primary abnormality may be in components of the innate immune system, at different stages of lymphocyte maturation, or in the responses of mature lymphocytes to antigenic stimulation. Inherited abnormalities affecting innate immunity generally affect the complement pathway or phagocytes. Abnormalities in lymphocyte development may be caused by mutations in genes encoding a variety of molecules, including enzymes and transcription factors. These inherited defects, and the corresponding targeted disruptions in mice, have been useful in elucidating the mechanisms of lymphocyte development (see Chapter 8). Abnormalities in B lymphocyte development and function result in deficient antibody production and increased susceptibility to infection by extracellular microbes, particularly encapsulated bacteria. B cell immunodeficiencies are diagnosed by reduced levels of serum immunoglobulin (Ig), defective antibody responses to vaccination, and, in some cases, reduced numbers of B cells in the circulation or lymphoid tissues or absent plasma cells in tissues (see Table 20–1). Abnormalities in T lymphocyte maturation and function lead to deficient cell-mediated immunity and an increased incidence of infection with intracellular microbes. Deficiencies of helper T cells may also result in reduced antibody production. Primary T cell immunodeficiencies are diagnosed by reduced numbers of peripheral blood T cells, low proliferative responses of blood lymphocytes to polyclonal T cell activators such as phytohemagglutinin, and deficient cutaneous delayed-type hypersensitivity (DTH) reactions to ubiquitous microbial antigens, such as *Candida* antigens. In the following sections, we describe immunodeficiencies caused by inherited mutations in genes encoding components of the innate immune system, or of genes required for lymphocyte development and activation. We conclude with a brief discussion of therapeutic strategies for these diseases.

Defects in Innate Immunity

Innate immunity constitutes the first line of defense against infectious organisms. Two important mediators of innate immunity are phagocytes and complement, both of which also participate in the effector phases of adaptive immunity. Therefore, congenital disorders of phagocytes and the complement system result in recurrent infections. Complement deficiencies were described in Chapter 14 (see Box 14–2). They typically present with recurrent bacterial infections, particularly by *Neisseriae* species, and often also contribute to susceptibility to autoimmune disorders, particularly systemic lupus erythematosus. Deficiencies have been described in the classical and alternative complement pathways, as well as in the lectin pathway. Mannose-binding lectin (MBL) is absent in a high frequency of individuals (up to 5% in some studies), and while some MBL-deficient patients present with recurrent infections, most are asymptomatic.

In this section of the chapter, we discuss some examples of congenital phagocyte disorders (Table 20–2).

Defective Microbicidal Activities of Phagocytes: Chronic Granulomatous Disease

Chronic granulomatous disease (CGD) is a rare disease, estimated to affect about 1 in 1 million individuals in the United States. About two thirds of cases show an X-linked recessive pattern of inheritance, and the remainder are autosomal recessive. CGD is caused by mutations in components of the phagocyte oxidase (phox) enzyme complex. The most common X-linked form of the disease is caused by a mutation in the gene encoding the 91-kD α subunit of cytochrome b_{558}, an integral membrane protein also known as phox-91. This mutation results in defective production of superoxide anion, a reactive oxygen species that constitutes a major microbicidal mechanism of phagocytes (see Chapter 2). Mutations in other components of the phox complex contribute to autosomal-recessive variants of CGD. Defective production of reactive oxygen species results in a failure to kill phagocytosed microbes. The disease is characterized by recurrent infections with catalase-producing intracellular bacterial and fungi, usually from early childhood. (Many of the organisms that are particularly troublesome in CGD patients produce catalase, which destroy the microbicidal hydrogen peroxide that may be produced by the microbes themselves or by host cells.) Because the infections are not controlled by phagocytes, they stimulate chronic cell-mediated

Table 20–2. Congenital Disorders of Innate Immunity

Disease	Functional deficiencies	Mechanism of defect
Chronic granulomatous disease	Defective production of reactive oxygen species by phagocytes; recurrent intracellular bacterial and fungal infections	Mutation in genes of phagocyte oxidase complex; phox-91 (cytochrome $b_{558}\alpha$ subunit) is mutated in X-linked form
Leukocyte adhesion deficiency type 1	Defective leukocyte adhesion and migration linked to decreased or absent expression of β2 integrins; recurrent bacterial and fungal infections	Mutations in gene encoding the β chain (CD18) of β2 integrins
Leukocyte adhesion deficiency type 2	Defective leukocyte adhesion and migration linked to decreased or absent expression of leukocyte ligands for endothelial E- and P-selectins causing failure of leukocyte migration into tissues; recurrent bacterial and fungal infections	Mutations in gene encoding a GDP-fucose transporter required for the synthesis of the sialyl Lewis^x component of E- and P-selectin ligands
Chédiak-Higashi syndrome	Defective vesicle fusion and lysosomal function in neutrophils, macrophages, dendritic cells, natural killer cells, cytotoxic T cells, and many other cell types; recurrent infections by pyogenic bacteria	Mutation in LYST leading to defect in secretory granule exocytosis and lysosomal function
Toll-like receptor signaling defects	Recurrent infections because of defects in TLR and CD40 signaling	Mutations in NEMO, IκBα, and IRAK4 compromise NF-κB activation downstream of Toll-like receptors

Abbreviations: IRAK4, IL-1 receptor associated kinase 4; LYST, lysosomal trafficking regulator protein; NEMO, NF-κB essential modulator.

immune responses resulting in T cell–mediated macrophage activation and the formation of granulomas composed of activated macrophages. Presumably, these activated macrophages try to limit or eliminate the microbes despite defective production of reactive oxygen species. This histologic appearance is the basis for the name of the disorder. The disease is often fatal, even with aggressive antibiotic therapy.

The cytokine interferon-γ (IFN-γ) enhances transcription of the phox-91 gene and also stimulates other components of the phagocyte oxidase enzyme complex. Therefore, IFN-γ stimulates the production of superoxide by normal neutrophils, as well as CGD neutrophils, especially in cases in which the phox-91 gene is intact but its transcription is reduced. Once neutrophil superoxide production is restored to about 10% of normal levels, resistance to infection is greatly improved. IFN-γ therapy is now commonly used for the treatment of X-linked CGD.

Leukocyte Adhesion Deficiencies

Leukocyte adhesion deficiency type 1 (LAD-1) is a rare autosomal-recessive disorder characterized by recurrent bacterial and fungal infections and impaired wound healing. In these patients, most adhesion-dependent functions of leukocytes are abnormal. These functions include adherence to endothelium, neutrophil aggregation and chemotaxis, phagocytosis, and cytotoxicity mediated by neutrophils, natural killer (NK) cells, and T lymphocytes. The molecular basis of the defect is absent or deficient expression of the β_2 integrins (heterodimers of CD18 and the CD11 family of glycoproteins) due to various mutations in the CD18 gene. The β_2 integrins include leukocyte function-associated antigen-1 (LFA-1 or CD11aCD18), Mac-1 (CD11bCD18), and p150,95 (CD11cCD18). These proteins participate in the adhesion of leukocytes to other cells, notably endothelial cells, and the binding of T lymphocytes to APCs (see Chapter 2, Box 2–3).

LAD-2 is another rare disorder that is clinically similar to LAD-1 but is not due to integrin defects. In contrast, LAD-2 results from an absence of sialyl Lewis X, the tetrasaccharide carbohydrate ligand on neutrophils that is required for binding to E-selectin and P-selectin on cytokine-activated endothelium (see Chapter 2, Box 2–2). This defect is caused by a mutation in a fucose transporter gene. The failure to transport fucose into the Golgi complex results in failure to synthesize sialyl Lewis X. The result is defective binding of neutrophils to endothelium and defective recruitment of the leukocytes to sites of infection.

Defects in NK Cells and Other Leukocytes: The Chédiak-Higashi Syndrome

The **Chédiak-Higashi syndrome** is a rare autosomal-recessive disorder characterized by recurrent infections by pyogenic bacteria, partial oculocutaneous albinism, and infiltration of various organs by non-neoplastic lymphocytes. The neutrophils, monocytes, and lymphocytes of these patients contain giant lysosomes. This disease is caused by mutations in the gene encoding the lysosomal-trafficking regulator protein LYST, resulting in defective phagosome-lysosome fusion in neutrophils and macrophages (causing reduced resistance to infection), defective melanosome formation in melanocytes (causing albinism), and lysosomal abnormalities in cells of the nervous system (causing nerve defects) and platelets (leading to bleeding disorders). The giant lysosomes found in neutrophils form during the maturation of these cells from myeloid precursors. Some of these neutrophil precursors die prematurely, resulting in moderate leukopenia. Surviving neutrophils may contain reduced levels of the lysosomal enzymes that normally function in microbial killing. These cells are also defective in chemotaxis and phagocytosis, further contributing to their deficient microbicidal activity. NK cell function in these patients is impaired, probably because of an abnormality in the cytoplasmic granules that store proteins mediating cytotoxicity. The defect in cytotoxic T lymphocyte (CTL) function seen in some patients is relatively mild, but other patients have a more pronounced CTL defect. A mutant mouse strain called the **beige mouse** is an animal model for the Chédiak-Higashi syndrome. This strain is characterized by deficient NK cell function and giant lysosomes in leukocytes. The beige mutation has been mapped to the mouse *LYST* locus.

Other mutations that affect both CTL and NK cell function will be considered below when we discuss defects in T lymphocyte activation and function. A mutation in CD16/FcγRIII, the Fc receptor on NK cells that is required for antibody-dependent cellular cytotoxicity (see Chapter 14), has been described in a subject with recurrent viral infections.

Inherited Defects in Toll-like Receptor Pathways and Nuclear Factor κB Signaling

A naturally occurring mutation in Toll-like receptor 4 (TLR4) has been described in *Lps* mice. In humans, more global inherited defects in TLR signaling have been described. Some immune deficiencies are caused by defects in signaling pathways downstream of TLRs. Mutations in the inhibitor of κB kinase γ (IKKγ), also known as nuclear factor κB essential modulator (NEMO), a component of the IκB kinase complex, contribute to the X-linked recessive condition known as *anhidrotic ectodermal dysplasia with immunodeficiency (EDA-ID)*. IKKγ/NEMO is required for NF-κB activation, and point mutations that partially impair NEMO function contribute to a disorder in which differentiation of ectoderm-derived structures is abnormal and immune function is impaired in a number of ways. Responses to TLR signals as well as CD40 signals are compromised. These patients suffer from infections with encapsulated pyogenic bacteria, as well as with intracellular bacterial pathogens including mycobacteria, viruses, and fungi such as *Pneumocystis jiroveci* (previously known as *Pneumocystis carinii*). An autosomal-recessive form of EDA-ID has been described in which a hypermorphic point mutation in IκBα prevents the phosphorylation, ubiquitinlation, and degradation of IκBα, thus leading to impaired NF-κB activation.

Another immunodeficiency state in which recurrent bacterial infections are observed is linked to mutations in the *IRAK-4* gene. Interleukin-1 receptor–associated kinase 4 (IRAK-4) is a critical kinase downstream of TLRs and the interleukin-1 (IL-1) receptor (see Chapter 2). Defective TLR and IL-1 receptor signaling presumably contributes to the relatively mild immunodeficiency in these patients.

Severe Combined Immunodeficiencies

In this section, we focus on congenital immunodeficiencies in humans that are known to result from impaired progression at various checkpoints during T lymphocyte development with or without defects in B cell maturation (Fig. 20–1). Disorders that affect both humoral and cell-mediated immunity are called **severe combined immunodeficiencies** (SCIDs) (Table 20–3). These diseases are characterized by deficiencies of both B and T cells, or only T cells; in the latter cases, the defect in humoral immunity is due to the absence of T cell help. Children with SCID usually have infections during the first year of life and succumb to these infections unless they are treated. The process of T (and B) lymphocyte maturation from hematopoietic stem cells to functionally competent mature lymphocytes involves proliferation of early lymphocyte progenitors, rearrangement of the locus encoding one chain of the antigen receptor followed by selection of cells that have made in-frame productive rearrangements at a pre-antigen receptor checkpoint, expression of both chains of the antigen receptor, and selection of cells with useful specificities (see Chapter 8). Defects in many of these steps have been described in different forms of SCID.

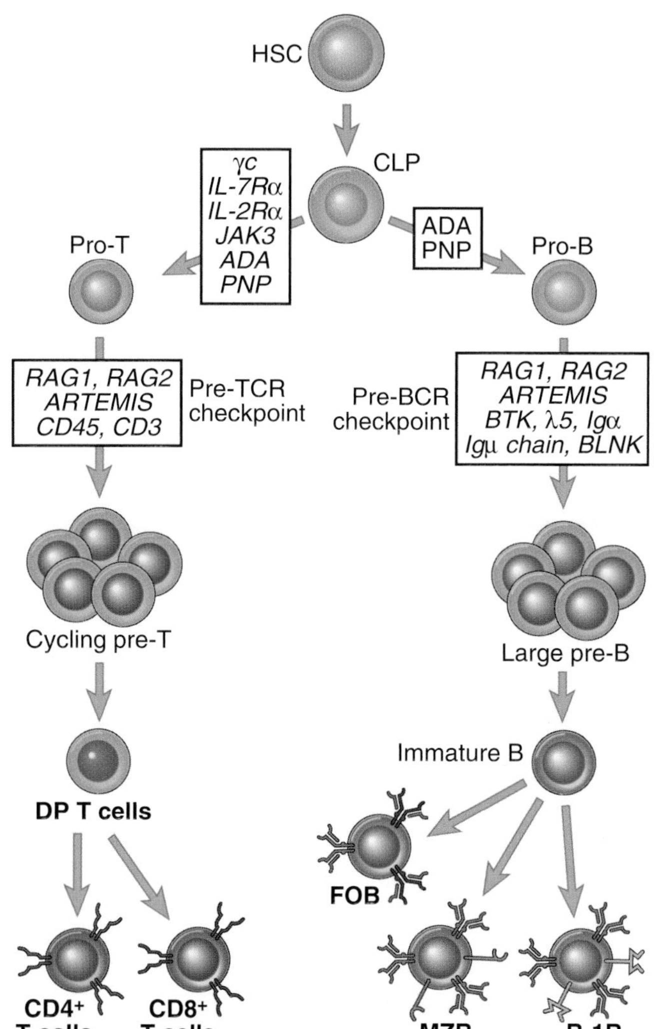

FIGURE 20–1 Immunodeficiency caused by defects in B and T cell maturation. Primary immunodeficiencies caused by genetic defects in lymphocyte maturation are shown. These defects (in italics) may affect T cell maturation alone, B cell maturation alone, or both. The survival of all lymphocyte progenitor populations requires the purine salvage pathway enzymes, ADA, and PNP. IL-7R signaling (γ_C, IL-7Rα, and JAK3) is required for human pro-T cell generation. The V(D)J recombination machinery (RAG-1, RAG-2, and ARTEMIS) is required for generating pre-B and pre-T cells, as is signaling through the pre-TCR (CD45, CD3) specifically for pre-T cells and the pre-BCR (Igμ chain, λ5, Igα, and BLNK) for pre-B cells. DP, double-positive; FoB, follicular B cells; HSC, hematopoietic stem cell; MZB, marginal zone B cells.

Immunodeficiencies Linked to Defective Cytokine Receptor Signaling: X-Linked SCID Caused by Mutations in the Cytokine Receptor Common γ Chain

Approximately 50% of SCID cases are X-linked and due to mutations in the gene encoding the **common γ (γ_C) chain** shared by the receptors for the interleukins IL-2, IL-4, IL-7, IL-9, and IL-15 (see Chapter 12). These mutations are recessive, so heterozygous females are usually phenotypically normal carriers, whereas males who inherit the abnormal X chromosome manifest the disease. Because developing cells in females randomly inactivate one of the two X chromosomes, the normal allele encoding a functional γ_C protein will not be expressed in half the lymphocyte precursors in a female carrier. These cells will fail to mature, and consequently, all the mature lymphocytes in a female carrier will have inactivated the same X chromosome (carrying the mutant allele). In contrast, half of all nonlymphoid cells will have inactivated one X chromosome, and half the other. A comparison of X chromosome inactivation in lymphoid cells versus nonlymphoid cells may be used to identify carriers of the mutant allele. The nonrandom use of X chromosomes in mature lymphocytes is also characteristic of female carriers of other X-linked mutations of genes that affect lymphocyte development, as discussed later.

X-linked SCID is characterized by impaired maturation of T cells and NK cells and greatly reduced numbers of mature T cells and NK cells, but the number of B cells is usually normal or increased. The humoral immunodeficiency in this disease is due to a lack of T cell help

Table 20–3. Severe Combined Immunodeficiencies

Disease	Functional deficiencies	Mechanism of defect
A. Defects in cytokine signaling		
X-linked SCID	Marked decrease in T cells; normal or increased B cells; reduced serum Ig	Cytokine receptor common γ chain mutations; defective T cell development in the absence of IL-7 derived signals
Autosomal recessive forms	Marked decrease in T cells; normal or increased B cells; reduced serum Ig	Mutations in IL-2Rα chain, IL-7Rα chain, JAK3
B. Defects in nucleotide salvage pathways		
ADA deficiency	Progressive decrease in T, B, and NK cells; reduced serum Ig	ADA deficiency leading to accumulation of toxic metabolites in lymphocytes
PNP deficiency	Progressive decrease in T, B, and NK cells; reduced serum Ig	PNP deficiency leading to accumulation of toxic metabolites in lymphocytes
C. Defects in V(D)J recombination		
RAG1 or RAG2 deficiency*	Decreased T and B cells; reduced serum Ig; absence or deficiency of T and B cells	Cleavage defect during V(D)J recombination; mutations in RAG1 or RAG2
ARTEMIS defects*	Decreased T and B cells; reduced serum Ig; absence or deficiency of T and B cells	Failure to resolve hairpins during V(D)J recombination; mutations in ARTEMIS
D. Defective thymus development		
Defective pre-TCR checkpoint	Decreased T cells; normal or reduced B cells; reduced serum Ig	Mutations in CD45, CD3δ, CD3ε, Orai1 (CRAC channel component)
DiGeorge syndrome	Decreased T cells; normal B cells; normal or reduced serum Ig	22q11 deletion; T box-1 (TBX1) transcription factor mutations
E. Other defects		
Reticular dysgenesis	Decreased T, B, and myeloid cells	Mutation not identified

Abbreviations: ADA, adenosine deaminase; CRAC, calcium release activated channel; PNP, purine nucleoside phosphorylase.

*Hypomorphic mutations in RAG genes and in ARTEMIS can contribute to Omenn syndrome.

for antibody production. This disease is a result of the inability of the lymphopoietic cytokine IL-7, whose receptor uses the γ_C chain for signaling, to stimulate the growth of immature thymocytes. In addition, the receptor for IL-15, which is a potent stimulus for the proliferation of NK cells, also uses the γ_C signaling chain, and the failure of IL-15 function accounts for the deficiency of NK cells.

Autosomal-Recessive Mutations in Cytokine Signaling that Lead to Impaired T Cell Development

Some patients with a disease identical to X-linked SCID show an autosomal-recessive inheritance. These patients have mutations in the IL-7 receptor α chain or the JAK3 kinase, which associates with the γ_C chain and is required for signaling by this protein (see Chapter 12, Box 12–2). Knockout mice lacking the γ_C chain, IL-7, the cytokine-binding α chain of the IL-7 receptor, or JAK3 develop a disease similar to human X-linked SCID, although B cell maturation is decreased more in mutant mice than in human SCID patients.

Severe Combined Immunodeficiency Linked to Defects in Purine Salvage Pathways

About 50% of patients with SCID show an autosomal-recessive pattern of inheritance, and many of these cases are due to deficiency of an enzyme called **adenosine deaminase** (ADA). ADA functions in the salvage pathway of purine synthesis and catalyzes the irreversible deamination of adenosine and 2′-deoxyadenosine to inosine and 2′-deoxyinosine, respectively. Deficiency of the enzyme leads to the accumulation of deoxyadenosine and its precursors *S*-adenosylhomocysteine and deoxyadenosine triphosphate (dATP). These by-products have many toxic effects, including inhibition of DNA synthesis. Although ADA is present in most cells, developing lymphocytes are less efficient than most other cell types at degrading dATP into 2′-deoxyadenosine, and therefore lymphocyte maturation is particularly sensitive to ADA deficiency. ADA deficiency leads to reduced numbers of B and T cells; lymphocyte cell numbers are usually normal at birth but fall off precipitously during the first year of life. A few patients may have a nearly normal number of T cells, but these cells do not proliferate in response to antigenic stimulation. A rarer autosomal-recessive form of SCID is due to the deficiency of another enzyme, called purine nucleoside phosphorylase (PNP), that is also involved in purine catabolism. PNP catalyzes the conversion of inosine to hypoxanthine and guanosine to guanine, and deficiency of PNP leads to the accumulation of deoxyguanosine and deoxyguanosine triphosphate, with toxic effects on immature lymphocytes, mainly T cells.

Severe Combined Immunodeficiency Linked to Defects in V(D)J Recombination

Mutations in the *RAG1* or *RAG2* genes [whose protein products mediate the cleavage step during V(D)J recombination] or the *ARTEMIS* gene, which encodes an endonuclease that resolves coding-end hairpins during V(D)J recombination, account for a large number of the autosomal-recessive forms of SCID. The normal functions of these genes are discussed in Chapter 8. In children with these mutations, B and T lymphocytes are absent and immunity is severely compromised. Hypomorphic mutations in the *RAG* genes, in *ARTEMIS,* and in IL-7Rα can contribute to a disorder characterized by restricted generation of T and B cells, immunodeficiency and immune dysregulation. This disorder is known as Omenn's syndrome. It is possible that this immune dyscrasia, in which immunodeficiency coexists with exaggerated immune activation and autoimmunity, may reflect the relative absence of regulatory T cells.

An instructive experimental model is the **SCID mouse,** in which B and T cells are absent because of an early block in maturation from bone marrow precursors. The defect in SCID mice is a mutation in the catalytic subunit of a DNA-dependent protein kinase, which is required for double-stranded break repair during V(D)J recombination (see Chapter 8). This defect results in the failure of B and T cell development.

Defective Pre-TCR Checkpoint Signaling

Although most autosomal-recessive forms of SCID are linked to mutations in *ADA, RAG1, RAG2,* and *ARTEMIS,* rare forms of this syndrome have been linked to mutations in the genes encoding CD45 and the CD3 δ or ε chains. Another rare form of SCID is caused by mutation in a gene encoding Orai1, a component of CRAC channels (see Chapter 9). Activation of antigen receptors as well as pre-antigen receptors leads to the activation of the γ isoform of phospholipase C (PLCγ) and the inositol triphosphate (IP_3)-dependent release of calcium ions from the endoplasmic reticulum and mitochondria (see Chapter 9). The released calcium is replenished by store-operated CRAC channels that facilitate an influx of extracellular calcium, and this process is crucial for lymphocyte activation, and it is defective in cells with mutant Orai1.

Defective Thymic Development: DiGeorge's Syndrome

This selective T cell deficiency is due to a congenital malformation that results in defective development of the thymus and the parathyroid glands as well as other structures that develop from the third and fourth pharyngeal pouches during fetal life. The congenital defect is manifested by hypoplasia or agenesis of the thymus leading to deficient T cell maturation, absent parathyroid glands causing abnormal calcium homeostasis and muscle twitching (tetany), abnormal development of the great vessels, and facial deformities. Different patients may show varying degrees of these abnormalities. The disease is caused by a deletion in chromosome 22q11.2. Mutations in a gene encoding a transcription factor called T box-1 (TBX1), which lies within the deleted region, also result in a similar defect in thymic development. It is likely that the immunodeficiency associated with DiGeorge's syndrome can be explained, at least in part, by the deletion of the *TBX1* gene. In this syndrome, peripheral blood T lymphocytes are absent or greatly reduced in number, and the cells do not respond to polyclonal T cell activators or in mixed leukocyte reactions. Antibody levels are usually normal but may be reduced in severely affected patients. As in other severe T cell deficiencies, patients are susceptible to mycobacterial, viral, and fungal infections.

The immunodeficiency associated with DiGeorge's syndrome can be corrected by fetal thymic transplantation or by bone marrow transplantation. Such treatment is usually not necessary, however, because T cell function tends to improve with age and is often normal by 5 years. Improvement with age probably occurs because of the presence of some thymic tissue or because some as yet undefined extrathymic sites assume the function of T cell maturation. It is also possible that as these patients grow older, thymus tissue develops at ectopic sites (i.e., other than the normal location).

An animal model of T cell immunodeficiency resulting from abnormal development of the thymus is the **nude (athymic) mouse.** These mice have an inherited defect of certain types of epithelial cells in the skin, leading to hairlessness, and in the lining of the third and fourth pharyngeal pouches, causing thymic hypoplasia. The disorder is due to a mutation in the *FoxN1* gene encoding a Forkhead family transcription factor that is required for the normal development of certain ectoderm-derived cell types. Affected mice have rudimentary thymuses in which T cell maturation cannot occur normally. As a result, few or no mature T cells are present in peripheral lymphoid tissues, and cell-mediated immune reactions cannot occur.

Reticular Dysgenesis and SCID

A particularly severe form of SCID is seen in a disease called **reticular dysgenesis.** This disorder is characterized by the absence of T and B lymphocytes and most myeloid cells, including granulocytes, and is presumably due to a defect in the hematopoietic stem cell. This disease is rare, and neither its molecular basis nor its mode of inheritance is known.

Antibody Deficiencies: Defects in B Cell Development and Activation

While defects in T cell development or in both T and B cell development contribute to the SCID phenotype, more circumscribed defects in B cell development or function result in disorders in which the primary abnormality is in antibody synthesis (Table 20–4 and Fig. 20–2). However, in one subset of hyper-IgM syndromes discussed below, antibody deficiencies are also accompanied by defects in macrophage and antigen-presenting cell (APC) activation, which in turn result in attenuated cell-mediated immunity.

An X-linked Pre-B Cell Receptor Signaling Defect: X-Linked Agammaglobulinemia

X-linked agammaglobulinemia, also called Bruton's agammaglobulinemia, is characterized by the absence of gamma globulin in the blood, as the name implies. It is one of the most common congenital immunodeficiencies and the prototype of a failure of B cell maturation. The defect in X-linked agammaglobulinemia is a failure of B cells to mature beyond the pre-B cell stage in the bone marrow (see Fig. 20–1). This failure is caused by

Table 20–4. Antibody Deficiencies

Disease	Functional deficiencies	Mechanism of defect
A. Agammaglobulinemias		
X-linked	Decrease in all serum Ig isotypes; reduced B cell numbers	Pre-B receptor checkpoint defect; Btk mutation
Autosomal recessive forms	Decrease in all serum Ig isotypes; reduced B cell numbers	Pre-B receptor checkpoint defect; mutations in IgM heavy chain (μ), surrogate light chains (λ5), Igα, BLNK
B. Hypogammaglobulinemias/isotype defects		
Selective IgA deficiency	Decreased IgA; may be associated with increased susceptibility to bacterial infections and protozoa such as *Giardia lamblia*	Mutations in TACI in some patients
Selective IgG2 deficiency	Increased susceptibility to bacterial infections	Small subset have deletion in IgH γ2 locus
Common Variable Immunodeficiency (CVID)	Hypogammaglobulinemia; normal or decreased B cell numbers	Mutations in ICOS and TACI in some patients
ICF syndrome	Hypogammaglobulinemia, occasional mild T cell defects	Mutations in DNMT3B
C. Hyper-IgM syndromes		
X-linked	Defects in T helper cell–mediated B cell, macrophage and dendritic cell activation; defects in somatic mutation, class switching, and germinal center formation; defective cell–mediated immunity	Mutation in CD40L
Autosomal recessive with cell-mediated immune defects	Defects in T helper cell–mediated B cell, macrophage and dendritic cell activation; defects in somatic mutation, class switching, and germinal center formation; defective cell–mediated immunity	Mutations in CD40, NEMO
Autosomal recessive with antibody defect only	Defects in somatic mutation and isotype switching	Mutations in AID, UNG

Abbreviations: AID, Activation-induced cytidine deaminase; DNMT3B, DNA methyl transferase 3B; ICOS, inducible costimulator; NEMO, NFκB essential modulator; TACI, transmembrane activator and calcium modulator and cyclophilin ligand interactor; UNG, uracil N-glycosylase.

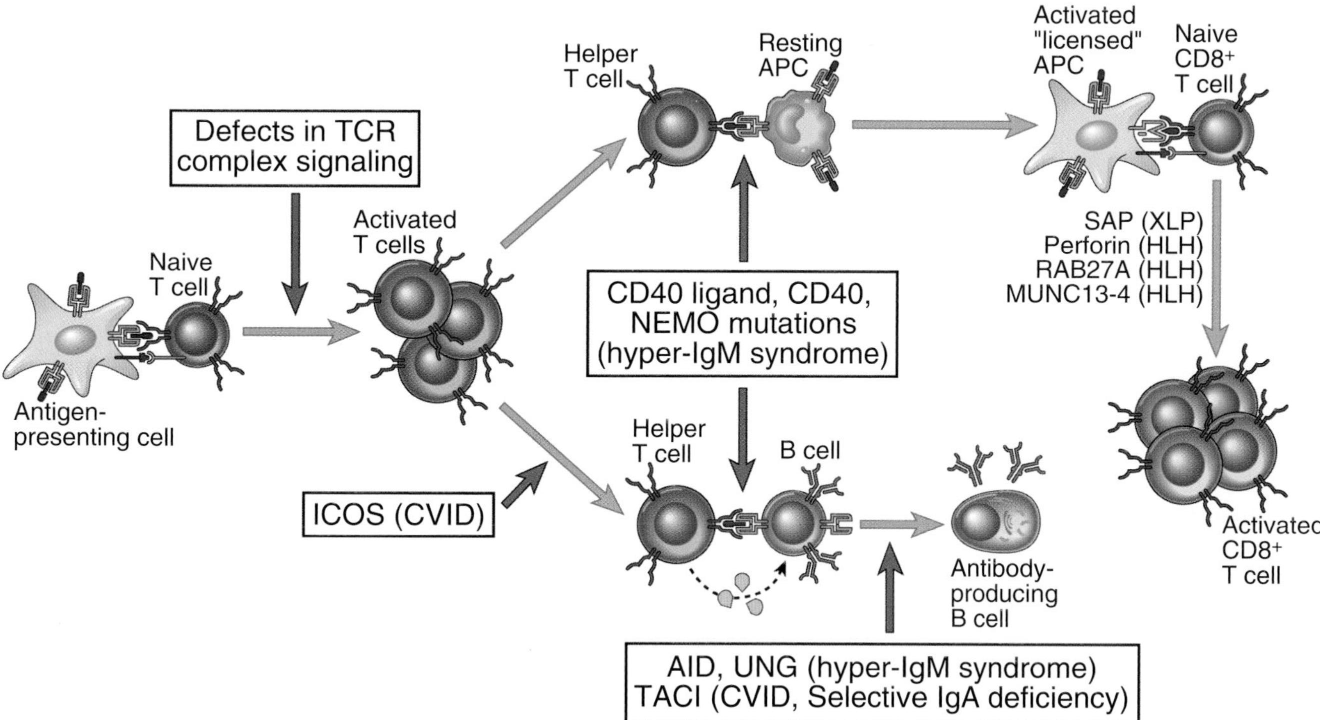

FIGURE 20–2 Immunodeficiency caused by defects in B and T cell activation. Primary immunodeficiencies may be caused by genetic defects in molecules required for T or B lymphocyte antigen receptor signaling, for helper T cell–mediated activation of B cells and antigen presenting cells (APCs), or for the activation of cytotoxic T lymphocytes and NK cells. Common variable immunodeficiency (CVID) has a number of causes, including mutations in ICOS (inducible costimulator) and TACI (transmembrane activator and calcium modulator and cyclophilin ligand interactor). TACI mutations are also a frequent cause of selective IgA deficiency. Patients with hyper-IgM syndrome who harbor mutations in the CD40 signaling pathway (CD40 ligand [CD40L], CD40, or NEMO) have defects in both T helper cell–mediated B cell activation and the activation of APCs and cell-mediated immunity. The most frequently mutated gene causing the hyper-IgM syndrome is the CD40L gene, which is X-linked. Mutations in the enzymes AID and in UNG cause hyper-IgM syndromes that only affect B cells. Mutations in a signaling molecule (SAP), in perforin, and in genes encoding proteins involved in granule exocytosis, such as Rab27A, and the Rab27A binding protein MUNC13-4, are all causes of hemophagocytic lymphohistiocytosis (HLH).

mutations or deletions in the gene encoding an enzyme called **Bruton tyrosine kinase** (Btk). Btk is involved in transducing signals from the pre-B cell receptor (pre-BCR) that are required for the survival and differentiation of pre-B cells (see Chapter 8). In female carriers of this disease, only B cells that have inactivated the X chromosome carrying the mutant allele mature. Unlike the case with X-linked SCID, described earlier, this nonrandom X chromosome inactivation is not seen in T cells. Patients with X-linked agammaglobulinemia usually have low or undetectable serum Ig, reduced or absent B cells in peripheral blood and lymphoid tissues, no germinal centers in lymph nodes, and no plasma cells in tissues. The maturation, numbers, and functions of T cells are generally normal. Some studies have revealed reduced numbers of activated T cells in patients, which may be a consequence of reduced antigen presentation caused by the lack of B cells. Autoimmune disorders develop in almost 20% of patients, for unknown reasons. The infectious complications of X-linked agammaglobulinemia are greatly reduced by periodic (e.g., weekly or monthly) injections of pooled gamma globulin preparations. Such preparations contain preformed antibodies against common pathogens and provide effective passive immunity.

Autosomal-Recessive Pre-B Cell Receptor Checkpoint Defects

Autosomal-recessive forms of agammaglobulinemia have been described, most of which can be linked to defects in pre-BCR signaling. Mutant genes that have been identified in this context include the μ (IgM heavy chain) gene, the $\lambda 5$ surrogate light chain gene, the *Igα* gene, which encodes a signaling component of the pre-BCR and BCR, and the *BLNK* gene, which encodes an important adapter downstream of the pre-BCR and BCR.

Knockout mice lacking Btk, as well as naturally Btk-mutant *Xid* mice, show a less severe defect in B cell maturation than humans do because a Btk-like tyrosine kinase called Tec is active in mouse pre-B cells that lack Btk. The main abnormalities in *Xid* mice are defective antibody responses to some polysaccharide antigens and a deficiency in mature follicular and B-1 B cells.

Selective Immunoglobulin Isotype Deficiencies

Many immunodeficiencies that selectively involve one or a few Ig isotypes have been described. The most common is **selective IgA deficiency,** which affects about 1 in 700 caucasian individuals and is thus the most common primary immunodeficiency known. IgA deficiency usually occurs sporadically, but many familial cases with either autosomal-dominant or recessive patterns of inheritance are also known. The clinical features are variable. Many patients are entirely normal; others have occasional respiratory infections and diarrhea; and rarely, patients have severe, recurrent infections leading to permanent intestinal and airway damage, with associated autoimmune disorders. IgA deficiency is characterized by low serum IgA, usually less than 50 μg/mL (normal, 2 to 4 mg/mL), with normal or elevated levels of IgM and IgG. The defect in these patients is a block in the differentiation of B cells to IgA antibody–secreting plasma cells. The α heavy chain genes and the expression of membrane-associated IgA are normal. No gross abnormalities in the numbers, phenotypes, or functional responses of T cells have been noted in these patients. In a small proportion of patients with selective IgA deficiency, mutations have been described in *TACI* (transmembrane activator and calcium modulator and cyclophilin ligand interactor), one of the three types of receptors for the cytokines BAFF (B cell activating factor) and APRIL (a proliferation-inducing ligand). *TACI* mutations are also an important cause of common variable immunodeficiency (CVID), discussed below. IgA deficiency may represent a *forme fruste* of CVID.

Selective IgG subclass deficiencies have been described in which total serum IgG levels are normal but concentrations of one or more subclasses are below normal. Deficiency of IgG3 is the most common subclass deficiency in adults, and IgG2 deficiency associated with IgA deficiency is the most common in children. Some individuals with these deficiencies have recurrent bacterial infections, but many do not have any clinical problems. Selective IgG subclass deficiencies are usually due to abnormal B cell differentiation and rarely to homozygous deletions of various constant region (C_γ) genes.

Defects in B Cell Differentiation: Common Variable Immunodeficiency

Common variable immunodeficiency is a group of heterogeneous disorders defined by reduced levels of serum Ig, impaired antibody responses to infection or vaccines, and increased incidence of infections. The diagnosis is usually one of exclusion when other primary immunodeficiency diseases are ruled out. The presentation and pathogenesis are, as the name implies, highly variable. Although Ig deficiency and associated pyogenic infections are major components of these disorders, autoimmune diseases, including pernicious anemia, hemolytic anemia, and rheumatoid arthritis, may be just as significant. A high incidence of malignant tumors is also associated with common variable immunodeficiency. These disorders may be diagnosed early in childhood or late in life. Both sporadic and familial cases occur, the latter with both autosomal-dominant and -recessive inheritance patterns. Mature B lymphocytes are present in these patients, but plasma cells are absent in lymphoid tissues, which suggests a block in B cell differentiation to antibody-producing cells. The defective antibody production has been attributed to multiple abnormalities, including intrinsic B cell defects, deficient T cell help, and excessive "suppressor cell" activity. A small proportion of patients with CVID have a shared deletion in the *ICOS* (inducible T cell costimulator) gene. A more common cause of this syndrome is the existence of mutations in *TACI,* described above in the context of selective IgA deficiency.

Hypogammaglobulinemia is also a feature of a distinct syndrome of *immunodeficiency, centromeric instability, and facial anomalies (ICF)* linked to mutations in the *DNA methyltransferase 3B* gene, which is a major participant in the de novo methylation of DNA. How DNA hypomethylation contributes to immunodeficiency is not understood.

Defects in T Cell–Dependent B Cell Activation: Hyper-IgM Syndromes

The **X-linked hyper-IgM syndrome** is a rare disorder associated with defective switching of B cells to the IgG and IgA isotypes; these antibodies are therefore reduced, and a compensatory increase in IgM in the blood occurs. The defect is caused by mutations in the gene encoding the T cell effector molecule **CD40 ligand.** The mutant forms of CD40 ligand produced in these patients do not bind to or transduce signals through CD40 and therefore do not stimulate B cells to undergo heavy chain isotype switching, which requires T cell help (see Chapter 10). Patients suffer from infections similar to those seen in other hypogammaglobulinemias. Patients with X-linked hyper-IgM syndrome also show defects in cell-mediated immunity (see Chapter 13), with a striking susceptibility to infection by the intracellular fungal microbe *Pneumocystis jiroveci.* This defective cell-mediated immunity occurs because CD40 ligand is also involved in T cell–dependent activation of macrophages and dendritic cells (see Chapter 13). Knockout mice lacking CD40 or CD40 ligand have a phenotype similar to that of the human disease.

Rare cases of hyper-IgM syndrome show an autosomal-recessive inheritance pattern. In these patients, the genetic defects may be in CD40 or in the enzyme activation-induced deaminase (AID) that is involved in heavy chain isotype switching and somatic mutation (see Chapter 10). One form of the hyper-IgM syndrome is caused by autosomal-recessive mutations in *uracil N glycosylase* (UNG; see Chapter 10), an enzyme that removes U residues from Ig genes during class switching and somatic mutation. An inherited disorder, EDA-ID, in which hypomorphic NEMO mutations contribute to a hyper-IgM state as well as defects in ectodermal structures, is described above in the section on TLR signaling defects.

Defects in T Lymphocyte Activation and Function

Congenital abnormalities in the activation of T lymphocytes are being increasingly recognized as our under-

Table 20–5. Defects in T Cell Activation

Disease	Functional deficiencies	Mechanism of defect
A. Defects in MHC expression		
Bare lymphocyte syndrome	Defective MHC class II expression and deficiency in CD4+ T cells; defective cell-mediated immunity, and T-dependent humoral immune responses	Defects in transcription factors regulating MHC class II gene expression, including CIITA, RFXANK, RFX5, and RFXAP
MHC class I deficiency	Decreased MHC class I levels; reduced CD8+ T cells	Mutations in TAP1, TAP2, and tapasin
B. Defective T cell signaling		
Proximal TCR signaling defects	Defects in cell-mediated immunity and T-dependent humoral immunity	Mutations in CD3 genes, CD45
Wiskott-Aldrich syndrome	Defective T cell activation, leukocyte mobility	TCR dependent actin-cytoskeletal rearrangements are defective because of mutations in WASP
C. Familial hemophagocytic lymphohistiocytoses		
X-linked lymphoproliferative syndrome	Uncontrolled EBV induced B cell proliferation, uncontrolled macrophage and CTL activation, defective NK cell and CTL function	Mutations in SAP
Perforin deficiencies	Uncontrolled macrophage and CTL activation, defective NK cell and CTL function	Mutations in perforin
Granule fusion defects	Uncontrolled macrophage and CTL activation, defective NK cell and CTL function	Defective cytotoxic granule exocytosis; mutations in RAB27A, MUNC13-4 (and in LYST in Chédiak-Higashi syndrome – see Table 20-2)

Abbreviations: LYST, lysosomal trafficking regulator protein; SAP, SLAM-associated protein; TAP, transporter associated with antigen processing; WASP, Wiskott-Aldrich syndrome protein.

standing of the molecular basis of lymphocyte activation improves (Table 20–5). Included in this broad category are some disorders of CTL and NK cell granule composition or exocytosis.

Defective Class II MHC Expression: The Bare Lymphocyte Syndrome

Class II major histocompatibility complex (MHC) deficiency, also called **bare lymphocyte syndrome,** is a rare heterogeneous group of autosomal-recessive diseases in which patients express little or no HLA-DP, HLA-DQ, or HLA-DR on B lymphocytes, macrophages, and dendritic cells and fail to express class II MHC molecules in response to IFN-γ. They express normal or only slightly reduced levels of class I MHC molecules and β_2-microglobulin. Most cases of the bare lymphocyte syndrome are due to mutations in genes encoding proteins that regulate class II MHC transcription. For example, mutations in the constitutively expressed transcription factor RFX5 or the IFN-γ-inducible transcriptional activator CIITA lead to reduced class II MHC expression and a failure of APCs to activate CD4⁺ T lymphocytes. Failure of antigen presentation may result in defective positive selection of T cells in the thymus with a reduction in the number of mature CD4⁺ T cells or defective activation of cells in the periphery. Affected individuals are deficient in DTH responses and in antibody responses to T cell–dependent protein antigens. The disease appears within the first year of life and is usually fatal unless it is treated by bone marrow transplantation.

Defective Class I MHC Expression

Autosomal-recessive class I MHC deficiencies have also been described and are characterized by decreased CD8⁺ T cell numbers and function. In some cases, the failure to express class I MHC molecules is due to mutations in the gene encoding the TAP-1 or TAP-2 subunit of the TAP (transporter associated with antigen processing) complex, which normally transports peptides from the cystol into the endoplasmic reticulum, where they are required for class I MHC assembly (see Chapter 6). These TAP-deficient patients express few cell surface class I MHC molecules, a phenotype similar to *TAP* gene knockout mice. Such patients suffer mainly from respiratory tract bacterial infections and not viral infections, which is surprising considering that a principal function of CD8⁺ T cells is defense against viruses. A similar deficiency of class I MHC expression has been observed in patients with mutations in the gene encoding the tapasin protein (see Chapter 6).

Defects in TCR Signal Transduction

Many examples of rare immunodeficiency diseases caused by defects in the expression of molecules required for T cell activation and function have been identified. Modern biochemical and molecular analyses of affected individuals have revealed mutations in the genes encoding various T cell proteins. Examples include impaired TCR complex expression or function caused by mutations in the CD3 ε or γ genes, defective TCR-mediated signaling caused by mutations in the *ZAP-70* gene, reduced synthesis of cytokines such as IL-2 and IFN-γ (in some cases caused by defects in transcription factors), and lack of expression of IL-2 receptors. These defects are often found in only a few isolated cases or in a few families, and the clinical features and severity vary widely. Patients with these abnormalities may have deficiencies predominantly in T cell function or have mixed T cell and B cell immunodeficiencies despite normal or even elevated numbers of blood lymphocytes. Some of these defects are associated with abnormal ratios of $CD4^+$ and $CD8^+$ T cell subsets, which may reflect impaired development of one subset in the thymus or impaired expansion of one subset in the peripheral immune system. For example, patients with ZAP-70 deficiency have reduced $CD8^+$ T cells but not $CD4^+$ T cells; the reason for the selective loss is not clear.

Wiskott-Aldrich Syndrome

Variable degrees of T and B cell immunodeficiency occur in certain congenital diseases with a wide spectrum of abnormalities involving multiple organ systems. One such disorder is **Wiskott-Aldrich syndrome,** an X-linked disease characterized by eczema, thrombocytopenia (reduced blood platelets), and susceptibility to bacterial infection. Some of the abnormalities in this disorder can be traced to defective T cell activation, though intrinsic loss of B cell function also contributes to the pathogenesis. In the initial stages of the disease, lymphocyte numbers are normal, and the principal defect is an inability to produce antibodies in response to T cell–independent polysaccharide antigens, because of which these patients are especially susceptible to infections with encapsulated pyogenic bacteria. The lymphocytes (and platelets) are smaller than normal. With increasing age, the patients show reduced numbers of lymphocytes and more severe immunodeficiency. The defective gene responsible for Wiskott-Aldrich syndrome encodes a cytoplasmic protein called WASP (Wiskott-Aldrich syndrome protein), expressed exclusively in bone marrow–derived cells, which interacts with several proteins, including adapter molecules downstream of the antigen receptor, such as Grb-2 (see Chapter 9), the Arp2/3 complex involved in actin polymerization, and small G proteins of the Rho family that regulate actin cytoskeletal rearrangement. Defective activation and synapse formation in lymphocytes, and defective mobility of all leukocytes, may account for the immunodeficiency observed in this syndrome.

The X-linked Lymphoproliferative Syndrome

X-linked lymphoproliferative disease is a disorder characterized by an inability to eliminate Epstein-Barr virus (EBV), eventually leading to fulminant infectious mononucleosis and the development of B cell tumors and associated hypogammaglobulinemia. In about 80% of cases, the disease is due to mutations in the gene encoding an adapter molecule called SAP (SLAM-associated protein) that binds to a family of cell surface molecules involved in the activation of NK cells and T and B lymphocytes, including the prototypic signaling lymphocyte activation molecule (SLAM). SAP links the membrane-associated proteins SLAM and 2B4 (see Chapter 8) to the Src-family kinase FynT. Defects in SAP contribute to attenuated NK and T cell activation and result in increased susceptibility to viral infections. In about 20% of cases, the genetic defect resides not in SAP but in the gene encoding XIAP (X-linked inhibitor of apoptosis). The resulting enhanced apoptosis of T cells and NK-T cells leads to a marked depletion of these cell types in the patients. This immunodeficiency is most commonly manifested by severe EBV infections, which probably arise opportunistically because of the ubiquitous nature of EBV.

Defective CTL and NK Cell Activation: the Familial Hemophagocytic Lymphohistiocytosis Syndromes

The hemophagocytic lymphohistiocytosis (HLH) syndromes are a group of life-threatening immunodeficiency disorders characterized by uncontrolled CTL and macrophage activation in which NK cell and CTL granule secretion is defective. A late but striking feature of these disorders is the ingestion of red blood cells by activated macrophages (hemophagocytosis). Mutations in the perforin gene, as well as mutations in genes encoding the cellular machinery involved in granule exocytosis, can contribute to the phenotypes observed in this syndrome. Specifically, mutations in *RAB27A,* a small guanosine triphosphatase involved in vesicular fusion, and in *MUNC13-4,* which encodes an adapter that participates in granule exocytosis, compromise the fusion of lytic granules with the plasma membrane and thus contribute to various subtypes of HLH. Similarly, mutations in the gene for one component of the AP-3 cytosolic adapter protein complex can also disrupt intracellular transport and contribute to a form of HLH. It is believed that T cells and macrophages respond strongly to microbes to compensate for the CTL and NK cell defects, and these responses are manifested by hemophagocytosis and lymphadenopathy in the context of immunodeficiency.

Multisystem Disorders with Immunodeficiency: Ataxia Telangiectasia

Immunodeficiency is often one of a constellation of symptoms in a number of inherited disorders. Examples of such syndromes discussed above include Chédiak-

Higashi syndrome, Wiskott-Aldrich syndrome, and DiGeorge's syndrome. **Ataxia telangiectasia** is an autosomal-recessive disorder characterized by abnormal gait (ataxia), vascular malformations (telangiectases), neurologic deficits, increased incidence of tumors, and immunodeficiency. The immunologic defects are of variable severity and may affect both B and T cells. The most common humoral immune defects are IgA and IgG2 deficiency. The T cell defects, which are usually less pronounced, are associated with thymic hypoplasia. Patients experience upper and lower respiratory tract bacterial infections, multiple autoimmune phenomena, and increasingly frequent cancers with advancing age. The gene responsible for this disorder is located on chromosome 11 and encodes a protein called ATM (ataxia telangiectasia mutated) that is related structurally to phosphatidylinositol-3 (PI-3) kinase, but is a protein kinase. The ATM protein can activate cell cycle checkpoints and apoptosis in response to double-stranded DNA breaks and has also been shown to contribute to the stability of DNA double-strand break complexes during V(D)J recombination. Because of these abnormalities in DNA repair, the generation of antigen receptors may also be abnormal.

Therapeutic Approaches for Congenital Immunodeficiencies

The current treatment of immunodeficiencies has two aims: to minimize and control infections and to replace the defective or absent components of the immune system by adoptive transfer or transplantation. **Passive immunization** with pooled gamma globulin is enormously valuable for agammaglobulinemic patients and has been lifesaving for many boys with X-linked agammaglobulinemia. **Bone marrow transplantation** is currently the treatment of choice for many immunodeficiency diseases and has been successful in the treatment of SCID with ADA deficiency, Wiskott-Aldrich syndrome, bare lymphocyte syndrome, and LAD. It is most successful with careful T cell depletion from the marrow and HLA matching to prevent graft-versus-host disease (see Chapter 16). Enzyme replacement therapy for ADA and PNP deficiencies has been attempted, with red blood cell transfusions used as a source of the enzymes. This approach has produced temporary clinical improvement in several patients with autosomal SCID. Injection of bovine ADA conjugated to polyethylene glycol to prolong its serum half-life has proved successful in some cases, but the benefits are usually short lived.

In theory, the therapy of choice for congenital disorders of lymphocytes is to replace the defective gene in self-renewing stem cells. Gene replacement remains a distant goal for most human immunodeficiencies at present, despite considerable effort. The main obstacles to this type of gene therapy are difficulties in purifying self-renewing stem cells, which are the ideal target for introduction of the replacement gene, and the lack of a method for introducing genes into cells to achieve stable, long-lived, and high-level expression. A small number of patients with X-linked SCID have been successfully treated by transplantation of autologous bone marrow cells engineered to express a normal γ_C chain gene. However, a few treated patients have developed leukemia, apparently because the introduced γ_C gene inserted adjacent to an oncogene and activated this gene. As a result, the future of gene therapy for this disease is uncertain. For unknown reasons, gene therapy has not been as successful in treating patients with autosomal SCID caused by ADA mutations.

Acquired (Secondary) Immunodeficiencies

Deficiencies of the immune system often develop because of abnormalities that are not genetic but acquired during life (Table 20–6). The most prominent of these abnormalities is HIV infection, and this is described in the next section. Acquired immunodeficiency diseases are caused by two main types of pathogenic mechanisms. First, immunosuppression may occur as a biologic complication of another disease process. Second, so-called iatrogenic immunodeficiencies may develop as complications of therapy for other diseases.

Diseases in which immunodeficiency is a common complicating element include malnutrition, neoplasms, and infections. Protein-calorie malnutrition is extremely common in developing countries and is associated with impaired cellular and humoral immunity to microorganisms. Much of the morbidity and mortality that afflict

Table 20–6. Acquired Immunodeficiencies

Cause	Mechanism
Human immunodeficiency virus infection	Depletion of $CD4^+$ helper T cells
Protein-calorie malnutrition	Metabolic derangements inhibit lymphocyte maturation and function
Irradiation and chemotherapy treatments for cancer	Decreased bone marrow lymphocyte precursors
Cancer metastases and leukemia involving bone marrow	Reduced site of leukocyte development
Immunosuppression for transplants, autoimmune diseases	Reduced lymphocyte activation
Removal of spleen	Decreased phagocytosis of microbes

malnourished people is due to infections. The basis for the immunodeficiency is not well defined, but it is reasonable to assume that the global metabolic disturbances in these individuals, caused by deficient intake of protein, fat, vitamins, and minerals, will adversely affect maturation and function of the cells of the immune system.

Patients with advanced widespread cancer are often susceptible to infection because of impaired cell-mediated and humoral immune responses to a variety of organisms. Bone marrow tumors, including cancers metastatic to marrow and leukemias that arise in the marrow, may interfere with the growth and development of normal lymphocytes and other leukocytes. In addition, tumors may produce substances that interfere with lymphocyte development or function. An example of malignancy-associated immunodeficiency is the impairment in T cell function commonly observed in patients with a type of lymphoma called Hodgkin's disease. This defect was first characterized as an inability to mount a DTH reaction on intradermal injection of various common antigens to which the patients were previously exposed, such as *Candida* or tetanus toxoid. Other *in vitro* measures of T cell function, such as proliferative responses to polyclonal activators, are also impaired in patients with Hodgkin's disease. Such a generalized deficiency in DTH responses is called **anergy.** The cause of these T cell abnormalities is unknown.

Various types of infections lead to immunosuppression. Viruses other than HIV are known to impair immune responses; examples include the measles virus and human T cell lymphotropic virus 1 (HTLV-1). Both viruses can infect lymphocytes, which may be a basis for their immunosuppressive effects. Like HIV, HTLV-1 is a retrovirus with tropism for CD4$^+$ T cells; however, instead of killing helper T cells, it transforms them and produces an aggressive T cell malignancy called adult T cell leukemia/lymphoma (ATL). Patients with ATL typically have severe immunosuppression with multiple opportunistic infections. Chronic infections with *Mycobacterium tuberculosis* and various fungi frequently result in anergy to many antigens. Chronic parasitic infections may also lead to immunosuppression. For example, African children with chronic malarial infections have depressed T cell function, which may be important in the pathogenesis of EBV-associated malignant tumors (see Chapter 17, Box 17–2).

Iatrogenic immunosuppression is most often due to drug therapies that either kill or functionally inactivate lymphocytes. Some drugs are given intentionally to immunosuppress patients, either for the treatment of inflammatory diseases or to prevent rejection of tissue allografts. The most commonly used anti-inflammatory and immunosuppressive drugs are corticosteroids and cyclosporine, respectively. Various chemotherapeutic drugs are administered to patients with cancer, and these drugs are usually cytotoxic to both mature and developing lymphocytes as well as to granulocyte and monocyte precursors. Thus, cancer chemotherapy is almost always accompanied by a period of immunosuppression and risk for infection. Iatrogenic immunosuppression and tumors involving the bone marrow are the most common causes of immunodeficiency in developed countries.

One other form of acquired immunosuppression results from the absence of a spleen caused by surgical removal of the organ after trauma and as treatment of certain hematologic diseases or by infarction in sickle cell disease. Patients without spleens are more susceptible to infection by some organisms, particularly encapsulated bacteria such as *Streptococcus pneumoniae.* This enhanced susceptibility is partly due to defective phagocytic clearance of opsonized blood-borne microbes, an important physiologic function of the spleen, and partly because of defective antibody responses resulting from the absence of marginal zone B cells.

Human Immunodeficiency Virus and the Acquired Immunodeficiency Syndrome

AIDS is the disease caused by infection with HIV and is characterized by profound immunosuppression with associated opportunistic infections and malignant tumors, wasting, and central nervous system (CNS) degeneration. HIV infects a variety of cells of the immune system, including CD4$^+$ helper T cells, macrophages, and dendritic cells. HIV evolved as a human pathogen very recently relative to most other known human pathogens, and the HIV epidemic was first identified only in the 1980s. However, the degree of morbidity and mortality caused by HIV and the global impact of HIV infection on health care resources and economics are already enormous and continue to grow. HIV has infected 50 to 60 million people and has caused the death of over 22 million adults and children. More than 42 million people are living with HIV infection and AIDS, of which approximately 70% are in Africa and 20% in Asia, and almost 3 million die of the disease every year. It is estimated that there are approximately 14,000 new infections every day, and by the year 2010, 50 to 75 million infected people will be added to the already staggering pool of cases worldwide. The disease is especially devastating because about half of the approximately 5 million new cases every year occur in young adults (15–24 years old). As a result, AIDS has left approximately 14 million orphans, and this number may climb to 25 million by 2010. Currently, there is no effective vaccine or cure for AIDS, although new anti-retroviral therapies have been developed. In this section of the chapter, we describe the molecular and biologic properties of HIV, the pathogenesis of HIV-induced immunodeficiency, and the clinical and epidemiologic features of HIV-related diseases.

Molecular and Biologic Features of HIV

HIV is a member of the lentivirus family of animal retroviruses. Lentiviruses, including visna virus of sheep and the bovine, feline, and simian immunodeficiency viruses (SIVs), are capable of long-term latent infection of cells and short-term cytopathic effects, and they all produce slowly progressive, fatal diseases that include wasting syndromes and CNS degeneration. Two closely related types of HIV, designated HIV-1 and HIV-2, have been identified. HIV-1 is by far the most common cause of AIDS, but HIV-2, which differs in genomic structure and antigenicity, causes a similar clinical syndrome.

HIV Structure and Genes

An infectious HIV particle consists of two identical strands of RNA packaged within a core of viral proteins and surrounded by a phospholipid bilayer envelope derived from the host cell membrane but including virally encoded membrane proteins (Fig. 20–3). The RNA genome of HIV is approximately 9.2 kb long and has the basic arrangement of nucleic acid sequences characteristic of all known retroviruses (Fig. 20–4). Long terminal repeats (LTRs) at each end of the genome regulate viral gene expression, viral integration into the host genome, and viral replication. The *gag* sequences encode core structural proteins. The *env* sequences encode the envelope glycoproteins gp120 and gp41, which are required for infection of cells. The *pol* sequences encode reverse transcriptase, integrase, and viral protease enzymes required for viral replication. In addition to these typical retrovirus genes, HIV-1 also includes six other regulatory genes, namely, the *tat, rev, vif, nef, vpr,* and *vpu* genes, whose products regulate viral reproduction in various ways. The functions of these genes are summarized in Figure 20–4.

Viral Life Cycle

HIV infection of cells begins when the envelope glycoprotein (Env) of a viral particle binds to both CD4 and a coreceptor that is a member of the chemokine receptor family (Fig. 20–5). The viral particles that initiate infection are usually in the blood, semen, or other body fluids of one individual and are introduced into another individual by sexual contact, needle stick, or transplacental passage. Env is a complex composed of a transmembrane gp41 subunit and an external, noncovalently associated gp120 subunit. These subunits are produced by proteolytic cleavage of a gp160 precursor. The Env complex is expressed as a trimeric structure of three gp120/gp41 pairs. This complex mediates a multistep process of fusion of the virion envelope with the membrane of the target cell (Fig. 20–6). The first step of this process is the binding of gp120 subunits to CD4 molecules, which induces a conformational change that promotes secondary gp120 binding to a chemokine coreceptor. Coreceptor binding induces a conformational change in gp41 that exposes a hydrophobic region, called the fusion peptide, that inserts into the cell membrane and enables the viral membrane to fuse with the target cell membrane. After the virus completes its life cycle in the infected cell (described later), free viral particles are released from one infected cell and bind to an uninfected cell, thus propagating the infection. In addition, gp120 and gp41, which are expressed on the plasma membrane of infected cells before virus is released, can mediate cell-cell fusion with an uninfected cell that

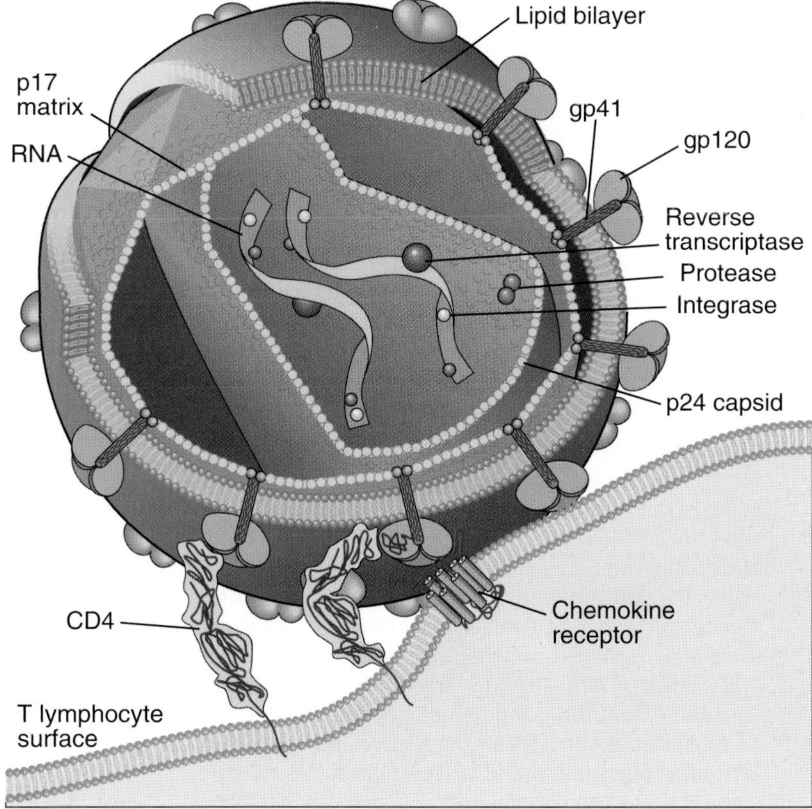

FIGURE 20–3 Structure of HIV-1. An HIV-1 virion is shown next to a T cell surface. HIV-1 consists of two identical strands of RNA (the viral genome) and associated enzymes, including reverse transcriptase, integrase, and protease, packaged in a cone-shaped core composed of p24 capsid protein with a surrounding p17 protein matrix, all surrounded by a phospholipid membrane envelope derived from the host cell. Virally encoded membrane proteins (gp41 and gp120) are bound to the envelope. CD4 and chemokine receptors on the host cell surface function as HIV-1 receptors. (© 2000 Terese Winslow.)

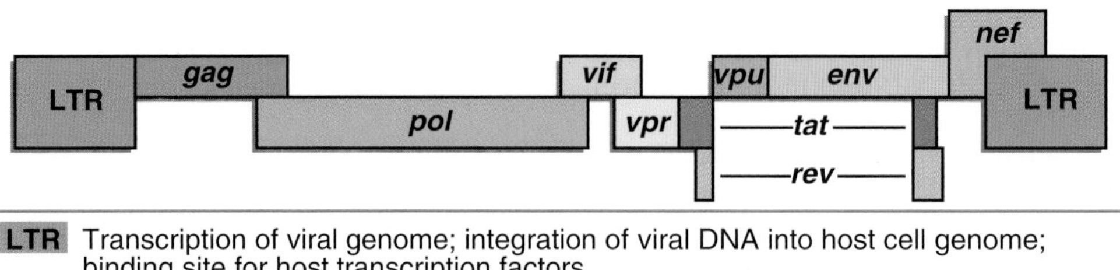

LTR	Transcription of viral genome; integration of viral DNA into host cell genome; binding site for host transcription factors
gag	Nucleocapsid core and matrix proteins
pol	Reverse transcriptase, protease, integrase, and ribonuclease
env	Viral coat proteins (gp120 and gp41)
vif	Overcomes inhibitory effect of host cell enzyme (APOBEC3G), promotes viral replication
vpr	Increases viral replication; promotes HIV infection of macrophages
tat	Required for elongation of viral transcripts
rev	Promotes nuclear export of incompletely spliced viral RNAs
vpu	Down-regulates host cell CD4 expression; enhances release of virus from cells
nef	Down-regulates host cell CD4 and class I MHC expression; enhances release of infectious virus

Abbreviations: LTR, long terminal repeat; pol, polymerase; env, envelope; vif, viral infectivity factor; vpr, viral protein R; tat, transcriptional activator; rev, regulator of viral gene expression; vpu, viral protein u; nef, negative effector

FIGURE 20–4 HIV-1 genome. The genes along the linear genome are indicated as differently colored blocks. Some genes use some of the same sequences as other genes, as shown by overlapping blocks, but are read differently by host cell RNA polymerase. Similarly shaded blocks separated by lines indicate genes whose coding sequences are separated in the genome and require RNA splicing to produce functional mRNA. (Adapted from Greene W. AIDS and the immune system. Copyright 1993 by Scientific American, Inc. All rights reserved.)

expresses CD4 and coreceptors, and HIV genomes can then be passed between the fused cells directly.

The identification of CD4 and chemokine receptors as HIV receptors came from several different experimental approaches and clinical observations.

- CD4 was first suspected as a viral receptor because of the selective destruction of $CD4^+$ T cells in HIV-infected individuals and the subsequent demonstration that HIV infects only $CD4^+$ cells in vitro. Receptor-binding studies using purified recombinant molecules have established that gp120 specifically binds to CD4, and mutational and x-ray crystallographic studies have identified the regions of both molecules that interact physically.
- The requirement for a coreceptor in addition to CD4 in HIV infection was first suspected because expression of recombinant human CD4 in many nonhuman cell lines did not render the cells susceptible to HIV infection but subsequent fusion with human cells did. The formal demonstration that a chemokine receptor can act as a cofactor for HIV entry into a cell was accomplished by screening human complementary DNA (cDNA) libraries for the ability to make a human CD4-expressing mouse cell line infectable by a T cell line–tropic HIV strain. A cDNA isolated by this strategy encoded the CXCR4 chemokine receptor, which binds the chemokines SDF-1α and SDF-1β.
- Concurrent with these studies, investigators discovered that soluble factors released by $CD8^+$ T cells could suppress HIV infection of macrophages by some isolates of HIV. These factors were identified as the chemokines RANTES (regulated by activation, normal T cell expressed and secreted), MIP-1α (macrophage inflammatory protein-1α), and MIP-1β, all of which bind to the CCR5 receptor and competitively inhibit virus binding. (The modern nomenclature of these chemokines is in Chapter 12.)

The most important chemokine receptors that act as coreceptors for HIV are CXCR4 and CCR5. More than seven different chemokine receptors have been shown to serve as coreceptors for HIV entry into cells, and several other proteins belonging to the seven-membrane-spanning G protein–coupled receptor family, such as the leukotriene B_4 receptor, can also mediate HIV infection of cells. Different isolates of HIV have distinct tropisms for different cell populations that are related to the specificity of gp120 variants for different chemokine receptors. All HIV strains can infect and replicate in freshly isolated human $CD4^+$ T cells that are activated in vitro. In contrast, some strains will infect primary cultures of human macrophages but not continuous T cell lines (macrophage-tropic, or M-tropic, virus), whereas other strains will infect T cell lines but not macrophages (T-tropic virus). Some virus strains

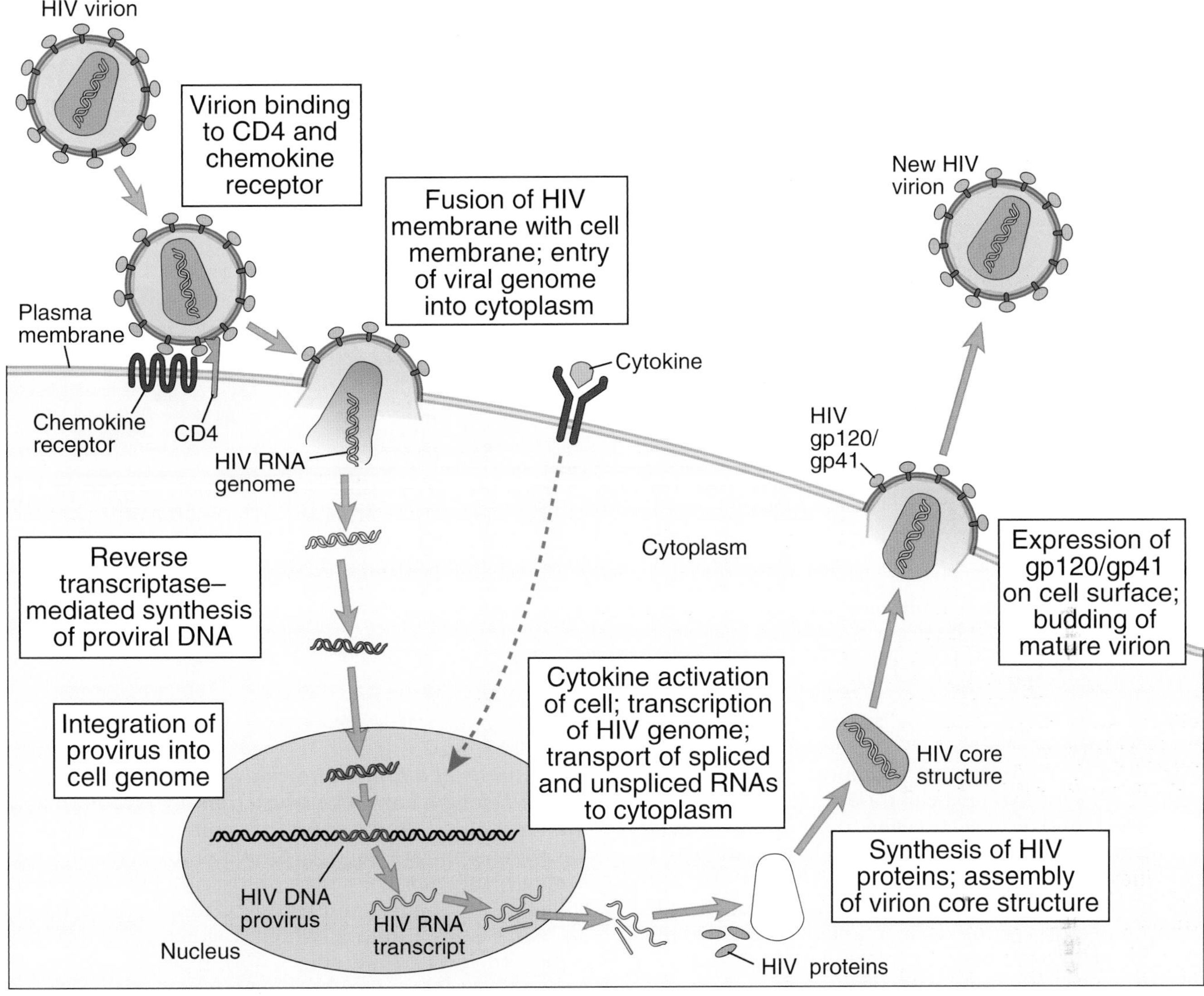

FIGURE 20–5 HIV life cycle. The sequential steps in the life cycle of HIV are shown, from initial infection of a host cell to viral replication and release of a new virion. For the sake of clarity, the production and release of only one new virion are shown. An infected cell actually produces many virions, each capable of infecting cells, thereby amplifying the infectious cycle.

also infect both T cell lines and macrophages (dual-tropic virus). Macrophage-tropic virus isolates express a gp120 that binds to CCR5, which is expressed on macrophages (and some memory T cells), whereas T cell–tropic viruses bind to CXCR4, which is expressed on T cell lines. HIV variants are described as X4 for CXCR4 binding, R5 for CCR5 binding, or R5X4 for the ability to bind to both chemokine receptors. In many HIV-infected individuals, there is a change from the production of virus that uses CCR5 and is predominantly macrophage tropic early in the disease to virus that binds to CXCR4 and is T cell line tropic late in the disease. The T-tropic strains tend to be more virulent, presumably because they infect and deplete T cells more than do M-tropic strains. The importance of CCR5 in HIV infection in vivo is supported by the finding that individuals who do not express this receptor because of genetic mutations are resistant to HIV infection.

Once an HIV virion enters a cell, the enzymes within the nucleoprotein complex become active and begin the viral reproductive cycle (see Fig. 20–5). The nucleoprotein core of the virus becomes disrupted, the RNA genome of HIV is transcribed into a double-stranded DNA form by viral reverse transcriptase, and the viral DNA enters the nucleus. The viral integrase also enters the nucleus and catalyzes the integration of viral DNA into the host cell genome. The integrated HIV DNA is called the **provirus.** The provirus may remain transcriptionally inactive for months or years, with little or no production of new viral proteins or virions, and in this way HIV infection of an individual cell can be latent.

Transcription of the genes of the integrated DNA provirus is regulated by the LTR upstream of the viral structural genes, and cytokines or other physiologic stimuli to T cells and macrophages enhance viral gene transcription. The LTRs contain polyadenylation signal

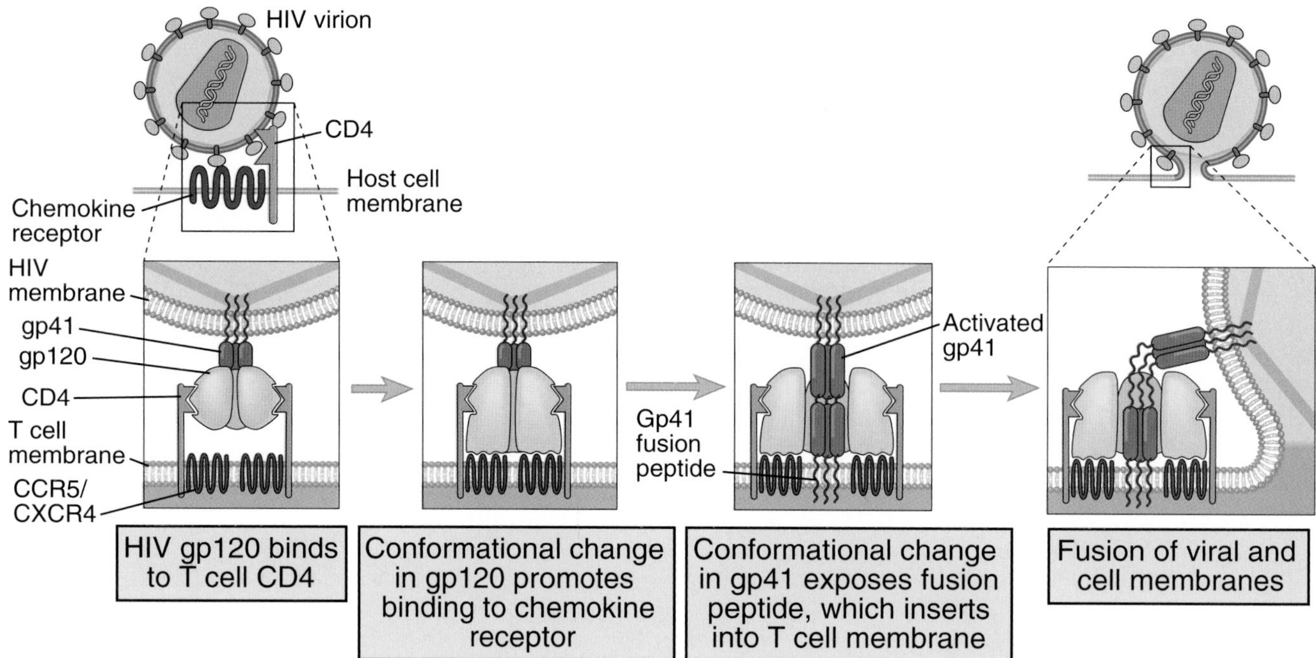

FIGURE 20–6 Mechanism of HIV entry into a cell. In the model depicted, sequential conformational changes in gp120 and gp41 are induced by binding to CD4. These changes promote binding of the virus to the coreceptor (a chemokine receptor) and fusion of the HIV-1 and host cell membranes. The fusion peptide of activated gp41 contains hydrophobic amino acid residues that mediate insertion into the host cell plasma membrane.

sequences, the TATA box promoter sequence, and binding sites for two host cell transcription factors, NF-κB and SP1. Initiation of HIV gene transcription in T cells is linked to activation of the T cells by antigen or cytokines. For example, polyclonal activators of T cells, such as phytohemagglutinin, and cytokines such as IL-2, tumor necrosis factor (TNF), and lymphotoxin stimulate HIV gene expression in infected T cells, and IL-1, IL-3, IL-6, TNF, lymphotoxin, IFN-γ, and granulocyte-macrophage colony-stimulating factor (GM-CSF) stimulate HIV gene expression and viral replication in infected monocytes and macrophages. TCR and cytokine stimulation of HIV gene transcription probably involves the activation of NF-κB and its binding to sequences in the LTR. This phenomenon is significant to the pathogenesis of AIDS because the normal response of a latently infected T cell to a microbe may be the way in which latency is ended and virus production begins. The multiple infections that AIDS patients acquire thus stimulate HIV production and infection of additional cells.

The Tat protein is required for HIV gene expression and acts by enhancing the production of complete viral messenger RNA (mRNA) transcripts. Even in the presence of optimal signals to initiate transcription, few if any HIV mRNA molecules are actually synthesized because transcription of HIV genes by mammalian RNA polymerase is inefficient and the polymerase complex usually stops before the mRNA is completed. Tat protein binds to the nascent mRNA and increases the "processivity" of RNA polymerase by several hundred-fold, which allows transcription to be completed to produce a functional viral mRNA.

Synthesis of mature, infectious viral particles begins after full-length viral RNA transcripts are produced and the viral genes are expressed as proteins. The mRNAs encoding the various HIV proteins are derived from a single full-genome-length transcript by differential splicing events. HIV gene expression may be divided into an early stage, during which regulatory genes are expressed, and a late stage, during which structural genes are expressed and full-length viral genomes are packaged. The Rev, Tat, and Nef proteins are early gene products encoded by fully spliced mRNAs that are exported from the nucleus and translated into proteins in the cytoplasm soon after infection of a cell. Late genes include *env, gag,* and *pol,* which encode the structural components of the virus and are translated from singly spliced or unspliced RNA. The Rev protein initiates the switch from early to late gene expression by promoting the export of these incompletely spliced late gene RNAs out of the nucleus. The *pol* gene product is a precursor protein that is sequentially cleaved to form reverse transcriptase, protease, ribonuclease, and integrase enzymes. As mentioned before, reverse transcriptase and integrase proteins are required for producing a DNA copy of the viral RNA genome and integrating it as a provirus into the host genome. The *gag* gene encodes a 55-kD protein that is proteolytically cleaved into p24, p17, and p15 polypeptides by the action of the viral protease encoded by the *pol* gene. These polypeptides are the core proteins that are required for assembly of infectious viral particles. The primary product of the *env* gene is a 160-kD glycoprotein (gp160) that is cleaved by cellular proteases within the endoplasmic reticulum into the gp120 and gp41 proteins required for HIV binding to cells, as discussed earlier. Current antiviral drug therapy for HIV disease includes inhibitors of the enzymes reverse transcriptase, protease, and integrase.

After transcription of various viral genes, viral proteins are synthesized in the cytoplasm. Assembly of infectious viral particles then begins by packaging full-length RNA transcripts of the proviral genome within a nucleoprotein complex that includes the *gag* core proteins and the *pol*-encoded enzymes required for the next cycle of integration. This nucleoprotein complex is then enclosed within a membrane envelope and released from the cell by a process of budding from the plasma membrane. The rate of virus production can reach sufficiently high levels to cause cell death, as discussed later.

Naive T cells are resistant to HIV infection because these cells contain an active form of an enzyme that introduces mutations in the HIV genome. This enzyme has been given the rather cumbersome name APOBEC3G (apolipoprotein B mRNA-editing enzyme catalytic polypeptide-like editing complex 3). It is a member of a family of cytidine deaminases that inhibit retroviral replication. APOBEC3G introduces cytosine to uracil mutations in the viral DNA that is produced by reverse transcription, and these mutations inhibit further DNA replication by mechanisms that are not fully defined. Activation of T cells converts cellular APOBEC3G into an inactive, high molecular mass complex. HIV has evolved to counteract this cellular defense mechanism—the viral protein Vif binds to APOBEC3G and promotes its degradation by cellular proteases.

Pathogenesis of HIV Infection and AIDS

HIV disease begins with acute infection, which is only partly controlled by the adaptive immune response, and advances to chronic progressive infection of peripheral lymphoid tissues (Fig. 20–7). Virus typically enters through mucosal epithelia. The subsequent events in the infection can be divided into several phases.

Acute (early) infection is characterized by infection of memory CD4⁺ T cells (which express CCR5) in mucosal lymphoid tissues, and death of many infected cells. Because the mucosal tissues are the largest reservoir of T cells in the body, and the major site of residence of memory T cells, this local loss is reflected in considerable depletion of lymphocytes. In fact, within 2 weeks of infection, the majority of $CD4^+$ T cells may be destroyed.

- Studies of simian immunodeficiency virus infection in macaques have shown that within 4 days of infec-

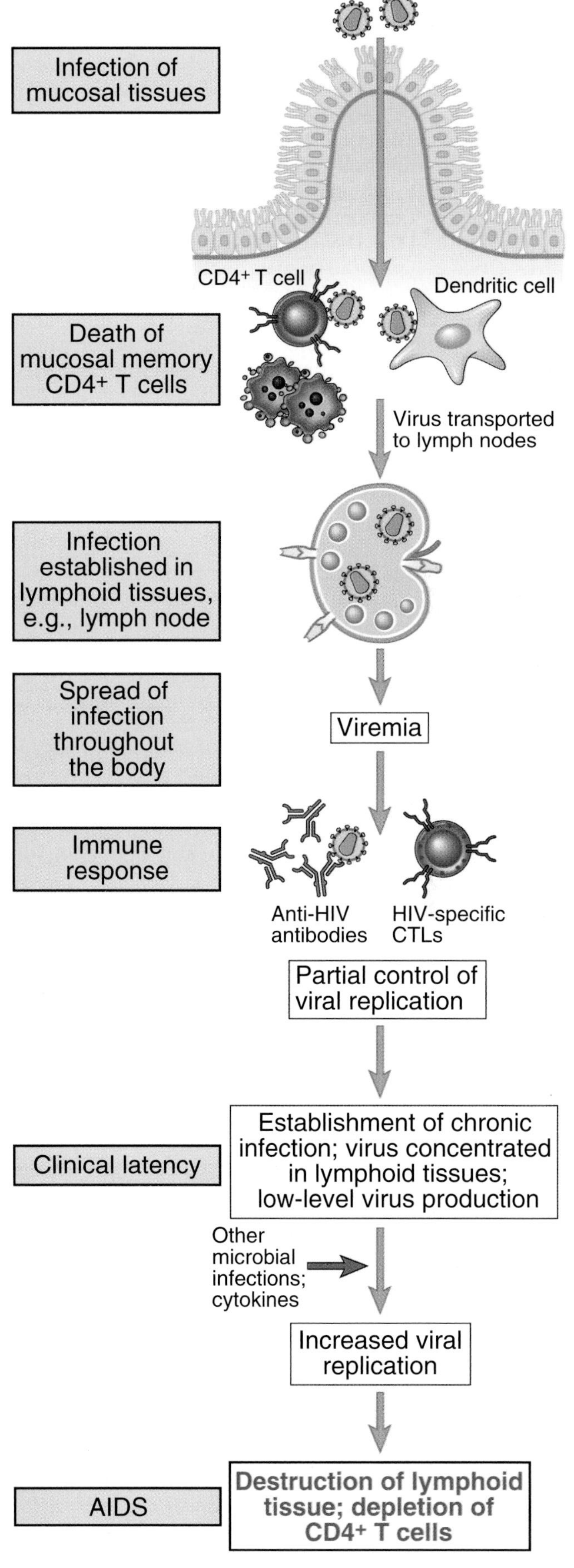

FIGURE 20–7 Progression of HIV infection. The progression of HIV infection correlates with spread of the virus from the initial site of infection to lymphoid tissues throughout the body. The immune response of the host temporarily controls acute infection but does not prevent the establishment of chronic infection of cells in lymphoid tissues. Cytokine stimuli induced by other microbes serve to enhance HIV production and progression to AIDS.

tion, about 60% of mucosal memory CD4⁺ T cells are infected, and 80% of these cells die in the first week.

The transition from the acute phase to a chronic phase of infection is characterized by dissemination of the virus, viremia, and the development of host immune responses. Dendritic cells in epithelia at sites of virus entry capture the virus and then migrate into the lymph nodes. Dendritic cells express a protein with a mannose-binding lectin domain that may be particularly important in binding the HIV envelope and transporting the virus. Once in lymphoid tissues, dendritic cells may pass HIV on to CD4⁺ T cells through direct cell-cell contact. Within days after the first exposure to HIV, viral replication can be detected in the lymph nodes. This replication leads to viremia, during which large numbers of HIV particles are present in the patient's blood, accompanied by an acute HIV syndrome that includes a variety of nonspecific signs and symptoms typical of many viral diseases (described below). The viremia allows the virus to disseminate throughout the body and to infect helper T cells, macrophages, and dendritic cells in peripheral lymphoid tissues. As the HIV infection spreads, the adaptive immune system mounts both humoral and cell-mediated immune responses directed at viral antigens, which we will describe later. These immune responses partially control the infection and viral production, and such control is reflected by a drop in viremia to low but detectable levels by approximately 12 weeks after the primary exposure.

In the next, chronic phase of the disease, lymph nodes and the spleen are sites of continuous HIV replication and cell destruction (see Fig. 20–7). During this period of the disease, the immune system remains competent at handling most infections with opportunistic microbes, and few or no clinical manifestations of the HIV infection are present. Therefore, this phase of HIV disease is called the clinical latency period. Although the majority of peripheral blood T cells do not harbor the virus, destruction of CD4⁺ T cells within lymphoid tissues steadily progresses during the latent period, and the number of circulating blood CD4⁺ T cells steadily declines (Fig. 20–8). More than 90% of the body's approximately 10^{12} T cells are normally found in peripheral and mucosal lymphoid tissues, and it is estimated that HIV destroys up to 1 to 2×10^9 CD4⁺ T cells every day. Early in the course of the disease, the body may continue to make new CD4⁺ T cells, and therefore CD4⁺ T cells can be replaced almost as quickly as they are destroyed. At this stage, up to 10% of CD4⁺ T cells in lymphoid organs may be infected, but the number of circulating CD4⁺ T cells that are infected at any one time may be less than 0.1% of the total CD4⁺ T cells in an individual. Eventually, during a period of years, the continuous cycle of virus infection, T cell death, and new infection leads to a steady decline in the number of CD4⁺ T cells in the lymphoid tissues and the circulation.

Mechanisms of Immunodeficiency Caused by HIV

HIV infection ultimately results in impaired function of both the adaptive and innate immune systems. The most prominent defects are in cell-mediated immunity, and they can be attributed to several mechanisms, including direct cytopathic effects of the virus and indirect effects.

An important cause of the loss of CD4⁺ T cells in HIV-infected people is the direct cytopathic effect of infection of these cells by HIV. Death of CD4⁺ T cells is associated

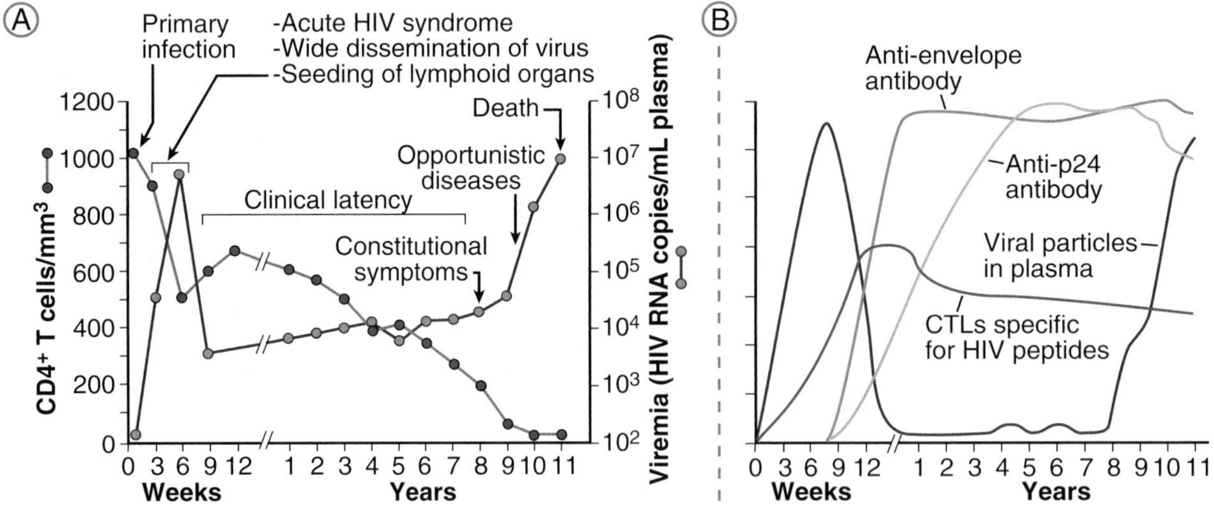

FIGURE 20–8 Clinical course of HIV disease. A. Plasma viremia, blood CD4⁺ T cell counts, and clinical stages of disease. About 12 weeks after infection, blood-borne virus (plasma viremia) is reduced to very low levels (detectable only by sensitive reverse-transcriptase polymerase chain reaction assays) and stays this way for many years. Nonetheless, CD4⁺ T cell counts steadily decline during this clinical latency period because of active viral replication and T cell infection in lymph nodes. When CD4⁺ T cell counts drop below a critical level (about 200/mm³), the risk for infection and other clinical components of AIDS is high. (From Pantaleo G, C Graziosi, and AS Fancim. The immunopathogenesis of human immunodeficiency virus infection. New England Journal of Medicine 328:327–335, 1993. Copyright © 1993 Massachusetts Medical Society. All rights reserved.) B. Immune response to HIV infection. A CTL response to HIV is detectable by 2 to 3 weeks after the initial infection and peaks by 9 to 12 weeks. Marked expansion of virus-specific CD8⁺ T cells occurs during this time, and up to 10% of a patient's CTLs may be HIV specific at 12 weeks. The humoral immune response to HIV peaks at about 12 weeks.

with production of virus in infected cells and is a major cause of the decline in the numbers of these cells, especially in the early (acute) phase of the infection. Several direct toxic effects of HIV on infected $CD4^+$ cells have been described:

- The process of virus production, with expression of gp41 in the plasma membrane and budding of viral particles, may lead to increased plasma membrane permeability and the influx of lethal amounts of calcium, which induces apoptosis, or osmotic lysis of the cell caused by the influx of water.
- Viral production can interfere with cellular protein synthesis and thereby lead to cell death.
- The plasma membranes of HIV-infected T cells fuse with uninfected $CD4^+$ T cells by virtue of gp120-CD4 interactions, and multinucleated giant cells or syncytia are formed. The process of HIV-induced syncytia formation can be lethal to HIV-infected T cells as well as to uninfected $CD4^+$ T cells that fuse to the infected cells. However, this phenomenon has largely been observed in vitro, and syncytia are rarely seen in the tissues of patients with AIDS.

Mechanisms in addition to direct lysis of infected $CD4^+$ T cells by virus have been proposed for the depletion and loss of function of these cells in HIV-infected individuals. One mechanism that has been suggested is related to chronic activation of uninfected cells by the infections that are common in patients infected with HIV and also by cytokines produced in response to these infections. Chronic activation of the T cells may predispose the cells to apoptosis; the molecular pathway involved in this type of apoptosis is not yet defined (see Chapter 11, Box 11–2). Apoptotic death of activated lymphocytes may account for the observation that the loss of T cells greatly exceeds the numbers of HIV-infected cells. HIV-specific CTLs are present in many patients with AIDS, and these cells can kill infected $CD4^+$ T cells. In addition, antibodies against HIV envelope proteins may bind to HIV-infected $CD4^+$ T cells and target the cells for antibody-dependent cell-mediated cytotoxicity (ADCC). Binding of gp120 to newly synthesized intracellular CD4 may interfere with normal protein processing in the endoplasmic reticulum and block cell surface expression of CD4, making the cells incapable of responding to antigenic stimulation. Other proposed mechanisms include defective maturation of $CD4^+$ T cells in the thymus. The relative importance of these indirect mechanisms in $CD4^+$ T cell depletion in HIV-infected patients is uncertain and controversial.

Functional defects in the immune system of HIV-infected individuals exacerbate the immune deficiency caused by depletion of $CD4^+$ T cells. These functional defects include a decrease in T cell responses to antigens and weak humoral immune responses even though total serum Ig levels may be elevated. The defects may be a result of the direct effects of HIV infection on $CD4^+$ T cells, including the effects of soluble gp120 released from infected cells binding to uninfected cells. For example, CD4 that has bound gp120 may not be available to interact with class II MHC molecules on APCs, and thus T cell responses to antigens would be inhibited. Alternatively, gp120 binding to CD4 may deliver signals that down-regulate helper T cell function. HIV-infected T cells are unable to form tight synapses with APCs, and this may also interfere with T cell activation. Some studies have demonstrated that the proportion of IL-2- and IFN-γ-secreting (T_H1) T cells decreases in HIV-infected patients and the proportion of IL-4- and IL-10-secreting (T_H2-like) T cells increases. This altered balance of T_H1 and T_H2 responses may partially explain the susceptibility of HIV-infected individuals to infection by intracellular microbes because IFN-γ activates and T_H2 cytokines may inhibit macrophage-mediated killing of such microbes. Patients with HIV infection may have increased numbers of $CD4^+$ $CD25^+$ regulatory T cells, but it is not yet clear if this is a consistent finding or if these cells actually contribute to defective immunity.

The Tat protein may play some role in the pathogenesis of immunodeficiency caused by HIV. Within T cells, Tat can interact with a variety of regulatory proteins, such as the p300 coactivator of transcription, and these interactions can interfere with normal T cell functions such as cytokine synthesis. Remarkably, Tat not only enters the nucleus of infected T cells but can also escape across the plasma membrane and enter neighboring cells, thus interfering with activation of uninfected T cells in a paracrine fashion.

Macrophages, dendritic cells, and follicular dendritic cells also play important roles in HIV infection and the progression of immunodeficiency.

- Macrophages express much lower levels of CD4 than helper T lymphocytes do, but they do express CCR5 coreceptors and are susceptible to HIV infection. However, macrophages are relatively resistant to the cytopathic effects of HIV. Macrophages may also be infected by a gp120/gp41-independent route, such as phagocytosis of other infected cells or Fc receptor–mediated endocytosis of antibody-coated HIV virions. Because macrophages can be infected but are not generally killed by the virus, they may become a reservoir for the virus. In fact, the quantity of macrophage-associated HIV exceeds T cell–associated virus in most tissues from patients with AIDS, including the brain and lung. HIV-infected macrophages may be impaired in antigen presentation functions and cytokine secretion.
- Dendritic cells can also be infected by HIV. Like macrophages, dendritic cells are not directly injured by HIV infection. However, these cells form intimate contact with naive T cells during the course of antigen presentation. It is proposed that dendritic cells infect naive T cells during these encounters and may thus be an important pathway for T cell injury.
- Follicular dendritic cells (FDCs) in the germinal centers of lymph nodes and the spleen trap large

amounts of HIV on their surfaces, in part by Fc receptor–mediated binding of antibody-coated virus. Although FDCs are not efficiently infected, they contribute to the pathogenesis of HIV-associated immunodeficiency in at least two ways. First, the FDC surface is a reservoir for HIV that can infect macrophages and $CD4^+$ T cells in the lymph nodes. Second, the normal functions of FDCs in immune responses are impaired, and they may eventually be destroyed by the virus. Although the mechanisms of HIV-induced death of FDCs are not understood, the net result of loss of the FDC network in the lymph nodes and spleen is a profound dissolution of the architecture of the peripheral lymphoid system.

HIV Reservoirs and Viral Turnover

The virus detected in patients' blood is produced mostly by short-lived infected $CD4^+$ T cells and in smaller amounts by other infected cells. Three phases of decay of plasma viremia have been observed in patients treated with anti-retroviral drugs, or predicted by mathematical modeling, and these decay curves have been used to surmise the distribution of HIV in different cellular reservoirs. Over 90% of plasma virus is believed to be produced by short-lived cells (half-lives of ~1 day), which are most likely activated $CD4^+$ T cells that are major reservoirs and sources of the virus in infected patients. About 5% of plasma virus is produced by macrophages, which have a slower turnover (half-life of about 2 weeks). It is hypothesized that a small fraction of the virus, perhaps as little as 1%, is present in latently infected memory T cells. Because of the long life span of memory cells, it could take decades for this reservoir of virus to be eliminated even if all new rounds of infection were blocked.

Clinical Features of HIV Disease

A vast amount of information has accumulated about the epidemiology and clinical course of HIV infection. As anti-retroviral drug therapy is improving, many of the clinical manifestations are changing. In the following section we describe the "classical" features of HIV infection, and refer to the changing pictures when relevant.

Transmission of HIV and Epidemiology of AIDS

HIV is transmitted from one individual to another by three major routes:

- Sexual contact is the most frequent mode of transmission, either between heterosexual couples (the most frequent mode of transmission in Africa and Asia) or between homosexual male partners. In sub-Saharan Africa, where the infection rate is the highest in the world (estimated to be about 10,000 new cases every day), more than half the infected individuals are women.
- Mother-to-child transmission of HIV accounts for the majority of pediatric cases of AIDS. This type of transmission occurs most frequently *in utero* or during childbirth, although transmission through breast milk is also possible.
- Inoculation of a recipient with infected blood or blood products is also a frequent mode of HIV transmission. Needles shared by intravenous drug abusers account for most cases of this form of transmission. With the advent of routine laboratory screening, transfusion of blood or blood products in a clinical setting accounts for a small portion of HIV infections.

Major groups at risk for the development of AIDS in the United States include homosexual or bisexual males, intravenous drug abusers, heterosexual partners of members of other risk groups, and babies born of infected mothers. Health care workers have a small increased risk for infection.

Clinical Course of HIV Infection

The course of HIV disease can be followed by measuring the amount of virus in the patient's plasma and by the blood $CD4^+$ T cell count (see Fig. 20–8).

The acute phase of the illness, also called the acute HIV syndrome, is the period of viremia characterized by nonspecific symptoms of infection. It develops in 50%

Table 20–7. Clinical Features of HIV Infection

Phase of disease	Clinical feature
Acute HIV disease	Fever, headaches, sore throat with pharyngitis, generalized lymphadenopathy, rashes
Clinical latency period	Declining blood $CD4^+$ T cell amount
AIDS	**Opportunistic infections:** Protozoa *(Toxoplasma Cryptosporidium)* Bacteria *(Mycobacteruim avium, Nocardia, Salmonella)* Fungi *(Candida, Cryptococcus neoformans, Coccidioides immitis, Histoplasma capsulatum, Pneumocystis)* Viruses *(cytomegalovirus, herpes simplex, varicella-zoster)* **Tumors:** Lymphomas (including EBV-associated B cell lymphomas) Kaposi's sarcoma Cervical carcinoma **Encephalopathy** **Wasting syndrome**

Abbreviations: AIDS, aquired immune deficiency syndrome; EBV, Epstein-Barr virus.

to 70% of infected adults typically 3 to 6 weeks after infection. There is a spike of plasma virus and a modest reduction in $CD4^+$ T cell counts, but the number of blood $CD4^+$ T cells often returns to normal. In many patients, however, the infection is occult and there are no symptoms.

The chronic phase of clinical latency may last for many years. During this time, the virus is contained within lymphoid tissues, and the loss of $CD4^+$ T cells is corrected by replenishment from progenitors. Patients are asymptomatic or suffer from minor infections. Within 2 to 6 months after infection, the concentration of plasma virus stabilizes at a particular set-point, which differs among patients. The level of the viral set-point and the number of blood $CD4^+$ T cells are clinically useful predictors of the progression of disease. As the disease progresses, patients become susceptible to other infections, and immune responses to these infections may stimulate HIV production and accelerate the destruction of lymphoid tissues. As discussed earlier, HIV gene transcription can be enhanced by stimuli that activate T cells, such as antigens and a variety of cytokines. Cytokines, such as TNF, that are produced by the innate immune system in response to microbial infections are particularly effective in boosting HIV production. Thus, as the immune system attempts to eradicate other microbes, it brings about its own destruction by HIV.

HIV disease progresses to the final and almost invariably lethal phase, called AIDS, when the blood $CD4^+$ T cell count drops below 200 cells/mm^3. HIV viremia may climb dramatically as viral replication in other reser-voirs accelerates unchecked. Patients with AIDS suffer from combinations of opportunistic infections, neoplasms, cachexia (HIV wasting syndrome), kidney failure (HIV nephropathy), and CNS degeneration (AIDS encephalopathy) (see Table 20–7). Because $CD4^+$ helper T cells are essential for both cell-mediated and humoral immune responses to various microbes, the loss of these lymphocytes is the main reason that patients with AIDS become susceptible to many different types of infections. Furthermore, many of the tumors that arise in patients with AIDS have a viral etiology, and their prevalence in the setting of AIDS reflects an inability of the HIV-infected patient to mount an effective immune response against oncogenic viruses. Most of the opportunistic infections and neoplasms associated with HIV infection occur after the blood $CD4^+$ T cell count drops below 200 cells/mm^3. Cachexia is often seen in patients with chronic inflammatory diseases and may result from effects of inflammatory cytokines (such as TNF) on appetite and metabolism. The CNS disease in AIDS may be due to neuronal damage by the virus or by shed viral proteins such as gp120 and Tat as well as to the effects of cytokines elaborated by infected microglial cells. Many of these devastating consequences of HIV infection, including opportunistic infections and tumors, have been significantly reduced by highly active antiretroviral therapy.

Although this summary of the clinical course is true for the most severe cases, the rate of progression of the disease is highly variable, and some individuals are long-term nonprogressors. The immunologic correlates of variable progression remain unknown. Also, recent antiretroviral therapy has changed the course, and greatly reduced the incidence, of severe opportunistic infections (such as *Pneumocystis*) and tumors (such as Kaposi's sarcoma).

Immune Responses to HIV

HIV-specific humoral and cell-mediated immune responses develop following infection but generally provide limited protection. The early response to HIV infection is, in fact, similar in many ways to the immune response to other viruses and serves effectively to clear most of the virus present in the blood and in circulating T cells. Nonetheless, it is clear that these immune responses fail to eradicate all virus, and the infection eventually overwhelms the immune system in most individuals. Despite the poor effectiveness of immune responses to the virus, it is important to characterize them for three reasons. First, the immune responses may be detrimental to the host, for example, by stimulating the uptake of opsonized virus into uninfected cells by Fc receptor–mediated endocytosis or by eradication of $CD4^+$ T cells expressing viral antigens by $CD8^+$ CTLs. Second, antibodies against HIV are diagnostic markers of HIV infection that are widely used for screening purposes. Third, the design of effective vaccines for immunization against HIV requires knowledge of the types of immune responses that are most likely to be protective (the "correlates of protection").

Many innate immune responses against HIV have been described. These include anti-microbial peptides (defensins), NK cells, dendritic cells (particularly plasmacytoid dendritic cells producing type I IFNs), and the complement system. The role of these responses in combating the infection are not established.

The initial adaptive immune response to HIV infection is characterized by expansion of $CD8^+$ T cells specific for HIV peptides. As many as 10% or more of circulating $CD8^+$ T cells may be specific for HIV during the early stages of infection. These CTLs control infection in the acute phase (see Fig. 20–8), but ultimately prove ineffective because of the emergence of viral escape mutants (variants with mutated antigens). Although $CD4^+$ T cells also respond to the virus, the importance of this response is unclear.

Antibody responses to a variety of HIV antigens are detectable within 6 to 9 weeks after infection. The most immunogenic HIV molecules that elicit antibody responses appear to be the envelope glycoproteins, and high titers of anti-gp120 and anti-gp41 antibodies are present in most HIV-infected individuals. Other anti-HIV antibodies found frequently in patients' sera include antibodies to p24, reverse transcriptase, and *gag* and *pol* products (see Fig. 20–8). The effect of these antibodies on the clinical course of HIV infection is uncertain. The early antibodies are not neutralizing, and are generally poor inhibitors of viral infectivity or cytopathic effects. Neutralizing antibodies against gp120 develop 2 to 3 months after primary infection, but even these antibodies cannot cope with a virus that is able to rapidly change the most immunodominant epitopes of its envelope glycoproteins.

Mechanisms of Immune Evasion by HIV

The failure of cell-mediated and humoral immune responses to eradicate HIV infection is probably due to several factors. Importantly, because of the depletion and functional inhibition of the $CD4^+$ T cells, the immune responses may be too compromised to eliminate the virus. In addition, several features of HIV may help the virus to evade host immunity.

- ***HIV has an extremely high mutation rate because of error-prone reverse transcription, and in this way it may evade detection by antibodies or T cells generated in response to viral proteins.*** It has been estimated that in an infected person, every possible point mutation in the viral genome occurs every day. A region of the gp120 molecule, called the V3 loop, is one of the most antigenically variable components of the virus; it varies in HIV isolates taken from the same individual at different times. Furthermore, the regions of the V3 loop that are critical for viral entry and therefore are less frequently mutated are not readily exposed to the humoral immune system. It is possible that the host immune response may work as a selective pressure that promotes survival of the most genetically variable viruses.
- ***HIV-infected cells may evade CTLs through down-regulation of class I MHC molecule expression.*** The HIV Nef protein inhibits expression of class I MHC molecules, mainly by promoting internalization of these molecules.
- ***HIV infection may inhibit cell-mediated immunity.*** We have mentioned previously that in infected individuals, T_H2 cells specific for HIV and other microbes may expand relative to T_H1 cells. Because T_H2 cytokines inhibit cell-mediated immunity, the net result of this imbalance is a form of dysregulation (called immune deviation) that increases host susceptibility to infection by intracellular microbes, including HIV itself. Along the same vein, increased numbers of regulatory T cells may inhibit host defenses.

Treatment and Prevention of AIDS and Vaccine Development

Active research efforts have been aimed at developing reagents that interfere with the viral life cycle. Treatment of HIV infection and AIDS now includes the administration of three classes of antiviral drugs, used in combination, that target viral molecules for which no human homologues exist. The first type of drug to be widely used consists of nucleoside analogues that inhibit reverse-transcriptase activity. These drugs include deoxythymidine nucleoside analogues such as 3′-azido-3′-deoxythymidine (AZT), deoxycytidine nucleoside analogues, and deoxyadenosine analogues. When these drugs are used alone, they are often effective in significantly reducing plasma HIV RNA levels for several months to years. They usually do not halt progression of HIV-induced disease, largely because of the evolution of virus with mutated forms of reverse transcriptase that are resistant to the drugs. More recently, viral protease inhibitors have been developed that block the processing of precursor proteins into mature viral capsid and core proteins. When these protease inhibitors are used alone, mutant viruses resistant to their effects rapidly emerge. However, protease inhibitors are now being used in combination with two different reverse-transcriptase inhibitors. This new triple-drug therapy, commonly referred to as HAART (highly active anti-retroviral therapy), has proved to be remarkably effective in reducing plasma viral RNA to undetectable levels in most treated patients for up to 3 years. An integrase inhibitor is also now used as part of anti-viral therapy. Although anti-retroviral therapy has reduced viral titers to below detection for up to 10 years in some patients, it is unlikely that such treatment can eliminate the virus from all reservoirs (especially long-lived infected cells), and resistance to the drugs may ultimately develop. Other formidable problems associated with these new drug therapies, which will impair their effective use in many parts of the world, include high expense, complicated administration schedules, and serious side effects.

The individual infections experienced by patients with AIDS are treated with the appropriate prophylaxis, antibiotics, and support measures. More aggressive antibiotic therapy is often required than for similar infections in less compromised hosts.

Efforts at preventing HIV infection are extremely important and potentially effective in controlling the HIV epidemic. In the United States, the routine screening of blood products for evidence of donor HIV infection has already reduced the risk of this mode of transmission to negligible levels. Various public health measures to increase condom use and to reduce the use of contaminated needles by intravenous drug users are now widespread. Perhaps the most effective efforts at prevention are campaigns to increase public awareness of HIV.

The development of an effective vaccine against HIV is a priority for biomedical research institutions worldwide. The task has been complicated by the ability of the virus to mutate and vary many of its immunogenic antigens. It is likely that an effective vaccine will have to stimulate both humoral and cell-mediated responses to viral antigens that are critical for the viral life cycle. To achieve this goal, several approaches are being tried for HIV vaccine development. Much of the preliminary work has involved SIV infection of macaques, and effective vaccines against SIV have already been developed. This success is encouraging because SIV is molecularly closely related to HIV and causes a disease similar to AIDS in macaques. Various live virus vaccines have been tested in the hope that they will induce strong CTL responses. Such vaccines include nonvirulent recombinant hybrid viruses composed of part SIV and part HIV sequences or viruses that have been attenuated by deletions in one or more parts of the viral genome, such as the *nef* gene. One concern with live virus vaccines is their potential to cause disease if they are not completely attenuated and possibly after recombination in vivo with wild-type HIV to produce a pathogenic variant. Another approach that avoids this safety concern but retains efficacy in inducing CTL-mediated immunity is the use of live recombinant non-HIV viral vectors carrying HIV genes. Preliminary trials in human volunteers have already shown that canarypox vaccines expressing several HIV-1 genes can induce strong CTL responses to the HIV antigens. Many DNA vaccines have also been studied; these vaccines are composed of combinations of structural and regulatory genes of SIV or HIV packaged in mammalian DNA expression vectors. Combinations of vaccines, such as initial immunization with a DNA vaccine followed by boosting with a canarypox vector expressing HIV genes, have yielded some of the most promising results to date. Recombinant protein or peptide subunit vaccines that elicit antibodies are of limited value by themselves because the antibodies often do not neutralize clinical isolates of HIV. It is possible that such vaccines may be useful given with live virus vaccines.

SUMMARY

- Immunodeficiency diseases are caused by congenital or acquired defects in lymphocytes, phagocytes, and other mediators of adaptive and innate immunity. These diseases are associated with an increased susceptibility to infection, the nature and severity of which depend largely on which component of the immune system is abnormal and the extent of the abnormality.

- Disorders of innate immunity include defects in microbial killing by phagocytes (e.g., CGD or Chédiak-Higashi syndrome), in leukocyte migration and adhesion (e.g., LAD), and in TLR signaling. Complement deficiencies were described in Chapter 14.

- Severe combined immunodeficiencies include defects in lymphocyte development that affect both T and B cells, and are caused by defective cytokine signaling, abnormal purine metabolism, defective V(D)J recombination, and mutations that affect T cell maturation.

- Antibody immunodeficiencies include diseases caused by defective B cell maturation or activation, and defects in T cell–B cell collaboration (X-linked hyper-IgM syndrome).

- T cell immunodeficiencies include diseases in which the expression of MHC molecules is defective, T cell signaling disorders, and rare diseases involving CTL and NK cell functions.

- Treatment of congenital immunodeficiencies involves transfusions of antibodies, bone marrow or stem cell transplantation, or enzyme replacement. Gene therapy may offer improved treatments in the future.

- Acquired immunodeficiencies are caused by infections, malnutrition, disseminated cancer, and immunosuppressive therapy for transplant rejection or autoimmune diseases.

- AIDS is a severe immunodeficiency caused by infection with HIV. This RNA virus infects $CD4^+$ T lymphocytes, macrophages, and dendritic cells, and causes massive dysfunction of the immune system. Most of the immunodeficiency in AIDS can be ascribed to the depletion of $CD4^+$ T cells.

- HIV enters cells by binding to both the CD4 molecule and a coreceptor of the chemokine receptor family. Once inside the cell, the viral genome is reverse-transcribed into DNA and incorporated into the cellular genome. Viral gene transcription and viral reproduction are stimulated by signals that normally activate the host cell. Production of virus is accompanied by cell death.

- The acute phase of infection is characterized by death of memory $CD4^+$ T cells in mucosal tissues and dissemination of the virus to lymph nodes. In the subsequent latent phase, there is low level virus replication in lymphoid tissues and slow, progressive loss of T cells. Persistent activation of T cells promotes their death, leading to rapid loss and immune deficiency in the chronic phase of the infection.

- $CD4^+$ T cell depletion in HIV-infected individuals is due to direct cytopathic effects of the virus, toxic effects of viral products such as shed gp120, and indirect effects such as activation-induced cell death or CTL killing of infected $CD4^+$ cells.

- Several reservoirs of HIV exist in infected individuals, including short-lived activated $CD4^+$ T cells, longer-lived macrophages, and very long lived, latently infected memory T cells.

- HIV-induced depletion of $CD4^+$ T cells results in increased susceptibility to infection by a number of opportunistic microorganisms. In addition, HIV-infected patients have an increased incidence of tumors, particularly Kaposi's sarcoma and EBV-associated B cell lymphomas, and encephalopathy frequently develops, the mechanism of which is not fully understood.

- HIV has a high mutation rate, which allows the virus to evade host immune responses and become resistant to drug therapies. Genetic variability also poses a problem for the design of an effective vaccine against HIV. HIV infection can be treated by a combination of inhibitors of viral enzymes.

Selected Readings

Barouch DH. Challenges in the development of an HIV-1 vaccine. Nature 455:613–619, 2008.

Blackburn MR, and RE Kellems. Adenosine deanimase deficiency: metabolic basis of immune deficiency and pulmonary inflammation. Advances in Immunology 86:1–4, 2005.

Bonilla FA, and RS Geha. Update on primary immunodeficiency diseases. Journal of Allergy and Clinical Immunology 117(Suppl):435–441, 2006.

Brenchley JM, DA Price, and DC Douek. HIV disease: fallout from a mucosal catastrophe? Nature Immunology 7:235–239, 2006.

Buckley RH. Molecular defects in human severe combined immunodeficiency and approaches to immune reconstitution. Annual Review of Immunology 22:625–655, 2004.

Bustamante J, S Boisson-Dupuis, E Jouanguy, C Picard, A Puel, L Abel, and JL Casanova. Novel primary immunodeficiencies revealed by the investigation of paediatric infectious diseases. Current Opinion in Immunology 20:39–48, 2008.

Casanova JL, and L Abel. Inborn errors of immunity to infection: the rule rather than the exception. Journal of Experimental Medicine 202:197–201, 2005.

Castigli E, and RS Geha. Molecular basis of common variable immunodeficiency. Journal of Allergy and Clinical Immunology 117:740–746, 2006.

Chen X, and PE Jensen. MHC class II antigen presentation and immunological abnormalities due to deficiency of MHC class II and its associated genes. Experimental and Molecular Pathology 85:40–44, 2008.

Chiu Y-L, and WC Greene. Multifaceted antiviral actions of APOBEC3 cytidine deaminase. Trends in Immunology 27:291–297, 2006.

Cunningham-Rundles C, and PP Ponda. Molecular defects in T- and B-cell primary immunodeficiency diseases. Nature Reviews Immunology 5:880–892, 2005.

Derdeyn CA, and G Silvestri. Viral and host factors in the pathogenesis of HIV infection. Current Opinion in Immunology 17:366–373, 2005.

Fauci AS, D Mavilio, and S Kottilil. NK cells in HIV infection: paradigm for protection or targets for ambush. Nature Reviews Immunology 5:835–843, 2005.

Fischer A. Human primary immunodeficiency diseases. Immunity 28:835–846, 2008.

Greene WC, and BM Peterlin. Charting HIV's remarkable voyage through the cell: basic science as a passport to future therapy. Nature Medicine 8:673–680, 2002.

Groneberg DA, D Quarcoo, N Frossard, and A Fischer. Gene therapy for severe combined immunodeficiency. Annual Review of Medicine 56:585–602, 2005.

Grossman Z, M Meier-Schellersheim, AE Sousa, RM Victorino, and WE Paul. CD4+ T-cell depletion in HIV infection: are we closer to understanding the cause? Nature Medicine 8:319–323, 2002.

Haase AT. Perils at mucosal front lines for HIV and SIV and their hosts. Nature Reviews Immunology 5:783–792, 2005.

Hladik F, and MJ McElrath. Setting the stage: host invasion by HIV. Nature Reviews Immunology 8:447–457, 2008.

Janka GE. Hemophagocytic lymphohistiocytosis. Hematology 10 Suppl 1:104–107, 2005.

Johnston MI, and AS Fauci. An HIV vaccine–evolving concepts. New England Journal of Medicine 356:2073–2081, 2007.

Lavin MF. Ataxia-telangiectasia: from a rare disorder to a paradigm for cell signalling and cancer. Nature Reviews Molecular and Cell Biology 9:759–769, 2008.

Letvin NL. Progress and obstacles in the development of an AIDS vaccine. Nature Reviews Immunology 6:930–939, 2006.

Letvin NL, and BD Walker. Immunopathogenesis and immunotherapy in AIDS virus infections. Nature Medicine 9:861–866, 2003.

Lusso P. HIV and the chemokine system: 10 years later. EMBO Journal 25:447–456, 2006.

McCune JM. The dynamics of CD4+ T-cell depletion in HIV disease. Nature 410:974–979, 2001.

McMichael AJ. HIV vaccines. Annual Review of Immunology 24:227–255, 2006.

McMichael AJ, and SL Rowland-Jones. Cellular immune responses to HIV. Nature 410:980–987, 2001.

Morra M, D Howie, M Simarro, et al. X-linked lymphoproliferative disease: a progressive immunodeficiency. Annual Review of Immunology 19:657–682, 2001.

Nixon DF, EM Aandahl, and J Michaelsson. CD4+CD25+ regulatory T cells in HIV infection. Microbes and Infection 7:1063–1065, 2005.

Ochs HD, and AJ Thrasher. The Wiskott-Aldrich Syndrome. Journal of Allergy and Clinical Immuology 117:725–738, 2006.

Peterlin MB, and D Trono. Hide, shield, and strike back: how HIV-infected cells avoid immune eradication. Nature Reviews Immunology 3:97–107, 2003.

Puel A, K Yang, CL Ku, et al. Heritable defects of the human TLR signaling pathways. Journal of Endotoxin Research 11:220–224, 2005.

Reith W, and B Mach. The bare lymphocyte syndrome and the regulation of MHC expression. Annual Review of Immunology 19:331–373, 2001.

Simon V, and DD Ho. HIV-1 dynamics in vivo: implications for therapy. Nature Reviews Microbiology 1:181–190, 2003.

Stebbing J, B Gazzard, and DC Douek. Where does HIV live? New England Journal of Medicine 350:1872–1880, 2004.

Stevenson M. HIV-1 pathogenesis. Nature Medicine 9:853–860, 2003.

Villa A, V Marrella, F Rucci, and LD Notarangelo. Genetically determined lymphopenia and autoimmune manifestations. Current Opinion in Immunology 20:318–324, 2008.

Appendix I

GLOSSARY

αβ T cell receptor (αβ TCR). The most common form of TCR, expressed on both $CD4^+$ and $CD8^+$ T cells. The αβ TCR recognizes peptide antigen bound to an MHC molecule. Both α and β chains contain highly variable (V) regions that together form the antigen-binding site as well as constant (C) regions. TCR V and C regions are structurally homologous to the V and C regions of Ig molecules.

ABO blood group antigens. Glycosphingolipid antigens present on many cell types, including red blood cells. These antigens differ between different individuals, depending on inherited alleles encoding the enzymes required for synthesis of the antigens. The ABO antigens act as alloantigens responsible for blood transfusion reactions and hyperacute rejection of allografts.

Accessory molecule. A lymphocyte cell surface molecule distinct from the antigen receptor complex that mediates adhesive or signaling functions important for activation or migration of the lymphocyte.

Acquired immunodeficiency. A deficiency in the immune system that is acquired after birth, usually because of infection (e.g., AIDS), and that is not related to a genetic defect.

Acquired immunodeficiency syndrome (AIDS). A disease caused by human immunodeficiency virus (HIV) infection that is characterized by depletion of $CD4^+$ T cells leading to a profound defect in cell-mediated immunity. Clinically, AIDS includes opportunistic infections, malignant tumors, wasting, and encephalopathy.

Activation protein-1 (AP-1). A family of DNA-binding transcription factors composed of dimers of two proteins that bind to one another through a shared structural motif called a leucine zipper. The best-characterized AP-1 factor is composed of the proteins Fos and Jun. AP-1 is involved in transcriptional regulation of many different genes important in the immune system, such as cytokine genes.

Active immunity. The form of adaptive immunity that is induced by exposure to a foreign antigen and activation of lymphocytes and in which the immunized individual plays an active role in responding to the antigen. This type contrasts with passive immunity, in which an individual receives antibodies or lymphocytes from another individual who was previously actively immunized.

Acute-phase reactants. Proteins, mostly synthesized in the liver, whose plasma concentrations increase shortly after infection as part of the systemic inflammatory response syndrome. Examples include C-reactive protein, fibrinogen, and serum amyloid A protein. Hepatic synthesis of these molecules is up-regulated by inflammatory cytokines, especially IL-6 and TNF. The acute-phase reactants play various roles in the innate immune response to microbes.

Acute-phase response. The increase in plasma concentrations of several proteins, called acute-phase reactants, that occurs as part of the early innate immune response to infections.

Acute rejection. A form of graft rejection involving vascular and parenchymal injury mediated by T cells, macrophages, and antibodies that usually begins after the first week of transplantation. Differentiation of effector T cells and production of antibodies that mediate acute rejection occur in response to the graft, thus the delay in onset.

Adapter protein. Proteins involved in intracellular signal transduction pathways by serving as bridge molecules or scaffolds for the recruitment of other signaling molecules. During lymphocyte antigen receptor or cytokine receptor signaling, adapter molecules may be phosphorylated on tyrosine residues to enable them to bind other proteins containing Src homology 2 (SH2) domains. Adapter molecules involved in T cell activation include LAT, SLP-76, and Grb-2.

Adaptive immunity. The form of immunity that is mediated by lymphocytes and stimulated by exposure to infectious agents. In contrast to innate immunity, adaptive immunity is characterized by exquisite specificity for distinct macromolecules and memory, which is the ability to respond more vigorously to repeated exposure to the same microbe. Adaptive immunity is also called specific immunity.

Addressin. Molecules expressed on endothelial cells in different anatomic sites that bind to counterreceptors on lymphocytes called homing receptors and that direct organ-specific lymphocyte homing. Mucosal addressin cell adhesion molecule-1 (MadCAM-1) is an example of an addressin expressed in Peyer's patches in the intestinal wall that binds to the integrin $\alpha_4\beta_7$ on gut-homing T cells.

Adhesion molecule. A cell surface molecule whose function is to promote adhesive interactions with other cells or the extracellular matrix. Leukocytes express various types of adhesion molecules, such as selectins, integrins, and members of the Ig superfamily, and these molecules play crucial roles in cell migration and cellular activation in innate and adaptive immune responses.

Adjuvant. A substance, distinct from antigen, that enhances T cell activation by promoting the accumulation and activation of antigen presenting cells (APCs) at a site of antigen exposure. Adjuvants enhance APC expression of T cell–activating costimulators and cytokines and may also prolong the expression of peptide-MHC complexes on the surface of APCs.

Adoptive transfer. The process of transferring lymphocytes from one, usually immunized, individual into another individual. Adoptive transfer is used in research to define the role of a particular cell population (e.g., $CD4^+$ T cells) in an immune response. Clinically, adoptive transfer of tumor-reactive T lymphocytes is used in experimental cancer therapy.

Affinity. The strength of the binding between a single binding site of a molecule (e.g., an antibody) and a ligand (e.g., an antigen). The affinity of a molecule X for a ligand Y is represented by the dissociation constant (K_d), which is the concentration of Y that is required to occupy the combining sites of half the X molecules present in a solution. A smaller K_d indicates a stronger or higher-affinity interaction, and a lower concentration of ligand is needed to occupy the sites.

Affinity maturation. The process that leads to increased affinity of antibodies for a particular protein antigen as a humoral response progresses. Affinity maturation takes place in germinal centers of lymphoid tissues, and is the result of somatic mutation of Ig genes, followed by selective survival of the B cells producing the highest affinity antibodies.

Allele. One of different forms of a gene present at a particular chromosomal locus. An individual who is heterozygous at a locus has two different alleles, each on a different member of a pair of chromosomes, one inherited from the mother and one from the father. If a particular gene in a population has many different alleles, the gene or locus is said to be polymorphic. The MHC locus is extremely polymorphic.

Allelic exclusion. The exclusive expression of only one of two inherited alleles encoding Ig heavy and light chains and TCR β chains. Allelic exclusion occurs when the protein product of one productively recombined antigen receptor locus on one chromosome blocks rearrangement of the corresponding locus on the other chromosome. This property ensures that all the antigen receptors expressed by one clone of lymphocytes will have the identical antigen specificities. Because the TCR α chain locus does not show allelic exclusion, some T cells do express two different types of TCR.

Allergen. An antigen that elicits an immediate hypersensitivity (allergic) reaction. Allergens are proteins or chemicals bound to proteins that induce IgE antibody responses in atopic individuals.

Allergy. A form of atopy or immediate hypersensitivity disease, often referring to the type of antigen that elicits the disease, such as food allergy, bee sting allergy, and penicillin allergy. All these conditions are related to antigen-induced mast cell or basophil activation.

Alloantibody. An antibody specific for an alloantigen (i.e., an antigen present in some individuals of a species but not in others).

Alloantigen. A cell or tissue antigen that is present in some members of a species and not in others and that is recognized as foreign on an allograft. Alloantigens are usually products of polymorphic genes.

Alloantiserum. The alloantibody-containing serum of an individual who has previously been exposed to one or more alloantigens.

Allogeneic graft. An organ or tissue graft from a donor who is of the same species but genetically nonidentical to the recipient (also called an allograft).

Alloreactive. Reactive to alloantigens; describes T cells or antibodies from one individual that will recognize antigens on cells or tissues of another genetically nonidentical individual.

Allotype. The property of a group of antibody molecules defined by their sharing a particular antigenic determinant found on the antibodies of some individuals but not others. Such determinants are called allotopes. Antibodies that share a particular allotope belong to the same allotype. Allotype is also often used synonymously with allotope.

Altered peptide ligands (APLs). Peptides with altered TCR contact residues that elicit responses different from the responses to native peptide ligands. Altered peptide ligands may be important in the regulation of T cell activation in physiologic, pathologic, or therapeutic situations.

Alternative pathway of complement activation. An antibody-independent pathway of activation of the complement system that occurs when the C3b protein binds to microbial cell surfaces. The alternative pathway is a component of the innate immune system and mediates inflammatory responses to infection as well as direct lysis of microbes.

Anaphylactic shock. Cardiovascular collapse occurring in the setting of a systemic immediate hypersensitivity reaction.

Anaphylatoxins. The C5a, C4a, and C3a complement fragments that are generated during complement activation. The anaphylatoxins bind specific cell surface receptors and promote acute inflammation by stimulating neutrophil chemotaxis and activating mast cells. At high concentrations, anaphylatoxins activate enough mast cells to mimic anaphylaxis.

Anaphylaxis. An extreme systemic form of immediate hypersensitivity in which mast cell or basophil mediators cause bronchial constriction, massive tissue edema, and cardiovascular collapse.

Anchor residues. The amino acid residues of a peptide whose side chains fit into pockets in the peptide-binding cleft of an MHC molecule. The side chains bind to complementary amino acids in the MHC molecule and therefore serve to anchor the peptide in the cleft of the MHC molecule.

Anergy. A state of unresponsiveness to antigenic stimulation. Clinically, anergy describes the lack of T cell–dependent cutaneous delayed-type hypersensitivity reactions to common antigens. Lymphocyte anergy (also called clonal anergy) is the failure of clones of T or B cells to react to antigen and may be a mechanism of maintaining immunologic tolerance to self.

Angiogenesis. New blood vessel formation regulated by a variety of protein factors elaborated by cells of the innate and adaptive immune systems and often accompanying chronic inflammation.

Antagonist peptide. Variant peptide ligands of a TCR in which one or two TCR contact residues have been changed and in which negative signals are delivered to specific T cells that inhibit responses to native peptides.

Antibody. A type of glycoprotein molecule, also called immunoglobulin (Ig), produced by B lymphocytes that binds antigens, often with a high degree of specificity and affinity. The basic structural unit of an antibody is composed of two identical heavy chains and two identical light chains. N-terminal variable regions of the heavy and light chains form the antigen-binding sites, whereas the C-terminal constant regions of the heavy chains functionally interact with other molecules in the immune system. Every individual has millions of different antibodies, each with a unique antigen-binding site. Secreted antibodies perform various effector functions, including neutralizing antigens, activating complement, and promoting leukocyte-dependent destruction of microbes.

Antibody-dependent cell-mediated cytotoxicity (ADCC). A process by which NK cells are targeted to IgG-coated cells, resulting in lysis of the antibody-coated cells. A specific receptor for the constant region of IgG, called FcγRIII (CD16), is expressed on the NK cell membrane and mediates binding to the IgG.

Antibody feedback. The down-regulation of antibody production by secreted IgG antibodies that occurs when antigen-antibody complexes simultaneously engage B cell membrane Ig and Fcγ receptors (FcγRII). Under these conditions, the cytoplasmic tails of the Fcγ receptors transduce inhibitory signals inside the B cell.

Antibody repertoire. The collection of different antibody specificities expressed in an individual.

Antibody-secreting cell. A B lymphocyte that has undergone differentiation and produces the secretory form of Ig. Antibody-secreting cells are produced in response to antigen and reside in the spleen and lymph nodes as well as in the bone marrow.

Antigen. A molecule that binds to an antibody or a TCR. Antigens that bind to antibodies include all classes of molecules. TCRs bind only peptide fragments of proteins complexed with MHC molecules; both the peptide ligand and the native protein from which it is derived are called T cell antigens.

Antigen presentation. The display of peptides bound by MHC molecules on the surface of an APC that permits specific recognition by TCRs and activation of T cells.

Antigen-presenting cell (APC). A cell that displays peptide fragments of protein antigens, in association with MHC molecules, on its surface and activates antigen-specific T cells. In addition to displaying peptide-MHC complexes, APCs must also express costimulatory molecules to activate T lymphocytes optimally.

Antigen processing. The intracellular conversion of protein antigens derived from the extracellular space or the cytosol into peptides and loading of these peptides onto MHC molecules for display to T lymphocytes.

Antiserum. Serum from an individual previously immunized against an antigen that contains antibody specific for that antigen.

Apoptosis. A process of cell death characterized by DNA cleavage, nuclear condensation and fragmentation, and plasma membrane blebbing that leads to phagocytosis of the cell without inducing an inflammatory response. This type of cell death is important in lymphocyte development, regulation of lymphocyte responses to foreign antigens, and maintenance of tolerance to self antigens.

Arthus reaction. A localized form of experimental immune complex–mediated vasculitis induced by injection of an antigen subcutaneously into a previously immunized animal or into an animal that has been given intravenous antibody specific for the antigen. Circulating antibodies bind to the injected antigen and form immune complexes that are deposited in the walls of small arteries at the injection site and give rise to a local cutaneous vasculitis with necrosis.

Atopy. The propensity of an individual to produce IgE antibodies in response to various environmental antigens and to develop strong immediate hypersensitivity (allergic) responses. People who have allergies to environmental antigens, such as pollen or house dust, are said to be atopic.

Autoantibody. An antibody produced in an individual that is specific for a self antigen. Autoantibodies can cause damage to cells and tissues and are produced in excess in systemic autoimmune diseases, such as systemic lupus erythematosus.

Autocrine factor. A molecule that acts on the same cell that produces the factor. For example, IL-2 is an autocrine T cell growth factor that stimulates mitotic activity of the T cell that produces it.

Autoimmune disease. A disease caused by a breakdown of self-tolerance such that the adaptive immune system responds to self antigens and mediates cell and tissue damage. Autoimmune diseases can be organ specific (e.g., thyroiditis or diabetes) or systemic (e.g., systemic lupus erythematosus).

Autoimmune regulator (AIRE). A gene or its encoded protein, which functions to stimulate expression of peripheral tissue protein antigens in thymic epithelial cells. Mutations in the *AIRE* gene in humans and mice lead to tissue specific autoimmune disease, consistent with a role for AIRE in central T cell tolerance.

Autoimmunity. The state of adaptive immune system responsiveness to self antigens that occurs when mechanisms of self-tolerance fail.

Autologous graft. A tissue or organ graft in which the donor and recipient are the same individual. Autologous bone marrow and skin grafts are commonly performed in clinical medicine.

Avidity. The overall strength of interaction between two molecules, such as an antibody and antigen. Avidity depends on both the affinity and the valency of interactions. Therefore, the avidity of a pentameric IgM antibody, with 10 antigen-binding sites, for a multivalent antigen may be much greater than the avidity of a dimeric IgG molecule for the same antigen. Avidity can be used to describe the strength of cell-cell interactions, which are mediated by many binding interactions between cell surface molecules.

B-1 B lymphocytes. A subset of B lymphocytes, which develop earlier during ontogeny than do conventional B cells, and express a limited repertoire of V genes with little junctional diversity, and secrete IgM antibodies that bind T-independent antigens. Many B-1 cells express the CD5 (Ly-1) molecule.

B cell tyrosine kinase (Btk). A tyrosine kinase of the Src family that plays an essential role in B cell maturation. Mutations in the gene encoding Btk cause X-linked agammaglobulinemia, a disease characterized by failure of B cells to mature beyond the pre-B cell stage.

B lymphocyte. The only cell type capable of producing antibody molecules and therefore the central cellular component of humoral immune responses. B lymphocytes, or B cells, develop in the bone marrow, and mature B cells are found mainly in lymphoid follicles in secondary lymphoid tissues, in bone marrow, and in low numbers in the circulation.

BCR (B cell receptor) complex. A multiprotein complex expressed on the surface of B lymphocytes that recognizes antigen and transduces activating signals into the cell. The BCR includes membrane Ig, which is responsible for binding antigen, and Igα and Igβ proteins, which initiate signaling events.

Bare lymphocyte syndrome. An immunodeficiency disease characterized by a lack of class II MHC molecule expression that leads to defects in antigen presentation and cell-mediated immunity. The disease is caused by mutations in genes encoding factors that regulate class II MHC gene transcription.

Basophil. A type of bone marrow–derived, circulating granulocyte with structural and functional similarities to mast cells that has granules containing many of the same inflammatory mediators as mast cells and expresses a high-affinity Fc receptor for IgE. Basophils that are recruited into tissue sites where antigen is present may contribute to immediate hypersensitivity reactions.

β_2-Microglobulin. The light chain of a class I MHC molecule. β_2-Microglobulin is an extracellular protein encoded by a nonpolymorphic gene outside the MHC, is structurally homologous to an Ig domain, and is invariant among all class I molecules.

Biogenic amines. Low molecular weight, nonlipid compounds, such as histamine, that share the structural feature of an amine group, are stored in and released from the cytoplasmic granules of mast cells, and mediate many of the biologic effects of immediate hypersensitivity (allergic) reactions. (Biogenic amines are sometimes called vasoactive amines.)

Biologic response modifiers. Molecules, such as cytokines, used clinically as modulators of inflammation, immunity, and hematopoiesis.

Bone marrow. The central cavity of bone that is the site of generation of all circulating blood cells in adults, including immature lymphocytes, and the site of B cell maturation.

Bone marrow transplantation. The transplantation of bone marrow, including stem cells that give rise to all mature blood cells and lymphocytes; it is performed clinically to treat hematopoietic or lymphopoietic disorders and malignant diseases and is also used in various immunologic experiments in animals.

Bronchial asthma. An inflammatory disease usually caused by repeated immediate hypersensitivity reactions in the lung that leads to intermittent and reversible airway obstruction, chronic bronchial inflammation with eosinophils, and bronchial smooth muscle cell hypertrophy and hyperreactivity.

Burkitt's lymphoma. A malignant B cell tumor that is defined by histologic features but almost always carries a reciprocal chromosomal translocation involving Ig gene loci and the cellular *myc* gene on chromosome 8. Many cases of Burkitt's lymphoma are associated with Epstein-Barr virus infection.

C (constant region) gene segments. The DNA sequences in the Ig and TCR gene loci that encode the nonvariable portions of Ig heavy and light chains and TCR α, β, γ, and δ chains.

C1. A serum complement system protein composed of several polypeptide chains that initiates the classical pathway of complement activation by attaching to the Fc portions of IgG or IgM antibody that has bound antigen.

C1 inhibitor (C1 INH). A plasma protein inhibitor of the classical pathway of complement activation. C1 INH is a serine protease inhibitor (serpin) that mimics the normal substrates of the C1r and C1s components of C1. A genetic deficiency in C1 INH causes the disease hereditary angioneurotic edema.

C3. The central and most abundant complement system protein; it is involved in both the classical and alternative pathway cascades. C3 is proteolytically cleaved during complement activation to generate a C3b fragment, which covalently attaches to cell or microbial surfaces, and a C3a fragment, which has various proinflammatory activities.

C3 convertase. A multiprotein enzyme complex generated by the early steps of either the classical or alternative pathway of complement activation. C3 convertase cleaves C3, which gives rise to two proteolytic products called C3a and C3b.

C5 convertase. A multiprotein enzyme complex generated by C3b binding to C3 convertase. C5 convertase cleaves C5 and initiates the late steps of complement activation leading to formation of the membrane attack complex and lysis of cells.

Calcineurin. A cytoplasmic serine/threonine phosphatase that dephosphorylates and thereby activates the transcription factor NFAT. Calcineurin is activated by calcium signals generated through TCR signaling in response to antigen recognition, and the immunosuppressive drugs cyclosporine and FK-506 work by blocking calcineurin activity.

Carcinoembryonic antigen (CEA, CD66). A highly glycosylated membrane protein; increased expression of CEA in many carcinomas of the colon, pancreas, stomach, and breast results in a rise in serum levels. The level of serum CEA is used to monitor the persistence or recurrence of metastatic carcinoma after treatment. Because CEA expression is normally high in many tissues during fetal life but is suppressed in adults except in tumor cells, it is called an oncofetal tumor antigen.

Caspases. Intracellular proteases with cysteines in their active sites that cleave substrates at the C-terminal sides of aspartic acid residues and are components of enzymatic cascades that cause apoptotic death of cells. Lymphocyte caspases may be activated by two pathways; one is associated with mitochondrial permeability changes in growth factor–deprived cells, and the other is associated with signals from death receptors in the plasma membrane.

Cathelicidins. Polypeptides produced by neutrophils and various barrier epithelia that serve various functions in innate immunity including direct toxicity to microorganisms, activation of leukocytes, and neutralization of lipopolysaccharide.

Cathepsins. Thiol and aspartyl proteases with broad substrate specificities. The most abundant proteases of endosomes in APCs, cathepsins play an important role in generating peptide fragments from exogenous protein antigens that bind to class II MHC molecules.

CD molecules. Cell surface molecules expressed on various cell types in the immune system that are designated by the "cluster of differentiation" or CD number. See Appendix II for a list of CD molecules.

Cell-mediated immunity (CMI). The form of adaptive immunity that is mediated by T lymphocytes and serves as the defense mechanism against microbes that survive within phagocytes or infect nonphagocytic cells. CMI responses include $CD4^+$ T cell–mediated activation of macrophages that have phagocytosed microbes and $CD8^+$ CTL killing of infected cells.

Central tolerance. A form of self-tolerance induced in generative (central) lymphoid organs as a consequence of immature self-reactive lymphocytes recognizing self antigens and subsequently leading to their death or inactivation. Central tolerance prevents the emergence of lymphocytes with high-affinity receptors for the ubiquitous self antigens that are likely to be present in the bone marrow or thymus.

Chédiak-Higashi syndrome. A rare autosomal-recessive immunodeficiency disease caused by a defect in the cytoplasmic granules of various cell types that affects the lysosomes of neutrophils and macrophages as well as the granules of CTLs and NK cells. Patients show reduced resistance to infection with pyogenic bacteria.

Chemokine receptors. Cell surface receptors for chemokines that transduce signals stimulating the migration of leukocytes. These receptors are members of the seven-transmembrane α-helical, G protein-linked family of receptors.

Chemokines. A large family of structurally homologous, low molecular weight cytokines that stimulate leukocyte movement and regulate the migration of leukocytes from the blood to tissues.

Chemotaxis. Movement of a cell directed by a chemical concentration gradient. The movement of lymphocytes, polymorphonuclear leukocytes, monocytes, and other leukocytes into various tissues is often directed by gradients of low molecular weight cytokines called chemokines.

Chromosomal translocation. A chromosomal abnormality in which a segment of one chromosome is transferred to another. Many malignant diseases of lymphocytes are associated with chromosomal translocations involving an Ig or TCR locus and a chromosomal segment containing a cellular oncogene.

Chronic granulomatous disease. A rare inherited immunodeficiency disease caused by a defect in the gene encoding a component of the phagocyte oxidase enzyme that is needed for microbial killing by polymorphonuclear leukocytes and macrophages. The disease is characterized by recurrent intracellular bacterial and fungal infections, often accompanied by chronic cell-mediated immune responses and the formation of granulomas.

Chronic rejection. A form of allograft rejection characterized by fibrosis with loss of normal organ structures occurring during a prolonged period. In many cases, the major pathologic event in chronic rejection is graft arterial occlusion, which is caused by proliferation of intimal smooth muscle cells and is called graft arteriosclerosis.

c-Kit ligand (stem cell factor). A protein required for hematopoiesis, early steps in T cell development in the thymus, and mast cell development. c-Kit ligand is produced in membrane-bound and soluble forms by stromal cells in the bone marrow and thymus and binds to the c-Kit tyrosine kinase membrane receptor on pluripotent stem cells.

Class I major histocompatibility complex (MHC) molecule. One of two forms of polymorphic, heterodimeric membrane proteins that bind and display peptide fragments of protein antigens on the surface of APCs for recognition by T lymphocytes. Class I MHC molecules usually display peptides derived from the cytoplasm of the cell.

Class II–associated invariant chain peptide (CLIP). A peptide remnant of the invariant chain that sits in the class II MHC peptide-binding cleft and is removed by action of the HLA-DM molecule before the cleft becomes accessible to peptides produced from extracellular protein antigens.

Class II major histocompatibility complex (MHC) molecule. One of two major classes of polymorphic, heterodimeric membrane proteins that bind and display peptide fragments of protein antigens on the surface of APCs for recognition by T lymphocytes. Class II MHC molecules usually display peptides derived from extracellular proteins that are internalized into phagocytic or endocytic vesicles.

Class II vesicle (CIIV). A membrane-bound organelle identified in murine B cells that is important in the class II MHC pathway of antigen presentation. The CIIV is similar to the MHC class II compartment (MIIC) identified in other cells and contains all the components required for the formation of complexes of peptide antigens and class II MHC molecules, including the enzymes that degrade protein antigens, class II molecules, invariant chain, and HLA-DM.

Classical pathway of complement activation. The pathway of activation of the complement system that is initiated by binding of antigen-antibody complexes to the C1 molecule and induces a proteolytic cascade involving multiple other complement proteins. The classical pathway is an effector arm of the humoral immune system that generates inflammatory mediators, opsonins for phagocytosis of antigens, and lytic complexes that destroy cells.

Clonal anergy. A state of antigen unresponsiveness of a clone of T lymphocytes experimentally induced by recognition of antigen in the absence of additional signals (costimulatory signals) required for functional activation. Clonal anergy is considered a model for one mechanism of tolerance to self antigens and may be applicable to B lymphocytes as well.

Clonal deletion. A mechanism of lymphocyte tolerance in which an immature T cell in the thymus or an immature B cell in the bone marrow undergoes apoptotic death as a consequence of recognizing an abundant antigen in the generative organ.

Clonal expansion. The increase in number of lymphocytes specific for an antigen that results from antigen stimulation and proliferation of naive T cells. Clonal expansion occurs in lymphoid tissues and is required to generate enough antigen-specific effector lymphocytes from rare naive precursors to eradicate infections.

Clonal ignorance. A form of lymphocyte unresponsiveness in which self antigens are ignored by the immune system even though lymphocytes specific for those antigens remain viable and functional.

Clonal selection hypothesis. A fundamental tenet of the immune system (no longer a hypothesis) stating that every individual possesses numerous clonally derived lymphocytes, each clone having arisen from a single precursor and being capable of recognizing and responding to a distinct antigenic determinant. When an antigen enters, it selects a specific preexisting clone and activates it.

c-*myc*. A cellular proto-oncogene that encodes a nuclear factor involved in cell cycle regulation. Translocations of the c-*myc* gene into Ig gene loci are associated with B cell malignant neoplasms.

Collectins. A family of proteins, including mannose-binding lectin, that are characterized by a collagen-like domain and a lectin (i.e., carbohydrate-binding) domain. Collectins play a role in the innate immune system by acting as microbial pattern recognition receptors, and they may activate the complement system by binding to C1q.

Colony-stimulating factors (CSFs). Cytokines that promote the expansion and differentiation of bone marrow progenitor cells. CSFs are essential for the maturation of red blood cells, granulocytes, monocytes, and lymphocytes. Examples of CSFs are granulocyte-monocyte colony-stimulating factor (GM-CSF), c-Kit ligand, IL-3, and IL-7.

Combinatorial diversity. Combinatorial diversity describes the many different combinations of variable, diversity, and joining segments that are possible as a result of somatic recombination of DNA in the Ig and TCR loci during B cell or T cell development. Combinatorial diversity is one mechanism for the generation of large numbers of different antigen receptor genes from a limited number of DNA gene segments.

Complement. A system of serum and cell surface proteins that interact with one another and with other molecules of the immune system to generate important effectors of innate and adaptive immune responses. The classical and alternative pathways of the complement system are activated by antigen-antibody complexes or microbial surfaces, respectively, and consist of a cascade of proteolytic enzymes that generate inflammatory mediators and opsonins. Both pathways lead to the formation of a common terminal cell lytic complex that is inserted in cell membranes.

Complement receptor type 1 (CR1). A high-affinity receptor for the C3b and C4b fragments of complement. Phagocytes use CR1 to mediate internalization of C3b- or C4b-coated particles. CR1 on erythrocytes serves in the clearance of immune complexes from the circulation. CR1 is also a regulator of complement activation.

Complement receptor type 2 (CR2). A receptor expressed on B cells and follicular dendritic cells that binds proteolytic fragments of the C3 complement protein, including C3d, C3dg, and iC3b. CR2 functions to stimulate humoral immune responses by enhancing B cell activation by antigen and by promoting the trapping of antigen-antibody complexes in germinal centers. CR2 is also the receptor for Epstein-Barr virus.

Complementarity-determining region (CDR). Short segments of Ig and TCR proteins that contain most of the sequence differences among different antibodies or TCRs and that make contact with antigen. Three CDRs are present in the variable domain of each antigen receptor polypeptide chain and six CDRs in an intact Ig or TCR molecule. These hypervariable segments assume loop structures that together form a surface that is complementary to the three-dimensional structure of the bound antigen.

Congenic mouse strains. Inbred mouse strains that are identical to one another at every genetic locus except the one for which they are selected to differ; such strains are created by repetitive back-crossbreeding and selection for a particular trait. Congenic strains that differ from one another only at a particular MHC allele have been useful in defining the function of MHC molecules.

Constant (C) region. The portion of Ig or TCR polypeptide chains that does not vary in sequence among different clones and is not involved in antigen binding.

Contact sensitivity. The propensity for a T cell–mediated, delayed-type hypersensitivity reaction to develop in the skin on contact with a particular chemical agent. Chemicals that elicit contact hypersensitivity bind to and modify self proteins or molecules on the surfaces of APCs, which are then recognized by $CD4^+$ or $CD8^+$ T cells.

Coreceptor. A lymphocyte surface receptor that binds to an antigen complex at the same time that membrane Ig or TCR binds the antigen and delivers signals required for optimal lymphocyte activation. CD4 and CD8 are T cell coreceptors that bind nonpolymorphic parts of an MHC molecule concurrently with the TCR binding to polymorphic residues and the bound peptide. CR2 is a coreceptor on B cells that binds to complement-opsonized antigens at the same time that membrane Ig binds another part of the antigen.

Costimulator. A molecule on the surface of or secreted by an APC that provides a stimulus (or second signal) required for the activation of naive T cells, in addition to antigen. The best defined costimulators are the B7 molecules on professional APCs that bind to the CD28 molecule on T cells.

CpG nucleotides. Unmethylated cytidine-guanine sequences found in microbial DNA that stimulate innate immune responses. CpG nucleotides are recognized by TLR-9, have adjuvant properties in the mammalian immune system, and may be important to the efficacy of DNA vaccines.

C-reactive protein (CRP). A member of the pentraxin family of plasma proteins involved in innate immune responses to bacterial infections. CRP is an acute-phase reactant, and it binds to the capsule of pneumococcal bacteria. CRP also binds to C1q and may thereby activate complement or act as an opsonin by interacting with phagocyte C1q receptors.

Crossmatching. A screening test performed to minimize the chance of graft rejection in which a patient in need of an allograft is tested for the presence of preformed antibodies against donor cell surface antigens (usually MHC antigens). The test involves mixing the recipient serum with leukocytes from potential donors, adding complement, and observing whether cell lysis occurs.

Cross-priming. A mechanism by which a professional APC activates (or primes) a naive $CD8^+$ CTL specific for the antigens of a third cell (e.g., a virus-infected or tumor cell). Cross-priming occurs, for example, when an infected (often apoptotic) cell is ingested by a professional APC and the microbial antigens are processed and presented in association with class I MHC molecules, just like any other phagocytosed antigen. The professional APC also provides costimulation for the T cells. Also called **cross-presentation.**

Cutaneous immune system. The components of the innate and adaptive immune system found in the skin that function together in a specialized way to detect and respond to environmental antigens. Components of the cutaneous immune system include keratinocytes, Langerhans cells, intraepithelial lymphocytes, and dermal lymphocytes.

Cyclosporine. An immunosuppressive drug used to prevent allograft rejection that functions by blocking T cell cytokine gene transcription. Cyclosporine (also called cyclosporin A) binds to a cytosolic protein called cyclophilin, and cyclosporine-cyclophilin complexes bind to and inhibit calcineurin, thereby inhibiting activation and nuclear translocation of the transcription factor NFAT.

Cytokines. Proteins produced by many different cell types that mediate inflammatory and immune reactions. Cytokines are principal mediators of communication between cells of the immune system.

Cytopathic effect of viruses. Harmful effects of viruses on host cells that are caused by any of a variety of biochemical or molecular mechanisms and are independent of the host immune response to the virus. Some viruses have little cytopathic effect but still cause disease because the immune system recognizes and destroys the infected cells.

Cytotoxic (or cytolytic) T lymphocyte (CTL). A type of T lymphocyte whose major effector function is to recognize and kill host cells infected with viruses or other intracellular microbes. CTLs usually express CD8 and recognize microbial peptides displayed by class I MHC molecules. CTL killing of infected cells involves the release of cytoplasmic granules whose contents include membrane pore-forming proteins and enzymes that initiate apoptosis of the infected cell.

Defensins. Cysteine-rich peptides present in the skin and in neutrophil granules that act as broad-spectrum antibiotics to kill a wide variety of bacteria and fungi. The synthesis of defensins is increased in response to inflammatory cytokines such as IL-1 and TNF.

Delayed-type hypersensitivity (DTH). An immune reaction in which T cell–dependent macrophage activation and inflammation cause tissue injury. A DTH reaction to the subcutaneous injection of antigen is often used as an assay for cell-mediated immunity (e.g., the purified protein derivative skin test for immunity to *Mycobacterium tuberculosis*). DTH is a frequent accompaniment of protective cell-mediated immunity against microbes.

Delayed xenograft rejection. A frequent form of rejection of xenografts that occurs within 2 to 3 days of transplantation and is characterized by intravascular thrombosis and fibrinoid necrosis of vessel walls. Delayed xenograft rejection is likely to be caused by antibody- and cytokine-mediated endothelial activation and damage.

Dendritic cells. Bone marrow–derived immune accessory cells found in epithelial and lymphoid tissues that are morphologically characterized by thin membranous projections. Dendritic cells function as APCs for naive T lymphocytes and are important for initiation of adaptive immune responses to protein antigen.

Desensitization. A method of treating immediate hypersensitivity disease (allergies) that involves repetitive administration of low doses of an antigen to which individuals are allergic. This process often prevents severe allergic reactions on subsequent environmental exposure to the antigen, but the mechanisms are not well understood.

Determinant. The specific portion of a macromolecular antigen to which an antibody binds. In the case of a protein antigen recognized by a T cell, the determinant is the peptide portion that binds to an MHC molecule for recognition by the TCR. Synonymous with **epitope.**

Determinant selection model. A model to explain MHC-linked immune responses that was proposed before the demonstration of peptide-MHC molecule binding. The model states that the products of MHC genes in each individual select which determinants of protein antigens will be immunogenic in that individual.

Diacylglycerol (DAG). A membrane-bound signaling molecule generated by phospholipase C (PLCγ1)-mediated hydrolysis of the plasma membrane phospholipid phosphatidylinositol 4,5-bisphosphate (PIP_2) during antigen activation of lymphocytes. The main function of DAG is to activate an enzyme called protein kinase C that participates in the generation of active transcription factors.

DiGeorge's syndrome. A selective T cell deficiency caused by a congenital malformation that results in defective development of the thymus, parathyroid glands, and other structures that arise from the third and fourth pharyngeal pouches.

Direct antigen presentation (or direct allorecognition). Presentation of cell surface allogeneic MHC molecules by graft cells to a graft recipient's T cells that leads to T cell activation, with no requirement for processing. Direct recognition of foreign MHC molecules is a cross-reaction in which a normal TCR that recognizes a self MHC molecule plus foreign peptide cross-reacts with an allogeneic MHC molecule plus peptide. Direct presentation is partly responsible for strong T cell responses to allografts.

Diversity. The existence of a large number of lymphocytes with different antigenic specificities in any individual (i.e., the lymphocyte repertoire is large and diverse). Diversity is a fundamental property of the adaptive immune system and is the result of variability in the structures of the antigen-binding sites of lymphocyte receptors for antigens (antibodies and TCRs).

Diversity (D) segments. Short coding sequences between the variable (V) and constant (C) gene segments in the Ig heavy chain and TCR β and γ loci that together with J segments are somatically recombined with V segments during lymphocyte development. The resulting recombined VDJ DNA codes for the carboxy-terminal ends of the antigen receptor V regions, including the third hypervariable (CDR) regions. Random use of D segments contributes to the diversity of the antigen receptor repertoire.

DNA vaccine. A vaccine composed of a bacterial plasmid containing a complementary DNA encoding a protein antigen. DNA vaccines presumably work because professional APCs are transfected *in vivo* by the plasmid and express immunogenic peptides that elicit specific responses. Furthermore, the plasmid DNA contains CpG nucleotides that act as potent adjuvants. DNA vaccines may elicit strong CTL responses.

Double-negative thymocyte. A subset of developing T cells (thymocytes) in the thymus that express neither CD4 nor CD8. Most double-negative thymocytes are at an early developmental stage and do not express antigen receptors. They will later express both CD4 and CD8 during the intermediate double-positive stage before further maturation to single-positive T cells expressing only CD4 or CD8.

Double-positive thymocyte. A subset of developing T cells (thymocytes) in the thymus at an intermediate developmental stage that express both CD4 and CD8. Double-positive thymocytes also express TCRs and are subject to selection processes, the survivors of which mature to single-positive T cells expressing only CD4 or CD8.

Ectoparasites. Parasites that live on the surface of an animal, such as ticks and mites. Both the innate and adaptive immune systems may play a role in protection against ectoparasites, often by destroying the larval stages of these organisms.

Effector cells. The cells that perform effector functions during an immune response, such as secreting cytokines (e.g., helper T cells), killing microbes (e.g., macrophages), killing microbe-infected host cells (e.g., CTLs), or secreting antibodies (e.g., differentiated B cells).

Effector phase. The phase of an immune response, after the recognition and activation phases, in which a foreign antigen is actually destroyed or inactivated. For example, in a humoral immune response, the effector phase may be characterized by antibody-dependent complement activation and phagocytosis of antibody- and complement-opsonized bacteria.

Endosome. An intracellular membrane–bound vesicle into which extracellular proteins are internalized during antigen processing. Endosomes have an acidic pH and contain proteolytic enzymes that degrade proteins into peptides that bind to class II MHC molecules. A subset of class II MHC-rich endosomes, called MIIC, play a special role in antigen processing and presentation by the class II pathway.

Endotoxin. A component of the cell wall of gram-negative bacteria, also called **lipopolysaccharide** (LPS), that is released from dying bacteria and stimulates many innate immune responses, including the secretion of cytokines, induction of microbicidal activities of macrophages, and expression of leukocyte adhesion molecules on endothelium. Endotoxin contains both lipid components and carbohydrate (polysaccharide) moieties.

Enhancer. A regulatory nucleotide sequence in a gene that is located either upstream or downstream of the promoter, binds transcription factors, and increases the activity of the promoter. In cells of the immune system, enhancers are responsible for integrating cell surface signals that lead to induced transcription of genes encoding many of the effector proteins of an immune response, such as cytokines.

Envelope glycoprotein (Env). A membrane glycoprotein encoded by a retrovirus that is expressed on the plasma membrane of infected cells and on the host cell–derived membrane coat of viral particles. Env proteins are often required for viral infectivity. The Env proteins of HIV include gp41 and gp120, which bind to CD4 and chemokine receptors, respectively, on human T cells and mediate fusion of the viral and T cell membranes.

Enzyme-linked immunosorbent assay (ELISA). A method of quantifying an antigen immobilized on a solid surface by use of a specific antibody with a covalently coupled enzyme. The amount of antibody that binds the antigen is proportional to the amount of antigen present and is determined by spectrophotometrically measuring the conversion of a clear substrate to a colored product by the coupled enzyme.

Eosinophil. A bone marrow–derived granulocyte that is abundant in the inflammatory infiltrates of immediate hypersensitivity late-phase reactions and that contributes to many of the pathologic processes in allergic diseases. Eosinophils are important in defense against extracellular parasites, including helminths.

Epitope. The specific portion of a macromolecular antigen to which an antibody binds. In the case of a protein antigen recognized by a T cell, an epitope is the peptide portion that binds to an MHC molecule for recognition by the TCR. Synonymous with **determinant.**

Epstein-Barr virus (EBV). A double-stranded DNA virus of the herpesvirus family that is the etiologic agent of infectious mononucleosis and is associated with some B cell malignant tumors and nasopharyngeal carcinoma. EBV infects B lymphocytes and some epithelial cells by specifically binding to CR2 (CD21).

Experimental autoimmune encephalomyelitis. An animal model of autoimmune demyelinating disease of the central nervous system (e.g., multiple sclerosis) that is induced in rodents by immunization with components of the myelin sheath (e.g., myelin basic protein) of nerves, mixed with an adjuvant. The disease is mediated in large part by cytokine-secreting $CD4^+$ T cells specific for the myelin sheath proteins.

Extravasation. Escape of the fluid and cellular components of blood from a blood vessel into tissues.

Fab (fragment, antigen-binding). A proteolytic fragment of an IgG antibody molecule that includes one complete light chain paired with one heavy chain fragment containing the variable domain and only the first constant domain. Fab fragment retains the ability to monovalently bind an antigen but cannot interact with IgG Fc receptors on cells or with complement. Therefore, Fab preparations are used in research and therapeutic applications when antigen binding is desired without activation of effector functions. (The Fab′ fragment retains the hinge region of the heavy chain.)

$F(ab')_2$ fragment. A proteolytic fragment of an IgG molecule that includes two complete light chains but only the variable domain, first constant domain, and hinge region of the two heavy chains. $F(ab')_2$ fragments retain the entire bivalent antigen-binding region of an intact IgG molecule but cannot bind complement or IgG Fc receptors. They are used in research and therapeutic applications when antigen binding is desired without antibody effector functions.

Fas (CD95). A member of the TNF receptor family that is expressed on the surface of T cells and many other cell types and initiates a signaling cascade leading to apoptotic death of the cell. The death pathway is initiated when Fas binds to Fas ligand expressed on activated T cells. Fas-mediated killing of T cells, called activation-induced cell death, is important for the maintenance of self-tolerance. Mutations in the Fas gene cause systemic autoimmune disease.

Fas ligand (CD95 ligand). A membrane protein that is a member of the TNF family of proteins expressed on activated T cells. Fas ligand binds to Fas, thereby stimulating a signaling pathway leading to apoptotic cell death of the Fas-expressing cell. Mutations in the Fas ligand gene cause systemic autoimmune disease in mice.

Fc (fragment, crystalline). A proteolytic fragment of IgG that contains only the disulfide-linked carboxy-terminal regions of the two heavy chains. Fc is also used to describe the corresponding region of an intact Ig molecule that mediates effector functions by binding to cell surface receptors or the C1q complement protein. (Fc fragments are so named because they tend to crystallize out of solution.)

Fc receptor. A cell surface receptor specific for the carboxy-terminal constant region of an Ig molecule. Fc receptors are typically multichain protein complexes that include signaling components and Ig-binding components. Several types of Fc receptors exist, including those specific for different IgG isotypes, IgE, and IgA. Fc receptors mediate many of the cell-dependent effector functions of antibodies, including phagocytosis of antibody-bound antigens, antigen-induced activation of mast cells, and targeting and activation of NK cells.

FcεRI. A high-affinity receptor for the carboxy-terminal constant region of IgE molecules that is expressed on mast cells and basophils. FcεRI molecules on mast cells are usually occupied by IgE, and antigen-induced cross-linking of these IgE-FcεRI complexes activates the mast cell and initiates immediate hypersensitivity reactions.

Fcγ receptor (FcγR). A specific cell surface receptor for the carboxy-terminal constant region of IgG molecules. There are several different types of Fcγ receptors, including a high-affinity FcγRI that mediates phagocytosis by macrophages and neutrophils, a low-affinity FcγRIIB that transduces inhibitory signals in B cells, and a low-affinity FcγRIIIA that mediates targeting and activation of NK cells.

First-set rejection. Allograft rejection in an individual who has not previously received a graft or otherwise been exposed to tissue alloantigens from the same donor. First-set rejection usually takes about 7 to 10 days.

FK-506. An immunosuppressive drug used to prevent allograft rejection that functions by blocking T cell cytokine gene transcription, similar to cyclosporine. FK-506 binds to a cytosolic protein called FK-506-binding protein, and the resulting complex binds to calcineurin, thereby inhibiting activation and nuclear translocation of the transcription factor NFAT.

Flow cytometry. A method of analysis of the phenotype of cell populations requiring a specialized instrument (flow cytometer) that can detect fluorescence on individual cells in a suspension and thereby determine the number of cells expressing the molecule to which a fluorescent probe binds. Suspensions of cells are incubated with fluorescently labeled antibodies or other probes, and the amount of probe bound by each cell in the population is measured by passing the cells one at a time through a fluorimeter with a laser-generated incident beam.

Fluorescence-activated cell sorter (FACS). An adaptation of the flow cytometer that is used for the purification of cells from a mixed population according to which and how much fluorescent probe the cells bind. Cells are first stained with fluorescently labeled probe, such as an antibody specific for a surface antigen of a cell population. The cells are then passed one at a time through a fluorimeter with a laser-generated incident beam and are differentially deflected by electromagnetic fields whose strength and direction are varied according to the measured intensity of the fluorescence signal.

Follicle. See **Lymphoid follicle.**

Follicular dendritic cells. Cells found in lymphoid follicles that express complement receptors, Fc receptors, and CD40 ligand and have long cytoplasmic processes that form a meshwork integral to the architecture of a lymphoid follicle. Follicular dendritic cells display antigens on their surface for B cell recognition and are involved in the activation and selection of B cells expressing high-affinity membrane Ig during the process of affinity maturation.

***N*-Formylmethionine.** An amino acid that initiates all bacterial proteins and no mammalian proteins (except those synthesized within mitochondria) and serves as a signal to the innate immune system of infection. Specific receptors for *N*-formylmethionine-containing peptides are expressed on neutrophils and mediate activation of the neutrophils.

FoxP3. A forkhead family transcription factor expressed by, and required for the development of, $CD4^+$ regulatory T cells. Mutations in FoxP3 in mice and humans result in an absence of $CD25^+$ regulatory T cells and multisystem autoimmune disease.

γδ T cell receptor (γδ TCR). A form of TCR that is distinct from the more common αβ TCR and is expressed on a subset of T cells found mostly in epithelial barrier tissues. Although structurally similar to the αβ TCR, the forms of antigen recognized by γδ TCRs are poorly understood; they do not recognize peptide complexes bound to polymorphic MHC molecules.

G protein–coupled receptor family. A diverse family of receptors for hormones, lipid inflammatory mediators, and chemokines that use associated trimeric G proteins for intracellular signaling.

G proteins. Proteins that bind guanyl nucleotides and act as exchange molecules by catalyzing the replacement of bound guanosine diphosphate (GDP) by guanosine triphosphate (GTP). G proteins with bound GTP can activate a variety of cellular enzymes in different signaling cascades. Trimeric GTP-binding proteins are associated with the cytoplasmic portions of many cell surface receptors, such as chemokine receptors. Other small soluble G proteins, such as Ras and Rac, are recruited into signaling pathways by adapter proteins.

GATA3. A transcription factor that promotes the differentiation of T_H2 cells from naive T cells.

Generative lymphoid organ. An organ in which lymphocytes develop from immature precursors. The bone marrow and thymus are the major generative lymphoid organs in which B cells and T cells develop, respectively.

Germinal center. A lightly staining region within a lymphoid follicle in spleen, lymph node, or mucosal lymphoid tissue that forms during T cell–dependent humoral immune responses and is the site of B cell affinity maturation.

Germline organization. The inherited arrangement of variable, diversity, joining, and constant region gene segments of the antigen receptor loci in nonlymphoid cells or in immature lymphocytes. In developing B or T lymphocytes, the germline organization is modified by somatic recombination to form functional Ig or TCR genes.

Glomerulonephritis. Inflammation of the renal glomeruli, often initiated by immunopathologic mechanisms such as deposition of circulating antigen-antibody complexes in the glomerular basement membrane or binding of antibodies to antigens expressed in the glomerulus. The antibodies can activate complement and phagocytes, and the resulting inflammatory response can lead to renal failure.

Graft. A tissue or organ that is removed from one site and placed in another site, usually in a different individual.

Graft arteriosclerosis. Occlusion of graft arteries caused by proliferation of intimal smooth muscle cells. This process is evident within 6 months to a year after transplantation and is responsible for chronic rejection of vascularized organ grafts. The mechanism is likely to be a result of a chronic immune response to vessel wall alloantigens. Graft arteriosclerosis is also called accelerated arteriosclerosis.

Graft rejection. A specific immune response to an organ or tissue graft that leads to inflammation, damage, and possibly graft failure.

Graft-versus-host disease. A disease occurring in bone marrow transplant recipients that is caused by the reaction of mature T cells in the marrow graft with alloantigens on host cells. The disease most often affects the skin, liver, and intestines.

Granulocyte colony-stimulating factor (G-CSF). A cytokine made by activated T cells, macrophages, and endothelial cells at sites of infection that acts on bone marrow to increase the production of and mobilize neutrophils to replace those consumed in inflammatory reactions.

Granulocyte-monocyte colony-stimulating factor (GM-CSF). A cytokine made by activated T cells, macrophages, endothelial cells, and stromal fibroblasts that acts on bone marrow to increase the production of neutrophils and monocytes. GM-CSF is also a macrophage-activating factor and promotes the differentiation of Langerhans cells into mature dendritic cells.

Granuloma. A nodule of inflammatory tissue composed of clusters of activated macrophages and T lymphocytes, often with associated necrosis and fibrosis. Granulomatous inflammation is a form of chronic delayed-type hypersensitivity, often in response to persistent microbes, such as *Mycobacterium tuberculosis* and some fungi, or in response to particulate antigens that are not readily phagocytosed.

Granzyme. A serine protease enzyme found in the granules of CTLs and NK cells that is released by exocytosis, enters target cells, and proteolytically cleaves and activates caspases, which in turn cleave several substrates and induce target cell apoptosis.

H-2 molecule. An MHC molecule in the mouse. The mouse MHC was originally called the H-2 locus.

Haplotype. The set of MHC alleles inherited from one parent and therefore on one chromosome.

Hapten. A small chemical that can bind to an antibody but must be attached to a macromolecule (carrier) to stimulate an adaptive immune response specific for that chemical. For example, immunization with dinitrophenol (DNP) alone will not stimulate an anti-DNP antibody response, but immunization with a protein with covalently bonded DNP hapten will.

Heavy chain class (isotype) switching. The process by which a B lymphocyte changes the class, or isotype, of the antibodies that it produces, from IgM to IgG, IgE, or IgA, without changing the antigen specificity of the antibody. Heavy chain class switching is regulated by helper T cell cytokines and CD40 ligand and involves recombination of B cell VDJ segments with downstream heavy chain gene segments.

Helminth. A parasitic worm. Helminthic infections often elicit T_H2-regulated immune responses characterized by eosinophil-rich inflammatory infiltrates and IgE production.

Helper T cells. The functional subset of T lymphocytes whose main effector functions are to activate macrophages in cell-mediated immune responses and to promote B cell antibody production in humoral immune responses. These effector functions are mediated by secreted cytokines and by T cell CD40 ligand binding to macrophage or B cell CD40. Most helper T cells express the CD4 molecule.

Hematopoiesis. The development of mature blood cells, including erythrocytes, leukocytes, and platelets, from pluripotent stem cells in the bone marrow and fetal liver. Hematopoiesis is regulated by several different cytokine growth factors produced by bone marrow stromal cells, T cells, and other cell types.

Hematopoietic stem cell. An undifferentiated bone marrow cell that divides continuously and gives rise to additional stem cells and cells of multiple different lineages. A hematopoietic stem cell in the bone marrow will give rise to cells of the lymphoid, myeloid, and erythrocytic lineage.

High endothelial venules (HEVs). Specialized venules that are the sites of lymphocyte extravasation from the blood into the stroma of a peripheral lymph node or mucosal lymphoid tissue. HEVs are lined by plump endothelial cells that protrude into the vessel lumen and express unique adhesion molecules involved in binding naive T cells.

Highly active antiretroviral therapy (HAART). Combination chemotherapy for HIV infection consisting of reverse transcriptase inhibitors and a viral protease inhibitor. HAART can reduce plasma virus titers to below detectable levels for more than 1 year and slow the progression of HIV disease.

Hinge region. A region of Ig heavy chains between the first two constant domains that can assume multiple conformations, thereby imparting flexibility in the orientation of the two antigen-binding sites. Because of the hinge region, an antibody molecule can simultaneously bind two epitopes that are anywhere within a range of distances from one another.

Histamine. A biogenic amine stored in the granules of mast cells that is one of the important mediators of immediate hypersensitivity. Histamine binds to specific receptors in various tissues and causes increased vascular permeability and contraction of bronchial and intestinal smooth muscle.

HLA. See **Human leukocyte antigens.**

HLA-DM. A peptide exchange molecule that plays a critical role in the class II MHC pathway of antigen presentation. HLA-DM is found in the specialized MIIC endosomal compartment and facilitates removal of the invariant chain-derived CLIP peptide and the binding of other peptides to class II MHC molecules. HLA-DM is encoded by a gene in the MHC and is structurally similar to class II MHC molecules, but it is not polymorphic.

Homeostasis. In the adaptive immune system, the maintenance of a constant number and diverse repertoire of lymphocytes, despite the emergence of new lymphocytes and tremendous expansion of individual clones that may occur during responses to immunogenic antigens. Homeostasis is achieved by several regulated pathways of lymphocyte death and inactivation.

Homing receptor. Adhesion molecules expressed on the surface of lymphocytes that are responsible for the different pathways of lymphocyte recirculation and tissue homing. Homing receptors bind to ligands (addressins) expressed on endothelial cells in particular vascular beds.

Human immunodeficiency virus (HIV). The etiologic agent of AIDS. HIV is a retrovirus that infects a variety of cell types, including CD4-expressing helper T cells, macrophages, and dendritic cells, and causes chronic progressive destruction of the immune system.

Human leukocyte antigens (HLAs). MHC molecules expressed on the surface of human cells. Human MHC molecules were first identified as alloantigens on the surface of white blood cells (leukocytes) that bound serum antibodies from individuals previously exposed to other individuals' cells (e.g., mothers or transfusion recipients).

Humanized antibody. A monoclonal antibody encoded by a recombinant hybrid gene and composed of the antigen-binding sites from a murine monoclonal antibody and the constant region of a human antibody. Humanized antibodies are less likely than mouse monoclonal antibodies to induce an anti-antibody response in humans; they are used clinically in the treatment of tumors and transplant rejection.

Humoral immunity. The type of adaptive immune response mediated by antibodies produced by B lymphocytes. Humoral immunity is the principal defense mechanism against extracellular microbes and their toxins.

Hybridoma. A cell line derived by cell fusion, or somatic cell hybridization, between a normal lymphocyte and an immortalized lymphocyte tumor line. B cell hybridomas created by fusion of normal B cells of defined antigen specificity with a myeloma cell line are used to produce monoclonal antibodies. T cell hybridomas created by fusion of a normal T cell of defined specificity with a T cell tumor line are commonly used in research.

Hyperacute rejection. A form of allograft or xenograft rejection that begins within minutes to hours after transplantation and that is characterized by thrombotic occlusion of the graft vessels. Hyperacute rejection is mediated by preexisting antibodies in the host circulation that bind to donor endothelial antigens, such as blood group antigens or MHC molecules, and activate the complement system.

Hypersensitivity diseases. Disorders caused by immune responses. Hypersensitivity diseases include autoimmune diseases, in which immune responses are directed against self antigens, and diseases that result from uncontrolled or excessive responses against foreign antigens, such as microbes and allergens. The tissue damage that occurs in hypersensitivity diseases is due to the same effector mechanisms used by the immune system to protect against microbes.

Hypervariable loop (hypervariable region). Short segments of about 10 amino acid residues within the variable regions of antibody or TCR proteins that form loop structures that contact antigen. Three hypervariable loops, also called CDRs, are present in each antibody heavy chain and light chain and in each TCR chain. Most of the variability between different antibodies or TCRs is located within these loops.

Idiotype. The property of a group of antibodies or TCRs defined by their sharing a particular idiotope; that is, antibodies that share a particular idiotope belong to the same idiotype. *Idiotype* is also used to describe the collection of idiotopes expressed by an Ig molecule, and it is often used synonymously with *idiotope.*

Idiotypic network. A network of complementary interactions involving idiotypes and anti-idiotypic antibodies (or T cells) that, according to the network hypothesis, reach a steady state at which the immune system is at homeostasis. Theoretically, when one or a few clones of lymphocytes respond to a foreign antigen, their idiotypes are expanded and anti-idiotype responses are triggered that function to shut off the antigen-specific response.

Igα and Igβ. Proteins that are required for surface expression and signaling functions of membrane Ig on B cells. Igα and Igβ pairs are disulfide linked to one another, noncovalently associated with the cytoplasmic tail of membrane Ig, and form the BCR complex. The cytoplasmic domains of Igα and Igβ contain ITAMs that are involved in early signaling events during antigen-induced B cell activation.

IL-1 receptor antagonist (IL-1ra). A natural inhibitor of IL-1 produced by mononuclear phagocytes that is structurally homologous to IL-1 and binds to the same receptors but is biologically inactive. Attempts to use IL-1 inhibitors to reduce inflammation in diseases such as rheumatoid arthritis are ongoing.

Immature B lymphocyte. A membrane IgM^+, IgD^- B cell, recently derived from marrow precursors, that does not proliferate or differentiate in response to antigens but rather may undergo apoptotic death or become functionally unresponsive. This property is important for the negative selection of B cells that are specific for self antigens present in the bone marrow.

Immediate hypersensitivity. The type of immune reaction responsible for allergic diseases and dependent on IgE plus antigen-mediated stimulation of tissue mast cells and basophils. The mast cells and basophils release mediators that cause increased vascular permeability, vasodilation, bronchial and visceral smooth muscle contraction, and local inflammation.

Immune complex. A multimolecular complex of antibody molecules with bound antigen. Because each antibody molecule has a minimum of two antigen-binding sites and many antigens are mutivalent, immune complexes can vary greatly in size. Immune complexes activate effector mechanisms of humoral immunity, such as the classical complement pathway and Fc receptor–mediated phagocyte activation. Deposition of circulating immune complexes in blood vessel walls or renal glomeruli can lead to inflammation and disease.

Immune complex disease. An inflammatory disease caused by the deposition of antigen-antibody complexes in blood vessel walls resulting in local complement activation and phagocyte recruitment. Immune complexes may form because of overproduction of antibodies to microbial antigens or as a result of autoantibody production in the setting of an autoimmune disease such as systemic lupus erythematosus. Immune complex deposition in the specialized capillary basement membranes of renal glomeruli can cause glomerulonephritis and impair renal function. Systemic deposition of immune complexes in arterial walls can cause thrombosis and ischemic damage to various organs.

Immune deviation. The conversion of a T cell response associated with one set of cytokines, such as T_H1 cytokines that stimulate cell-mediated immunity, to a response associated with other cytokines, such as T_H2 cytokines that stimulate the production of selected antibody isotypes.

Immune inflammation. Inflammation that is a result of an adaptive immune response to antigen. The cellular infiltrate at the inflammatory site may include cells of the innate immune system such as neutrophils and macrophages, which are recruited as a result of the actions of T cell cytokines.

Immune response. A collective and coordinated response to the introduction of foreign substances in an individual mediated by the cells and molecules of the immune system.

Immune response (Ir) genes. Originally defined as genes in inbred strains of rodents that were inherited in a dominant mendelian manner and that controlled the ability of the animals to make antibodies against simple synthetic polypeptides. We now know that Ir genes are polymorphic MHC genes that encode peptide-binding molecules required for the activation of T lymphocytes and are therefore also required for helper T cell–dependent B cell (antibody) responses to protein antigens.

Immune surveillance. The concept that a physiologic function of the immune system is to recognize and destroy clones of transformed cells before they grow into tumors and to kill tumors after they are formed. The term *immune surveillance* is sometimes used in a general sense to describe the function of T lymphocytes to detect and destroy any cell, not necessarily a tumor cell, that is expressing foreign (e.g., microbial) antigens.

Immune system. The molecules, cells, tissues, and organs that collectively function to provide immunity, or protection, against foreign organisms.

Immunity. Protection against disease, usually infectious disease, mediated by a collection of molecules, cells, and tissues collectively called the immune system. In a broader sense, immunity refers to the ability to respond to foreign substances, including microbes or molecules.

Immunoblot. An analytical technique in which antibodies are used to detect the presence of an antigen bound to (i.e., blotted on) a solid matrix such as filter paper (also known as a Western blot).

Immunodominant epitope. A linear amino acid sequence of a multideterminant protein antigen for which most of the responding T cells in any individual are specific. Immunodominant epitopes correspond to the peptides proteolytically generated within APCs that bind most avidly to MHC molecules and are most likely to stimulate T cells.

Immunofluorescence. A technique in which a molecule is detected by use of an antibody labeled with a fluorescent probe. For example, in immunofluorescence microscopy, cells that express a particular surface antigen can be stained with a fluorescein-conjugated antibody specific for the antigen and then visualized with a fluorescent microscope.

Immunogen. An antigen that induces an immune response. Not all antigens are immunogens. For example, small molecular weight compounds may not stimulate an immune response unless they are linked to macromolecules.

Immunoglobulin (Ig). Synonymous with antibody (see **Antibody**).

Immunoglobulin domain. A three-dimensional globular structural motif found in many proteins in the immune system, including Igs, TCRs, and MHC molecules. Ig domains are about 110 amino acid residues in length, include an internal disulfide bond, and contain two layers of β-pleated sheets, each layer composed of three to five strands of antiparallel polypeptide chain. Ig domains are classified as V-like or C-like on the basis of closest homology to either the Ig V or C domains.

Immunoglobulin heavy chain. One of two types of polypeptide chains in an antibody molecule. The basic structural unit of an antibody includes two identical, disulfide-linked heavy chains and two identical light chains. Each heavy chain is composed of a variable (V) Ig domain and three or four constant (C) Ig domains. The different antibody isotypes, including IgM, IgD, IgG, IgA, and IgE, are distinguished by structural differences in their heavy chain constant regions. The heavy chain constant regions also mediate effector functions, such as complement activation or engagement of phagocytes.

Immunoglobulin light chain. One of two types of polypeptide chains in an antibody molecule. The basic structural unit of an antibody includes two identical light chains, each disulfide linked to one of two identical heavy chains. Each light chain is composed of one variable (V) Ig domain and one constant (C) Ig domain. There are two light chain isotypes, called κ and λ, both functionally identical. About 60% of human antibodies have κ light chains and 40% have λ light chains.

Immunoglobulin superfamily. A large family of proteins that contain a globular structural motif called an Ig domain, or Ig fold, originally described in antibodies. Many proteins of importance in the immune system, including antibodies, TCRs, MHC molecules, CD4, and CD8, are members of this superfamily.

Immunohistochemistry. A technique to detect the presence of an antigen in histologic tissue sections by use of an enzyme-coupled antibody that is specific for the antigen. The enzyme converts a colorless substrate to a colored insoluble substance that precipitates at the site where the antibody and thus the antigen are localized. The position of the colored precipitate, and therefore the antigen, in the tissue section is observed by conventional light microscopy. Immunohistochemistry is a routine technique in diagnostic pathology and various fields of research.

Immunological tolerance. See **Tolerance.**

Immunologically privileged site. A site in the body that is inaccessible to or constitutively suppresses immune responses. The anterior chamber of the eye, the testes, and the brain are examples of immunologically privileged sites.

Immunoperoxidase technique. A common immunohistochemical technique in which a horseradish peroxidase–coupled antibody is used to identify the presence of an antigen in a tissue section. The peroxidase enzyme converts a colorless substrate to an insoluble brown product that is observable by light microscopy.

Immunoprecipitation. A technique for the isolation of a molecule from a solution by binding it to an antibody and then rendering the antigen-antibody complex insoluble, either by precipitation with a second anti-antibody or by coupling the first antibody to an insoluble particle or bead.

Immunoreceptor tyrosine-based activation motif (ITAM). A conserved motif composed of two copies of the sequence tyrosine-X-X-leucine (where X is an unspecified amino acid) found in the cytoplasmic tails of various membrane proteins in the immune system that are involved in signal transduction. ITAMs are present in the ζ and CD3 proteins of the TCR complex, in Igα and Igβ proteins in the BCR complex, and in several Ig Fc receptors. When these receptors bind their ligands, the tyrosine residues of the ITAMs become phosphorylated and form docking sites for other molecules involved in propagating cell-activating signal transduction pathways.

Immunoreceptor tyrosine-based inhibition motif (ITIM). A six–amino acid (isoleucine-X-tyrosine-X-X-leucine) motif found in the cytoplasmic tails of various inhibitory receptors in the immune system, including FcγRIIB on B cells and killer cell Ig-like receptors (KIR) on NK cells. When these receptors bind their ligands, the ITIMs become phosphorylated on their tyrosine residue and form a docking site for protein tyrosine phosphatases, which in turn function to inhibit other signal transduction pathways.

Immunosuppression. Inhibition of one or more components of the adaptive or innate immune system as a result of an underlying disease or intentionally induced by drugs for the purpose of preventing or treating graft rejection or autoimmune disease. A commonly used immunosuppressive drug is cyclosporine, which blocks T cell cytokine production.

Immunotherapy. The treatment of a disease with therapeutic agents that promote or inhibit immune responses. Cancer immunotherapy, for example, involves promoting active immune responses to tumor antigens or administering anti-tumor antibodies or T cells to establish passive immunity.

Immunotoxins. Reagents that may be used in the treatment of cancer and consist of covalent conjugates of a potent cellular toxin, such as ricin or diphtheria toxin, with antibodies specific for antigens expressed on the surface of tumor cells. It is hoped that such reagents can specifically target and kill tumor cells without damaging normal cells, but safe and effective immunotoxins have yet to be developed.

Inbred mouse strain. A strain of mice created by repetitive mating of siblings that is characterized by homozygosity at every genetic locus. Every mouse of an inbred strain is genetically identical (syngeneic) to every other mouse of the same strain.

Indirect antigen presentation (or indirect allorecognition). In transplantation immunology, a pathway of presentation of donor (allogeneic) MHC molecules by recipient APCs that involves the same mechanisms used to present microbial proteins. The allogeneic MHC proteins are processed by recipient professional APCs, and peptides derived from the allogeneic MHC molecules are presented, in association with recipient (self) MHC molecules, to host T cells. In contrast to indirect antigen presentation, direct antigen presentation involves recipient T cell recognition of unprocessed allogeneic MHC molecules on the surface of graft cells.

Inflammation. A complex reaction of vascularized tissue to infection, toxin exposure, or cell injury, which involves extravascular accumulation of plasma proteins and leukocytes. Acute inflammation is a common result of innate immune responses, and local adaptive immune responses can also promote inflammation. Although inflammation serves a protective function in controlling infections and promoting tissue repair, it can also cause tissue damage and disease.

Inflammatory bowel disease (IBD). A group of disorders, including ulcerative colitis and Crohn's disease, characterized by chronic inflammation in the gastrointestinal tract. The etiology of IBD is not known, but some evidence indicates that immune mechanisms may be involved. IBD develops in gene knockout mice lacking IL-2, IL-10, or the TCR α chain.

Innate immunity. Protection against infection that relies on mechanisms that exist before infection, are capable of a rapid response to microbes, and react in essentially the same way to repeated infections. The innate immune system includes epithelial barriers, phagocytic cells (neutrophils, macrophages), NK cells, the complement system, and cytokines, largely made by mononuclear phagocytes, that regulate and coordinate many of the activities of the cells of innate immunity.

Inositol 1,4,5-triphosphate (IP_3). A cytoplasmic signaling molecule generated by phospholipase C (PLCγ1)-mediated hydrolysis of the plasma membrane phospholipid PIP_2 during antigen activation of lymphocytes. The main function of IP_3 is to stimulate the release of intracellular stores of calcium from membrane-bound compartments such as the endoplasmic reticulum.

Insulin-dependent diabetes mellitus. A disease characterized by a lack of insulin that leads to various metabolic and vascular abnormalities. The insulin deficiency results from autoimmune destruction of the insulin-producing β cells of the islets of Langerhans in the pancreas, usually during childhood. $CD4^+$ and $CD8^+$ T cells, antibodies, and cytokines have been implicated in the islet cell damage. Also called type 1 diabetes mellitus.

Integrins. Heterodimeric cell surface proteins whose major functions are to mediate the adhesion of leukocytes to other leukocytes, endothelial cells, and extracellular matrix proteins. Integrins are important for T cell interactions with APCs and for migration of leukocytes from blood into tissues. The ligand-binding affinity of the integrins can be regulated by various stimuli, and the cytoplasmic domains of integrins bind to the cytoskeleton. There are two main subfamilies of integrins; the members of each family express a conserved β chain ($β_1$, or CD29, and $β_2$, or CD18) associated with different α chains. VLA-4 (very late activation protein-4) is a $β_1$ integrin expressed on T cells, and LFA-1 (leukocyte function-associated antigen-1) is a $β_2$ integrin expressed on T cells and phagocytes.

Interferon-γ (IFN-γ). A cytokine produced by T lymphocytes and NK cells whose principal function is to activate macrophages in both innate immune responses and adaptive cell-mediated immune responses. (IFN-γ is also called immune or type II interferon.)

Interleukin (IL). Another name for a cytokine originally used to describe a cytokine made by leukocytes that acts on leukocytes. The term is now generally used with a numerical suffix to designate a structurally defined cytokine regardless of its source or target.

Interleukin-1 (IL-1). A cytokine produced mainly by activated mononuclear phagocytes whose principal function is to mediate host inflammatory responses in innate immunity. The two forms of IL-1 (α and β) bind to the same receptors and have identical biologic effects, including induction of endothelial cell adhesion molecules, stimulation of chemokine production by endothelial cells and macrophages, stimulation of the synthesis of acute-phase reactants by the liver, and fever.

Interleukin-2 (IL-2). A cytokine produced by antigen-activated T cells that acts in an autocrine manner to stimulate T cell proliferation and also potentiates the apoptotic cell death of antigen-activated T cells. Thus, IL-2 is required for both the induction and self-regulation of T cell–mediated immune responses. IL-2 also stimulates the proliferation and effector functions of NK cells and B cells.

Interleukin-3 (IL-3). A cytokine produced by $CD4^+$ T cells that promotes the expansion of immature marrow progenitors of all known mature blood cell types. IL-3 is also known as multilineage colony-stimulating factor.

Interleukin-4 (IL-4). A cytokine produced mainly by the T_H2 subset of $CD4^+$ helper T cells whose functions include induction of differentiation of T_H2 cells from naive $CD4^+$ precursors, stimulation of IgE production by B cells, and suppression of IFN-γ-dependent macrophage functions.

Interleukin-5 (IL-5). A cytokine produced by $CD4^+$ T_H2 cells and activated mast cells that stimulates the growth and differentiation of eosinophils and activates mature eosinophils.

Interleukin-6 (IL-6). A cytokine produced by many cell types, including activated mononuclear phagocytes, endothelial cells, and fibroblasts, that functions in both innate and adaptive immunity. IL-6 stimulates the synthesis of acute-phase proteins by hepatocytes as well as the growth of antibody-producing B lymphocytes.

Interleukin-7 (IL-7). A cytokine secreted by bone marrow stromal cells that stimulates survival and expansion of immature, but lineage-committed, precursors of B and T lymphocytes.

Interleukin-10 (IL-10). A cytokine produced by activated macrophages and some helper T cells whose major function is to inhibit activated macrophages and therefore to maintain homeostatic control of innate and cell-mediated immune reactions.

Interleukin-12 (IL-12). A cytokine produced by mononuclear phagocytes and dendritic cells that serves as a mediator of the innate immune response to intracellular microbes and is a key inducer of cell-mediated immune responses to these microbes. IL-12 activates NK cells, promotes IFN-γ production by NK cells and T cells, enhances the cytolytic activity of NK cells and CTLs, and promotes the development of T_H1 cells.

Interleukin-15 (IL-15). A cytokine produced by mononuclear phagocytes and other cells in response to viral infections whose principal function is to stimulate the proliferation of NK cells. It is structurally similar to IL-2.

Interleukin-17 (IL-17). A family of structurally related pro-inflammatory cytokines, some of which cause tissue damage in autoimmune disease, and others which protect against bacterial infections. IL-17–producing $CD4^+$ effector T cells are a distinct lineage from T_H1 or T_H2 cells, called T_H17.

Interleukin-18 (IL-18). A cytokine produced by macrophages in response to LPS and other microbial products that functions together with IL-12 as an inducer of cell-mediated immunity. IL-18 synergizes with IL-12 in stimulating the production of IFN-γ by NK cells and T cells. IL-18 is structurally homologous to but functionally different from IL-1.

Intracellular bacterium. A bacterium that survives or replicates within cells, usually in endosomes. The principal defense against intracellular bacteria, such as *Mycobacterium tuberculosis,* is cell-mediated immunity.

Intraepidermal lymphocytes. T lymphocytes found within the epidermal layer of the skin. In the mouse, most of the intraepidermal T cells express the $\gamma\delta$ form of TCR (see **Intraepithelial T lymphocytes**).

Intraepithelial T lymphocytes. T lymphocytes present in the epidermis of the skin and in mucosal epithelia that typically express a limited diversity of antigen receptors. Some of these lymphocytes may recognize microbial products, such as glycolipids, associated with nonpolymorphic class I MHC-like molecules. Intraepithelial T lymphocytes may be considered effector cells of innate immunity and function in host defense by secreting cytokines and activating phagocytes and by killing infected cells.

Invariant chain (I_i). A nonpolymorphic protein that binds to newly synthesized class II MHC molecules in the endoplasmic reticulum. The invariant chain prevents loading of the class II MHC peptide-binding cleft with peptides present in the endoplasmic reticulum, and such peptides are left to associate with class I molecules. The invariant chain also promotes folding and assembly of class II molecules and directs newly formed class II molecules to the specialized endosomal MIIC compartment, where peptide loading takes place.

Isotype. One of five types of antibodies, determined by which of five different forms of heavy chain are present. Antibody isotypes include IgM, IgD, IgG, IgA, and IgE, and each isotype performs a different set of effector functions. Additional structural variations characterize distinct subtypes of IgG and IgA.

J chain. A small polypeptide that is disulfide bonded to the tail pieces of multimeric IgM and IgA antibodies.

JAK/STAT signaling pathway. A signaling pathway initiated by cytokine binding to type I and type II cytokine receptors. This pathway sequentially involves activation of receptor-associated Janus kinase (JAK) tyrosine kinases, JAK-mediated tyrosine phosphorylation of the cytoplasmic tails of cytokine receptors, docking of signal transducers and activators of transcription (STATs) to the phosphorylated receptor chains, JAK-mediated tyrosine phosphorylation of the associated STATs, dimerization and nuclear translocation of the STATs, and STAT binding to regulatory regions of target genes causing transcriptional activation of those genes.

Janus kinases (JAK kinases). A family of tyrosine kinases that associate with the cytoplasmic tails of several different cytokine receptors, including the receptors for IL-2, IL-4, IFN-γ, IL-12, and others. In response to cytokine binding and receptor dimerization, JAKs phosphorylate the cytokine receptors to permit the binding of STATs, and then the JAKs phosphorylate and thereby activate the STATs. Different JAK kinases associate with different cytokine receptors.

Joining (J) segments. Short coding sequences, between the variable (V) and constant (C) gene segments in all the Ig and TCR loci, that together with D segments are somatically recombined with V segments during lymphocyte development. The resulting recombined VDJ DNA codes for the carboxy-terminal ends of the antigen receptor V regions, including the third hypervariable (CDR) regions. Random use of different J segments contributes to the diversity of the antigen receptor repertoire.

Junctional diversity. The diversity in antibody and TCR repertoires that is attributed to the random addition or removal of nucleotide sequences at junctions between V, D, and J gene segments.

Kaposi's sarcoma. A malignant tumor of vascular cells that frequently arises in patients with AIDS. Kaposi's sarcoma is associated with infection by the Kaposi's sarcoma–associated herpesvirus (human herpesvirus 8).

Killer Ig-like receptors (KIRs). Ig superfamily receptors expressed by NK cells that recognize different alleles of HLA-A, HLA-B, and HLA-C molecules. Some KIRs have signaling components with ITIMs in their cytoplasmic tails, and these deliver inhibitory signals to inactivate the NK cells. Some members of the KIR family have short cytoplasmic tails without ITIMs, but associate with other ITAM-containing polypeptides and function as activating receptors.

Knockout mouse. A mouse with a targeted disruption of one or more genes that is created by homologous recombination techniques. Knockout mice lacking functional genes encoding cytokines, cell surface receptors, signaling molecules, and transcription factors have provided extensive information about the roles of these molecules in the immune system.

Langerhans cells. Immature dendritic cells found as a continuous meshwork in the epidermal layer of the skin whose major function is to trap and transport protein antigens to draining lymph nodes. During their migration to the lymph nodes, Langerhans cells mature into lymph node dendritic cells, which can efficiently present antigen to naive T cells.

Large granular lymphocyte. Another name for an NK cell based on the morphologic appearance of this cell type in the blood.

Late-phase reaction. A component of the immediate hypersensitivity reaction that ensues 2 to 4 hours after mast cell and basophil degranulation and that is characterized by an inflammatory infiltrate of eosinophils, basophils, neutrophils, and lymphocytes. Repeated bouts of this late-phase inflammatory reaction can cause tissue damage.

Lck. An Src family nonreceptor tyrosine kinase that noncovalently associates with the cytoplasmic tails of CD4 and CD8 molecules in T cells and is involved in the early signaling events of antigen-induced T cell activation. Lck mediates tyrosine phosphorylation of the cytoplasmic tails of CD3 and ζ proteins of the TCR complex.

Lectin pathway of complement activation. A pathway of complement activation triggered, in the absence of antibody, by the binding of microbial polysaccharides to circulating lectins such as MBL. MBL is structurally similar to C1q and activates the C1r-C1s enzyme complex (like C1q) or activates another serine esterase, called mannose-binding protein-associated serine esterase. The remaining steps of the lectin pathway, beginning with cleavage of C4, are the same as the classical pathway.

Leishmania. An obligate intracellular protozoan parasite that infects macrophages and can cause a chronic inflammatory disease involving many tissues. *Leishmania* infection in mice has served as a model system for study of the effector functions of several cytokines and the helper T cell subsets that produce them. T_H1 responses to *Leishmania major* and associated IFN-γ production control infection, whereas T_H2 responses with IL-4 production lead to disseminated lethal disease.

Lethal hit. A term used to describe the events that result in irreversible damage to a target cell when a CTL binds to it. The lethal hit includes CTL granule exocytosis, perforin polymerization in the target cell membrane, and entry of calcium ions and apoptosis-inducing enzymes (granzymes) into the target cell cytoplasm.

Leukemia. A malignant disease of bone marrow precursors of blood cells in which large numbers of leukemic cells usually occupy the bone marrow and often circulate in the blood stream. Lymphocytic leukemias are derived from B or T cell precursors, myelogenous leukemias are derived from granulocyte or monocyte precursors, and erythroid leukemias are derived from red blood cell precursors.

Leukocyte adhesion deficiency (LAD). One of a rare group of immunodeficiency diseases with infectious complications that is caused by defective expression of the leukocyte adhesion molecules required for tissue recruitment of phagocytes and lymphocytes. LAD-1 is due to mutations in the gene encoding the CD18 protein, which is part of β_2 integrins. LAD-2 is caused by mutations in a gene that encodes a fucose transporter involved in the synthesis of leukocyte ligands for endothelial selectins.

Leukotrienes. A class of arachidonic acid–derived lipid inflammatory mediators produced by the lipoxygenase pathway in many cell types. Mast cells make abundant leukotriene C_4 (LTC_4) and its degradation products LTD_4 and LTE_4, which bind to specific receptors on smooth muscle cells and cause prolonged bronchoconstriction. Leukotrienes contribute to the pathologic processes of bronchial asthma. Collectively, LTC_4, LTD_4, and LTE_4 constitute what was once called slow-reacting substance of anaphylaxis.

Lipopolysaccharide. Synonymous with **endotoxin.**

Live viral vaccine. A vaccine composed of a live but nonpathogenic (attenuated) form of a virus. Attenuated viruses carry mutations that interfere with the viral life cycle or pathogenesis. Because live virus vaccines actually infect the recipient cells, they can effectively stimulate immune responses, such as the CTL response, that are optimal for protecting against wild-type viral infection. A commonly used live virus vaccine is the Sabin poliovirus vaccine, and there is much interest in development of an attenuated live virus vaccine to protect against HIV infection.

LMP-2 and LMP-7. Two catalytic subunits of the proteasome, the organelle that degrades cytosolic proteins into peptides in the class I MHC pathway of antigen presentation. LMP-2 and LMP-7 are encoded by genes in the MHC, are up-regulated by IFN-γ, and are particularly important for generating class I MHC-binding peptides.

Lymph node. Small nodular, encapsulated aggregates of lymphocyte-rich tissue situated along lymphatic channels throughout the body where adaptive immune responses to lymph-borne antigens are initiated.

Lymphatic system. A system of vessels throughout the body that collects tissue fluid called lymph, originally derived from the blood, and returns it, through the thoracic duct, to the circulation. Lymph nodes are interspersed along these vessels and trap and retain antigens present in the lymph.

Lymphocyte homing. The directed migration of subsets of circulating lymphocytes into particular tissue sites. Lymphocyte homing is regulated by the selective expression of adhesion molecules, called homing receptors, on the lymphocytes and the tissue-specific expression of endothelial ligands for these homing receptors, called addressins, in different vascular beds. For example, some T lymphocytes preferentially home to intestinal lymphoid tissue (e.g., Peyer's patches), and this directed migration is regulated by binding of the VLA-4 integrin on the T cells to the MadCAM addressin on Peyer's patch endothelium.

Lymphocyte maturation. The process by which pluripotent bone marrow precursor cells develop into mature, antigen receptor–expressing naive B or T lymphocytes that populate peripheral lymphoid tissues. This process takes place in the specialized environments of the bone marrow (for B cells) and the thymus (for T cells).

Lymphocyte migration. The movement of lymphocytes from the blood stream into peripheral tissues.

Lymphocyte recirculation. The continuous movement of lymphocytes through the blood stream and lymphatics, between the lymph nodes or spleen, and, if activated, to peripheral inflammatory sites.

Lymphocyte repertoire. The complete collection of antigen receptors and therefore antigen specificities expressed by the B and T lymphocytes of an individual.

Lymphoid follicle. A B cell–rich region of a lymph node or the spleen that is the site of antigen-induced B cell proliferation and differentiation. In T cell–dependent B cell responses to protein antigens, a germinal center forms within the follicles.

Lymphokine. An old name for a cytokine (soluble protein mediator of immune responses) produced by lymphocytes.

Lymphokine-activated killer (LAK) cells. NK cells with enhanced cytolytic activity for tumor cells as a result of exposure to high doses of IL-2. LAK cells generated *in vitro* have been adoptively transferred back into patients with cancer to treat their tumors.

Lymphoma. A malignant tumor of B or T lymphocytes usually arising in and spreading between lymphoid tissues but that may spread to other tissues. Lymphomas often express phenotypic characteristics of the normal lymphocytes from which they were derived.

Lymphotoxin (LT, TNF-β). A cytokine produced by T cells that is homologous to and binds to the same receptors as TNF. Like TNF, LT has proinflammatory effects, including endothelial and neutrophil activation. LT is also critical for the normal development of lymphoid organs.

Lysosome. A membrane-bound, acidic organelle abundant in phagocytic cells that contains proteolytic enzymes that degrade proteins derived both from the extracellular environment and from within the cell. Lysosomes are involved in the class II MHC pathway of antigen processing.

M cells. Specialized epithelial cells overlying Peyer's patches in the gut that play a role in delivering antigens to Peyer's patches.

Macrophage. A tissue-based phagocytic cell derived from blood monocytes that plays important roles in innate and adaptive immune responses. Macrophages are activated by microbial products such as endotoxin and by T cell cytokines such as IFN-γ. Activated macrophages phagocytose and kill microorganisms, secrete proinflammatory cytokines, and present antigens to helper T cells. Macrophages may assume different morphologic forms in different tissues, including the microglia of the central nervous system, Kupffer cells in the liver, alveolar macrophages in the lung, and osteoclasts in bone.

Major histocompatibility complex (MHC). A large genetic locus (on human chromosome 6 and mouse chromosome 17) that includes the highly polymorphic genes encoding the peptide-binding molecules recognized by T lymphocytes. The MHC locus also includes genes encoding cytokines, molecules involved in antigen processing, and complement proteins.

Major histocompatibility complex (MHC) molecule. A heterodimeric membrane protein encoded in the MHC locus that serves as a peptide display molecule for recognition by T lymphocytes. Two structurally distinct types of MHC molecules exist. Class I MHC molecules are present on most nucleated cells, bind peptides derived from cytosolic proteins, and are recognized by $CD8^+$ T cells. Class II MHC molecules are restricted largely to professional APCs, bind peptides derived from endocytosed proteins, and are recognized by $CD4^+$ T cells.

Mannose receptor. A carbohydrate-binding receptor (lectin) expressed by macrophages that binds mannose and fucose residues on microbial cell walls and mediates phagocytosis of the organisms.

Mannose-binding lectin (MBL). A plasma protein that binds to mannose residues on bacterial cell walls and acts as an opsonin by promoting phagocytosis of the bacterium by macrophages. Macrophages express a surface receptor for C1q that can also bind MBL and mediate uptake of the opsonized organisms.

Marginal zone. A peripheral region of splenic lymphoid follicles containing macrophages that are particularly efficient at trapping polysaccharide antigens. Such antigens may persist for prolonged periods on the surfaces of marginal zone macrophages, where they are recognized by specific B cells, or they may be transported into follicles.

Marginal zone B lymphocytes. A subset of B lymphocytes, found exclusively in the marginal zone of the spleen, which respond rapidly to blood borne microbial antigens by producing IgM antibodies with limited diversity.

Mast cell. The major effector cell of immediate hypersensitivity (allergic) reactions. Mast cells are derived from the marrow, reside in most tissues adjacent to blood vessels, express a high-affinity Fc receptor for IgE, and contain numerous mediator-filled granules. Antigen-induced cross-linking of IgE bound to the mast cell Fc receptors causes release of their granule contents as well as new synthesis and secretion of other mediators, leading to an immediate hypersensitivity reaction.

Mature B cell. IgM- and IgD-expressing, functionally competent naive B cells that represent the final stage of B cell maturation in the bone marrow and that populate peripheral lymphoid organs.

Membrane attack complex (MAC). A lytic complex of the terminal components of the complement cascade, including multiple copies of C9, that forms in the membranes of target cells. The MAC causes lethal ionic and osmotic changes in cells.

Memory. The property of the adaptive immune system to respond more rapidly, with greater magnitude, and more effectively to a repeated exposure to an antigen, compared with the response to the first exposure.

Memory lymphocytes. B or T lymphocytes that mediate rapid and enhanced (i.e., memory or recall) responses to second and subsequent exposures to antigens. Memory B and T cells are produced by antigen stimulation of naive lymphocytes and survive in a functionally quiescent state for many years after the antigen is eliminated.

MHC class II (MIIC) compartment. A subset of endosomes (membrane-bound vesicles involved in cell trafficking pathways) found in macrophages and human B cells that are important in the class II MHC pathway of antigen presentation. The MIIC contains all the components required for formation of peptide–class II MHC molecule complexes, including the enzymes that degrade protein antigens, class II molecules, invariant chain, and HLA-DM.

MHC restriction. The characteristic of T lymphocytes that they recognize a foreign peptide antigen only when it is bound to a particular allelic form of an MHC molecule.

MHC-tetramer. A reagent used to identify and enumerate T cells that specifically recognize a particular MHC-peptide complex. The reagent consists of four recombinant, biotinylated MHC molecules (usually class I) bound to a fluorochrome-labeled avidin molecule and loaded with a peptide. T cells that bind the MHC-tetramer can be detected by flow cytometry.

Mitogen-activated protein (MAP) kinase cascade. A signal transduction cascade initiated by the active form of the Ras protein and involving the sequential activation of three serine/threonine kinases, the last one being MAP kinase. MAP kinase in turn phosphorylates and activates other enzymes or transcription factors. The MAP kinase pathway is one of several signal pathways activated by antigen binding to the TCR.

Mixed leukocyte reaction (MLR). An *in vitro* reaction of alloreactive T cells from one individual against MHC antigens on blood cells from another individual. The MLR involves proliferation of and cytokine secretion by both CD4$^+$ and CD8$^+$ T cells and is used as a screening test to assess the compatibility of a potential graft recipient with a potential donor.

Molecular mimicry. A postulated mechanism of autoimmunity triggered by infection with a microbe containing antigens that cross-react with self antigens. Immune responses to the microbe result in reactions against self tissues.

Monoclonal antibody. An antibody that is specific for one antigen and is produced by a B cell hybridoma (a cell line derived by the fusion of a single normal B cell and an immortal B cell tumor line). Monoclonal antibodies are widely used in research and clinical diagnosis and therapy.

Monocyte. A type of bone marrow–derived circulating blood cell that is the precursor of tissue macrophages. Monocytes are actively recruited into inflammatory sites, where they differentiate into macrophages.

Monocyte colony-stimulating factor (M-CSF). A cytokine made by activated T cells, macrophages, endothelial cells, and stromal fibroblasts that stimulates the production of monocytes from bone marrow precursor cells.

Monokine. An old name for a cytokine produced by mononuclear phagocytes.

Mononuclear phagocytes. Cells with a common bone marrow lineage whose primary function is phagocytosis. These cells function as accessory cells in the recognition and activation phases of adaptive immune responses and as effector cells in innate and adaptive immunity. Mononuclear phagocytes circulate in the blood in an incompletely differentiated form called monocytes, and once they settle in tissues, they mature into macrophages.

Mucosa-associated lymphoid tissue. Lymphocytes and accessory cells within the mucosa of the gastrointestinal and respiratory tracts that are sites of adaptive immune responses to environmental antigens. Mucosa-associated lymphoid tissues include intraepithelial lymphocytes, mainly T cells, and organized collections of lymphocytes, often rich in B cells, below mucosal epithelia, such as Peyer's patches in the gut or pharyngeal tonsils.

Mucosal immune system. A part of the immune system that responds to and protects against microbes that enter the body through mucosal surfaces, such as the gastrointestinal and respiratory tracts. The mucosal immune system is composed of mucosa-associated lymphoid tissues, which are collections of lymphocytes and accessory cells in the epithelia and lamina propria of mucosal surfaces.

Multiple myeloma. A malignant tumor of antibody-producing B cells that often secretes Igs or parts of Ig molecules. The monoclonal antibodies produced by multiple myelomas were critical for early biochemical analyses of antibody structure.

Mycobacterium. A genus of aerobic bacteria, many species of which can survive within phagocytes and cause disease. The principal host defense against mycobacteria such as *Mycobacterium tuberculosis* is cell-mediated immunity.

N nucleotides. The name given to nucleotides randomly added to the junctions between V, D, and J gene segments in Ig or TCR genes during lymphocyte development. The addition of up to 20 of these nucleotides, which is mediated by the enzyme terminal deoxyribonucleotidyl transferase, contributes to the diversity of the antibody and TCR repertoires.

Naive lymphocyte. A mature B or T lymphocyte that has not previously encountered antigen, nor is it the progeny of an antigen-stimulated mature lymphocyte. When naive lymphocytes are stimulated by antigen, they differentiate into effector lymphocytes, such as antibody-secreting B cells or helper T cells and CTLs. Naive lymphocytes have surface markers and recirculation patterns that are distinct from those of previously activated lymphocytes. ("Naive" also refers to an unimmunized individual.)

Natural antibodies. IgM antibodies, largely produced by B-1 cells, specific for bacteria that are common in the environment and gastrointestinal tract. Normal individuals contain natural antibodies without any evidence of infection, and these antibodies serve as a preformed defense mechanism against microbes that succeed in penetrating epithelial barriers. Some of these antibodies cross-react with ABO blood group antigens and are responsible for transfusion reactions.

Natural killer (NK) cells. A subset of bone marrow–derived lymphocytes, distinct from B or T cells, that function in innate immune responses to kill microbe-infected cells by direct lytic mechanisms and by secreting IFN-γ. NK cells do not express clonally distributed antigen receptors like Ig receptors or TCRs, and their activation is regulated by a combination of cell surface stimulatory and inhibitory receptors, the latter recognizing self MHC molecules.

Natural killer T cells (NKT cells). A numerically small subset of lymphocytes that express surface molecules characteristic of both NK cells and T cells. They express $\alpha\beta$ T cell antigen receptors with very little diversity, and perform various effector functions typical of helper T cells. NKT cells are considered as part of both adaptive and innate immune systems. Some NKT cells recognize lipid antigens presented by CD1 molecules.

Negative selection. The process by which developing lymphocytes that express self-reactive antigen receptors are eliminated, thereby contributing to the maintenance of self-tolerance. Negative selection of developing T lymphocytes (thymocytes) is best understood and involves high-avidity binding of a thymocyte to self MHC molecules with bound peptides on thymic APCs leading to apoptotic death of the thymocyte.

Neonatal Fc receptor (FcRn). An IgG-specific Fc receptor that mediates the transport of maternal IgG across the placenta and the neonatal intestinal epithelium. FcRn resembles a class I MHC molecule. An adult form of this receptor functions to protect plasma IgG antibodies from catabolism.

Neonatal immunity. Passive humoral immunity to infections in mammals in the first months of life, before full development of the immune system. Neonatal immunity is mediated by maternally produced antibodies transported across the placenta into the fetal circulation before birth or derived from ingested milk and transported across the gut epithelium.

Neutrophil (also polymorphonuclear leukocyte, PMN). A phagocytic cell characterized by a segmented lobular nucleus and cytoplasmic granules filled with degradative enzymes. PMNs are the most abundant type of circulating white blood cells and are the major cell type mediating acute inflammatory responses to bacterial infections.

Nitric oxide. A biologic effector molecule with a broad range of activities that in macrophages functions as a potent microbicidal agent to kill ingested organisms.

Nitric oxide synthase. A member of a family of enzymes that synthesize the vasoactive and microbicidal compound nitric oxide from l-arginine. Macrophages express an inducible form of this enzyme on activation by various microbial or cytokine stimuli.

Nuclear factor κB (NF-κB). A family of transcription factors composed of homodimers or heterodimers of proteins homologous to the c-Rel protein. NF-κB proteins are important in the transcription of many genes in both innate and adaptive immune responses.

Nuclear factor of activated T cells (NFAT). A transcription factor required for the expression of IL-2, IL-4, TNF, and other cytokine genes. The four different NFATs are each encoded by separate genes; NFATp and NFATc are found in T cells. Cytoplasmic NFAT is activated by calcium/calmodulin-dependent, calcineurin-mediated dephosphorylation that permits NFAT to translocate into the nucleus and bind to consensus binding sequences in the regulatory regions of IL-2, IL-4, and other cytokine genes, usually in association with other transcription factors such as AP-1.

Nude mouse. A strain of mice that lacks development of the thymus, and therefore T lymphocytes, as well as hair follicles. Nude mice have been used experimentally to define the role of T lymphocytes in immunity and disease.

Oncofetal antigen. Proteins that are expressed at high levels on some types of cancer cells and in normal developing (fetal) but not adult tissues. Antibodies specific for these proteins are often used in histopathologic identification of tumors or to monitor the progression of tumor growth in patients. CEA (CD66) and α-fetoprotein are two oncofetal antigens commonly expressed by certain carcinomas.

Opsonin. A macromolecule that becomes attached to the surface of a microbe and can be recognized by surface receptors of neutrophils and macrophages and that increases the efficiency of phagocytosis of the microbe. Opsonins include IgG antibodies, which are recognized by the Fcγ receptor on phagocytes, and fragments of complement proteins, which are recognized by CR1 (CD35) and by the leukocyte integrin Mac-1.

Opsonization. The process of attaching opsonins, such as IgG or complement fragments, to microbial surfaces to target the microbes for phagocytosis.

Oral tolerance. The suppression of systemic humoral and cell-mediated immune responses to an antigen after the oral administration of that antigen as a result of anergy of antigen-specific T cells or the production of immunosuppressive cytokines such as transforming growth factor-β. Oral tolerance is a possible mechanism for preventing immune responses to food antigens and to bacteria that normally reside as commensals in the intestinal lumen.

P nucleotides. Short inverted repeat nucleotide sequences in the VDJ junctions of rearranged Ig and TCR genes that are generated by RAG-1- and RAG-2-mediated asymmetric cleavage of hairpin DNA intermediates during somatic recombination events. P nucleotides contribute to the junctional diversity of antigen receptors.

Paracrine factor. A molecule that acts on cells in proximity to the cell that produces the factor. Most cytokines act in a paracrine fashion.

Partial agonist. A variant peptide ligand of a TCR that induces only a subset of the functional responses by the T cell or responses entirely different from responses to the unaltered (native) peptide. For instance, a partial agonist may stimulate production of only some of the many cytokines that are induced by the native peptide or quantitatively smaller responses. Partial agonist peptides are usually synthetic peptides in which one or two TCR contact residues have been changed; they are also called APLs.

Passive immunity. The form of immunity to an antigen that is established in one individual by transfer of antibodies or lymphocytes from another individual who is immune to that antigen. The recipient of such a transfer can become immune to the antigen without ever having been exposed to or having responded to the antigen. An example of passive immunity is the transfer of human sera containing antibodies specific for certain microbial toxins or snake venom to a previously unimmunized individual.

Pathogenicity. The ability of a microorganism to cause disease. Multiple mechanisms may contribute to pathogenicity, including production of toxins, stimulation of host inflammatory responses, and perturbation of host cell metabolism.

Pattern recognition receptors. Receptors of the innate immune system that recognize frequently encountered structures called molecular patterns produced by microorganisms and that facilitate innate immune responses against the microorganisms. Examples of pattern recognition receptors include CD14 receptors on macrophages, which bind bacterial endotoxin leading to macrophage activation, and the mannose receptor on phagocytes, which binds microbial glycoproteins or glycolipids.

Pentraxins. A family of plasma proteins that contain five identical globular subunits; includes the acute-phase reactant C-reactive protein.

Peptide-binding cleft. The portion of an MHC molecule that binds peptides for display to T cells. The cleft is composed of paired α-helices resting on a floor made up of an eight-stranded β-pleated sheet. The polymorphic residues, which are the amino acids that vary among different MHC alleles, are located in and around this cleft.

Perforin. A protein that is homologous to the C9 complement protein and is present as a monomer in the granules of CTLs and NK cells. When perforin is released from the granules of activated CTLs or NK cells, it forms a complex with granzymes and proteoglycans that binds to the target cell plasma membrane and promotes entry of the granzymes into the target cell. This channel can cause osmotic lysis of the target cell and serve as a channel for the influx of enzymes derived from the CTL granules.

Periarteriolar lymphoid sheath (PALS). A cuff of lymphocytes surrounding small arterioles in the spleen, adjacent to lymphoid follicles. A PALS contains mainly T lymphocytes, about two thirds of which are $CD4^+$ and one third $CD8^+$. In humoral immune responses to protein antigens, B lymphocytes are activated at the interface between the PALS and follicles and then migrate into the follicles to form germinal centers.

Peripheral lymphoid organs and tissues. Organized collections of lymphocytes and accessory cells, including the spleen, lymph nodes, and mucosa-associated lymphoid tissues, in which adaptive immune responses are initiated.

Peripheral tolerance. Physiologic unresponsiveness to self antigens that are present in peripheral tissues and not usually in the generative lymphoid organs. Peripheral tolerance is induced by the recognition of antigens without adequate levels of the costimulators required for lymphocyte activation or by persistent and repeated stimulation by these self antigens.

Peyer's patches. Organized lymphoid tissue in the lamina propria of the small intestine in which immune responses to ingested antigens may be initiated. Peyer's patches are composed mostly of B cells, with smaller numbers of T cells and accessory cells, all arranged in follicles similar to those found in lymph nodes, often with germinal centers.

Phagocytosis. The process by which certain cells of the innate immune system, including macrophages and neutrophils, engulf large particles (>0.5 μm in diameter) such as intact microbes. The cell surrounds the particle with extensions of its plasma membrane by an energy- and cytoskeleton-dependent process; this process results in the formation of an intracellular vesicle called a phagosome, which contains the ingested particle.

Phagosome. A membrane-bound intracellular vesicle that contains microbes or particulate material from the extracellular environment. Phagosomes are formed during the process of phagocytosis, and fusion with other vesicular structures such as lysosomes leads to enzymatic degradation of the ingested material.

Phosphatase (protein phosphatase). An enzyme that removes phosphate groups from the side chains of certain amino acid residues of proteins. Protein phosphatases in lymphocytes, such as CD45 or calcineurin, regulate the activity of various signal transduction molecules and transcription factors. Some protein phosphatases may be specific for phosphotyrosine residues and others for phosphoserine and phosphothreonine residues.

Phospholipase Cγ (PLCγ). An enzyme that catalyzes hydrolysis of the plasma membrane phospholipid PIP_2 to generate two signaling molecules, IP_3 and DAG. PLCγ becomes activated in lymphocytes by antigen binding to the antigen receptor.

Phytohemagglutinin (PHA). A carbohydrate-binding protein, or lectin, produced by plants that cross-links human T cell surface molecules, including the T cell receptor, thereby inducing polyclonal activation and agglutination of T cells. PHA is frequently used in experimental immunology to study T cell activation. In clinical medicine, PHA is used to assess whether a patient's T cells are functional or to induce T cell mitosis for the purpose of generating karyotypic data.

Plasma cell. A terminally differentiated antibody-secreting B lymphocyte with a characteristic histologic appearance, including an oval shape, eccentric nucleus, and perinuclear halo.

Platelet-activating factor (PAF). A lipid mediator derived from membrane phospholipids in several cell types, including mast cells and endothelial cells. PAF can cause bronchoconstriction and vascular dilatation and leak and may be an important mediator in asthma.

Polyclonal activators. Agents that are capable of activating many clones of lymphocytes, regardless of their antigen specificities. Examples of polyclonal activators include anti-IgM antibodies for B cells and anti-CD3 antibodies, bacterial superantigens, and PHA for T cells.

Poly-Ig receptor. An Fc receptor expressed by mucosal epithelial cells that mediates the transport of IgA and

IgM through the epithelial cells into the intestinal lumen.

Polymerase chain reaction (PCR). A rapid method of copying and amplifying specific DNA sequences up to about 1 kb in length that is widely used as a preparative and analytical technique in all branches of molecular biology. The method relies on the use of short oligonucleotide primers complementary to the sequences at the ends of the DNA to be amplified and involves repetitive cycles of melting, annealing, and synthesis of DNA.

Polymorphism. The existence of two or more alternative forms, or variants, of a gene that are present at stable frequencies in a population. Each common variant of a polymorphic gene is called an allele, and one individual may carry two different alleles of a gene, each inherited from a different parent. The MHC genes are the most polymorphic genes in the mammalian genome.

Polyvalency. The presence of multiple identical copies of an epitope on a single antigen molecule, cell surface, or particle. Polyvalent antigens, such as bacterial capsular polysaccharides, are often capable of activating B lymphocytes independent of helper T cells.

Positive selection. The process by which developing T cells in the thymus (thymocytes) whose TCRs bind to self MHC molecules are rescued from programmed cell death, whereas thymocytes whose receptors do not recognize self MHC molecules die by default. Positive selection ensures that mature T cells are self MHC restricted and that $CD8^+$ T cells are specific for complexes of peptides with class I MHC molecules and $CD4^+$ T cells for complexes of peptides with class II MHC molecules.

Pre-B cell. A developing B cell present only in hematopoietic tissues that is at a maturational stage characterized by expression of cytoplasmic Ig μ heavy chains and surrogate light chains but not Ig light chains. Pre-B cell receptors composed of μ chains and surrogate light chains deliver signals that stimulate further maturation of the pre-B cell into an immature B cell.

Pre-B cell receptor. A receptor expressed on maturing B lymphocytes at the pre-B cell stage that is composed of an Ig μ heavy chain and an invariant surrogate light chain. The surrogate light chain is composed of two proteins, including the λ5 protein, which is homologous to the λ light chain C domain, and the V pre-B protein, which is homologous to a V domain. The pre-B cell receptor associates with the Igα and Igβ signal transduction proteins to form the pre-B cell receptor complex. Pre-B cell receptors are required for stimulating the proliferation and continued maturation of the developing B cell. It is not known whether the pre-B cell receptor binds a specific ligand.

Pre-cytolytic T lymphocyte (pre-CTL). A mature, naive $CD8^+$ T lymphocyte that cannot perform effector functions but, on activation by antigen and costimulators, will differentiate into a CTL capable of lysing target cells and secreting cytokines.

Pre-T cell. A developing T lymphocyte in the thymus at a maturational stage characterized by expression of the TCR β chain, but not the α chain or CD4 or CD8. In pre-T cells, the TCR β chain is found on the cell surface as part of the pre-T cell receptor.

Pre-T cell receptor. A receptor expressed on the surface of pre-T cells that is composed of the TCR β chain and an invariant pre-Tα protein. This receptor associates with CD3 and ζ molecules to form the pre-T cell receptor complex. The function of this complex is similar to that of the pre-B cell receptor in B cell development, namely, the delivery of signals that stimulate further proliferation, antigen receptor gene rearrangements, and other maturational events. It is not known whether the pre-T cell receptor binds a specific ligand.

Pre-Tα. An invariant transmembrane protein with a single extracellular Ig-like domain that associates with TCR β chain in pre-T cells to form the pre-T cell receptor.

Primary immune response. An adaptive immune response that occurs after the first exposure of an individual to a foreign antigen. Primary responses are characterized by relatively slow kinetics and small magnitude compared with the responses after a second or subsequent exposure.

Primary immunodeficiency. A genetic defect in which an inherited deficiency in some aspect of the innate or adaptive immune system leads to an increased susceptibility to infections. Primary immunodeficiency is frequently manifested early in infancy and childhood but is sometimes clinically detected later in life.

Pro-B cell. A developing B cell in the bone marrow that is the earliest cell committed to the B lymphocyte lineage. Pro-B cells do not produce Ig, but they can be distinguished from other immature cells by the expression of B lineage–restricted surface molecules such as CD19 and CD10.

Professional antigen-presenting cells (professional APCs). APCs for naive helper T lymphocytes, used to refer to dendritic cells, mononuclear phagocytes, and B lymphocytes, all of which are capable of expressing class II MHC molecules and costimulators. The most important professional APCs for initiating primary T cell responses are dendritic cells.

Programmed cell death. A pathway of cell death by apoptosis that occurs in lymphocytes deprived of necessary survival stimuli, such as growth factors or costimulators. Programmed cell death, also called death by neglect or passive cell death, is characterized by the release of mitochondrial cytochrome *c* into the cytoplasm, activation of caspase-9, and initiation of the apoptotic pathway.

Promoter. A DNA sequence immediately 5′ to the transcription start site of a gene where the proteins that initiate transcription bind. The term *promoter* is often used to mean the entire 5′ regulatory region of a gene, including enhancers, which are additional sequences that bind transcription factors and interact with the basal transcription complex to increase the rate of transcriptional initiation. Other enhancers may be located at a significant distance from the promoter, either 5′ of the gene, in introns, or 3′ of the gene.

Prostaglandins. A class of lipid inflammatory mediators derived from arachidonic acid in many cell types through the cyclooxygenase pathway. Activated mast cells make prostaglandin D_2 (PGD_2), which binds to receptors on smooth muscle cells and acts as a vasodilator and a bronchoconstrictor. PGD_2 also promotes neutrophil chemotaxis and accumulation at inflammatory sites.

Pro-T cell. A developing T cell in the thymic cortex that is a recent arrival from the bone marrow and does not express TCRs, CD3, ζ chains, or CD4 or CD8 molecules. Pro-T cells are also called double-negative thymocytes.

Protease. An enzyme that cleaves peptide bonds and thereby breaks proteins down into peptides. Different kinds of proteases have different specificities for bonds between particular amino acid residues. Proteases inside phagocytes are important for killing ingested microbes during innate immune responses, and proteases released from phagocytes at inflammatory sites can cause tissue damage. Proteases in APCs are critical for generating peptide fragments of protein antigens that bind to MHC molecules during T cell–mediated immune responses.

Proteasome. A large multiprotein enzyme complex with a broad range of proteolytic activity that is found in the cytoplasm of most cells and generates from cytosolic proteins the peptides that bind to class I MHC molecules. Proteins are targeted for proteasomal degradation by covalent linkage of ubiquitin molecules.

Protein kinase C (PKC). Any of several isoforms of an enzyme that mediates the phosphorylation of serine and threonine residues in many different protein substrates and thereby serves to propagate various signal transduction pathways leading to transcription factor activation. In T and B lymphocytes, PKC is activated by DAG, which is generated in response to antigen receptor ligation.

Protein tyrosine kinases (PTKs). Enzymes that mediate the phosphorylation of tyrosine residues in proteins and thereby promote phosphotyrosine-dependent protein-protein interactions. PTKs are involved in numerous signal transduction pathways in cells of the immune system.

Protozoa. Single-celled eukaryotic organisms, many of which are human parasites and cause diseases. Examples of pathogenic protozoa include *Entamoeba histolytica,* which causes amebic dysentery; *Plasmodium,* which causes malaria; and *Leishmania,* which causes leishmaniasis. Protozoa stimulate both innate and adaptive immune responses. It has proved difficult to develop effective vaccines against many of these organisms.

Provirus. A DNA copy of the genome of a retrovirus that is integrated into the host cell genome and from which viral genes are transcribed and the viral genome is reproduced. HIV proviruses can remain inactive for long periods and thereby represent a latent form of HIV infection that is not accessible to immune defense.

Purified antigen (subunit) vaccine. A vaccine composed of purified antigens or subunits of microbes. Examples of this type of vaccine include diphtheria and tetanus toxoids, pneumococcus and *Haemophilus influenzae* polysaccharide vaccines, and purified polypeptide vaccines against hepatitis B and influenza virus. Purified antigen vaccines may stimulate antibody and helper T cell responses, but they do not generate CTL responses.

Pyogenic bacteria. Bacteria, such as the gram-positive staphylococci and streptococci, that induce inflammatory responses rich in polymorphonuclear leukocytes (giving rise to pus). Antibody responses to these bacteria greatly enhance the efficacy of innate immune effector mechanisms to clear infections.

Rac. A small guanine nucleotide-binding protein that is activated by the GDP-GTP exchange factor Vav during the early events of T cell activation. GTP·Rac triggers a three-step protein kinase cascade that culminates in activation of the stress-activated protein (SAP) kinase, c-Jun N-terminal kinase (JNK), and p38 kinase, which are similar to the MAP kinases.

Radioimmunoassay. A highly sensitive and specific immunologic method of quantifying the concentration of an antigen in a solution that relies on a radioactively labeled antibody specific for the antigen. Usually, two antibodies specific for the antigen are used. The first antibody is unlabeled but attached to a solid support, where it binds and immobilizes the antigen whose concentration is being determined. The amount of the second, labeled antibody that binds to the immobilized antigen, as determined by radioactive decay detectors, is proportional to the concentration of antigen in the test solution.

Ras. A member of a family of 21-kD guanine nucleotide-binding proteins with intrinsic GTPase activity that are involved in many different signal transduction pathways in diverse cell types. Mutated *ras* genes are associated with neoplastic transformation. In T cell activation, Ras is recruited to the plasma membrane by tyrosine-phosphorylated adapter proteins, where it is activated by GDP-GTP exchange factors. GTP·Ras then initiates the MAP kinase cascade, which leads to expression of the *fos* gene and assembly of the AP-1 transcription factor.

Reactive oxygen intermediates (ROIs). Highly reactive metabolites of oxygen, including superoxide anion, hydroxyl radical, and hydrogen peroxide, that are produced by activated phagocytes. ROIs are used by the phagocytes to form oxyhalides that damage ingested bacteria. ROIs may also be released from cells and promote inflammatory responses or cause tissue damage.

Reagin. IgE antibody that mediates an immediate hypersensitivity reaction.

Receptor editing. A process by which some immature B cells that recognize self antigens in the bone marrow may be induced to change their Ig specificities. Receptor editing involves reactivation of the *RAG* genes, additional light chain VJ recombinations, and new Ig light chain production, which allows the cell to express a different Ig receptor that is not self-reactive.

Recombination-activating gene 1 and 2 (*RAG1* and *RAG2*). The genes encoding RAG-1 and RAG-2 proteins, which are the lymphocyte-specific components of V(D)J recombinase and are expressed in developing B and T cells. RAG proteins bind to recombination recognition sequences and are critical for DNA recombination events that form functional Ig and TCR genes. Therefore, RAG proteins are required for expression of antigen receptors and for the maturation of B and T lymphocytes.

Recombination signal sequences. Specific DNA sequences found adjacent to the V, D, and J segments in the antigen receptor loci and recognized by the RAG-1/RAG-2 component of V(D)J recombinase. The recognition sequences consist of a highly conserved stretch of 7 nucleotides, called the heptamer, located adjacent to the V, D, or J coding sequence, followed by a spacer of exactly 12 or 23 nonconserved nucleotides and a highly conserved stretch of 9 nucleotides, called the nonamer.

Red pulp. An anatomic and functional compartment of the spleen composed of vascular sinusoids, scattered among which are large numbers of erythrocytes, macrophages, dendritic cells, sparse lymphocytes, and plasma cells. Red pulp macrophages clear the blood of microbes, other foreign particles, and damaged red blood cells.

Regulatory T cells. A population of T cells that regulates the activation of other T cells and is necessary to maintain peripheral tolerance to self antigens. Most regulatory T cells are CD4$^+$ and many constitutively express CD25, the α chain of the IL-2 receptor, and the transcription factor FoxP3.

Respiratory burst. The process by which reactive oxygen intermediates such as superoxide anion, hydroxyl radical, and hydrogen peroxide are produced in macrophages and polymorphonuclear leukocytes. The respiratory burst is mediated by the enzyme phagocyte oxidase and is usually triggered by inflammatory mediators, such as LTB_4, PAF, and TNF, or by bacterial products, such as *N*-formylmethionyl peptides.

Reverse transcriptase. An enzyme encoded by retroviruses, such as HIV, that synthesizes a DNA copy of the viral genome from the RNA genomic template. Purified reverse transcriptase is used widely in molecular biology research for purposes of cloning complementary DNAs encoding a gene of interest from messenger RNA. Reverse transcriptase inhibitors are used as drugs to treat HIV-1 infection.

Reverse-transcriptase polymerase chain reaction (RT-PCR). An adaptation of the polymerase chain reaction (PCR) used to amplify a complementary DNA (cDNA) of a gene of interest. In this method, RNA is isolated from a cell expressing the gene, and cDNAs are synthesized by use of the reverse-transcriptase enzyme. The cDNA of interest is then amplified by conventional PCR techniques with gene-specific primers.

Rh blood group antigens. A complex system of protein alloantigens expressed on red blood cell membranes that are the cause of transfusion reactions and hemolytic disease of the newborn. The most clinically important Rh antigen is designated D.

Rheumatoid arthritis. An autoimmune disease characterized primarily by inflammatory damage to joints and sometimes inflammation of blood vessels, lungs, and other tissues. CD4$^+$ T cells, activated B lymphocytes, and plasma cells are found in the inflamed joint lining (synovium), and numerous proinflammatory cytokines, including IL-1 and TNF, are present in the synovial (joint) fluid.

RNase protection assay. A sensitive method of detecting and quantifying messenger RNA (mRNA) copies of particular genes based on hybridization of the mRNA to radiolabeled RNA probes and digestion of unhybridized RNA with the enzyme RNase. The double-stranded RNA duplexes created during the hybridization reaction resist degradation by RNase and are of a particular size determined by the length of the probe. They can be separated by gel electrophoresis and are detected and quantitated by radioautography.

Scavenger receptors. A family of cell surface receptors expressed on macrophages, originally defined as receptors that mediate endocytosis of oxidized or acetylated low-density lipoprotein particles but that also bind and mediate the phagocytosis of a variety of microbes.

SCID mouse. A mouse strain in which B and T cells are absent because of an early block in maturation from bone marrow precursors. SCID mice carry a mutation in a component of the enzyme DNA-dependent protein kinase, which is required for double-stranded DNA break repair. Deficiency of this enzyme results in abnormal joining of Ig and TCR gene segments during recombination and therefore failure to express antigen receptors.

Secondary immune response. An adaptive immune response that occurs on second exposure to an antigen. A secondary response is characterized by more rapid kinetics and greater magnitude relative to the primary immune response, which occurs on first exposure.

Second-set rejection. Allograft rejection in an individual who has previously been sensitized to the donor's tissue alloantigens by having received another graft or transfusion from that donor. In contrast to first-set rejection, which occurs in an individual who has not previously been sensitized to the donor alloantigens, second-set rejection is rapid and occurs in 2 to 3 days as a result of immunologic memory.

Secretory component. The proteolytically cleaved portion of the extracellular domain of the poly-Ig receptor that remains bound to an IgA molecule in mucosal secretions.

Selectin. Any one of three separate but closely related carbohydrate-binding proteins that mediate adhesion of leukocytes to endothelial cells. Each of the selectin molecules is a single-chain transmembrane glycoprotein with a similar modular structure, including an extracellular calcium-dependent lectin domain. The selectins include L-selectin (CD62L), expressed on leukocytes; P-selectin (CD62P), expressed on platelets and activated endothelium; and E-selectin (CD62E), expressed on activated endothelium.

Selective immunoglobulin deficiency. Immunodeficiencies characterized by a lack of only one or a few Ig classes or subclasses. Selective IgA deficiency is the most common selective Ig deficiency, followed by IgG3 and IgG2 deficiencies. Patients with these disorders may be at increased risk for bacterial infections, but many are normal.

Self MHC restriction. The limitation (or restriction) of antigens that can be recognized by an individual's T cells to complexes of peptides bound to major histocompatibility complex (MHC) molecules that were present in the thymus during T cell maturation (i.e., self MHC molecules). The T cell repertoire is self MHC restricted as a result of the process of positive selection.

Self-tolerance. Unresponsiveness of the adaptive immune system to self antigens, largely as a result of inactivation or death of self-reactive lymphocytes induced by exposure to those self antigens. Self-tolerance is a cardinal feature of the normal immune system, and failure of self-tolerance leads to autoimmune diseases.

Septic shock. An often lethal complication of severe gram-negative bacterial infection with spread to the blood stream (sepsis) that is characterized by vascular collapse, disseminated intravascular coagulation, and metabolic disturbances. This syndrome is due to the effects of bacterial LPS and cytokines, including TNF, IL-12, and IL-1. Septic shock is also called endotoxin shock.

Seroconversion. The production of detectable antibodies in the serum specific for a microorganism during the course of an infection or in response to immunization.

Serology. The study of blood (serum) antibodies and their reactions with antigens. The term *serology* is often used to refer to the diagnosis of infectious diseases by detection of microbe-specific antibodies in the serum.

Serotype. An antigenically distinct subset of a species of an infectious organism that is distinguished from other subsets by serologic (i.e., serum antibody) tests. Humoral immune responses to one serotype of microbes (e.g., influenza virus) may not be protective against another serotype.

Serum. The cell-free fluid that remains when blood or plasma forms a clot. Blood antibodies are found in the serum fraction.

Serum amyloid A (SAA). An acute-phase protein whose serum concentration rises significantly in the setting of infection and inflammation, mainly because of IL-1- and TNF-induced synthesis by the liver. SAA activates leukocyte chemotaxis, phagocytosis, and adhesion to endothelial cells.

Serum sickness. A disease caused by the injection of large doses of a protein antigen into the blood and characterized by the deposition of antigen-antibody (immune) complexes in blood vessel walls, especially in the kidneys and joints. Immune complex deposition leads to complement fixation and leukocyte recruitment and subsequently to glomerulonephritis and arthritis. Serum sickness was originally described as a disorder that occurred in patients receiving injections of serum containing antitoxin antibodies to prevent diphtheria.

Severe combined immunodeficiency (SCID). Immunodeficiency diseases in which both B and T lymphocytes do not develop or do not function properly, and therefore both humoral and cell-mediated immunity are impaired. Children with SCID usually have infections during the first year of life and succumb to these infections unless the immunodeficiency is treated. SCID has several different genetic causes.

Shwartzman reaction. An experimental model of the pathologic effects of bacterial LPS and TNF in which two intravenous injections of LPS are administered to a rabbit 24 hours apart. After the second injection, the rabbit suffers disseminated intravascular coagulation and neutrophil and platelet plugging of small blood vessels.

Signal transducer and activator of transcription (STAT). A member of a family of proteins that function as signaling molecules and transcription factors in response to binding of cytokines to type I and type II cytokine receptors. STATs are present as inactive monomers in the cytoplasm of cells and are recruited to the cytoplasmic tails of cross-linked cytokine receptors, where they are tyrosine phosphorylated by JAKs. The phosphorylated STAT proteins dimerize and move to the nucleus, where they bind to specific sequences in the promoter regions of various genes and stimulate their transcription. Different STATs are activated by different cytokines.

Simian immunodeficiency virus. A lentivirus closely related to HIV-1 that causes disease similar to AIDS in monkeys.

Single-positive thymocyte. A maturing T cell precursor in the thymus that expresses CD4 or CD8 molecules but not both. Single-positive thymocytes are found mainly in the medulla and have matured from the double-positive stage, during which thymocytes express both CD4 and CD8 molecules.

Smallpox. A disease caused by variola virus. Smallpox was the first infectious disease shown to be preventable by vaccination and the first disease to be completely eradicated by a worldwide vaccination program.

Somatic hypermutation. High-frequency point mutations in Ig heavy and light chains that occur in germinal center B cells. Mutations that result in increased affinity of antibodies for antigen impart a selective survival advantage to the B cells producing those antibodies and lead to affinity maturation of a humoral immune response.

Somatic recombination. The process of DNA recombination by which the functional genes encoding the variable regions of antigen receptors are formed during lymphocyte development. A relatively limited set of inherited, or germline, DNA sequences that are initially separated from one another are brought together by enzymatic deletion of intervening sequences and religation. This process occurs only in developing B or T lymphocytes. This process is sometimes referred to as somatic rearrangement.

Southern blot. A technique used to determine the organization of genomic DNA around a particular gene. The DNA is cut into fragments by restriction endonucleases, different-sized fragments are electrophoretically separated in a gel, and the DNA is then immobilized (blotted) onto a sheet of nitrocellulose or nylon. The position and therefore the size of a particular DNA fragment can then be detected by use of a radioactively labeled DNA probe with a homologous sequence. (See Appendix III for a detailed description.)

Specificity. A cardinal feature of the adaptive immune system, namely, that immune responses are directed toward and able to distinguish between distinct antigens or small parts of macromolecular antigens. This fine specificity is attributed to lymphocyte antigen receptors that may bind to one molecule but not to another with only minor structural differences from the first.

Spleen. A secondary lymphoid organ in the left upper quadrant of the abdomen. The spleen is the major site of adaptive immune responses to blood-borne antigens. The red pulp of the spleen is composed of blood-filled vascular sinusoids lined by active phagocytes that ingest opsonized antigens and damaged red blood cells. The white pulp of the spleen contains lymphocytes and lymphoid follicles where B cells are activated.

Src homology 2 (SH2) domain. A three-dimensional domain structure of about 100 amino acid residues present in many signaling proteins that permits specific noncovalent interactions with other proteins by binding to phosphotyrosines. Each SH2 domain has a unique binding specificity that is determined by the amino acid residues adjacent to the phosphotyrosine on the target protein. Several proteins involved in early signaling events in T and B lymphocytes interact with one another through SH2 domains.

Src homology 3 (SH3) domain. A three-dimensional domain structure of about 60 amino acid residues present in many signaling proteins that mediates protein-protein binding. SH3 domains bind to proline residues and function cooperatively with the SH2 domains of the same protein. For instance, Sos, the guanine nucleotide exchange factor for Ras, contains both SH2 and SH3 domains, and both are involved in Sos binding to the adapter protein Grb-2.

Stem cell. An undifferentiated cell that divides continuously and gives rise to additional stem cells and to cells of multiple different lineages. For example, all blood cells arise from a common hematopoietic stem cell.

Superantigens. Proteins that bind to and activate all the T cells in an individual that express a particular set or family of V_β TCR genes. Superantigens are presented to T cells by binding to nonpolymorphic regions of class II MHC molecules on APCs, and they interact with conserved regions of TCR V_β domains. Several staphylococcal enterotoxins are superantigens. Their importance lies in their ability to activate many T cells, which results in large amounts of cytokine production and a clinical syndrome that is similar to septic shock.

Suppressor T cell. T cells that block the activation and function of other effector T lymphocytes. Suppressor function may be attributed to a still poorly defined population of T cells currently called **regulatory T cells.**

Surrogate light chain. A complex of two nonvariable proteins that associate with Ig μ heavy chains in pre-B cells to form the pre-B cell receptor. The two surrogate light chain proteins include V pre-B protein, which is homologous to a light chain V domain, and λ5, which is covalently attached to the μ heavy chain by a disulfide bond.

Switch recombination. The molecular mechanism underlying Ig isotype switching in which a rearranged VDJ gene segment in an antibody-producing B cell recombines with a downstream C gene and the intervening C gene is deleted. DNA recombination events in switch recombination are triggered by CD40 and cytokines and involve nucleotide sequences called switch regions located in the introns at the 5′ end of each C_H locus.

Syngeneic. Genetically identical. All animals of an inbred strain and monozygotic twins are syngeneic.

Syngeneic graft. A graft from a donor who is genetically identical to the recipient. Syngeneic grafts are not rejected.

Synthetic vaccine. Vaccines composed of recombinant DNA-derived antigens. Synthetic vaccines for hepatitis B virus and herpes simplex virus are now in use.

Systemic inflammatory response syndrome (SIRS). The systemic changes observed in patients who have disseminated bacterial infections. In its mild form, SIRS consists of neutrophilia, fever, and a rise in acute-phase reactants in the plasma. These changes are stimulated by bacterial products such as LPS and are mediated by cytokines of the innate immune system. In severe cases, SIRS may include disseminated intravascular coagulation, adult respiratory distress syndrome, and septic shock.

Systemic lupus erythematosus (SLE). A chronic systemic autoimmune disease that affects predominantly women and is characterized by rashes, arthritis, glomerulonephritis, hemolytic anemia, thrombocytopenia, and central nervous system involvement. Many different autoantibodies are found in patients with SLE, particularly anti-DNA antibodies. Many of the manifestations of SLE are due to the formation of immune complexes composed of autoantibodies and their specific antigens, with deposition of these complexes in small blood vessels in various tissues. The underlying mechanism for the breakdown of self-tolerance in SLE is not understood.

T-bet. A T-box family transcription factor that promotes the differentiation of T_H1 cells from naïve T cells.

T cell receptor (TCR). The clonally distributed antigen receptor on $CD4^+$ and $CD8^+$ T lymphocytes that recognizes complexes of foreign peptides bound to self MHC molecules on the surface of APCs. The most common form of TCR is composed of a heterodimer of two disulfide-linked transmembrane polypeptide chains, designated α and β, each containing one N-terminal Ig-like variable (V) domain, one Ig-like constant (C) domain, a hydrophobic transmembrane region, and a short cytoplasmic region. (Another less common type of TCR, composed of γ and δ chains, is found on a small subset of T cells and recognizes different forms of antigen.)

T cell receptor complex. A multiprotein plasma membrane complex on T lymphocytes that is composed of the highly variable, antigen-binding TCR heterodimer and the invariant signaling proteins CD3 δ, ε, and γ and the ζ chain.

T lymphocyte. The cell type that mediates cell-mediated immune responses in the adaptive immune system. T lymphocytes mature in the thymus, circulate in the blood, populate secondary lymphoid tissues, and are recruited to peripheral sites of antigen exposure. They express antigen receptors (TCRs) that recognize peptide fragments of foreign proteins bound to self MHC molecules. Functional subsets of T lymphocytes include $CD4^+$ helper T cells and $CD8^+$ CTLs.

T-dependent antigen. An antigen that requires both B cells and helper T cells to stimulate an antibody response. T-dependent antigens are protein antigens that contain some epitopes recognized by T cells and other epitopes recognized by B cells. Helper T cells produce cytokines and cell surface molecules that stimulate B cell growth and differentiation into antibody-secreting cells. Humoral immune responses to T-dependent antigens are characterized by isotype switching, affinity maturation, and memory.

T_H1 cells. A functional subset of $CD4^+$ helper T cells that secrete a particular set of cytokines, including IFN-γ, and whose principal function is to stimulate phagocyte-mediated defense against infections, especially with intracellular microbes.

T_H2 cells. A functional subset of $CD4^+$ helper T cells that secrete a particular set of cytokines, including IL-4 and IL-5, and whose principal functions are to stimulate IgE and eosinophil/mast cell–mediated immune reactions and to down-regulate T_H1 responses.

T_H17 cells. A functional subset of $CD4^+$ helper T cells that secrete a particular set of inflammatory cytokines, including IL-17, which are protective against certain bacterial infections and also mediate pathogenic responses in autoimmune diseases.

Thymic epithelial cells. Epithelial cells abundant in the cortical and medullary stroma of the thymus that play a critical role in T cell development. Thymic epithelial cells secrete factors, such as IL-7, that are required for the early stages of T cell development. In the process of positive selection, maturing T cells must recognize self peptides bound to MHC molecules on the surface of thymic epithelial cells to be rescued from programmed cell death.

Thymocyte. A precursor of a mature T lymphocyte present in the thymus.

Thymus. A bilobed organ situated in the anterior mediastinum that is the site of maturation of T lymphocytes from bone marrow–derived precursors. Thymic tissue is divided into an outer cortex and an inner medulla and contains stromal thymic epithelial cells, macrophages, dendritic cells, and numerous T cell precursors (thymocytes) at various stages of maturation.

T-independent antigen. Nonprotein antigens, such as polysaccharides and lipids, that can stimulate antibody responses without a requirement for antigen-specific helper T lymphocytes. T-independent antigens usually contain multiple identical epitopes that can cross-link membrane Ig on B cells and thereby activate the cells. Humoral immune responses to T-independent antigens show relatively little heavy chain isotype switching or affinity maturation, two processes that require signals from helper T cells.

Tissue typing. The determination of the particular MHC alleles expressed by an individual for the purpose of matching allograft donors and recipients. Tissue typing, also called HLA typing, is usually done by testing whether sera known to be reactive with certain MHC gene products mediate complement-dependent lysis of an individual's lymphocytes. PCR techniques are now also used to determine whether an individual carries a particular MHC allele.

TNF receptor–associated factors (TRAFs). A family of adapter molecules that interact with the cytoplasmic domains of various receptors in the TNF receptor family, including TNF-RII, lymphotoxin (LT)-β receptor, and CD40. Each of these receptors contains a cytoplasmic motif that binds different TRAFs, which in turn engage other signaling molecules leading to activation of the transcription factors AP-1 and NF-κB. A transforming gene product of Epstein-Barr virus encodes a protein with a domain that binds TRAFs, and therefore infection by the virus mimics TNF- or CD40-induced signals.

Tolerance. Unresponsiveness of the adaptive immune system to antigens, as a result of inactivation or death of antigen-specific lymphocytes, induced by exposure to the antigens. Tolerance to self antigens is a normal feature of the adaptive immune system, but tolerance to foreign antigens may be induced under certain conditions of antigen exposure.

Tolerogen. An antigen that induces immunologic tolerance, in contrast to an immunogen, which induces an immune response. Many antigens can be either tolerogens or immunogens, depending on how they are administered. Tolerogenic forms of antigens include large doses of the proteins administered without adjuvants, APLs, and orally administered antigens.

Toll-like receptors. Cell surface molecules on phagocytes and other cell types that are involved in recognition of microbial structures, such as endotoxin, and the generation of signals that lead to the activation of innate immune responses. Toll-like receptors share structural homology and signal transduction pathways with the type I IL-1 receptor.

Toxic shock syndrome. An acute illness characterized by shock, skin exfoliation, conjunctivitis, and diarrhea that is associated with tampon use and caused by a *Staphylococcus aureus* superantigen.

Transforming growth factor-β (TGF-β). A cytokine produced by activated T cells, mononuclear phagocytes, and other cells whose principal actions are to inhibit the proliferation and differentiation of T cells, to inhibit the activation of macrophages, and to counteract the effects of proinflammatory cytokines.

Transfusion. Transplantation of circulating blood cells, platelets, or plasma from one individual to another. Transfusions are performed to treat blood loss from hemorrhage or to treat a deficiency in one or more blood cell types resulting from inadequate production or excess destruction.

Transfusion reactions. An immunologic reaction against transfused blood products, usually mediated by preformed antibodies in the recipient that bind to donor blood cell antigens, such as ABO blood group antigens or histocompatibility antigens. Transfusion reactions can lead to intravascular lysis of red blood cells and, in severe cases, kidney damage, fever, shock, and disseminated intravascular coagulation.

Transgenic mouse. A mouse that expresses an exogenous gene that has been introduced into the genome by injection of a specific DNA sequence into the pronuclei of fertilized mouse eggs. Transgenes insert randomly at chromosomal break points and are subsequently inherited as simple mendelian traits. By the design of transgenes with tissue-specific regulatory sequences, mice can be produced that express a particular gene only in certain tissues. Transgenic mice are used extensively in immunology research to study the functions of various cytokines, cell surface molecules, and intracellular signaling molecules.

Transplantation. The process of transferring cells, tissues, or organs (i.e., grafts) from one individual to another or from one site to another in the same individual. Transplantation is used to treat a variety of diseases in which there is a functional disorder of a tissue or organ. The major barrier to successful transplantation between individuals is immunologic reaction (rejection) to the transplanted graft.

Transporter associated with antigen processing (TAP). An adenosine triphosphate (ATP)-dependent peptide transporter that mediates the active transport of peptides from the cytosol to the site of assembly of class I MHC molecules inside the endoplasmic reticulum. TAP is a heterodimeric molecule composed of TAP-1 and TAP-2 polypeptides, both encoded by genes in the MHC. Because peptides are required for stable assembly of class I MHC molecules, TAP-deficient animals express few cell surface class I MHC molecules, which results in diminished development and activation of $CD8^+$ T cells.

Tumor immunity. Protection against the development of tumors by the immune system. Although immune responses to naturally occurring tumors can frequently be demonstrated, true immunity may occur only in the case of a subset of these tumors that express immunogenic antigens (e.g., tumors that are caused by oncogenic viruses and therefore express viral antigens). Research efforts are under way to enhance weak immune responses to other tumors by a variety of approaches.

Tumor-infiltrating lymphocytes (TILs). Lymphocytes isolated from the inflammatory infiltrates present in and around surgical resection samples of solid tumors that are enriched with tumor-specific CTLs and NK cells. In an experimental mode of cancer treatment, TILs are grown *in vitro* in the presence of high doses of IL-2 and are then adoptively transferred back into patients with the tumor.

Tumor necrosis factor (TNF). A cytokine produced mainly by activated mononuclear phagocytes that functions to stimulate the recruitment of neutrophils and monocytes to sites of infection and to activate these cells to eradicate microbes. TNF stimulates vascular endothelial cells to express new adhesion molecules, induces macrophages and endothelial cells to secrete chemokines, and promotes apoptosis of target cells. In severe infections, TNF is produced in large amounts and has systemic effects, including induction of fever, synthesis of acute-phase proteins by the liver, and cachexia. The production of large amounts of TNF can cause intravascular thrombosis and shock. (TNF-β, or lymphotoxin, is a closely related cytokine with biologic effects identical to those of TNF-α but is produced by T cells.)

Tumor necrosis factor (TNF) receptors. Cell surface receptors for TNF-α and TNF-β (LT), present on most cell types. There are two distinct TNF receptors, TNF-RI and TNF-RII, but most biologic effects of TNF are mediated by TNF-RI. TNF receptors are members of a family of homologous receptors with cysteine-rich extracellular motifs that include Fas and CD40.

Tumor-specific antigen. An antigen whose expression is restricted to a particular tumor and is not expressed by normal cells. Tumor-specific antigens may serve as target antigens for antitumor immune responses.

Tumor-specific transplantation antigen (TSTA). An antigen expressed on experimental animal tumor cells that can be detected by induction of immunologic rejection of tumor transplants. TSTAs were originally defined on chemically induced rodent sarcomas and shown to stimulate CTL-mediated rejection of transplanted tumors.

Two-signal hypothesis. A now proven hypothesis that states that the activation of lymphocytes requires two distinct signals, the first being antigen and the second either microbial products or components of innate immune responses to microbes. The requirement for antigen (so-called signal 1) ensures that the ensuing immune response is specific. The requirement for additional stimuli triggered by microbes or innate immune reactions (signal 2) ensures that immune responses are induced when they are needed, that is, against microbes and other noxious substances and not against harmless substances, including self antigens. Signal 2 is referred to as costimulation and is often mediated by membrane molecules on professional APCs, such as B7 proteins.

Type I cytokine receptors. A family of cytokine receptors, also called hemopoietin receptors, that contain conserved structural motifs in their extracellular domains and bind cytokines that fold into four α-helical strands, including growth hormone, IL-2, IL-3, IL-4, IL-5, IL-6, IL-7, IL-9, IL-11, IL-13, IL-15, GM-CSF, and G-CSF. Some of these receptors consist of a ligand-binding chain and one or more signal-transducing chains, and all of these chains have the same structural motifs. Type I cytokine receptors are dimerized on binding their cytokine ligands, and they signal through JAK/STAT pathways.

Type I interferons (IFN-α, IFN-β). A family of cytokines, including several structurally related IFN-α proteins and a single IFN-β protein, all of which have potent antiviral actions. The major source of IFN-α is mononuclear phagocytes; IFN-β is produced by many cells, including fibroblasts. Both IFN-α and IFN-β bind to the same cell surface receptor and induce similar biologic responses. Type I IFNs inhibit viral replication, increase the lytic potential of NK cells, increase expression of class I MHC molecules on virus-infected cells, and stimulate the development of T_H1 cells, especially in humans.

Ubiquitination. Covalent linkage of several copies of a small polypeptide called ubiquitin to a protein. Ubiquitination serves to target the protein for proteolytic degradation by proteasomes, a critical step in the class I MHC pathway of antigen processing and presentation.

Urticaria. Localized transient swelling and redness of the skin caused by leakage of fluid and plasma proteins from small vessels into the dermis during an immediate hypersensitivity reaction.

V gene segments. A DNA sequence that encodes the variable domain of an Ig heavy chain or light chain or a TCR α, β, γ, or δ chain. Each antigen receptor locus contains many different V gene segments, any one of which may recombine with downstream D or J segments during lymphocyte maturation to form functional antigen receptor genes.

V(D)J recombinase. A collection of enzymes that together mediate the somatic recombination events that form functional antigen receptor genes in developing B and T lymphocytes. Some of the enzymes, such as RAG-1 and RAG-2, are found only in developing lymphocytes, and others are ubiquitous DNA repair enzymes.

Vaccine. A preparation of microbial antigen, often combined with adjuvants, that is administered to individuals to induce protective immunity against microbial infections. The antigen may be in the form of live but avirulent microorganisms, killed microorganisms, purified macromolecular components of a microorganism, or a plasmid that contains a complementary DNA encoding a microbial antigen.

Variable region. The extracellular, N-terminal region of an Ig heavy or light chain or a TCR α, β, γ, or δ chain that contains variable amino acid sequences that differ between every clone of lymphocytes and that are responsible for the specificity for antigen. The antigen-binding variable sequences are localized to extended loop structures or hypervariable segments.

Virus. A primitive obligate intracellular parasitic organism or infectious particle that consists of a simple nucleic acid genome packaged in a protein capsid, sometimes surrounded by a membrane envelope. Many pathogenic animal viruses cause a wide range of diseases. Humoral immune responses to viruses can be effective in blocking infection of cells, and NK cells and CTLs are necessary to kill cells already infected.

Western blot. An immunologic technique to determine the presence of a protein in a biologic sample. The method involves separation of proteins in the sample by electrophoresis, transfer of the protein array from the electrophoresis gel to a support membrane by capillary action (blotting), and finally detection of the protein by binding of an enzymatically or radioactively labeled antibody specific for that protein.

Wheal and flare reaction. Local swelling and redness in the skin at a site of an immediate hypersensitivity reaction. The wheal reflects increased vascular permeability and the flare results from increased local blood flow, both changes resulting from mediators such as histamine released from activated dermal mast cells.

White pulp. The part of the spleen that is composed predominantly of lymphocytes, arranged in periarteriolar lymphoid sheaths, and follicles and other leukocytes. The remainder of the spleen contains sinusoids lined with phagocytic cells and filled with blood, called the **red pulp.**

Wiskott-Aldrich syndrome. An X-linked disease characterized by eczema, thrombocytopenia (reduced blood platelets), and immunodeficiency manifested as susceptibility to bacterial infections. The defective gene encodes a cytosolic protein involved in signaling cascades and regulation of the actin cytoskeleton.

Xenoantigen. An antigen on a graft from another species.

Xenogeneic graft (xenograft). An organ or tissue graft derived from a species different from the recipient. Transplantation of xenogeneic grafts (e.g., from a pig) to humans is not yet practical because of special problems related to immunologic rejection.

Xenoreactive. Describing a T cell or antibody that recognizes and responds to an antigen on a graft from another species (a xenoantigen). The T cell may recognize an intact xenogeneic MHC molecule or a peptide derived from a xenogeneic protein bound to a self MHC molecule.

X-linked agammaglobulinemia. An immunodeficiency disease, also called Bruton's agammaglobulinemia, characterized by a block in early B cell maturation and absence of serum Ig. Patients suffer from pyogenic bacterial infections. The disease is caused by mutations or deletions in the gene encoding Btk, an enzyme involved in signal transduction in developing B cells.

X-linked hyper-IgM syndrome. A rare immunodeficiency disease caused by mutations in the CD40 ligand gene and characterized by failure of B cell heavy chain isotype switching and cell-mediated immunity. Patients suffer from both pyogenic bacterial and protozoal infections.

ζ Chain. A transmembrane protein expressed in T cells as part of the TCR complex that contains ITAMs in its cytoplasmic tail and binds the ZAP-70 protein tyrosine kinase during T cell activation.

Zeta-associated protein of 70kD (ZAP-70). An Src family cytoplasmic protein tyrosine kinase that is critical for early signaling steps in antigen-induced T cell activation. ZAP-70 binds to phosphorylated tyrosines in the cytoplasmic tails of the ζ chain of the TCR complex and in turn phosphorylates adapter proteins that recruit other components of the signaling cascade.

Appendix II

PRINCIPAL FEATURES OF SELECTED CD MOLECULES

The table below includes selected CD molecules that are referred to in the text. We have not included cytokine receptors and Toll-like receptors, many of which have been assigned CD numbers, because we refer to these molecules by the more descriptive names throughout the book. Many other molecules that have CD number designations are not described in the text, and therefore they are not included in this selected list. A complete and up-to-date listing of CD molecules may be found on the WWW at http://www.hlda8.org.

CD designation	Common synonyms	Molecular structure, family	Main cellular expression	Known or proposed functions
CD1a*	T6	49 kD; class I MHC family; β_2 microglobulin-associated	Thymocytes, dendritic cells (including Langerhans cells)	Presentation of nonpeptide (lipid and glycolipid) antigens to some T cells
CD1b	T6	45 kD; class I MHC family; β_2 microglobulin-associated	Same as CD1a	Same as CD1a
CD1c	T6	43 kD; class I MHC family; β_2 microglobulin-associated	Thymocytes, dendritic cells (including Langerhans cells), some B cells	Same as CD1a
CD1d	—	49 kD; class I MHC family; β_2 microglobulin associated	Thymocytes, dendritic cells (including Langerhans cells), intestinal epithelial cells, some B cells	Same as CD1a
CD1e	—	28 kD; class I MHC family; β_2 microglobulin-associated	Dendritic cells	Same as CD1a
CD2	T11; LFA-2; sheep red blood cell receptor	50 kD; Ig superfamily; CD2/CD48/CD58 family	T cells, NK cells	Adhesion molecule (binds CD58); T cell activation; CTL- and NK cell–mediated lysis
CD3γ	T3; Leu-4	25–28 kD; associated with CD3δ and CD3ε in TCR complex; Ig superfamily; ITAM in cytoplasmic tail	T cells	Cell surface expression of and signal transduction by the T cell antigen receptor
CD3δ	T3; Leu-4	20 kD; associated with CD3δ and CD3ε in TCR complex; Ig superfamily; ITAM in cytoplasmic tail (Chapter 6)	T cells	Cell surface expression of and signal transduction by the T cell antigen receptor

The complete listing of CD molecules, called Human Cell Differentiation Markers (HCDM), formerly called Human Leukocyte Differentiation Antigens, is compiled by the Collaborative Research on Cellular Markers workshop. The HCDM website, http://www.hlda8.org/, includes links to various gene and protein databases, which contain information about each molecule.

CD designation	Common synonyms	Molecular structure, family	Main cellular expression	Known or proposed functions
CD3ε	T3; Leu-4	20 kD; associated with CD3δ and CD3ε in TCR complex; Ig superfamily; ITAM in cytoplasmic tail	T cells	Cell surface expression of and signal transduction by the T cell antigen receptor
CD4	T4; Leu-3; L3T4	55 kD; Ig superfamily	Class II MHC–restricted T cells, monocytes and macrophages	Signaling and adhesion coreceptor in class II MHC–restricted antigen-induced T cell activation (binds to class II MHC molecules); receptor for HIV
CD5	T1; Ly-1	67 kD; scavenger receptor family	T cells, B cell subset	Signaling molecule; binds CD72
CD8α	T8; Leu2; Lyt2	34 kD; expressed as homodimer or heterodimer with CD8 β	Class I MHC–restricted T cells	Signaling and adhesion coreceptor in class I MHC–restricted antigen-induced T cell activation (binds to class I MHC molecules); thymocyte development
CD8β	T8; Leu2; Lyt2	34 kD; expressed as heterodimer with CD8 α; Ig superfamily	Same as CD8α	Same as CD8α
CD10	Common acute lymphoblastic leukemia antigen (CALLA); neutral endopeptidase. metalloendopeptidase; enkephalinase	100 kD; type II membrane protein	Immature and some mature B cells; lymphoid progenitors, granulocytes	Metalloproteinase; B cell development
CD11a	LFA-1 α chain; α_L integrin subunit	180 kD; noncovalently linked to CD18 to form LFA-1 integrin	Leukocytes	Cell:cell adhesion; binds to ICAM-1 (CD54), ICAM-2 (CD102), and ICAM-3 (CD50)
CD11b	Mac-1; Mo1; CR3 (iC3b receptor); αM integrin chain	165 kD; noncovalently linked to CD18 to form Mac-1 integrin	Granulocytes, monocytes/ macrophages, dendritic cells, NK cells	Phagocytosis of iC3b-coated particles; neutrophil and monocyte adhesion to endothelium (binds CD54) and extracellular matrix proteins
CD11c	p150,95; CR4 α chain; α_X integrin chain	145 kD; noncovalently linked to CD18 to form p150,95 integrin	Monocytes/macrophages, granulocytes, NK cells	Similar functions to CD11b; major CD11CD18 integrin on macrophages
CD14	Mo2; LPS receptor	53 kD; GPI-linked	Monocytes, macrophages, granulocytes	Binds complex of LPS and LPS-binding protein; required for LPS-induced macrophage activation
CD16a	FcγRIIIA	50–70 kD; transmembrane protein; Ig superfamily	NK cells, macrophages	Binds Fc region of IgG; phagocytosis and antibody-dependent cellular cytotoxicity
CD16b	FcγRIIIB	50–70 kD; GPI linked; Ig superfamily	Neutrophils	Binds Fc region of IgG; synergy with FcγRII in immune complex-mediated neutrophil activation
CD18	β chain of LFA-1 family; β_2 integrin subunit	95 kD; noncovalently linked to CD11a, CD11b, or CD11c to form β_2 integrins	Leukocytes	See CD11a, CD11b, CD11c
CD19	B4	95 kD; Ig superfamily	Most B cells	B cell activation; forms a coreceptor complex with CD21 and CD81 which delivers signals that synergize with signals from B cell antigen receptor complex
CD20	B1	35–37 kD; tetraspan (TM4SF) family	Most or all B cells	? Role in B cell activation or regulation; calcium ion channel
CD21	CR2; C3d receptor; B2	145 kD; regulators of complement activation	Mature B cells, follicular dendritic cells	Receptor for complement fragment C3d; forms a coreceptor complex with CD19 and CD81 which delivers activating signals in B cells; Epstein-Barr virus receptor

CD designation	Common synonyms	Molecular structure, family	Main cellular expression	Known or proposed functions
CD22	BL-CAM; Lyb8	130–140 kD; Ig superfamily; sialadhesin family; ITIM in cytoplasmic tail	B cells	Regulation of B cell activation; adhesion molecule
CD23	FcεRIIb; low-affinity IgE receptor	45 kD; c-type lectin	Activated B cells, monocytes, macrophages	Low-affinity Fcε receptor, induced by IL-4; ? regulation of IgE synthesis; ? triggering of monocyte cytokine release
CD25	IL-2 receptor α chain; TAC; p55	55 kD; regulators of complement activation family; noncovalently associates with IL-2Rβ (CD122) and IL-2Rγ (CD132) chains to form high-affinity IL-2 receptor	Activated T and B cells; regulatory T cells; activated macrophages	Binds IL-2; subunit of IL-2R
CD28	Tp44	Homodimer of 44 kD chains; Ig superfamily	T cells (most CD4, some CD8 cells)	T cell receptor for costimulator molecules CD80 (B7-1) and CD86 (B7-2)
CD29	β chain of VLA antigens; β1 integrin subunit; platelet GPIIa	130 kD; noncovalently linked with CD49a-d chains to form VLA (β1) integrins	T cells, B cells, monocytes, granulocytes	Leukocyte adhesion to extracellular matrix proteins and endothelium (see CD49)
CD30	Ki-1	120 kD; TNF-R family	Activated T and B cells; NK cells, monocytes, Reed-Sternberg cells in Hodgkin's disease	Role in activation-induced cell death of CD8+ T cells; binds to CD153 (CD30L) on neutrophils, activated T cells, and macrophages
CD31	PECAM-1; platelet GPIIa	130–140 kD; Ig superfamily	Platelets; monocytes, granulocytes, B cells, endothelial cells	Adhesion molecule involved in the leukocyte transmigration through endothelium
CD32	FcγRIIA; FcγRIIB; FcγRIIC	40 kD; Ig superfamily; ITIM in cytoplasmic tail; A, B, and C forms products of different but homologous genes	Macrophages, granulocytes, B cells, eosinophils, platelets	Fc receptor for aggregated IgG; binds C-reactive protein; role in phagocytosis, ADCC; acts as inhibitory receptor that terminates activation signals initiated by the B cell antigen receptor
CD34	gp105–120	105–120 kD; sialomucin	Precursors of hematopoietic cells, endothelial cells in high endothelial venules	Cell-cell adhesion; binds CD62L (L-selectin)
CD35	CR1; C3b receptor	190–285 kD (four products of polymorphic alleles); regulators of complement activation family	Granulocytes, monocytes, erythrocytes, B cells, T cell subsets, follicular dendritic cells	Binds C3b and C4b; promotes phagocytosis of C3b- or C4b-coated particles and immune complexes; regulates complement activation
CD36	Platelet GPIIIb; GPIV	85–90 kD	Platelets, monocytes, and macrophages, microvascular endothelial cells	Scavenger receptor for oxidized low-density lipoprotein; platelet adhesion; phagocytosis of apoptotic cells
CD40	—	Homodimer of 44–48 kD chains; TNF-R family	B cells, macrophages, dendritic cells, endothelial cells	Binds CD154 (CD40 ligand); role in T cell–dependent B cell, activation, and macrophage, dendritic cell, and endothelial cell activation
CD43	Sialophorin; leukosialin	95–135 kD; sialomucin	Leukocytes (except circulating B cells)	Adhesive and anti-adhesive functions
CD44	Pgp-1; Hermes	80 to >100 kD, highly glycosylated; cartilage link protein family	Leukocytes, erythrocytes	Binds hyaluronan; involved in leukocyte adhesion to endothelial cells and extracellular matrix; leukocyte aggregation
CD45	Leukocyte common antigen (LCA); T200; B220	Multiple isoforms, 180–220 kD (see CD45R); protein tyrosine phosphatase receptor family; fibronectin type III family	Hematopoietic cells	Tyrosine phosphatase which plays critical role in regulating T and B cell antigen receptor-mediated signaling
CD45R	Forms of CD45 with restricted cellular expression	CD45RO: 180 kD CD45RA: 220 kD CD45RB: 190, 205, and 220 kD isoforms	CD45RO: memory T cells, subset of B cells, monocytes, macrophages CD45RA: naive T cells, B cells, monocytes CD45RB: B cells, subset of T cells	See CD45

CD designation	Common synonyms	Molecular structure, family	Main cellular expression	Known or proposed functions
CD46	Membrane cofactor protein (MCP)	52–58 kD; regulators of complement activation family	Leukocytes, epithelial cells, fibroblasts	Regulation of complement activation
CD49a	α_1 integrin subunit	210 kD; noncovalently linked to CD29 to form VLA-1 (β1 integrin)	Activated T cells, monocytes	Leukocyte adhesion to extracellular matrix; binds collagens, laminin
CD49b	α_2 integrin subunit; platelet GPIa	165 kD; noncovalently linked to CD29 to form VLA-2 (β1 integrin)	Platelets, activated T cells, monocytes, some B cells	Leukocyte adhesion to extracellular matrix; binds collagen, laminin
CD49c	α_3 integrin subunit	Dimer of 130 and 25 kD chains; noncovalently linked to CD29 to form VLA-3 (β1 integrin)	T cells, some B cells, monocytes	Leukocyte adhesion to extracellular matrix; binds fibronectin, collagens, laminin
CD49d	α_4 integrin subunit	150 kD; noncovalently linked to CD29 to form VLA-4 ($\alpha_4\beta_1$) integrin	T cells, monocytes, B cells, NK cells, eosinophils, dendritic cells, thymocytes	Leukocyte adhesion to endothelium and extracellular matrix; binds to VCAM-1 and MAdCAM-1; binds fibronectin and collagens
CD49e	α_5 integrin subunit	Heterodimer of 135 and 25 kD chains; noncovalently linked to CD29 to form VLA-5 (β1 integrin)	T cells; few B cells and monocytes, thymocytes	Adhesion to extracellular matrix; binds fibronectin
CD49f	α_6 integrin subunit	Heterodimer of 125 and 25 kD chains; noncovalently linked to CD29 to form VLA-6 (β1 integrin)	Platelets, megakaryocytes, activated T cells, monocytes	Adhesion to extracellular matrix; binds fibronectin
CD54	ICAM-1	75–114 kD; Ig superfamily	Endothelial cells, T cells, B cells, monocytes, endothelial cells (cytokine inducible)	Cell-cell adhesion; ligand for CD11aCD18 (LFA-1) and CD11bCD18 (Mac-1); receptor for rhinovirus
CD55	Decay-accelerating factor (DAF)	55–70 kD; GPI linked; regulators of complement activation family	Broad	Regulation of complement activation; binds C3b, C4b
CD58	Leukocyte function-associated antigen-3 (LFA-3)	55–70 kD; GPI linked or integral membrane protein; CD2/CD48/CD58 family	Broad	Leukocyte adhesion; binds CD2
CD59	Membrane inhibitor of reactive lysis (MIRL)	18–20 kD; GPI linked; Ly-6 superfamily	Broad	Binds C9; inhibits formation of complement membrane attack complex
CD62E	E-selectin; ELAM-1	115 kD; selectin family	Endothelial cells	Leukocyte-endothelial adhesion
CD62L	L-selectin; LAM-1; MEL-14	74–95 kD; selectin family	B cells, T cells, monocytes, granulocytes, some NK cells	Leukocyte-endothelial adhesion; homing of naive T cells to peripheral lymph nodes
CD62P	P-selectin; gmp140; PADGEM	140 kD; selectin family	Platelets, endothelial cells (present in granules, translocated to cell surface upon activation)	Leukocyte adhesion to endothelium, platelets; binds CD162 (PSGL-1)
CD64	FcγRI	72 kD; Ig superfamily; noncovalently associated with the common FcR γ chain	Monocytes, macrophages, activated neutrophils	High-affinity Fcγ receptor; role in phagocytosis, ADCC, macrophage activation
CD66e	Carcinoembryonic antigen (CEA)	180–220 kD; Ig superfamily; carcinoembryonic antigen (CEA) family	Colonic and other epithelial cells	? Adhesion; clinical marker of carcinoma burden
CD74	Class II MHC invariant (γ) chain; I_i	33, 35, and 41 kD isoforms	B cells, monocytes, macrophage, other class II MHC–expressing cells	Binds to and directs intracellular sorting of newly synthesized class II MHC molecules
CD79a	Igα, MB1	32, 45 kD; forms dimer with CD79β; Ig superfamily; ITAM in cytoplasmic tail	Mature B cells	Required for cell surface expression of and signal transduction by the B cell antigen receptor complex
CD79b	Igβ, B29	37–39 kD; forms dimer with CD79α; Ig superfamily; ITAM in cytoplasmic tail	Mature B cells	Required for cell surface expression of and signal transduction by the B cell antigen receptor complex

CD designation	Common synonyms	Molecular structure, family	Main cellular expression	Known or proposed functions
CD80	B7-1; BB1	60 kD; Ig superfamily	Dendritic cells, activated B cells and macrophages	Costimulator for T lymphocyte activation; ligand for CD28 and CD152 (CTLA-4)
CD81	Target for antiproliferative antigen-1 (TAPA-1)	26 kD; tetraspan (TM4SF)	T cells, B cells, NK cells, dendritic cells, thymocytes, endothelium	B cell activation; forms a coreceptor complex with CD19 and CD21 which delivers signals that synergize with signals from B cell antigen receptor complex
CD86	B7-2	80 kD; Ig superfamily	B cells, monocytes, dendritic cells; some T cells	Costimulator for T lymphocyte activation; ligand for CD28 and CD152 (CTLA-4)
CD88	C5a receptor	43 kD; G protein–coupled, 7-membrane–spanning receptor family	Granulocytes, monocytes, dendritic cells, mast cells	Receptor for C5a complement fragment; role in complement-induced inflammation
CD89	Fcα receptor (FcαR)	55–75 kD; Ig superfamily; noncovalently associated with the common FcR γ chain	Granulocytes, monocytes, macrophages, T cell subset, B cell subset	Binds IgA; mediates IgA-dependent cellular cytotoxicity
CD90	Thy-1	25–35 kD; GPI linked; Ig superfamily	Thymocytes, peripheral T cells (mice), CD34$^+$ hematopoietic progenitor cells, neurons	Marker for T cells; ? role in T cell activation
CD94	Kp43; KIR	43 kD; C-type lectin; on NK cells, covalently assembles with other C-type lectin molecules (NKG2)	NK cells; subset of CD8$^+$ T cells	CD94/NKG2 complex functions as an NK cell inhibitory receptor; binds HLA-E class I MHC molecules
CD95	Fas antigen, APO-1	Homotrimer of 45 kD chains; TNF receptor family	Multiple cell types	Binds Fas ligand; mediates signals leading to activation-induced cell death
CD102	ICAM-2	55–65 kD; Ig superfamily	Endothelial cells, lymphocytes, monocytes, platelets	Ligand for CD11aCD18 (LFA-1); cell-cell adhesion
CD103	HML-1; α_E integrin subunit	Dimer of 150 and 25 kD subunits; noncovalently linked to β_7 integrin subunit to form $\alpha_E\beta_7$ integrin	Intraepithelial lymphocytes, other cell types	Role in T cell homing to and retention in mucosa; binds E-cadherin
CD106	Vascular cell adhesion molecule-1 (VCAM-1); INCAM-110	100–110 kD; Ig superfamily	Endothelial cells, macrophages, follicular dendritic cells, marrow stromal cells	Adhesion; receptor for CD49dCD29 (VLA-4) integrin; role in lymphocyte trafficking, activation; role in hematopoiesis
CD150	Signaling lymphocyte activation molecule (SLAM); IPO-3	75–95 kD; Ig superfamily	Thymocytes, activated lymphocytes, dendritic cells, endothelial cells	Regulation of B cell–T cell interactions and proliferative signals in B lymphocytes; binds itself as a self ligand
CD152	Cytotoxic T lymphocyte-associated protein-4 (CTLA-4)	33, 50 kD; Ig superfamily	Activated T lymphocytes	Inhibitory signaling in T cells; binds CD80 (B7-1) and CD86 (B7-2) on antigen-presenting cells
CD153	CD30 ligand (CD30L)	40 kD; TNF family	Activated T cells, resting B cells, granulocytes, macrophages, thymocytes	Role in activation-induced cell death of CD8$^+$ T cells; binds to CD30
CD154	CD40 ligand (CD40L); TNF-related activation protein (TRAP); gp39	Homotrimer of 32–39 kD chains; TNF receptor family	Activated CD4$^+$ T cells	Activates B cells, macrophages, and endothelial cells; ligand for CD40
CD158	Killer Ig receptor (KIR)	50, 58 kD; Ig superfamily; killer Ig-like receptor (KIR) family; ITIMS in cytoplasmic tail	NK cells, T cell subsets	Inhibition or activation of NK cells upon interaction with the appropriate class I HLA molecules
CD159a	NKG2A	43 kD; C-type lectin; forms heterodimer with CD94	NK cells, T cell subsets	Inhibition or activation of NK cells upon interaction with the appropriate class I HLA molecules

CD designation	Common synonyms	Molecular structure, family	Main cellular expression	Known or proposed functions
CD159c	NKG2C	40 kD; C-type lectin; forms heterodimer with CD94	NK cells	Activation of NK cells upon interaction with the appropriate class I HLA molecules
CD162	PSGL-1	Homodimer of 120 kD chains; sialomucin	T cells, monocytes, granulocytes, some B cells	Ligand for selectins (CD62P, CD62L); adhesion of leukocytes to endothelium
CD247	Zeta chain; TCR ζ	17 kD; ITAMs in cytoplasmic tail	T cells, NK cells	Signaling chain of TCR and NK cell–activating receptors
CD273	B7-DC, PD-L2	25 kD; Ig superfamily; B7 costimulator family	Dendritic cells, monocytes, macrophages	Binds PD-1; inhibition of T cell activation
CD274	B7-H1, PD-L1	33 kD; Ig superfamily; B7 costimulator family	Leukocytes	Binds PD-1; inhibition of T cell activation
CD275	B7-H2, ICOS ligand, B7-RP1	60 kD; Ig superfamily; B7 costimulator family	B cells, dendritic cells, monocytes	Binds ICOS (CD278); T cell costimulation
CD276	B7-H3	40–45 kD; Ig superfamily; B7 costimulator family	Dendritic cells, monocytes, activated T cells	T cell costimulation
CD278	ICOS, AILIM	55–60 kD; Ig superfamily; CD28 costimulator family	Activated T cells	Binds ICOS-L (CD275); T cell costimulation
CD279	PD1, SLEB2	55 kD; Ig superfamily; CD28 costimulator family	Activated T cells, activated B cells	Binds B7-H1 (CD274) and B7-DC (CD273); regulation of T cell activation
CD280	ENDO180, UPARAP	180 kD; C-type lectin	Macrophages, chondrocytes, fibroblasts, endothelial cells	Mannose receptor; endocytic pattern recognition of innate immunity receptor
CD314	NKG2D, KLR	42 kD; C-type lectin	NK cells, activated $CD8^+$ T cells, NK1.1 T cells, some myeloid cells	Binds MHC class I, MICA, MICB, Rae1 and ULBP4; NK cell and CTL activation

* The lowercase letters affixed to some CD numbers refer to complex CD molecules that are encoded by multiple genes or that belong to families of structurally related proteins. For instance, CD1a, CD1b, CD1c, and CD1d are structurally related but distinct forms of a β_2 microglobulin-associated nonpolymorphic protein.

Abbreviations: ADCC, antibody-dependent cell-mediated cytotoxicity; GP, glycoprotein; ICAM, intercellular adhesion molecule; Ig, immunoglobulin; IL, interleukin; ITAM, immunoreceptor tyrosine-based activation motif; ITIM, immunoreceptor tyrosine-based inhibition motif; kD, kilodalton; LFA, lymphocyte function-associated antigen; LPS, lipopolysaccharide; MHC, major histocompatibility complex; NK, natural killer; GPI, glycophosphatidylinositol; VCAM, vascular cell adhesion molecule; VLA, very late antigen.

Appendix III

LABORATORY TECHNIQUES COMMONLY USED IN IMMUNOLOGY

Many laboratory techniques that are routine in research and clinical settings are based on the use of antibodies. In addition, many of the techniques of modern molecular biology have provided invaluable information about the immune system. We have mentioned these techniques often throughout the book. In this appendix, we describe the principles underlying some of the most commonly used laboratory methods in immunology. In addition, we summarize how B and T lymphocyte responses are studied using laboratory techniques. Details of how to carry out various assays may be found in laboratory manuals.

LABORATORY METHODS USING ANTIBODIES

The exquisite specificity of antibodies for particular antigens makes antibodies valuable reagents for detecting, purifying, and quantitating antigens. Because antibodies can be produced against virtually any type of macromolecule and small chemical, antibody-based techniques may be used to study virtually any type of molecule in solution or in cells. The method for producing monoclonal antibodies (see Chapter 4, Box 4–1) has greatly increased our ability to generate antibodies of almost any desired specificity. Historically, many of the uses of antibody depended on the ability of antibody and specific antigen to form large immune complexes, either in solution or in gels, that could be detected by various optical methods. These methods were of great importance in early studies but have now been replaced almost entirely by simpler methods based on immobilized antibodies or antigens.

Quantitation of Antigen by Immunoassays

Immunologic methods of quantifying antigen concentration provide exquisite sensitivity and specificity and have become standard techniques for both research and clinical applications. All modern immunochemical methods of quantitation are based on having a pure antigen or antibody whose quantity can be measured by an indicator molecule. When the indicator molecule is labeled with a radioisotope, as first introduced by Rosalyn Yalow and colleagues, it may be quantified by instruments that detect radioactive decay events; the assay is called a **radioimmunoassay (RIA).** When the

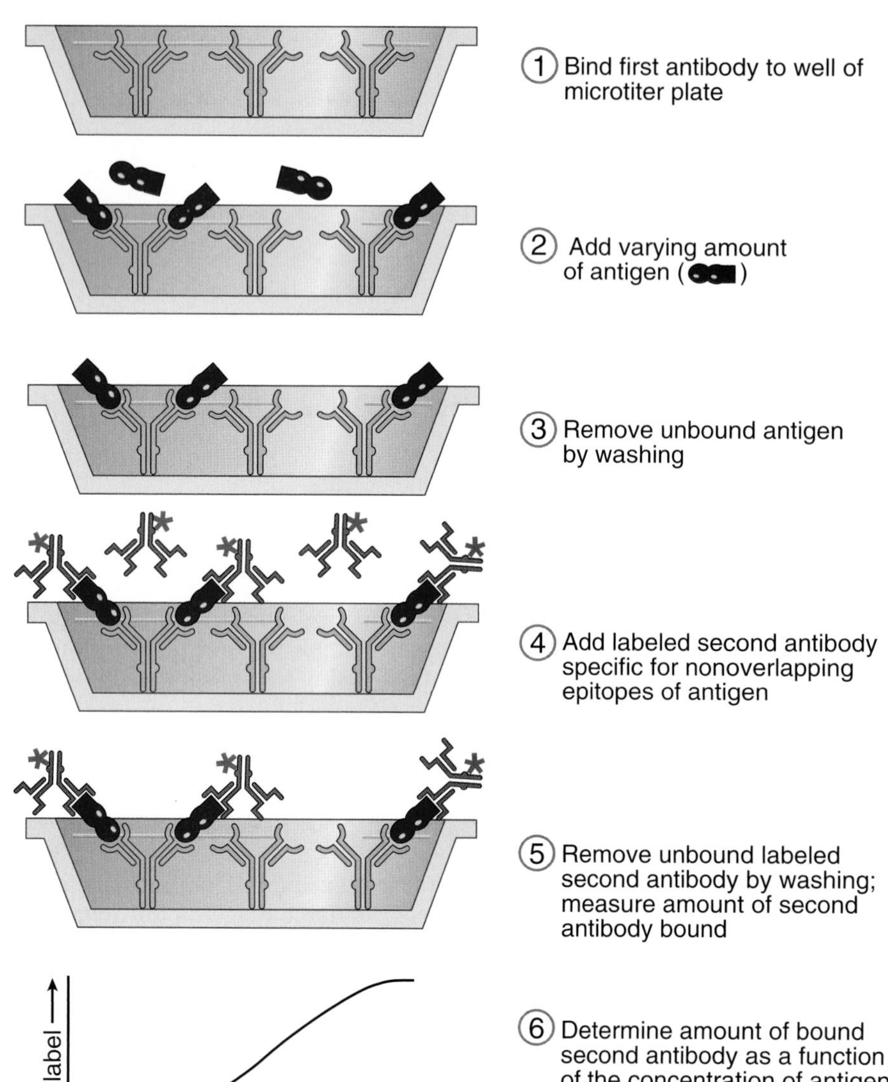
1 Bind first antibody to well of microtiter plate
2 Add varying amount of antigen ( )
3 Remove unbound antigen by washing
4 Add labeled second antibody specific for nonoverlapping epitopes of antigen
5 Remove unbound labeled second antibody by washing; measure amount of second antibody bound
6 Determine amount of bound second antibody as a function of the concentration of antigen added (construction of a standard curve)
Bound label
Concentration of antigen

FIGURE A–1 Sandwich enzyme-linked immunosorbent assay or radioimmunoassay. A fixed amount of one immobilized antibody is used to capture an antigen. The binding of a second, labeled antibody that recognizes a nonoverlapping determinant on the antigen will increase as the concentration of antigen increases and thus allow quantification of the antigen.

indicator molecule is covalently coupled to an enzyme, it may be quantified by determining with a spectrophotometer the rate at which the enzyme converts a clear substrate to a colored product; the assay is called an **enzyme-linked immunosorbent assay (ELISA).** Several variations of RIA and ELISA exist, but the most commonly used version is the sandwich assay (Fig. A–1). The sandwich assay uses two different antibodies reactive with different epitopes on the antigen whose concentration needs to be determined. A fixed quantity of one antibody is attached to a series of replicate solid supports, such as plastic microtiter wells. Test solutions containing antigen at an unknown concentration or a series of standard solutions with known concentrations of antigen are added to the wells and allowed to bind. Unbound antigen is removed by washing, and the second antibody, which is enzyme linked or radiolabeled, is allowed to bind. The antigen serves as a bridge, so the more antigen in the test or standard solutions, the more enzyme-linked or radiolabeled second antibody will bind. The results from the standard solutions are used to construct a binding curve for second antibody as a function of antigen concentration, from which the quantities of antigen in the test solutions may be inferred. When this test is performed with two monoclonal antibodies, it is essential that these antibodies see nonoverlapping determinants on the antigen; otherwise, the second antibody cannot bind.

In an important clinical variant of immunobinding assays, samples from patients may be tested for the presence of antibodies that are specific for a microbial antigen (e.g., antibodies reactive with proteins from human immunodeficiency virus [HIV] or hepatitis B virus) as indicators of infection. In this case, a saturating quantity of antigen is added to replicate wells containing plate-bound antibody, or the antigen is attached directly to the plate, and serial dilutions of the patient's serum are then allowed to bind. The amount of the patient's antibody bound to the immobilized antigen is determined by use of an enzyme-linked or radiolabeled second antihuman immunoglobulin (Ig) antibody.

Purification and Identification of Proteins

Antibodies can be used to purify proteins from solutions and to identify and characterize proteins. Two commonly used methods to purify proteins are immunoprecipitation and affinity chromatography. Western blotting is a widely used technique to determine the presence and size of a protein in a biologic sample.

Immunoprecipitation and Affinity Chromatography

Immunoprecipitation is a technique in which an antibody specific for one protein antigen in a mixture of proteins is used to isolate the specific antigen from the mixture (Fig. A–2A). In most modern procedures, the antibody is attached to a solid-phase particle (e.g., an agarose bead) either by direct chemical coupling or indi-

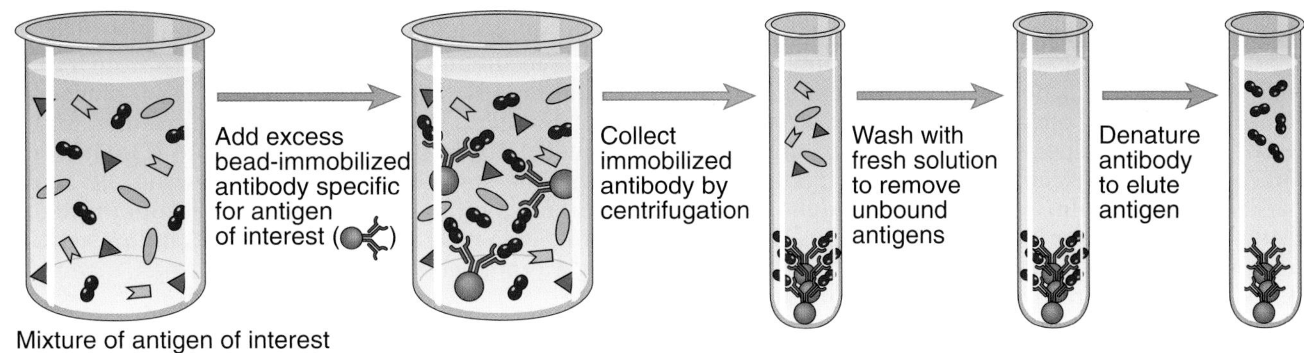
A Immunoprecipitation
Add excess bead-immobilized antibody specific for antigen of interest ( )
Collect immobilized antibody by centrifugation
Wash with fresh solution to remove unbound antigens
Denature antibody to elute antigen
Mixture of antigen of interest ( ) with other antigens

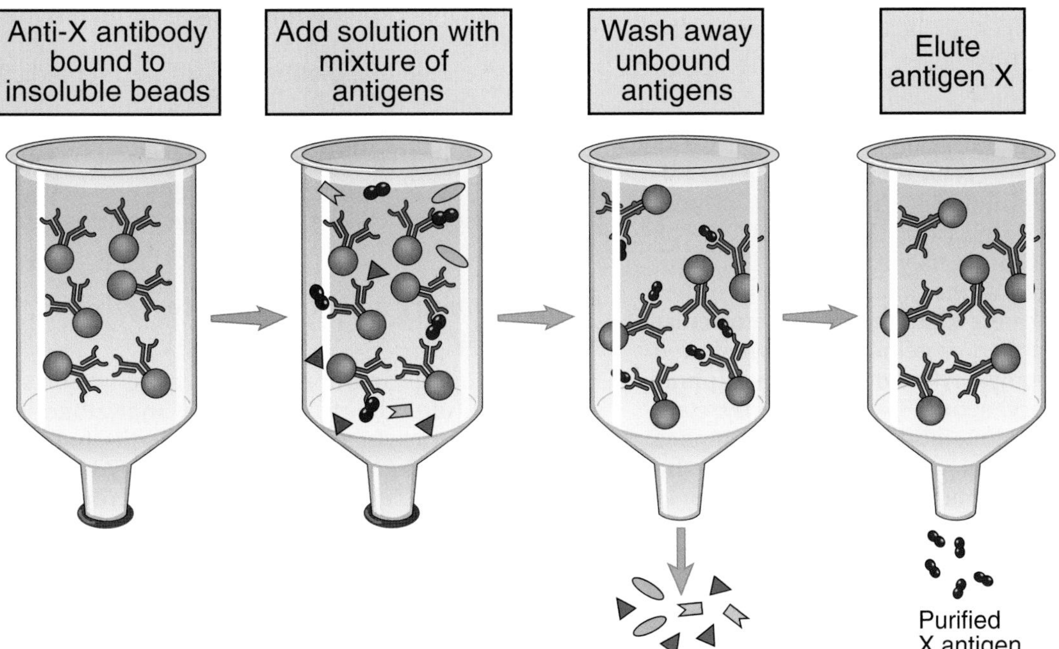
B Affinity chromatography
Anti-X antibody bound to insoluble beads
Add solution with mixture of antigens
Wash away unbound antigens
Elute antigen X
Purified X antigen

FIGURE A–2 Isolation of an antigen by immunoprecipitation or affinity chromatography. A. A particular antigen can be purified from a mixture of antigens in serum or other solutions by adding antibodies specific to the antigen, which are bound to insoluble beads. Unbound antigens are then washed away, and the desired antigen is recovered by changing the pH or ionic strength of the solution so that the affinity of antibody-antigen binding is lowered. Immunoprecipitation can be used as a means of purification, as a means of quantification, or as a means of identification of an antigen. Antigens purified by immunoprecipitation are often analyzed by sodium dodecyl sulfate–polyacrylamide gel electrophoresis. B. Affinity chromatography is based on the same principle as immunoprecipitation, except that the antibody is fixed to an insoluble matrix or beads, usually in a column. The method is often used to isolate soluble antigens (shown) or antibodies specific for an immobilized antigen.

rectly. Indirect coupling may be achieved by means of an attached anti-antibody, such as rabbit antimouse Ig antibody, or by means of some other protein with specific affinity for the Fc portion of Ig molecules, such as protein A or protein G from bacteria. After the antibody-coated beads are incubated with the solution of antigen, unbound molecules are separated from the bead-antibody-antigen complex by washing. Specific antigen is then released (eluted) from the antibody by changing the pH or by other solvent conditions that reduce the affinity of binding. The purified antigen can then be analyzed by conventional chemical techniques. Alternatively, a small amount of radiolabeled protein can be purified and the characteristics of the macromolecule inferred from the behavior of the radioactive label in analytical separation techniques, such as sodium dodecyl sulfate–polyacrylamide gel electrophoresis (SDS-PAGE) or isoelectric focusing.

Affinity chromatography, like immunoprecipitation, uses antibodies attached to an insoluble support to remove and thereby purify antigens from a solution (Fig. A–2B). Antibodies specific for the desired antigen are attached to a solid support, such as agarose beads packed into a column, either by direct coupling or indirectly, as described for immunoprecipitation. A complex mixture of antigens is passed through the beads to allow the antigen that is recognized by the antibody to bind. Unbound molecules are washed away, and the bound antigen is eluted by changing the pH or by exposure to a chemical that breaks the antigen-antibody bonds. The same method may be used to purify antibodies from culture supernatants or natural fluids, such as serum, by first attaching the antigen to beads and passing the supernatants or serum through.

Western Blotting

Western blotting (Fig. A–3) is used to determine the relative quantity and the molecular weight of a protein within a mixture of proteins or other molecules. The mixture is first subjected to analytical separation, typically by SDS-PAGE, so that the final positions of different proteins in the gel are a function of their molecular size. The array of separated proteins is then transferred from the separating polyacrylamide gel to a support membrane by capillary action (blotting) or by electrophoresis such that the membrane acquires a replica of the array of separated macromolecules present in the gel. SDS is displaced from the protein during the transfer process, and native antigenic determinants are often regained as the protein refolds. The position of the protein antigen on the membrane can then be detected by binding of labeled antibody specific for that protein, thus providing information about antigen size and quantity. If radiolabeled antibody probes are used, the proteins on the blot are visualized by autoradiographic exposure of film. More recently, antibody probes are labeled with enzymes that generate chemiluminescent signals and leave images on photographic film. The sensitivity and specificity of this technique can be increased by starting with immunoprecipitated proteins instead of crude protein mixtures. This sequential technique is especially useful for detecting protein-protein interactions. For example, the physical association of two different proteins in the membrane of a lymphocyte can be established by immunoprecipitating a membrane extract by use of an antibody specific for one of the proteins and probing a Western blot of the immunoprecipitate by use of a labeled antibody specific for the second protein that may have been co-immunoprecipitated along with the first protein. A variation of the Western blot technique is routinely used to detect the presence of anti-HIV antibodies in patients' sera. In this case, a defined mixture of HIV proteins is separated by SDS-PAGE and blotted onto a membrane, and the membrane is incubated with dilutions of the test serum. The blot is then probed with a second labeled antihuman Ig to detect the presence of HIV-specific antibodies that were in the serum and bound to the HIV proteins.

The technique of transferring proteins from a gel to a membrane is called Western blotting as a biochemist's joke. Southern is the last name of the scientist who first blotted DNA from a separating gel to a membrane, a technique since called Southern blotting. By analogy, Northern blotting was applied to the technique of transferring RNA from a gel to a membrane, and Western blotting was applied to protein transfer.

Labeling and Detection of Antigens in Cells and Tissues

Antibodies specific for antigens expressed on or in particular cell types are commonly used to identify these cells in tissues or cell suspensions and to separate these cells from mixed populations. In these methods, the antibody can be radiolabeled, enzyme linked, or, most commonly, fluorescently labeled, and a detection system is used that can identify the bound antibody. Antibodies attached to magnetic beads can be used to physically isolate cells expressing specific antigens.

Flow Cytometry and Fluorescence-Activated Cell Sorting

The tissue lineage, maturation stage, or activation status of a cell can often be determined by analyzing the cell surface or intracellular expression of different molecules. This technique is commonly done by staining the cell with fluorescently labeled probes that are specific for those molecules and measuring the quantity of fluorescence emitted by the cell (Fig. A–4). The flow cytometer is a specialized instrument that can detect fluorescence on individual cells in a suspension and thereby determine the number of cells expressing the molecule to which a fluorescent probe binds. Suspensions of cells are incubated with fluorescently labeled probes, and the amount of probe bound by each cell in the population is measured by passing the cells one at a time through a fluorimeter with a laser-generated incident beam. The relative amounts of a particular molecule on different cell populations can be compared by staining each pop-

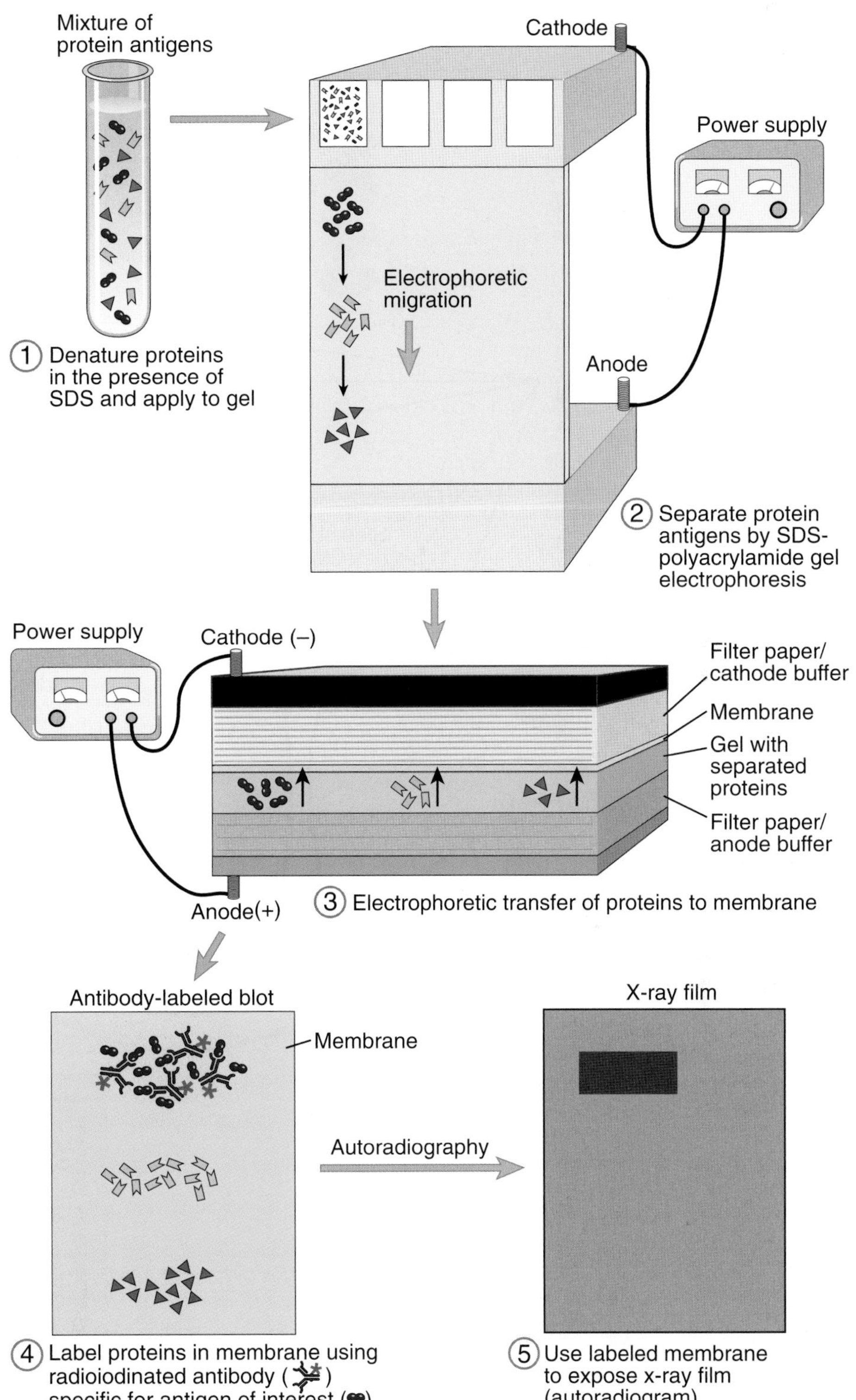
Mixture of protein antigens
Cathode
Power supply
Electrophoretic migration
Anode
1 Denature proteins in the presence of SDS and apply to gel
2 Separate protein antigens by SDS-polyacrylamide gel electrophoresis
Power supply
Cathode (–)
Filter paper/ cathode buffer
Membrane
Gel with separated proteins
Filter paper/ anode buffer
Anode(+)
3 Electrophoretic transfer of proteins to membrane
Antibody-labeled blot
Membrane
Autoradiography
X-ray film
4 Label proteins in membrane using radioiodinated antibody ( ) specific for antigen of interest ( )
5 Use labeled membrane to expose x-ray film (autoradiogram)

FIGURE A–3 Characterization of antigens by Western blotting. Protein antigens, separated by sodium dodecyl sulfate (SDS)-polyacrylamide gel electrophoresis and transferred to a membrane, can be labeled with radioactive or (not shown) enzyme-coupled antibodies. Analysis of an antigen by Western blotting provides information similar to that obtained from immunoprecipitation followed by polyacrylamide gel electrophoresis. Some antibodies work only in one or the other technique.

ulation with the same probe and determining the amount of fluorescence emitted. In preparation for flow cytometric analysis, cell suspensions are stained with the fluorescent probes of choice. Most often, these probes are fluorochrome-labeled antibodies specific for a cell surface molecule. Alternatively, cytoplasmic molecules can be stained by temporarily permeabilizing cells and permitting the labeled antibodies to enter through the plasma membrane. In addition to antibodies, various fluorescent indicators of cytoplasmic ion concentrations and reduction-oxidation potential can be detected by flow cytometry. Cell cycle studies can be performed by flow cytometric analysis of cells stained with fluorescent DNA-binding probes such as propidium

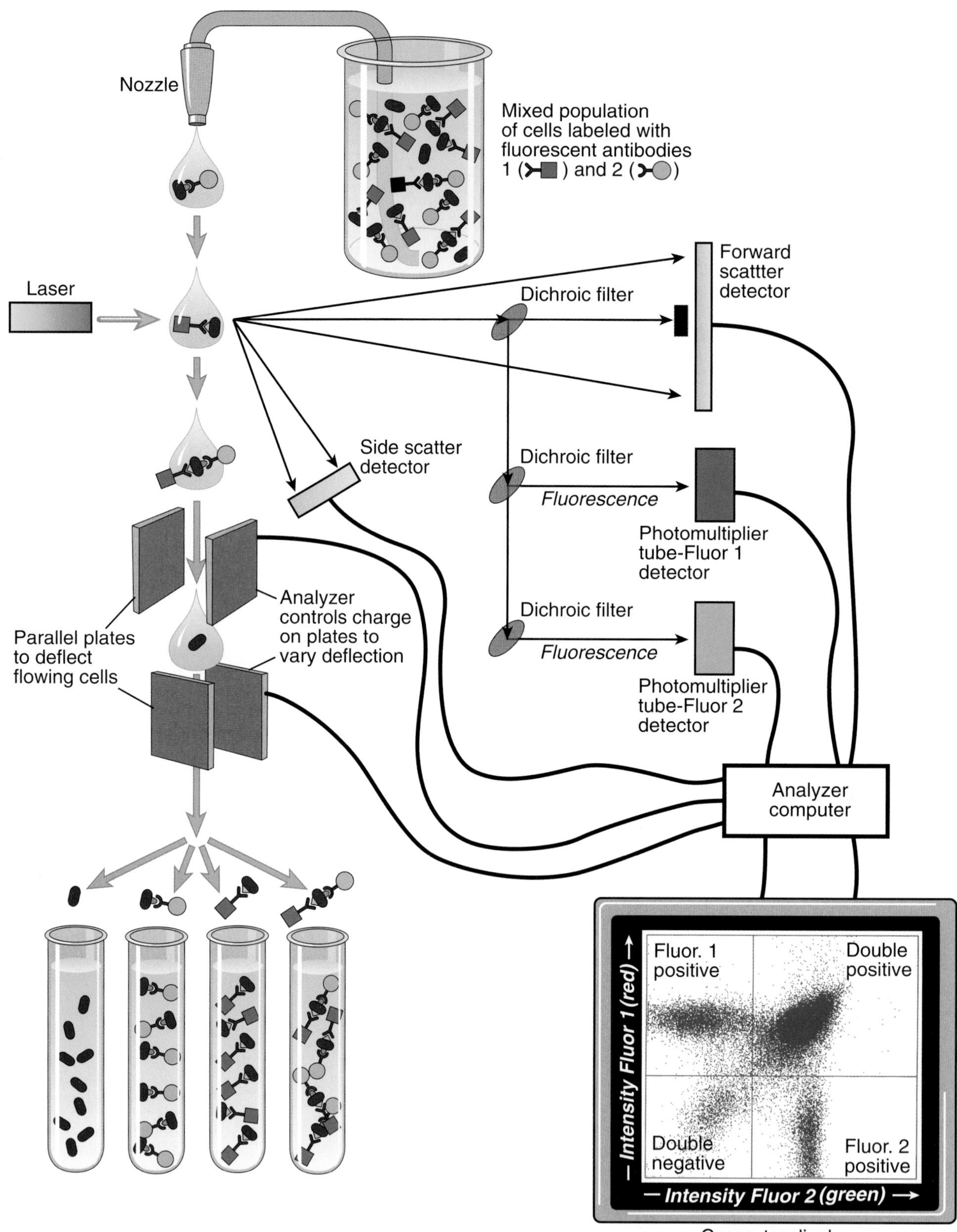

FIGURE A–4 Principle of flow cytometry and fluorescence-activated cell sorting. The incident laser beam is of a designated wavelength, and the light that emerges from the sample is analyzed for forward and side scatter as well as fluorescent light of two or more wavelengths that depend on the fluorochrome labels attached to the antibodies. The separation depicted here is based on two antigenic markers (two-color sorting). Modern instruments can routinely analyze and separate cell populations on the basis of three or more different colored probes.

iodide. Apoptotic cells can be identified using fluorescent probes, such as Annexin V, that bind to abnormally exposed phospholipids on the surface of the dying cells. Modern flow cytometers can routinely detect three or more different-colored fluorescent signals, each attached to a different antibody or other probe. This technique permits simultaneous analysis of the expression of many different combinations of molecules by a cell. In addition to detecting fluorescent signals, flow cytometers also measure the forward and side light-scattering properties of cells, which reflect cell size and internal complexity, respectively. This information is often used to distinguish different cell types. For example, compared with lymphocytes, neutrophils cause greater side scatter because of their cytoplasmic granules, and monocytes cause greater forward scatter because of their size.

Purification of Cells

A fluorescent-activated cell sorter (FACS) is an adaptation of the flow cyotmeter that allows one to separate cell populations according to which and how much fluorescent probe they bind. This technique is accomplished by differentially deflecting the cells with electromagnetic fields whose strength and direction are varied according to the measured intensity of the fluorescent signal (Fig. A–4). The cells may be labeled with fluorescently tagged antibodies ex vivo, or, in the case of experimental animal studies, labeling may be accomplished in vivo by expression of transgenes that encode fluorescent proteins, such as green fluorescent protein (GFP). (Transgenic technology is described later in this appendix.)

Another commonly used technique to purify cells with a particular phenotype relies on antibodies that are attached to magnetic beads. These "immunomagnetic reagents" will bind to certain cells, depending on the specificity of the antibody used, and the bound cells can then be pulled out of suspension using a strong magnet.

Immunofluorescence and Immunohistochemistry

Antibodies can be used to identify the anatomic distribution of an antigen within a tissue or within compartments of a cell. To do so, the tissue or cell is incubated with an antibody that is labeled with a fluorochrome or enzyme, and the position of the label, determined with a suitable microscope, is used to infer the position of the antigen. In the earliest version of this method, called immunofluorescence, the antibody was labeled with a fluorescent dye and allowed to bind to a monolayer of cells or to a frozen section of a tissue. The stained cells or tissues were examined with a fluorescence microscope to locate the antibody. Although sensitive, the fluorescence microscope is not an ideal tool for identifying the detailed structures of the cell or tissue because of a low signal-to-noise ratio. This problem has been overcome by new technologies including confocal microscopy, which uses optical sectioning technology to filter out unfocused fluorescent light, and two-photon microscopy, which prevents out-of-focus light from forming. Alternatively, antibodies may be coupled to enzymes that convert colorless substrates to colored insoluble substances that precipitate at the position of the enzyme. A conventional light microscope may then be used to localize the antibody in a stained cell or tissue. The most common variant of this method uses the enzyme horseradish peroxidase, and the method is commonly referred to as the immunoperoxidase technique. Another commonly used enzyme is alkaline phosphatase. Different antibodies coupled to different enzymes may be used in conjunction to produce simultaneous two-color localizations of different antigens. In other variations, antibody can be coupled to an electron-dense probe such as colloidal gold, and the location of antibody can be determined subcellularly by means of an electron microscope, a technique called immunoelectron microscopy. Different-sized gold particles have been used for simultaneous localization of different antigens at the ultrastructural level.

In all immunomicroscopic methods, signals may be enhanced by use of sandwich techniques. For example, instead of attaching horseradish peroxidase to a specific mouse antibody directed against the antigen of interest, it can be attached to a second anti-antibody (e.g., rabbit antimouse Ig antibody) that is used to bind to the first, unlabeled antibody. When the label is attached directly to the specific, primary antibody, the method is referred to as direct; when the label is attached to a secondary or even tertiary antibody, the method is indirect. In some cases, molecules other than antibody can be used in indirect methods. For example, staphylococcal protein A, which binds to IgG, or avidin, which binds to primary antibodies labeled with biotin, can be coupled to fluorochromes or enzymes.

Measurement of Antigen-Antibody Interactions

In many situations, it is important to know the affinity of an antibody for an antigen. For example, the usefulness of a monoclonal antibody as an experimental or therapeutic reagent depends on its affinity. Antibody affinities for antigen can be measured directly for small antigens (e.g., haptens) by a method called **equilibrium dialysis** (Fig. A–5). In this method, a solution of antibody is confined within a "semipermeable" membrane of porous cellulose and immersed in a solution containing the antigen. (Semipermeable in this context means that small molecules, such as antigen, can pass freely through the membrane pores but that macromolecules, such as antibody, cannot.) If no antibody is present within the membrane-bound compartment, the antigen in the bathing solution enters until the concentration of antigen within the membrane-bound compartment becomes exactly the same as that outside. Another way to view the system is that at dynamic equilibrium, antigen enters and leaves the membrane-bound compartment at exactly the same rate. However, when antibody is present inside the membrane, the net amount of

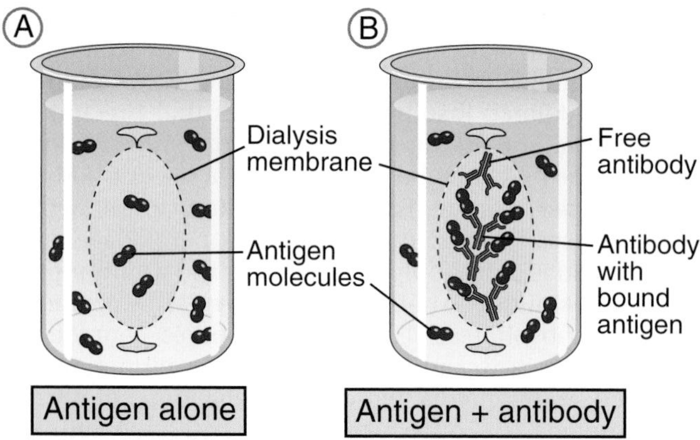

FIGURE A–5 Analysis of antigen-antibody binding by equilibrium dialysis. In the presence of antibody (B), the amount of antigen within the dialysis membrane is increased compared with the absence of antibody (A). As described in the text, this difference, caused by antibody binding of antigen, can be used to measure the affinity of the antibody for the antigen. This experiment can be performed only when the antigen is a small molecule (e.g., a hapten) capable of freely crossing the dialysis membrane.

antigen inside the membrane at equilibrium increases by the quantity that is bound to antibody. This phenomenon occurs because only unbound antigen can diffuse across the membrane, and at equilibrium, it is the unbound concentration of antigen that must be identical inside and outside the membrane. The extent of the increase in antigen inside the membrane depends on the antigen concentration, on the antibody concentration, and on the dissociation constant (K_d) of the binding interaction. By measuring the antigen and antibody concentrations, by spectroscopy or by other means, K_d can be calculated.

An alternative way to determine K_d is by measuring the rates of antigen-antibody complex formation and dissociation. These rates depend, in part, on the concentrations of antibody and antigen and on the affinity of the interaction. All parameters except the concentrations can be summarized as rate constants, and both the **on-rate constant** (K_{on}) and the **off-rate constant** (K_{off}) can be calculated experimentally by determining the concentrations and the actual rates of association or dissociation, respectively. The ratio of K_{off}/K_{on} allows one to cancel out all the parameters not related to affinity and is exactly equal to the dissociation constant K_d. Thus, one can measure K_d at equilibrium by equilibrium dialysis or calculate K_d from rate constants measured under nonequilibrium conditions.

Transgenic Mice and Targeted Gene Knockouts

Two important methods for studying the functional effects of specific gene products in vivo are the creation of transgenic mice that overexpress a particular gene in a defined tissue and the creation of gene knockout mice, in which a targeted disruption is used to ablate the function of a particular gene. Both techniques have been widely used to analyze many biologic phenomena, including the maturation, activation, and tolerance of lymphocytes.

To create transgenic mice, foreign DNA sequences, called transgenes, are introduced into the pronuclei of fertilized mouse eggs, and the eggs are implanted into the oviducts of pseudopregnant females. Usually, if a few hundred copies of a gene are injected into pronuclei, about 25% of the mice that are born are transgenic. One to 50 copies of the transgene insert in tandem into a random site of breakage in a chromosome and are subsequently inherited as a simple mendelian trait. Because integration usually occurs before DNA replication, most (about 75%) of the transgenic pups carry the transgene in all their cells, including germ cells. In most cases, integration of the foreign DNA does not disrupt endogenous gene function. Also, each founder mouse carrying the transgene is a heterozygote, from which homozygous lines can be bred.

The great value of transgenic technology is that it can be used to express genes in particular tissues by attaching coding sequences of the gene to regulatory sequences that normally drive the expression of genes selectively in that tissue. For instance, lymphoid promoters and enhancers can be used to overexpress genes, such as rearranged antigen receptor genes, in lymphocytes, and the insulin promoter can be used to express genes in the β cells of pancreatic islets. Examples of the utility of these methods for studying the immune system are mentioned in many chapters of this book. Transgenes can also be expressed under the control of promoter elements that respond to drugs or hormones, such as tetracycline or estrogens. In these cases, transcription of the transgene can be controlled at will by administration of the inducing agent.

A powerful method for developing animal models of single-gene disorders, and the most definitive way of establishing the obligatory function of a gene in vivo, is the creation of knockout mice by targeted mutation or disruption of the gene. This technique relies on the phenomenon of homologous recombination. If an exogenous gene is inserted into a cell, for instance, by electroporation, it can integrate randomly into the cell's genome. However, if the gene contains sequences that are homologous to an endogenous gene, it will preferentially recombine with and replace endogenous sequences. To select for cells that have undergone homologous recombination, a drug-based selection strategy is used. The fragment of homologous DNA to be inserted into a cell is placed in a vector typically containing a neomycin resistance gene and a viral thymidine kinase *(tk)* gene (Fig. A–6A). This targeting vector is constructed in such a way that the neomycin resistance gene is always inserted into the chromosomal DNA, but the *tk* gene is lost whenever homologous recombination (as opposed to random insertion) occurs. The vector is introduced into cells, and the cells are grown in neomycin and ganciclovir, a drug that is metabolized by thymidine kinase to generate a lethal product. Cells in which the gene is integrated randomly will be resistant to neomycin but will be killed by ganciclovir, whereas cells in which homologous recombination has occurred will be resistant to both drugs because the *tk* gene will not be incorporated. This positive-negative selection ensures that the inserted gene in surviving cells has undergone homologous recombination with endogenous sequences. The presence of the inserted DNA in the middle of an endogenous gene usually disrupts the coding sequences and ablates expression or function of that gene. In addition, targeting vectors can be designed such that homologous recombination will lead to the deletion of one or more exons of the endogenous gene.

To generate a mouse carrying a targeted gene disruption or mutation, a targeting vector is used to first disrupt the gene in a murine embryonic stem (ES) cell line. ES cells are pluripotent cells derived from mouse embryos that can be propagated and induced to differentiate in culture or that can be incorporated into a mouse blastocyst, which may be implanted in a pseudopregnant mother and carried to term. Importantly, the progeny of the ES cells develop normally into mature tissues that will express the exogenous genes that have been transfected into the ES cells. Thus, the targeting vector designed to disrupt a particular gene is inserted into ES cells, and colonies in which homologous recombination has occurred (on one chromosome) are selected with drugs, as described before (Fig. A–6B). The presence of the desired recombination is verified by analysis of DNA with techniques such as Southern blot hybridization or PCR. The selected ES cells are injected into blastocysts, which are implanted into pseudopregnant females. Mice that develop will be chimeric for a heterozygous disruption or mutation, that is, some of the tissues will be derived from the ES cells and others from the remainder of the normal blastocyst. The germ cells are also usually chimeric, but because these cells are haploid, only some will contain the chromosome copy with the disrupted (mutated) gene. If chimeric mice are mated with normal (wild-type) animals and either sperm or eggs containing the chromosome with the mutation fuse with the wild-type partner, all cells in the offspring derived from such a zygote will be heterozygous for the mutation (so-called germline transmission). Such heterozygous mice can be mated to yield animals that will be homozygous for the mutation with a frequency that is predictable by simple mendelian segregation. Such knockout mice are deficient in expression of the targeted gene.

Homologous recombination can also be used to replace a normal gene sequence with another gene, thereby creating a knock-in mouse strain. In a sense, knock-in mice are mice carrying a transgene at a defined site in the genome rather than in a random site as in conventional transgenic mice. This strategy is used when it is desirable to have the expression of the transgene regulated by certain endogenous DNA sequences, such as a particular enhancer or promoter region. In this case, the targeting vector contains an exogenous gene encoding a desired product as well as sequences homologous to an endogenous gene that are needed to target the site of recombination.

Although the conventional gene-targeting strategy has proved to be of great usefulness in immunology research, the approach has some potentially significant

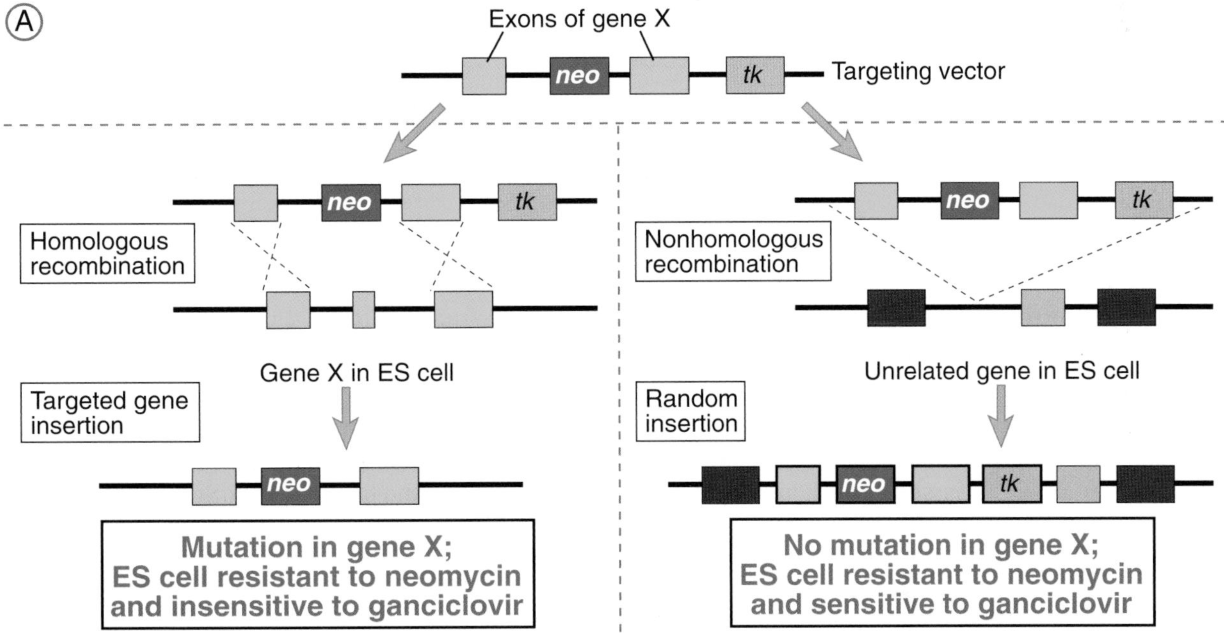

FIGURE A–6 Generation of gene knockout. A. The disruption of gene X in an embryonic stem (ES) cell is accomplished by homologous recombination. A population of ES cells is transfected with a targeting vector that contains sequences homologous to two exons of gene X flanking a neomycin resistance *(neo)* gene. The *neo* gene replaces or disrupts one of the exons of gene X on homologous recombination. The thymidine kinase *(tk)* gene in the vector will be inserted into the genome only if random, nonhomologous recombination occurs.

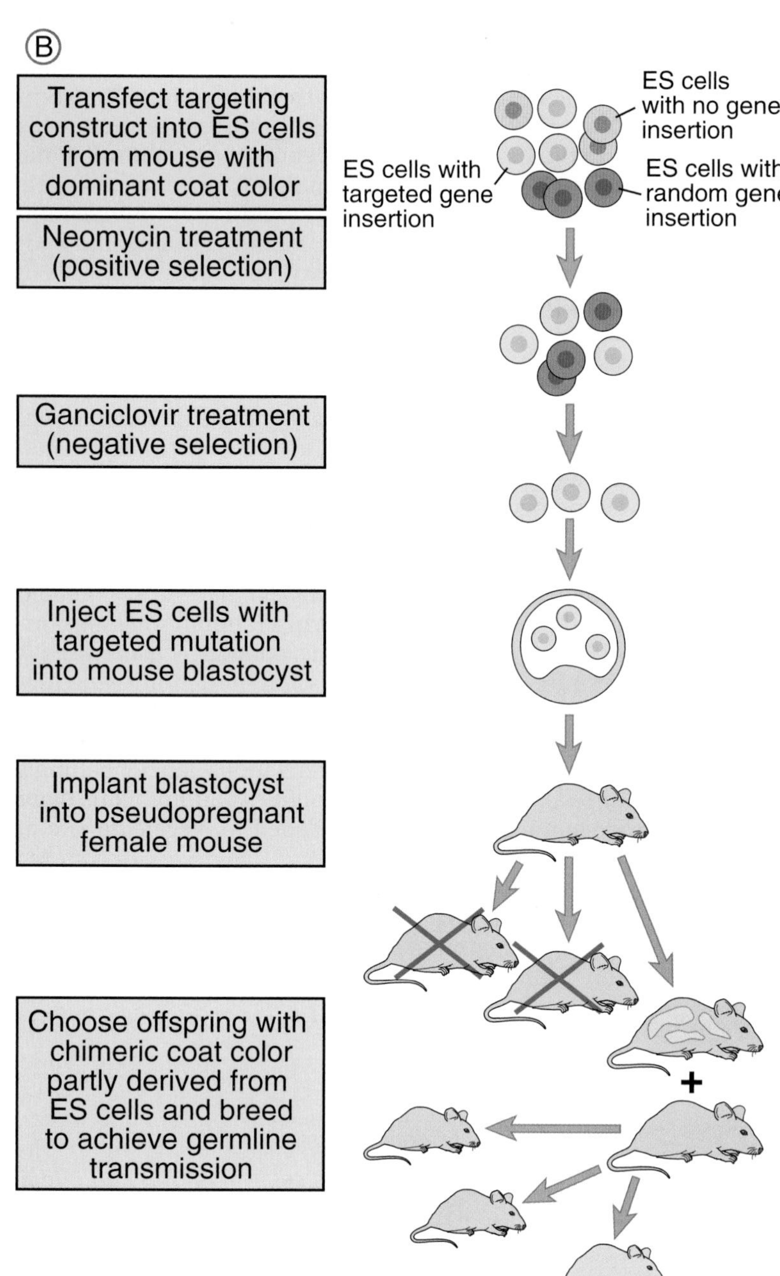
B
Transfect targeting construct into ES cells from mouse with dominant coat color
Neomycin treatment (positive selection)
ES cells with no gene insertion
ES cells with targeted gene insertion
ES cells with random gene insertion
Ganciclovir treatment (negative selection)
Inject ES cells with targeted mutation into mouse blastocyst
Implant blastocyst into pseudopregnant female mouse
Choose offspring with chimeric coat color partly derived from ES cells and breed to achieve germline transmission
+

FIGURE A–6—Cont'd B. The ES cells that were transfected by the targeting vector are selected by neomycin and ganciclovir so that only those cells with targeted insertion (homologous recombination) survive. These cells are then injected into a blastocyst, which is then implanted into the uterus of a pseudopregnant mouse. A chimeric mouse will develop in which some of the tissues are derived from the ES cell carrying the targeted mutation in gene X. These chimeric mice are identified by a mixed-color coat, including the color of the mouse strain from which the ES cells were derived and the color of the mouse strain from which the blastocyst was derived. If the mutation is present in germ cells, it can be propagated by further breeding.

drawbacks. First, the mutation of one gene during development may be compensated for by altered expression of other gene products, and therefore the function of the targeted gene may be obscured. Second, in a conventional gene knockout mouse, the importance of a gene in only one tissue or at only one time during development cannot be easily assessed. Third, a functional selection marker gene, such as the neomycin resistance gene, is permanently introduced into the animal genome, and this alteration may have unpredictable results on the phenotype of the animal. An important refinement of gene knockout technology that can overcome many of these drawbacks takes advantage of the bacteriophage-derived Cre/*loxP* recombination system. The Cre enzyme is a DNA recombinase that recognizes a 34-bp sequence motif called *loxP,* and the enzyme mediates the deletion of gene segments flanked by two *loxP* sites in the same orientation. To generate mice with *loxP*-tagged genes, targeting vectors are constructed with one *loxP* site flanking the neomycin resistance gene at one end and a second *loxP* site flanking the sequences homologous to the target at the other end. These vectors are transfected into ES cells, and mice carrying the *loxP*-flanked but still functional target gene are generated as described for conventional knockout mice. A second strain of mice carrying a *cre* transgene is then bred with the strain carrying the *loxP*-flanked target gene. In the offspring, expression of Cre recombinase will mediate deletion of the target gene. Both the normal gene sequences and the neomycin resistance gene will be deleted. Importantly, expression of the *cre* gene, and therefore deletion of the targeted gene, can be restricted to certain tissues or specified times by the use of *cre* transgene constructs with different promoters. For example, selective deletion of a gene only in helper T cells can be accomplished by using a *cre* transgenic mouse in which *cre* is driven by a CD4 promoter. Alternatively, a steroid-inducible promoter can be used so that Cre expression and subsequent gene deletion occur only after mice are given a dose of dexamethasone. Many other variations on this technology have been devised to create conditional mutants. Cre/*loxP* technology can also be used to create knock-in mice. In this case, *loxP* sites are placed in the targeting vector to flank the neomycin resistance gene and the homologous sequences, but they do not flank the replacement (knock-in) gene sequences. Therefore, after *cre*-mediated deletion, the exogenous gene remains in the genome at the targeted site.

METHODS FOR STUDYING T LYMPHOCYTE RESPONSES

Our current knowledge of the cellular events in T cell activation is based on a variety of experimental techniques in which different populations of T cells are activated by defined stimuli and functional responses are measured. In vitro experiments have provided a great deal of information on the changes that occur in a T cell when it is stimulated by antigen. More recently, several techniques have been developed to study T cell proliferation, cytokine expression, and anatomic redistribution in response to antigen activation in vivo. The new experimental approaches have been particularly useful for the study of naive T cell activation and the localization of antigen-specific memory T cells after an immune response has waned.

Polyclonal Activation of T Cells

Polyclonal activators of T cells bind to many or all TCR complexes regardless of specificity and activate the T cells in ways similar to peptide-MHC complexes on APCs. Polyclonal activators are mostly used in vitro to activate T cells isolated from human blood or the lymphoid tissues of experimental animals. Polyclonal activators can also be used to activate T cells with unknown antigen specificities, and they can evoke a detectable response from mixed populations of naive T cells, even though the frequency of cells specific for any one antigen would be too low to elicit a detectable response. The polymeric plant proteins called lectins, such as concanavalin-A (Con-A) and phytohemagglutinin (PHA), are one commonly used group of polyclonal T cell activator. Lectins bind specifically to certain sugar residues on T cell surface glycoproteins, including the TCR and CD3 proteins, and thereby stimulate the T cells. Antibodies specific for invariant framework epitopes on TCR or CD3 proteins also function as polyclonal activators of T cells. Often, these antibodies need to be immobilized on solid surfaces or beads or cross-linked with secondary anti-antibodies to induce optimal activation responses. Because soluble polyclonal activators do not provide costimulatory signals that are normally provided by APCs, they are often used together with stimulatory antibodies to receptors for costimulators, such as anti-CD28 or anti-CD2. Superantigens, another kind of polyclonal stimulus, bind to and activate all T cells that express particular types of TCR β chain (see Chapter 15, Box 15–2). T cells of any antigen specificity can also be stimulated with pharmacologic reagents, such as the combination of the phorbol ester PMA and the calcium ionophore ionomycin, that mimic signals generated by the TCR complex.

Antigen-Induced Activation of Polyclonal T Cell Populations

Polyclonal populations of normal T cells that are enriched for T cells specific for a particular antigen can be derived from the blood and peripheral lymphoid organs of individuals after immunization with the antigen. The immunization serves to expand the number of antigen-specific T cells, which can then be restimulated in vitro by adding antigen and MHC-matched APCs to the T cells. This approach can be used to study antigen-induced activation of a mixed population of previously activated ("primed") T cells expressing many different TCRs, but the method does not permit analysis of responses of naive T cells.

Antigen-Induced Activation of T Cell Populations with a Single Antigen Specificity

Monoclonal populations of T cells, which express identical TCRs, have been useful for functional, biochemical, and molecular analyses. The limitation of these monoclonal populations is that they are maintained as long-term tissue culture lines and therefore may have phenotypically diverged from normal T cells in vivo. One type of monoclonal T cell population that is frequently used in experimental immunology is an antigen-specific T cell clone. Such clones are derived by isolating T cells from immunized individuals, as described for polyclonal T cells, followed by repetitive in vitro stimulation with the immunizing antigen plus MHC-matched APCs and cloning of single antigen-responsive cells in semisolid media or in liquid media by limiting dilution. Antigen-specific responses can easily be measured in these populations because all the cells in a cloned cell line have the same receptors and have been selected for growth in response to a known antigen-MHC complex. Both helper and CTL clones have been established from mice and humans. Other monoclonal T cell populations used in the study of T cell activation include antigen-specific T cell hybridomas, which are produced like B cell hybridomas (see Box 3–1, Chapter 3), and tumor lines derived from T cells have been established in vitro after removal of malignant T cells from animals or humans with T cell leukemias or lymphomas. Although some tumor-derived lines express functional TCR complexes, their antigen specificities are not known, and the cells are usually stimulated with polyclonal activators for experimental purposes. The Jurkat line, derived from a human T cell leukemia cell, is an example of a tumor line that is widely used as a model to study T cell signal transduction.

TCR transgenic mice are a source of homogeneous, phenotypically normal T cells with identical antigen specificities that are widely used for in vitro and in vivo experimental analyses. If the rearranged α and β chain genes of a single TCR of known specificity are expressed as a transgene in mice, a majority of the mature T cells in the mice will express that TCR. If the TCR transgene is crossed onto a RAG-1– or RAG-2–deficient background, no endogenous TCR gene expression occurs and 100% of the T cells will express only the transgenic TCR. TCR transgenic T cells can be activated in vitro or in vivo with a single peptide antigen, and they can be identified by antibodies specific for the transgenic TCR. One of the unique advantages of TCR transgenic mice is that they permit the isolation of sufficient numbers of naive T cells of defined specificity to allow one to study functional responses to the first exposure to antigen. This advantage has allowed investigators to study the in vitro conditions under which antigen activation of naive T cells leads to differentiation into functional subsets such as T_H1 and T_H2 cells (see Chapter 12). Naive T cells from TCR transgenic mice can also be injected into normal syngeneic recipient mice, where they home to lymphoid tissues. The recipient mouse is then exposed to the antigen for which the transgenic TCR is specific. By use of antibodies that label the TCR transgenic T cells, it is possible to follow their expansion and differentiation *in vivo* and to isolate them for analyzing recall (secondary) responses to antigen ex vivo.

Methods to Enumerate and Study Functional Responses of T Cells

Proliferation assays for T lymphocytes, like that of other cells, are conducted *in vitro* by determining the amount of 3H-labeled thymidine incorporated into the replicating DNA of cultured cells. Thymidine incorporation provides a quantitative measure of the rate of DNA synthesis, which is usually directly proportional to the rate of cell division. Cellular proliferation in vivo can be measured by injecting the thymidine analogue bromodeoxyuridine (BrdU) into animals and staining cells with anti-BrdU antibody to identify and enumerate nuclei that have incorporated BrdU into their DNA during DNA replication.

Fluorescent dyes can be used to study proliferation of T cells in vivo. T cells are first labeled with chemically reactive lipophilic fluorescent esters and then adoptively transferred into experimental animals. The dyes enter cells, form covalent bonds with cytoplasmic proteins, and then cannot leave the cells. One commonly used dye of this type is 5,6-carboxyfluorescein diacetate succinimidyl ester (CFSE), which can be detected in cells by standard flow cytometric techniques. Every time a T cell divides, its dye content is halved, and therefore it is possible to determine whether the adoptively transferred T cells present in lymphoid tissues of the recipient mouse have divided in vivo and to estimate the number of doublings each T cell has gone through.

Peptide-MHC tetramers are used to enumerate T cells with a single antigen specificity isolated from blood or lymphoid tissues of experimental animals or humans. These tetramers contain four of the peptide-MHC complexes that the T cell would normally recognize on the surface of APCs. The tetramer is made by producing a class I MHC molecule to which is attached a small molecule called biotin by use of recombinant DNA technology. Biotin binds with high affinity to a protein called avidin, and each avidin molecule binds four biotin molecules. Thus, avidin forms a substrate for assembling four biotin-conjugated MHC proteins. The MHC molecules can be loaded with a peptide of interest and thus stabilized, and the avidin molecule is labeled with a fluorochrome, such as FITC. This tetramer binds to T cells specific for the peptide-MHC complex with high enough avidity to label the T cells even in suspension. This method is the only feasible approach for identifying antigen-specific T cells in humans. For instance, it is possible to identify and enumerate circulating HLA-A2–restricted T cells specific for an HIV peptide by staining blood cells with a tetramer of HLA-A2 molecules loaded with the peptide. The same technique is being used to enumerate and isolate T cells specific for self antigens in normal individuals and in patients with autoimmune diseases. Peptide-MHC tetramers that bind to a particular transgenic TCR can also be used to quantify the transgenic T cells in different tissues after adoptive transfer and antigen stimulation. The technique is now widely used with class I MHC molecules; in class I molecules, only one polypeptide is polymorphic, and stable molecules can be produced in vitro. This is more difficult for class II molecules, because both chains are polymorphic and required for proper assembly, but class II–peptide tetramers are also being produced.

Cytokine secretion assays can be used to quantify cytokine-secreting effector T cells within lymphoid tissues. The most commonly used methods are cytoplasmic staining of cytokines and single-cell enzyme-linked immunosorbent assays (ELISPOT). In these types of studies, antigen-induced activation and differentiation of T cells take place in vivo, and then T cells are isolated and tested for cytokine expression in vitro. Cytoplasmic staining of cytokines requires permeabilizing the cells so that fluorochrome-labeled antibodies specific for a particular cytokine can gain entry into the cell, and the stained cells are analyzed by flow cytometry. Cytokine expression by T cells specific for a particular antigen can be determined by additionally staining T cells with peptide-MHC tetramers or, in the case of TCR-transgenic T cells, antibodies specific for the transgenic TCR. By use of a combination of CFSE and anticytokine antibodies, it is possible to examine the relationship between cell division and cytokine expression. In the ELISPOT assay, T cells freshly isolated from blood or lymphoid tissues are cultured in plastic wells coated with antibody specific for a particular cytokine. As cytokines are secreted from individual T cells, they bind to the antibodies in discrete spots corresponding to the location of individual T cells. The spots are visualized by adding secondary enzyme-linked anti-immunoglobulin, as in a standard ELISA (see Appendix III), and the number of spots is counted to determine the number of cytokine-secreting T cells.

METHODS FOR STUDYING B LYMPHOCYTE REPONSES

Activation of Polyclonal B Cell Populations

It is technically difficult to study the effects of antigens on normal B cells because, as the clonal selection hypothesis predicted, very few lymphocytes in an individual are specific for any one antigen. An approach to circumventing this problem is to use anti-Ig antibodies as analogues of antigens, with the assumption that anti-Ig will bind to constant (C) regions of membrane Ig molecules on all B cells and will have the same biologic effects as an antigen that binds to the hypervariable regions of membrane Ig molecules on only the antigen-specific B cells. To the extent that precise comparisons are feasible, this assumption appears generally correct, indicating that anti-Ig antibody is a valid model for antigens. Thus, anti-Ig antibody is frequently used as a polyclonal activator of B lymphocytes, similar to the use of anti- CD3 antibodies as polyclonal activators of T lymphocytes discussed earlier.

Antigen-Induced Activation of B Cell Populations with a Single Antigen-Specificity

To examine the effects of antigen binding to B cells, investigators have attempted to isolate antigen-specific B cells from complex populations of normal lymphocytes or to produce cloned B cell lines with defined antigenic specificities. These efforts have met with little success. However, transgenic mice have been developed in which virtually all B cells express a transgenic Ig of known specificity, so that most of the B cells in these mice respond to the same antigen. A somewhat more sophisticated approach has been to generate antigen receptor knockin mice, in which rearranged Ig H and L chain genes have been homologously recombined into their endogenous loci. Such knockin animals have proved particularly useful in the examination of receptor editing.

Assays to Measure B Cell Proliferation and Antibody Production

Much of our knowledge of B cell activation is based on in vitro experiments, in which different stimuli are used to activate B cells and their proliferation and differentiation can be measured accurately. The same assays may be done with B cells recovered from mice exposed to different antigens or with homogeneous B cells expressing transgene-encoded antigen receptors.

B cell proliferation is measured using 3H-labeled thymidine incorporation in vitro and BrdU labeling in vivo, a described for T cell proliferation, above.

Antibody production is measured in two different ways: with assays for cumulative Ig secretion, which measure the amount of Ig that accumulates in the supernatant of cultured lymphocytes or in the serum of an immunized individual and with single-cell assays, which determine the number of cells in an immune population that secrete Ig of a particular specificity or isotype. The most accurate, quantitative, and widely used techniques for measuring the total amount of Ig in a culture supernatant or serum sample is ELISA. By use of antigens bound to solid supports, it is possible to use ELISA to quantify the amount of antibody in a sample specific for a particular antigen. In addition, the availability of anti-Ig antibodies that detect Igs of different heavy or light chain classes allows measurement of the quantities of different isotypes in a sample. Other techniques for measuring antibody levels include hemagglutination for antierythrocyte antibodies and complement-dependent lysis for antibodies specific for known cell types. Both assays are based on the demonstration that if the amount of antigen (i.e., cells) is constant, the concentration of antibody determines the amount of antibody bound to cells, and this is reflected in the degree of cell agglutination or subsequent binding of complement and cell lysis. Results from these assays are usually expressed as antibody titers, which are the dilution of the sample giving half-maximal effects or the dilution at which the end point of the assay is reached.

A single-cell assay for antibody secretion is the ELISPOT assay. In this method, antigen is bound to the bottom of a well, antibody-secreting cells are added, and antibodies that have been secreted and are bound to the antigen are detected by an enzyme-linked anti-Ig antibody, as in an ELISA, in a semisolid medium. Each spot represents the location of an antibody-secreting cell. Single-cell assays provide a measure of the numbers of Ig-secreting cells, but they cannot accurately quantify the amount of Ig secreted by each cell or by the total population. The ELISA and ELISPOT techniques can be adapted to assess affinity of antibodies, by the use of antigens with differing numbers of hapten moieties. IN this way affinity maturation can be assessed by testing serum or B cells sampled at different times during an immune response.

Index

Note: Page numbers followed by f indicate figures; those followed by t indicate tables; and those followed by b indicate boxed material.